2025/2026

THE NEXT STEP
Advanced Medical Coding and Auditing

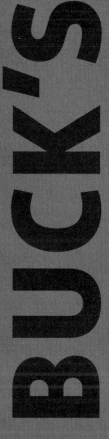

BUCK'S

ELSEVIER

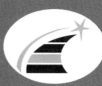

2025/2026

THE NEXT STEP
Advanced Medical Coding and Auditing

BUCK'S

Jackie L. Koesterman, CPC
Coding and Reimbursement Specialist
JDK Medical Coding EDU
Grand Forks, North Dakota

ELSEVIER

Elsevier
3251 Riverport Lane
St. Louis, Missouri 63043

BUCK'S THE NEXT STEP: ADVANCED MEDICAL CODING
AND AUDITING, 2025/2026 EDITION

ISBN: 978-0-443-24880-1

Access to the 2026 coding updates can be found in the "Content Updates" section located in your Evolve Resources.

NOTE: The *2025 ICD-10-CM* and *2025 ICD-10-PCS* were used in preparing this text.

NOTE: *Current Procedural Terminology, 2025,* was used in updating this text.

Current Procedural Terminology (CPT) is copyright 2024 American Medical Association. All Rights Reserved. No fee schedules, basic units, relative values, or related listings are included in CPT. The AMA assumes no liability for the data contained herein. Applicable FARS/DFARS restrictions apply to government use.

Previous editions copyrighted: 2023, 2021, 2019, 2017, 2016, 2015, 2014, 2013, 2012, 2011, 2010, 2009, 2008, 2006, 2004.

International Standard Book Number: 978-0-443-24880-1

Senior Content Strategist: Luke E. Held
Content Development Manager: Danielle Frazier
Senior Content Development Specialist: Joshua S. Rapplean
Publishing Services Manager: Deepthi Unni
Project Manager: Nayagi Anandan
Senior Book Designer: Maggie Reid

Printed in Canada

Last digit is the print number: 9   8   7   6   5   4   3   2   1

Working together
to grow libraries in
developing countries

www.elsevier.com • www.bookaid.org

Dedication

To all the students, whose abilities to surmount tremendous obstacles to achieve their goals have been a source of unending inspiration.

To the teachers, who give of their talent, time, and knowledge to help the students who enter their classrooms, may this work make your load just a little lighter as we travel the same road, toward the same goal.

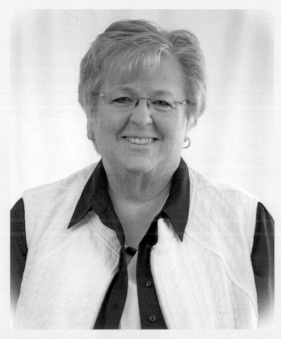

Carol J. Buck

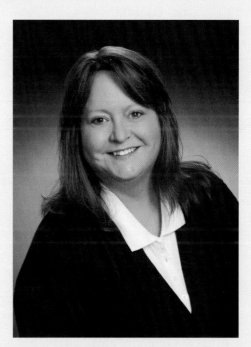

Jackie L. Koesterman

About the Author

Carol J. Buck, MS, is a leading coding author and educator. Her *Step* series of textbooks were the first in the market to help coders and coding students develop their skills to advanced and specialized levels. Carol has dedicated herself to the growth and advancement of the coding profession.

Carol has a Master's degree in Education. She began authoring textbooks when she was the Program Director of the Medical Secretarial programs at the Northwest Technical College in Minnesota and recognized the need for classroom texts that could be used to teach medical coding. It was then that she began developing classroom lectures, abstracting medical reports, and compiling materials to prepare her students for careers as medical coders. These materials later became *Step-by-Step Medical Coding*.

Carol has expanded on the original text with a line of annual products for advanced coding, certification, specialization, and reference manuals, providing quality educational materials from the first day of a coding program to preparation for national certification.

To meet the needs of practicing coders, Carol and Elsevier produce professional editions of ICD-10-CM, ICD-10-PCS, and HCPCS references, designed by coders for coders, with unique features such as color tables and the Official Guidelines for Coding and Reporting.

From the classroom to the workplace, from application to certification, Carol J. Buck and Elsevier are the trusted names for coding education, practice, and professionalism.

Jackie L. Koesterman, CPC, has been a Certified Professional Coder and Medical Assistant for over 25 years. Jackie has also served as an instructor at the Minnesota Northland Technical College in the medical clerical and medical assistant programs. Jackie is employed by a large medical health system as a Senior Coder III and Reimbursement Specialist, specializing in multi-specialty coding and multi-payer denial review in both the inpatient and outpatient settings. She also serves as a trainer and mentor to the coders. Jackie performs audits for multi-specialties for private practice clinics in her area.

Since the inception of *Step-by-Step Medical Coding*, Jackie has been involved in the development and review of the texts serving as technical collaborator, reviewer, and author.

Acknowledgments

This text was developed through a team effort. Each member of the team was vital for the completion of this volume of work. Each person shared the vision for an advanced coding text that would enable the learner to be better prepared to meet the exciting challenge presented by medical coding.

Special thanks goes to the team of wonderful people at Elsevier. Your professionalism, amazing skill, and genuine desire to assist in the educational process by providing high-quality texts are readily apparent and greatly appreciated.

Rachel E. Briggs, Subject Matter Expert, who graciously lends her amazing knowledge and attention to detail. Her dedication to excellence consistently improves this work.

Luke Held, Senior Content Strategist, who has tremendous enthusiasm for our mission. **Josh Rapplean,** Senior Content Development Specialist, who has shouldered the huge task of seeing this text to completion with an exceptional level of professionalism. He is the consummate professional who improves all projects with his involvement. **Nayagi Anandan,** Project Manager, who has assumed responsibility while maintaining a high degree of professionalism.

Preface

Thank you for purchasing *The Next Step Advanced Medical Coding and Auditing.* This 2025/2026 edition has been carefully reviewed and updated with the latest content, making it the most current textbook for your class. The author and publisher have made every effort to equip you with skills and tools you will need to succeed on the job. *The Next Step Advanced Medical Coding and Auditing* presents essential applications and real-world patient cases to explain coding services. Hands-on practice with physician documentation provides the auditing skills needed to be a successful medical coder. No other text on the market brings together such thorough coverage of the coding systems in one source.

Organization of this Textbook

Developed in collaboration with employers and educators, *Next Step Advanced Medical Coding and Auditing* takes an advanced approach to training and coding for a successful career. The text is divided into chapters covering ICD-10-CM, CPT, and HCPCS. Auditing Review questions are found at the end of each chapter.

Chapter 1, Evaluation and Management Services, is an in-depth overview of the three factors and medical decision making component of E/M coding.

Chapter 2, Medicine, provides information on the codes throughout the Medicine section of the CPT, along with reports and modifier information.

Chapter 3, Radiology, begins with the positions and placement for radiology services. The text covers information on CT Scans, Ultrasound, X-rays and Radiation Oncology.

Chapter 4, Pathology and Laboratory, provides an overview of the types of services and includes drug assays and panels from the CPT manual. Information is presented on the lab/path superbill/requisition form and labeled figures of the forms are included.

Chapters 5-13, Surgical Chapters, begin with information and reports covering the Integumentary System. Each chapter provides in-depth information and reports for all remaining Body Systems.

Chapter 14, Anesthesia, begins with an introduction to the types of anesthesia. Information is provided on Base Units, Physical Status Modifiers, and Concurrent Care Modifiers. Reports within the chapter cover the different types of anesthesia used with procedures and services.

List of Physicians

A list of physicians is located at the end of the "Introduction" piece ahead of the Table of Contents. The list contains names of the physicians that provide services to the patients in this text. The list is displayed in alphabetic order by physician last name and by specialty. There are two physicians who are employed by the hospital (Dr. Hart and Dr. Sutton), and the remaining physicians are employed at the local clinic. The coder will be assigning codes for all the physicians.

Some of the CPT code descriptions for physician services include physician extender services. Physician extenders, such as nurse practitioners, physician assistants, and nurse anesthetists, etc., provide medical services typically performed by a physician. Within this educational material the term "physician" may include "and other qualified health care professionals" depending on the code. Refer to the official CPT® code descriptions and guidelines to determine codes that are appropriate to report services provided by non-physician practitioners.

Abbreviations and Acronyms

Select abbreviations and acronyms used in the cases in each chapter are displayed at the beginning of each chapter. **Appendix C** contains a compilation of these abbreviations and acronyms.

Glossary

There is a main glossary of terms that is a compilation of the more complex words from the text.

Evaluation

The tests contain at least two reports that are similar to ones that appeared in the chapter.

Distinctive Features of our Approach

This book was designed to be the second step in your coding career, and it has unique features to help you along the way.
- The repetition of skills in each chapter reinforces the material and creates a logical progression for learning and applying each skill!
- In-text cases further reinforce important concepts and allow you to check your comprehension as you read (answers to every other case are located in Appendix D).
- Throughout this text material has been highlighted to call attention to the importance of this information. The Physical Examination below has highlighted words that call out each body and organ system that will assist in coding E/M services. Other highlighted areas include details in reports and critical information that will aid in reporting the correct diagnosis codes and selecting accurate CPT codes.

PHYSICAL EXAMINATION

The patient is very sluggish,(general appearance/constitutional) although he does answer questions. Blood pressure 96/76,(constitutional) pulse 130, and regular(constitutional) respirations 22.(constitutional) Eyes: Sunken significantly. Fundi are not visualized.(OS/ophthalmologic) Ears: Negative.(OS/otolaryngologic) Carotids are 4/4 without bruits.(OS/cardiovascular) Neck: supple,(BA/neck) nodes are negative. Thyroid is normal to palpation. Axillary nodes negative.(OS/lymphatic) Chest: Clear to auscultation.(OS/respiratory) Heart: Tachycardic but no extra heart sounds heard. No murmur is appreciated.(OS/cardiovascular) Abdomen: Some minimal tenderness in the right mid abdomen and left upper abdomen.(BA/abdomen) Genital/Rectal: Not performed. Peripheral extremities reveal good pulses in the legs with no edema.(OS/also cardiovascular) Respiratory: Negative.(OS/respiratory) GI: Negative.(OS/gastrointestinal)

(Highlighted terms will appear underlined in eBook format due to technical requirements.)

- A full-color design brings a fresh look to the material, visually reinforcing new concepts and examples.
- Medical procedures or conditions are illustrated and discussed in the text to help you understand the services being coded.

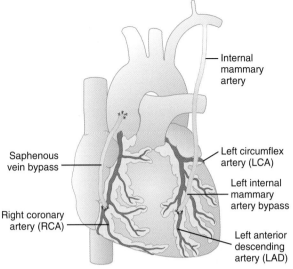

FIGURE 6–3 Coronary artery bypass.

- *From the Trenches* boxes highlight a different real-life medical coding practitioner in each chapter, with photographs throughout the chapter alongside quotes that offer practical advice or motivational comments.

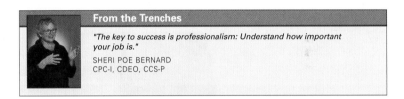

From the Trenches

"The key to success is professionalism: Understand how important your job is."

SHERI POE BERNARD
CPC-I, CDEO, CCS-P

Supplemental Resources

Considering the broad range of students, programs, and institutions in which this textbook is used, we have developed supplements designed to complement *The Next Step Advanced Medical Coding and Auditing*. Each of these comprehensive supplements has been developed with the needs of both students and instructors in mind.

TEACH Instructor Resources on Evolve

No matter what your level of teaching experience, this total-teaching solution will help you plan your lessons with ease, and the author has developed all the curriculum materials necessary to use *The Next Step Advanced Medical Coding and Auditing* in the classroom. Instructors can download:

- All auditing review answers with rationales.
- Course calendar and syllabus.
- Curriculum guides and TEACH lesson plans.
- Abstracting cases and question answers.
- Test Banks that include a wide variety of multiple choice, true/false, matching, and completion questions that correlate to each chapter of the text.
- Comprehensive PowerPoint collection that can be easily customized to support your lectures, formatted with PowerPoint as overhead transparencies, or formatted as handouts for student note-taking.

ICD-10-CM Chapters
(Slide 1 of 2)

- Chapter 1: Certain Infectious and Parasitic Disease (A00 – B99)
- Chapter 2: Neoplasms (C00 – D49)
- Chapter 3: Disease of the Blood and Blood-Forming Organs and Certain Disorders Involving the Immune Mechanism (D50 – D89)
- Chapter 4: Endocrine, Nutritional, and Metabolic Disorders (E00 – E89)
- Chapter 5: Mental, Behavioral, and Neurodevelopmental Disorders (F01 – F99)
- Chapter 6: Diseases of the Nervous System (G00-G99)
- Chapter 7: Diseases of the Eye and Adnexa (H00 – H59)
- Chapter 8: Diseases of the Ear and Mastoid Process (H60 – H95)
- Chapter 9: Diseases of the Circulatory System (I00 – I99)
- Chapter 10: Diseases of the Respiratory System (J00 – J99)
- Chapter 11: Diseases of the Digestive System (K00 – K95)
- Chapter 12: Diseases of the Skin and Subcutaneous Tissue (L00 – L99)
- Chapter 13: Diseases of the Musculoskeletal System and Connective Tissue (M00– M99)
- Chapter 14: Diseases of the Genitourinary System (N00 – N99)

Copyright © 2021 by Elsevier Inc.   Slide 6

Evolve Learning Resources

The Evolve Learning Resources offer helpful material that will extend your studies beyond the classroom.

Official Guidelines for Coding and Reporting, Content Updates, and Coding links help you stay current with this ever-changing field. Online Activities and Chapter Review applications provide electronic assessment options (though answers are still only provided at the discretion of the instructor).

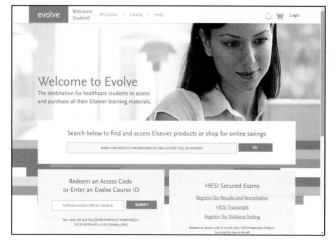

A Course Management System is also available free to instructors who adopt this textbook. This web-based platform gives instructors yet another resource to facilitate learning and to make medical coding content accessible to students.

To access this comprehensive online resource, simply go to the Evolve home page at http://evolve.elsevier.com and enter the user name and password provided by your instructor. If your instructor has not set up a Course Management System, you can still access the free Evolve Learning Resources at http://evolve.elsevier.com/Buck/next/.

A Special Note

Coders are a very special group of individuals. They have keen minds and tend to be gifted with great patience for the detail-oriented process of medical coding. They have immense professionalism and seek to do an exemplary job of the most difficult task of translating services and diagnoses into codes and ensuring appropriate reimbursement. They are exemplified by a statement made many years ago by Orison Swett Marden:

> *People who have accomplished work worthwhile have had a very high sense of the way to do things. They have not been content with mediocrity. They have not confined themselves to the beaten tracks; they have never been satisfied to do things just as others do them, but always a little better. They always pushed things that came to their hands a little higher up, a little farther on. It is this little higher up, this little farther on, that counts in the quality of life's work. It is the constant effort to be first class in everything one attempts that conquers the heights of excellence.*

Medical coding is a fine profession that has the ability to intrigue and captivate you for a lifetime. Practice your craft carefully, with due diligence, patience for the process, and always the highest ethical standards.

Carol J. Buck, MS
Jackie L. Koesterman, CPC

Development of This Edition

Introduction

Types of Codes

This text presents cases that are to be coded with **service codes** (CPT and HCPCS) and **diagnosis codes** (ICD-10-CM) in the outpatient settings of the clinic and inpatient or outpatient services at the hospital for the physician (professional). Answer lines are provided for the ICD-10-CM codes, along with rationales within the textbook.

Appendix B of this text displays the website to reference the 1995 and 1997 Documentation Guidelines for Evaluation and Management Services. Each medical facility chooses one of the documentation guidelines and submits all Medicare and Medicaid E/M charges using that specific set of guidelines. This text has been developed using the 1995 guidelines, as that tends to be the more popular version. Private third-party payers (not Medicare, Medicaid, or any other government program) may not require adherence to a specific set of E/M documentation guidelines.

Unlike the inpatient facility coder, who has all of the documentation from a hospital stay available when assigning diagnoses codes, the outpatient coder reports diagnoses based on the information present in the one report being coded. In this text, a case may contain numerous reports that chronicle the patient's care. When coding each of the reports in the case, the coder is to consider only the diagnoses information present in that report, because this is the way the reports are coded in outpatient settings. For example, a physician admits a patient to the hospital for possible pneumonia with chief complaint of shortness of breath and wheezing. The coder reporting the physician's admit service would report the symptoms of shortness of breath and wheezing, even though on a subsequent report within that case the physician does diagnose the patient's condition as pneumonia. One exception to this rule would be when coding an operative report in which a specimen was sent to the pathology department for analysis. The pathologist's diagnosis would be used as the diagnosis when coding the operative report, because the findings are usually more current and definitive than the diagnosis stated by the surgeon.

Clarification regarding the reporting guidelines for diagnostic tests, such as pathology reports, is located in AB-01-144. The Centers for Medicare and Medicaid, Program Memorandum (PM), Transmittal AB-01-144 is displayed in **Appendix A** of this text and outlines current coding guidelines for reporting the diagnosis for diagnostic tests. The PM provides direction on coding diagnostic tests and coordinates with the *Official Guidelines for Coding and Reporting*. Although there is no specific memorandum for ICD-10-CM, the content of the ICD-9-CM memorandum is still applicable. The PM is an important document to read before beginning to use this text, because it outlines the guidelines used when this text was developed. The coder is introduced to this document in Chapter 1 of the text under the heading Diagnosis Coding. This document has foundational information that must be carefully read and thoroughly understood by the coder prior to assigning diagnosis codes. The links to the *Official Guidelines for Coding and Reporting* are also displayed in Appendix B.

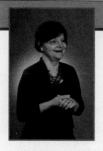

From the Trenches

"The continuing education process will always be essential since compliance regulations and coding elements are always changing."

PATRICIA HENRICKSEN
MS, CPC-I, CPC, CHCA, CCP-P, ACS-PM

The number of cases in each chapter was determined by the complexity of coding and the most common services in the specialty. For example, Chapter 6, Cardiovascular System, is quite lengthy, as this is a very complex area to code and many of the basic cardiovascular services, such as ECG and cardiac event monitoring, are commonly provided in most outpatient settings. There are many coding challenges in cardiology, such as coronary artery bypass graft, and only through repeated cases can the coder gain understanding and then confidence in his/her cardiology coding skill.

Case Numbering System

The cases are numbered by chapter, case, and report. For example, in 7-15A, the "7" indicates that the case appears within Chapter 7. The "15" indicates that the case is the 15th case in Chapter 7. The "A" indicates that the report is the first report in the case. Subsequent reports within 7-15 are identified by B, C, etc.

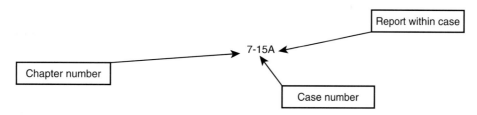

Tests are identified by a "T" preceding the case. For example, T7-1A indicates that the test (T) is from Chapter 7, is the first case (1), and is the first report (A) in the case. The web cases are numbered in the same way, but with a "W" preceding the case. For example, W7-1A indicates that this is a web case from Chapter 7, is the first case (1), and is the first report (A) in the case.

Each chapter has an outline that lists all the cases and reports at the beginning of the chapter, as illustrated in the following:

Evaluation and Management Services

CASE 6-1

6-1A   Cardiothoracic Surgery Consultation

Cardiac Artery Bypass Grafts

CASE 6-2

6-2A   Coronary Artery Bypass

Pacemaker

CASE 6-3

6-3A   Cardiology Follow-Up Note

CASE 6-7

6-7A   Cardiology Consultation
6-7B   Hospital Service
6-7C   Radiography Report, Chest
6-7D   Cardiothoracic Surgical Consultation
6-7E   Radiography Report, Chest

CASE 6-8

6-8A   Echo Doppler Report

CASE 6-9

6-9A   Cardiology Consultation

CASE 6-12

6-12C   Radiology Report, Chest
6-12D   Cardiac Catheterization Report
6-12E   Radiology Report, GI

Miscellaneous Reports

CASE 6-13

6-13A   Cardioversion

CASE 6-14

6-14A   Transesophageal Echocardiogram Report

Report Format

Information is provided regarding a coding concept, such as pacemaker implantation:

Pacemaker

A pacemaker is an electrical device that is inserted into the body to shock the heart electrically into regular rhythm. The two parts of a pacemaker are the battery and electrode. The electrode is the device that emits the electrical charge. The electrode is also called the *lead* and is a flexible, thin tube. The battery is also called a *pulse generator*. Some generators are programmable and have a wide range of programming options. The pulse generator is placed into a pocket either under the clavicle, as illustrated in **Figure 6-4,** or under the muscle of the abdomen below the rib cage.

Either an epicardial or a transvenous approach can be used to implant the electrode portion of the pacemaker. The epicardial approach involves opening the chest to the view of the surgeon and placing the device on the heart. The transvenous approach is most commonly used because it is the least traumatic to the patient; it involves inserting a needle with a wire attached (guidewire) into a vein. The guidewire then directs the placement of the electrode into the heart while the surgeon views the progression using a fluoroscope. The electrode is then attached to the pulse generator.

The pacemaker can be a single- or dual-chamber unit. A single-chamber pacemaker uses one pulse generator and one electrode that is placed in either the atrium or the ventricle. A dual-chamber pacemaker uses a pulse generator and two electrodes—one placed in the atrium and the other placed in the ventricle.

Pacemakers can be permanent or temporary. A temporary pacemaker can be used when the heart needs only short-term pacing support, for example, when a patient is waiting for placement of a permanent pacemaker or a patient is experiencing postsurgical cardiac instability. After the pacemaker is placed, the physician will test the device to ensure that it is operating correctly. The pacemaker implantation report will indicate a statement such as "thresholds were obtained and were adequate." The testing and setting are included in the implantation service and are not reported separately. Special or extensive pacing, if noted in the report as those above the usual service, can be reported separately.

As the text progresses, the coder is assigned more complex cases with fewer directives and less information to ensure the development of the ability to transfer previously learned knowledge, thereby strengthening confidence in his/her coding and auditing abilities. The **goal of this text** is to present the coder with a wide array of cases from across the major medical specialties. These reports are the "real thing" from clinics and hospitals. The reports were selected to give you a realistic picture of the type and scope of reports you will be coding on the job.

The format of the text is two columns to save space and contain the cost of production. Although the coder will not see a two-column report on the job, it is the documentation that is important, in whatever format that information is presented. For example, the pathology reports may be in the front of the medical record at one facility; at another facility, the reports may be in the back of the record, or the coder may work exclusively with online records and never use the printed format.

The coder assigns the service and diagnosis codes to reports. The following is an example of a report from the text:

6-5C Operative Report, Pacemaker Implantation

LOCATION: Outpatient, Hospital

PATIENT: Herbert Gillford

SURGEON: Marvin Elhart, MD

PROCEDURE PERFORMED: Dual-chamber pacemaker implantation

INDICATION: Bradyarrhythmia

BRIEF HISTORY: This patient has been experiencing recurrent syncope. He was evaluated in the last year or so. Because of the presence of first-degree AV (atrioventricular) block, sinus bradycardia, and bundle-branch block, the cause for his syncope most likely is his bradyarrhythmia; for that reason, a dual-chamber pacemaker implantation was recommended after discussion with his cousin, who consented to the procedure. The cousin was informed of all potential complications, including infection, hematoma, pneumothorax, hemothorax, myocardial infarction, and even death. He agreed to proceed.

PROCEDURE: The patient was brought to the cardiac catheterization laboratory. He was placed on the catheterization table, where he was prepped and draped in the usual fashion. The procedure was extremely difficult to perform as a result of the patient's agitation despite adequate sedation. With reasonable hemostasis, the pacemaker pocket was performed in the left infraclavicular area after anesthetizing the area with 0.5 cc (cubic centimeter) of Xylocaine. Hemostasis was secured with cautery. The patient had excessive venous oozing from Valsalva and straining, and that was controlled with pressure. A single stick was performed because of the patient's agitation. Using a 9-French peel-away sheath, we introduced an atrial and a ventricular lead and placed them in an excellent position.

Thresholds were obtained adequately. The leads were sutured using 0 silk over their sleeves and secured. The pulse generator was connected. The pacemaker pocket was flushed with antibiotic solution. The pacemaker and leads were placed in the pocket and the pocket closed in two layers.

COMPLICATION: None

EQUIPMENT USED: Pulse generator was Medtronic model 60 Thera DRI, serial B28H. The ventricular lead was Medtronic serial L420V, model 4524 Link. The atrial lead was Medtronic 24-58, serial 326V.

The following parameters were obtained after implantation: Pacing threshold in the atrium was excellent at 0.5 msec and 0.5 V, and impedance was 445 ohms and sensing 2.1 mV. In the ventricle, 0.5 msec and 0.3 V with R wave of 19.9 mV and impedance 668 (device evaluation).

The following parameters were left at implantation: DDDR with lower rate limit of 70 and an upper rate limit of 120. The amplitude was 3.5 V in the atrium at 0.4 msec with a sensitivity of 0.5 mV. The ventricle was 3.5 V and 0.4 msec at 2.8-mV sensitivity (device evaluation).

CONCLUSION: Successful implantation of dual-chamber pacemaker without immediate complications.

PLAN: Patient to return to recovery unit and to be discharged late this evening to the nursing home with routine postpacemaker care.

6-5C:

SERVICE CODE(S): _____

ICD-10-CM DX CODE(S): _____

Auditing Review

An audit review evaluates service and diagnosis codes and is necessary to provide efficient and accurate documentation. The format of each audit review guides the coder in the development of coding abilities.

Audit Report 6.5 Adenosine Cardiolite Stress Test

LOCATION: Outpatient, Hospital

PATIENT: Matt Arman

PHYSICIAN: Marvin Elhart, MD

INDICATIONS: The patient is status post heart catheterization and stent placement × 3 and now has recurring chest pain.

IDENTIFICATION: 61-year-old male, 5′ 8″, 210 pounds.

The patient underwent stress test according to Bruce protocol with Myoview injection.

HEMODYNAMIC RESPONSE: Heart rate at rest was 68 and at peak exercise was 132. Blood pressure at rest was 138/78 and at peak was 168/78.

During the stress test, the patient had no chest pain. The test was stopped due to fatigue. At baseline, the patient had a normal sinus rhythm with

no ST segment changes. At peak exercise, the patient had no ST segment changes noted.

The patient exercised for a total of 10 minutes, achieving 11.3 METS.

CONCLUSION:

1. Excellent exercise tolerance.
2. Good hemodynamic response to exercise.
3. This EKG stress test is not suggestive for significant obstructive disease. No chest pain clinically. The Myoview part of the stress test will be reported separately.

One or more of the following codes are reported incorrectly for this case. Indicate the incorrect code or codes.

SERVICE CODE(S):   Cardiovascular stress test. **93015-26**

ICD-10-CM DX CODE(S):   Chest pain. **R07.9**

INCORRECT/MISSING CODE(S): _____

- Answer blank for one or more service codes
- Answer blank for one or more diagnosis codes
- Answer blank for Incorrect/Missing codes for Audit Report

Multiple Modifiers

Multiple modifiers are added to codes by placing the numbers first in descending order, followed by the lettered modifiers in alphabetic order. For example, if the code were to be reported with -55 and -RT, the -55 would be placed first, followed by the -RT. As another example, if the code were to be reported with -50 and -52, the -52 would be placed first, followed by the -50. This is the format that is followed in this text.

Use of Modifiers -26 and -TC

- Modifier -26 requests payment from the third-party payer for the professional component percentage of the fee only.
- Modifier -TC requests payment for the technical component percentage of the fee only.

These modifiers are usually used with radiology and pathology services. An example is an independent radiology facility that takes the x-rays (technical component) and sends them to a private radiologist who reads the x-rays and writes a report of the findings (professional component). The independent radiology facility would report the service with the x-ray code with modifier -TC added to indicate that only the technical component was provided. The physician's services would be reported with modifier -26 added to the x-ray code to indicate that only the professional component of the x-ray service was provided. If both the technical and professional services of the x-ray were provided at the same place, such as the clinic, no modifiers would be added, since both components of the service were provided at the same place and reporting the x-ray code without a modifier requests the full fee from the carrier. Provision of both technical and professional services is called a global service.

For the purposes of this text, the radiologist and pathologists are employed by the facility unless specifically stated otherwise.

Pathology and Laboratory

Chapter 4, Pathology and Laboratory, guides the coder in the use of a standard laboratory requisition or superbill as illustrated on the following page.

When the coders have finished the activities within the chapter, they will have a completed laboratory requisition that contains the codes for the tests listed. The coder will then be familiar with the most frequently ordered laboratory tests.

From the Trenches

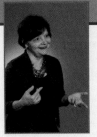

"Certified coders are in high demand, not only as coders and auditors for physicians, but for claims review by insurance companies, contract auditing, outsource billing, and as educators."

PATRICIA HENRICKSEN
MS, CPC-I, CPC, CHCA, CCP-P, ACS-PM

Order Date: _____ Order Time: _____

General Laboratory Requisition

PRIORITY (Routine unless otherwise specified)
☐ ASAP   ☐ STAT   All tests: ☐ Yes   ☐ No
If No, Specify Tests: _____

☐ **RECURRING ORDER** (not to exceed 12 months)
Frequency: _____   Start Date: _____   End Date: _____

SPECIAL INSTRUCTIONS

FOR PHYSICIAN OFFICE COLLECTION ONLY:
Collected: Date: _____   Time: _____ By: _____

FOR LAB COLLECTION ONLY:
Collected: Date: _____   Time: _____ By: _____

Code	CHEMISTRY	DX
	Albumin/Serum	
	Alkaline phosphatase	
	ALT/SGPT	
	Amylase	
	Arterial Blood Gas	
	AST/SGOT	
	Bilirubin, direct	
	Bilirubin, total	
	BUN, Quant	
	Calcium, total	
	Carbon dioxide (CO_2)	
	CEA	
	Chloride, blood	
	Cholesterol, serum	
	CK (creatine kinase)	
	Creatinine, blood	
	FSH	
	Ferritin	
	Folic Acid (Folate), blood	
	GGT	
	Glucose, blood non-reag	
	Glycated Hgb (Hgb A1C)	
	HCG-Qualitative	
	HCG-Quantitative	
	HDL Cholesterol	
-90	Immun. Electrophoresis	
	Iron	
	Iron Binding Capacity	
NC	% saturation requires iron & IBC to be ordered	
	LDH (lactate dehydrogenase)	
	LH (luteinizing hormone)	
	Magnesium	
	Phosphorus, blood	
	Potassium, blood	
	Prolactin, blood	
	Protein, total	
-90	Protein Electrophoresis, serum	
	PSA, total	
	Sodium, serum	
	T4, free (thyroxine)	
	TSH	
	Triglycerides	
	Uric Acid, blood	
	Vitamin B12	
	CALCULATIONS	
NC	LDL requires Chol & HDL to be ordered	
NC	CHOL/HDL requires Chol & HDL to be ordered	

Code	TOXICOLOGY/ THERAPEUTIC DRUGS	DX
Last Dose:		
	Carbamazepine	
	Digoxin	
	Lithium	
	Phenobarbital	
	Phenytoin (Dilantin)	
	Salicylate	
	Valproic Acid	
	Theophylline	

Code	IMMUNOLOGY (Blood)	DX
	ANA (FANA) Screen if ANA positive, 86039 titer performed, if titer >1:160 cascade performed (anti-ds DNA, ENA I & ENA II)	
	Anti-ds DNA	
	ENA I (Sm, RNP)	
	ENA II (SSA, SSB)	
	ASO screen (ASO titer if screen positive 86060)	
	Rheumatoid factor (qual)	
	RPR (Syphilis Serology), quant	
	Cold Agglutinin titer	
	Hep B surface antigen	
-90	Hep B surface antigen OB (PHL)	
-90	HIV	
	Mono test	
	Rubella Antibody	

Code	PANELS	DX
	Electrolytes CO_2, Cl, K, Na	
	Bas Met, cal ion	
	Bas Met, cal tot	
	Comprehensive metabolic Alb, Bili tot, Ca tot, Cl, Creat, Glu, Alk phos, K, Prot tot, Na, AST, ALT, BUN, CO_2	
	Hepatic Function Alb, Bili tot and dir, Alk phos, AST, ALT, Prot tot	
	Lipid Chol tot, HDL, Trig., calc, LDL, Chol/HDL ratio	
	Gen health, Comp met, CBC, TSH	

Code	HEMATOLOGY	DX
	Hemogram WBC, auto WBC diff	
	Hemogram micro exam, WBC diff	
	Hemogram micro exam, w/o diff	
	Hemogram manual WBC diff, buffy	
	Hematocrit	
	Hemoglobin	
	Platelet count, auto	
	Reticulocyte count, manual	
	Sedimentation Rate, auto	
	WBC, automated	
	CBC, with diff Hgb, Hct, RBC, WBC, Platelet	
	CBC, w/o diff Hgb, Hct, RBC, WBC, Platelet	

Code	COAGULATION	DX
☐ Coumadin ☐ Heparin		
	APTT	
	Prothrombin time	
	Bleeding time	

Code	OFFICE TESTING	DX
	UA, Dipstick in Office	

Code	URINE/STOOL	DX
	UA, Routine	
	UA SAVE (for possible urine culture if requested)	
	UA with microscopic	
	Urinalysis, Dipstick, Lab	
	Occult Blood	
	Urine HCG	
	Diabetic urine cascade	

Code	TIMED URINE	DX
Hours:		
	Creatinine Clearance	
	Calcium, Urine, Quant.	
	Uric acid	

Code	BODY FLUID	DX
Fluid Source:		
	Cell Count w/o Diff	
	Protein	
	Glucose	
	Semen Analysis	
	Semen Analysis, Comp	

Code	IMMUNOHEMATOLOGY	DX
	Blood type ABO, Rh(D)	
	Weak D performed if Rh negative	
	Antibody Screen Identification, if positive, titer if indicated	
	Direct Coombs additional testing if positive	

WRITE-IN TESTS		DX	Lab Use

Medical Necessity Statement: Tests ordered on Medicare patients must follow CMS rules regarding medical necessity and FDA approval guidelines and must include diagnosis, symptoms, or reason for testing as indicated on the medical record. For any patient of any payor (including Medicare and Medicaid) that has a medical necessity requirement, order only those tests which are medically necessary for the diagnosis and treatment of the patient.

DX	CODE	WRITTEN INDICATION/DIAGNOSIS	(Match Diagnosis # to Test)
1			
2			
3			
4			

LAB USE ONLY
Arterial Puncture
Venipuncture
Venipuncture MC/MA
Handling Fee
Urine Volume Measurement
-90 PKU

Chart #: _____   Date: _____
Name: _____   M/F
DOB: _____
Physician: _____

Medicare #: _____   Medicaid #: _____
☐ No ABN needed   ☐ Patient refused to sign ABN
Nursing Home Part A Medicare: ☐ Yes ☐ No
Worker's Comp: ☐ Yes ☐ No
Company Account: _____

The Top 10 List for Coders

Contributed by Karen D. Lockyer

10. Abstracting is getting the essence of the relevant facts.
 9. When in doubt, ASK—don't assume anything.
 8. Never be afraid to question a physician.
 7. Work with good reference books.
 6. Always use current code books.
 5. Make notes in your coding manuals—it saves time later on.
 4. Good coders are always learning.
 3. Speed of record reading comes with practice; never sacrifice accuracy.
 2. If it isn't documented, it didn't happen.
 1. **NEVER CODE DIRECTLY FROM THE INDEX OF A CODE MANUAL!**

Some of the CPT code descriptions for physician services include physician extender services. Physician extenders, such as nurse practitioners, physician assistants, and nurse anesthetists, etc., provide medical services typically performed by a physician. Within this educational material, the term "physician" may include "and other qualified health care professionals," depending on the code. Refer to the official CPT® code descriptions and guidelines to determine codes that are appropriate to report services provided by nonphysician practitioners.

List of Physicians

Physicians by Name

Alanda, MD, Leslie	Internal Medicine & Vascular
Aljabar, MD, Alfa	Nuclear Medicine
Almaz, MD, Mohomad	Orthopedics
Avila, MD, Ira	Urology
Barneswell, MD, Mary	Physical Therapy
Barton, MD, David	Cardiothoracic Surgery
Brown, MD, Robert	Critical Care
Dawson, MD, Gregory	Respiratory Care
Doron, MD, Phil	Endocrinology
Eagle, MD, James	Radiation Oncology
Elhart, MD, Marvin	Cardiology
Erickson, MD, Mark	Plastic Surgery
Friendly, MD, Larry P.	Gastroenterology
Gaul, MD, Frank	Family Practice
Green, MD, Ronald	Internal Medicine & Critical Care
Hamilton, MD, Monica J.	Interventional Radiology
Hart, MD, Phillip	Neuroradiology—Hospital Employee
Hodgson, MD, John	Surgical Neurosurgery
Jayco, MD, Gordon	Endocrinology & Nephrology
King, MD, Jeff	Otorhinolaryngology
Larson, MD, Janice E.	Anesthesia
Lauer, MD, Elmer	Dermatology
Lin, MD, Lou	Infectious Diseases
Lonewolf, MD, Grey	Pathology
Lorabi, MD, Gerald	Hematology
Lovejoy, MD, Noah	Dermatology
Martinez, MD, Andy	Obstetrics & Gynecology
Monson, MD, Morton	Radiology
Munoz, MD, Orland	Psychiatry
Naraquist, MD, Alma	Internal Medicine
Nelson, MD, Jerome	Neuropsychology
Noonar, MD, James	Cardiology
Noss, MD, Laddie N.	Diabetes & Internal Medicine
Olanka, MD, Daniel G.	Gastroenterology
Orbitz, MD, George	Nephrology
Ortez, MD, Rolando	Pediatrics & Neonatology
Peterson, MD, Rush K.	Allergy & Immunology
Pleasant, MD, Timothy L.	Neurology
Riddle, MD, Edward	Interventional Radiology
Ripple, MD, Ronald	Thoracic Surgery
Sanchez, MD, Gary I.	General Surgery
Smithson, MD, Paula	Urology
Sutton, MD, Paul	Emergency Medicine—Hospital Employee
Warner, MD, Samuel	Podiatry
White, MD, Loren	General Surgery
White, MD, Rapheal	Oncology
Wimer, MD, Rita	Ophthalmology

Physicians by Specialty

Allergy & Immunology	Peterson, MD, Rush K.
Anesthesia	Larson, MD, Janice E.
Cardiology	Elhart, MD, Marvin
Cardiology	Noonar, MD, James
Cardiothoracic Surgery	Barton, MD, David
Critical Care	Brown, MD, Robert
Dermatology	Lauer, MD, Elmer
Dermatology	Lovejoy, MD, Noah
Diabetes & Internal Medicine	Noss, MD, Laddie N.
Emergency Medicine—Hospital Employee	Sutton, MD, Paul
Endocrinology	Doron, MD, Phil
Endocrinology & Nephrology	Jayco, MD, Gordon
Family Practice	Gaul, MD, Frank
Gastroenterology	Friendly, MD, Larry P.
Gastroenterology	Olanka, MD, Daniel G.
General Surgery	Sanchez, MD, Gary I.
General Surgery	White, MD, Loren
Hematology	Lorabi, MD, Gerald
Infectious Diseases	Lin, MD, Lou
Internal Medicine	Naraquist, MD, Alma
Internal Medicine & Critical Care	Green, MD, Ronald
Internal Medicine & Vascular	Alanda, MD, Leslie
Interventional Radiology	Hamilton, MD, Monica J.
Interventional Radiology	Riddle, MD, Edward
Nephrology	Jayco, MD, Gordon
Nephrology	Orbitz, MD, George
Neurology	Pleasant, MD, Timothy L.
Neuropsychology	Nelson, MD, Jerome
Neuroradiology—Hospital Employee	Hart, MD, Phillip
Nuclear Medicine	Aljabar, MD, Alfa
Obstetrics & Gynecology	Martinez, MD, Andy
Oncology	White, MD, Raphael
Ophthalmology	Wimer, MD, Rita
Orthopedics	Almaz, MD, Mohomad
Otorhinolaryngology	King, MD, Jeff
Pathology	Lonewolf, MD, Grey
Pediatrics & Neonatology	Ortez, MD, Rolando
Physical Therapy	Barneswell, MD, Mary
Plastic Surgery	Erickson, MD, Mark
Podiatry	Warner, MD, Samuel
Psychiatry	Munoz, MD, Orland
Radiation Oncology	Eagle, MD, James
Radiology	Monson, MD, Morton
Respiratory Care	Dawson, MD, Gregory
Surgical Neurosurgery	Hodgson, MD, John
Thoracic Surgery	Ripple, MD, Ronald
Urology	Avila, MD, Ira
Urology	Smithson, MD, Paula

Contents

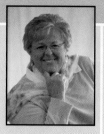

"Your willingness to expand your coding skills by advanced study is remarkable! Coders that have that drive are always great additions to the coding team."

Evaluation and Management Services

http://evolve.elsevier.com/Buck/next

(Answers to every other Case are located in Appendix D, with the full answer key only available in the TEACH Instructor Resources on Evolve)
(Auditing Review answers with rationales are only available in the TEACH Instructor Resources on Evolve)

The most often reported codes in the CPT manual are those in the Evaluation and Management (E/M) section. These codes can also be the most troublesome for the new coder to assign because there are so many variables; but once you learn all the intricacies of E/M coding, you will be able to assign E/M codes with complete confidence that you have assigned the correct code. The first step is to review some of the basics of E/M code assignment. If you are comfortable with the basics of E/M code assignment begin applying E/M codes to physician services.

Within this text, the American Medical Association® Evaluation and Management (E/M) Services Guidelines have been referenced when coding E/M services.

Let us begin with some basics.

E/M Review—The Basics

Three Factors of E/M Code

The codes in the E/M section are based on three factors:
1. Place of service
2. Type of service
3. Patient status

Place of Service The first step in choosing the correct E/M code is to identify the place or setting in which the service was provided. Codes vary based on the place of service. For example, there are different codes for outpatient and inpatient settings.

Type of Service The second step in choosing the correct E/M code is to identify the type of service. The type of service is the kind of service. Examples of types of service are consultation, hospital admission, or an office visit. Codes are divided based on the type of service.

Patient Status The third step in choosing the correct E/M code is to identify the patient status correctly. There are four types of patient status:
1. **New patient**—has not received professional service from the physician or another physician of the exact same specialty and subspecialty in the same group practice within the past 3 years.
2. **Established patient**—has received professional service from the physician or another physician of the exact same specialty and subspecialty in the same group practice within the past 3 years.

3. **Outpatient**—has not been formally admitted to a health care facility.
4. **Inpatient**—has been formally admitted to a health care facility.

Office or Other Outpatient Code Guidelines

As of January 1, 2021 the American Medical Association incorporated new CPT Guidelines for Office or Other Outpatient codes 99202-99215, and also deleted new patient code 99201. The new Guidelines eliminate the history and physical exam portion as key component for code selection, the physician now bases their code selection on only the medical decision-making (MDM) component, or total time spent.

Medical Decision Making (MDM) The elements of Medical Decision Making (MDM) remove the focus of adding up tasks and now focus on the element that affect the management of a patient's condition that include the number and complexity of problems addressed, amount and/or complexity of data reviewed, and risk of complications and/or morbidity or mortality of patient management. Table 1-1 illustrates basic elements of MDM.

Time Total Time may be used to report office or other outpatient services instead of MDM. Total time is used to report the code. Total time includes face-to-face time as well as non-face-to-face time spent on the date of service with the patient and performing other activities, such as pre-visit reviewing and charting. Tables 1-2 and 1-3 display Time.

Time includes performing the following activities, when performed by the physician or other qualified health care professional:*

- Preparing to see the patient (eg, review of tests)
- Obtaining and/or reviewing separately obtained history
- Performing a medically appropriate exam and/or evaluation
- Counseling and educating the patient/family/caregiver
- Ordering medications, tests, or procedures
- Referring and communicating with other health care professionals
- Documenting clinical information in the electronic or other health record

---

* Definitions from 2024 CPT, Evaluation and Management Guidelines, p. 14. CPT codes, descriptions, and materials only are © 2023 American Medical Association.

TABLE 1-1

BASIC ELEMENTS OF MEDICAL DECISION MAKING

Code	Level of MDM	Number and Complexity of Problems Addressed	Amount and/or Complexity of Data	Risk of Complications and/or Morbidity or Mortality
99211	N/A	N/A	N/A	N/A
99202, 99212	Straightforward	Minimal	Minimal or none	Minimal risk
99203, 99213	Low	Low	Limited	Low risk
99204, 99214	Moderate	Moderate	Moderate	Moderate risk
99205, 99215	High	High	Extensive	High risk

*To qualify, two of the three elements of MDM must be met or exceeded.

TABLE 1-2

TIME TABLE - NEW PATIENT

99201	**Deleted. To report, use 99202**
99202	15 minutes
99203	30 minutes
99204	45 minutes
99205	60 minutes
(For services 75 minutes or longer, see Prolonged Services code 99417)	

TABLE 1-3

TIME TABLE - ESTABLISHED PATIENT

99211	N/A
99212	10 minutes
99213	20 minutes
99214	30 minutes
99215	40 minutes
(For service 55 minutes or longer, see Prolonged Service code 99417)	

- Independently interpreting results (not separately reported) and communicating results to the patient/family/caregiver
- Care coordination (not separately reported)

Prolonged Service codes (99417, 99418, G2212) are only reported when Level 5 codes are selected on the basis of time alone. One unit of service reports a full 15 minutes of additional time.

When clinical staff performs the face-to-face time with the patient and the physician or other qualified health care professional performs only supervision, report 99211.

Once you have identified the place of service, type of service, and patient status, you are ready to locate the information in the medical record that identifies the medical decision-making complexity.

Medical Decision Making Complexity The key component of MDM is based on the complexity of the decision the physician must make regarding the patient's diagnosis and care. Complexity of decision making is based on three elements:

1. Number of diagnoses. The options can be minimal, low, moderate, or high.
2. Amount and/or complexity of **data to review**. The data can be minimal or none, limited, moderate, or extensive.
3. **Risk** of complication and/or death if the condition goes untreated. Risk can be minimal, low, moderate, or high.

Although the level of the MDM is most subjective in establishing the level of E/M services, characteristics of the MDM can indicate complexity. The information that follows will provide you with foundational information regarding the MDM.

Number and Complexity of Problems. Some basic guidelines for documentation of management options in the medical record are as follows:

1. For each encounter, an assessment, clinical impression, or diagnosis should be documented. It may be explicitly stated or implied in documented decisions regarding management plans or further evaluation.
   - For a presenting problem with an established diagnosis, the record should reflect whether the problem is (a)

From the Trenches

"Medical coding is such an exciting career. There is so much to learn, and things change all the time, so there is never a chance to get bored with your job. Dive in and you'll see how this profession keeps you on your toes - in a good way!"

JENNA PRICE

improved, well controlled, resolving, or resolved; or (b) inadequately controlled, worsening, or failing to respond as expected.

- ■ For a presenting problem without an established diagnosis, the assessment or clinical impression may be stated in the form of differential diagnoses or as a "possible," "probable," or "rule out" (R/O) diagnosis.

2. The initiation of, or changes in, treatment should be documented. Treatment includes a wide range of management options, including patient instructions, nursing instructions, therapies, and medications.

3. If referrals are made, consultations requested, or advice sought, the record should indicate to whom or where the referral or consultation is made or from whom the advice is requested.

Data to Be Reviewed. The following are some basic documentation guidelines for the amount and complexity of data to be reviewed:

1. If a diagnostic service (test or procedure) is ordered, planned, scheduled, or performed at the time of the E/M encounter, the type of service (e.g., laboratory or radiology) should be documented.

2. The review of laboratory, radiology, or other diagnostic tests should be documented. An entry in a progress note such as "WBC elevated" or "chest x-ray unremarkable" is acceptable. Alternatively, the review may be documented by initializing and dating the report containing the test results.

3. A decision to obtain old records or to obtain additional history from the family, caregiver, or other source to supplement that obtained from the patient should be documented.

4. Relevant findings from the review of old records or the receipt of additional history from the family, caregiver, or other source should be documented. If there is no relevant information beyond that already obtained, that fact should be documented. A notation of "old records reviewed" or "additional history obtained from family" without elaboration is insufficient.

5. The results of discussion of laboratory, radiology, or other diagnostic tests with the physician who performed or interpreted the study should be documented.

6. The direct visualization and independent interpretation of an image, tracing, or specimen previously interpreted by another physician should be documented.

Risk. Some basic documentation guidelines for risk of significant complications, morbidity, or mortality include the following:

1. Comorbidities, underlying diseases, or other factors that increase the complexity of MDM by increasing the risk of complications, morbidity, or mortality should be documented.

2. If a surgical or invasive diagnostic procedure is ordered, planned, or scheduled at the time of the E/M encounter, the type of procedure (e.g., laparoscopy) should be documented.

3. If a surgical or invasive diagnostic procedure is performed at the time of the E/M encounter, the specific procedure should be documented.

4. The referral for or decision to perform a surgical or invasive diagnostic procedure on an urgent basis should be documented or implied.

Examples of the levels of risk are found in Table 1-4.

The extent to which each of these elements is considered determines the levels of MDM complexity:

1. **Straightforward:** Minimal diagnosis and/or management options, minimal or none for the amount and complexity of data to be reviewed, and minimal risk to the patient of complications or death if untreated.

2. **Low complexity:** Limited number of diagnoses and/or management options, limited data to be reviewed, and low risk to the patient of complications or death if untreated.

3. **Moderate complexity:** Multiple diagnoses and/or management options, moderate amount and complexity of data to be reviewed, and moderate risk to the patient of complications or death if untreated.

4. **High complexity:** Extensive diagnoses and/or management options, extensive amount and complexity of data to be reviewed, and high risk to the patient for complications or death if the problem is untreated.

When you select one of the four types of MDM complexity—straightforward, low, moderate, or high—the documentation in the medical record must support the selection in terms of the number of diagnoses or management options, amount or complexity of data to be reviewed, and risks.

Given the information in the medical record, you would consider the information in the context of the complexity of the diagnosis and management options, data to be reviewed, and risks to the patient to choose the complexity of MDM. An example of MDM is illustrated in **Figure 1-1**. To qualify for a given level of MDM complexity, two or three elements must be met or exceeded.

Time Time was not included in the CPT manual before 1992 but was incorporated to assist with selection of the most appropriate level of E/M services. The times indicated with the codes are only averages and represent simple estimates of the possible duration of a service.

Face-to-face time and **non face-to-face time** are two descriptions of time. Face-to-face time is the time a physician spends directly with a patient during an office visit obtaining the history, performing an examination, and discussing results. Non face-to-face time describes the time a physician spends reviewing test results, obtaining additional history from family members, ordering medications or tests, and performing other activities to care for the patient without the patient present.

MDM ELEMENTS	Documented
# OF DIAGNOSIS	
1. Minimal	
2. Low	
3. Moderate	✗
4. High	
LEVEL	3
AMOUNT AND/OR COMPLEXITY OF DATA TO REVIEW	Documented
1. Minimal/None	
2. Limited	
3. Moderate	✗
4. Extensive	
LEVEL	3
RISK OF COMPLICATION OR DEATH IF NOT TREATED	Documented
1. Minimal	
2. Low	
3. Moderate	✗
4. High	
MDM LEVEL	3

FIGURE 1-1 Medical Decision Making (MDM).

Time in the E/M section is referred to in statements such as this one, which is located with code 99222:

When using total time on the date of the encounter for code selection, 55 minutes must be met or exceeded.

This means that instead of assigning the code level based on medical decision making, you can assign it based on the total time.

Watch for reports that indicate the time the physician spent with the patient. However, just because time is documented, it does not mean that the time is in excess of any given code. Some physicians always document the time spent with a patient in the medical record, so you cannot assume the indication of time calls for an increase in code assignment. You need to check the time statements in the codes to ensure that it is appropriate to assign a higher-level code.

Hospital Inpatient and Observation Care Services

Hospital Inpatient and Observation Care Services codes (99221-99239) are reported to indicate a patient's status as an inpatient in a hospital or partial hospital setting; therefore, these codes are reported to identify the hospital setting as the place where the physician renders service to the patient. An inpatient is one who has been formally admitted to an acute health care facility.

Note that within the subsection Hospital Inpatient and Observation Care Services, all the subheadings except Hospital Discharge Services are divided primarily on the basis of MDM complexity and total time. **Discharge** services are based on time. The Initial Hospital Inpatient or Observation Care codes and the Subsequent Hospital Inpatient or Observation Care codes are all reported based on MDM or the total time documented. For example, code 99222 is a moderate level of MDM complexity. If the case you are coding has a low MDM complexity, you cannot assign code 99222; instead, you would assign the lower-level code 99221.

The subsection of Hospital Inpatient and Observation Care Services is divided into:
1. Initial Hospital Inpatient or Observation Care
2. Subsequent Hospital Inpatient or Observation Care
3. Hospital Inpatient or Observation Care Services (Including Admission and Discharge Services)
4. Hospital Inpatient or Observation Discharge Services

Initial Hospital Inpatient or Observation Care

Initial Hospital Inpatient or Observation Care codes (99221-99223) report the initial service of admission to the hospital (inpatient or observation) by the admitting physician. Only the admitting physician can use the Initial Hospital Inpatient or Observation Care codes. These codes reflect not only the admission but also the services in any setting (office, emergency department, nursing home) provided in conjunction with the admission. For example, if the patient is seen in the office and is immediately admitted to the hospital, the office visit is bundled into the initial hospital care service and not reported separately. These services provided in the office may be taken into account when selecting the appropriate code for the hospital admission. The hospital admission includes the patient's admitting diagnosis, history, physical, and orders directing the nursing and ancillary staff regarding the patient's care.

Subsequent Hospital Inpatient or Observation Care

Subsequent Hospital Inpatient or Observation Care (99231-99233) is the second subheading of codes in the Hospital Inpatient and Observation Services subsection. The Subsequent Hospital Inpatient or Observation Care codes are used by physicians to report daily hospital visits while the patient is hospitalized. These codes indicate the status of the patient, such as stable/unstable or recovering/unresponsive.

The first Subsequent Hospital Inpatient or Observation Care code is 99231, and it typically implies that the patient is in stable condition and responding well to treatment.

When using total time on the date of the encounter for code selection, 25 minutes must be met or exceeded.

More than one physician can use the subsequent care codes on the same day. This is called **concurrent care**. Concurrent care is being provided when more than one physician provides service to a patient on the same day for different conditions. An example of concurrent care is a circumstance in which physician A, a cardiologist, treats a patient for a heart condition, and at the same time physician B, an oncologist, treats the patient for a lung neoplasm. The patient's **attending physician** maintains the primary responsibility for the overall care of the patient, no matter how many other physicians are providing services to the patient, unless a formal transfer of care has occurred.

An **attending physician** is a physician who, on the basis of education, training, and experience, is granted medical staff membership and clinical privileges by a health care organization to perform diagnostic or therapeutic procedures. An attending physician is legally responsible for the care and treatment provided to a patient. The attending physician may be a patient's personal physician or may be a physician assigned to a patient who has been admitted to a hospital through the emergency department or by another physician who assumed responsibility for the patient. The attending physician is usually a provider of primary care, such as a family practitioner, internist, or pediatrician, but may also be a surgeon or other type of specialist. In an academic medical center, the attending physician may be a member of the academic or medical school staff who is responsible for the supervision of medical residents, interns, and students and oversees the care these individuals provide to patients.

Hospital Inpatient or Observation Care Services (Including Admission and Discharge Services)

These codes are reported for either observation status or inpatients who are admitted and discharged on the same day. In these cases, the admit and discharge codes are not separately reported. Hospital Inpatient or Observation Care Services (Including Admission and Discharge Services).

Hospital Inpatient or Observation Discharge Services

Inpatient Hospital Discharge Services (99238, 99239) are reported on the final day of services for a **multiple-day stay** in a hospital setting. The service reflects the final examination of the patient as appropriate, follow-up instructions to the patient, and arrangements for discharge, including completion of discharge records. The Hospital Inpatient or Observation Discharge Services codes are based on the time spent by the physician in handling the final discharge of the patient as 99238 for 30 minutes or less and 99239 for more than 30 minutes.

The Hospital Inpatient or Observation Discharge Services codes are not reported if the physician is a **consultant**. If a consulting physician is seeing the patient for a separate condition, those services would require a subsequent hospital care code. Only the attending physician is responsible for completion of the final examination, follow-up instructions, and arrangements for discharge and discharge records, and therefore only the attending physician can report services using the discharge codes.

Diagnosis Coding

The *ICD-10-CM Official Guidelines for Coding and Reporting* are displayed on the Evolve website. See Appendix B for instructions. These *Guidelines* assist the coder in assignment of ICD-10-CM codes. Review the *Guidelines* if you need a refresher on code assignment and to ensure that you are up-to-date on the changes that have taken place within the *Guidelines*. Updates to the *Guidelines* are located at www.cdc.gov/nchs/icd.htm.

As with all diagnosis coding, the coder is to report the most definitive diagnosis available at the time of the report. However, before assigning a code, the coder must identify the correct diagnosis to ensure coding the correct diagnostic statement. It is always tempting to report what you know about the patient from previous documentation in the medical record, but it is important to remember that you must not use information from any other area of the chart except the report you are coding (except in operative reports, for which the pathology report is considered). In the first case in this text you are going to code the CC of the patient, which is recurrent nausea and vomiting, reported with R11.0. On reading the report, however, you find that the physician indicated the patient has nausea and vomiting due to early diabetic ketoacidosis. The first-listed (primary) diagnosis would not then be the symptoms of nausea and vomiting but would be the diabetic ketoacidosis because it is the most definitive diagnosis.

Another area of challenge is the coding of diagnostic tests. The *Program Memorandum* from the Centers for Medicare and Medicaid Services (CMS) dated September 26, 2001, (AB-01-144) addressed the issue of diagnostic testing and diagnosis (see box on p. 7).

The reason for the diagnostic test is to be documented in the patient's medical record by the physician ordering the test. This order is then faxed, mailed, delivered, e-mailed, or telephoned to the testing facility. This order would include the diagnostic information that indicates the **reason** the test was requested. This establishes medical necessity and is a very important concept for justification of the test.

Incidental findings are findings that were not the reason for the test. For example, a patient is sent to a radiologist for a chest x-ray because of wheezing. The chest x-ray is negative, but a degenerative joint disease of the spine is visualized on the examination. The radiologist would report the wheezing (symptom) as the primary diagnosis and may then list the degenerative joint disease as a secondary diagnosis. This incidental finding is unrelated to the reason the test was ordered.

If a test is ordered for screening (no signs or symptom exists), an ICD-10-CM screening code, such as Z11-Z13.9, would be assigned as the reason for the test.

The coder is directed to report the diagnosis code that most precisely explains the **reason** the test was ordered. This

The following are excerpts from the Program Memorandum of the CMS:[1]

The ICD-9-CM Coding Guidelines for Outpatient Services (hospital-based and physician office) have instructed physicians to report diagnoses based on test results. The Coding Clinic for ICD-9-CM confirms this long-standing coding guideline. CMS agrees with these long-standing official coding and reporting guidelines.

"Following are instructions for contractors, physicians, hospitals, and other health care providers to use in determining the use of ICD-9-CM codes for coding diagnostic test results. The instructions below provide guidance on the appropriate assignment of ICD-9-CM diagnoses codes to simplify coding for diagnostic tests consistent with the ICD-9-CM Guidelines for Outpatient Services (hospital-based and physician office). Note that physicians are responsible for the accuracy of the information submitted on the bill.

A. Determining the Appropriate Primary ICD-9-CM Diagnosis Code for Diagnostic Tests Ordered Due to Signs and/or Symptoms.

1. If the physician has confirmed a diagnosis based on the results of the diagnostic test, the physician interpreting the test should report that diagnosis. The signs and/or symptoms that prompted ordering the test may be reported as additional diagnoses if they are not fully explained or related to the confirmed diagnosis.

    Example 1: A surgical specimen is sent to a pathologist with a diagnosis of "mole." The pathologist personally reviews the slides made from the specimen and makes a diagnosis of "malignant melanoma." The pathologist should report a diagnosis of "malignant melanoma" as the primary diagnosis.

    Example 2: A patient is referred to a radiologist for an abdominal CT scan with a diagnosis of abdominal pain. The CT scan reveals the presence of an abscess. The radiologist should report a diagnosis of "intra-abdominal abscess."

    Example 3: A patient is referred to a radiologist for a chest x-ray with a diagnosis of "cough." The chest x-ray reveals a 3-cm peripheral pulmonary nodule. The radiologist should report a diagnosis of "pulmonary nodule" and may sequence "cough" as an additional diagnosis.

2. If the diagnostic test did not provide a diagnosis or was normal, the interpreting physician should report the sign(s) or symptom(s) that prompted the treating physician to order the study.

    Example 1: A patient is referred to a radiologist for a spine x-ray due to complaints of "back pain." The radiologist performs the x-ray, and the results are normal. The radiologist should report a diagnosis of "back pain" since this was the reason for performing the spine study.

    Example 2: A patient is seen in the ER for chest pain. EKG is normal, and the final diagnosis is chest pain due suspected gastroesophageal reflux disease (GERD). The patient was told to follow up with his primary care physician for further evaluation of the suspected GERD. The primary diagnosis code for the EKG should be chest pain. Although the EKG was normal, a definitive cause for the chest pain was not determined.

3. If the results of the diagnostic test are normal or nondiagnostic, and the referring physician records a diagnosis preceded by words that indicate uncertainty (e.g., probable, suspected, questionable, rule out, or working), the interpreting physician should not report the referring diagnosis. Rather, the interpreting physician should report the signs(s) or symptom(s) that prompted the study. Diagnoses labeled as uncertain are considered by the ICD-9-CM Coding Guidelines as unconfirmed and should not be reported. This is consistent with the requirement to report the diagnosis to the highest degree of certainty.

    Example: A patient is referred to a radiologist for a chest x-ray with a diagnosis of "rule out pneumonia." The radiologist performs a chest x-ray, and the results are normal. The radiologist should report the sign(s) or symptom(s) that prompted the test (e.g., cough).

A copy of the full program memorandum is included as Appendix A.

---

[1]Although this memorandum is for ICD-9-CM and there is currently no such memorandum for ICD-10-CM, the content is applicable to ICD-10-CM.

---

is often referred to as the greatest level of specificity. What this means is that the diagnosis code should match the reason the test was ordered as closely as possible. For example, if you are reporting a chest x-ray for malignancy of the left lower lobe of the lung, C34.32 most closely matches the diagnosis or the reason for the test. It would be incorrect to assign C34.00 for other parts of the bronchus or lung or C34.90 for unspecified bronchus or lung. The greatest level of specificity also means that all available characters/digits must be assigned for the code to be complete.

Any report that has been prepared or interpreted by a physician can be the basis of a diagnosis. This would include a radiology report and a pathology report because both are written and interpreted by physicians. A routine laboratory report is prepared by a laboratory technician and is not to be used for the diagnostic statement until a physician has interpreted the report. For example, the surgical specimen is sent to the pathology department for analysis. The diagnosis statement on the operative report indicates skin lesion. The pathology report is available at the time of code assignment with a diagnosis of basal cell carcinoma. The code assigned would indicate basal cell carcinoma, not skin lesion, because the pathologist is a physician and as such is qualified to make the assessment. If, however, a patient is sent to the laboratory for a urine analysis based on the CC of frequent urination and the analysis indicated a bacterial infection, the diagnosis of bacterial infection is not reported until a physician has interpreted the report, even if the report is available at the time of code assignment. This is because a laboratory technician, not a physician, performed the laboratory analysis.

Inpatient and Outpatient Coders

There is a difference between the medical record documentation available to the inpatient and outpatient coder at the time of code assignment. The **inpatient coder** reports the services provided to the patient at the end of the hospital stay and has all of the medical documentation for that stay available at the time of code assignment. The diagnoses are based on all information compiled during the stay. The **outpatient coder** has only the latest service available at the time of code assignment. The services to that patient may or may not be concluded at the time of code assignment. For example, a patient presents to the physician's office with the symptom of wheezing. The physician examines the patient and orders a chest x-ray for the clinical indication of "wheezing." The results probably will not have been returned when the coder assigns a code for the physician's office visit service, and as such the diagnosis would be reported as "wheezing" (R06.2). On a later date, the x-ray report for the patient comes back with the radiologist's diagnosis of "pneumonia" (J18.9) based on the results of the x-ray. When the coder reports the radiologist's services, the diagnosis of pneumonia (J18.9) would be reported. Upon reviewing the radiologist's report, the patient's physician orders a pathology examination of the patient's sputum to determine the organism responsible for the pneumonia. The results are returned from the pathologist with a diagnosis of "streptococcus, type B" (J15.3, pneumonia due to streptococcus, Group B). The coder would report the pathologist's services using J15.3, streptococcus Group B pneumonia. At each step in the process, the diagnosis for the patient became more definitive, and the coder reported the most definitive diagnosis available at the time based on the documentation available in the report being coded. Had this wheezing patient been an inpatient, the inpatient coder would have had the final definitive diagnosis of pneumonia due to streptococcus, Group B, and would have assigned J15.3 as the diagnosis when reporting the services for that inpatient stay.

The medical coder employed by a hospital to assign codes to services provided in its outpatient departments, such as the ambulatory or same-day surgery center, reports those outpatient services provided by the facility. For example, a patient presents to the ambulatory surgery center at the hospital for a surgical procedure that is performed by a clinic-employed general surgeon. The clinic outpatient coder would report the service provided by the surgeon. The hospital outpatient coder would report the facility portion of the same service. Both coders report outpatient services, one employed by the clinic and the other employed by the hospital. The clinic coder reports the physician (professional) portion of the service on the CMS-1500 Universal Claim Form, and the hospital (facility) coder reports the facility portion of the service on the CMS-1450 (UB-04). Both coders assign codes based on the documentation available at the time of code assignment.

All tissue removed during an operative procedure requires pathological examination and becomes a specimen. The pathologist analyzes the tissue and prepares a written report of the findings. To ensure reporting of the most definitive diagnosis, the operative report service is not usually reported until the results of the pathological examination are known.

If you are a hospital coder and the hospital employs a physician, you report the physician's professional services on the CMS-1500. If you are a hospital coder reporting the hospital services provided to an inpatient, you report these facility services on a CMS-1450 after the patient is discharged. Again, as the inpatient coder, you have available all of the documentation

compiled during the hospital stay and assign diagnoses codes based on the entire stay. You will not be assigning or auditing codes to inpatient services (facility) in this text.

When you are assigning diagnoses codes to the reports within this text, **you are functioning as the outpatient coder and will assume that you have only the current report available to you and on which you will assign a code for the diagnosis**. For example, if a case contains three reports and you are assigning a diagnosis code for the first report, you have only the first report available and on which to base code assignment. If you are assigning a diagnosis code for the second report, you will assume you have only the second report available and on which to assign the most precise code. If you are assigning a diagnosis code to the third of three reports, you will assume you have only the third report available and on which to base code assignment. Each report, in the outpatient setting, stands on its own, and the coding is based on the information in just that report. There are two major exceptions to this rule. The first exception is an operative report that indicates a specimen was removed. The diagnosis for the operative report is reported only after reviewing the pathology report that indicates the results of the specimen analysis (because the result of benign or malignant will determine the code choice). Within this text each operative report will be followed by the pathology report, or a note at the end of the operative report will indicate "Pathology Report Later Indicated," followed by the pathology results. The second exception to the "each report stands on its own" rule is when the directions for the case indicate that you are to report the services in a particular way. For example, Case 1-16 requires you to report the critical care services that a physician provided to a patient during a 24-hour period. Because critical care services are reported once for each 24 hours, you will be using all three reports in that case when assigning a code.

All medical reports in this text are printed as dictated by the physician. Also, the physician gives direction on the format he or she wants used when the report is transcribed and, as such, report formats vary. For example, some physicians want each major element of an examination in capital letters, such as ENDOCRINE, CARDIOVASCULAR, and RESPIRATORY. Therefore, the coder should anticipate that the formats within this text will vary to reflect the real world of coding.

Time To Code!

You will be assigning diagnosis codes and can find the latest *Official Guidelines for Coding and Reporting* in your Evolve Learning Resources.

The most important thing about abstracting a medical record, whether it is an operative report or inpatient/outpatient record, is knowing what you are looking for and understanding what you are reading. As you work through this text, read with a highlighter in your hand and a medical dictionary close by. The following steps were developed by Karen Lockyer and contain excellent advice to help you build your coding skills.

Steps to Building Your Coding and Auditing Skills

Step 1 Read the record for the first time for content and the second time for understanding.

Step 2 During the second reading, highlight important words that may apply to either the diagnosis (acute, chronic, malignant, etc.) or procedure (with or without, internal, external). Words a physician or surgeon uses to further document relevant aspects of the procedure may necessitate the use of modifiers. Look for words and phrases such as "heavily obstructed" or "severely impacted."

Step 3 This is a fundamental skill coders build upon by practice. For example, there is a big difference between nephrectomy and nephrostomy, and the difference affects the code choice.

Step 4 When tips are given in this text, consider transferring them to your coding manual for instant reference when you are coding or auditing a service or diagnosis in the future.

Now, let's put the information that you have just learned about coding E/M services to work by coding and auditing services using CPT, diagnosis, and HCPCS codes.

Let's do Case 1-1 A together. First, read the report carefully.

It is customary to assign the diagnoses codes before assigning the CPT code. Assign the diagnosis code(s) for Case 1-1A, then return to review the diagnosis information that follows.

Diabetic Ketoacidosis

The physician indicates in the Impression section of the report that the symptoms of nausea and vomiting are due to Type 1 diabetic ketoacidosis (accumulation of acid in the blood). Ketoacidosis is very serious if left untreated, and there is a high risk of death.

The ICD-10-CM requires the indication of the type of diabetes; therefore, in the Index, under the main term "Diabetes," you must reference the subterm "type 1" and then the subterms "with, ketoacidosis," to be directed to E10.10.

The symptoms of nausea and vomiting are not reported, as the etiology (cause) is identified as diabetic ketoacidosis. The second statement under the Impression section is "Diabetes mellitus type 1 with a history of recurrent ketoacidosis," and is not reported separately, as it is included in the E10.10.

Asthma

Asthma is also documented as a diagnosis. Asthma is a disease of the airways in which the airways are hypersensitive. The typical manifestations of an acute asthma attack are wheezing, rapid and labored breathing, and cough with marked dyspnea. In the Index under the main term "Asthma," the coder is directed to J45.909.

In the Index, locate "Asthma." Since no other description or exacerbation is documented, J45.909 is referenced in the Tabular, "Unspecified asthma, uncomplicated."

Medical Decision Making Complexity (MDM)

In the opinion of many coders, the identification of MDM level is the most difficult part of E/M coding. This is because it is the most abstract, which means the coder can't just check off a list and add the items to arrive at the level. Rather, the coder must assess the complexity, which takes time and practice to learn. Think about the report in total, identify the level of MDM, and then return here.

Level of Diagnoses

Here are some questions you need to ask yourself to assess the level of diagnoses/management options for this case:

■ Was there an established diagnosis when the patient presented? *(At this time, the patient presents with nausea and vomiting, cause unknown at presentation.)*

■ Does the report reflect whether the problem was improved, well controlled, resolving or resolved, or was the problem inadequately controlled, worsening, or was the patient failing to respond? *(This patient's problem was inadequately controlled; without care she would have continued to worsen.)*

■ Could there be multiple causes of nausea and vomiting? *(Yes, there could be, and the physician will have to identify the causes from a wide range of possibilities in a patient with known multiple health problems.)*

This is an example of extensive diagnoses and management options, or a level 4.

Level of Data to Review

Did the physician review data? *(There was no indication that data from old records were requested or reviewed, and if it is not documented, it didn't happen. So, there were no data reviewed, except the fingerstick documented before the Impression section of the report.)*

This is a minimal/none level of data review or a level 1.

Level of Risk

Does the patient have other conditions that could affect the management and treatment of the condition? *(Yes, the patient is a diabetic with reoccurring ketoacidosis and in addition has asthma. The report indicates ketoacidosis in the diagnosis section of the report.)*

There is a high level of risk of death or complication for this patient or a level 4.

The MDM level is based on 2 of 3 elements. You do not need all 3 elements of the MDM to be at the same level to assign that level. There are two elements at a level 4, so this is a level 4 MDM.

This report contained a high MDM complexity. CPT code 99223 requires a high MDM complexity.

Time

Time may be used to report initial inpatient or observation services instead of MDM. Total time is used to report the code. Total time includes face-to-face time as well as non-face-to-face time spent on the date of service with the patient and performing other activities, such as pre-visit reviewing and charting.

CASE 1-1A   *Initial Hospital Care*

Report Dr. Alanda's professional services for Sally Jacobson's initial hospital care.

LOCATION: Inpatient, Hospital

PATIENT: Sally Jacobson

PHYSICIAN: Leslie Alanda, MD

CHIEF COMPLAINT: Recurrent nausea and vomiting.

HISTORY OF PRESENT ILLNESS: The patient is a 17-year-old female with type 1 diabetes mellitus who has had several admissions for ketoacidosis. The patient indicates that she was feeling quite good last night and ate her evening meal without problems. She had a blood sugar of about 168 mg/dL sometime yesterday. This morning she woke about 5:00 AM and had sugar that was over 500 mg/dL. This was associated with emesis, which has continued on a recurrent basis since that time. The patient did take Humalog 10 units and Ultralente 14 units when she awoke with the high sugar. She also apparently took an additional dose of possibly 20 units of Humalog around 9:00 AM.

Because of the persistence of vomiting, her mother called in at noon and was advised to bring her in. She indicates that the daughter has been a little bit confused. In addition, she states that the daughter is having some abdominal discomfort, ongoing nausea, and cramping in her legs.

The patient's mother indicates she has been very good with her diet and has not had any recent problems with skipped shots or high sugars. She has been testing anywhere from two to four times per day. The patient denies that she has had any cough, although she has had a slightly sore throat today. No other symptoms, such as diarrhea, have been noted.

MEDICATIONS:

1. Humalog 7 units, Ultralente 14 units at breakfast and suppertime, and Humalog 7 units at noon.
2. Albuterol nebulizer treatments p.r.n. (as needed).

ALLERGIES: None.

PAST MEDICAL HISTORY:

SURGICAL: None.

MEDICAL:

1. Diabetes mellitus type 1 with history of recurrent ketoacidosis.
2. Asthma, p.r.n albuterol.

SOCIAL HISTORY: The patient lives with her parents. She has two brothers, both of whom now have type 1 diabetes. Her oldest brother was recently diagnosed with diabetes. She is going into the senior grade in high school. She states that she does not smoke or use drugs.

FAMILY HISTORY: Strongly positive for diabetes in a cousin and an uncle. There is also a history of coronary artery disease and stroke.

REVIEW OF SYSTEMS: Eyes: Negative. Ears: Negative. Mouth: As noted above. Chest: As noted above. Cardiac: As noted above. Hematologic: Negative. Infectious disease: Negative. Neurologic: Negative. Psychiatric: As noted above. Musculoskeletal: Negative. GU (genitourinary): The patient generally has nocturia.

PHYSICAL EXAMINATION: The patient is very sluggish, although she does answer questions. Blood pressure 96/76, pulse 130 and regular, respirations normal. EYES: Sunken significantly. Fundi are not visualized. EARS: Negative. MOUTH: Tongue is dry and throat looked all right. Carotids are 4/4 without bruits. Thyroid is normal to palpation. NECK: supple, nodes are negative. Axillary nodes negative. CHEST: Symmetrical. Clear to auscultation. HEART: Tachycardic but no extra heart sounds heard. No murmur is appreciated. ABDOMEN: Some minimal tenderness in the right midabdomen and left upper abdomen. GENITAL/RECTAL: Not performed. Peripheral extremities reveal good pulses in the legs with no edema.

Fingerstick in the office was 110 mg/dL.

IMPRESSION:

1. Nausea and vomiting due to diabetic ketoacidosis.
2. Diabetes mellitus type 1 with a history of recurrent ketoacidosis.
3. Asthma.

PLAN: The patient will need intravenous fluids and low doses of insulin along with intravenous glucose for her rehydration. She has been sluggish in the past when hospitalized, so I suspect she will have a slow recovery time but should be able to go home tomorrow.

There is no apparent etiology for the onset of the acidosis.

The situation has been discussed frankly with the patient's mother, and she understands the objectives and our treatment plan.

Total of 45 minutes was spent with the patient today.

SERVICE CODE(S): _____

ICD-10-CM DX CODE(S): _____

(Answers to every other Case are located in Appendix D . The full answer key is only available in the TEACH Instructor Resources on Evolve.)

Hospital Inpatient or Observation Discharge Services

The hospital discharge services are based on the time the physician spends in the final discharge of the patient. The service may or may not include an examination of the patient. If the physician does not indicate the time spent in discharge of the patient, the lowest level of discharge would be reported (99238). Physician education about documentation is very important to ensure appropriate reimbursement since only if the physician records the amount of time can the coder assign a discharge code for a higher-level discharge service. The time must be documented in the medical record with the beginning and ending time, and the time does not have to be consecutive. The physician may spend time on preparation of the final discharge and then return and spend additional time on the discharge documentation.

At the time of discharge, the physician will indicate the discharge diagnoses, usually in a "Discharge Diagnosis" section of the report. However, the full report must be carefully read to ensure that other diagnoses pertinent to the service provided are also reported.

Recall that you do not report symptoms when there is a more definitive diagnosis available, but note that in report 1-1B, the discharge diagnosis indicates "Vomiting with dehydration, secondary to early diabetic ketoacidosis." The vomiting is a symptom of the ketoacidosis; however, the dehydration is not a symptom of the ketoacidosis but a separate, distinct condition and is therefore assigned a code. Although there is a combination code for vomiting with nausea, there is no combination code for vomiting with dehydration.

CASE 1-1B *Discharge Summary*

Report Dr. Alanda's professional services for Sally's discharge from the hospital.

LOCATION: Inpatient, Hospital

PATIENT: Sally Jacobson

PHYSICIAN: Leslie Alanda, MD

DISCHARGE DIAGNOSES:

1. Vomiting with dehydration, secondary to early diabetic ketoacidosis.
2. Diabetes mellitus type 1.
3. Asthma.

HOSPITAL COURSE: The patient was admitted with recurrent vomiting and clinical evidence for dehydration. Earlier on the day of admission, the patient had sugar over 500 mg/dL but was able to get this down to about 120 mg/dL around the time of admission. Nonetheless, she was also confused on admission, and with rehydration and intravenous insulin, she gradually rehydrated and returned to her normal status. It is unclear why the patient developed this problem because there was no other evidence for any gastroenteritis or intestinal problems. The patient's measured bicarbonate level on admission was 22.2, which is slightly low. Blood sugars while hospitalized ranged from 77 to 328 mg/dL.

DISCHARGE ACTIVITY: Regular.

DISCHARGE DIET: 2400 calories ADA.

DISCHARGE FOLLOW-UP: The patient will see me in 1 week's time at the clinic. She is to continue testing her sugars four times a day and taking regular meals.

LABORATORY STUDIES: Hemoglobin 15.9 with an MCV (mean corpuscular volume) of 78. Platelet count was 491,000. White count was 12,550. BUN (blood urea nitrogen) was 27, bicarb 22.2, and glucose 154 on admission.

DISCHARGE CONDITION: The patient is eating, ambulatory, and alert.

DISCHARGE MEDICATION: Ultralente 14 units, Humalog 7 units at breakfast, and Humalog 7 units at noon, albuterol, p.r.n. (as needed).

SERVICE CODE(S): _____

ICD-10-CM DX CODE(S): _____

Discussion

The physician made no note of the length of time spent providing the discharge service, so the lowest level discharge service is reported (99238). The diagnoses are type 1 diabetes with ketoacidosis (E10.10), dehydration (E86.0 is a separate, distinct condition), and asthma without mention of the status (J45.909).

From the Trenches

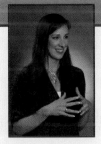

"Anyone who enjoys problem-solving and critical thinking will be successful in the medical coding arena. It's a lot like a puzzle - finding the various pieces and fitting them together. Attention to detail and perseverance are a must."

JENNA PRICE
CPC

CASE 1-2 *Emergency Department Services*

The patient in Case 1-2 is the same patient in Case 1-1. The patient presents to the emergency department with nausea and recurrent vomiting.

LOCATION: Hospital Emergency Department

PATIENT: Sally Jacobson

PHYSICIAN: Paul Sutton, MD

CHIEF COMPLAINT: Nausea and recurrent vomiting with dehydration.

HISTORY OF PRESENT ILLNESS: The patient is a 17-year-old girl with type 1 diabetes mellitus since age 11 who has had pharyngitis for about the past 5 days. She was seen by her regular internist 2 days ago, and throat culture was negative. The feeling was she had a viral pharyngitis because her brother had similar symptoms. The patient indicates that she has had nausea with some vomiting for the past 3 days and has really not eaten anything for the past 2 days. She also indicates she has had some fever and chills and some cough. Generally, she feels poorly and indicates that she has been running to

Continued

CASE 1-2—*cont'd*

the bathroom quite frequently. She does indicate that she has taken all of her insulin shots as noted below, but she has not been able to eat. She does indicate that she has had an associated headache but no other symptoms. Blood sugar at noon today was about 190 mg/dL by Accu-Chek.

ALLERGIES: None known.

MEDICATIONS:

1. Ultralente 16 units, morning and evening.
2. Humalog 14 units in the morning, 7 units at noon, and 14 units at supper.
3. Albuterol nebulizer treatments p.r.n. (as needed).

PAST MEDICAL HISTORY: Asthma, presently albuterol p.r.n. Diabetes mellitus type 1 with several admissions for ketoacidosis.

PAST SURGICAL HISTORY: None.

FAMILY HISTORY: Positive in two brothers with type 1 diabetes mellitus. She also has a cousin and uncle with diabetes. There is also positive family history for coronary artery disease. An uncle has lung cancer.

SOCIAL HISTORY: The patient is a senior in high school.

REVIEW OF SYSTEMS: Eyes: Blurred double vision. Ears: Hearing is okay. GI (gastrointestinal): As noted above. GU (genitourinary): As noted above. Cardiac: Negative. Chest: As noted above. She has had no SOB (shortness of breath) or heavy breathing. Hematologic: Negative. Infectious disease: As noted above. Neurologic: Negative. Psychiatric:

Negative. Sleep pattern has been off in the past, and she has been treated with amitriptyline. This has not been such a significant problem of late.

EXAMINATION: The patient appears dehydrated with sunken eyeballs and a flushed face. Blood pressure 102/70, pulse 120 and regular, and temperature 97.8° F. Tongue is mildly dry. Eyes: Good range of motion of the eyes, but the eyeballs are sunken. Neck: Supple. Nodes are negative. Carotids are 4/4 without bruits. Thyroid is normal to palpation. Chest: Clear to auscultation. Heart: Tachycardia is present, but no murmurs or extra sounds appreciated. No Kussmaul breathing is noted. Abdomen: Soft, nontender without palpable masses. Genitorectal: Not performed. Peripheral extremities reveal good pulses and normal reflexes. No edema is present.

IMPRESSION:

1. Dehydration secondary to #2 with possible ketoacidosis.
2. Viral pharyngitis with gastroenteritis component.
3. Diabetes mellitus type 1, 6 years without complication.
4. Asthma, presently stable.

PLAN: The patient will be treated with intravenous fluids and insulin as indicated. Once she is able to eat and is ambulatory, she will be able to go home.

SERVICE CODE(S): _____

ICD-10-CM DX CODE(S): _____

(Answers to every other Case are located in Appendix D. The full answer key is only available in the TEACH Instructor Resources on Evolve.)

CASE 1-3A   *Initial Hospital Service*

The patient in Cases 1-1 and 1-2 is again admitted, at a later time, to the hospital, this time for abdominal pain.

LOCATION: Inpatient, Hospital

PATIENT: Sally Jacobson

ATTENDING PHYSICIAN: Leslie Alanda, MD

CHIEF COMPLAINT: Abdominal pain for 48 hours.

HISTORY OF PRESENT ILLNESS: This is a 17-year-old female who presents with a 24- to 48-hour history of right lower-quadrant abdominal pain. The patient has a history of diabetes mellitus. The patient states that nothing has made it better and nothing has made the pain any more tolerable. She states that the pain is becoming gradually worse. She states she has taken Advil to no avail. The patient does have positive nausea with no vomiting. No diarrhea and no constipation. No dysuria. The patient states that she has eaten very little today because of the pain and is not hungry at this time.

PAST MEDICAL HISTORY:

1. Diabetes mellitus.
2. Sinusitis.
3. Asthma.

MEDICATIONS:

1. Humalog 7 units in the morning, noon, and q.h.s. (each bedtime).
2. Ultralente 14 units q.a.m. (every morning) and 14 units q.p.m. (every afternoon or evening).
3. Elavil 100 mg (milligram) p.o. (by mouth) q.h.s.

ALLERGIES: None.

SOCIAL HISTORY: The patient now states that she has drunk in the past. She does smoke three to five cigarettes daily. She is otherwise a normal, healthy senior high school student.

FAMILY HISTORY: Neither of her parents has diabetes mellitus; however, there is a history of diabetes in that her two brothers have it and that a cousin and uncle have it. There is also a history of CVAs (stroke/cardiovascular accident), myocardial infarctions, and cancer.

REVIEW OF SYSTEMS: General: The patient states she has been in good health other than the right abdominal pain.

HEENT (head, ears, eyes, nose, throat): The patient denies any headache, diplopia, blurred vision, eye pain, redness, cataracts, glaucoma, loss of vision, hearing loss, tinnitus, or epistaxis. Cardiovascular: The patient denies any chest pain, chest pressure, orthopnea, or PND (paroxysmal nocturnal dyspnea). Respiratory: The

CASE 1-3A—*cont'd*

patient denies any coughing, wheezing, and hemoptysis. She does complain of the history of asthma as stated in the past medical history. She does not take medications for that. GI (gastrointestinal): The patient complains of right lower-quadrant pain and nausea but denies vomiting, constipation, or diarrhea. GU (genitourinary): The patient denies dysuria, hematuria, nocturia, or changes in frequency. Extremities: The patient has a good range of motion and states that she has no complications of gait. Neurologic: The patient denies any paresthesias or paralysis complications. Psychiatric: She denies any agitation, increased depression, or personality disorders.

PHYSICAL EXAMINATION: Vitals: Blood pressure 123/67, pulse 115, respirations 20, and temperature 35.0° C. HEENT: Head is normocephalic with no contusion or abrasions. Eyes: EOMS (extraocular movements) are intact. Ears: Tympanic membranes are visualized with no erythema. Nose: Nares are patent. Mucosa pink and moist. Throat: Mucosa pink and moist. Tongue and uvula midline. Cardiovascular: S1 (first heart sound) and S2 (second heart sound) with a regular rate and rhythm. No murmurs are audible. No bruits evident on examination. Respiratory: Lungs are clear to auscultation bilaterally. No wheezing or rhonchi. Abdomen: There are positive bowel sounds. There is right lower-quadrant pain, which she rates 8/10. There is also positive Rovsing's sign and negative rebound tenderness. There are no masses palpable

on examination. Extremities: The patient has good range of motion and peripheral pulses are intact.

LABORATORY: White cell count of 5.46, with a hemoglobin of 14.0 and a hematocrit of 40.9.

ASSESSMENT:

1. Rule out appendicitis.
2. Diabetes mellitus, type 1.
3. Sinusitis, acute.
4. Asthma.

PLAN: Admit the patient to the hospital. The patient will be n.p.o. (nothing by mouth). Will get her vitals q.4h. (every 4 hours). Will start IV (intravenous) fluids of D5 (dextrose 5% water) LR 125 cc (cubic centimeters) per hour. Will give Accu-Cheks q.i.d. (four times a day). Will get a CBC (complete blood count) and basic metabolic panel in the morning. We will continue the patient on her regular insulin regimen. We will also give her Demerol for pain, and we will re-evaluate in the morning. We will hold the Demerol at 4 AM so that our evaluation in the morning is adequate.

Total time spent on the admit today was 60 minutes.

SERVICE CODE(S): _____

ICD-10-CM DX CODE(S): _____

Discussion

The physician coder reports the reason for the service or encounter as presented in the report that is being coded, not on diagnoses stated previously in the patient record. You will have only the report you are currently coding to reference.

Rule Out Diagnosis

There were many diagnoses referred to in the 1-3A report of initial hospital services. In the HPI section of the report, the "right lower-quadrant abdominal pain" is stated. In the Assessment section of the report, "rule out appendicitis" is stated. Because physician coders do not report "rule out" statements, you report the symptom of abdominal pain rather than the appendicitis. Note that in the HPI section, the statement

is made that the patient has nausea. Some coders consider the nausea to be an integral part of the abdominal pain and would not report the nausea separately; however, other coders would report the nausea with a separate code (R11.0).

The type 1 diabetes mellitus and asthma would need to be reported, as these conditions would have implications for the medications and treatment ordered for the patient. The acute sinusitis should probably be reported as it may be significant in the care of an asthmatic patient (although in the Physical Examination section of the report, there is no mention of the symptoms of sinusitis). The physician should be queried as to the sinusitis. On the paper CMS-1500, there is space for 12 diagnoses. The diagnoses for this report are abdominal pain (R10.31), diabetes (E10.9), acute sinusitis (J01.90), and asthma (J45.909).

CASE 1-3B *Consultation*

You will find detailed information regarding coding a consultation in the information that follows Case 1-9. You will begin to code an assortment of consultative services there. Dr. Alanda requested a consultation from Dr. Jayco, an endocrinologist, prior to the planned appendectomy. Report the professional consultation services of Dr. Jayco.

LOCATION: Inpatient, Hospital

PATIENT: Sally Jacobson

ATTENDING PHYSICIAN: Leslie Alanda, MD

CONSULTANT: Gordon Jayco, MD

REASON FOR CONSULTATION: Preoperative diabetes management.

HISTORY: The patient is a 17-year-old girl with type 1 diabetes, history of asthma, sinusitis, and migraine headache. She was in good health until approximately 1 to 2 days ago, when she developed right lower-quadrant pain with decreased appetite. She states that the intensity of the pain is 6/10. She had no change in bowel habits and no fevers or chills. No other viral symptoms. She was admitted to the hospital with a concern of possible acute appendicitis. She was kept n.p.o. (nothing by mouth), and admission blood sugar was approximately 270. I had been asked to evaluate her diabetes and manage if needed. The patient normally is on a basal bolus insulin regimen at home with 14 Ultralente b.i.d. (twice a day) and 7 units Humalog with meals. Her past level of glycemic control has been fair with her hemoglobin A1Cs (glycated hemoglobin) ranging from about 8.5 to 10%. She did have a mild degree of microalbuminuria when last tested but no other diabetes complications.

Continued

CASE 1-3B—cont'd

PAST MEDICAL HISTORY:

1. Type 1 diabetes as discussed above.
2. History of asthma.
3. History of sinusitis.
4. History of migraine headaches.

ALLERGIES: None.

HABITS: The patient does occasionally smoke. No alcohol use.

CURRENT MEDICATIONS:
1. Ultralente 14 units b.i.d. and 7 units Humalog with meals.
2. Elavil 100 mg (milligram) p.o. (by mouth) q.h.s. (each bedtime).

FAMILY HISTORY: She has two brothers with type 1 diabetes as well as a cousin and uncle. Father's side of family has coronary artery disease. Another uncle had lung cancer.

SOCIAL HISTORY: The patient is a senior in high school.

REVIEW OF SYSTEMS: As discussed above.

PHYSICAL EXAMINATION: The patient is in no acute distress. Weight is 151 pounds. Height 5 feet 3 inches. Vital signs are stable. She was afebrile. Lungs are clear to auscultation. Cardiac exam shows a regular rate and rhythm with a normal S1 (first heart sound) and S2 (second heart sound) without murmurs. Abdomen is notable for some mild hypertrophy. There is some tenderness in the right lower quadrant. No guarding or rebound. Bowel sounds are present. Extremities are unremarkable.

LABORATORY STUDIES: Admission blood sugar was 276. White count was normal.

ASSESSMENT AND PLAN:

1. Type 1 diabetes. The patient admitted with presumptive diagnosis of acute appendicitis, now n.p.o. with hyperglycemia. I recommend continuing dextrose-containing IV (intravenous) fluids, but we will add 15 units of insulin per liter. Total fluids to run at 125 cc (cubic centimeters) per hour. We will monitor blood sugars q.4h. (every 4 hours) and q.1h. perioperatively with a target range of 100 to 200. Once her diet is resumed, we will get her back on her usual outpatient insulin regimen.
2. Abdominal pain. Plans for monitoring and possible exploratory surgery per surgical team.

Total time spent with patient for consultation today was 60 minutes.

SERVICE CODE(S): _____

ICD-10-CM DX CODE(S): _____

Discussion

The reason for this service is the first-listed (primary) diagnosis, and in this case the diabetes management is the primary reason Dr. Jayco is providing a consultation. In the Assessment and Plan section of the report, the physician also indicates the abdominal pain and discusses this pain in the History section of the report; therefore, the abdominal pain is listed second. The asthma, sinusitis, and migraine headaches mentioned in the Past Medical History section of the report would not usually be reported. If you were to report any of the other conditions, the asthma would be the most significant and would therefore be reported.

(Answers to every other Case are located in Appendix D . The full answer key is only available in the TEACH Instructor Resources on Evolve.)

CASE 1-3C   *Radiology Report*

Report Dr. Monson's radiology service. Remember to report only the physician portion of the service.

LOCATION: Inpatient, Hospital

PATIENT: Sally Jacobson

ATTENDING PHYSICIAN: Leslie Alanda, MD

RADIOLOGIST: Morton Monson, MD

ULTRASOUND OF RIGHT LOWER QUADRANT: The patient has right lower-quadrant pain and a normal white blood count. Ultrasound views of the right lower quadrant are submitted. We did image a tubular structure. This tubular structure is, however, compressible, and that is not the usual case with an appendix that is inflamed. This could be a loop of bowel, but the technologist indicates that this area did not show peristalsis throughout the examination. This tubular structure measures 1.4 cm (centimeter) × 7.6 mm (millimeter). In cross-section, it does not show the typical target sign. There are no fluid collections. There is no free fluid. Technologist indicates that the patient was tender over this tubular structure.

IMPRESSION:

1. We do demonstrate a tubular structure in the right lower quadrant that is tender when the technologist presses on it.
2. This tubular structure is, however, compressible, which would not be the usual case in an inflamed appendix.
3. It could be that we are dealing with very early appendicitis. It could also be that the structure we are seeing is simply a loop of bowel, which did not happen to peristalse during the course of the evaluation. Overall, this does not demonstrate a structure that fits all the criteria of inflamed appendix.
4. No free fluid or fluid collections.

SERVICE CODE(S): _____

ICD-10-CM DX CODE(S): _____

(Answers to every other Case are located in Appendix D . The full answer key is only available in the TEACH Instructor Resources on Evolve.)

CASE 1-3D *Radiology Report*

Report Dr. Monson's radiology service.

LOCATION: Inpatient, Hospital
PATIENT: Sally Jacobson
ATTENDING PHYSICIAN: Leslie Alanda, MD
RADIOLOGIST: Morton Monson, MD
INDICATIONS: Cough and fever

PA (POSTERIOR/ANTERIOR) & LATERAL CHEST, 9:15 AM: The previous film is from last month. There is no pneumonia. The lung fields are clear. There are no effusions. The heart and vascular markings are normal. Bony structures are unremarkable.

IMPRESSION: Normal chest x-ray.

SERVICE CODE(S): _____

ICD-10-CM DX CODE(S): _____

Discussion

Dr. Alanda requests radiology services for Sally because of her cough and fever. Again, no more definitive diagnosis is stated, and as such the presenting symptoms of cough and fever are reported as the diagnoses.

CASE 1-4 *Initial Hospital Care*

The patient in Case 1-4 is a 32-year-old male who was seen by his physician, Dr. Green, at the outpatient clinic. Dr. Green immediately admitted the patient to the hospital. Report Dr. Green's service.

LOCATION: Inpatient, Hospital
PATIENT: Jonathan Harley
ATTENDING PHYSICIAN: Ronald Green, MD

The patient, along with his wife, comes in today as he relates issues with worsening of his dyspepsia/GERD (gastroesophageal reflux disease). He relates that his medications are not working as previously noted since he has been removed from a proton pump inhibitor, Prevacid, to the Protonix secondary to insurance issues. He also relates to me issues of his worsening shortness of breath beyond his chronic status. This is more predominant with exertion. He has had worsening of daytime somnolence and sleep issues. He has had persisting fatigue over the course of the past 2 months as well as mild fluid gain.

SURGICAL HISTORY: The patient's past surgical history is positive for an appendectomy as a youth.

MEDICAL HISTORY:

1. Hypertension that has been under good control currently.
2. Asthma that is under fair control; the asthma is of chronic obstructive nature.
3. Chronic back pain, treated with a TENS (transcutaneous electrical nerve stimulator) unit.
4. Diverticulosis.
5. Dysphagia.

CURRENT MEDICATIONS:

1. Albuterol inhaler 4 puffs q.i.d. (four times a day).
2. Allegra 180 mg (milligram) q.d. (every day).
3. Aspirin 325 mg, 6 tablets q.d. on a p.r.n. (as needed) basis.
4. Flovent inhaler 4 puffs b.i.d. (twice a day).
5. Labetalol 300 mg b.i.d.
6. Nasacort AQ 2 sprays b.i.d.
7. Norvasc 5 mg q.d.
8. Protonix 40 mg 1 tablet per day. He has been using 2 recently.
9. Serevent inhaler 2 puffs q.i.d.

ALLERGIES: Ultram.

FAMILY HISTORY: Positive for emphysema in his father, who died at a young age from an accident. Mother is age 67, has had abdominal issues and surgery from noncarcinoma issues, about which he is nonspecific. The patient is the second of five children, having three brothers and one sister, all of whom are in good health.

SOCIAL HISTORY: The patient is disabled secondary to his chronic back pain. He is married. He relates eating a non–heart-healthy diet, high in fatty products. He is a nonsmoker. He averages 4 to 5 glasses of wine and 10 to 12 beers a week in alcohol intake. He has very limited exercise, including any active walking, secondary to his chronic back pain.

REVIEW OF SYSTEMS: No worsening of his headache issues. No change in mentation (activity of the mind). Hearing is gone in the right ear and diminished some in the left. His vision has been intact. Appetite has been good. He shows positive weight gain. He has no difficulty swallowing. He relates his dyspepsia/GERD has been worsening with some abdominal discomfort, postprandial specifically. He has had a nontender lower abdomen, predominantly the upper bothering him more. This radiates upward somewhat, specifically in his sleep. His sleep pattern has been disturbed. He relates chronic fatigue issues in the past month and has had worsening of the dyspepsia and GERD despite the use of proton pump inhibitor. No constipation; regular bowel movements. No dysuria or polyuria. Occasional nocturia. No aches or pains in the extremities but notes slight swelling of his legs. He has had some shortness of breath on exertion, specifically on stairways, but denies any type of chest pain of a cardiac nature. He relates immobility issues secondary to chronic pain as well as worsening shortness of breath.

PHYSICAL EXAMINATION: His examination today shows he is age 32 and is in no apparent distress. Slightly pale in color. Weight is 202 pounds. Height is 5 feet 5 inches. Blood pressure is 118/78. Pulse is 80 and regular. Respiratory rate is 20. He is afebrile at 96.4º F. HEENT (head, ears, eyes, nose, throat): Negative for discharge or deformity. The right tympanic membrane is severely scarred. The left shows a bolus-type effusion. No tenderness to the tragus, auricle, or mastoid process. Pupils are equal,

Continued

CASE 1-4—cont'd

round, and light accommodating. Nondilated funduscopy reveals no nicking or scarring. No tenderness of sinuses. Nasal and oral mucosa is pink and moist. There is extreme gag reflex elicited on attempt to view the posterior oropharynx. Neck is soft and supple. No lymphadenopathy. No supraclavicular nodes are noted. There are no carotid bruits. Cranial nerves II–XII are grossly intact. Lateralization Weber to the left as well as air-to-bone conduction being normal on the left and extremely reduced hearing on the right. Thorax: Scattered wheezes throughout; no crackles are noted. Cardiac: S1 (first heart sound) and S2 (second heart sound) with a 1/6 systolic murmur, best heard at the base on the right side of the sternum at the second and third intercostal space. This does not seem to change during inhalation, exhalation, or positioning. Abdomen is round, obese, with tenderness of the upper right quadrant with palpation as well as the epigastric region, which promotes some issue of reflux to the esophagus on deep palpation. The lower part of the abdomen is nontender. No rebound tenderness. Bowel sounds are present throughout. Normal-appearing male genitalia. Negative for inguinal hernia. Rectal exam reveals sphincter tone intact. Prostate is firm, mildly tender but more of a pressure sensation. Stool is guaiac negative for occult blood. There is 2× edema of the lower extremities. Skin is warm and dry. Sensation is intact.

LABORATORY DATA: Laboratory analysis conducted at this time for an amylase, lipase, comprehensive metabolic panel, CBC (complete blood count), TSH (thyroid stimulating hormone), T₄ (thyroxine), lipid panel, PSA (prostate specific antigen) for screening, and *H. pylori*. Results at this time show his triglycerides to be 1410, total cholesterol 266. His hepatic panel shows his bilirubin total at 0.4. His AST (aspartate aminotransferase [formerly SGOT]) is 69 with ALT (alanine transaminase [formerly SGPT]) of 75. Total protein is 7.4. BUN (blood urea nitrogen) is 18, sodium 137, chloride 102, creatinine 0.8, glucose mildly elevated at 117. His albumin is 3.7, alkaline phosphatase 79. Amylase is 40. WBC (white blood count) 4.67, hemoglobin 14.6, hematocrit 42.2; monocytes elevated at 12.8. He is negative for *H. pylori* antibody.

PLAN: The patient will be admitted to general medical, with pancreatitis and shortness of breath with exertion. Vital signs will be q.4h. (every 4 hours) times three, then q. shift. He will have bathroom privileges. The patient will be n.p.o. (nothing by mouth). Will establish an IV (intravenous) of D5W (dextrose 5% water) half normal saline at 100 cc per hour. He will have sequentials on while in bed. I&Os (intake and output) will be done with daily weights on his chart. Will obtain an echocardiogram for Dr. Elhart to read and obtain a 1-day stress test if possible, and if the patient is in stable condition secondary to his shortness of breath on Monday or Tuesday at the time of his discharge. He will be on O₂ (oxygen) on a p.r.n. basis per nasal cannula to keep saturations greater than 90%. He will receive albuterol nebs q.i.d. and p.r.n.; Flovent inhaler 4 puffs b.i.d. (twice a day); Serevent inhaler 2 puffs b.i.d. We will place him on Labetalol 20 mg IV b.i.d.; Nasacort AQ 2 sprays b.i.d.; and Protonix 40 mg IV q.d. Consideration for implementation of Tricor 160 mg as soon as the amylase and lipase are both showing negative.

Secondary to the patient's intense gag reflex, we will refrain from placing an NG (nasogastric) or Cor-Flo at this time and see whether adequate hydration and n.p.o. status will help resolve.

Chest x-ray was obtained via the dictation line, showing a stable appearance from the previous film, which had been done here in the clinic, free of any acute infiltrates.

His right upper quadrant underwent ultrasound, which was negative for cholelithiasis or cholecystitis, and the head of the pancreas appeared to be near normal from what was able to be visualized with the rest obscured secondary to bowel gas.

The patient will be admitted to the hospital. Discussion in the event of blood and blood products revealed that the patient has no religious beliefs contraindicating the aspect of the blood transfusion. The risks and benefits were explained, including transfusion reaction, hepatitis, HIV (human immunodeficiency virus), incompatibility, and other risks. The patient does agree to this, and I explained to him that unless it was an emergent situation, that discussion would be held again at the time if something did arise where he required blood, that there would be a further explanation discussing the risks and benefits of that being held. Both he and his wife agreed with this. He will be admitted at this time to the floor as a code level I.

SERVICE CODE(S): _____

ICD-10-CM DX CODE(S): _____

Discussion

Pancreatitis

In the Plan section of the report, the physician indicates that he is admitting the patient with "pancreatitis and shortness of breath with exertion." Pancreatitis is an inflammation of the pancreas and can be either in an acute (K85.9-) or chronic form (K86.1) **(Figure 1-2)**. The ultrasound was

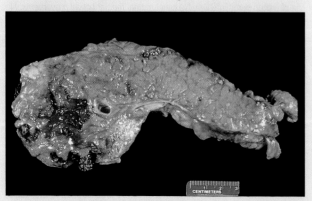

FIGURE 1–2 Pancreatitis.

performed to determine the status of the pancreas. The shortness of breath on exertion is often a symptom of a problem with the heart, and the physician ordered a stress test be conducted by Dr. Elhart (under the Plan section). A chest x-ray was also done to assist in the diagnosis as to the origin of the shortness of breath. The code for shortness of breath is used to substantiate the medical necessity for the stress test.

This patient has numerous other conditions, such as hypertension, asthma, chronic back pain, diverticulosis, and dysphagia. These were not the primary reasons the service was provided, nor is there an indication that tests are going to be done for any of these additional diagnoses. The physician did order medications for some of these conditions, such as the patient's asthma (albuterol, Flovent, Serevent, Nasacort), hypertension (labetalol), and GERD (gastroesophageal reflex disease, Protonix); additionally, the physician has ordered Tricor after laboratory workup. Tricor is prescribed for patients with primary hypercholesterolemia (excess cholesterol in the blood). In the inpatient setting, all of these conditions would be reported for the facility; but for the physician services, the focus is on reporting the condition(s) that prompted the encounter, which are pancreatitis and shortness of breath.

CASE 1-5A *Initial Hospital Care*

The patient in Case 1-5 is an 87-year-old female who is to be admitted by her nephrologist, Dr. Pleasant, after the patient had been seen in Dr. Pleasant's office that morning. The physician also went to the emergency department to care for the patient.

LOCATION: Inpatient, Hospital

PATIENT: Rosie Hovett

ATTENDING PHYSICIAN: Timothy L. Pleasant, MD

I am admitting this patient primarily because of symptomatic bradycardia secondary to medications. The patient is an 87-year-old woman who was recently discharged from the hospital after being diagnosed with new-onset atrial fibrillation with rapid ventricular response. The patient was started on medications digoxin, labetalol, Cardizem, and metoprolol.

Since discharge from the hospital back on May 20, the patient has related that she has had some episodes of weakness. There were also some episodes when she was noted to be significantly hypotensive and feeling generally weak with some diaphoresis. Because these symptoms persisted, the patient then decided to come into the emergency room, where she was found to be in bradycardia, with a heart rate in the 40s to 50s. I think this is primarily brought about by the combination of digoxin, labetalol, Cardizem, and metoprolol. Therefore, at this time, the plan is to admit the patient to the telemetry unit and rule her out for MI (myocardial infarction) because she is also at risk for that problem. At this time, I am going to hold the digoxin, labetalol, Cardizem, and metoprolol. Obviously we cannot hold the clonidine patch because this may lead to rebound hypertension. I will continue the rest of her medications except for the ones that I have mentioned above.

We will also check her cardiac enzymes to rule out MI.

The patient has a past medical and past surgical history that consists of the following:

1. Hypertension.
2. New-onset atrial fibrillation.
3. Thoracic abdominal aortic aneurysm.
4. Hyperthyroidism. I am not exactly sure which one she has—hyperthyroidism or hypothyroidism—because the discharge summary indicates the presence of hypothyroidism, whereas the admission history and physical per Dr. Green indicated hyperthyroidism. Nevertheless, she is not on any thyroid supplements. If she indeed is hypothyroid, this certainly could contribute to her present situation as well. We need to review her old medical records for this particular issue.

SOCIAL HISTORY: The patient is currently retired. She does have family here in town. She is widowed and lives on her own. She has an 86-pack-a-year smoking history. She denies any current or previous use of alcohol or intravenous or recreational drugs.

FAMILY HISTORY is positive for cancer and diabetes and negative for heart disease, hypertension, stroke, kidney disease, bleeding disorder, or dyscrasia. A sister has been diagnosed with breast cancer, and her two other sisters have been diagnosed with uterine cancer. There is a strong family history of diabetes in the immediate family.

MEDICATIONS currently being taken at home include the following:

1. Clonidine patch.
2. Digoxin 0.125 mg (milligram) q.d. (every day).
3. Diltiazem CD 240 mg q.d.
4. Vasotec 10 mg q.d.
5. Labetalol 200 mg b.i.d. (twice a day).
6. Maalox extra strength 15 ml (milliliter) q.h.s. (each bedtime).
7. Metoprolol 25 mg q.h.s.
8. Nitroglycerin sublingual 0.4 mg p.r.n. (as needed).

ALLERGIES: No known drug allergies.

Latest laboratory results are as follows: Hemogram shows an H&H (hematocrit and hemoglobin) of 10.6/31.4, WBC (white blood count) 7.5, normochromic/normocytic indices, platelets 182. There is no left shift as neutrophils are only 63.6%. Chemistries are as follows: sodium 141, potassium 4.3, chloride 105, CO_2 (carbon dioxide) 27.2, BUN (blood urea nitrogen) and creatinine 19.1/1, glucose 146, calcium 9.1. Digoxin level is 0.3, which is low. Magnesium level is 1.6. Cardiac enzymes are essentially unremarkable, as troponin is less than 0.3 and CK-MB (creatine kinase-methylene blue) is less than 1 and total CPK (creatine phosphokinase) is 36. Thyroid function tests done on previous admission were well within normal limits, as TSH (thyroid stimulating hormone) was measured to be 4.53.

REVIEW OF SYSTEMS: Constitutional: No fever or chills. No recent weight change. She appears to be fairly weak. No night sweats. Skin: No skin lesions. No active dermatosis. Eyes: No eye discharge. No eye itching. No visual changes. No diplopia. ENT: No ear discharge. No hearing difficulty. No pharyngeal hyperemia, congestion, or exudates. Lymph nodes: No lymphadenopathy in the neck, axillary, or groin. Neurologic: Positive headaches. Positive gait instability. No falls. No seizures. Psychiatric: No behavioral changes. Neck: No thyromegaly. Respiratory: Positive cough. No colds. No hemoptysis. Positive for shortness of breath with strenuous exertion only. No colds. No hemoptysis. Cardiovascular: No chest pain. Positive palpitations. No orthopnea. No paroxysmal nocturnal dyspnea. Gastrointestinal: Positive anorexia. No nausea, vomiting, dysphagia, odynophagia, constipation, or diarrhea. No abdominal pain. No fecal incontinence. No hematemesis. No hematochezia. No melena. Genitourinary: No urgency, frequency, dysuria, hematuria, urinary incontinence, nocturia, vaginal discharge, vaginal lesions, or vaginal bleeding. Musculoskeletal: Positive joint pains. Positive occasional muscle pains/weaknesses. Hematologic: No bleeding tendencies. No purpura. No petechiae. No ecchymosis. Endocrinologic: No heat or cold intolerance.

PHYSICAL EXAMINATION: Vital signs are stable. Blood pressure is 117/80. Heart rate is in the 50s. Respirations 20. She is afebrile. Normocephalic, atraumatic. Pink palpebral conjunctivae, anicteric sclerae. No nasal or aural discharge. Moist tongue and buccal mucosa. No pharyngeal hyperemia, congestion, or exudate. Supple neck. No lymphadenopathy. Symmetrical chest expansion. No retractions. Positive rhonchi. A few bibasilar crackles. No wheezes. S1 (first heart sound) and S2 (second heart sound) are distinct. No S3 (third heart sound) or S4 (fourth heart sound). Regular rate and rhythm. Abdomen: Positive bowel sounds. Soft, nontender. Both upper and lower extremities reveal arthritic changes. Pulses are fair.

ASSESSMENT/PLAN:

1. Symptomatic bradycardia secondary to medications, namely, digoxin, labetalol, Cardizem, and metoprolol. Admit to telemetry. Check cardiac enzymes to rule out MI. Start enteric-coated aspirin 325 mg q.d.

   Please note this patient also had a recent 2-D echocardiogram performed by Dr. Monson showing a normal overall LV (left ventricle) systolic function, 3+ mitral insufficiency, 1–2+ aortic insufficiency, 2–3+ tricuspid insufficiency, 1+ pulmonic valve insufficiency, and moderate pulmonary hypertension.

Continued

CASE 1-5A—*cont'd*

2. Anemia, questionable etiology. Would need to review old medical records to see whether this has been worked up already. Anemia in this elderly age group needs to be evaluated more closely because the possibility of malignancy runs high on the list.

3. History of hypothyroidism, stable. She is not requiring thyroid supplements. As noted above, the latest TSH (thyroid stimulating hormone) level was well within normal limits.

4. Thoracic abdominal aortic aneurysm, stable.

5. Hypertension. Blood pressure right now is well controlled with a systolic blood pressure ranging from 117 to 120. There may be a possibility of her blood pressure going up because we are withholding three of her blood pressure medications, namely, labetalol, Cardizem, and metoprolol. At this time, we just have to continue to observe the patient, and if blood pressure goes up to higher levels, then we may consider starting the patient on either labetalol or Norvasc.

6. Atrial fibrillation. I am wondering why this patient was not placed on anticoagulation. We will check PT (prothrombin time) and INR (International Normalized Ration). We will discuss with Dr. Green on Monday whether or not the patient needs to be anticoagulated or whether there is a contraindication that was noted in the past.

Unit time was 2 hours and 20 minutes. We will continue to follow up on this patient from the critical care standpoint.

SERVICE CODE(S): _____

ICD-10-CM DX CODE(S): _____

Discussion

Well-Controlled or Stable Conditions

This report is an excellent example of how you can identify the most important and, therefore, reportable diagnoses. Note that under the Assessment/Plan section of the report there are 6 diagnoses stated and 3 are stated to be well controlled or stable. These controlled or stable conditions are not usually reported for physician coding—hypothyroidism, aortic aneurysm, and hypertension. This leaves the bradycardia secondary to medications, anemia, and atrial fibrillation as the reason this service was provided.

Cardiac Dysrhythmia

The cardiac dysrhythmia (I49.9) of bradycardia (R00.1) is also known as bradyarrhythmia and is defined as fewer than 60 beats per minute. (Tachyarrhythmia or tachycardia is a condition in which the heart beats in excess of 100 per minute.) Bradycardia can have many origins, such as central nervous system disease, infectious disease, or vascular disease. The cause of the bradycardia in this report is identified as being secondary to the patient's medications.

Another cardiac dysrhythmia is fibrillation. Fibrillation is an involuntary contraction of a muscle. Atrial fibrillation (I48.91) is a cardiac dysrhythmia of the atrial myocardium in which the atria quivers continuously in an irregular pattern. This is also known as AFib or AF (also A Fib). Vfib or VF is a ventricular fibrillation (I49.01) involving the ventricular muscle of the heart. Note that the codes are different for A/V fibrillation or flutter, as these are two different conditions.

Anemia

Anemia is a reduction in number of erythrocytes or decrease in quality of hemoglobin. There are many types of anemia such as:

- Iron-deficiency anemia (D50)
- Other deficiency anemias (D51-D53, pernicious, vitamin B_{12}, folate deficiency, etc.)
- Hereditary hemolytic anemias (D55-D56, thalassemias, sickle-cell, etc.)
- Acquired hemolytic anemias (D59, autoimmune, non-autoimmune, hemoglobinuria, etc.)
- Aplastic anemia (D60, constitutional, other specified, unspecified)
- Other and unspecified anemias (D85 and D63-D64, in chronic illness)

CASE 1-5B   *Progress Report*

Dr. Pleasant, as the attending physician, continues to monitor Rosie Hovett's progress while she is in the hospital. Report his services.

LOCATION: Inpatient, Hospital

PATIENT: Rosie Hovett

ATTENDING PHYSICIAN: Timothy L. Pleasant, MD

She states she feels much better today compared with yesterday, although she has some nausea. The patient was seen and examined and chart reviewed. The patient appears to be hemodynamically stable, not in any form of respiratory distress or compromise. No specific complaints. No chest pain. No shortness of breath. No diaphoresis. No nausea or vomiting. No palpitations. No diarrhea or constipation. No frequency, urgency, or dysuria.

PHYSICAL EXAMINATION: Vital signs are stable. Blood pressure is 133/54. Heart rate is 59. Respirations 20. She is saturating 96% on 2 liters O_2 (oxygen) nasal cannula. Temperature is 36.2° C (Celsius).

Normocephalic, atraumatic. Pink palpebral conjunctivae, anicteric sclerae. No nasal or aural discharge. Moist tongue and buccal mucosa. No pharyngeal hyperemia, congestion, or exudate. Supple neck. No lymphadenopathy. Symmetrical chest expansion. No retractions. Positive rhonchi. No crackles. No wheezes. S1 (first heart sound) and S2 (second heart sound) are indistinct. Regular rate and irregular rhythm. Abdomen: Positive bowel sounds. Soft, nontender. Both upper and lower extremities reveal arthritic changes. Pulses are fair.

Latest laboratory tests are as follows: sodium 144, potassium 4.9, chloride 107, CO_2 (carbon dioxide) 31.2, BUN (blood urea nitrogen) and creatinine 15/0.8, glucose 94, calcium 8.8. Hemogram shows H&H (hematocrit and hemoglobin) of 10.7/32.2, WBC (white blood count) 7.28, normochromic/normocytic indices, and platelets 174. Cardiac enzymes have remained negative in the past 16 hours. Latest PT (prothrombin time) and INR (International Normalized Ration) are 12.5 and 1.1, respectively. It must be noted that this patient was discharged home and was not sent home on Coumadin. I am suspecting that

CASE 1-5B—cont'd

this has something to do with her thoracic aortic aneurysm. I think this patient would still benefit, however, from anticoagulation because of her underlying atrial fibrillation. Her anemia is improving.

IMPRESSION/PLAN:

1. Symptomatic bradycardia secondary to medications, namely, labetalol, Cardizem, digoxin, and metoprolol. Cardiac enzymes remain negative, suggesting MI (myocardial infarction) has been ruled out. Will check 12-lead ECG (electrocardiogram). Her blood pressure right now appears to be well controlled with the Clonidine patch, Vasotec

10 mg (milligram) q.d. (every day), and nitroglycerin sublingual p.r.n. (as needed). At this time, she does not require initiation of the other antihypertensive medications, which were held at the time of admission.

Await cardiology consult. I did speak with Dr. Elhart from cardiology yesterday, who feels that because most of the recent clinical scenario resulted from overzealous use of heart rate-lowering medications, it is worthwhile to keep this medication on hold before reconsidering the issue of a pacemaker.

SERVICE CODE(S): _____

ICD-10-CM DX CODE(S): _____

Discussion

Report 1-5B is a good example of the type of report that does not contain all of the diagnoses within the Impression/Plan section of the report. Again, you must focus on the primary reason the service is being provided to this patient. Remember that you only have this one progress report available to you when the service is coded. According to the Impression/Plan section, the patient has bradycardia due to previously prescribed medications. It is not until the entire report is read that the additional

diagnoses of atrial fibrillation (second-to-last sentence of Physical Examination section) and "Her anemia is improving" (last sentence of Physical Examination section) are noted. Both the atrial fibrillation and anemia are reported. There is mention of nausea in the first line of the report, which could be reported with (R11.0), although the physician made no mention of a treatment for the condition nor correlated it to any current condition.

CASE 1-6   *Progress Report*

Dr. Pleasant has been the attending physician for the patient in Case 1-6 while the patient's physician, Dr. Alanda, was out of town on a personal emergency. Dr. Pleasant is providing the last service to the patient because Dr. Alanda is returning this evening from out of town and will assume responsibility for the patient. Report Dr. Pleasant's service.

LOCATION: Inpatient, Hospital

PATIENT: Kyle Ottegard

ATTENDING PHYSICIAN: Timothy L. Pleasant, MD

The patient was seen and examined and chart reviewed. The patient appears to be hemodynamically stable, not in any form of respiratory distress or compromise. No abdominal pain today and no dyspepsia noted. One of other complaints he had on admission is that of left otalgia pain. Since we started him on empiric antibiotic coverage with IV (intravenous) Claforan, this has not been bothering him anymore. We are still awaiting ENT consultation at this time.

PHYSICAL EXAMINATION: Vital signs are stable. Blood pressure is 143/82. Heart rate is 82. Respirations 24. Saturating 97% on room air. Temperature is 36.6° C (Celsius). Normocephalic, atraumatic. Pink palpebral conjunctivae, anicteric sclerae. No nasal or aural discharge. Moist tongue and buccal

mucosa. No pharyngeal hyperemia, congestion, or exudate. Supple neck. No JVD (jugular vein distention). No lymphadenopathy. No bruits. Symmetrical chest expansion. No retractions. No rhonchi. No crackles. No wheezes. S1 (first heart sound) and S2 (second heart sound) are distinct. No S3 (third heart sound) or S4 (fourth heart sound). Regular rate and irregular rhythm. Abdomen: Positive bowel sounds. Soft, nontender, obese. Both upper and lower extremities reveal no gross deformities or edema. Pulses are full and equal.

ASSESSMENT/PLAN:

1. Abdominal pain. Pancreatitis, ruled out. Severe hypertriglyceridemia of 1410 mg/dl (milligram/deciliter). Continue low-fat, low-cholesterol diet. Continue Tricor 160 mg q.d. (every day) with meals.
2. Left ear infection, questionable. The patient has been started on IV Claforan and has been clinically responsive to that medication.

At this time, we are awaiting the ENT consultation. It is hoped that the patient can be discharged by Dr. Alanda's service and be followed up in 6 weeks for recheck of his cholesterol and triglyceride profile.

Dr. Alanda will reassume care tomorrow.

SERVICE CODE(S): _____

ICD-10-CM DX CODE(S): _____

Discussion
Hypertriglyceridemia

The first numbered item of the Assessment/Plan section of the report indicates diagnoses of abdominal pain and hypertriglyceridemia. Hypertriglyceridemia is a condition in which there are excessive triglycerides and very low-density lipoproteins in the blood. A lipoprotein is a protein wrapped around cholesterol (E78.0-), lipids (E78.2), or triglycerides (E78.1).

- HDL (high-density lipoproteins) are the "good" cholesterol.
- LDL (low-density lipoproteins) are the "bad" cholesterol.

- VLDL (very low-density lipoproteins, primarily triglyceride and protein) are the "very bad" cholesterol.

Pancreatitis has been "ruled out" as a diagnosis and, as such, will not be reported in the outpatient setting. The ear infection is only "suspected" and not confirmed, and as such cannot be reported. The ear pain (otalgia H92.02) can be reported as it is mentioned.

"Rule out" means the condition is going to be either proven to exist or not to exist. "Ruled out" means that the diagnosis has already been proven not to exist.

CASE 1-7   *Progress Report*

Dr. Pleasant is the attending physician for Arnold Gonzalez. Report Dr. Pleasant's service.

LOCATION: Inpatient, Hospital

PATIENT: Arnold Gonzalez

ATTENDING PHYSICIAN: Timothy L. Pleasant, MD

The patient was seen and the chart reviewed. The patient appears to be hemodynamically stable, not in respiratory distress or compromise.

PHYSICAL EXAMINATION: Vital signs are stable. Blood pressure is 132/72. Heart rate is 108. Respirations 20s. Saturating 94% on room air. Input and output in the last 24 hours is 3796/1925. Normocephalic, atraumatic. Pink palpebral conjunctivae, anicteric sclerae. Symmetrical chest expansion. Positive rhonchi. Positive crackles. No wheezes. S1 (first heart sound) and S2 (second heart sound) are indistinct. No S3 (third heart sound) or S4 (fourth heart sound). Irregular rhythm, tachycardiac rate, no rubs. Abdomen: Decreased bowel sounds, soft and nontender. Both upper and lower extremities reveal arthritic changes. Pulses are fair.

Latest labs are as follows: Sodium 141, potassium 4.6, chloride 115, CO_2 (carbon dioxide) 17.4, BUN (blood urea nitrogen) and creatinine 50/1.4, glucose 112, calcium and phosphorus are 8.1 and 2.2, respectively, magnesium 1.4, and albumin 1.1. Digoxin level is 2.4. Latest hemogram shows H&H (hematocrit and hemoglobin) of 10.5/33.2, WBC (white blood count) 13.32, platelets 108. PT (prothrombin time) and INR (International Normalized Ration) are 13 and 1.2, respectively.

ASSESSMENT/PLAN:

1. Acute renal failure/chronic renal failure. The patient has had improved urine output.
2. Status post ruptured appendix with cecectomy.
   a. Nutrition. After reviewing patient's electrolytes, I would recommend resuming the same tube feedings except with additives of 10 mEq (milliequivalent) potassium phosphate/L and 10 mEq sodium plus citrate/L. Recommend checking chemistries again in the morning.
3. Status post tracheostomy. Continue inhaler treatments.
4. Anemia of chronic illness/chronic renal disease.
5. Questionable small bowel obstruction.
6. New onset atrial fibrillation. The patient is now day two of Coumadin 5 mg (milligram) q.d. (every day). Target INR is 2–3. It was decided not to heparinize this patient anymore but to proceed with Coumadin anticoagulation outright.

Yesterday afternoon I was called in because the patient was due to receive a fourth dose of 0.25 mg digoxin IV (intravenous) push, but his heart rate was already in the 80s. Therefore, I recommended decreasing the dose to 0.125 instead of the previously ordered 0.25 mg. This morning his digoxin level turned out to be 2.4; therefore, we are going to hold the digoxin today. His heart rate, however, remains in the 90s to 100 range.

SERVICE CODE(S): _____

ICD-10-CM DX CODE(S): _____

Discussion
Renal Failure

Acute renal failure (N17.9) is sudden onset of renal failure. It can be caused by trauma, infection, inflammation, or exposure to a toxic substance (toxicity). There are several types of acute renal failure:

- Prerenal
- Associated with poor systemic perfusion
- Decreased renal blood flow
- Such as with congestive heart failure
- Intrarenal
- Associated with renal parenchyma disease (functional tissue of kidney)
- Such as acute interstitial nephritis
- Postrenal
- Resulting from urine flow obstruction out of kidney

The symptoms of acute renal failure are uremia (excess of urea in the blood), oliguria (decreased output) or anuria (no output), hyperkalemia (high potassium in the blood), and pulmonary edema. Treatment involves resolution of the underlying condition, dialysis, and monitoring the patient's fluid and electrolyte balance. Acute renal failure is usually a reversible condition.

Chronic renal failure (N17.9) is a gradual loss of function that involves progressively more severe renal insufficiency until the end stage of ESRD (end-stage renal disease) or irreversible kidney failure is reached. The cause is often exposure to nephrotoxins. The symptoms are polyuria, nausea or anorexia, dehydration, and neurological manifestations.

Unspecified renal failure (N19) is renal failure that is not documented as acute or chronic.

Chronic kidney disease is referred to as a specific stage (1, 2, 3, 4, 5) end-stage, or unspecified chronic kidney disease. The stages are based on the glomerular filtration rate (GFR). In Stage 1 the kidney is damaged, but the GFR is normal or near normal. In Stage 2 there is a mild decrease in the GFR; in Stage 3 there is a moderate decrease in the GFR; in Stage 4 there is a severe decrease in the GFR; and in Stage 5 there is kidney failure or the patient is on dialysis. In each of the stages, the patient may recover kidney function, but in end-stage renal disease the patient will not recover without a kidney transplant. If the stage is documented, report the diagnosis that corresponds to that stage (N18.1-N18.5). If the documentation indicates end-stage renal disease, end-stage kidney disease, or Stage 5 CKD requiring chronic dialysis, assign N18.6. If the documentation indicates nonspecific diagnostic statements such as "chronic renal disease" or "chronic renal insufficiency," report N18.9.

According to the *ICD-10-CM Official Guidelines for Coding and Reporting*, Section I.B.8., the coder is to report both an acute and chronic condition if there are separate subentries in the Alphabetic Index of the ICD-10-CM

CASE 1-7—cont'd

at the same indentation level. The acute condition is sequenced first, and the chronic condition is sequenced second.

Circumstances of the Encounter

In Case 1-5B, you were presented information about anemia, and the anemia in this case is that in a chronic illness. The code for the anemia is reported in conjunction with the code(s) that describe the underlying chronic illness and are sequenced according to the circumstances of the encounter. If the patient encounter is primarily for the anemia in end-stage renal disease, the anemia code would be reported first, but if the anemia is not the primary reason for the encounter, it is not reported first.

Again, questionable, probable, suspected, or rule out are not reported by outpatient and physician coders.

The following was prepared by Karla Lovaasen to clarify coding chronic renal failure (CRF), chronic renal insufficiency (CRI), and chronic kidney disease (CKD):

- CKD + hypertension = I12.9 + N18.9 (unspecified)
- CRI + hypertension = I12.9 + N18.9
- CKD/CRF/CRI + hypertension = I12.9 + N18.9
- CKD Stage 1 + hypertension = I12.9 + N18.1
- CKD Stage 2 + hypertension = I12.9 + N18.2
- CKD Stage 3 + hypertension = I12.9 + N18.30-N18.32
- CKD Stage 4 + hypertension = I12.9 + N18.4
- CKD Stage 5 + hypertension = I12.0 + N18.5
- CKD Stage 6/ESRD or on dialysis + hypertension = I12.0 + N18.6
- Patient with CRF on any type of dialysis is I12.0 + N18.6 + Z99.2.

(Answers to every other Case are located in Appendix D . The full answer key is only available in the TEACH Instructor Resources on Evolve.)

CASE 1-8 *Progress Report*

Dr. Pleasant provides a follow-up service to a patient he admitted to the hospital to rule out pancreatitis.

LOCATION: Inpatient, Hospital

PATIENT: Corrbet Zornomba

ATTENDING PHYSICIAN: Timothy L. Pleasant, MD

The patient was seen and examined and chart reviewed. The patient appears to be hemodynamically stable, not in any form of respiratory distress or compromise. No specific complaints. No abdominal pain or dyspepsia since admission to the hospital.

Amylase and lipase values have been obtained, and both are within normal limits.

PHYSICAL EXAMINATION: Vital signs are stable. Blood pressure is 126/61. Heart rate is 63. Respirations 18. Saturating 96% on room air. Temperature is 35.7° C (Celsius).

Normocephalic, atraumatic. Pink palpebral conjunctivae, anicteric sclerae. No nasal or aural discharge. Moist tongue and buccal mucosa. No pharyngeal hyperemia, congestion, or exudate. Supple neck. No JVD (jugular vein distention). No lymphadenopathy. No bruits. Symmetrical chest expansion. No retractions. No rhonchi. No crackles. No wheezes. S1 (first heart sound) and S2 (second heart sound) are distinct. No S3 (third heart sound) or S4 (fourth heart sound). Regular rate and rhythm. Abdomen: Positive bowel sounds. Soft and nontender. Both upper and lower extremities reveal no gross deformities or edema. Pulses are full and equal.

ASSESSMENT/PLAN:

1. Abdominal pain. Pancreatitis ruled out. Severe hypertriglyceridemia at 1410 mg/dl (milligram/deciliter). The plan right now is to start him on clear liquids and then to advance his feedings as tolerated to a low-fat, low-cholesterol diet. We will start him on Tricor 160 mg daily with his evening meal.
2. Hypothyroidism. We will restart Synthroid p.o. (by mouth). May discontinue IV (intravenous) Synthroid.
3. Hypertension, fairly controlled. We will start Labetalol and Norvasc p.o.
4. We will discontinue all IV medications at this time as he is going to be started on oral feedings.

Continued

CASE 1-8—cont'd

At this time, we will continue to monitor the patient's progress and plan for discharge sometime on Monday with subsequent follow-up with Dr. Alanda.

We will continue to follow this patient from the critical care standpoint.

SERVICE CODE(S): _____

ICD-10-CM DX CODE(S): _____

Discussion

In the Assessment/Plan section of the report, the diagnoses listed are abdominal pain, hypertriglyceridemia, hypothyroidism, and hypertension, and these conditions are being treated. Note that pancreatitis was ruled out and would therefore not be reported.

(Answers to every other Case are located in Appendix D . The full answer key is only available in the TEACH Instructor Resources on Evolve.)

CASE 1-9   *Discharge Summary*

Today, Dr. Pleasant is discharging the patient. Report Dr. Pleasant's service.

LOCATION: Inpatient, Hospital

PATIENT: Frances Miley

ATTENDING PHYSICIAN: Timothy L. Pleasant, MD

REASON FOR ADMISSION: Chronic duodenal ulcer

SUMMARY OF HOSPITAL COURSE: The patient is a 60-year-old female with a history of ulcer disease that failed medical management. She was subsequently referred to Dr. Friendly for partial duodenectomy. On Monday, the patient was admitted and taken to the operating room, where she underwent exploratory laparotomy with partial duodenectomy. All pathology reports were benign. The patient tolerated the procedure well. She had an epidural in place following this, and she was transferred to the ICU (intensive care unit) for observation postoperatively. *(The epidural was "in place" in her back for pain control.)*

The patient did well in the ICU, and by Thursday the patient was ready for transfer to the floor. By Saturday, her ileus was resolving, her NG discontinued, and she was started on a diet. By Monday, the patient was tolerating a regular diet. Her Jackson-Pratts were removed. She was afebrile with stable vital signs and was ready for discharge home.

DISCHARGE INSTRUCTIONS: Activity as tolerated. Diet as tolerated.

DISCHARGE MEDICATIONS: Tylenol no. 3, 1 or 2 tablets p.o. (by mouth) q.4h. (every 4 hours) p.r.n. (as needed) pain.

FOLLOW-UP: The patient is to call for an appointment with Dr. Friendly.

CONDITION ON DISCHARGE: Improved.

DISCHARGE DIAGNOSIS:

1. Chronic duodenal ulcer

PROCEDURE PERFORMED: Duodenectomy

SERVICE CODE(S): _____

ICD-10-CM DX CODE(S): _____

(Answers to every other Case are located in Appendix D . The full answer key is only available in the TEACH Instructor Resources on Evolve.)

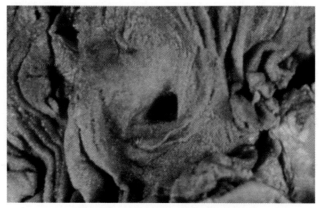

FIGURE 1–3 Chronic duodenal ulcer.

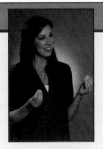

From the Trenches

"I have never seen another field where people are so willing to share their knowledge and help their colleagues. Coders want coders to succeed, and you will no doubt feel that camaraderie in this profession."

JENNA PRICE
CPC

Consultations, Prolonged Services, Standby, and Critical Care Services

Consultation Services

When physicians need opinions and advice, they ask another physician for an opinion or advice on the treatment, diagnosis, or management of a patient. This is different from a referral where a physician asks another physician to treat the problem. The physician asking for the advice or opinion is making a **request for consultation** and is the **requesting physician**. The physician giving the advice is providing a consultation and is the **consultant**. "Request for consultation" used to be termed "referral"; making a referral meant that the referring physician was asking for the advice or opinion of another physician (a consultation). Some third-party payers have chosen to define "referral" to mean a total transfer of the care of a patient. In other words, if a patient is referred by physician A to physician B, physician A is expecting physician B to evaluate and treat the patient for the condition for which the patient is being referred. The services of physician B would *not* be reported using consultation codes. On the other hand, if physician A makes a request for a consultation to physician B, it is expected that physician B will provide physician A with his or her advice or opinion and that the patient will return to physician A for any necessary treatment. Physician B would then report his or her services using consultation codes. Although these semantics (uses of words) may seem unimportant, they make a difference in the codes you use to report the services.

In the Consultation subsection, the two subheadings of consultations are:
1. Office or Other Outpatient Consultations (99242-99245)
2. Inpatient Consultations (99252-99255)

Office or Other Outpatient Consultations and Inpatient Consultations define the location in which the service is rendered; the patient is either an outpatient or an inpatient. Both subheadings are for new or established patients.

Only one initial consultation is reported by a consultant for the patient on each admission, and any subsequent service is reported using codes from the Subsequent Hospital Inpatient or Observation Care codes (99231-99233).

A **consultation** is a service provided by a physician whose opinion or advice regarding the management or diagnosis of a specific problem has been requested. The consultant provides a written report of the opinion or advice to the attending physician and documents the opinion and services provided in the medical record; the care of the patient is thus complete.

Sometimes the attending physician will request the consultant to assume responsibility for a specific area of the patient's care. For example, a consultant may be asked by the attending physician to see an inpatient regarding the care of the patient's diabetes while the patient is hospitalized for gallbladder surgery. After the initial consultation, the attending physician may ask the consultant to continue to monitor the patient's diabetic condition. The consultant assumes responsibility for management of the patient in the specific area of diabetes. Subsequent visits made by the consultant would then be reported using the codes from the subheading Subsequent Hospital Care.

Documentation in the medical record for a consultation must show a request from the attending physician for an opinion or the advice of a consultant on a specific condition. A request from the attending physician to have the consultant continue caring for the patient for that specific condition must also be documented in the medical record. Findings and treatments rendered during the consultation must be documented in the medical record by the consultant and communicated to the attending physician. A consultant can order tests and services for an inpatient, but the medical necessity of all tests and services must be indicated in the medical record.

CMS doesn't recognize CPT consultation codes (ranges 99242-99245 and 99252-99255) for inpatient facility and office/outpatient settings where consultation codes were previously billed. When an inpatient consultation is requested by the admitting provider, the consultant would report the appropriate admit code (99221-99223). The admitting physician reports 99221-99223 with modifier -AI appended.

Office or Other Outpatient Consultations

The Office or Other Outpatient Consultations codes (99242-99245) are used to report consultative services provided a patient in an office or other ambulatory patient setting, including hospital observation services, home services, custodial care, and services that are provided in a home or emergency department. Outpatient consultations include consultations provided in the emergency department because the patient is considered an outpatient in the emergency department setting. The codes are for both new and established patients and are of increasing complexity, based on the MDM or total time.

Inpatient Consultations The codes in the Inpatient Consultations subheading (99252-99255) are used to report services by physicians in inpatient settings. This subheading is used for both new and established patients and can be reported only one time per patient admission per consulting physician. After the initial consultation report, the subsequent inpatient or observation hospital visit codes would be used to report services.

A patient may have more than one concurrent (at the same time) consultant during an admission. For example, the attending physician may request a consultant, an endocrinologist, to render an opinion on a patient's diabetes, while at the same time another consultant, a cardiologist, is rendering an opinion on the patient's heart murmur.

Critical Care Services

Critical Care Services codes (99291, 99292) are used to identify services that are provided during medical emergencies to patients 72 months of age and over who are either critically ill or injured. Critical care provided in outpatient settings (ER or office) for neonates and pediatric patients up through 71 months is also coded with 99291 or 99292. These service codes require the physician to be constantly available to the patient and providing services exclusively to that patient. For example, a patient who is in shock or cardiac arrest would require the physician to provide bedside critical care services. Critical care is often, but not required to be, provided in an acute care setting of a hospital. Acute care settings are intensive care units, coronary care units, emergency departments, pediatric intensive care units, and similar critical care units of a hospital. Codes in this subsection are listed according to the total time the physician spends providing critical care to the patient.

The total critical care time, per day, the physician spends in care of the patient is stated in one amount of time, even if the time was not concurrent. Code 99291 is reported only once a day. As an example, if a physician attends to a critical care patient for 74 minutes and then leaves and returns for 30 minutes of critical care at a later time in the same day, the coding would be for 104 minutes of care. The coding for 104 minutes would be:

99291 for the 74 minutes

99292 for the additional 30 minutes

The physician must document the times in the medical record. Code 99291 is reported for the first 30 to 74 minutes of critical care, and code 99292 is reported for each additional 30 minutes beyond 74 minutes. If the critical care is less than 30 minutes, an E/M code would be used to report the service.

There are service codes that are bundled into the Critical Care Services codes. These services are normally provided to

stabilize the patient. An example of this bundling is as follows: A physician starts ventilation management (94002) while providing critical care services to a patient in the intensive care unit of a hospital. The ventilator management is not reported separately but, instead, is considered to be bundled into the Critical Care Services code. The notes preceding the critical care codes in the CPT manual list the services and procedures bundled into the codes. If the physician provided a service at the same time as critical care and that service is not bundled into the code, the service could be reported separately; however, the time for the service should not be included in the critical care time. You will know what is bundled into the codes because this information is listed either in the extensive description of the code or in the notes preceding the code. Be certain to read these notes, as they contain many exclusions and inclusions for these codes. For example, a parenthetical note directs the coder to not assign ventilator management codes 94002-94004 with E/M codes (99202-99499).

If the patient is in a critical care unit but is stable, you report the services using codes from the Hospital Inpatient Services subsection, Subsequent Hospital Care subheading or from the Inpatient Consultations subsection.

Prolonged Services

In the Prolonged Services subsection, there are four subheadings:

■ Prolonged Service on the Date Other than the Face-to-Face Evaluation and Management Service Without Direct Patient Contact

■ Prolonged Clinical Staff Services with Physician or Other Qualified Health Care Professional Supervision

■ Prolonged Service With or Without Direct Patient Contact on the Date of an Evaluation and Mangement Service

■ Standby Services

Prolonged Services codes are mostly add-on codes. Note the plus symbol (+) beside the codes in the range 99415-99418. Because add-on codes can be reported only with another code, Prolonged Services codes are intended to be reported only in addition to other codes to show an addition to some other service. As the instructional notes indicate, if the service is prolonged but is less than 30 minutes, it may not be separately reported. The prolonged services code may be assigned after the first 30 minutes of the prolonged services have been provided. The physician, therefore, has to spend at least 30 minutes beyond the typical time with the patient before it is possible to code 99415 (30-74 minutes of prolonged services). The following example illustrates the use of these codes.

EXAMPLE: An established patient with a history of COPD presents in an office visit with moderate respiratory distress. The physician conducts a history followed by an examination, which shows a respiratory rate of 30, and labored breathing and wheezing are heard in all lung fields. Office treatment is initiated; it includes intermittent bronchial dilation and subcutaneous epinephrine. The service requires the physician to have intermittent direct contact with the patient over a 2-hour period. The MDM complexity is low.

The office visit service would be reported using the office visit code 99215, which is a 40 minute service. The additional time the physician spent providing service to the patient would have to be reported using a prolonged services code.

This service was 120 minutes in length. This is 80 minutes beyond the typical time for a 99215. In this case, 99417 is assigned for each additional 15 minutes of total time.

The coding for the case is 99215 for the office visit, 99417 for each 15 minutes of prolonged services so 99417 ×5 for each additional 15 minutes.

The time the physician spends providing the prolonged services does not have to be continuous, as is the situation in this example; the physician monitored the patient on an intermittent basis, coming into the room to check on the patient and then leaving the room. However, the time must be documented in the patient record.

For help in applying these codes, note the table preceding the Prolonged Services codes; there you can locate the total time your physician spent with the patient and see an example of the correct coding.

Prolonged Services with Direct Patient Contact codes describe services that require the physician to have direct contact with the patient. However, the Prolonged Physician Services without Direct Patient Contact codes describe services during which the physician is not in direct contact with the patient. For example, a physician evaluates an established patient, a 70-year-old female with dementia, in an office visit. The physician then spends an extensive amount of time discussing the patient's condition, her treatment plan, and other recommendations with the patient's daughter. The services are reported using an office visit code for the patient evaluation and the appropriate Prolonged Services with or without Direct Patient Contact code for the time spent with the daughter.

Prolonged Services with or without Direct Patient Contact codes are divided on the basis of whether the services were provided to an outpatient or an inpatient.

Standby Services

The code 99360 for Standby Services is reported when a physician, at the request of the attending physician, is standing by in case his or her services are needed. The standby physician cannot be rendering services to another patient during this time. The standby codes are reported in increments of 30 minutes. If the total time for the standby service was less than 30 minutes, the service is not reported separately. The 30-minute increments refer to the 1st to 30th minute and do not have any of the complicated rules for reporting time that exist for reporting prolonged or critical services.

An important note concerning the standby codes is that these codes are assigned only when no service is performed and there is no direct contact with the patient. These codes are *not* assigned when a standby status ends with the physician providing a service to a patient. The service the physician provides is reported as any other service would be, even though it began as a standby service. For example, a cardiac surgeon may "stand by" during a cardiac catheterization in case the procedure needs to be converted to open heart surgery. This standby time is reported for each increment of 30 minutes. If the surgeon must then perform an open heart surgery, the surgeon would not report the time spent in standby but would instead report the open heart procedure.

CASE 1-10   *Consultation*

Report Dr. Lauer's professional service.

Consultation

LOCATION: Outpatient, Clinic

PATIENT: Gloria Freeman

PRIMARY CARE PHYSICIAN: Leslie Alanda, MD

CONSULTANT: Elmer Lauer, MD

The patient is a 37-year-old female I am asked to see by Dr. Alanda to render an opinion regarding painful varicose veins located on her lower left thigh posteriorly. These developed after her pregnancies. She works in a nursing home and does get rather severe pain when she is up on her feet for long periods. She does use support hose but has not used any Jobst support stockings. She has had no previous pelvic radiation. She has had no previous deep vein thrombosis. She has had a hysterectomy in July for endometriosis.

CURRENT MEDICATIONS: Premarin q.d.

PHYSICAL EXAMINATION: On examination there are no obvious varicosities involving the saphenous vein of either leg. The only area of varicosities is located in the posterior surface of the lower left thigh. These are small to moderate-sized veins.

Continued

CASE 1-10—cont'd

We discussed in detail indications for vein stripping as well as sclerotherapy. I talked about the risks of sclerotherapy, including skin slough, induration, pigmentation, as well as recurrence. She wanted to have the veins injected. I explained to her that I have stopped injecting veins mainly because of patients' high expectations with venous sclerotherapy. The other problem is that at this time we are not able to get 3% sodium tetradecyl sulfate. Given the location of these veins in the upper leg, I think that if any injection were to be done, I would recommend using the 3% solution just because of the location. It is not

known when this solution will become available again. We have been contacting the company periodically, and they are still not sure when they will have 3% solution on the market again.

We decided to give her a prescription for Jobst waist-high moderate support stockings to see if they work. I told her she could call us in 3 months to see whether we have gotten the solution.

SERVICE CODE(S): _____

ICD-10-CM DX CODE(S): _____

Discussion

This patient presents with the CC of varicose veins, which are veins in which blood has pooled. Usually, varicose veins occur in the saphenous veins of the leg and become distended. People who stand for long periods of time, cross their legs at the knees, or wear constricting garments are more prone to developing varicose veins. Conservative treatment for varicose veins is antiembolism stockings (such as Jobst) and the avoidance of other contributory factors, such as standing and crossing of legs. If the conservative treatment is not effective, saphenous vein stripping would be considered. If left untreated, varicose veins can develop and lead to venous stasis ulcers, which are susceptible to infection. ICD-10-CM codes for varicose veins are divided based on the location of the vein; lower extremities (I83.90), with bleeding or rupture (I83.899) and other sites (I86.8). There are specific codes for lower extremities when there is an ulcer (I83.009); inflammation (I83.10); ulcer and inflammation (I83.209); other complications, such as edema, pain, and swelling (I83.899/I83.819); and asymptomatic (I83.90), which are those without any symptoms.

Note that category I84 is hemorrhoids, which technically are varicose veins of the anus.

Varicose veins of other sites are specific as to the location, such as esophageal (I85.01 with bleeding, I85.00 without bleeding), sublingual (I86.0), scrotal (I86.1), pelvic (I86.2), and varices of other sites (I86.8).

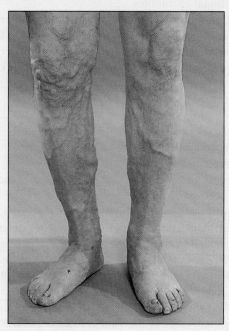

FIGURE 1-4 Varicose veins.

(Answers to every other Case are located in Appendix D . The full answer key is only available in the TEACH Instructor Resources on Evolve.)

CASE 1-11   *Consultation*

Report Dr. Alanda's professional service.

Consultation

LOCATION: Outpatient, Clinic

PATIENT: Gilda Spellhurst

PHYSICIAN: Leslie Alanda, MD

PRIMARY: Elmer Lauer, MD

I was asked to evaluate the patient by the patient's primary to render an opinion for preparation for pending gastric resection. The patient was examined and the chart reviewed.

HISTORY OF PRESENT ILLNESS: She has been having problems with recurrent peptic ulcer disease despite therapy with Zantac and Prilosec. She had undergone several endoscopies, which revealed a large ulcer that was reported to be benign. The patient was also noted to have a slightly elevated CEA (carcinoembryonic antigen) of 11. On June 30, the

CASE 1-11—cont'd

patient underwent laparoscopy, which turned out to be normal as well and benign. There were no signs of any lymphadenopathy.

PAST SURGICAL HISTORY:

1. Hysterectomy
2. Tubal ligation

The patient never has problems with surgery or anesthesia.

SOCIAL HISTORY: Positive for smoking. The patient denies alcohol abuse. She smokes about a pack per day.

FAMILY HISTORY: Negative for colonic carcinoma and premature coronary artery disease, but positive for severe peptic ulcer disease in her mother.

ALLERGIES: NONE.

REVIEW OF SYSTEMS: Negative for melena, hematochezia, and hematemesis.

PHYSICAL EXAMINATION demonstrates a slender Hispanic female in no acute distress. She is uncomfortable, however, because of epigastric discomfort. Her neck is supple. There is no thyromegaly or regional lymphadenopathy. No subclavicular or supraclavicular lymph nodes. ENT is within normal limits. Eyes: Sclerae anicteric. Conjunctivae are pale. Funduscopic exam shows no AV (arteriovenous) nicking, hemorrhages, exudates, or papilledema. Chest is barrel-shaped without dullness to percussion but with rhonchi scattered throughout the lung fields. Prolonged expiratory phase was noted. Cardiac exam: Regular rhythm. Distant heart sounds, 1/6 systolic ejection murmur at the base. Abdomen is soft and tender to palpation. Epigastric area without rebound, tenderness, or guarding. Liver span is 7 cm (centimeter); edge at right costal margin. Aorta diameter is normal. Extremities: Upper and lower show no edema, cyanosis, or clubbing. Neurologic exam is nonfocal.

REVIEW OF LABORATORY ANALYSIS revealed hypercalcemia of 10.3, which is probably exaggerated by a low albumin and likely is to be more significant than that. Creatinine is 0.5. AST is 15. Cancer embryonic antigen is 11.5. *H. pylori* is 4.8.

IMPRESSION/PLAN: Nonhealing peptic ulcer disease. Patient's doctor increased her Prilosec to 2 a day and continued Zantac at the present dose. In fact, one might increase it to 300 mg (milligram) b.i.d. (twice a day) if necessary. There is certainly a need to rule out Zollinger-Ellison and hyperparathyroidism as the sources of the patient's nonhealing ulcer. C-terminal PTH (parathyroid hormone) will be checked along with ionized calcium. One might plan parahyperthyroidectomy simultaneous with gastrectomy if patient has high PTH, which I suspect will be the case, although in the case of treatment with H_2 blockers and Prilosec, a gastrin level might be elevated. Anyhow, we will check it and make sure that it is not extreme. If the gastrin level is high, one might consider complete gastrectomy rather than a partial one on the presumption of Z-E syndrome. The patient will be re-evaluated after results of the aforementioned tests are available and will be scheduled for surgery. Elevated CEA is bothersome. She has not had colonoscopy for some time and should it again be elevated, one might consider simultaneous colonoscopy during the same admission. The patient will be sent to Dr. Dawson. I am concerned with her pulmonary status. She is advised to curtail her cigarette consumption to as low as possible and switch to low-tar nicotine cigarettes in the interim. Once she is admitted, therapy with beta agonists and Atrovent will be immediately initiated, and the patient will be started on incentive spirometry.

Thank you for allowing me to assist you in this interesting case. We discussed the aforementioned problem with the patient's primary, who will hold surgery for 1 week until all laboratory analyses are completed. A total of 80 minutes was spent with patient, and 55 minutes were spent going over the data in the patient's medical record.

SERVICE CODE(S): _____

ICD-10-CM DX CODE(S): _____

Discussion
Ulcer

An ulcer is an erosive area or a break. The term "peptic" pertains to pepsin or to digestion. A peptic ulcer occurs on the mucosal lining of the stomach (K25.9) or duodenum (K26.9) that results in the submucosal areas being exposed to gastric secretions. The site may be unspecified (K27.9) in the medical record.

Tobacco Dependence

In Case 1-11A, note that the physician indicates her concern for the patient's pulmonary status and has advised the patient to stop her cigarette consumption or to keep the number of cigarettes smoked as low as possible. She also indicates that once the patient was admitted, pulmonary therapy was to be initiated (beta agonists, Atrovent, incentive spirometry). Given these statements in the medical documentation, the patient's dependency on tobacco will have to be reported (F17.210).

(Answers to every other Case are located in Appendix D . The full answer key is only available in the TEACH Instructor Resources on Evolve.)

CASE 1-12A   *Consultation*

Report Dr. Pleasant's service.

LOCATION: Inpatient, Hospital

PATIENT: Gladys Hanson

ATTENDING PHYSICIAN: Alma Naraquist, MD

CONSULTANT: Timothy L. Pleasant, MD

I am being asked by Dr. Naraquist to render an opinion on this patient primarily because of azotemia.

The patient is a 74-year-old white woman who had been admitted primarily because of right-sided hemiparesis secondary to a presumed cerebrovascular accident.

The patient has been followed up in the hospital by Dr. Naraquist.

She had laboratory work done recently, which showed the following results: sodium 139, potassium 4.8, chloride 108, CO_2 (carbon dioxide) 21.3, BUN (blood urea nitrogen) and creatinine 89/4.6 (71/4.1 yesterday; 46/2.4 on April 6, creatinine baseline of 0.8 to 1.2 as far back as October), glucose 162, calcium 9. Hemogram shows H&H (hematocrit and hemoglobin) of 10.9/33.2, WBC (white blood count) 15.99, normochromic/normocytic indices, and platelets 384.

This patient has also been seen by Dr. Green over the weekend while Dr. Green was covering for Dr. Naraquist and has been given a working diagnosis of acute renal failure secondary to severe intravascular volume depletion. Postrenal causes have likewise been ruled out by ultrasound, which did not reveal any hydronephrosis but did reveal an unobstructing calculus 4 mm in the left renal system. Review of the patient's medical record does not really reveal any obvious culprit as far as her underlying renal failure is concerned, but gentamicin/aminoglycoside nephrotoxicity seems to be an attractive consideration. Eosinophils were also checked because of the possibility of an acute interstitial nephritis, but this turned out to be negative. Nevertheless, the patient has been placed on a course of intravenous steroids.

The patient has a past medical and past surgical history that consists of the following:

1. Hypertension.
2. Hyperlipidemia.
3. Degenerative joint disease; questionable osteoporosis.
4. Coronary artery disease, congestive heart failure.
5. Cerebrovascular accident.
6. History of gastric ulcer/duodenal bulb, complicated by anemia.
7. History of Sjögren syndrome.

SOCIAL HISTORY: She is married and retired. She lives with her husband and is accompanied by her husband during hospital visit today. She denies any current use of alcohol, tobacco, IV (intravenous) or recreational drugs.

FAMILY HISTORY: Noncontributory.

LABORATORY RESULTS: As noted above.

REVIEW OF SYSTEMS: Constitutional: No fever or chills. Positive recent weight loss. She appears to be fairly well nourished. No night sweats. Skin: No skin lesions. No active dermatosis. Eyes: No eye discharge or itching. No visual changes or diplopia. ENT (ears, nose, throat): No ear discharge. No difficulty hearing. No pharyngeal hyperemia, congestion, or exudates. Lymph nodes: No lymphadenopathy in the neck, axillary, or groin. Neurological: Positive occasional headache. Positive gait instability. No recent falls. No seizures. Psychiatric: No behavior changes. Neck: No thyromegaly. Respiratory: Positive occasional cough. No cold. No hemoptysis. No shortness of breath. Cardiovascular: No chest pain. No palpitations. No orthopnea. No paroxysmal nocturnal dyspnea. Gastrointestinal: Positive anorexia. Positive nausea. No vomiting. No dysphagia. No odynophagia. No constipation or diarrhea. No abdominal pain. No fecal incontinence. No hematemesis, hematochezia, or melena. Genitourinary: No urgency, frequency, or dysuria. No hematuria. No urinary incontinence. No nocturia. No vaginal discharge. No vaginal lesion. No vaginal bleeding. Musculoskeletal: Positive joint pain. Positive muscle weakness/pain. Hematologic: No bleeding tendencies. No purpura. No petechiae. No ecchymosis. Endocrine: No heat or cold intolerance.

CURRENT MEDICATIONS:

1. Iron sulfate.
2. Vasotec 10 mg (milligram) q.h.s. (each bedtime), 20 mg q.a.m. (every morning).
3. Lacrisert eye drops.
4. Synthroid 0.125 q.d. (every day).
5. Tegretol 200 t.i.d. (three times a day).
6. Plavix 75 mg q.d.
7. Digoxin 0.125 q.d.

ALLERGIES: Tetracycline.

PHYSICAL EXAMINATION: Vital signs stable. Blood pressure 137/76, heart rate 81, respirations 20, and saturating 93% on room air. Input and output in the last 24 hours is 2969/1479. Pink palpebral conjunctivae and anicteric sclerae. Positive weakness of the right extraocular muscles. No pharyngeal hyperemia, congestion, or exudates. Somewhat dry tongue and buccal mucosa related to mouth breathing. Supple neck. No lymphadenopathy. Symmetrical chest expansion. Poor inspiratory effort with decreased breath sounds in both lung fields. Occasional rhonchi. No crackles. No wheezes. S1 (first heart sound) and S2 (second heart sound) are distinct. No S3 (third heart sound) or S4 (fourth heart sound). Regular rate and rhythm. Positive 3/6 systolic murmur over the apex radiating to the carotid, most likely suggestive of an aortic stenosis. Abdomen obese. Positive bowel sounds, soft and nontender. No abdominal bruits. Both upper and lower extremities reveal arthritic changes. Pulses are fair.

ASSESSMENT/PLAN:

1. Acute renal failure (baseline creatinine is 0.8–1.2 past 4 months), secondary to the following:
    A. Intravascular volume depletion brought about by decreased p.o. (by mouth) intake/decreased IV (intravenous) fluids.
    B. Nephrotoxic ATN (acute tubular necrosis)/ aminoglycoside/ gentamicin.
    C. Acute interstitial nephritis probably related to cephalosporin antibiotics. The patient is on IV steroids per Dr. Naraquist.

At this time, patient continues to make a fair amount of urine output even though she is off diuretic medications. Assuming that this is primarily secondary to nephrotoxic effects of aminoglycoside antibiotics, one should expect full to partial recovery of renal function in this particular lady. Per chart notes, the patient and her husband vehemently have expressed their lack of desire to pursue any dialysis treatment if it is ever required.

CASE 1-12A—cont'd

Today I had a brief discussion with the patient's husband, and I explained to him that I think her renal failure is primarily acute in nature, although the possibility of a chronic renal failure cannot be undermined despite a normal baseline creatinine, considering her significant hypoalbuminemia. Nevertheless, because she continues to make an excellent amount of urine output, and the possible culprit medications have been withdrawn, one should expect her creatinine to plateau and stabilization followed by a subsequent declining trend, which should be observed within at least the next 3 weeks.

At this point, the patient does not require dialysis or any form of renal replacement therapy. If the time comes that she does, however, we will discuss these options again with the patient and her husband and proceed from there on.

At this time, I am going to continue with the patient as requested by Dr. Naraquist.

SERVICE CODE(S): _____

ICD-10-CM DX CODE(S): _____

Discussion

Dr. Pleasant is providing an initial consultation for Gladys Hanson because of azotemia. Azotemia, also known as uremia, is an excess of urea or other nitrogenous wastes in the blood, and is a symptom of renal dysfunction. In the Assessment/Plan section of the report, Dr. Pleasant states a diagnosis of acute renal failure. (For information regarding renal failure, refer to the information following Case 1-7.) The dehydration,

ATN (acute tubular necrosis) and nephritis are not reported because the physician states that each of these conditions is caused by (secondary to) the acute renal failure.

The attending physician, Dr. Naraquist, has requested that Dr. Pleasant continue treating the patient, so Dr. Pleasant's future visits would be subsequent hospital care.

(Answers to every other Case are located in Appendix D . The full answer key is only available in the TEACH Instructor Resources on Evolve.)

CASE 1-12B   *Progress Report*

Report Dr. Pleasant's service.

LOCATION: Inpatient, Hospital

PATIENT: Gladys Hanson

ATTENDING PHYSICIAN: Alma Naraquist, MD

CONSULTANT: Timothy L. Pleasant, MD

The patient is seen and examined, chart reviewed.

I have had a lengthy discussion with the patient and her husband today regarding issues pertaining to renal functioning.

Latest labs performed on April 9: Sodium 138, potassium of 4.6, chloride of 107, CO_2 (carbon dioxide) of 19.6, BUN (blood urea nitrogen) and creatinine 107/5.4, glucose 138, calcium 9.3. Hemogram shows an H&H (hematocrit and hemoglobin) of 9.6/29.2, WBC (white blood count) 19.84, normochromic/normocytic indices. Platelets are 380. There is a significant left shift of 90% neutrophils. Magnesium is 2.3. Phosphorus is 4.5.

Several issues have been brought forth this morning. Because the patient's renal functioning is worsening, the issue of renal replacement therapy in the form of dialysis has been brought forth again.

According to the chart notes, it has been assumed that this patient's acute renal failure is secondary to nephrotoxic acute tubular necrosis secondary to aminoglycoside/gentamicin nephrotoxicity. There are, however, some components of this patient's clinical scenario that may or may not be consistent with either nephrotoxic ATN (acute tubular necrosis) or even acute interstitial nephritis. Because of this, the issue of performing a renal biopsy was considered. In my opinion, a renal biopsy would be a good definitive way of determining her diagnosis. As far as the interstitial nephritis is concerned, it may not yield significant findings,

primarily because of the patient being on at least 5 to 7 days of steroid therapy. On the other hand, if it turns out to be a vasculitis or one of those glomerular diseases, it must be noted that this patient has already been on steroids, and she should show some form of response already. Finally, I do not believe that the patient would eventually be a candidate for any form of cytotoxic therapy with cyclophosphamide or chlorambucil or the like. Therefore, renal biopsy may not be an option at this point.

On the other hand, what is clear from this present examination is that the patient does require renal replacement therapy or dialysis. The patient's husband has expressed concern that because of her other comorbid illnesses pertaining to her cardiac status, he has expressed reservations about proceeding with dialysis. I have spent a great deal of time explaining to him and the patient that if the patient's kidney function continues to decline and dialysis is not chosen as an option, then she will certainly die from the complications of uremia. If we choose to proceed with intermittent hemodialysis, however, and if it turns out that her underlying renal disease is secondary to nephrotoxic causes, then we should see at least some improvement in renal function.

PHYSICAL EXAMINATION: On examination, vital signs are stable. Blood pressure is 145/69, heart rate 106, respirations 20, and saturations 93%. Temperature is 36.4° C (Celsius). Pink palpebral conjunctivae and anicteric sclerae. No nasal or aural discharge. Moist tongue and buccal mucosa. No pharyngeal hyperemia, congestion, or exudates. Supple neck. No lymphadenopathy. Symmetrical chest expansion. Decreased breath sounds in both lung fields related to poor inspiratory effort. Positive rhonchi. No crackles. No wheezes. S1 (first heart sound) and S2 (second heart sound) are distinct. No S3 (third heart sound) or S4 (fourth heart sound). Regular rate and rhythm. Abdomen: Positive bowel sounds, soft and nontender. Both upper and lower extremities reveal arthritic changes. Pulses are fair.

Continued

CASE 1-12B—cont'd

ASSESSMENT/PLAN:

1. Acute renal failure (baseline creatinine was 0.8-1.2 since October), secondary to the following:
   A. Intravascular volume depletion brought about by decreased p.o. (by mouth) intake/decreased fluids.
   B. Nephrotoxic ATN/aminoglycoside/gentamicin.
   C. Acute interstitial nephritis, probably related to cephalosporins.
   D. Questionable glomerular/vascular disorder.

Please refer to the above for more detailed discussion.

I am going to schedule the patient for a tentative hemodialysis catheter placement tomorrow morning and eventual dialysis. If the patient's family decides not to proceed with dialysis, then my recommendation is to proceed with possible do-not-resuscitate status or code III.

I have spent a total of 40 minutes evaluating and reviewing this patient's medical record. I have spent an additional 45 minutes discussing the case with the patient and her husband. The counseling of the patient took over 50% of the time of this service.

SERVICE CODE(S): _____

ICD-10-CM DX CODE(S): _____

(Answers to every other Case are located in Appendix D . The full answer key is only available in the TEACH Instructor Resources on Evolve.)

CASE 1-12C   *Progress Report*

Report Dr. Pleasant's service.

LOCATION: Inpatient, Hospital
PATIENT: Gladys Hanson
ATTENDING PHYSICIAN: Alma Naraquist, MD
CONSULTANT: Timothy L. Pleasant, MD

The patient is seen and examined, chart reviewed. Today I had a discussion with the patient's husband, and it has been finally decided that the patient will not be subjected to any form of renal replacement therapy or dialysis. The pros and cons of this decision have been discussed once again, and the patient's husband understands.

Latest labs are as follows: Hemogram: Hemoglobin 9.3, hematocrit 28.7, WBC (white blood count) 17.67, normochromic/normocytic indices, and platelets 411. There is a significant left shift of 90% neutrophils. The rest of the chemistries are as follows: Sodium 141, potassium 5.1, chloride 108, CO_2 (carbon dioxide) 18.8, BUN (blood urea nitrogen) 114, and creatinine 6 (89 and 4.6 yesterday; 71 and 4.1 on April 7), glucose 115, and calcium 9.3.

EXAMINATION: Vital signs are stable. Blood pressure 130s/50s. Heart rate is in the 90s. Respirations 20s. She is febrile. HEENT (head, ears, eyes, nose, throat): Normocephalic and atraumatic. Pink palpebral conjunctivae and anicteric sclerae. No nasal or aural discharge. Moist tongue and buccal mucosa. No pharyngeal hyperemia, congestion, or exudates. Supple neck. No lymphadenopathy. Symmetrical chest expansion. Decreased breath sounds in both lung fields related to poor inspiratory effort. Positive rhonchi. No crackles. No wheezes. S1 (first heart sound) and S2 (second heart sound) are distinct. No S3 (third heart sound) or S4 (fourth heart sound). Regular rate and rhythm. Abdomen: Positive bowel sounds, soft and nontender. Both upper and lower extremities reveal arthritic changes. Pulses are fair.

ASSESSMENT/PLAN:

1. Acute renal failure (baseline creatinine 0.8 and 0.2 since November), secondary to the following:
   A. Intravascular volume depletion brought about by decreased p.o. (by mouth) intake.
   B. Nephrotoxicity ATN (acute tubular necrosis)/aminoglycoside/gentamicin.
   C. Acute interstitial nephritis, probably related to cephalosporins.
   D. Questionable glomerular/vascular disorder.

Please refer to my progress note from yesterday for more details.

At this time, because it has been decided not to consider dialysis, I am going to withdraw from this case. I have informed the husband as well. At the same time, I would recommend that the patient be considered a code III level status/palliative/comfort care. Dr. Naraquist is taking over the case from here.

SERVICE CODE(S): _____

ICD-10-CM DX CODE(S): _____

(Answers to every other Case are located in Appendix D . The full answer key is only available in the TEACH Instructor Resources on Evolve.)

CASE 1-13   *Critical Care*

The physician in this case is being requested to provide a consultation for the tachypnea (excessive, rapid breathing) as indicated in the first paragraph by the statement "The main reason for consultation is that of possible mechanical ventilation primarily for airway protection due to tachypnea." Report Dr. Dawson's service.

LOCATION: Inpatient, Hospital
PATIENT: Peter Gluzinski
ATTENDING PHYSICIAN: Ronald Green, MD
CONSULTANT: Gregory Dawson, MD

CASE 1-13—cont'd

I am being asked by Dr. Green to render an opinion on this patient from the critical care standpoint because the patient is in acute alcohol intoxication. The main reason for consultation is that of possible mechanical ventilation primarily for airway protection due to tachypnea.

The patient is a 62-year-old white man who has had multiple admissions in the past for multiple acute alcohol intoxications/detoxifications.

The patient was initially brought to the emergency room, where patient was noted to be significantly intoxicated. His blood alcohol level is 400 mg/dl (milligram/deciliter), and this was drawn at 4 o'clock this morning.

The patient was then placed on intermittent dosing of Ativan with no success. And so Dr. Green decided to contact me, and we have agreed to have the anesthesia service intubate the patient.

The patient is being placed on an initial mechanical ventilation setup consisting of FiO_2 (forced inspiration oxygen) of 100%, SIMV (synchronized intermittent mandatory ventilation) of 14, tidal volume of 600, PEEP (positive end-expiratory pressure) of 5, and pressure support of 10. Blood gases are to be drawn in 30 minutes, and chest x-rays are to be done to reassess placement of the endotracheal tube.

Latest laboratory tests performed on this patient are as follows: Sodium 141, potassium 3.9, chloride 100, CO_2 (carbon dioxide) 25.4, BUN (blood urea nitrogen) and creatinine 10/1, glucose 113, calcium 8.5, ALT (alanine transaminase [formerly SGPT]) 54. Alcohol level is 400 mg/dl as noted above.

Hemogram shows H&H (hematocrit and hemoglobin) of 16/45.2, WBC (white blood count) 7.46, normochromic/normocytic indices, and platelets 202. There is no left shift, as neutrophils are only 46.7%.

PAST MEDICAL/SURGICAL HISTORY:

1. Hypertension.
2. Nicotine dependence.
3. Alcohol abuse/dependence with multiple admissions for acute intoxications; alcohol withdrawal/alcohol withdrawal seizures; alcohol rehabilitation/detoxifications.
4. Questionable coronary artery disease (per medical records).

FAMILY HISTORY: According to the medical records, it is positive for diabetes. Negative for hypertension, stroke, kidney disease, bleeding disorder/dyscrasia.

SOCIAL HISTORY: He works at the local automobile factory, and he smokes two packs per day. As noted above, he does have a history of significant alcohol binges. He denies any previous or current use of intravenous or recreational drugs. His daughter has terminal liver disease/illness.

MEDICATIONS: Lotensin 10 mg q.d. (every day)

ALLERGIES: No known drug allergies.

LABORATORY RESULTS: As noted above.

REVIEW OF SYSTEMS: Unobtainable at this time as patient is intubated, mechanically ventilated (96 hours), and sedated with an Ativan drip.

PHYSICAL EXAMINATION: On examination, vital signs are stable. Blood pressure 137/69, heart rate 89, respirations 16, and saturation 94%. Latest blood gases are as follows: 7.34/4 5.7/92.4/24.1/97.6% on setting of FiO_2 of 80%, SIMV of 14, tidal volume of 600, PEEP of

5, and pressure support of 10. Normocephalic and atraumatic. Pink palpebral conjunctivae and anicteric sclerae. Intubated and mechanically ventilated. Supple neck. No lymphadenopathy. Symmetrical chest expansion. No retractions. No rhonchi. No crackles. No wheezes. S1 (first heart sound) and S2 (second heart sound) are distinct. No S3 (third heart sound) or S4 (fourth heart sound). Regular rate and rhythm. Abdomen: Obese. Positive bowel sounds, soft and nontender. No abdominal bruits appreciated. Both upper and lower extremities reveal arthritic changes. No edema on both lower extremities. Pulses are fair.

ASSESSMENT/PLAN:

1. Acute alcohol intoxication. It must be noted that the toxicity of ethanol is dose-related but tolerance has a wide variation. In this case, with levels in excess of 400 mg/dl, respiratory depression is common and death is possible from such a problem; hence, the patient has been intubated and mechanically ventilated. At this time, the plan is as follows:
   a. Admit to medical ICU (intensive care unit).
   b. Monitor vital signs q.4h. (every 4 hours).
   c. Monitor daily weights, inputs, and outputs.
   d. Nasogastric tube, Foley catheter.
   e. IV (intravenous) fluids D5 (dextrose 5% water) $^1/_2$ normal saline with 100% thiamine plus multivitamin 1 ampule plus folic acid 1 mg at a rate of 150 ml (milliliter)/hour followed by D5$^1/_4$ normal saline to infuse at a maintenance IV fluid rate of 150 ml/hour.

I do not believe that charcoal would be helpful at this time because of rapid absorption of alcohol from the stomach. At this time, he does not really require hemodialysis. Based on my clinical examination and evaluation of this patient, there is indeed presence of alcohol intoxication; however, there does not seem to be any underlying illness or significant alcoholic ketoacidosis. At this time, we will continue ventilator support as required and also will continue to observe him until he is sober, that is, until blood alcohol level is less than 100 mg/dl, at which time he can be transferred to the medical floor. At that time, I would recommend consultation with psychiatry and an alcohol guidance counselor.

After reviewing his blood gases, I would recommend that we try to wean his oxygen down while maintaining a saturation of greater than or equal to 90%. Likewise, I am going to recommend increasing SIMV to 16. Blood gases will be repeated in the morning.

2. Hypertension, fairly controlled. At this time, blood pressure appears to be relatively well controlled. If he does develop a hypertensive crisis in relation to alcohol withdrawal, my recommendation would be to place him on either atenolol or clonidine for blood pressure control.
3. History of tobacco abuse; questionable chronic obstructive pulmonary disease.
4. Psychiatric issues.

I will continue to follow up on this patient from the critical care standpoint, and Dr. Green will take over in the morning as far as management of his ventilation is concerned. I spent a total of 90 minutes evaluating and reviewing this patient's medical record. I spent another 10 minutes discussing the case with Dr. Green.

SERVICE CODE(S): _____

ICD-10-CM DX CODE(S): _____

Continued

CASE 1-13—cont'd

Discussion

Acute Alcohol Intoxication

You did a fine job if you reported the tachypnea, acute alcohol intoxication, and hypertension. The hypertension is reported because the report indicated that it was "fairly controlled," and as such, is a consideration in treatment. In Point 2 in the Assessment/Plan section of the report, the physician indicates that he is concerned that the patient may develop a hypertensive crisis in relation to the alcohol withdrawal. The report indicates that the patient was admitted many times for acute alcohol intoxications/detoxifications. When an alcohol-dependent patient is acutely intoxicated and presents for care, report F10.2-, with additional characters/digits assigned to indicate the type of dependency.

The COPD (chronic obstructive pulmonary disease) was questionable and would not be reported in an outpatient setting. The history of tobacco abuse and psychiatric issues do not have a direct involvement in the service being provided, so they are not reported.

(Answers to every other Case are located in Appendix D . The full answer key is only available in the TEACH Instructor Resources on Evolve.)

Cerebral Hemorrhage

The three protective membranes that surround the brain and spinal cord are the dura mater, arachnoid, and pia mater (as illustrated in **Figure 1-5**). Intracranial hemorrhage can be extradural (outside the dura), subdural (between the dura and arachnoid), subarachnoid (between the arachnoid and pia mater), or cerebral (parenchymatous or within the tissues of the brain).

In the Index of the ICD-10-CM, locate the main term "Hemorrhage," subterm "brain (miliary) (nontraumatic)." ("Miliary" means resembling a small seed and is an area of minute lesion.) You are directed to "*see* Hemorrhage, intracranial, intracerebral," which directs you to I61.9. Within the Tabular for **nontraumatic** intracerebral hemorrhage, I61 is the code for **intracerebral** hemorrhage of various anatomical areas, such as intraventricular and cerebellar (see Figure 1-5). Nontraumatic intracerebral hemorrhage can be caused by any number of conditions such as leukemia, hemophilia, liver disease, or hypertension.

Subarachnoid hemorrhage is reported with I60.9 and includes congenital cerebral aneurysm and berry aneurysm. (An aneurysm is a sac formed by dilatation of a vessel wall.) A berry aneurysm is one that forms in the cerebral artery, usually at a junction of a vessel. It is termed a berry aneurysm because the neck of the aneurysm is smaller than the body of the aneurysm. It is also known as a cerebral aneurysm. A nonruptured berry aneurysm is reported with I67.1.

Nontraumatic **subdural** hemorrhage is reported with I62.00, nontraumatic extradural hemorrhage is reported with I62.1, and unspecified intracranial hemorrhage that is not further specified is reported with I62.9.

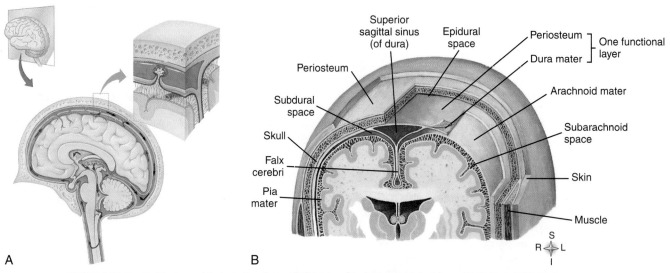

FIGURE 1–5 Meninges of the brain. From Patton KE, Thibodeau GA: *Anatomy and physiology*, ed 7, St. Louis, 2010, Mosby.

CASE 1-14 *ICU Report*

Report Dr. Naraquist's service.

LOCATION: Inpatient, Hospital
PATIENT: Morley Overmoe
ATTENDING PHYSICIAN: Alma Naraquist, MD

I am admitting this patient to the medical ICU (intensive care unit) because of a recent hemorrhagic stroke involving the left frontal area.

The patient is a 49-year-old white, obese, known hypertensive patient who was found to be unresponsive in his home. The history of present illness started a few hours before admission this morning when he started to have acute onset of headache involving the right temporal area. He started becoming weak afterward, and he self-medicated with two enteric-coated aspirins, 81 mg (milligram) per day. The patient did not have any seizure episodes, but was later noted by his wife to manifest suddenly a staggering gait later followed by unresponsiveness.

The patient then was brought to the hospital, where subsequent CT (computerized tomography) scan showed a significant large left frontal lobe hemorrhage.

The patient was evaluated in the emergency room and was noted to have 2-mm (millimeter) pupils, nonreactive, positive cornealis, with no appreciable spontaneous breaths, at least during my examination.

LABORATORY TESTS that were performed in the hospital include the following: Electrocardiogram primary shows sinus bradycardia with first-degree AV (arteriovenous) block, rate of 51 beats per minute, no ST (sinus tachycardia) or T wave changes. Hemogram shows an H&H (hematocrit and hemoglobin) of 16.5/48.8, WBC (white blood count) of 11.8, normochromic/normocytic indices, and platelets 252. Sodium is 127, potassium 3.1, chloride 102, CO_2 (carbon dioxide) 28, BUN (blood urea nitrogen) and creatinine 18/1.2, glucose 251, and calcium is 9.1.

In the hospital, the patient is also intubated and mechanically ventilated. Latest blood gases prior to intubation are as follows: 7.37/47.3/115/27/29/98% Venti mask.

PAST MEDICAL/SURGICAL HISTORY:

1. Hypertension.
2. Obesity.
3. Questionable congestive heart failure.

MEDICATIONS taken at home including the following:

1. Atenolol 75 mg q.d. (every day).
2. Norvasc 5 mg q.d.
3. Digoxin 0.25 mg q.d.
4. Quinapril 40 mg q.d.
5. Doxazosin 4 mg q.d.
6. Aspirin 1 tab q.d.
7. Hydrochlorothiazide 25 mg q.d.

ALLERGIES: Penicillin.

FAMILY HISTORY: Positive for hypertension and cancer. Father and mother have been afflicted with hypertension and heart disease. Negative history of diabetes, stroke, kidney disease, bleeding disorder, or dyscrasia.

SOCIAL HISTORY: According to the wife, the patient has not had any usage of alcohol, tobacco, or intravenous or recreational drugs.

REVIEW OF SYSTEMS: Unobtainable.

NEUROLOGICAL EXAMINATION: Please refer to Sutton's note for more details.

PHYSICAL EXAMINATION: On examination, vital signs are stable. Blood pressure is 180s/80s. Heart rate is in the 60s to 70s. Respirations are 12. He is afebrile, normocephalic, and atraumatic. Pink palpebral conjunctivae, anicteric sclerae. Supple neck. No lymphadenopathy. Intubated and mechanically ventilated. Symmetrical chest expansion. No retractions. Positive rhonchi. No crackles or wheezes. S1 (first heart sound) and S2 (second heart sound) are distinct. No S3 (third heart sound) or S4 (fourth heart sound). Regular rate and rhythm. Abdomen is obese. Positive bowel sounds. Soft and nontender. No abdominal bruits. Both upper and lower extremities reveal no gross deformities; positive arthritic changes. Pulses are fair.

ASSESSMENT/PLAN: Left frontal lobe hemorrhage. A neurosurgeon, Dr. Hodgson, has been consulted. The patient's poor prognosis has been discussed with the patient's wife. The patient is actually a code level III according to the wife.

Plan right now is to render conservative medical management with antihypertensive regimen consisting of nitroprusside drip. Dr. Pleasant also has suggested giving the patient a dose of mannitol. We will continue to monitor the patient's daily weights, inputs, and outputs.

We will try to do neuro checks on an hourly basis. We will also check the patient's lab values. I am also going to order cardiac enzymes on this patient.

Target systolic blood pressure is 140s to 160s, so that we do not precipitate any ischemic deficit as a result of overzealous antihypertensive medication use.

A lengthy discussion with the patient's wife was held, during which it was explained that surgery is an option; however, the results may not necessarily be encouraging. The wife has expressed her understanding and appreciation of our explanations.

The patient is going to be admitted to medical ICU and monitored with re-evaluation in the morning.

I spent a total of 60 minutes evaluating and reviewing this patient's medical records.

SERVICE CODE(S): _____

ICD-10-CM DX CODE(S): _____

Discussion
Code Levels
Hospitals have pre-established resuscitation levels. These levels specify the conditions under which a patient is or is not to be resuscitated.

The patient has agreed to the conditions of this level, usually stated in terms such as "Code 1," "Code 2," etc. The higher the level, the more conditions that have to be met before the patient is resuscitated should that situation arise. Note that this patient is a code level 3, which

Continued

CASE 1-14—cont'd

means that the patient or his wife has recognized the severity of the patient's condition and has chosen a code level that is less likely to result in resuscitation.

Critical Care

The physician has indicated the time he spent with this patient providing critical care service, which is necessary to accurately report the service. If the physician does not indicate the time, you cannot report the critical

care service. You would need to assign an E/M code based on the location in which the service was provided (i.e., ED, inpatient unit) and the key components (history, exam, and MDM). It is important to educate the physician regarding the need for indicating time on the medical record in order to correctly report critical care services.

Remember that critical care is the type of service rendered, not necessarily the place (e.g., the critical care unit) it was provided.

(Answers to every other Case are located in Appendix D . The full answer key is only available in the TEACH Instructor Resources on Evolve.)

CASE 1-15 *Critical Care*

Report Dr. Dawson's service.

LOCATION: Inpatient, Hospital

PATIENT: Sebastian Gunther

ATTENDING PHYSICIAN: Alma Naraquist, MD

CONSULTANT: Gregory Dawson, MD

I am being consulted primarily because of acute onset of hypotension.

The patient is a 76-year-old white, obese man who had been admitted to his hometown hospital around 2 days ago, primarily because of mild degree of shortness of breath. The patient has had a long-standing history of alcohol abuse in the past and continues to abuse alcohol on a regular basis.

On admission, he was started on diuretic medications in the form of Bumex for what I suppose is pulmonary congestion/fluid overload, questionable. The patient was likewise empirically started on Levaquin for a questionable pneumonia.

In the past 24 hours, the patient has been stable; however, he has had some episodes of hypotension earlier today. This evening, he once again had an episode of hypotension, with the systolic blood pressure running in the 60s to 70s range. He was likewise noted to be somewhat obtunded. On further review of the patient's medical records, the patient continues to receive Bumex and lisinopril as well as Ativan on a continuous basis, and I think this can probably account for the patient's hypotension. With regard to the alleged pneumonia, I do not think based on my clinical examination that the patient is actually septic. Nevertheless, the patient is already empirically started on Levaquin, which was later changed to moxifloxacin/Avelox.

At this time, with the patient's hypotension, the plan is to admit the patient to the medical ICU (intensive care unit) with cultures to be drawn, namely, blood culture times two, urinalysis, urine culture, sputum culture, and Gram stain. We will check a CBC (complete blood count) with manual differential count, basic metabolic panel, phosphorus, magnesium, and albumin.

A blood gas was performed this evening, which showed the following results: 7.442/40.4/56.6/27/98.6% on 2 liters O_2 (oxygen) nasal cannula.

I will also change the patient's IV (intravenous) fluids to D5 (dextrose 5% water) half normal saline with incorporations of multivitamins 1 ampule, thiamine 100 mg (milligram), and folic acid 1 mg on a daily

basis followed by a maintenance fluid of D5 normal saline infusing at a rate of 65 ml (milliliter)/hour. The reason why we are going to start off with a low intravenous fluid rate is primarily because the patient may have some degree of congestive heart failure and is the reason why he was receiving Bumex earlier on. If he has any bouts of hypotension in the next few hours, plan would be either to increase IV fluids rate or change them to 0.9% normal saline/isotonic solution and/or start the patient on dopamine infusion. At this point, these measures do not seem to be necessary; hence we are going to hold off on them.

I still believe that a significant contribution to this patient's hypotensive episode is that of the combination of medications, namely Bumex, lisinopril, and Ativan.

The patient has a past medical history and past surgical history that consists of the following:

1. Alcoholic cardiomyopathy, congestive heart failure, history of atrial fibrillation, status postatrial fibrillation.
2. Pulmonary hypertension/chronic obstructive pulmonary disease.
3. Alcohol abuse.
4. Hypertension.
5. Chronic renal insufficiency, questionable, probably related to long-standing cardiac history as well as hypertension.
6. Depression.

He continues to drink alcohol on a regular basis. He claims to have not drunk any alcohol in the 4 days before admission. He denies any use of tobacco or intravenous or recreational drugs.

FAMILY HISTORY: Negative for heart disease, hypertension, diabetes, stroke, cancer, kidney disease, bleeding disorder, or dyscrasia.

Although the patient denies significant history of tobacco, according to medical records, he has a history of smoking a cigar on a daily basis.

MEDICATIONS:

1. Aspirin.
2. Lisinopril 40 q.d. (every day).
3. Atrovent and albuterol metered dose inhaler.
4. Bumex.
5. Protonix.

I think the patient was on Lasix at home, but when he was admitted this was changed to Bumex.

CASE 1-15—cont'd

Past laboratory tests on this patient are as follows: Sodium 132, potassium 4.4, chloride 94, CO_2 (carbon dioxide) 32.9, BUN (blood urea nitrogen) and creatinine 75/1.2, glucose 94, and calcium 8. Hemogram shows an H&H (hematocrit and hemoglobin) of 12.1/36.5, WBC (white blood count) 5.82, normochromic/normocytic indices, and platelets 88. There is a slight left shift of neutrophils measured at 78.2%.

Latest blood gases are as noted above.

REVIEW OF SYSTEMS: (Primarily based on patient's medical records as the patient is quite confused and disoriented at this time): Constitutional: No fever or chills. No recent weight change. He appears to be fairly disheveled. No night sweats. Skin: No skin lesions. No active dermatosis. Eyes: No eye discharge. No eye itching. No visual changes. No diplopia. ENT: No ear discharge. No hearing difficulty. No pharyngeal hyperemia, congestion, or exudates. Lymph nodes: No lymphadenopathy in the neck, axillae, or groin. Neurologic: No headaches. Positive gait instability. No falls. No seizures. Psychiatric: No behavioral changes. Neck: No thyromegaly. Respiratory: Positive cough. No colds. No hemoptysis. Positive shortness of breath. Cardiovascular: No chest pain, questionable palpitations. No orthopnea. No paroxysmal nocturnal dyspnea. Gastrointestinal: Positive anorexia. Positive nausea. No vomiting. No dysphagia. No odynophagia. No constipation. No diarrhea. No abdominal pain or fecal incontinence. No hematemesis, hematochezia, or melena. Genitourinary: No urgency, frequency, dysuria, or hematuria. No urinary incontinence. No nocturia. No penile discharge. No penile lesions. Musculoskeletal: Positive joint pains. Positive muscle pains/weaknesses. Hematologic: No bleeding tendencies. No purpura. No petechiae. No ecchymosis. Endocrinologic: No heat or cold intolerance.

PHYSICAL EXAMINATION: Vital signs are stable. Blood pressure 120s/70s. Heart rate is in the 70s. Respirations 20s. He is afebrile. Since the patient was brought to the medical ICU, his blood pressure has been in the 120s to 130s systolic. Normocephalic and atraumatic. Pink palpebral conjunctivae. Anicteric sclerae. No nasal or aural discharge. Somewhat dry tongue and buccal mucosa. Supple neck. No lymphadenopathy. No obvious JVD (jugular vein distention). Symmetrical chest expansion. No retractions. Positive rhonchi. A few basilar crackles. No wheezes. S1 (first heart sound) and S2 (second heart sound) are distinct. No S3 (third heart sound) or S4 (fourth heart sound). A 3/6 systolic murmur heard throughout the precordium.

Abdomen: Positive bowel sounds; soft and nontender. No abdominal bruits. Morbidly obese. Both upper and lower extremities reveal arthritic changes. Positive edema on both lower extremities. Positive retrosacral edema. Pulses are fair.

ASSESSMENT/PLAN:

1. Alcoholic cardiomyopathy.
2. Congestive heart failure.
3. Pulmonary hypertension.
4. Chronic renal insufficiency.

At this time, the plan is as dictated above. Admit to medical ICU. Hold lisinopril and Bumex until further orders. Monitor daily weights, inputs, and outputs. Follow-up plan cultures. Continue empiric antibiotic coverage.

I am also going to check for cardiac enzymes primarily to rule out the possibility of an acute myocardial infarction, which may have had some temporal relation with the hypotensive episode.

If the patient remains stable and all the labs are satisfactory, the patient could probably be transferred to the medical floor for subsequent management by primary service/family practice teaching service.

Code-level issues have apparently been addressed by the primary physician with the patient's relatives and the patient, and this patient is currently code level I. I would also recommend that long-term plans be made for this patient. Apparently this patient lives alone, but the way things are going, I think he is probably better off living in an assisted-living situation, such as a nursing home or the like.

Would also consider the possibility of rehabilitation medicine, physical therapy/occupational therapy following up on this patient's care.

Tomorrow, we are also going to check for the patient's CBC (complete blood count) and manual differential, basic metabolic panel, and chest x-ray. We may also need to check blood gases if he continues to show signs of respiratory compromise.

As noted above, I have recommended holding off the diuretics because I think this is significantly contributing to the patient's intravascular volume depletion/hypotension.

I have spent a total of 90 minutes evaluating and reviewing this patient's medical records. Again, this is a critical care consultation note.

SERVICE CODE(S): _____

ICD-10-CM DX CODE(S): _____

Discussion

This is a long and complicated report that must be carefully read. The physician who prepared this report did two things that assist the coder in accurate coding: He listed the complete diagnoses in the Assessment/Plan section of the report, and he indicated the time for his critical care services. If all physicians were this careful in their documentation, it would greatly help the coders.

Cardiomyopathy

This patient has alcoholic cardiomyopathy, which is thought to be brought on by the toxic effect of alcohol, nutritional deficiencies, and the toxic effect of the additives in alcohol (such as cobalt).

Cardiomyopathy affects the myocardium and is categorized as dilated, hypertropic, restrictive, or obliterative, depending on the effects. Alcoholic cardiomyopathy is a dilated type that is characterized by ventricular dilation and impaired systolic function. This means the heart does not contract sufficiently and therefore does not eject blood with the force it should.

Congestive Heart Failure

Congestive heart failure is a condition in which the heart is unable to generate adequate output. When the heart has lost its ability to pump effectively, blood may back up into other organs, such as the

Continued

CASE 1-15—*cont'd*

liver or lungs. When the organs do not get a sufficient blood supply, they can be damaged and lose their ability to function properly. In the Index of the ICD-10-CM, one way to locate the code is under the entry "Failure, heart, congestive." You are then directed to the Tabular to read the full description and all notes regarding the code.

Pulmonary Hypertension

Pulmonary hypertension occurs when the blood pressure in the arteries of the lungs is too high. The arteries narrow, which increases the resistance to blood flow. This makes the heart work harder to pump, and eventually the right side of the heart becomes enlarged for the additional workload. There is no known cure, only treatment of the symptoms, such as shortness of breath. Pulmonary hypertension is also known as primary pulmonary hypertension, idiopathic (unknown cause) pulmonary arteriosclerosis, and essential pulmonary hypertension.

Chronic Renal Insufficiency

Chronic renal insufficiency is a progressive condition in which the renal tissue is destroyed through sclerosis and loss of nephrons over time **(Figure 1-6).** The designation as chronic renal insufficiency is assessed by the glomerular filtration rate (GFR) that progressively decreases with the loss of nephrons. **Chronic renal failure** is the term used for patients whose GFR is less than 30 cc/min. **Chronic renal insufficiency** is the preferred term for patients with mild-to-moderate renal impairment, those whose GFR is at 30–70 cc/min. **End-stage renal disease** (ESRD), is often associated with uremia and is the term used for patients whose GFR has declined to levels of less than 10 cc/min.

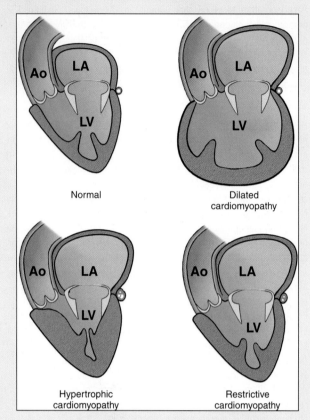

FIGURE 1–6 Cardiomyopathy.

(Answers to every other Case are located in Appendix D . The full answer key is only available in the TEACH Instructor Resources on Evolve.)

CASE 1-16A   *Critical Care*

The services in 1-16A, B, and C were all provided on the same day. You will report services for Dr. Orbitz based on all three reports within this case.

Report Dr. Orbitz's service.

LOCATION: Inpatient, Hospital

PATIENT: Ann Danube

ATTENDING PHYSICIAN: George Orbitz, MD

The emergency room physician called me in primarily because this patient was transferred from Anytown after being noted to have gone into a cardiopulmonary arrest. I was informed that advanced cardiac support measures were rendered, and the patient was revived; hence, the patient was transferred here.

The patient is a 56-year-old white woman who is well known to me because she is one of my chronic renal failure patients whom I had last

seen last year. The patient apparently had a recent episode of congestive heart failure/fluid overload, during which time the patient was noted to have severe mitral valve disease. The patient was then subjected to a mitral valve replacement surgery per cardiothoracic surgery.

The patient was discharged improved 90 days ago. According to the patient's daughters, she was not doing well; she had significant limitation in her activities because she would easily get short of breath since the time of discharge. Furthermore, they noticed she has been having significant fluid retention/worsening edema since that time. On the day of admission, the patient was noted to have gone into a state of cardiopulmonary arrest and was subjected to ACLS (Advanced Cardiac Life Support) measures by EMS team, and the patient was brought into the emergency room, already intubated and Ambu-bagged.

During my evaluation, the patient was subjected to a transthoracic echocardiogram, which confirmed the presence of some fluid in the pericardium but was not consistent with that of a pericardial tamponade.

CASE 1-16A—cont'd

This issue was actually discussed by the echocardiogram technician and Dr. Monson as well as Dr. Sutton. Furthermore, Dr. Monson's opinion was also obtained by the ED (emergency department) physician.

At this time, the patient appears to be hemodynamically stable, and she is intubated and mechanically ventilated. My plan right now is to admit her to medical ICU (intensive care unit) and stabilize her. We will work her up for a rule-out myocardial infarction. Her blood pressure right now is stable at 110 to 120 systolic. I have also discussed the issue of putting her on heparin with Dr. Elhart of cardiology, and he agreed.

The patient has a past medical history and past surgical history that consists of the following:

1. Coronary artery disease, congestive heart failure, bilateral pleural effusions with severe mitral regurgitation/stenosis, status post mitral valve replacement, aortic insufficiency, and hypertension.
2. Chronic renal insufficiency—latest creatinine clearance is 93 ml (milliliter)/min. with a creatinine of 0.8, total volume of 2550 ml with undetermined proteinuria performed, most likely secondary to the following:
   a. Hypertension.
   b. Type 2 diabetes.
   c. History of bilateral renal artery stenosis, status post bilateral stent placements in April.
   d. Coronary artery disease. See note above.
3. Chronic obstructive pulmonary disease/pulmonary hypertension/? cor pulmonale.
4. Anxiety/depression.
5. Hyperlipidemia.
6. Degenerative joint disease.
7. Peptic ulcer disease.
8. Status post previous cataract surgery (questionable retinopathy).
9. Status post previous finger amputation (questionable related to diabetic vascular neuropathies).

SOCIAL HISTORY: The patient smoked one to two packs of cigarettes per day for at least 40 to 50 years. She occasionally drank alcohol but denies any current use of tobacco, alcohol, intravenous or recreational drugs.

FAMILY HISTORY: Positive for diabetes and heart disease. Negative history for stroke, cancer, kidney disease, bleeding disorder, or dyscrasia. Her mother died at age 76 because of diabetes complications. Her father died at age 65 because of cardiac complications.

ALLERGIES: She has no known drug allergies.

CURRENT MEDICATIONS:

1. Albuterol metered dose inhaler 2 puffs b.i.d. (twice a day).
2. Combivent metered dose inhaler 2 puffs q.i.d. (four times a day).
3. Bumex 1 mg (milligram) b.i.d.
4. Calcium carbonate 650 mg 1 tablet q.d. (every day).
5. Diltiazem CD 180 mg b.i.d.
6. Sodium docusate 100 mg b.i.d.
7. Amitriptyline 10 mg at bedtime.
8. Lorazepam 1 mg q.8h. (every 8 hours) p.r.n. (as needed) anxiety.
9. Propoxyphene 1–2 tablets q.3–4h. p.r.n.
10. Novolin NPH 15 units b.i.d.
11. Regular Novolin R as directed.
12. Lisinopril 10 mg q.d.
13. Metoprolol 25 b.i.d.
14. Coumadin 2 mg q.d.

REVIEW OF SYSTEMS: Unobtainable because the patient is intubated and mechanically ventilated.

EXAMINATION: Vital signs are stable. Blood pressure is 120s/60s. Heart rate is in the 70s. Respirations are 20s. Saturating 95%. Normocephalic and atraumatic. Pink palpebral conjunctivae. Anicteric sclerae. Intubated and mechanically ventilated. Symmetrical chest expansion. Positive rhonchi. Positive basilar crackles. No wheezes. S1 (first heart sound) and S2 (second heart sound) are distinct. No S3 (third heart sound) or S4 (fourth heart sound). Regular rate and rhythm. Positive history of pacemaker placement? Abdomen is obese. Positive bowel sounds. Soft and nontender. No abdominal bruits appreciated at this time. Both upper and lower extremities reveal arthritic changes. Positive edema on both lower extremities. Positive retrosacral edema. Pulses are fair.

ASSESSMENT/PLAN:

1. Status post cardiopulmonary arrest. Rule out myocardial infarction. Admit to medical ICU. Mechanical ventilation as ordered. Heparin as ordered. Cardiology consultation by Dr. Elhart. Cardiothoracic consultation by Dr. Barton. Check chemistries, CBC (complete blood count), PT (prothrombin time), INR (International Normalized Ration), 12-lead ECG (electrocardiogram), chest x-ray, and cardiac enzymes q.8h. times three. Monitor I's (inputs) and O's (outputs), daily weights. NGT (nasogastric tube). Foley catheter. Aspirin 325 p.o. (by mouth) now and then q.d.
2. Respiratory failure, intubated and on ventilator. We will check the chest x-ray to see if this patient has any evidence of congestive heart failure/fluid overload, which may necessitate the use of intravenous diuretics for preload reduction.
3. Acute renal failure (latest creatinine clearance is 93 ml/min with a creatinine of 0.8, total volume 2,550 ml/min, and undetermined proteinuria previously performed), secondary to the following:
   a. Hypertension, fairly controlled. Hold blood pressure medications right now because her blood pressure is tethering from 100 to 120 systolic range.
   b. Type 2 diabetes mellitus, fairly controlled. Novolin R sliding scale as ordered. Check blood sugars every 6 hours.
   c. History of bilateral renal artery stenosis, status post bilateral renal artery stent placement.
   d. Coronary artery disease. See note above.
4. Chronic obstructive pulmonary disease/pulmonary hypertension/? cor pulmonale. Mechanical ventilation setup FiO₂ (forced inspiration oxygen) 100%, SIMV (synchronized intermittent mandatory ventilation) 14, tidal volume 500, PEEP (positive end expiratory pressure) of 5, and pressure support of 10. Dr. Dawson will follow up from the pulmonary/critical care standpoint starting tomorrow. Albuterol/Atrovent nebulization treatments q.4h. (every 4 hours) p.r.n. Check ABGs (arterial blood gases).
5. Anxiety disorder/depression.
6. Hyperlipidemia.
7. Degenerative joint disease.

Continued

CASE 1-16A—cont'd

LATEST LABORATORY TESTS PERFORMED AS FOLLOWS: Hemogram shows an H&H (hematocrit and hemoglobin) of 9.1/29.9, WBC (white blood count) 11.11, hyperchromic indices, and platelets of 283. There is a left shift of 93.4 neutrophils. Chemistries are as follows: Sodium 138, potassium 6.2, chloride 98, CO_2 (carbon dioxide) 22.2, BUN (blood urea nitrogen) and creatinine 41/1.6 (24/0.9 two months ago), glucose 213, and calcium 8.4. PT and INR are 14.6 and 1.5, respectively,

suggesting undercoagulation. The latest blood gases are as follows: 7.573/32.4/306.8/29.2, and this is while the patient is being Ambu-bagged. First set of cardiac enzymes are as follows: Troponin less than 0.04, CK-MB 5, and total CPK (creatine phosphokinase) of 72.

I have spent a total of 90 minutes evaluating and reviewing this patient's medical record and formulating the treatment strategy.

CASE 1-16B   *Progress Report-Same Day as Case 1-16A*

Report Dr. Orbitz's service.

LOCATION: Inpatient, Hospital

PATIENT: Ann Danube

ATTENDING PHYSICIAN: George Orbitz, MD

Review of the labs reveals several abnormalities, the most important of which is that of an acute renal failure, most likely superimposed on top of an underlying chronic renal insufficiency. Evidence of this is the acute rise in BUN (blood urea nitrogen) and creatinine, 41/1.6 (from 24/0.9), and accompanying hyperkalemia of 6.2. This is most likely explained by the recent cardiopulmonary arrest/decreased myocardial pump function, which leads to renal underperfusion and is manifested by azotemia.

At this time, I am going to order 30 g (gram) of Kayexalate to be given per nasogastric tube to decrease the patient's potassium. I am also going to order for around-the-clock albuterol nebulization treatments, which may help in shifting potassium levels in between cells.

One has to be very cautious in the overzealous use of diuretics in this patient as the patient may be pushed into a state of intravascular volume depletion, especially now that there is some semblance of prerenal state. The patient is also significantly anemic, and this has to be monitored closely.

We will continue to follow this patient from the critical care standpoint.

I have spent an additional 40 minutes re-evaluating and reassessing this patient's labs and making adjustments in the medications.

CASE 1-16C   *Progress Report-Same Day as Case 1-16A and 1-16B*

Report Dr. Orbitz's service.

LOCATION: Inpatient, Hospital

PATIENT: Ann Danube

ATTENDING PHYSICIAN: George Orbitz, MD

I am re-evaluating the patient for hypotension with systolic blood pressure in the 60s range.

At this time the plan is to:

1. Start her on dopamine 5 mg/kg (milligram/kilogram) per minute.
2. We are going to bolus her with 1 liter of normal saline now.
3. Withhold intravenous diuretic as ordered earlier.

I have also obtained the patient's latest blood gases as follows: 7.341/56.5/110.4/96.% on setting of FiO_2 (forced inspiration oxygen) of 50%, SIMV (synchronized intermittent mandatory ventilation) of 14, tidal volume of 500, PEEP (positive end expiratory pressure) of 5, and pressure support of 10.

PLAN:

1. Decreased SIMV to 12.
2. Decreased FiO_2 to 40%.

A few minutes since starting the dopamine and giving her around 250 ml (milliliter) of normal saline, the patient's blood pressure was noted to have recovered to 160–170 systolic. At this time, we are going to try to cut down on the dopamine to titrate MAP (mean arterial pressure) to greater than or equal to 60. I am also going to cut down on her normal saline infusion to 100 ml (milliliter)/hour. Again, for her

hyperkalemia, I have ordered 30 mg of Kayexalate p.o. (by mouth) as well as albuterol nebulization treatments q.2h × four.

At this time, I have spent another 45 minutes re-evaluating and reassessing the situation and formulating the above treatment plan. During this examination also, there was some concern brought about that she had some ecchymosis noted on her lower abdominal area. I spoke with the family concerning this particular problem, but they relay to me this has been there since her recent hospitalization when she had her mitral valve replacement surgery. Therefore, I think it is okay to start her on heparin anticoagulation at this time.

Another issue noted is that of some abdominal distention. I suspect the patient may have had a misintubation in the field such that there was some abdominal distention brought by the Ambu bagging of the gastrointestinal tract. Based on the patient's clinical situation right now and her latest blood gases as well as review of the patient's portable chest x-ray performed in the emergency room, I am pretty sure that the endotracheal tube is in the right place, that is, in the airway. I am also going to drop a nasogastric tube for decompression purposes. We will also use this for administration of the 30 g (gram) of Kayexalate.

The patient has had a 225 ml urine output from the emergency room. We will send a sample of this urine sodium and urine creatinine.

1-16A, 1-16B, 1-16C:

SERVICE CODE(S): _____

ICD-10-CM DX CODE(S): _____

CASE 1-16C—cont'd

Discussion

This is a very challenging set of reports, but they are the types of reports that you need to know how to code. Let's go through them one step at a time and analyze how these services and diagnoses are reported.

Critical Care Services

Read each report carefully with your attention on the diagnoses and indications of time spent in care of the patient, as these are all critical care reports. The three reports in 1-16 are considered together for reporting purposes because they are all critical care services provided on the same day. Do not complete an E/M audit form for critical care services, as it is assumed the patient is in a life-threatening situation with a high risk for death. The services provided involved a very high level of complexity to assess, manipulate, and support the patient's vital functions. This patient had multiple vital OS failure (heart, respiratory, kidneys). Time spent with the patient must be recorded in the critical care note. In this case, add together the time indicated on each report, and report the total time with critical care codes 99291 and 99292, based on the total time of 175 minutes.

Cardiac Arrest

The diagnoses reported for this critical care service (1-16A, B, and C) are considered together. When there are many diagnoses stated in the reports, it is difficult to identify which ones should be reported. Dr. Orbitz treated the patient last year. In the Assessment/Plan section of the report, Dr. Orbitz indicates in point 1 that the patient has experienced cardiac arrest (the heart stopped beating). The patient was mechanically resuscitated (as mentioned in paragraph 1 of 1-16A). When referencing the term "Arrest, cardiac" in the Index of the ICD-10-CM, the coder is referred to I46.9. Read the full description of the code in the Tabular.

Respiratory Failure

In 1-16A, point 2 indicates respiratory failure. The underlying reason for the failure has yet to be determined. If the underlying reason had been indicated to be, for example, the congestive heart failure, the respiratory failure would be considered a symptom of the diagnosis of congestive heart failure and would not be reported separately. In this case, however, the physician is considering multiple diagnoses that could be the cause of the respiratory failure, so the condition that is reported is acute respiratory failure NOS (not otherwise specified). Reference "Failure, respiration, respiratory, acute" in the Index of the ICD-10-CM, and review the code information in the Tabular to assign a code to this second diagnosis.

Chronic Renal Failure

In 1-16A, point 3 indicates acute renal failure. Previously, information regarding reporting renal failure was presented (after 1-7A). There is mention in paragraph 2 of 1-16A that this patient was "... well known to me because she is one of my chronic renal failure patients ..." Chronic renal failure is a permanent condition that worsens over time, which means that this patient currently has CRF and it is a diagnosis that must be reported. The physician should have stated that the patient had CRF in the Assessment/Plan section of the report. Remember to sequence the acute and chronic renal failure according to the *Official Guidelines for Coding and Reporting*.

Questionable Diagnosis

In 1-16A, point 4 indicates "Chronic obstructive pulmonary disease/ pulmonary hypertension/? cor pulmonale." Cor pulmonale is a chronic heart disease characterized by hypertrophy that is also known as chronic pulmonary heart disease (there is also an acute cor pulmonale). This condition is secondary to pulmonary hypertension caused by a disorder of the chest wall or lungs. The "?" before cor pulmonale indicates questionable diagnoses that the physician is considering at the time the report was dictated, and as such, are not reported in the outpatient setting. The COPD (chronic obstructive pulmonary disease) was treated and is therefore reported.

Diagnoses Not Reported

In 1-16A, points 5, 6, and 7, the physician indicates that the patient has anxiety disorder/depression, hyperlipidemia (excess fat in the blood), and degenerative joint disease; but at this time these conditions are not affecting care, nor were there treatments undertaken. These diagnoses are, therefore, not reported.

Hyperkalemia

In 1-16B, paragraph 1, the physician discusses the rise in some of the laboratory values. In an effort to decrease the level of potassium in the patient's blood serum, the physician orders Kayexalate, which is an antihyperkalemic medication. Because the physician diagnosed and treated the hyperkalemia, the diagnosis is reported. The physician reports that the patient is "significantly anemic," but since no treatment was undertaken, this diagnosis is not reported.

Hypotension

In 1-16C, the physician states that he is re-evaluating the patient for hypotension (low blood pressure) and is ordering medication and treatment for the condition, so the diagnosis is reported.

How was that for a complex case? You can see that if you analyze the case one line and one report at a time, you will arrive at a reason for the inclusion or exclusion of each diagnosis. This is a time-consuming process at the beginning, but it goes more quickly as you work through the various reports.

(Answers to every other Case are located in Appendix D . The full answer key is only available in the TEACH Instructor Resources on Evolve.)

CASE 1-17   *Critical Care Admission*

Report Dr. Dawson's service.

LOCATION: Inpatient, Hospital

PATIENT: Theodore Wilson

ATTENDING PHYSICIAN: Gregory Dawson, MD

The patient is being admitted primarily because of hypotension/respiratory failure.

The patient is a 75-year-old white man who is visiting from Texas. Today he had some strenuous exertion when he lifted heavy luggage on their way back to Texas; however, while at the airport, his wife noticed that he was having some diaphoresis and he did not feel well. This prompted him to be brought to the emergency room where he was noted to be in CHF (congestive heart failure)/fluid overload with chest x-rays. He was initially placed on BiPAP, but he continues to desaturate. Eventually, he was intubated and mechanically ventilated.

He was also given a dose of Lasix 80 mg (milligram) IV (intravenous) push and a p.o. (by mouth) dose of Lasix 60 mg. Accordingly, in the emergency room, his blood pressure has been in the 120s to 140s systolic; however, as soon as he hit the medical ICU (intensive care unit), his blood pressure was noted to start trending down, as it was in the 60s/40s. At this time, I have recommended starting the patient on dopamine drip, discontinued the nitroglycerin drip, and discontinued normal saline infusion. The patient's blood pressure started to improve to MAP (mean arterial pressure) of 60s to 70s.

I had a lengthy discussion with the patient's wife regarding the rest of his history. See note below. I have also consulted Dr. Elhart in cardiology for his expertise.

The patient has a past medical history and past surgical history that consists of the following:

1. Coronary artery disease, status post five-vessel CABG (coronary artery bypass graft); multiple stent/plasties in the past with most recent myocardial infarction requiring two stent placements.
2. Hypertension.
3. Type 2 diabetes (he was on Glucophage, but this was discontinued as his blood sugars were fairly controlled in the 110–120 range).
4. Degenerative joint disease.

MEDICATIONS:

1. Toprol 50 b.i.d. (twice a day).
2. Aspirin.
3. Plavix 75 q.d. (every day).
4. Lasix 80 b.i.d.
5. Imdur 60 q.d.
6. Lotensin 40 b.i.d.
7. Potassium chloride 20 mEq (milliequivalent).
8. Zocor 20 q.d.

SOCIAL HISTORY: He has not been using any tobacco or intravenous or recreational drugs currently. He used to smoke heavily in the past, one pack per day for at least 25+ years, but he is noted to have quit smoking for at least 25 years also. He drinks a couple of beers on a daily basis regularly.

FAMILY HISTORY: Positive for heart disease, hypertension, and stroke. Negative for kidney disease, cancer, bleeding disorder, or dyscrasia. Both parents died of heart disease complications.

REVIEW OF SYSTEMS: Unobtainable as the patient is intubated, mechanically ventilated, and sedated.

Latest LABS are as follows: Hemogram shows an H&H (hematocrit and hemoglobin) of 15.8/46, WBC (white blood count) 13.29, normochromic/normocytic indices. Platelets 196. There is no left shift as neutrophils are only 70.9%. Sodium 136, potassium 3.7, chloride 100, CO_2 (carbon dioxide) 25.7, BUN (blood urea nitrogen) and creatinine 38/2.2, glucose 287, calcium is 8, and magnesium is 1.9.

The latest blood gases prior to intubation are 7.116/61.1/53.9/19.2/71.3% on 100% nonrebreather.

PHYSICAL EXAMINATION: Vital signs are stable. Blood pressure is 101/40s, MAP in the 70s, respirations 20s. He is afebrile. Heart rate in the 50s. He has a pacemaker also. Normocephalic, atraumatic. Pink palpebral conjunctivae, anicteric sclerae. Intubated and mechanically ventilated. Supple neck. No lymphadenopathy. Symmetrical chest expansion. Positive rhonchi, positive crackles. No wheezes. S1 (first heart sound) and S2 (second heart sound) are noted. Positive pacemaker. No rubs appreciated. Abdomen: Positive bowel sounds. Soft, nontender. No abdominal bruits. Both upper and lower extremities reveal arthritic changes. Pulses are fair.

ASSESSMENT/PLAN:

1. Rule out myocardial infarction. Check cardiac enzymes. Cardiology consult. Check 12-lead ECG (electrocardiogram).
2. Congestive heart failure, fluid overload/pulmonary edema secondary to #1. Follow-up daily chest x-rays.
3. Acute renal failure, most likely superimposed on top of underlying chronic renal failure secondary to the following:
   A. Congestive heart failure/overload.
   B. Hypertension.
   C. History of type 2 diabetes.
4. Check blood sugars q.6h. We will also check urine sodium and urine creatinine. I suspect this patient has some degree of prerenal failure brought about by decreased renal perfusion secondary to cardiac pump dysfunction. At this time, we are going to continue the dopamine drip as ordered. We are still awaiting input from Dr. Elhart from a cardiology standpoint.
5. Code level I per discussion with the patient's wife.
6. Will continue to follow this patient from the critical care standpoint.

I have spent a total of 120 minutes evaluating and reviewing this patient's medical record, from 9 AM to 11 AM.

SERVICE CODE(S): _____

ICD-10-CM DX CODE(S): _____

(Answers to every other Case are located in Appendix D . The full answer key is only available in the TEACH Instructor Resources on Evolve.)

Office and Other Outpatient Services

You will recall that a new patient is defined as one who has not seen the physician or another physician with the same specialty in the same group practice within the past 3 years. A physician must spend more time with a new patient—obtaining the history, conducting the examination, and considering the data—than with an established patient. Consider that the established patient is probably known to the physician and the person's medical records are available. For these reasons, the cost of a new-patient office visit is higher, so third-party payers reimburse the physician at a higher rate for new-patient services than for the same type of service when it is provided to an established patient. An established patient is one who has received professional services from the physician or another physician of the same specialty in the same group practice within the past 3 years. The medical record of the patient is available to the physician.

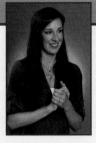

From the Trenches

"E/M coding can seem difficult and daunting, but if you look at it as trying to solve a puzzle, it makes it an exciting challenge instead of an impossible task. There are a number of resources that can help you gain the knowledge you need. Stay on top of the information out there, use the audit form (it's on Evolve!) and build your skills with practice."

JENNA PRICE
CPC

CASE 1-18 *Office Visit*

Report Dr. Naraquist's services for this case.

LOCATION: Outpatient, Clinic

PATIENT: Susan Oyez

PRIMARY CARE PHYSICIAN: Alma Naraquist, MD

CHIEF COMPLAINT: Dizziness.

SUBJECTIVE: This established patient is a 32-year-old female who reports she was feeling well until yesterday, when she developed some dizziness, which has persisted. She also feels like pills and food have been "sticking" in her throat. She is concerned that she may have a thyroid problem. She has a history of hypothyroidism for which she is on Synthroid 0.125 mg (milligram) q.d. (every day). Her last TSH (thyroid stimulating hormone) level was done in March and at that time was normal at 0.57.

OBJECTIVE: White female who appears to be in general good health. Her blood pressure is 118/82, respiratory 20s, afebrile. HEENT (head, ears, eyes, nose, throat) is unremarkable. Neck is supple. No masses. No palpable thyromegaly, nodules, or tenderness. TSH (thyroid stimulating hormone) level is elevated at 11.77.

ASSESSMENT: Hypothyroidism.

PLAN: We will increase Synthroid to 0.15 mg q.d. Recommend follow-up TSH level in 3 months.

SERVICE CODE(S): _____

ICD-10-CM DX CODE(S): _____

(Answers to every other Case are located in Appendix D . The full answer key is only available in the TEACH Instructor Resources on Evolve.)

CASE 1-19A *Office Visit*

LOCATION: Outpatient, Clinic

PATIENT: Sally Lin

PRIMARY CARE PHYSICIAN: Alma Naraquist, MD

This new patient is a 2½-year-old child seen today because of swelling on the right side of the neck. Nothing the mother has tried has reduced the swelling. It is the first time the patient has been seen here at the clinic. Mother has noticed this lump in her neck for the last week. She has had a little bit of an upper respiratory infection. They also have a dog at home, which the patient plays with infrequently.

PAST MEDICAL HISTORY: Pregnancy was complicated by gestational diabetes. It was a term, normal spontaneous vaginal delivery birth. No problems with jaundice. The patient has been developing normally. She sat at 6 months. Walked a little before a year. Past history is complicated by a recurrent otitis. The patient had PE (pressure equalization) tubes placed at 11 months of age.

Continued

CASE 1-19A—cont'd

ALLERGIC to SULFA–developed a rash. Currently, no medications.

Immunizations are up-to-date.

FAMILY HISTORY: Mother is 32. Dad is 35. Mother is 5 feet 5 inches, and father is 6 feet 2 inches. Both in good health. They have a 5-year-old daughter, a 1-year-old son, and the patient, who is 2½ years old. There is a family history of lung disease and also diabetes. Otherwise negative for renal, cystic fibrosis, asthma, Crohn's, ulcerative colitis, or childhood deaths.

REVIEW OF SYSTEMS: HEENT (head, ears, eyes, nose, throat) is otherwise negative other than the recurrent otitis. Lungs: Negative. Heart: Negative. GI (gastrointestinal): Negative. Neurologic: Negative.

PHYSICAL EXAMINATION: Happy, alert 2½-year-old child in no acute distress. Afebrile. Weight is 23 pounds. Length is 33¾ inches. Both at just below the 5th percentile. Mother states this is where she has been tracking for the last year and a half or so. HEENT: Head, nontraumatic. TMs (tympanic membrane): Both tubes are out, but they are clear. Pupils are equal and reactive to light and accommodation.

Extraocular movements are intact. Nose with some mild congestion. Throat mildly erythematous. Neck supple, with some shotty anterior cervical adenopathy. On the left side, there is a lymph node of about 0.8 mm (millimeter). No erythema. Easily movable. No supraclavicular nodes. No axillary nodes are felt. Lungs are clear. Cardiovascular: Regular rate and rhythm. Intermittent vibratory 1/6 murmur, left sternal border. Abdomen: Bowel sounds are positive. No hepatosplenomegaly. No masses. Nontender. GUR: Normal Tanner I female. Spine is straight. Neurologically intact.

IMPRESSION: Lymphadenopathy, secondary to URI (upper respiratory infection).

PLAN: Will go ahead and screen her with a CBC (complete blood count) and diff. We will also do a throat culture. Will begin Augmentin 125/5, 1 teaspoon p.o. (by mouth) t.i.d. (three times a day) for 10 days. Recheck in 2 weeks.

SERVICE CODE(S): _____

ICD-10-CM DX CODE(S): _____

CASE 1-19B   *Office Visit*

LOCATION: Outpatient, Clinic

PATIENT: Sally Lin

PRIMARY CARE PHYSICIAN: Alma Naraquist, MD

The patient comes in for a 2-week follow-up visit for lymphadenitis, which was treated with Augmentin. Mother states that the lump that was on the right side of her neck is still there; however, it is not sore, and she will allow them to check it with no problems. She did get some diarrhea with the antibiotic. She has not had any cold symptoms with congestion since finishing her antibiotics. The mother states that the patient has returned to herself being playful and eating well and being more interactive.

PHYSICAL EXAMINATION: HEENT (head, ears, eyes, nose, throat): TMs (tympanic membranes) have good landmarks and are pearly gray bilaterally. Sinus mucosa is pink and moist. Pharynx is unremarkable. There is some shotty lymphadenopathy on the left side of the neck. There

is a small, 0.5-cm (centimeter) enlarged lymph node underneath the right mandible. There is also a small, approximately 0.5-cm lymph node on the right side of the neck. Chest is clear to auscultation bilaterally. The heart has a regular sinus rhythm without clicks, rubs, or murmurs. Abdomen is soft with no organomegaly or masses.

IMPRESSION: Resolving lymphadenitis.

PLAN: We will not put the patient on antibiotics at this time; however, we will have her return to the clinic in 1 month to make sure the lymph node continues to get smaller. If there are any problems with high fever or increased cough or other health problems before the 1-month time, she is instructed to bring the patient in for evaluation. Total time spent with the patient today was 25 minutes.

SERVICE CODE(S): _____

ICD-10-CM DX CODE(S): _____

CASE 1-19C   *Clinic Progress Note*

LOCATION: Outpatient, Clinic

PATIENT: Sally Lin

PRIMARY CARE PHYSICIAN: Alma Naraquist, MD

HISTORY: This established patient came in with complaints of cold symptoms for the past couple of days. She had a couple of episodes of emesis this morning; however, nothing for the past 6 hours now. She has drunk fluids and eaten a little bit since then without difficulty. She has had a little bit of a low-grade temperature and occasional cough. She has also complained intermittently of a sore throat. No diarrhea. She is otherwise healthy, and her immunizations are up-to-date, according to Mom.

EXAMINATION: She is alert and in no distress. She is afebrile. Eyes are clear. Tympanic membranes are clear with good landmarks. Nose reveals some crusting to the nares. Mucous membranes are moist, and her pharynx shows some mild erythema but no exudate. Neck is supple

without significant lymphadenopathy. Lungs are clear to auscultation. Heart has a regular rate and rhythm without murmur. GI (gastrointestinal) is benign.

IMPRESSION: Upper respiratory infection with a little bit of pharyngitis.

PLAN: Symptomatic care is discussed. The possibility of this evolving into more of a gastroenteritis picture was discussed. If she starts vomiting more, they should place her on clear liquids and avoid dairy products. Push fluids, small amounts frequently. We will go ahead and get a throat culture, and if it comes back positive, we will start her on antibiotics. Otherwise, continue symptomatic care. They should return if her condition worsens or if they have other concerns. Total time spent with the patient today was 20 minutes.

SERVICE CODE(S): _____

ICD-10-CM DX CODE(S): _____

Hospital Observation Services

As of January 1, 2023, the codes in the Hospital Observation subsection are included with the Inpatient codes (99221-99239).

Observation Care Services

The Observation Care Discharge Services code includes the final examination of the patient on discharge from observation status. Discussion of the hospital stay, instructions for continued care, and preparation of discharge records are also bundled into the Observation Care Discharge Services code. The code is assigned only to patients who are discharged on a day that follows the first day of observation.

Initial and Subsequent Observation Care

Initial Observation Care codes (99221-99223) are assigned to designate the beginning of observation status in a hospital. The hospital does not need to have a formal observation area because the designation of observation status is dependent on the severity of illness of the patient. The codes also include development of a care plan for the patient and periodic reassessment while on observation status. Observation admission can be reported only for the first day of the service. If the patient is admitted and discharged on the same day, a code from the range 99234-99236, Observation or Inpatient Care Services, is used to report the service. If the patient is in the hospital overnight but remains there for a period that is less than 48 hours, the first day's service is reported with a code from 99221-99223. If the patient is on observation status for longer than 48 hours, the first day is reported with 99221-99223, Initial Observation Care; the subsequent day(s) is reported with 99231-99233, Subsequent Observation Care; and the discharge day is reported with 99238-99239.

Observation Care Discharge Services

Services performed in sites other than the observation area (e.g., clinic, nursing home, emergency department) and that precede admission to observation status are bundled into the Initial Observation Care codes and are not reported separately.

For example, an established patient was seen in the physician's office for frequent fainting of unknown origin. The MDM complexity was high. The code for the office visit is 99215, but the physician decided to admit the patient immediately on observation status until a further determination could be made as to the origin of the fainting. You would choose a code from the Hospital Observation Services subsection, Initial Observation Care subheading, in order to report the physician's service of admission on observation status (99222) and would not separately report the office visit.

CASE 1-20　*Observation*

Report Dr. Naraquist's service.

LOCATION: Hospital Observation Unit

PATIENT: Missy Lunde

ATTENDING PHYSICIAN: Alma Naraquist, MD

REASON FOR ADMISSION: Acute diarrhea and volume depletion.

HISTORY OF PRESENT ILLNESS: The patient is a 52-year-old white female who is known to have chronic renal failure, presumed to be related to lupus nephritis, who was vacationing in Jamaica and came back last night. She went out and had dinner at Mable's Castle here in town. Since 8:00 PM last night, she has been having diarrhea at least four times an hour. Her diarrhea increased until 6:00 in the morning. I received a call from her husband in the early morning, and I advised them to come to the emergency room. She was thought to be dehydrated in the ED (emergency department) and was admitted.

Her diarrhea is mostly loose. It does not seem to be explosive; minimal mucus, and no blood. It is associated with some cramping, especially after she passes a bowel movement. She denies any fever or chills. She has no night sweats. This seems all to be acute and she did not have any problems with diarrhea before.

She has no heartburn, nausea, or vomiting.

She has seen a physician in Jamaica, who added to her medications, Mavik 4 mg (milligram) q.d. (every day) and Catapres to treat her uncontrolled hypertension.

The patient seemed frustrated with her care because she is taking five medications for high blood pressure and she has been compliant with diet, but her blood pressure does not seem to be controlled.

PAST MEDICAL HISTORY: Significant for the following:

1. Systemic lupus erythematosus, which seems to be inactive.
2. Chronic renal failure requiring dialysis for a few weeks and then recovery of her renal function documented with a creatinine clearance of 23 ml (milliliter)/min with a serum creatinine of 2.9 and urine creatinine of 76 mg/dl (milligram/deciliter) last month. She continues to have a right IJ (internal jugular) tunneled dialysis catheter, but she has not been on dialysis for 3 weeks. The patient has been feeling good about that. She has been seen at the Jamaican Clinic and was started on CellCept 1 g (gram) b.i.d. (twice a day).
3. Also, the patient had a kidney biopsy done here under CT (computerized tomography) guidance. Unfortunately, no glomeruli were noted. Most of the two pieces of tissue submitted contained medulla. The patient had proteinuria up to 6 g in 24 hours. This is at the time when she had her kidney biopsy. She had only one kidney biopsy,

Continued

and this has never been followed up. We do not have any diagnosis, unfortunately, at this time, and she has been treated empirically.

4. Uncontrolled hypertension with multiple medications and regimens back and forth for the past few months without any benefit. The patient still runs 160–180 systolic over 90–100 diastolic.
5. History of BOOP (*Bronchiolitis obliterans* organizing pneumonia) in the past, status post thoracotomy.
6. Restrictive lung disease.
7. Chronic dry cough.
8. Chronic dry mouth.
9. Chronic anemia of kidney disease and probably of chronic disease.
10. History of bilateral flank pain of unclear etiology while she was on dialysis. It has never been worked up.
11. Multiple compression fractures with osteoporosis.
12. Hyperlipidemia.

ALLERGIES: Amoxicillin.

CURRENT MEDICATIONS:

1. Prednisone 10 mg q.d.
2. CellCept 500 mg 2 b.i.d.
3. Cozaar 50 mg 2 b.i.d.
4. Epogen 15,000 subcutaneously twice a week.
5. Nephrocaps 1 q.d.
6. Renagel 1 t.i.d with meals.
7. Norvasc 10 mg q.d.
8. Metoprolol XL 100 mg b.i.d.
9. Catapres patch 0.1 mg 2 patches once a week.
10. Tylenol PM.
11. Lasix 40 mg b.i.d.
12. Protonix 40 mg 1 q.d.
13. Mavik 4 mg 1 q.d. for the past week.

SOCIAL HISTORY: The patient is a nonsmoker and nondrinker. She lives with her husband.

FAMILY HISTORY: She has 2 sisters and 1 brother, and most of them are hypertensive. Otherwise, her family history is noncontributory.

REVIEW OF SYSTEMS: General: No fever, chills, night sweats, or recent weight change. ENT: Dryness in her mouth and nose, which is chronic. Eyes: Status post cataract surgeries. Neurologic: No numbness, tingling, headaches, or fainting spells. Respiratory: Chronic cough, occasional sputum production. No orthopnea or PNDs (paroxysmal nocturnal dyspnea). Occasional leg edema. Cardiac: No chest pain, orthopnea, PNDs, leg edema, or claudication. GI (gastrointestinal): As mentioned in the HPI. GU (genitourinary): No frequency, urgency, hematuria, or nocturia. Skin: No recent rashes or itching. Endocrine: No diabetes or thyroid problems, but she has been on chronic steroid therapy.

PHYSICAL EXAMINATION: On examination, the patient is lying in bed. She looks dry. She is not in any distress. Blood pressure is 180s/90s. She is afebrile. Respiratory rate is 16 per minute. Saturations are maintained on room air in the mid-90s. She has no increased jugular venous pressure. She has right IJ tunnel dialysis catheter. No cervical lymphadenopathy other than dry mucous membranes. ENT (ears, nose, throat) is negative. Lungs: Good air entry bilaterally without crackles. No sacral edema. 1+ leg edema bilaterally. Abdomen is very soft and nontender. I cannot hear any renal bruits. Cardiac exam: Regular S1 (first heart sound) and S2 (second heart sound) without any murmurs

or friction rubs. Neurologic: The patient is awake, alert, and oriented. Cranial nerves II–XII seem to be intact. Motor power is 5/5 bilaterally with normal gait. Spine straight.

LABORATORY STUDIES: Sodium 144, potassium 4.5, chloride 117, bicarb 13.3, glucose 94, creatinine 2.3, calcium 8.3, and BUN (blood urea nitrogen) 46.

Hemoglobin is 9.5, white count 7.1 thousand, and platelets were 111,000.

Her last bicarb last month was 25.1. At that time her last platelet count was 188,000.

Urinalysis showed no white or red cells. Rare hyaline casts, pH (potential of hydrogen) of 6.0, protein more than 300, and specific gravity of 1.020.

Stool was negative for PMNs.

Abdominal x-rays were negative.

IMPRESSION:

1. Acute diarrhea, probably infectious in etiology, and so far she does not have any loose stools since she has been admitted.
2. I do not know what her renal function is like. I suppose that her kidney function will improve with hydration.
3. Metabolic acidosis secondary to diarrhea.
4. Chronic renal failure, related to lupus nephritis, but no tissue diagnosis unfortunately in this relatively young woman.
5. Very uncontrolled hypertension with multiple medications.

PLAN:

1. The patient was admitted for observation.
2. We will give her D5W, 3 amp of bicarb at 150 cc an hour for a total of 3 liters.
3. We will repeat her labs in the morning.
4. After she gets fluids, I will check aldosterone and renin levels in the morning.
5. I will obtain a renal ultrasound.
6. I will hold her Cozaar and Mavik at this time.
7. I will hold her furosemide.
8. I will hold her CellCept and Protonix at this time.
9. We will continue with metoprolol and Norvasc for blood pressure.
10. I will check a phosphorus level on her and repeat labs in the morning.
11. I will check and also recheck her platelets in the morning.

I had a long discussion with the patient. I spent 60 minutes out of 85 minutes with the patient and her husband counseling on her kidney disease and uncontrolled hypertension. We also discussed her acute problem with diarrhea. We have discussed the possibilities of secondary causes of hypertension. She has been on chronic steroid therapy, but renal stenosis has never been pursued. She has never had an ultrasound of her kidneys. We do not have even a tissue diagnosis on her renal failure. This is all unfortunate. The patient needs to be followed up more closely, and we need to try and evaluate for possible treatable causes of hypertension.

I will probably discharge the patient by tomorrow if she is feeling better and her diarrhea has resolved. I will schedule her to have an MRA (Magnetic Resonance Angiogram) next week. I would also schedule her to have a kidney biopsy by myself under real time ultrasound guidance.

The patient is a candidate for kidney transplant if her kidney function is going to deteriorate and stays in the mid-20s; however, we need to look at her tissue, look at her glomeruli and interstitium, and see whether there is any possibility for reversibility.

CASE 1-20—cont'd

All the above was discussed with the patient and her husband. They both seem to understand and agree with the above plan. I also have stressed to them that only one physician should follow her blood pressure and manage it.

Both the patient and her husband seem to be satisfied and agreeable with the above plan.

SERVICE CODE(S): _____

ICD-10-CM DX CODE(S): _____

Discussion

This report contained several diagnoses. In addition to the other codes, the following are two coding situations that you may not have encountered. Section I.C.9.a.2. of the ICD-10-CM *Guidelines* directs the coder to assign codes from category I12 (hypertensive chronic kidney disease) when both hypertension and a condition classifiable to category N18, Chronic kidney disease (CKD), are present. This means that if hypertension is present along with chronic kidney disease, you report a hypertensive chronic kidney disease code (I12). The diagnoses of chronic kidney disease and hypertension become the one diagnosis of hypertensive chronic kidney. The instructional notes under I12 category indicate to report the stage of kidney disease if known. Since the stage is unknown in this case, you would report the unspecified stage (N18.9).

Lupus Nephritis

In the Impression section of the report, the physician stated the CRF is related to lupus nephritis. Lupus nephritis is inflammation of the kidney caused by systemic lupus erythematosus (SLE), a disease of the immune system.

ICD-10-CM: When referencing "Lupus, nephritis" in the Index of the ICD-10-CM, the coder is directed to one code for both the etiology (cause) and the manifestation (symptom), M32.14.

(Answers to every other Case are located in Appendix D . The full answer key is only available in the TEACH Instructor Resources on Evolve.)

Neonatal Care Services

A neonate is a newborn infant who is 0 to 28 days old. There are numerous categories of E/M codes that can be used to report services to neonates. There are two groups of E/M codes that are specific to neonatal care services:

- Newborn Care Services (99460-99465) include codes to report initial services for normal newborns, subsequent evaluation and management of normal newborns, and attendance at delivery for other than normal newborns to provide stabilization and/or resuscitation.
- Inpatient Neonatal Intensive Care Services and Pediatric and Neonatal Critical Care Services (99466-99486) report direct services during transport of a critically ill, neonatal/pediatric patient, critical care in the hospital setting, and intensive care services.

Neonatal coding is a bit more complex than other E/M services because not only does the neonate have a separate set of critical and intensive care codes, but also separate history and examination codes (Newborn Care Services) when the service is provided in the hospital setting. In addition to using these codes to report neonate services, you must also use codes from throughout the CPT manual to accurately report the services provided to the neonate.

When coding neonatal services, the status of the newborn, the location in which the service was provided, and the type of service must first be considered.

The first consideration is the **status** of the newborn:

- Normal Newborn Services—The normal newborn services are to be reported using the Newborn Care codes (99460-99463).
- Resuscitation—The newborn resuscitation is reported with 99465.

- Critically Ill—Services for a critically ill neonate are reported with 99468/99469 or 99291-99292 depending on the place of service. See below for further explanation.
- Intensive Care—Services to a non-critical neonate who requires intensive care are reported with either 99477-99480 or subsequent hospital inpatient or observation visit codes 99231-99233. See below for further explanation.

The second consideration is the **location** of the service:

- If the location of normal newborn care initial service was in the **hospital** setting, you would report 99460 (history and examination of normal newborn infant, initiation of diagnostic and treatment programs, and preparation of hospital records) and service on a subsequent day with 99462 (Subsequent hospital care, for the evaluation and management of a normal newborn, per day).
- Critical Care Services to a neonate in the outpatient setting (i.e., ED) are reported with 99291-99292. If this same service was performed in the inpatient setting, 99468, 99469 would be reported.
- If the initial newborn service is provided in the office or other **outpatient** setting, the established patient codes 99202-99205 (New Patient, Office or Other Outpatient Service) are used to report the service as you would for any new patient.

The third consideration is the **type** of service:

- If the first service was an outpatient **preventive medicine service,** use 99381 to report an initial comprehensive preventive medicine service provided to an infant (under 1 year).

With these considerations in mind, let's take a closer look at the specifics of neonatal critical care, continuing intensive care services, and newborn care.

Neonatal Critical Care (NCC)

The name of the critical or intensive care unit does not matter in the application of inpatient NCC. The services can be provided in an intensive care unit, neonatal critical care unit, or any of the many names that these types of intensive care units have. What is important in the use of inpatient NCC codes is that the neonate:

■ is 28 days of age or younger
■ is critically ill

Services for a critically ill neonate (28 days of age or younger) are to be reported with 99468 and 99469 or Critical Care codes 99291 and 99292 depending on the location of the service. Inpatient NCC codes (99468/99469) are critical care codes for neonates who are inpatients. If the service is provided to a neonate in the outpatient department (i.e., emergency room), then 99291-99292 codes are reported (for more information, see the section regarding critical care coding). The medical record must contain documentation that indicates that the neonate is in an acute, life-threatening situation. If the patient is not in a life-threatening situation, you would not use these codes.

The codes from the inpatient NCC are reported only once in every 24-hour period (same day). There are no hourly service codes as there are in other critical care codes. If a critically ill infant 29 days through 24 months of age is admitted to an intensive care unit, the services would be reported using the Pediatric Critical Care Service codes 99471-99472, which are also reported per day.

Bundled into the NCC codes are many services you would anticipate would be reported in the support of a critically ill neonate, for example, umbilical arterial catheters, nasogastric tube placement, endotracheal intubation, and invasive electronic monitoring of vital signs. The extensive notes preceding the NCC codes list bundled services. As you code NCC services, you will need to refer back to the list of services and codes that are bundled into the codes in this subsection. If the physician performed a service not listed in the notes, you would report for the service separately. You must carefully read all notes, parenthetical information, and code descriptions to accurately assign these codes.

Initial and Continuing Intensive Care codes (99477-99480) report services when a low birth weight (present weight of 5000 grams or less) or neonate (28 days of age or younger) is not critically ill but needs intensive services. Codes 99478-99480 are divided by the patient's present weight.

Report Initial and Continuing Intensive Care Services codes based on:

■ 99477, 28 days or younger
■ 99478, very low birth weight (VLBW) less than 1500 grams (less than 3.3 pounds)
■ 99479, low birth weight (LBW), 1500-2500 grams (3.3- 5.5 pounds)
■ 99480, normal birth weight, 2501-5000 grams (5.51- 11.01 pounds)

Services to a non-critical neonate weighing more than 5000 grams that does not require intensive or critical care services are reported with the subsequent hospital inpatient or observation codes (99231-99233).

Newborn Care (NC)

Newborn Care Services codes 99460 through 99465 report services provided to normal newborns from birth through 28 days of age. There are three history and examination codes; one is specifically for a newborn assessment and discharge from a hospital or birthing center on the same date (99463), one is for initial assessment **in** a hospital or birthing center (99460), and one is for initial assessment **in other than** a hospital or birthing center (99461). All of the codes report a "per day" service, which is a 24-hour period. Subsequent services are reported with 99462, also a per day service. If the physician provides a discharge service to a newborn on a date that is subsequent to the admission date, assign a code from Hospital Discharge Services (99238, 99239).

The obstetrician cares for the mother during delivery. Sometimes the obstetrician may request a pediatrician to be in attendance during delivery to stabilize and provide immediate care to the neonate. The pediatrician would report this service with 99464 (Attendance at delivery). If the pediatrician needs to resuscitate the newborn by means of chest compression or positive pressure ventilation (PPV), the resuscitation service would be reported with 99465 (Newborn resuscitation). A parenthetical note following the code description for 99464 (Attendance at delivery) indicates that 99464 and 99465 (Newborn resuscitation) cannot be reported at the same time. Because you can report only one of the services—either the attendance at delivery or the resuscitation—you should report the resuscitation (99465) since the resuscitation code has a higher reimbursement than the attendance code (99464).

When an infant is born, a slimy substance (mucilaginous material, meconium) is present in the esophagus, stomach, and intestines of the infant. This substance is a mixture of secretions from the liver, intestines, and amniotic fluid. It may be necessary for the pediatrician to suction this material from the trachea by **endotracheal intubation**. The intubation service would be reported separately with a Respiratory System code 31500 (Intubation, endotracheal, emergency procedure). The pediatrician in attendance may also need to **catheterize the umbilical vein** for blood sampling or administration of medication, and this service is reported separately with 36510 (Catheterization of umbilical vein).

When reporting services with the Neonatal Critical Care codes, recall that there were many services bundled into the codes, and a list of the bundled services appears in the notes preceding the codes. With the Newborn Care codes, that is not the case. With the NC codes, the services the physician provides are reported separately, such as central catheters (36510), peripheral vessel catheterization (36000), lumbar puncture (62270, 62328), bladder aspiration (51100-51102), and so on. See the list of services that are bundled into the

NCC codes for further examples of services that are not bundled into the NC.

Newborn Diagnosis Coding

Reporting the Liveborn Infant

Category Z38 is assigned to report liveborn infants.

The codes identify single, twin, other multiple, or unspecified births. These codes are only assigned to the newborn record, not the mother's record. If the infant's medical record indicated other significant conditions, these conditions would be reported in addition to the Z38 code.

Disorders Relating to Short Gestation and Low Birth Weight

The gestation of a fetus takes approximately 266 days or 40 weeks. Category P07 is used to report short gestation and low birth weight, with further characters/digits assigned to indicate the newborn weight.

CASE 1-21   *Newborn Care*

The newborn in Case 1-21 was a liveborn, full-term delivered by the obstetrician by means of cesarean section. You will code the services of Dr. Ortez, the pediatrician, which will include the daily services (1-1 through 1-4, a procedure, and a discharge service) based on the information in the Progress Notes section of the form. The first day, 1/1, services are indicated on the check-off portion of the form.

LOCATION: Inpatient, Hospital

PATIENT: Anthony Marcello

ATTENDING PHYSICIAN: Roland Ortez, MD

See **Figure 1-7**.

SERVICE CODE(S): _____

ICD-10-CM DX CODE(S): _____

(Answers to every other Case are located in Appendix D . The full answer key is only available in the TEACH Instructor Resources on Evolve.)

	Normal	Abnormal	NEWBORN EXAM RECORD ADMISSION EXAM Date: 1/1	Normal	Abnormal	DISCHARGE EXAM Date: 1/5
Head/Fontanels		✓	1cm area between fontanels left of sagittal suture	✓		Head healing well
Eyes	✓		✓	✓		
Ears/Nose/Throat	✓		✓			
Heart	✓		✓			
Lungs	✓		✓			
Abdomen	✓		✓			
Trunk/Spine	✓		✓			
Anus	✓		✓			
Genitalia	✓		✓			
Negative Barlow Test	✓		✓			
Negative Ortolani Test	✓		✓			
Extremities/Clavicles	✓		✓			
Skin	✓		✓			
Neurological/Tone	✓		✓			

PROGRESS NOTES:

1/2 Exam on 1 x top of head, which is clean and dry. Color good. Wt down 2.5%. Nursing poorly. GJH	
1/3 Exam: head healing well. Color good. Nursing better. Wt down 6.8%. Circumcised with ring block per parent request. GJH	
1/4 Exam: wt down 8.9%. Nursing poorly. Color good. GJH	
1/5 Exam: wt down 9.2%. Nursing poorly. Discharge from the hospital and I will see on Monday in the office. GJH	
	Hearing Exam: Passed AZ

FIGURE 1-7 Newborn examination record.

CASE 1-22A   *Hospital Services*

Report Dr. Ortez's services for Case 1-22, which includes both the delivery and the NICU care.

LOCATION: Inpatient, Hospital, Delivery Room and Neonatal Intensive Care Unit

PATIENT: Robert Zimmerman

ATTENDING PHYSICIAN: Roland Ortez, MD

CHIEF COMPLAINT: Prematurity with respiratory difficulty.

HISTORY: This is a 30-week gestation male infant with a birth weight of 1808 g (gram). Mom is a 27-year-old gravida 2, now para 2 mom. Her blood type is B, antibody negative, RPR (rapid reagin plasma) nonreactive, rubella immune, hepatitis B surface antigen negative, HIV (human immunodeficiency virus) negative, GC (gonorrhea) negative, *Chlamydia* negative, group B strep status unknown. No neural tube defect. No amniocentesis performed. She was on prenatal vitamins.

First pregnancy went without complications. She is doing well at 3 years of age; however, she does have Noonan syndrome. Mom presented with

CASE 1-22A—cont'd

questionable rupture of membranes in preterm labor 4 weeks ago. It was found that her membranes were intact, and she continued throughout the rest of her pregnancy to have a high AFI (amniotic fluid index). Preterm labor was stopped with magnesium sulfate. Mom's magnesium level today is 7.5. She was also on penicillin G ½ 48 hours. She received two doses of betamethasone.

Mom was noted to have increased urinary frequency today, and labs were obtained, which showed elevation of her AST (aspartate aminotransferase [formerly SGOT]) and ALT (alanine transaminase [formerly SGPT]) into the 300s. Also, elevation of her bilirubin to 2.6 with concerns for her developing fatty liver of pregnancy. Her platelet count was 178,000 today and hemoglobin 11.6. Coagulation studies were normal on the mom. Because of concern for fatty liver of pregnancy, an emergent cesarean section was performed.

I did attend the delivery, and the infant was delivered at 2:01 PM today. Spontaneous cry noted and Apgar scores were 7 at 1 minute with points off for color, tone, and grimace. Then at 5 minutes, an Apgar score of 8 with points off for grimace and tone. The infant was brought back to the NICU (neonatal intensive care unit) for further management.

The infant's face does look somewhat dysmorphic with concerns of Noonan syndrome. A very small posterior pharyngeal space was noted with difficult intubation, and after several attempts, anesthesia was called and came up and intubated the infant. Throughout the intubation attempts, standard procedure was followed, and the infant tolerated the attempts very well. The intubation was performed because of concerns of hypoventilation noted on exam with decreased breath sounds bilaterally as well as increased work of breathing.

Umbilical artery catheter was also placed without difficulty. First blood sugar did come back at 23, and a peripheral IV (intravenous) was placed promptly and 2 cc (cubic centimeter)/ kilo of D10 was given along with placing the infant on D10 at 80 cc/kilo. Second blood sugar has come back elevated.

Chest x-ray is obtained as well as abdominal films and shows good placement of the UAC (umbilical artery catheter) at T7, and the endotracheal tube is also in good placement and is 3.02. The OG has been advanced. The lung fields do show significant granularity present. No pneumothorax. No cardiomegaly. Blood gas is 7.32, PCO_2 (partial pressure of carbon dioxide) of 50, PO_2 (partial pressure of oxygen) of 100, and that is on a setting of 22/4, rate of 60, and 80% FiO_2 (forced inspiration oxygen).

PHYSICAL EXAMINATION: Currently is intubated. His weight is 1808 g. His OFC is 30.5 cm (centimeter). Length is 39.4 cm. Heart rate is in the 130s to 140s. Respiratory rate is 60 on the ventilator. O_2 (oxygen)

saturation is in the mid 90s. Blood pressure in right arm 67/34 with a mean of 46 and right leg 67/32 with a mean of 44.

Mild splitting of the cranial sutures is noted along with open posterior and anterior fontanel. Red reflex times two. The eyes appear to have hypertelorism present and questionable epicanthal folds along with some down-slanting palpebral fissures. Ears appear to be low set and posteriorly rotated. Palate is intact. Small retropharyngeal space. Clavicles are intact. I do not appreciate any webbing on the neck. Nipples questionably mildly wide-spaced. Lungs at this time are clear to auscultation. He has good symmetric aeration, minimal chest rise noted. Prior to that, lungs were remarkable for decreased aeration with crackles. Heart is regular rate and rhythm; no murmurs noted. Femoral pulses palpable. Capillary refill less than 2 seconds. Abdomen without hepatosplenomegaly. Three-vessel cord. Genitourinary: Normal external male. Testes are not descended. Extremities: Adequate range of motion. No contractures or hip abnormalities noted. The skin is ruddy in complexion. Neurologic exam: Hypotonia diffusely.

Developmental assessment: No breast buds. Soft pinna with minimal recoil. No creases on the feet. No rugae on the testes. All consistent with a 30-week preterm infant.

IMPRESSION:

1. Premature male infant.
2. Respiratory distress consistent with hyaline membrane disease as well as a component of hypoventilation secondary to maternal elevated magnesium.
3. Observation for sepsis.
4. Maternal hypermagnesemia with elevated magnesium in the infant as well.

PLAN: Admission to the NICU. Intubation has been performed, and he is on mechanical ventilation. Will go ahead with the surfactant therapy per protocol. Close cardiorespiratory monitoring and monitoring of blood gases and chest x-rays. NPO (nothing by mouth) status, and he will be on D10 with 0.94 mEq (milliequivalent) of calcium gluconate added to run at 80 cc/kilo per day. Ampicillin and gentamicin per protocol. Blood cultures have been obtained as well as a CBC (complete blood count), magnesium level, and further glucose monitoring. He will also need chromosomal testing, and that will be drawn in the near future. Also head ultrasound at 6 days of life will need to be performed. I have not talked with the mother. Her condition has deteriorated post cesarean section and is not available at this time. I have talked in detail with the father in regard to the above, including the possibility of further deterioration, prompting transfer to another facility. All his questions were answered.

SERVICE CODE(S): _____

ICD-10-CM DX CODE(S): _____

Discussion

Hyaline Membrane Disease

The primary reason this service is being provided is that the newborn has hyaline membrane disease, which is a respiratory syndrome of a newborn. As such, this is the first-listed diagnosis.

Gestation and Birth Weight

This is a premature infant, so you will need to assign two codes, one for the gestation and one for the birth weight (refer back to the information before case 1-21A).

Continued

CASE 1-22A—cont'd

Observation

Note that in this report the physician indicated that the newborn was being placed on observation for sepsis. Sepsis is a condition in which pathogenic microorganisms and/or their toxins are in the blood. This status of "observation" would be reported with Z05.1 code to indicate observation for a suspected condition in a newborn (first 28 days of life) for an infectious disease not found if blood work indicates sepsis not found. No signs or symptoms were provided to indicate why sepsis was suspected.

Hypermagnesemia

In point 4 of the Impression section of this report, the physician indicated that the infant has hypermagnesemia, which is a high level of magnesium in the blood.

Outcome of Delivery

The Z code is reported on all newborn deliveries.

CASE 1-22B   *NICU Progress Report*

On a subsequent day, Dr. Ortez provided the following service.

LOCATION: Inpatient, Hospital, Neonatal Intensive Care Unit

PATIENT: Robert Zimmerman

ATTENDING PHYSICIAN: Roland Ortez, MD

SUBJECTIVE: Baby boy is slightly under 24 hours old.

OBJECTIVE: Weight today is 1.851 kg (kilogram) (increased 43 g [gram] over birth weight). OFC (occipitofrontal circumference) is 30.5 cm (centimeter) (unchanged). Intake and output from yesterday do appear adequate, although it is less than 24 hours. He has had no stool since birth. Vital signs reveal his temperature to be acceptable while being maintained on an open radiant warmer. Heart rate is generally in the 110s to 140s. Respiratory rate is generally equal to the IMV (intermittent mandatory ventilation). Mean blood pressures had decreased last night to the low 30s but are now in the low to mid-40s while on dopamine infusion.

PHYSICAL EXAMINATION: In general, he is pink on current ventilator settings. He does appear slightly dysmorphic with eyes wide set and slightly down-slanting palpebral fissures. Ears appear low-set and posteriorly rotated. Endotracheal tube is in place. Chest reveals symmetric expansion, and the lungs are clear to auscultation on current ventilator settings. Cardiac exam reveals a regular rate without murmur or click. Peripheral pulses are 2× and symmetric. Abdominal exam reveals an umbilical arterial catheter in place. Liver is palpable 1 cm below the right costal margin. No splenomegaly or masses are noted. Genital examination reveals normal male; testes are not palpable. Extremity examination reveals no fixed decreased range of motion, deformity, or joint abnormality. Neurologic exam reveals diffuse hypotonia. No focal deficits are appreciated.

CURRENT MEDICATIONS:

1. Ampicillin 90.4 mg (milligram) IV (intravenous) q.12h.
2. Gentamicin 5.4 mg IV q.18h.
3. Morphine sulfate 0.18 mg IV q.6h and q.1h. p.r.n. (as needed).
4. Dopamine 5 mcg/kg (microgram/kilogram) per minute.
5. Vecuronium 0.18 mg IV q.1-2h. p.r.n.

LABORATORY STUDIES: Last arterial blood gas was obtained on ventilator settings of IMV (intermittent mandatory ventilation) 60, pressure 22/4, and FiO_2 (forced inspiration oxygen) 0.53 and revealed pH (potential of hydrogen) 7.3, PCO_2 (partial pressure of carbon dioxide) 46.6, PO_2 52.7, and bicarbonate 22.7. Chemistry panel this AM revealed sodium 123, potassium 5.7, chloride 93, glucose 66, BUN (blood urea nitrogen) 12, creatinine 0.9, calcium 7.3, magnesium 5.4, phosphorus 6.8, bilirubin 4.4, alkaline phosphatase 200, ALT (alanine transaminase [formerly SGPT]) 14, AST (aspartate aminotransferase [formerly SGOT]) 38, albumin 1.7, and total protein 3.6. Electrolytes were repeated and were unchanged. CBC (complete blood count) with differential this AM revealed a white count of 8230 with 7 bands, 46 neutrophils, 33 lymphocytes, 8 monocytes, and 6 eosinophils. H&H (hematocrit and hemoglobin) was 20.7 and 61.8 with an MCV (mean corpuscular volume) of 113. Platelet count was 98,000. Chest x-ray continues to show significant evidence of hyaline membrane disease.

IMPRESSIONS/RECOMMENDATIONS:

1. Less than 24-hour-old infant who was born at 30 weeks' gestation. Based on clinical examination, he may have Noonan syndrome.
2. RESPIRATORY: He has evidence of hyaline membrane disease with respiratory distress. He has received two doses of surfactant and will receive a third dose soon. We will adjust his ventilator setting based on serial clinical examinations, pulse oximetry, arterial blood gas determinations, and chest x-rays. Will continue sedation and paralysis at this time. Would recommend a short course of steroids because of the intubation attempts when he is extubated.
3. CARDIOVASCULAR: Cardiovascular status is acceptable at this time while on dopamine 5 mcg/kg per minute. Blood pressure has improved on echocardiography to evaluated PDA (patent ductus arteriosus), depending on his clinical course.
4. GASTROINTESTINAL: Abdominal exam remains benign. He is NPO (nothing by mouth). He has mild hyperbilirubinemia, and Mom is noted to have O positive blood and Rh (rhesus factor). We are going to obtain a direct antibody test. Will follow with serial bilirubin determinations.
5. HEMATOLOGIC: He has developed a mild thrombocytopenia; will monitor.
6. INFECTIOUS DISEASE: Blood culture remains negative. He is on ampicillin and gentamicin. We will check closely.
7. NEUROLOGIC: Neurologic exam remains acceptable given his extreme prematurity. He will require screening intracranial ultrasounds and long-term neurodevelopmental follow-up.
8. RENAL/METABOLIC: Urine output remains adequate at this time. Metabolic parameters were acceptable. Will monitor closely.
9. FLUID/ELECTROLYTE/NUTRITION: He has gained some weight since birth. Multiple electrolyte dysfunctions are noted. This is partially due to dilution. We have restricted fluid somewhat and added various electrolytes/minerals to his TPN (total parenteral nutrition). We will monitor with serial chemistry panels.
10. APNEA/BRADYCARDIA: None since birth.
11. HEALTH CARE MAINTENANCE: None yet.
12. SOCIAL: Mom and Dad have been kept up-to-date in regard to their son's condition. Their questions have been answered, and they are in agreement with the outlined management plan.

SERVICE CODE(S): _____

ICD-10-CM DX CODE(S): _____

CASE 1-22C *NICU Progress Report*

LOCATION: Inpatient, Hospital, Neonatal Intensive Care Unit

PATIENT: Robert Zimmerman

ATTENDING PHYSICIAN: Roland Ortez, MD

SUBJECTIVE: Baby boy is currently 2 days old, slightly under 48 hours.

OBJECTIVE: Weight today is 1.716 kg (kilogram) (decreased by 135 g [gram]). He is down 5.1% of his weight since birth. OFC (occipitofrontal circumference) is 30 cm (centimeter) (decreased 0.5 cm). Intake yesterday was 152 cc, 82 cc/kg per day. Output was 170 cc, 3.8 cc/kg (cubic centimeter/kilogram) per hour. He has had no stools since birth. Vital signs reveal his temperature to be acceptable while on an open, radiant warmer. Heart rate is generally in the 110s–120s. Respiratory rate is generally equal to the IMV (intermittent mandatory ventilation). Mean blood pressures have generally been in the 40s to 50s. Oxygen saturations have remained in the high 90s.

PHYSICAL EXAMINATION: In general, he is pink on current ventilator settings. Endotracheal tube is in place. Neck is without masses. Chest reveals symmetric expansion, and the lungs are clear to auscultation on current ventilator settings. Cardiac exam reveals a regular rate without murmur or click. Peripheral pulses are 2+ and symmetric. Abdominal exam reveals an umbilical arterial catheter in place. Liver is palpable 1 cm below the right costal margin. No splenomegaly or masses are noted. Genital examination reveals a normal male; testes are not palpable. Extremity examination reveals no fixed decreased range of motion, deformity, or joint abnormality. Neurologic exam reveals mild diffuse hypotonia. No focal deficits are appreciated.

CURRENT MEDICATIONS:

1. Ampicillin 90.4 mg (milligram) IV (intravenous) q.12h.
2. Gentamicin 5.4 mg IV q.18h.
3. Morphine sulfate 0.18 mg IV q.6h and q.1h p.r.n. (as needed).
4. Dopamine 5 mcg/kg (microgram/kilogram) per minute.
5. Vecuronium 0.18 mg IV q.1-2h p.r.n.

LABORATORY STUDIES: Last arterial blood gas was obtained on ventilator settings of IMV 60, pressure 24/4, and FiO$_2$ (forced inspiration oxygen) 0.5 and revealed pH (potential of hydrogen) 7.27, PCO$_2$ (partial pressure of carbon dioxide) 51.1, PO$_2$ (partial pressure of oxygen) 66.5, and bicarbonate 22.5. Chemistry panel this AM revealed sodium 134, potassium 4.9, chloride 102, glucose 111, BUN (blood urea nitrogen) 18, creatinine 1.0, calcium 7.5, magnesium 3.8, phosphorus 7.5, and bilirubin 7.8. CBC (complete blood count) reveals a white count of 6,190. H&H (hematocrit and hemoglobin) is 17.6 and 54.3. Platelet count was 98,000. Chest x-ray continues to show significant evidence of hyaline membrane disease. Endotracheal tube is near the carina and has been withdrawn somewhat.

IMPRESSIONS/RECOMMENDATIONS:

1. Two-day-old infant who was born at 30 weeks' gestation. He does have clinical features suggestive of Noonan syndrome.
2. RESPIRATORY: Continues to show evidence of hyaline membrane disease with respiratory distress. He has received three doses of surfactant therapy. He does have echocardiographic evidence of PDA (patent ductus arteriosus), and we will be treating this at this time. We will attempt to decrease his ventilator settings based on serial clinical examination, pulse oximetry, arterial blood gas determinations, and chest x-ray.
3. CARDIOVASCULAR: Cardiovascular status is acceptable at this time while on dopamine at 5 mcg/kg per minute. Echocardiogram shows a patent ductus arteriosus. There also appears to be a slight abnormality to the pulmonary valve, which could be associated with his possible Noonan syndrome. He is going to receive indomethacin therapy.
4. GASTROINTESTINAL: Abdominal exam remains benign. He is NPO (nothing by mouth). He does have mild hyperbilirubinemia. Direct antibody test was negative. We will begin phototherapy at this time.
5. HEMATOLOGIC: Serial CBCs have been acceptable except for mild thrombocytopenia. We will continue to monitor, especially in light of the indomethacin therapy. He has not required any blood product transfusions since birth.
6. INFECTIOUS DISEASE: Blood culture remains negative at this time. We have discontinued his gentamicin, and he is being placed on cefotaxime because of the indomethacin.
7. NEUROLOGIC: Neurologic exam remains acceptable given his extreme prematurity. He will require screening intracranial ultrasound and also long-term neurodevelopmental follow-up.
8. RENAL/METABOLIC: Urine output remains adequate, and renal function studies are acceptable. Previous metabolic parameters are acceptable. We will repeat in the AM.
9. FLUIDS/ELECTROLYTES/NUTRITION: Weight loss is acceptable, and electrolytes are in the normal range today. We will adjust his TPN (total parenteral nutrition) accordingly.
10. APNEA/BRADYCARDIA: None since birth.
11. HEALTH CARE MAINTENANCE: None yet.
12. SOCIAL: The parents' questions have been answered, and they are in agreement with the outlined management plan.

SERVICE CODE(S): _____

ICD-10-CM DX CODE(S): _____

Discussion

The primary condition of this newborn is that he is in respiratory distress, so this will be the first listed diagnosis.

Noonan Syndrome

Although the physician mentioned Noonan syndrome, both in the Laboratory Study and the Impression/Recommendations (point 1) sections of the report, there is no definitive diagnosis of this condition. The physician uses "significant evidence" and "suggestive of" statements, but no definitive diagnostic statement; therefore it cannot be reported. Noonan syndrome is a condition in which the features of the infant are down-slanting eyes and webbed neck, and in which 25% of the newborns have intellectual disabilities. Half of the newborns have congenital heart disease, and usually there are physical deformities. So, without being able to review the entire medical record or query the physician, this would not be reported as it is not definitively stated in the record or confirmed by a chromosomal report.

Converting Kilograms to Grams

The physician indicated that the patient was premature, which means you need to assign a premature gestation diagnosis code with a

Continued

CASE 1-22C—cont'd

character/digit based on the weight of the newborn in grams. In the Objective section of the report, the physician refers to the weight of the newborn in kilograms. To convert kilograms into grams, multiply the kilograms by 1000: (1.851 kg × 1000 = 1851 g). You also need to report the weeks of gestation as stated in the report as 30 weeks.

Thrombocytopenia

In point 5 of the Impression/Recommendations section of the report, you can see that the physician diagnosed thrombocytopenia, which is a decrease in the number of platelets in the newborn's blood. A platelet transfusion was ordered.

Hyperbilirubinemia

In point 4 of the Impression/Recommendation section of the report, the physician indicated that the newborn has hyperbilirubinemia, which is excess bilirubin in the blood. The physician ordered phototherapy for the infant.

(Answers to every other Case are located in Appendix D . The full answer key is only available in the TEACH Instructor Resources on Evolve.)

CASE 1-22D   *NICU Progress Report*

LOCATION: Inpatient, Hospital, NICU (neonatal intensive care unit)

PATIENT: Robert Zimmerman

ATTENDING PHYSICIAN: Roland Ortez, MD

SUBJECTIVE: The patient is currently 4 days old.

OBJECTIVE: Weight today is 1.744 kg (kilogram) (decreased by 25 g [gram]). He is down 3.5% of his birth weight. OFC (occipitofrontal circumference) is 29 cm (centimeter) (no change from yesterday). Intake yesterday was 158 cc, 89.3 cc/kg (cubic centimeter/kilogram) per day. Output was 84 cc, 1.98 cc/kg per hour. He has had no stools since birth. Vital signs reveal his temperature to be acceptable while on the warmer. T-max 37.5 and T-current 36.8. Heart has been in the 110s to 130s. Respiratory rate is equal to IMV (intermittent mandatory ventilation) of 60. Mean blood pressures have been 40s to 50s, mean values were noted to be 27 and 36 yesterday, a couple in the 60s and 71. O_2 (oxygen) saturations remain in the high 90s. He does have occasional episodes when being examined where he desaturates.

PHYSICAL EXAMINATION: In general, he is pink on ventilator settings. Endotracheal tube is in place. Neck is without masses. Chest reveals symmetrical expansion. Lungs reveal crackles bilaterally. Cardiac exam: Regular rate without murmur or click. Peripheral pulses are 2+ and symmetric. Abdominal exam reveals a UAC (umbilical artery catheter) in place. Liver is palpable 1 cm below the right costal margin. No splenomegaly or masses noted. Genital examination reveals a normal male; testes nonpalpable. Extremity examination reveals no fixed decreased range of motion, deformity, or joint abnormality. Neurologic exam reveals a mild diffuse hypotonia. No focal deficits are appreciated.

CURRENT MEDICATIONS:

1. Ampicillin 90.4 mg (milligram) IV (intravenous) q.12h.
2. Cefotaxime 85 mg IV q.12h.
3. Morphine sulfate 0.1 mg/kg q.1h. p.r.n. (as needed).
4. Dopamine 5 mcg/kg per minute.
5. Lasix 0.18 mg times one dose at 3 PM on the 5th.
6. Zantac 0.858 mg IV q.6h.

LABORATORY STUDIES: Arterial blood gas was obtained on ventilator settings of IMV 60, PIP 22, PEEP (positive end-expiratory pressure) 4, and FiO_2 (forced inspiration oxygen) 42%. The pH (potential of hydrogen) was 7.298, PCO_2 (partial pressure of carbon dioxide) 46.6, PO_2 (partial pressure of oxygen) 91.4, and bicarbonate 22.1, base excess 3.3. Chemistry panel revealed sodium 139, potassium 4.0, chloride 105, CO_2 (carbon dioxide) 23.4, glucose 91, BUN (blood urea nitrogen) 34, creatinine 1.3, calcium 8.9, magnesium 3.0, and phosphorus 5.1. Hematology showed a white count of 5.98, hemoglobin 15.9, hematocrit 50.8, and platelets 74.

Chest x-ray continued to show evidence of hyaline membrane disease; however, he was slightly more improved today, with heart borders appearing clearer. There was a question of an enlarging cardiothymic silhouette; however, this may be related to poor inspiration. Supportive apparatuses were in place.

IMPRESSIONS/RECOMMENDATIONS:

1. Four-day-old infant born at 30 weeks' gestation does have clinical features of Noonan syndrome; chromosomal studies are pending.
2. RESPIRATORY: Patient continues to show evidence of hyaline membrane disease with respiratory distress. He has received three doses of surfactant therapy. He does have echocardiographic evidence of a small patent ductus arteriosus without a left-to-right shunt. We will continue to try to wean down on the ventilator settings based on serial clinical examination, pulse oximetry, arterial blood gas determinations, and chest x-rays.
3. CARDIOVASCULAR: We are continuing dopamine blood pressure support at 5 mcg/kg (microgram/kilogram) per minute. Mean blood pressures have slowly been rising, so we will continue to watch those. Echocardiogram showed a small patent ductus arteriosus without left-to-right shunt. The patient has been treated with indomethacin therapy times three doses. We will be repeating the echocardiogram today.
4. GASTROINTESTINAL: Abdominal exam remains benign. He is NPO (nothing by mouth). He does have mild hyperbilirubinemia, which has improved with phototherapy. We will continue with treatment. Direct antibody test was negative.
5. HEMATOLOGIC: Serial CBCs (complete blood count) have shown worsening thrombocytopenia today at 74,000. The patient will be transfused with one unit of platelets today, leukodepleted, and irradiated. Risks and benefits of transfusion were discussed with the mother, and an informed consent was obtained.
6. INFECTIOUS DISEASE: Blood cultures remain negative. We will continue with ampicillin and cefotaxime at this time.

CASE 1-22D—cont'd

7. NEUROLOGIC: Neurologic exam remains acceptable given his extreme prematurity. We will obtain screening intracranial ultrasound tomorrow. The patient will need long-term neurodevelopmental follow-up.

8. RENAL/METABOLIC: Renal output remains adequate, and renal function studies are acceptable. The patient received a dose of Lasix 0.18 mg times one yesterday with good diuresis. Metabolic parameters are acceptable.

9. FLUID/ELECTROLYTES/NUTRITION: Weight loss is currently 3.5% from birth weight. We would like to see more of a weight loss

because there is concern with fluid overload in this patient. We will adjust the patient's TPN (total parenteral nutrition) accordingly.

10. APNEA/BRADYCARDIA: None since birth.

11. HEALTH CARE MAINTENANCE: None yet.

12. SOCIAL: The mom and dad are up-to-date with regard to their son's condition.

SERVICE CODE(S): _____

ICD-10-CM DX CODE(S): _____

Discussion

Patent Ductus Arteriosus

All of the diagnoses in this report are ones that you have reported previously, except for the patent ductus arteriosus. **Patent ductus arteriosus** (PDA) is a heart defect in which the ductus arteriosus (blood

vessel) does not close after birth as it usually would. This open channel allows blood to bypass the lungs. A large PDA will lead to respiratory distress and can flood the lungs with blood, resulting in congestive heart failure.

(Answers to every other Case are located in Appendix D . The full answer key is only available in the TEACH Instructor Resources on Evolve.)

Preventive Medicine Services

Use Preventive Medicine Services codes to report the routine evaluation and management of a patient who is healthy and has no complaint or when the patient has a chronic condition or disease that is controlled but involves yearly routine physicals. The codes in this subsection would be used to report a routine physical examination done at the patient's request, such as a well-baby checkup. Preventive Medicine codes are intended to be used to identify comprehensive services, not a single-system examination, such as an annual gynecologic examination. The codes are assigned for infants, children, adolescents, and adults; they differ according to the age of the patient and whether the patient is a new or an established patient.

Note that in the code descriptions for both the New Patient and the Established Patient categories, the terms "comprehensive history" and "comprehensive examination" are used. These terms are not the same as the ones used with other E/M codes (99202-99350). Here, "comprehensive" means a complete history and a complete examination, as is conducted during an annual physical. The preventive service is not problem oriented; therefore, there is no HPI, but there is a complete ROS and PFSH. The comprehensive examination performed as part of the preventive medicine E/M service is a multisystem examination, but the extent of the examination is determined by the age of the patient and the risk factors identified for that individual.

You have done a super job of working through this difficult chapter. You will find that the reports that follow are not quite as complex as the ones you have been reviewing. The next few reports are commonly provided office services.

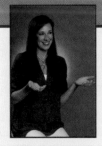

From the Trenches

"Coding is always evolving which means there are a number of opportunities to find a job that will keep you engaged and excited about what you do."

JENNA PRICE
CPC

Z Codes

Z codes are located in the Index under terms such as "admission," "examination," "history," "observation," and "problem." Z codes are assigned under the following circumstances:

- When a person who is **not currently sick** encounters health services for a specific purpose, such as to act as a donor or receive a vaccination
- When a person with a **known disease or injury** presents for specific treatment of that condition—such as dialysis, chemotherapy, or cast change
- When a circumstance **may influence** a patient's health status
- To indicate the **birth status and outcome** of delivery of a newborn

Several examples of assignment of these codes are:

1. When a person who is currently not sick encounters the health services for some specific purpose, such as to act as donor of an organ or tissue, to receive a preventive vaccination, or to discuss a problem that is in itself not a disease or injury. Occurrences such as these will be fairly rare among hospital inpatients but common among outpatients at health clinics. Examples are a kidney donor who is not ill but encounters health care (Z52.4), a well child who receives a polio vaccination (Z23), or a student who seeks health care to discuss a problem with school (Z55.9).

2. When a circumstance or problem is present that influences the person's health status but is not in itself a current illness or injury. For example, a family history of malignant gastrointestinal neoplasms (Z80.0) is significant to the patient's health care. The main term in this case is "History, **family,** malignant neoplasm, gastrointestinal tract." If, however, the diagnosis was a personal history of malignant neoplasm, the Index location would be History, **personal,** malignant, neoplasm, gastrointestinal tract, and the code would be Z85.00.

CASE 1-23A *Office Visit*

Report Dr. Alanda's service.

LOCATION: Outpatient, Clinic

PATIENT: Annabel Goth

PRIMARY CARE PHYSICIAN: Leslie Alanda, MD

CHIEF COMPLAINT: Pap and physical.

SUBJECTIVE: This 30-year-old married white female is an established patient who presents for routine annual exam and Pap. No particular concerns.

PAST MEDICAL HISTORY: Generally healthy. She has been treated for hypothyroidism for the past 4 years. Recent TSH (thyroid stimulating hormone) was normal at 1.30.

GYN HISTORY: Gravida 3, para (to bring forth) 3. Daughters aged 15 months, 4 and 5 years. No history of abnormal Pap smears. Husband has had a vasectomy. Menses regular q. month. LMP (last menstrual period): 3 weeks ago.

FAMILY HISTORY: Father—MI (myocardial infarction). Mother—high cholesterol and hypertension. Cancer, in grandparents.

SOCIAL/OCCUPATIONAL: She is a physical therapist working 3 days a week at the local rehabilitation hospital. Husband is a factory foreman at the local water-treatment plant.

HABITS: Tobacco: None. Alcohol: Rare. Diet: Watches fat. She daily drinks 8 cups of coffee. She has started a walking program to facilitate weight loss. Sleep is fair. Seatbelts are used consistently.

REVIEW OF SYSTEMS: Essentially negative. She would like to lose 50 pounds over the next several months.

EXAMINATION: Weight refused. Blood pressure of 118/68. General: Well-developed, well-nourished female. Skin is negative. HEENT (head, ears, eyes, nose, throat) is unremarkable. Neck is supple with no palpable nodes. Thyroid easily palpable but not enlarged. Breasts are symmetric and nontender with no palpable mass or discharge. Lungs clear to auscultation. Heart: Regular rate; no murmur. Abdomen is mildly obese, soft, and nontender with no palpable mass. No CVA (stroke/cardiovascular accident) tenderness. Pelvic: Normal female genitalia. No odor or discharge. Cervix is clear. No uterine or adnexal mass or tenderness.

IMPRESSION:

1. Normal gynecologic exam.
2. Hypothyroidism, on replacement therapy.
3. Overweight.

PLAN: Pap; will notify. Reinforced monthly BSE and positive lifestyle behaviors. Encourage weight-loss program. Refill Levothroid 0.125 mg (milligram) 1 q.d. (every day) for 1 year. Return to clinic annually and p.r.n. (as needed).

SERVICE CODE(S): _____

ICD-10-CM DX CODE(S): _____

(Answers to every other Case are located in Appendix D . The full answer key is only available in the TEACH Instructor Resources on Evolve.)

CASE 1-23B *Office Visit*

The patient returns to the clinic 1 year later. Report Dr. Alanda's service.

LOCATION: Outpatient, Clinic

PATIENT: Annabel Goth

PRIMARY CARE PHYSICIAN: Leslie Alanda, MD

CHIEF COMPLAINT: Checkup.

SUBJECTIVE: The patient is a 31-year-old married white female who is an established patient who presents today for her annual examination. She reports that she has been doing well except for some mild cold symptoms, which are now resolving. Over the past year, she has lost more than 50 pounds through an organized weight-loss program. She has been exercising on a regular basis. She is very pleased with the results and wishes to lose another 15 to 20 pounds.

PAST MEDICAL HISTORY: Significant for hypothyroidism for which she is on Synthroid 0.125 mg (milligram) q.d. (every day). She has otherwise enjoyed very good health. She is gravida 3, para (to bring forth) 3. She reports that her menstrual cycle is regular. Husband has had a vasectomy. No breast or pelvic complaints.

FAMILY HISTORY: Father—MI (myocardial infarction). Mother—high cholesterol and hypertension. Cancer, in grandparents.

SOCIAL HISTORY: The patient continues to work as a physical therapist at the local rehabilitation hospital. She is a nonsmoker. No alcohol problems.

OBJECTIVE: White female who appears to be in general good health. Her weight is down to 152 pounds. Blood pressure today somewhat elevated at 142/92. HEENT (head, ears, eyes, nose, throat) remarkable for a healing cold sore above her lips. Neck is supple; no masses. Lung fields are clear to auscultation. Heart is regular rate and rhythm; no audible murmurs. Breasts are symmetrical in size and shape. No masses, tenderness, or nipple discharge. Axillae negative. Abdomen is benign. Pelvic examination deferred due to menses. Extremities without edema. Skin is clear.

ASSESSMENT:

1. Healthy female.
2. History of hypothyroidism.
3. Obesity with weight loss of 50 pounds.

PLAN: Preventative health measures reviewed. The patient will have an annual TSH (thyroid stimulating hormone) level today as well as a screening cholesterol level. She will return in 2 weeks to complete pelvic examination and Pap smear, at which time we will also recheck her blood pressure. At that time, we will review her lab results and refill her Synthroid as indicated.

SERVICE CODE(S): _____

ICD-10-CM DX CODE(S): _____

CASE 1-23C *Office Visit*

The patient returns to the clinic 2 weeks later. Report Dr. Alanda's service.

LOCATION: Outpatient, Clinic

PATIENT: Annabel Goth

PRIMARY CARE PHYSICIAN: Leslie Alanda, MD

CHIEF COMPLAINT: College physical.

SUBJECTIVE: The patient is a 31-year-old married white female who presents today for a college physical. She is also due for her annual GYN (gynecology) exam. She denies any particular concerns. No recent illnesses or injuries. She was seen earlier this month with complaints of dizziness. She has a history of hypothyroidism, and her TSH (thyroid stimulating hormone) level is elevated at 11.77. Subsequently, her Synthroid has been increased to 0.15 mg (milligram) q.d. (every day). The patient reports that she is feeling fine at this time.

PAST MEDICAL HISTORY: Otherwise significant only for pregnancy and delivery. She is gravida 3, para (to bring forth) 3. No breast or pelvic complaints. Husband has had a vasectomy.

OBJECTIVE: White female who appears to be in general good health. Her weight is 151 pounds. Blood pressure is 100. HEENT (head, ears, eyes, nose, throat): Within normal limits. Neck: Supple. No masses. Normal thyroid. Lung fields are clear. Heart: Regular rate and rhythm. No audible murmurs. Breasts are symmetrical in size and shape. No tenderness, masses, or nipple discharge. Axillae: Negative. Abdomen: Benign. Pelvic exam is within normal limits. Pap smear was done. Extremities: Normal. Skin: Clear.

ASSESSMENT:

1. Healthy female.
2. Normal gynecologic exam.
3. Hypothyroidism, which is under good control with Synthroid.

PLAN: Preventative health measures reviewed. College forms completed with copies enclosed in chart. Return clinic visit in one year and p.r.n. (as needed).

SERVICE CODE(S): _____

ICD-10-CM DX CODE(S): _____

Discussion

In 1-23A, you reported a preventive medicine service at which a Pap was performed. If there are other conditions that the physician stated or treated, you would report the diagnosis codes for these conditions in addition to the Z code for the general medical examination. Note that when gynecological and physical examinations are completed at the same time, the physical examination (Z00.00) includes the gynecologic portion and is not separately reported.

In 1-23B, the patient again presented for a preventive medicine service, this time without Pap performed. A routine health examination is reported with a Z code. Any additional conditions indicated in the report and treated would be reported. (Z00.00) includes the gynecologic portion and is not separately reported.

In 1-23C, the patient presents for a college physical, and there is a special Z code for students. This code is for general medical exams and includes the gynecologic exam. Any diagnosis noted and treated would be reported.

CASE 1-24   *Office Visit*

Report Dr. Alanda's service.

LOCATION: Outpatient, Clinic

PATIENT: Lionel VanDoran

PRIMARY CARE PHYSICIAN: Leslie Alanda, MD

The patient is in for his annual checkup and is a 54-year-old established patient.

For past medical history, please see assessment.

CURRENT MEDICATIONS: Lotrel 5/20, #100 per day. Also takes Tylenol and ibuprofen on a p.r.n. (as needed) basis.

ALLERGIES to sulfa drugs and bees.

SOCIAL HISTORY: Two-pack-per-day smoker. He has not tried recently to quit smoking. Alcohol use has decreased from six to two beers per day. He works in the summertime as a pool cleaner and doing yard work.

HEALTH MAINTENANCE: The last lipid panel was good. Cholesterol was 203. He wears a seatbelt all the time.

FAMILY HISTORY: Mother, father, one brother, four daughters are all in good health. Denies family history of colon or prostate cancer, diabetes, or glaucoma.

REVIEW OF SYSTEMS: Complains of a sore throat in the morning, worse in the winter months when it is dry. He is a loud snorer. His wife states that he has had some bouts of apneic spells but not that prominent.

OBJECTIVE: Weight is stable at 220 pounds. Blood pressure is decreased to 142/88. Pulse is 84.

PERRLA (pupils equal, round, reactive to light, and accommodation): Normal extraocular movements. Tympanic membranes are benign.

Pharynx is erythematous. Nasal mucosa is erythematous, more so on the left. No areas that I can cauterize easily today. Neck is benign. Thyroid is not enlarged. Heart is S1 (first heart sound) and S2 (second heart sound). Lungs are clear. Abdomen is benign. There are no masses, tenderness, or organomegaly appreciated. There is no cervical, supraclavicular, axillary, or inguinal adenopathy appreciated. Reflexes are brisk. There is no pitting edema appreciated.

ASSESSMENT:

1. Physical examination.
2. Hypertension, under improved control on treatment.
3. Tobacco and alcohol use.
4. No hospitalizations, but did have foot injury in the past.
5. Sore throat in the morning. Question component of sleep apnea and loud snoring.

PLAN: Samples of Lotrel and prescription were given today. We will check a complete metabolic panel to check on his electrolytes, etc., and also his previous elevated liver enzymes. I discussed with him that we should reduce his alcohol use down to a maximum of two drinks per day because it is toxic to the heart and raises blood pressure. I also discussed again that smoking is definitely bad for his blood pressure as well, and he needs to quit. I discussed also increasing the humidity in the bedroom at nighttime and if he still has a sore throat after this, I would recommend an ENT referral. Health sheet was given along with standard recommendations. We will send a letter with his complete metabolic panel and cholesterol level return.

SERVICE CODE(S): _____

ICD-10-CM DX CODE(S): _____

(Answers to every other Case are located in Appendix D . The full answer key is only available in the TEACH Instructor Resources on Evolve.)

CASE 1-25   *Office Visit*

Report Dr. Alanda's service.

LOCATION: Outpatient, Clinic

PATIENT: Tiffany Hopman

PRIMARY CARE PHYSICIAN: Leslie Alanda, MD

PRESENTING COMPLAINT: Checkup

This girl is in for a checkup. She is now 1 year of age and an established patient. She is doing very well. Her birthday was April 21. She is cruising around furniture, but not quite walking. She eats well and sleeps well. Has no difficulties.

I examined this young girl and filled out the form for 1 year. Please see same. She has four lower and four upper teeth. Can say hi; waves bye-bye. Cruises here in the office.

ASSESSMENT: Healthy 1-year-old female.

Mom has diabetes and is pregnant. She is due in May. At that time, the patient will get a new sibling. We are certain this one will be born early. Mom will be going in for prenatal steroids. I will see her back at 15 months or p.r.n. (as needed).

SERVICE CODE(S): _____

ICD-10-CM DX CODE(S): _____

(Answers to every other Case are located in Appendix D . The full answer key is only available in the TEACH Instructor Resources on Evolve.)

CASE 1-26 *Office Visit*

Report Dr. Alanda's service.

LOCATION: Outpatient, Clinic

PATIENT: Marissa Glendale

PRIMARY CARE PHYSICIAN: Leslie Alanda, MD

CHIEF COMPLAINT: Pelvic exam and Pap smear.

SUBJECTIVE: This is a 41-year-old married white female who presents today to complete her pelvic exam and Pap smear. She was seen 2 weeks ago for her annual checkup.

OBJECTIVE: Blood pressure today is normal at 118/68. Pelvic exam: Normal external genitalia. Vagina without discharge. Cervix: Multiparous, clear. Pap smear done. Bimanual exam unremarkable.

ASSESSMENT:

1. Normal blood pressure.
2. Normal pelvic exam.

PLAN: Return clinic visit in 1 year and p.r.n. (as needed).

SERVICE CODE(S): _____

ICD-10-CM DX CODE(S): _____

(Answers to every other Case are located in Appendix D . The full answer key is only available in the TEACH Instructor Resources on Evolve.)

CHAPTER 1 *Auditing Review*

Audit the coding for the following reports.

Audit Report 1.1 Hospital Services

LOCATION: Inpatient, Hospital

PATIENT: Dana Obright

ATTENDING PHYSICIAN: Marvin Elhart, MD

REASON FOR ADMISSION: Congestive heart failure.

The patient is an 82-year-old Caucasian female who was getting ready to go to bed tonight and felt sudden shortness of breath. She had no chest pain, neck, or jaw pain. She could not take a deep breath. She presented to the emergency room where a chest x-ray was obtained, and she was in florid pulmonary edema, and her blood pressure was 180s-190s/110.

The patient has been having exertional dyspnea for some time. She usually sees Dr. Noonar. She recently had a pacemaker placed for sick sinus syndrome.

The patient had a recent echocardiogram, which showed normal left ventricular systolic function with severe mitral regurgitation and tricuspid regurgitation with moderate pulmonary hypertension.

PAST MEDICAL HISTORY:

1. Hypertension.
2. History of atrial fibrillation.
3. Thoracic aortic aneurysm.
4. Hysterectomy.
5. Bilateral cataract surgery.

ALLERGIES: No known drug allergies

SOCIAL HISTORY: Retired, lives in Manytown. She is widowed. She denies any alcohol or smoking.

FAMILY HISTORY: Positive for cancer and diabetes. She has an aunt who had breast cancer, otherwise negative.

MEDICATION

1. Clonidine patch 0.2.
2. Vasotec l0 mg q.d.
3. Premarin 0.625 mg q.d.
4. Labetalol 100 mg b.i.d.

REVIEW OF SYSTEMS: General: Pale. No fever, chills, or night sweats. No change in weight or loss of appetite. ENT: Negative. Eyes: Negative. Cardiovascular: No claudication. Occasional leg edema. The rest as mentioned in the HPI. GU: Negative. GI: Negative. Skin: Negative. Neuro: Negative. Musculoskeletal: Occasional arthralgias, otherwise negative. Respiratory: Cannot get her breath.

PHYSICAL EXAMINATION: I saw the patient after she received 1 mg of Bumex and after she diuresed more than 1000 cc. She was lying in bed not in any distress. Blood pressure went down to 102/90s. Heart rate 80s to 90s per minute. Respirations 22 per minute. She is pale and afebrile. There is increased jugular venous pressure and mild neck vein distention. Lungs show good air entry bilaterally with crackles in the bases. Abdomen: Obese, nontender. No organomegaly. Extremities: 1+ edema. She has a Foley catheter, which has light urine.

LABORATORY STUDIES: All her labs including CBC, basic metabolic panel, and troponin today were negative.

CHEST X-RAY: Cardiomegaly and florid pulmonary edema with edema in the right transverse fissure.

IMPRESSION:

1. Congestive heart failure, multifactorial. Probably she has left ventricular hypertrophy and also mitral regurgitation that tipped her over the edge.
2. Hypoxic with saturations of 86% on room air secondary to pulmonary edema.

PLAN: I will give her another 0.5 mg of Bumex IV. We will repeat her labs at 9 including troponins. The patient does not usually use salt in her diet, but we will fluid restrict her for 1500 cc.

One of the following codes is reported incorrectly for this case. Indicate the incorrect code.

PROFESSIONAL SERVICES: Evaluation and Management, **99222**

ICD-10-CM DX: Congestive heart failure, **I50.9**

INCORRECT CODE: _____

Audit Report 1.2 Consultation

LOCATION: Inpatient, Hospital

PATIENT: Raymond Hunt

REQUESTING PROVIDER: Mohamad Almaz, MD

CONSULTING PROVIDER Ronald Green, MD

REASON FOR CONSULTATION: Opinion regarding preoperative clearance.

HISTORY OF PRESENT ILLNESS: A 53-year-old male who has been admitted today to the hospital because of right tibia and fibula fracture. Patient tells me he was walking out when he slipped on the ice and fell. He complains of pain of 5/10 in the right leg, just below the knee joint. He has had a fracture. No history of radiation of pain. It is worse with movements. Patient works as a laborer, works on a farm. He says he does mostly physical labor. He tells me that he never gets any chest pain or shortness of breath. No history of any orthopnea or paroxysmal nocturnal dyspnea. No history suggestive of any angina. No history of any pain going to the left arm at any time with

exertion. No history of any headache or blurring of vision. No history of any cough. No history of fever, chills, or rigors. No history of any recent weight gain or weight loss. No history of any pain in abdomen. No history of any change in bowel habits. No history of any bleeding per rectum or melena. No history of dysuria, hematuria, or pyuria.

PAST MEDICAL HISTORY:

1. Hypertension.
2. Hyperlipidemia.

PAST SURGICAL HISTORY: History of hernia repair when he was 36 and 46.

SOCIAL HISTORY: Still smoking a pack per day. He has been smoking for more than 20 years. The last time he took alcohol was 22 months ago. He stated he didn't try really before that.

ALLERGIES:

1. Zetia. He could not tolerate the medication, had a rash.
2. He is allergic to latex.

CHAPTER 1—*cont'd*

FAMILY HISTORY: Father deceased from stroke at the age of 39. Also had hypertension. Mother passed away a couple of years ago. She had history of hypertension and what looks like a massive heart attack.

CURRENT MEDICATIONS:

1. Aspirin.
2. Lisinopril 10 mg daily.
3. He takes herbal medication, red rice yeast, 600 mg tablets twice a day.
4. Omega-3 capsules.

REVIEW OF SYSTEMS: A full review of systems which include CARDIAC, PULMONARY, GASTROINTESTINAL, MUSCULOSKELETAL, NEUROLOGIC, ENDOCRINE, RHEUMATOLOGY, IMMUNOLOGY, AND ONCOLOGY were performed and negative for symptoms except for as noted.

PHYSICAL EXAMINATION: Patient is alert and oriented to time, place, and person. PULSE: 138. RESPIRATORY RATE: 20. BLOOD PRESSURE: 120/76. HEAD: Atraumatic. EYES: Pupils are reactive. NOSE and THROAT: Oral mucosa is slightly dry. NECK: Supple. No JVD. No carotid bruit. HEART: S1 and S2, regular. LUNGS: Clear to auscultation. ABDOMEN: Soft. Bowel sounds are positive, nontender, nondistended. EXTREMITIES: Pulses are positive, no clubbing, no cyanosis, no edema in the left lower extremity. Right lower extremity is in cast. NEUROLOGICAL: Grossly, normal. No focal deficits. PSYCHIATRIC: Normal mood and affect. SKIN: No acute rashes.

LABORATORY STUDIES AND INVESTIGATIONS: He did have labs done in January, which show a BUN of 14, creatinine of 0.9, and calcium of 9.3. His cholesterol was 215 at the time with triglycerides of 32, HDL of 44, and LDL of 154.

I did an EKG and reviewed this. This shows normal sinus rhythm but slightly prominent T-waves.

ASSESSMENT:

1. Preoperative clearance.
2. Hypertension.

3. Hyperlipidemia.
4. Prominent T-waves on the electrocardiogram.

RECOMMENDATIONS:

1. Patient is a 53-year-old male with decent exercise tolerance. Patient does have risk factors including smoking, hypertension, hyperlipidemia, and age for his coronary artery disease but patient does not have any exertional angina or exertional shortness of breath. His EKG does not show any acute changes other than some changes in T-waves. At this time, I think he can proceed with surgery without any further work-up. He can be continued on his ACE inhibitor for high blood pressure. He will be a mild to moderate risk for intraoperative and postoperative risk of myocardial infarction and heart failure but, at this time, there is no acutely modifiable risk factors as such. I did discuss the risks with the patient too and he has consented for surgery.
2. Patient does have slightly prominent T-waves on the EKG. We will check a BMP at this time. Check on potassium levels, especially as he is on ACE inhibitor.
3. Patient does have hyperlipidemia and he may be continued on his current home medications.
4. I did discuss the plan with the patient and also my recommendations with Dr. Almaz. Some of the old charts are reviewed.
5. We also recommend keeping him on DVT prophylaxis.

One or more of the following codes are reported incorrectly for this case. Indicate the incorrect code or codes.

PROFESSIONAL SERVICES: Consultation, **99254**

ICD-10-CM DX: Traumatic tibia fracture, **S82.201A;** Traumatic fibula fracture, **S82.401A;** Hypertension, **I10;** Hyperlipidemia, **E78.5;** Abnormal electrocardiogram, **R94.31;** Preprocedural cardiovascular examination, **Z01.810**

INCORRECT CODE: _____

Audit Report 1.3 Neurology Consultation

LOCATION: Outpatient, Emergency Department

PATIENT: Kathryn Abbott

REFERRING PHYSICIAN: Paul Sutton, MD

CONSULTING PHYSICIAN: Timothy Pleasant, MD

Kathryn is a 22-year-old female whom I was asked to consult by Dr. Sutton regarding new-onset headache and double vision. The patient notes that she may get a mild bitemporal headache once every 3 months. However, 1 to 2 nights ago, she began developing a frontal headache which is a pressure type like someone was pushing on her head. She thought initially she had some problem with focusing and attributed this to the headache. However, last night, she began seeing double vision somewhat, one figure on top of another and worse if she looked over to the right interior vision. She denies any fever or chills. There has been no photo or photo sensitivity. She denies any nausea or vomiting. She has not had any recent trauma. She does note that she had some sinus congestion, maybe 2 weeks ago, but this resolved spontaneously. She scales the headache at approximately 6-7/10 currently.

REVIEW OF SYSTEMS: She does have some problems with anxiety. All other review of systems are negative.

ALLERGIES: No known drug allergies.

MEDICATIONS:

1. Very infrequent Ibuprofen.
2. Recent Claritin.
3. She has a script for Zoloft but is currently not taking this.
4. Depo-Provera, q. 3 months.

PAST MEDICAL HISTORY: History of anxiety as above.

FAMILY HISTORY: Mother has some cardiac valvular changes. She also has migraines. One sister has migraines. One brother and one other sister are healthy. Dad is healthy. He does have some increased cholesterol. SOCIAL HABITS: She smokes 1 pack every 2 to 3 days of cigarettes. No alcohol. SOCIAL HISTORY: She is single. She is a representative at Job Service. She has one son, 14 months of age. She lives in Tempe.

PHYSICAL EXAMINATION: T-max of 36.2 degrees. Pulse is 96. Respiratory rate is 20. Blood pressure was 138/85. In GENERAL, she appears comfortable. She has a normal affect initially and later on in the exam, she becomes somewhat anxious. SKIN is warm and dry. HEENT EXAM reveals an atraumatic head. There is no photophobia or meningismus. CHEST was clear to auscultation with a regular breathing rhythm. HEART: Regular rate and rhythm. ABDOMEN was soft and nontender. NEURO: Oriented to person, place, and time.

IMPRESSION:

1. Headache.
2. Double vision.

PLAN: The patient was observed for several hours in the emergency room. She was given Imitrex, and her headache has dissipated.

She will be observed for a few more hours. Her friend will drive her home.

One of the following codes is reported incorrectly for this case. Indicate the incorrect code.

PROFESSIONAL SERVICES: Consultation, **99243**

ICD-10-CM DX: Headache, **R51.9**; Double vision, **H53.2**

INCORRECT CODE: _____

Audit Report 1.4 Emergency Department Services

LOCATION: Hospital Emergency Department

PATIENT: Fran Green

PHYSICIAN: Paul Sutton, MD

CHIEF COMPLAINT: Level 3 trauma

SUBJECTIVE: A 44-year-old female was treating a sick calf when a cow attacked her and stomped her. She presents to the emergency room via ambulance complaining of an open ankle dislocation. She also is complaining of some abrasions on her chin and under her left leg. She specifically denies loss of consciousness or headache. No neck, back, chest, abdomen, or pelvic pain. She is quite stoic.

PAST MEDICAL HISTORY: Remarkable for some hypertension, depression, and migraine.

MEDICATIONS:

1. Premarin
2. Question Xanax

ALLERGIES: None

FAMILY HISTORY: Deemed noncontributory

SOCIAL HISTORY: She is married, I believe a nonsmoker, and is a laborer.

REVIEW OF SYSTEMS: As above. She says her foot is cold.

PHYSICAL EXAMINATION: Preliminary survey is benign. Secondary survey: Alert and Oriented × 3. Immobilized in a C-collar and long spine board. Head is normocephalic. There is no hemotympanum. Pupils are equal. There is an abrasion under her chin. Trachea is midline. She does

have a C-collar in place. Air entry is equal. Lungs are clear. Chest wall is nontender. Abdomen is soft. Pelvis is stable. Long bones are remarkable for an obvious open dislocation of the right ankle. The toes are all dusky, she has a strong posterior tibial pulse, and the nurse thinks she felt a faint dorsalis pedis. She has an abrasion under her left leg.

HOSPITAL COURSE: We did give her a tetanus shot and 1 g of Ancef. I immediately gave her some parenteral Fentanyl and Versed, and we were able to reduce the dislocation without difficulty. Postreduction film looks surprisingly good. There is perhaps a subtle fracture noted only on the lateral projection. C-spine shows some degenerative change, is of poor quality, but is negative; and upon re-examination she is not tender in that area. However, it was done because she had such a severe distracting injury and given the mechanism. Chest x-ray and left femur look fine.

ASSESSMENT: Level 3 trauma with an open right ankle dislocation, multiple abrasions.

PLAN: Plan to call Dr. Almaz, who graciously agreed to assume care. The patient is kept n.p.o.

One or more of the following codes is/are reported incorrectly or missing for this case. Indicate the incorrect or missing code or codes.

SERVICE CODE(S):   Evaluation and Management, **99283**

ICD-10-CM DX CODE(S):   Ankle dislocation, **S93.04XA**, Open wound, right ankle, **S91.001A**, Abrasion of head, **S00.81XA**, Abrasion, left lower leg, **S80.812**

INCORRECT/MISSING CODE(S): _____

Audit Report 1.5 Progress Note

LOCATION: Inpatient, Hospital

PATIENT: David R. Harris

ATTENDING PHYSICIAN: Timothy L. Pleasant, MD

SUBJECTIVE: The patient is doing very well today. His lower back pain is much better after he has had the epidural pump. He complains of increased secretions in the trachea and some rattling noise and pain in his chest when he breathes. He is not coughing up any secretions, and he has no other chest pain. He is not having any fever. No other complaints.

REVIEW OF SYSTEMS: Complete and negative other than what is mentioned above.

OBJECTIVE: He looks okay, in no acute distress. Vitals are stable and he is afebrile; temperature just for one time was 37.9° C, otherwise afebrile. Blood pressure this morning was 96/41. Ears, nose, and throat are unremarkable. Neck is supple, no JVD. Lungs clear to auscultation with a few rhonchi and no wheezing. The abdomen is benign. Extremities: There is trace edema, peripheral pulses palpated.

BLOOD WORK FOR TODAY: Gram stain of the pleural fluid showed a lot of RBCs, no growth. Bedside glucose was 108. Blood cultures are negative. Cell count, on the pleural effusion nucleated cells, were 520 and RBCs 2800. Sputum culture is pending.

ASSESSMENT:

1. Pleuritic chest pain, likely related to metastatic non–small cell carcinoma of the lungs and pain medication withdrawal

2. Lower back pain and lower extremity pain, resolved right now with epidural pain pump
3. Non–small cell carcinoma, lung
4. History of chronic smoking, and he is still smoking. He is on the nicotine patch.
5. Malnutrition
6. Hepatitis C
7. Depression
8. History of coronary artery disease
9. Hypertension
10. COPD

PLAN: Waiting for permanent pain pump, hopefully tomorrow morning. I will add Combivent and Allegra to help with secretions. Continue other management.

One or more of the following codes are reported incorrectly or missing for this case. Indicate the incorrect or missing code or codes.

SERVICE CODE(S): Evaluation and Management, **99232**

ICD-10-CM DX CODE(S): Other chest pain, **R07.81;** Low back pain, **M54.50;** Unspecified malignant neoplasm of bronchus and lung, **C34.90;** Chronic obstructive pulmonary disease, unspecified, **J44.9**

INCORRECT/MISSING CODE(S): _____

Audit Report 1.6 Consultation

LOCATION: Inpatient, Hospital

PATIENT: Shawn Peterson

PRIMARY CARE PHYSICIAN: Leslie Alanda, MD

CONSULTANT: Elmer Lauer, MD

The patient is a 60-year-old male who was transferred from Franklin Hospital for further management. He was admitted earlier today for what later was shown to be diabetic ketoacidosis. However, while he was there, he was noted to have some GI bleeding, having a black emesis and having passed black, tarry stools. Because they did not have the facilities for endoscopy, the patient was subsequently transferred here.

The patient apparently presented to the Emergency Room over at Franklin Hospital complaining of nausea and vomiting for the past 2 days. This was associated with some epigastric pain and tenderness and some coughing. He denies any dark stools or blood in his emesis prior to being seen in the Emergency Room. On admission to the ICU here, he was hemodynamically stable. He did not appear to be in any acute distress.

REVIEW OF SYSTEMS: He denies any other constitutional symptoms. He denies any recent fevers, chills, or night sweats. He also denies any recent dyspnea or chest pain even on exertion. Other than the abdominal pain that is associated with his nausea and vomiting for the past 2 days, he said he has not noticed any changes in his bowel habits. He also denies any changes in his voiding or urinary habits.

PAST MEDICAL HISTORY:

1. Type 1 diabetes, which he has had for more than 30 years now. When asked about his diabetes care, he did admit he often runs out of his medications. At home he says his blood sugar in the last several weeks has actually been consistently above 300 mg percent.
2. Hypertension, which he has also had for several years.
3. Hypothyroid.

MEDICATIONS:

Prior to transfer, the patient was on the following medications:

1. Arthrotec 50 mg twice a day.
2. Thiamine 100 mg twice a day.

The patient was on the following medications on transfer:

1. Arthrotec 50 mg twice a day.
2. Thiamine 100 mg twice a day.
3. Ecotrin 325 mg daily.
4. Maxzide 75/30 mg daily.
5. Tamsulosin 0.4 mg twice a day before meals.
6. Synthroid 0.125 mg daily.
7. Lisinopril 10 mg daily.
8. Multivitamins one tablet daily.
9. KCL 10 mEq three times a day.
10. Tylenol 325 mg as needed for pain.
11. Benadryl 25 mg as needed for sleep.
12. Prilosec 20 mg daily.
13. Lantus insulin 10 units in the morning and regular insulin four times a day as a sliding scale.

ALLERGIES: He has no known drug allergies.

FAMILY HISTORY: Significant for diabetes. The patient's father and brother both carry the disease. Both his brother and his mother are hypertensive. His mother also had cerebrovascular disease. Mother also was diagnosed with lung cancer after smoking for several decades. The patient is a widower and has four children, all of whom are alive and well.

SOCIAL HISTORY: He denies any recent tobacco or alcohol intake. He said he quit smoking in December of 2003 primarily for financial reasons. He does have about a 50 to 60 pack per year smoking history though. He did admit to significant alcohol use. He said that he is a binge drinker. He has had several problems with alcohol in the past. His last binge was about 4 or 5 months ago. During these binges the patient would often pass out. He is not aware of any liver complications from his alcohol intake.

PHYSICAL EXAMINATION: He was lying down in bed. He did not appear to be in any acute pain or distress. His blood pressure was 117/60, pulse rate 99, breathing about 16 to 18 times per minute on room air and was saturating 100%. HEAD/NECK: Showed pink palpebral conjunctivae with anicteric sclerae. He did not have any active nasal or ear discharge. His oropharynx was otherwise clear of any exudates or any lesions. His neck was supple and was nontender. He did not have any cervical or submandibular lymphadenopathy. His carotid upstroke was normal. CHEST: Shows lung fields to be essentially clear to auscultation

Continued

CHAPTER 1—*cont'd*

bilaterally; however, he did have some decreased breath sounds towards both bases. There were no distinct rales or wheezes. CARDIAC: Shows a regular rate and rhythm without any rubs. ABDOMEN: Showed it to be soft, slightly tender to deep palpation, particularly in the epigastric area. He did have normoactive bowel sounds. There were no palpable masses or any bruits appreciated. EXTREMITIES: Showed fair and equal pulses without any significant edema.

LABORATORY DATA: Today's hemoglobin is 16 with a white count of 17.6 and a platelet count of 320,000. Sodium is 134, potassium 5.3, chloride 92, and bicarb 19. His anion gap was 22 to 23. BUN 42, creatinine 1.9, glucose 605. His stool guaiac was positive for occult blood. He also had a blood gas that showed a pH of 7.29. His serum ketones were positive but were not quantified.

ASSESSMENT:

1. Diabetic ketoacidosis. I am not sure what the initiating or precipitating event was. The patient does not appear to have any clear focus of infection; however, we will need to rule out the more common causes, including pneumonia, urinary tract infection, and possible gastroenteritis.
2. GI bleeding. The patient currently is hemodynamically stable despite the bleeding episode.

PLAN:

1. Hydrate the patient with 0.9 normal saline. Switch the normal saline to D5 normal saline once his Accu-Cheks have dropped below 200.
2. Start on insulin drip. Accu-Cheks and adjustments of the drips per protocol.
3. Keep the patient NPO for now.
4. Keep the patient on IV proton pump inhibitors.
5. Start the bowel prep with magnesium citrate and Dulcolax in preparation for possible endoscopy tomorrow.
6. Will consult GI in the morning to evaluate the patient for possible endoscopic evaluation.
7. Will keep the patient on serial compression device boots for DVT prophylaxis.
8. Follow the patient's BMP and anion gap. Continue the insulin until the patient's anion gap acidosis has resolved.

Total time spent with patient tonight was 2 hours and 20 minutes.

One or more of the following codes are reported incorrectly or missing for this case. Indicate the incorrect or missing code or codes.

SERVICE CODE(S):   Evaluation and Management, **99255**

ICD-10-CM DX CODE(S):   Type 1 diabetes with DKA, **E10.10**; Type 1 diabetes with hyperglycemia, **E10.65**

INCORRECT/MISSING CODE(S):

(Auditing Review answers with rationales are only available in the TEACH Instructor Resources on Evolve.)

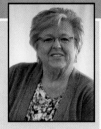

"Excellent coders always strive to be the best they can be by knowing as much as possible about the areas in which they code."

Medicine

http://evolve.elsevier.com/Buck/next

Immune Globulins/Immunizations/Vaccines/ Toxoids (90281-91322)

Operative Reports
- 2-1A   Chart Note
- 2-2A   Chart Note
- 2-3A   Chart Note

Hydration, (96360, 96361); and Therapeutic, Prophylactic, and Diagnostic Injections and Infusions (Excludes Chemotherapy and Other Highly Complex Drug or Highly Complex Biologic Agent Administration) (96365-96379)

Operative Reports
- 2-4A   Chart Note
- 2-5A   Chart Note

Psychiatry

Operative Reports
- 2-6A   Psychological Evaluation

Dialysis (90935-90999)

Operative Reports
- 2-7A   Hemodialysis Progress Report
- 2-8A   History and Physical Examination
- 2-8B   CAPD Progress Note
- 2-8C   Dialysis Progress Note
- 2-8D   Thoracic Medicine and CAPD Progress Note
- 2-8E   Dialysis Progress Note
- 2-8F   Dialysis Progress Note
- 2-8G   Discharge Summary

Noninvasive Vascular Diagnostic Studies

Operative Reports
- 2-9A   Duplex Carotid Artery Study
- 2-10A   Duplex Carotid Artery Study
- 2-11A   Arterial Doppler Test
- 2-12A   Vascular Laboratory Report, Arterial Doppler Test

Cardioversion

Operative Reports
- 2-13A   Electrical Cardioversion

Ultrasound

Operative Reports
- 2-14A   Ultrasound, Lower Extremities

Central Nervous System Assessments/Tests (e.g., Neurocognitive, Mental Status, Speech Testing) (96105-96146)

Operative Reports
- 2-15A   Cognitive Function Assessment

Health Behavior Assessment and Intervention

Operative Reports
- 2-16A   Behavior Assessment

Chemotherapy Administration (96401-96549)

Operative Reports
- 2-17A   Infusion

Photodynamic Therapy (96567-96574)

Operative Reports
- 2-18A   Photodynamic Therapy

Physical Medicine and Rehabilitation

Operative Reports
- 2-19A   Physical Therapy Evaluation
- 2-20A   Physical Therapy Evaluation
- 2-20B   Physical Therapy Evaluation
- 2-20C   Physical Therapy Evaluation

Medical Nutrition Therapy

Osteopathic and Chiropractic Manipulative Treatment

Special Services, Procedures, and Reports

Operative Reports
- 2-21A   Office Procedure
- 2-21B   Clinic Progress Note

(Answers to every other Case are located in Appendix D, with the full answer key only available in the TEACH Instructor Resources on Evolve)
(Auditing Review answers with rationales are only available in the TEACH Instructor Resources on Evolve)

The Medicine section has many subsections that encompass a broad range of services. Take a moment to review these subsections in the CPT and then review the Medicine Guidelines. The section contains diagnostic (determining nature of disease) and therapeutic (curative) services that are both invasive (entering the body) and noninvasive (not entering the body).

Immune Globulins/Immunizations/Vaccines/Toxoids (90281-91322)

When coding from this section, you will need to remember this is the one section in the CPT manual that actually has codes for both administration of the drug and the drug product. You would usually assign the drug product code from HCPCS National Level II manual. There are payer-specific rules that still may lead you to a HCPCS National Level II code, but there are drug codes in the medicine section for vaccines and immune globulins.

The codes are categorized as follows:

Vaccine Administration	90460-0174A
Vaccine/Toxoids	90476-90749
Immune Globulins	96365-96368,
Administration	96372, 96374,
	96375
Immune Globulins Products	90281-90399

The two types of immunizations are active and passive. **Active immunization** can be either a toxoid or a vaccine and is administered in anticipation that a patient will come into contact with a disease. **Toxoids** are the bacteria that cause the disease that have been made nontoxic. When the toxoid is injected, the body's immune system produces an immune response that builds protection from the disease. A **vaccine** is the injection of the actual virus in small doses to allow the body's immune system to produce an immune response. **Passive immunization** does not cause an immune response; rather, immune globulins (antibodies) are injected to protect the body from a specific disease. Within the Medicine section, the codes for active immunizations are Vaccines/Toxoids (90476-90749), and the codes for passive immunizations are Immune Globulins (90281-90399).

Whenever an immunization or immune globulin is administered, the substance (vaccine/toxoid or immune globulin) is reported along with an administration code (90460-0174A for vaccine/toxoid and 96365-96368, 96372, 96374, 96375 for immune globulins). For example, an immune globulin of diphtheria antitoxin (90296) for a patient over 19 years of age, injected intramuscularly, is reported as follows:

90296	Diphtheria antitoxin (substance)
96372	Therapeutic injection subcutaneously or intramuscularly (injection)
Z41.8	Prophylactic immunotherapy (diagnosis code)

The vaccination administration codes (90460-0174A) are divided by age and route of administration. Codes 90460/90461 (through 18 years of age) are reported for any method of administration of a vaccine when face-to-face counseling with the patient/family is provided. Assign codes 90471/90472 to report intradermal (ID), percutaneous (PERC), **subcutaneous (SQ),** or **intramuscular (IM)** administration for patients when the physician did not counsel the family and for all other patients over 18 years of age. Codes 90473/90474 are used to report administration by intranasal or oral methods. For codes 90471-90474, the type and number of administrations determines the type and number of codes reported, not the number of substances being administered. For example, if the patient received a tetanus toxoid, rubella virus, and diphtheria toxoid in three separate injections, the service would be reported as follows:

Substance (Drug Supply)	Administration (Service)
90749 Tetanus toxoid	90471 Administration, tetanus toxoid
90749 Rubella virus	90472 Administration, rubella virus
90749 Diphtheria toxoid	90472 Administration, diphtheria toxoid

If a 6-year-old child receives a combination of tetanus and diphtheria that was injected in one syringe, and the rubella in another syringe, with physician counseling, the service would be reported as follows:

Substance (Drug Supply)	Administration (Service)
90702 Tetanus and diphtheria toxoids	90460 Administration, tetanus toxoid
	90461 Administration, diphtheria toxoid
90749 Rubella virus	90461 Administration, rubella virus

The unlisted vaccine/toxoid code is reported when there is no listing for an individual vaccine or toxoid.

An E/M code is reported with an immunization service only when there is another separate, identifiable evaluation and management service provided and documented in the medical record. Report the E/M service with modifier -25 added to the code to indicate that the service was separate from the immunization service. If the only service provided was the injection, it is not appropriate to report an E/M service because administration of the injection is reported with the administration code (90460-0174A). The substance injected is reported with the toxoid, vaccine, or immune globulin code, so it is not correct to report a supply code (e.g., 99070) unless some other supply was provided in conjunction with another separate service in addition to the immunization.

Two vaccinations that are commonly provided are influenza and pneumococcal. Report a code for the substance injected (vaccine) and a code for the administration of the vaccine. The third-party payer may require you to submit CPT codes or CPT with HCPCS National Level II codes for the service. The following identifies the codes that are usually reported for influenza and pneumococcal immunizations.

CPT influenza **vaccine** codes:

90657	Influenza virus vaccine, trivalent (IIV3), split virus, 0.25 mL dosage, for intramuscular use
90658	Influenza virus vaccine, trivalent (IIV3), split virus, 0.5 mL dosage, for intramuscular use

HCPCS National Level II code used to report the **administration** of an influenza vaccine to a Medicare patient:

G0008	Administration of influenza virus vaccine

CPT codes used to report the administration of the influenza vaccine:

90471	Intramuscular administration, one vaccine
90472	Intramuscular administration, each additional vaccine

The diagnosis code assigned when the only reason for the encounter is an influenza vaccine (flu shot) is Z23, Influenza vaccination. The diagnosis and service codes must correlate (connect).

CPT pneumococcal **vaccine** code:

90732	Pneumococcal polysaccharide vaccine, 23-valent (PPSV23), adult or immunosuppressed patient dosage, when administered to individuals 2 years or older, for subcutaneous or intramuscular use

HCPCS National Level II code to report the administration of the pneumococcal vaccine to a Medicare patient:

G0009	Administration of pneumococcal vaccine

CPT codes used to report the administration of the pneumococcal vaccine:

90471	Intramuscular administration, one vaccine
90472	Intramuscular administration, each additional vaccine

The diagnosis code assigned when the only reason for the encounter is a pneumococcal vaccine (pneumonia shot) is Z23. The diagnosis and service codes must correlate.

Codes 91304, 91318-91322 report the vaccine for SARS-CoV-2, coronavirus disease COVID-19. Administration codes 90480 is also reported in conjunction with code 91304, 91318-91322.

Diagnosis Coding for Vaccinations and Immune Globulins

Vaccinations are reported with Z23 because there is no sign, symptom, or disease actually present. There is only one code to report vaccinations (Z23).

CASE 2-1 *Chart Note*

Mary Ann Roberts, a Medicare patient, presents for an influenza vaccination. A HCPCS National Level II administration code is used to report the vaccination of a Medicare patient.

Chart Note

LOCATION: Outpatient, Clinic
PATIENT: Mary Ann Roberts
PHYSICIAN: Alma Naraquist, MD

AGE: 72

COVERAGE: Medicare

Patient presents for administration of a trivalent IM (intramuscular) injection of split virus influenza vaccine, 0.5 mL administered by her nurse.

SERVICE CODE(S): _____

ICD-10-CM DX CODE(S): _____

(Answers to every other Case are located in Appendix D . The full answer key is only available in the TEACH Instructor Resources on Evolve.)

CASE 2-2   *Chart Note*

Gerald is a Medicare patient. Report the services provided by Dr. Naraquist's nurse.

Chart Note

LOCATION: Outpatient, Clinic

PATIENT: Gerald Parr

PHYSICIAN: Alma Naraquist, MD

AGE: 82

COVERAGE: Medicare

Patient presents for administration of a trivalent IM (intramuscular) injection of split virus influenza vaccine, 0.25 mL and a 23-valent pneumococcal vaccination administered by Dr. Naraquist's nurse.

SERVICE CODE(S): _____

ICD-10-CM DX CODE(S): _____

CASE 2-3   *Chart Note*

Use the CPT code for the administration and injection service for this non-Medicare patient. A Z code is assigned. There is a combination Z code for MMRV. There is only one administration; there are several substances in the one administration.

Chart Note

LOCATION: Outpatient, Clinic

PATIENT: Mindy O'Bright

PHYSICIAN: Rolando Ortez, MD

AGE: 10

Patient presents for administration of a subcutaneous injection of a combination injection of MMRV (measles, mumps, rubella, and varicella) that was ordered by Dr. Ortez and administered by Dr. Ortez's nurse.

SERVICE CODE(S): _____

ICD-10-CM DX CODE(S): _____

Hydration, (96360, 96361); and Therapeutic, Prophylactic, and Diagnostic Injections and Infusions (Excludes Chemotherapy and other Highly Complex Drug or Highly Complex Biologic Agent Administration) (96365-96379)

Codes 96360-96379 report the administration of drugs/substances for hydration and injection and infusion services other than chemotherapy. The physician's work related to these services usually involves the oversight of the treatment plan and staff supervision. When the physician provides a significant, separately identifiable E/M service, report the service with an appropriate E/M code and modifier -25. Sometimes third-party payers will require an E/M service provided on the same day as a hydration, injection, or infusion to have a different diagnosis than the condition for which the hydration, injection, or infusion is being provided, but that is not the case for reporting E/M services with these codes. However, modifier -25 must be added to the E/M code, or the E/M service will be thought to be related to the physician's service for the hydration, injection, or infusion service.

Bundled into the hydration, injection, and infusion services are local anesthesia, placing the intravenous line, accessing an indwelling access line/catheter/port, flushing at the end of the infusion, and all standard supplies.

Hydration

CPT codes 96360 and 96361 report intravenous hydration infusions that include the pre-packaged fluid and electrolytes (such as normal saline) for intravenous hydration infusion. These codes only include the administration and therefore the substance is always reported separately with a HCPCS National Level II code. If a substance other than pre-packaged fluid or electrolytes is infused, then codes 96360 and 96361 are not reported. Rather, the coder would assign Therapeutic, Prophylactic, and Diagnostic Infusion codes 96365-96371 (Intravenous and subcutaneous infusion), or 96379. The Hydration infusion codes include physician supervision and oversight of the staff providing the direct services. Code 96360 is reported for the first hour of intravenous infusion hydration service, and 96361 is used to report each additional hour. Each additional hour is defined as intervals greater than 30 minutes. Therefore, if a patient had 1 hour and 31 minutes of hydration, you would assign code 96360 for the first hour and 96361 for the additional 31 minutes. If the patient only had 1 hour and 30 minutes of hydration, you would only report 96360 because the additional minutes after the first hour were not greater than 30 minutes.

Therapeutic, Prophylactic, and Diagnostic Injections and Infusions (Excludes Chemotherapy and Other Highly Complex Drug or Highly Complex Biologic Agent Administration) (96365-96379)

Codes 96365-96379 are used to report the administration of a nonchemotherapy therapeutic, prophylactic, or diagnostic intravenous infusion or injection. Intravenous **infusions** are reported with 96365-96368 and are divided based on the time and type of infusion. The initial infusion is reported with 96365 (up to 1 hour) once per encounter, unless the protocol requires two different venous access sites, and each additional hour of the same drug/substance (up to 8 hours) with 96366. In order to report code 96366, there must be infusion intervals of greater than 30 minutes (up to 1 hour), beyond the initial 1-hour increment of infusion. Sometimes one infusion is provided followed by another infusion of a different drug/substance (sequential infusions). In this case, the initial infusion is reported first with 96365, and the additional sequential infusion is reported with add-on code 96367 for each separate infusate mix. When a sequential infusion runs for more than 1 hour, the CPT guidelines following code 96366 instruct you to report code 96366 for additional sequential hour(s). There are times when more than one infusion of a different drug/substance is provided at the same time, in which case the initial or sequential infusion is listed first, and then the additional **concurrent infusion** is listed (96368). Code 96368 can only be reported once per encounter. If multiple drugs are mixed together in the same bag, only one administration code can be reported, but all drugs should be billed separately.

Subcutaneous infusion for therapy is reported with codes 96369-96371. The initial subcutaneous infusion code 96369 reports up to 1 hour of infusion and includes the pump set-up and establishment of the site. Code 96370 is an add-on code that reports each additional hour, and 96371 is also an add-on code that reports an additional pump set-up with establishment of a new subcutaneous site.

Therapeutic, prophylactic, and diagnostic **injections** are divided based on the administration method. Subcutaneous and intramuscular injections are reported with 96372, along with a code to report the substance injected. For example, if 40 mg of Kenalog is injected subcutaneously, J3301 × 4 is reported for the substance, and 96372 is reported for the administration. You would not assign code 96372 to report subcutaneous or IM chemotherapy administration (see 96401-96402). Injections for allergen immunotherapy are reported with 95115-95117, not with therapeutic, prophylactic, or diagnostic injection codes. Intra-arterial injection is reported with 96373. Intravenous push is reported with 96374 and add-on codes 96375-96376. IV or intravenous push is defined as an infusion lasting 15 minutes or less or an injection in which the nurse is continually present to administer the injection and observe the patient. Code 96375 is used for additional IV pushes of different drugs/substances. Once again, all drugs are to be reported separately using HCPCS National Level II codes or CPT code 99070.

CASE 2-4   *Chart Note*

This is a Medicare patient.

Chart Note
LOCATION: Outpatient, Office
PATIENT: Connor Lunderquist
PHYSICIAN: Alma Naraquist, MD

AGE: 74
COVERAGE: Medicare
Therapeutic infusion of saline solution with pre-packaged 5% dextrose IV (intravenous) 500 mL (milliliter) for dehydration, lasting 50 minutes.

SERVICE CODE(S): _____

ICD-10-CM DX CODE(S): _____

CASE 2-5   *Chart Note*

Report the injection service for this Medicare patient using an HCPCS National Level II code to report the substance injected and a CPT code to report the intramuscular antibiotic injection.

Chart Note
LOCATION: Outpatient, Clinic
PATIENT: LuLu Busquet
PHYSICIAN: Alma Naraquist, MD

AGE: 81
COVERAGE: Medicare
Patient presents for an injection of tetracycline for an acute upper respiratory infection. She was seen in the clinic on Friday and returns on Tuesday after talking with Dr. Naraquist, who instructed the patient to come to the office for an injection. Dr. Naraquist's nurse administers an IM (intramuscular) injection of tetracycline, 200 mg (milligram).

SERVICE CODE(S): _____

ICD-10-CM DX CODE(S): _____

Psychiatry

A psychiatric diagnostic evaluation is an involved assessment to identify an emotional, developmental, or behavioral diagnosis and development of a treatment plan. The physician conducts an interview with the patient to collect information to establish the diagnosis and develop a treatment plan. The evaluation is reported with 90791 (evaluation) or 90792 (evaluation with medical service).

Psychotherapy is the therapeutic treatment of a psychological disorder or behavior and is reported with codes

90832-90838. The codes are time based (30, 45, or 60 minutes) and subdivided based on if the psychotherapy was provided in addition to another primary procedure. The medical record must identify the time spent providing the psychotherapy service. If the time spent providing the service is not recorded on the medical record, the physician should be queried. If no time can be identified, report the service with an E/M code, not a Psychotherapy code. The psychotherapy service may be provided to a patient and/or the patient's family member.

Crisis psychotherapy (90839, 90840) provides treatment to a patient experiencing an acute reaction to a more specific event or situation. For example, a drug overdose, attempted suicide, or an episode of severe depression. Crisis psychotherapy focuses on the immediate assessment and treatment of the patient in a crisis and is not intended to treat chronic psychological conditions.

The remainder of the codes in this subsection are for Other Psychotherapy (90845-90853) which describes psychoanalysis and individual, family, multiple-family, or group psychotherapy and Other Psychiatric Services or Procedures (90863-90899) which describes medication management, electroconvulsive therapy, biofeedback, hypnotherapy, evaluation of hospital records, consultation, and other services. Most of these codes are not time based, but several are, such as 90875, individual psychophysiological training.

For neuropsychological and cognitive, psychological, developmental, and neurobehavioral testing, you would use codes 96105-96146.

From the Trenches

"Because the coding profession is wide ranging and varied, it provides many opportunities to explore new areas, such as a new medical specialty or coding for facilities or physicians."

RACHEL E. BRIGGS
BA, CPC, CPMA, CENTC, CEMC

CASE 2-6   *Psychological Evaluation*

Joel Wall is an inpatient for whom Dr. Nelson provided an inpatient psychotherapy service. This is not a consultation.

Psychological Evaluation

LOCATION: Inpatient, Hospital

PATIENT: Joel Wall

PHYSICIAN: Jerome Nelson, MD

REASON FOR VISIT: Joel Wall is a 50-year-old right-handed gentleman who was seen for 65 minutes of interview and records review, in addition to 1.5 hours of testing, scoring, interpretation, and generation of documentation. He is being assessed primarily in regard to postconcussion syndrome.

HISTORY: The patient was involved in a motor vehicle accident on 04/07 of this year and sustained multiple injuries, including bilateral pulmonary contusions, bilateral pneumothorax, and multiple facial fractures, particularly on the left. He is currently on ventilation. The patient did have an alcohol level of .142 at the time of his admission. He has had some reactive depression. Reportedly, the patient has had several prior concussions and motor vehicle accidents. Previous medical history is also significant for chemical dependency treatment in 2000 and again in 2001. The patient had one prior hospitalization on the psychiatric unit last year with adjustment issues following the suicide of his daughter.

Previous medical history is also significant for rotator cuff repair 3 or 4 years ago. The patient is a chronic smoker at the rate of three packs a day. He has a history of borderline diabetes and hypertension. He has chronic arthritis and a history of peptic ulcer.

CURRENT MEDICATION: Mucomyst, albuterol, ipratropium, bacitracin, bisacodyl, Procrit, heparin, Mycostatin, PCS, morphine, Protonix, and Zosyn.

FAMILY HISTORY: Significant for heart disease in the patient's father who died at age 52; his mother died at age 65 from cardiovascular accident.

SOCIAL HISTORY: The patient lives in Manytown and is currently a widower. He has no surviving children, is a graduate of a 2-year vocational college in the East, and has completed military service.

INTERVIEW: The patient admits he feels somewhat reactively depressed; however, he states that this is nothing like the depression he had about 2 years ago. The patient states that this depression is primarily attributed to being laid off at his place of employment. He feels he is doing well with it. He does not have suicidal ideation. He states that several years ago he became a devoted Buddhist and that has been supportive for him during difficult times. He states that he could go home and stay with one of his nephews with whom he is close.

BEHAVIOR OBSERVATIONS: On interview, the patient is lying in his bed. He is on the ventilator and so has to communicate primarily by writing, which he does do quite efficiently. I do note, however, that the patient includes some extra letters or missequences his letters at times. When asked about this, the patient attributes it to not having his reading glasses. The patient is able to tell me about his accident, although we asked when it happened and he writes that it occurred "July 4"; and when asked whether he is sure about this, he insists that it is true and that it happened after he had been to the local theater to see an adventure show he had been looking forward to. He insists it was on July 4th. He seems surprised and embarrassed when told that, in fact, it happened in April. The patient states that prior to the accident he was actively employed as a carpenter and, when he had time, worked in the evenings and weekends as a painter.

TESTING: On testing, the patient is found to be alert, motivated, and cooperative. Good rapport was easily established. The patient was confident, relaxed, and focused. Of note is the fact that the patient was wearing wrist restraints, which did interfere slightly with some of the testing. The patient did not appear bothered by this. He displayed no difficulty with the comprehension or retention of test instructions. He was careful and reflective in his approach to testing tasks. Test results are believed to be a valid reflection of his current abilities.

The patient proves to be well oriented today (8/8). He has an excellent fund of personal and current information (6/6). He has excellent performance on a test of foresight and planning (Porteus Maze Test: 121/121). Immediate verbal span of concentration is average at 6 forward and 5 backward (50th percentile). Verbal block-tapping span is better yet at 6 forward and 6 backward (91st percentile).

Copying of simple figures is performed well (14/14), as is matching simple figures (4/4). Immediate memory for simple designs is average (58th percentile). After a delay, however, he is noted to lose one of the designs and invert another one. His recollection of the other two is as it was initially. With recognition cueing, he does well (3/4).

Learning of a 9-word categorized list (California Verbal Learning Test) reveals an identifiable learning curve (4, 6, 8, 9, 9). Introduction of a distractor list results in mild retroactive inhibitions (7/9), but the patient improves his performance with semantic cueing (8/9). After a delay he has retained this information. Semantic cueing is not helpful, but with recognition cueing, he is able to identify correctly all 9 of the 9 list items with no intrusive error.

The patient's response to the Beck Depression Inventory-II results in a score within the normal or nondepressed range (1/3). The patient relates only that he has less energy than he used to have. He denies feeling of dysphoria or sadness and denies any element of suicidal ideation.

IMPRESSION: Joel Wall was involved in a serious motor vehicle accident and received significant facial and upper-torso trauma; he also suffers from postconcussion syndrome. He has been on a ventilator and has had some reactive depression. Current testing would suggest that the patient is not experiencing significant depression at this time. From a cognitive standpoint, he seems to be doing quite well, and there is really minimal if any evidence of cognitive dysfunction.

I will work with Joel to help him with better understanding of the specific obstacles to his being discharged and any progress he might be making on these. When I spoke to him, he indicated that he had no idea of what the specific issues were and certainly had no sense of a timeline, which was a source of great frustration for him.

The patient also identifies that he has benefited from pastoral care from the local Buddhist monk, and hopefully they will be able to follow up with him on a regular basis to provide support.

SERVICE CODE(S): _____

ICD-10-CM DX CODE(S): _____

(Answers to every other Case are located in Appendix D . The full answer key is only available in the TEACH Instructor Resources on Evolve.)

Dialysis

Dialysis, cleansing of the blood, can be temporary or permanent, depending on the needs of the patient. End-stage renal disease (ESRD) is a condition from which the patient will not recover without a kidney transplant, so these patients require permanent dialysis support. Non-ESRD is a condition from which the patient may recover and needs dialysis support only temporarily.

The End Stage Renal Disease Services provided in the outpatient setting (90951-90962) are divided initially on the age of the patient and the number of visits in the 30-day period. These codes are used to report the physician portion of the dialysis service. The **monthly service** codes (90951-90962) cover all physician visits to the hemodialysis laboratory during that month to assess the patient while receiving hemodialysis as well as the establishment of a treatment plan (dialyzing cycle) and management of the patient during the month. Monthly service codes 90963-90966 cover all physician related services for home dialysis (peritoneal dialysis) during that full month of service. If less than a full month of service is provided to an ESRD patient in an outpatient setting, assign a code from code range 90967-90970 to report these per-day services.

Hemodialysis or other dialysis procedures are reported with 90935, 90937, 90945, or 90947 to report inpatient ESRD dialysis and inpatient non-ESRD dialysis. The codes are reported on the day of the dialysis procedure. If the physician provides EM services that are unrelated to dialysis, those services are reported separately by adding modifier -25 to the EM code.

Patients can be trained in self-dialysis, which can be performed at home (peritoneal dialysis). Training is reported with codes 90989 and 90993. Most third-party payers allow only one dialysis training course. If a patient is trained to receive peritoneal dialysis after receiving hemodialysis training or vice versa, documentation would need to be submitted to the third-party payer to support the additional dialysis training.

Hemodialysis is performed at the hospital as either an inpatient or outpatient procedure. The physician services are reported based on the **type** of dialysis the patient is receiving, the **complexity** of the service, and the **number** of visits the physician provides to the patient. As with all patients, dialysis patients must sometimes be admitted to the hospital for other medical problems, such as gallbladder disease, and while in the hospital must continue to receive dialysis treatments. When the physician provides an evaluation of the hemodialysis for an inpatient while the patient is receiving dialysis, you would report 90935 (single visit) or 90937 (multiple visits). The multiple visits are provided during the same dialysis session. Code 90937 requires repeated physician evaluations and may include a significant revision of the dialysis prescription. If a hospitalized patient receiving peritoneal dialysis is seen by the physician, the physician services are reported with 90945 (single visit) and 90947 (multiple visits). Code 90947 requires repeated physician evaluations and may include a significant revision of the dialysis prescription. Modifier -26 is not reported with dialysis codes to indicate the professional component of the service was provided because the code description already describes the physician service to the dialysis patient.

CASE 2-7 *Hemodialysis Progress Report*

The patient is seen in the dialysis unit, which is an outpatient unit. Report a Z/V code as the primary reason for the encounter followed by the ESRD diagnosis(es). The date of this service is the 30th day of services provided to this ESRD patient by Dr. Orbitz. Report the monthly ESRD service code (4+) for this 32-year-old patient.

Hemodialysis Progress Report

LOCATION: Outpatient, Hospital

PATIENT: Maryellen Menez

PHYSICIAN: George Orbitz, MD

This 32-year-old patient is seen, and I examined her hemodialysis chart. The patient appears to be hemodynamically stable and not in any form of respiratory distress or compromise. She is tolerating dialysis without any problems. Predialysis vital signs are noted. Blood pressure is 148/60, heart rate 58, respirations 16, temperature 36.3° C (Celsius), and today she weighs 62.7 kg (kilogram). Normocephalic and atraumatic. Pink palpebral conjunctivae, anicteric sclerae. No nasal or aural discharge. Moist tongue and buccal mucosa. No pharyngeal hyperemia, congestion, or exudate. Supple neck. No lymphadenopathy. Symmetrical chest. No retractions. No rhonchi, crackles, or wheezes. S1 (first heart sound) and S2 (second heart sound) are distinct. No S3 (third heart sound) or S4 (fourth heart sound). Regular rate and rhythm. Abdomen: Positive bowel sounds, soft and nontender. No laboratory tests are available today.

HEMODIALYSIS: Today we will dialyze her using her left-sided Perm-A-Cath for a total of 3 hours using an HP-150 dialyzer with a 2.0 potassium bath. Will give her a heparin loading dose of 2000 units and a maintenance dose of 1 mL (milliliter) per hour. Vital signs at present are stable. Blood pressure is 120/70, heart rate in the 70s, and she is tolerating a blood flow rate of 350 mL per minute.

ASSESSMENT/PLAN:

1. Chronic renal failure/end-stage renal disease (on maintenance hemodialysis Tuesday, Thursday, and Saturday), secondary to the following:
   a. Status post right-sided nephrectomy in 1996.
   b. Diabetes type 2.
   c. Diabetic nephropathy.
   d. Hypertension.
2. Multiple electrolyte abnormalities related to problem chronic renal failure/end-stage renal disease.
   a. Hyperphosphatemia. Continue Renagel and Phoslo.
   b. Hypocalcemia.
3. Hypothyroidism. Continue Synthroid.
4. Nutrition.
5. Analgesia.
6. Deconditioning.

At the end of the dialysis, we will give her a dose of Zemplar.

SERVICE CODE(S): _____

ICD-10-CM DX CODE(S): _____

Discussion

The physician provided 1 month of service with more than 4 encounters. Codes 90951-90962 are reported only once for each month of physician service and include patient management services and evaluations during that month. This 32-year-old patient was provided services for an entire month, and as such the physician's service is reported with 90960.

Diagnoses

The reason for the encounter was dialysis, and this is the first-listed (primary) diagnosis **(Z99.2)**.

Hypertension and Chronic Renal Failure

The Assessment/Plan section of the report indicates that the chronic renal failure is due to hypertension. When hypertension is present with renal failure (N18.-), the *Guidelines* direct the coder to assume a cause-and-effect relationship (the hypertension caused the kidney disease). Reference "hypertension" in the ICD-10-CM Index. The subterms "kidney, with, stage 5 chronic kidney disease (CKD) or end-stage renal disease (ESRD)" directs the coder to assign (I12.0) to report the hypertension and renal disease. The instructional note under I12.0 in the Tabular states that an additional code is to be assigned to report the stage of chronic kidney disease; therefore, a code from category N18 is also assigned for the chronic renal disease.

Diabetes

The next diagnosis is the diabetes, which also causes diabetic nephropathy.

ICD-10-CM Official Guidelines for Coding and Reporting

I.C.9.a.2. **Hypertensive Chronic Kidney Disease**. Assign codes from category I12, Hypertensive chronic kidney disease, when both hypertension and a condition classifiable to category N18, Chronic kidney disease (CKD), are present. CKD should not be coded as hypertensive if the provider indicates the CKD is not related to the hypertension.

The appropriate code from category N18 should be used as a secondary code with a code from category I12 to identify the stage of chronic kidney disease.

See Section I.C.14. Chronic kidney disease.

If a patient has hypertensive chronic kidney disease and acute renal failure, the acute renal failure should also be coded. Sequence according to the circumstances of the admission/encounter.

When referencing the Index under the main term "Diabetes" subterm "type 2, nephropathy," the coder is directed to E11.21. The Tabular indicates that the code is assigned to report "Type 2 diabetes mellitus with diabetic nephropathy."

Electrolyte Imbalance

The electrolyte imbalance is hyperphosphatemia and hypocalcemia reported with E83.39 and E83.51. It is not necessary to assign E87.8 for unspecified electrolyte imbalance.

The patient previously had a kidney removed, which is significant for this episode of care and is reported with **Z90.5**.

Peritoneal Dialysis

Peritoneal dialysis uses the **peritoneal cavity** as a filter. The dialysis fluid is introduced into the peritoneal cavity and left there for several hours as cleansing takes place, as illustrated in **Figure 2-1**. The fluid is then drained from the cavity. This dialysis service is reported on a full-month or per-day basis. Since patients do peritoneal dialysis at home every day alone, there is usually no physician service involved with the exception of the patients' monthly visit and labs that are drawn at the dialysis unit/clinic or unless a physician evaluation is required. In that case, the patient most likely would present to the office or be admitted to the hospital.

One of the risks of peritoneal dialysis is peritonitis, an infection of the peritoneal cavity. The treatment for the infection usually involves introduction of antibiotics into the peritoneal fluid, as you will see in the following case.

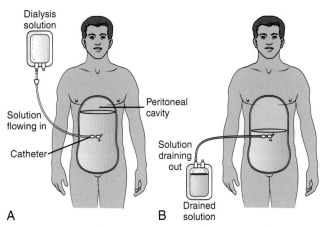

FIGURE 2-1 Peritoneal dialysis can be done by the patient. The dialysis solution enters the peritoneal cavity through a catheter. After the solution has remained within the patient for several hours, it is drained out through the catheter.

CASE 2-8A   *History and Physical Examination*

This patient has been receiving ambulatory peritoneal dialysis for several years. She has encountered a complication and is admitted to the hospital by Dr. Orbitz for treatment for the complication. The complication is the primary reason for the treatment. This patient has hypertensive renal disease, so review I.C.9.a.2. of the ICD-10-CM Official Guidelines for Coding and Reporting before assigning the diagnoses for this case.

LOCATION: Inpatient, Hospital

PATIENT: Grace Hargrove

PHYSICIAN: George Orbitz, MD

This 79-year-old woman is being admitted because of acute peritonitis due to peritoneal dialysis.

HISTORY OF PRESENT ILLNESS: This patient is a chronic ambulatory peritoneal dialysis patient who is currently on cycle PD (peritoneal dialysis) for 10 hours at night. She was started on dialysis last year and has been a model patient having done superbly with no episodes of peritonitis prior to now. Her husband died 6 months ago. Since then, she has had increasing depression and failure to thrive with decreased nutrition and of late has been complaining of 2/10 abdominal discomfort and/or bloating for the past few days. Her ESRD (end-stage renal disease) is multifactorial and/or idiopathic. She has a long history of hypertension. She also has coronary artery disease and history of an MI (myocardial infarction), CABG (coronary artery bypass graft) 3 years ago, and remote history of recurrent CHF (congestive heart failure). She also has hyperlipidemia and 4 years ago had a parathyroidectomy. She had a CVA (stroke/cardiovascular accident) 2 years ago, anemia of chronic disease, and degenerative arthritis. She is attended by her son.

SOCIAL HISTORY: She used to be a factory worker, currently retired. Catholic. Tenth-grade education. She was married for 58 years. She is a nonuser of alcohol, tobacco, or other medications. She has a remote history of smoking, 40-pack-a-year total.

FAMILY HISTORY: Positive for cardiovascular disease and complications thereafter, as well as cancer in the father with heart failure, who died at age 83.

MEDICATIONS: See Medications Admittance Record.

PHYSICAL EXAMINATION: Her lungs have decreased percussion note or dullness at the bases with decreased breath sounds. Some crackles, otherwise hyporesonant. PMI (point of maximal impulse) not well felt. Probably diffuse. Heart regular. She has no significant murmur at this time, rub, or S3 (third heart sound). Abdomen: Soft. Some discomfort diffusely. Fluid from the exit site looks okay. Extremities: No peripheral edema. No lateralizing neuro signs. Mental status normal. Skin: Normal. GYN (gynecology), breasts, and rectal exams deferred.

Fluid exam shows evidence of peritonitis. Her current hemoglobin is 9.7 as a result of cessation temporarily of Epogen.

CLINICAL IMPRESSION: Acute peritonitis resulting from peritoneal dialysis; end-stage renal failure due to hypertension.

OTHER DIAGNOSES: As above, including failure to thrive, recent depression because of the death of her husband, malnutrition with hypoalbuminemia, atherosclerotic heart disease, ASCVD (arteriosclerotic cardiovascular disease), etc.

SERVICE CODE(S): _____

ICD-10-CM DX CODE(S): _____

(Answers to every other Case are located in Appendix D . The full answer key is only available in the TEACH Instructor Resources on Evolve.)

Complications

Complications code assignment is based on the provider's documentation of the relationship between the condition and the procedure.

Reporting pain associated with devices, implants, or grafts is assigned a code from Chapter 19, Injury, Poisoning, and Certain Other Consequences of External Causes. Codes to report pain due to medical devices are located in the T code section. Use additional codes from category G89 to identify acute or chronic pain due to the presence of the device, implant, or graft.

Two codes are necessary to report a transplant complication, the appropriate code from category T86, Complications of transplanted organs and tissues, and a secondary code that identifies the complication.

Codes to report complications of pregnancy, abortion, labor, or delivery are located in Chapter 13, Pregnancy, childbirth, and the puerperium (O00-O9A). Complication codes that include the external cause do not require an additional external cause code.

Codes to report intraoperative and postoperative complication are located in the body system chapters with codes specific to organs and structures of that body system. These codes should be sequenced first, followed by a code for the specific complication, if applicable.

Let's look at an example of locating a complication in the Index of the ICD-10-CM. Using the diagnosis statement of "complication of intrauterine device causing excessive bleeding":

Contraception (ICD-10-CM)
  device (in situ) Z97.5
    causing menorrhagia T83.83--
or
Complications (ICD-10-CM)
  intrauterine, contraceptive device
    (subterms by type of complication)

CASE 2-8B   *CAPD Progress Note*

The complication is now being managed by means of antibiotics in the peritoneal fluid, so the complication diagnosis is now listed second and the hypertensive renal disease is listed first.

LOCATION: Inpatient, Hospital

PATIENT: Grace Hargrove

PHYSICIAN: George Orbitz, MD

CAPD PROGRESS NOTE: This patient with hypertensive end-stage renal disease was admitted and evaluated regarding her dialysis prescription. Because of her diagnosis of acute peritonitis due to peritoneal dialysis, the plan at this time is to use all of 1.5% Dianeal and 2-liter volumes and do CAPD (continuous ambulatory peritoneal dialysis) instead of cycler. The initial bag will contain antibiotic. The gent bag is next. Cultures are pending. We will proceed from there. The patient was evaluated after admission. She is empty at this point, and we have yet to place the first bag. Her abdomen is a little tender, and she is bloated. There is no doubt in my mind that we are seeing a developing peritonitis. The concern, of course, is the fact that she has been constipated and the worry is that this may represent a more serious colonic perforation.

SERVICE CODE(S): _____

ICD-10-CM DX CODE(S): _____

(Answers to every other Case are located in Appendix D . The full answer key is only available in the TEACH Instructor Resources on Evolve.)

CASE 2-8C   *Dialysis Progress Note*

The complication continues to be treated with antibiotics.

LOCATION: Inpatient, Hospital

PATIENT: Grace Hargrove

PHYSICIAN: George Orbitz, MD

DIALYSIS PROGRESS NOTE: The patient continues to be on peritoneal dialysis. She is doing well with that. She is using 1.5%. No ultrafiltration. In fact, ultrafiltration is negative. Her peritonitis seems to be doing better since she has no pain. Her appetite is better, and she is not having any more diarrhea.

Her vital signs are stable except that her pressure is a little high, 180s/90s. Temperature is 37° C (Celsius).

We will continue with antibiotic treatment and continue to watch her blood pressure. She has no edema right now and will continue to use 1.5%. We possibly could use 2.5% over the weekend.

The patient agrees with the plan. Will probably plan on discharging her on Monday.

SERVICE CODE(S): _____

ICD-10-CM DX CODE(S): _____

(Answers to every other Case are located in Appendix D . The full answer key is only available in the TEACH Instructor Resources on Evolve.)

CASE 2-8D   *Thoracic Medicine and CAPD Progress Note*

The infection is now known to be streptococcal, and as such this diagnosis must be added to the list of diagnoses for this patient. Place the code for the streptococcal infection immediately after the peritonitis code.

LOCATION: Inpatient, Hospital

PATIENT: Grace Hargrove

PHYSICIAN: George Orbitz, MD

THORACIC MEDICINE AND CRITICAL CARE PROGRESS NOTE: This is a CAPD (continuous ambulatory peritoneal dialysis) note. The patient is admitted for acute peritonitis with group A, not group D, streptococcal

peritonitis. She is getting her dialysis performed while she is here. She gets five exchanges in a day. She gets Kefzol 500 mg (milligram) in each dialyzing exchange. Also has gentamicin as dosed by pharmacy to each exchange, and she gets 2 liters of 1.5% 5 times a day. Abdomen today is still a little tender. She is, however, afebrile. We will make sure she has something for pain because she says it is somewhat uncomfortable. On reviewing her medications, she does not have anything ordered for pain, so I will make sure that she does.

SERVICE CODE(S): _____

ICD-10-CM DX CODE(S): _____

(Answers to every other Case are located in Appendix D . The full answer key is only available in the TEACH Instructor Resources on Evolve.)

CASE 2-8E   *Dialysis Progress Note*

The patient continues to receive treatment for the complication.

LOCATION: Inpatient, Hospital

PATIENT: Grace Hargrove

PHYSICIAN: George Orbitz, MD

THORACIC MEDICINE AND CAPD PROGRESS NOTE: The patient is in with acute peritonitis, group A streptococcus, and is undergoing peritoneal dialysis. The pain is less. She has only used 3 pain pills since yesterday. She remains afebrile. Abdomen is actually fairly benign on palpation today. The max temperature was 36.2° C (Celsius) in the last 24 hours. She has 5 exchanges in the day with CAPD (continuous ambulatory peritoneal dialysis), and we will not

change that. We used a 2-liter volume 1.5%, added Kefzol 500 mg (milligram) to each dialysis exchange, and then added gentamicin to be decided on by pharmacology. That will be done to each exchange. She has Tylenol no. 3 for pain, and it is controlling the pain fairly well.

No need to change anything at this point; dialysis is going fine. I do not need to change anything there. Her weight is stable, 129.3 pounds. It has been like that for 2 days now.

SERVICE CODE(S): _____

ICD-10-CM DX CODE(S): _____

(Answers to every other Case are located in Appendix D . The full answer key is only available in the TEACH Instructor Resources on Evolve.)

CASE 2-8F   *Dialysis Progress Note*

The patient is discharged from the hospital. The first-listed diagnosis continues to be the complication for which the admission was made.

LOCATION: Inpatient, Hospital

PATIENT: Grace Hargrove

PHYSICIAN: George Orbitz, MD

DIALYSIS PROGRESS NOTE: The patient had no more major events during the night. She has less pain. She is eating well. She denies any

complaints. She is tolerating peritoneal dialysis very well with 1.5%. Her vital signs are stable. She is afebrile at 36.5° C (Celsius). The plan is to send her home taking Kefzol. She will be discharged home today. Patient agrees with the plan.

SERVICE CODE(S): _____

ICD-10-CM DX CODE(S): _____

(Answers to every other Case are located in Appendix D . The full answer key is only available in the TEACH Instructor Resources on Evolve.)

CASE 2-8G *Discharge Summary*

LOCATION: Inpatient, Hospital

PATIENT: Grace Hargrove

PHYSICIAN: George Orbitz, MD

PRIMARY DIAGNOSIS: Acute peritonitis due to peritoneal dialysis.

SECONDARY DIAGNOSIS: End-stage renal disease, hypertensive, on chronic peritoneal dialysis for chronic renal failure.

HISTORY OF PRESENT ILLNESS: The patient is a 79-year-old white female who is known to have end-stage renal disease on CAPD (continuous ambulatory peritoneal dialysis).

HOSPITAL COURSE: She was admitted with abdominal pain and cloudy dialysate. She was found to have alpha streptococcal peritonitis. She was

given vancomycin, gentamicin, and Kefzol. The Group A strep was sensitive to cephalosporins. She did well during her hospitalization and felt better.

DISCHARGE PLAN: The patient will be discharged home today. Mario, from dialysis, will teach her how to add antibiotics to her peritoneal dialysis bags.

The patient agrees with the plan. She was advised to call us back if she has any more problems.

SERVICE CODE(S): _____

ICD-10-CM DX CODE(S): _____

Discussion

This is a short report, but it contains considerable diagnoses coding. The reason the patient received this care is primarily the complication of an infection from a catheter. The dialysis complication is, therefore, the first-listed diagnosis. Next, the complication led to peritonitis due to a streptococcal infection. The peritonitis is listed next, followed by the causative bacteria (streptococcal infection). The patient has hypertensive end-stage renal disease, which is why she is on CAPD. You assign a code from I12 (Hypertensive chronic kidney disease) when a condition classified to category N18 is present. Code N18 reports chronic kidney disease.

(Answers to every other Case are located in Appendix D . The full answer key is only available in the TEACH Instructor Resources on Evolve.)

Noninvasive Vascular Diagnostic Studies

Many of the codes in the Cardiovascular subsection (92920-93799) of Medicine are reviewed in Chapter 6, Cardiovascular System, because these codes predominantly refer to diagnostic and therapeutic services for heart conditions such as coronary thrombolysis, electrocardiogram, electrocardiography, cardiac catheterization, and electrophysiology. Noninvasive Vascular Diagnostic Studies codes (93880-93998) are used to report extracranial (outside the cranium) vascular studies, as well as vascular studies of the extremities, viscera, penis, etc. Noninvasive Vascular Diagnostic Studies codes include the supervision, interpretation, and written report of the results. Vascular flow analysis is the determination of the blood flow within arteries and veins. One analysis method used is a **duplex scan,** which uses ultrasound that bounces off the vessel and produces a color picture on a monitor showing the blood flow within veins and arteries. The duplex scan uses real-time and color-flow Doppler imaging to view the blood flow. Most of the codes within the Noninvasive Vascular Diagnostic Studies subsection are used to report services using a duplex scan. These scans are helpful in diagnosing a wide range of vascular diseases, such as varicose veins of the leg, which is a chronic venous disease. The duplex scan allows for the identification of a specific area(s) of restriction or blockage. **Cerebrovascular disease** is blockage of the arteries of the brain, which increases the risk of stroke. Cerebrovascular disease can be detected with transcranial Doppler (TCD) or carotid artery duplex scan; this is reported with 93880-93895. Subheading codes indicate the area of study, for example, cerebrovascular, renal, the extent of the study as bilateral (e.g., 93880), unilateral (e.g., 93882), complete (e.g., 93975), or limited (e.g., 93976). The subheadings of extremity study codes are arterial (93922-93931), venous (93970-93971), and arterial-venous hemodialysis access (93990).

Modifier -26 is added to the physician portion of these services to indicate that only the professional component of the service was provided.

CASE 2-9 *Duplex Carotid Artery Study*

The following arterial study was performed by a physician who specializes in vascular diseases for a 76-year-old female with suspected narrowing of the carotid artery, causing an increased heart rate.

LOCATION: Outpatient, Hospital

PATIENT: Elizabeth McConnell

REQUESTING PHYSICIAN: Alma Naraquist, MD

PHYSICIAN: Leslie Alanda, MD

CLINICAL SYMPTOMS: Rapid ventricular rate

DUPLEX CAROTID ARTERY TEST: Real-time (imaging) analysis: On the right side, there is a little "hard plaque" in the posterior wall of the internal carotid. On the left side, there is some hard plaque in the distal common carotid in the posterior wall.

CASE 2-9—cont'd

Doppler (flow) analysis is normal throughout both sides, indicating less than 50% stenosis. There is no spectral broadening, which if present, would indicate turbulence.

The vertebral arteries both show antegrade flow.

CONCLUSION: There is some atherosclerotic change, but it is not prominent.

SERVICE CODE(S): _____

ICD-10-CM DX CODE(S): _____

(Answers to every other Case are located in Appendix D . The full answer key is only available in the TEACH Instructor Resources on Evolve.)

Late Effects

Late effects codes are not assigned to a separate chapter in the Tabular. Instead, you must first identify a diagnosis as a late effect and then code it as such. You report late effects codes when the acute phase of the illness or injury has passed but a residual remains. Sometimes an acute illness or injury leaves a patient with a residual health problem that remains after the illness or injury has resolved.

A person cannot have both a current right hip fracture (S72.001A) and a late effect of the right hip fracture (S72.001S). The code is either a current injury or a condition caused by a prior injury; it cannot be both at the same time. (The only exception to this rule is in category I69, late effects of cerebrovascular disease, which is explained below.)

Codes from category I69 may be assigned on a health care record with codes from I60-I67 if the patient has a current cerebrovascular accident (CVA) and deficits from an old CVA. Assign code Z86.73, Personal history of transient ischemic attack (TIA), and cerebral infarction without residual deficits

(not a code from category I69) as an additional code for history of cerebrovascular disease when no neurologic deficits are present.

For example, using ICD-10-CM:

Diagnosis:	Dysphagia due to a previous cerebral infarct
Residual:	Dysphagia (The dysphagia is a problem that remains following the acute illness of the cerebral infarct.)
Cause:	Cerebral infarct (This patient had a previous cerebrovascular accident.)
Terms to code:	Dysphagia [residual], following, cerebrovascular disease, cerebral infarct [cause]. The late effect of cerebral infarct is reported with one code.

Locate the terms "Dysphagia, cerebrovascular disease, cerebral infarct," and you will be directed to I69.391, which reports both the residual and the cause in one code.

CASE 2-10   *Duplex Carotid Artery Study*

This patient has late effects (hemiparalysis and aphasia) of a cerebrovascular accident (stroke). These late effects are the reason for the encounter.

LOCATION: Outpatient, Hospital

PATIENT: Larry Smith

EXAMINATION OF: Duplex carotid artery outpatient study

CLINICAL SYMPTOMS: Previous stroke with right hemiparesis and aphasia.

ORDERING PHYSICIAN: Ronald Green, MD

PHYSICIAN: James Noonar, MD

DUPLEX CAROTID ARTERY STUDY: The patient is a 30-year-old male who suffered a massive stroke 1 month ago and has resultant right hemiparesis and aphasia.

Real-time (imaging) analysis: On the right side, there is some soft plaque on the anterior wall of the distal bulb/proximal internal carotid. On the

left side, there is soft plaque on the anterior wall of the bulb and on the anterior and posterior walls of the internal carotid.

Doppler (flow) analysis: On the right side, the peak systolic velocity of the internal carotid artery is 1.42 m/sec, indicating 50% to 75% stenosis. Peak diastolic velocity is 0.27, indicating a less than 50% stenosis, and the IC/CC ratio is 1.31. There is slight spectral broadening.

On the left side, we get extremely low velocities and then a "thud," indicating occlusion just downstream from the scanning area.

The vertebral arteries both show antegrade flow.

CONCLUSION: There is some stenosis on the right side. The left side implies occlusion distal to the area scanned. This would certainly fit with the above symptoms.

SERVICE CODE(S): _____

ICD-10-CM DX CODE(S): _____

(Answers to every other Case are located in Appendix D . The full answer key is only available in the TEACH Instructor Resources on Evolve.)

CASE 2-11   *Arterial Doppler Test*

The patient is a diabetic with pain in the left leg. The physician orders a Doppler arterial analysis (not a duplex scan) in which ultrasound is used to analyze the vessels.

LOCATION: Outpatient, Hospital

PATIENT: Gary Kettle

REQUESTING PHYSICIAN: Alma Naraquist, MD

PHYSICIAN: Leslie Alanda, MD

CLINICAL SYMPTOMS: Diabetes, pain in left leg

ARTERIAL DOPPLER TEST: The patient is a 72-year-old with diabetes and pain in the left leg.

The results of this limited bilateral study are abnormal. On the right side, despite normal ankle-to-brachial index at 1.22, the waveforms are monophasic. The digital pressure is only 70 for an index of 0.5. I believe there is disease in this leg throughout, but more distally than proximally.

In the left leg, the waveforms are even more abnormal. Again, an ankle-to-brachial index of 1.3 is erroneous due to calcified vessels. Waveforms are severely monophasic distally. The digital pressure is only 12 for an index of 0.09, which indicates severe ischemia.

CONCLUSION: I believe there is probably disease in both legs, but it is quite severe on the left, which would explain the pain. The disease level on the left would appear to be proximal to the popliteal and perhaps very proximal.

SERVICE CODE(S): _____

ICD-10-CM DX CODE(S): _____

(Answers to every other Case are located in Appendix D . The full answer key is only available in the TEACH Instructor Resources on Evolve.)

CASE 2-12   *Vascular Laboratory Report, Arterial Doppler Test*

Report Dr. Noonar's service.

LOCATION: Outpatient, Hospital

PATIENT: Ilene Sogla

ORDERING PHSYCIAN: Ronald Green, MD

PHYSICIAN: James Noonar, MD

INDICATION: Leg pain

The patient is a 65-year-old female with known coronary artery disease. She complains of some pain with walking.

She exercised for 5 minutes at 2 miles an hour at 10% grade. The resting ankle-to-brachial index is 1.23 on the right and left. The brachial pressure went up from 115 to 130. The right ankle pressure dropped minimally from 142 to 132, and the left ankle pressure remains stable.

CONCLUSION: There may be trivial arterial insufficiency, but nothing impressive here.

SERVICE CODE(S): _____

ICD-10-CM DX CODE(S): _____

(Answers to every other Case are located in Appendix D . The full answer key is only available in the TEACH Instructor Resources on Evolve.)

Cardioversion

Cardioversion is the restoration of the heart to normal rhythm. The electrical conversion of an arrhythmia may be performed externally by placing the paddles on the chest or internally by opening the chest and exposing the heart to the view of the surgeon with paddles being placed directly on the heart. The cardioversion codes are designated "separate procedure" and are reported only when the cardioversion is the only procedure performed. A cardiologist usually performs an elective cardioversion as a treatment for arrhythmia. You will be coding another cardioversion case in Chapter 6, Cardiovascular System.

From the Trenches

"A successful coder is well organized and able to absorb a significant amount of information in a short amount of time."

RACHEL E. BRIGGS

BA, CPC, CPMA, CENTC, CEMC

CASE 2-13 *Electrical Cardioversion*

Report the cardioversion provided by Dr. Elhart.

LOCATION: Inpatient, Hospital

PATIENT: Rick Eck

PREOPERATIVE DIAGNOSIS: Atrial flutter

POSTOPERATIVE DIAGNOSIS: Atrial flutter

PROCEDURE PERFORMED: Electrical cardioversion

SURGEON: Gary Sanchez, MD

PRIMARY PHYSICIAN: Ronald Green, MD

CONSULTING PHYSICIAN: Marvin Elhart, MD

BRIEF HISTORY: This is a 59-year-old patient with respiratory failure and on a ventilator. He was noted to have supraventricular tachycardia in the form of atrial flutter. Cardioversion was recommended. The patient is already anticoagulated. He has a low risk for embolization. Indication for cardioversion is to improve his hemodynamics and

control his rate. The procedure was explained to the wife, and she consents to it.

PROCEDURE: The patient was sedated with Versed and morphine. He was given a total of 5 mg (milligram) Versed. He was cardioverted with 50 joules into sinus tachycardia.

The patient was given 20 mcg (microgram) Cardizem IV (intravenous) push. His heart rate went down to 110s, and he was definitely in sinus tachycardia.

CONCLUSION: Successful electrical cardioversion of atrial flutter into sinus tachycardia.

PLAN: The patient will need to have his rate and blood pressure controlled. A Cardizem drip is an excellent choice until the patient can take p.o. (by mouth). He needs to have his TSH (thyroid stimulating hormone) and T_4 (thyroxine) levels assessed.

SERVICE CODE(S): _____

ICD-10-CM DX CODE(S): _____

(Answers to every other Case are located in Appendix D . The full answer key is only available in the TEACH Instructor Resources on Evolve.)

Ultrasound

Diagnostic ultrasound is the use of high-frequency sound waves to image anatomic structures and to detect the cause of illness and disease. It is used by the physician in the diagnosis process. Ultrasound moves at different speeds through tissue, depending on the density of the tissue. Forms and outlines of organs can be identified by ultrasound as the sound waves move through or bounce back (echo) from the tissues.

The ultrasound codes for heart and vessels are located in the Medicine section; all other ultrasound codes are located

in the Radiology section. Codes for ultrasound procedures are found in 3 locations:

■ Radiology section, Diagnostic Ultrasound subsection, 76506-76999, divided on the basis of the anatomic location of the procedure (chest, pelvis)

■ Medicine section, Non-Invasive Vascular Diagnostic Studies subsection, 93880-93990, divided on the basis of the anatomic location of the procedure (cerebrovascular, extremity)

■ Medicine section, Echocardiography (ultrasound of the heart and great arteries), 93303-93355

CASE 2-14 *Ultrasound, Lower Extremities*

Report the ultrasound service provided by Dr. Monson.

LOCATION: Outpatient, Hospital

PATIENT: Dennis Hooperman

REQUESTING PHYSICIAN: Alma Naraquist, MD

PHYSICIAN: Morton Monson, MD

EXAMINATION OF: Ultrasound of both lower extremities

CLINICAL SYMPTOMS: Bilateral edema

ULTRASOUND OF BOTH LOWER EXTREMITIES: FINDINGS: Ultrasound examination of the deep venous system of the lower extremities shows

no evidence of a deep venous thrombosis. Bilateral posterior tibial, greater saphenous, popliteal, and femoral veins are patent with no evidence of thrombus. The distal portion of both superficial femoral veins is not well seen because of patient body habitus but shows no gross evidence of DVT (deep vein thrombosis).

SERVICE CODE(S): _____

ICD-10-CM DX CODE(S): _____

(Answers to every other Case are located in Appendix D . The full answer key is only available in the TEACH Instructor Resources on Evolve.)

Codes Reviewed Elsewhere

Many of the codes in the Medicine section are reviewed elsewhere in this text because the codes are best studied in the specialties within which they are most often used. As with all codes within the CPT, any physician can report any code, but most often the codes are applicable to

specialty areas of practice, and therefore the following codes are presented in other chapters of the text as follows:

■ Gastroenterology codes 91010-91299, Chapter 7, Digestive System, Hemic/Lymphatic System, and Mediastinum/ Diaphragm

- Ophthalmology codes 92002-92499 and Special Otorhinolaryngologic Services 92502-92700, Chapter 13, Eye and Auditory Systems
- Pulmonary codes 94002-94799, Chapter 9, Respiratory System
- Endocrinology codes 95250-95251, Chapter 10, Urinary, Male Genital, and Endocrine Systems
- Neurology and Neuromuscular Procedures 95700-96020, Chapter 12, Nervous System
- Special Dermatological Procedures 96900-96999, Chapter 5, Integumentary System
- Qualifying Circumstances for Anesthesia add-on codes (99100-99140) and Sedation with or without Analgesia (Moderate [Conscious] Sedation) 99151-99157, Chapter 14, Anesthesia

Central Nervous System Assessments/ Tests (e.g., Neurocognitive, Mental Status, Speech Testing)

The codes in the Central Nervous System Assessment/Tests (96105-96146) are used to identify psychological testing, speech/language assessments, developmental progress assessments, and thinking/reasoning status examination (neurobehavioral). The codes are reported based on a per-hour basis except for the basic developmental assessments. The physician or other health care provider would interpret the test results and provide a written report of the assessment.

Cognitive (thinking) processes are assessed with a variety of testing instruments, such as MMPI (Minnesota Multiphasic Personality Inventory), which is an assessment of personality types. The Rorschach is an assessment in which inkblots are shown to the patient and the patient is asked to describe what he or she sees in the image.

Developmental testing is used to assess the psychomotor or cognitive abilities by means of assessment instruments such as the Early Language Milestone Screen or the Bayley Scales of Infant Development. Neurobehavioral status is an assessment of the thinking and reasoning abilities of the patient, for example, an elderly patient with Alzheimer's.

Dementia

Primary dementia is the most common type of dementia. It is a progressive disease that results in damage to neurons and is usually fatal within 3–20 years. There are many causes, such as infection, metabolic disorders, lesions, vascular disorders, toxins, and infarction. The symptoms are impaired memory, thinking, and behavior. There is no cure, only treatment of the symptoms. Secondary dementia (caused by another condition, and also known as nutritional degenerative disease) results from a deficiency of B vitamins, niacin, and pantothenic acid associated with alcoholism.

Let's take a look at how to report the diagnosis of "Alzheimer's with behavior disturbances" using ICD-10-CM:

Dementia
Alzheimer's type—*see* Disease, Alzheimer's
Disease
Alzheimer's G30.9 *[F02.80]*
with behavioral disturbance G30.9 *[F02.81-]*

The Index directs the coder to reference G30.9 and F02.81- in the Tabular, which displays the following:

G30	**Alzheimer's disease**
i	**Includes**: Alzheimer's dementia senile and presenile forms

Use additional code, if applicable, to identify:
dementia with behavioral disturbance (F02.81-)
dementia with anxiety (F02.84, F02.A4, F02.B4, F02.C4)
dementia with behavioral disturbance (F02.81-, F02.A1-, F02.B1-, F02.C1-)
dementia with mood disturbance (F02.83, F02.A3, F02.B3, F02.C3)
dementia with psychotic disturbance (F02.82, F02.A2, F02.B2, F02.C2)
dementia without behavioral disturbance (F02.80, F02.A0, F02.B0, F02.C0)
mild neurocognitive disorder due to known physiological condition (F06.7-)
Excludes1: senile degeneration of brain NEC (G31.1)
senile dementia NOS (F03)
senile NOS (R41.81)

G30.0 Alzheimer's disease with early onset

G30.1 Alzheimer's disease with late onset

G30.8 Other Alzheimer's disease

G30.9 Alzheimer's disease, unspecified

The Index directed you to report G30.9 followed by F02.81, and note that the Tabular note at G30 also directs the coder to "Use additional code, if applicable, to identify: dementia with behavior disturbances" with F08.81-. The Tabular indicates that F02.818 is to be reported with " . . . other diseases classified elsewhere . . .," which indicates the F02.818 is listed after the Alzheimer's code.

F02.81	*Dementia in other diseases classified elsewhere, unspecified severity, with behavioral disturbance*
F02.811	*Dementia in other diseases classified elsewhere, unspecified severity, with agitation*

Dementia in other diseases classified elsewhere, unspecified severity, with aberrant motor behavior such as restlessness, rocking, pacing, or exit-seeking

---

Dementia in other diseases classified elsewhere, unspecified severity, with verbal or physical behaviors such as profanity, shouting, threatening, anger, aggression, combativeness, or violence
Major neurocognitive disorder in other diseases classified elsewhere, unspecified severity, with aberrant motor behavior such as restlessness, rocking, pacing, or exit-seeking
Major neurocognitive disorder in other diseases classified elsewhere, unspecified severity, with verbal or physical behaviors such as profanity, shouting, threatening, anger, aggression, combativeness, or violence

F02.818 Dementia in other diseases classified elsewhere, unspecified severity, with other behavioral disturbance
Dementia in other diseases classified elsewhere with sleep disturbance, social disinhibition, or sexual disinhibition
Major neurocognitive disorder in other diseases classified elsewhere with sleep disturbance, social disinhibition, or sexual disinhibition
Use Additional code, if applicable, to identify wandering in dementia in conditions classified elsewhere (Z91.83)

If the dementia is stated without any underlying condition, such as "senile dementia," only the code for the dementia is reported (F03, Unspecified dementia).

CASE 2-15 *Cognitive Function Assessment*

Report Dr. Shongo's service.

LOCATION: Outpatient, Clinic

Dr. Leslie Alanda refers Sam Kaiser, an 83-year-old male patient with suspected dementia, to Dr. Fred Shongo for an assessment. The physician administered a battery of written and oral neurobehavioral tests to assess Sam's memory (cognitive function) that took 2 hours to complete. The diagnosis was stated as senile dementia with depression.

SERVICE CODE(S): _____
ICD-10-CM DX CODE(S): _____

Health Behavior Assessment and Intervention

The prevention, treatment, or management of a health problem that requires an assessment of psychological, behavioral, emotional, thinking, or social factors is reported with codes 96156-96171. An acute or chronic illness or prevention of an illness or maintenance of the patient's health is associated with the use of these codes.

Codes 96156-96171 are for services provided to patients who have an established illness or symptom and do not have symptoms or an established diagnosis of mental illness. The Health Behavior Assessment and Intervention codes are not used instead of Preventive Medicine Services, Counseling, and/or Risk Reduction Intervention (99401-99404) from the E/M section. The E/M codes are used to report services to a patient without symptoms or an established illness.

CASE 2-16 *Behavior Assessment*

Report Dr. Shongo's service.

LOCATION: Outpatient, Clinic

Dr. Alma Naraquist referred Beth Roy, a 13-year-old female patient, to Dr. Fred Shongo, a psychiatrist, for a behavior assessment regarding her chronic nail biting. She bites the nails until they bleed and further aggravates the situation by picking at the cuticles. Dr. Naraquist has treated the chronic infection present on Beth's fingers and asks Dr. Shongo to assess Beth's behavioral condition. Dr. Shongo provides an initial assessment of 45 minutes and schedules Beth to return the following week.

SERVICE CODE(S): _____
ICD-10-CM DX CODE(S): _____

Chemotherapy Administration (96401-96549)

Chemotherapy may be administered by several methods:
- **Subcutaneous** or **intramuscular** injection of a hormonal or non-hormonal anti-neoplastic.
- **Intralesional** or direct injection into a lesion.
- Intravenous or intra-arterial **push** (quick administration by forcing medication into the veins or arteries).
- Intravenous or intra-arterial **infusion** (administration over a long period, based on the time it takes to complete the infusion, e.g., 1, 2–8, or 9+ hours).
- Insertion into the **pleural cavity.**
- Insertion into the **peritoneal cavity.**
- **CNS** administration (e.g., intrathecal).
- **Subarachnoid** or **intraventricular** administration by means of a subcutaneous reservoir.

The medical record will indicate the method used for administration of the medicine, which will direct the choice of codes to report the service. Chemotherapy Administration codes (96401-96549) report only the **administration** and do not include the drug or an office service. If the patient requires a separate E/M code to report a significant office service in addition to the administration, the service is reported with modifier -25 (Significant, Separately

CASE 2-17   *Infusion*

Assign the diagnosis code, CPT code, plus the HCPCS National
Level II code for the drug.

SERVICE CODE(S): _____

ICD-10-CM DX CODE(S): _____

LOCATION: Outpatient, Clinic

Pat Strand is a 40-year-old patient with multiple myeloma. She
presents for 50 minutes of infusion of carmustine (100 mg [milligram])
chemotherapy administration.

(Answers to every other Case are located in Appendix D . The full answer key is only available in the TEACH Instructor Resources on Evolve.)

Identifiable Evaluation and Management Service by the Same
Physician or Other Qualified Health Care Professional on the
Same Day of the Procedure or Other Service). The provision
of the chemotherapy **agent** is reported separately with the
appropriate HCPCS National Level II J code(s).

If the patient is given an additional medication such as an
analgesic or antiemetic before or after chemotherapy, also report
the administration of the medication based on the method
of administration and the drug(s) reported with a HCPCS
National Level II J code (based on the type of medication).

The chemotherapy codes (96440-96549) are for services
such as refilling and maintaining portable and implantable
chemotherapy pumps or central nervous system, pleural, and
peritoneal cavity administration.

Diagnosis Coding for Chemotherapy

There are also encounter codes for chemotherapy (Z51.11)
and radiotherapy (Z51.0). When coding an encounter for
chemotherapy or radiotherapy, code the Z code first, followed
by the active code for the malignant neoplasm, even if that
neoplasm has already been removed. As long as the neoplasm
is being treated with adjunctive therapy following a surgical
removal of the cancer, you can code that neoplasm as if it still
exists. You would not assign a "history of" Z code, because
the neoplasm is the reason for the treatment. Instead, the
neoplasm is coded as a current or active disease.

Photodynamic Therapy

Photodynamic therapy (PDT) is a medical procedure in
which a photosensitive (light-activated) drug is injected,
infused, or applied to an area, as illustrated in **Figure 2-2**. The
drug accumulates in the diseased tissue at a higher rate than
the surrounding nondiseased tissue. Targeted irradiation of
the tissue is then administered with laser.

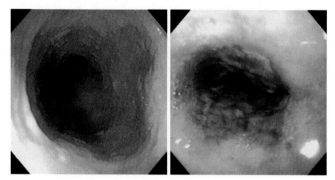

F I G U R E 2 – 2 Photodynamic therapy.

Porfimer sodium (Photofrin®, J9600, 75 mg) is a light-
sensitive drug that is used in PDT for esophageal cancer or
lung cancer. The drug is administered in a two-stage process.
In the first stage the drug is injected, and approximately
40 hours later the laser is applied. The second stage of the
procedure is performed through an esophagoscopy tube for
esophageal cancer and a bronchoscopy tube for lung cancer.
The procedure would be reported separately as:

31641	Bronchoscopy, with destruction of tumor
J9600 × 2	Photosensitive drug (Porfimer sodium 150 mg)
96570	Endoscopic application of laser (96570 [first 30 minutes] and 96571 [each additional 15 minutes])

Verteporfin (Visudyne®, J3396, 0.1 mg) is a light-activated
drug used to destroy lesions that occur as a result of age-
related macular degeneration. Fluorescein angiogram is
used to determine the extent of the degeneration and
demonstrate the medical necessity of the photodynamic
treatment(s). Verteporfin is intravenously injected, and laser
light is directed into the patient's eye(s) for about 90 seconds.
The injection of the drug is adequate for treatment of both

CASE 2-18   *Photodynamic Therapy*

LOCATION: Outpatient, Clinic

Dr. Barton provided service for Donna Sinne who has actinic
keratosis on her lip. The treatment provided entails 3 phototherapy
exposures over the course of several weeks using a 354-mg (milligram)

single-unit dose of aminolevulinic acid HCL during each session.
Report todays therapy only.

SERVICE CODE(S): _____

ICD-10-CM DX CODE(S): _____

(Answers to every other Case are located in Appendix D . The full answer key is only available in the TEACH Instructor Resources on Evolve.)

eyes. The procedure is reported with a code such as 67221 (Destruction of choroid lesion).

Aminolevulinic acid HCL (Levulan® Kerastick®, J7308, 354 mg) is a photosensitive topical drug used to treat nonhyperkeratotic actinic keratosis. Nonhyperkeratotic actinic keratosis is a cutaneous growth that may develop into squamous cell carcinoma. It is caused by excessive exposure to the sun and usually occurs in the middle-aged or elderly, especially those with fair skin. As a treatment for this condition, the photosensitive drug is applied, then blue light is delivered to the area approximately 16 hours later. The service is reported with a code such as 96567 (PDT, external application). Code 96567 is reported only once per day, for any number of PDT sessions provided.

Physical Medicine and Rehabilitation (97010-97799)

A physician or a therapist can report the Physical Medicine and Rehabilitation codes. Rehabilitation uses a variety of modalities for treatment (whirlpool, electrical stimulation).

Services are usually reported based on the time spent in the session. Unit coding (e.g., code × 2) is frequently used. For those services reported based on time, the time must be documented in the medical record.

Codes 97161-97164 are used to report a physical therapy evaluation or re-evaluation. The physician or physical therapist examines the patient and provides an assessment of the current status of the patient in the area or areas requested. This would include a prognosis and plan for interventional physical therapy that would improve the condition.

The codes in the Modalities category (97010-97028) specify that the provider does not need to be in constant attendance to report the service. For example, the provider may place hot packs (97010) on the patient's lower back and leave the treatment room to attend to other patients. The Constant Attendance category requires the provider to be in direct contact during the entire session. An example is a contrast bath (in which the patient is placed into a hot tub and then a cold tub for contrasting temperatures). For this service, the provider must be in attendance

CASE 2-19 *Physical Therapy Evaluation*

The patient presents for an after visit following musculoskeletal surgery; therefore, a Z code will be the first-listed diagnosis.

LOCATION: Outpatient, Rehabilitation Clinic

Nikki Fire is referred to the local rehabilitation center by her family physician for a physical therapy evaluation after a knee repair. Nikki has degenerative

osteoarthritis. The rehabilitation physician provided the evaluation, and a written report was developed. A total of 20 minutes was spent with patient. Report the rehabilitation physician's evaluative services.

SERVICE CODE(S): _____

ICD-10-CM DX CODE(S): _____

(Answers to every other Case are located in Appendix D . The full answer key is only available in the TEACH Instructor Resources on Evolve.)

CASE 2-20A *Physical Therapy Evaluation*

The following is a full-length physical therapy evaluation for which you are to report Dr. Barneswell's service. This is not a consultation, but a physical therapy evaluation. A Z code for the physical therapy is reported as the first-listed diagnosis, because that is the primary reason the patient is being evaluated. Next listed would be the quadriplegia.

LOCATION: Outpatient, Clinic

PATIENT: Terra Benson

REFERRING PHYSICIAN: Ronald Green, MD

PHYSICIAN: Mary Barneswell, MD

DIAGNOSIS: Congenital cerebral palsy spastic quadriplegia with intrathecal baclofen pump.

SUBJECTIVE: Terra is referred to Physical Therapy for evaluation for a session of intensive summer programming. The patient has participated in the summer programming in the past, and both the patient and her mother state that she has benefited from this programming, particularly in the area of balance. Terra states that at the time of her first summer session she was unable to sit independently on the toilet, and following the summer session, she has been able to sit independently on the toilet. The patient states that she uses both a

power and manual wheelchair for transportation. Her mother states that they switch on and off which one they use. Her mother is with her quite a bit of the time to assist her with activities. The patient is a 10th grader this year at Mother of Hope School. The patient states that she is not receiving any physical therapy programming at school. They are also not performing any type of home exercise program at this time. Both the patient and her mother state that both sitting balance and tightness of the adductor musculature are their primary concerns at this time. Patient/Family goal: Both the patient and her mother state that they would like to increase Terra's sitting balance.

OBJECTIVE: Observation: Terra does demonstrate a windswept posture to the right, indicating weakness of the left gluteal musculature compared to the right.

Range of Motion: Ankle dorsiflexion on the left is to the neutral position. The patient does report that she did have an injury to that leg a few weeks ago, which may be causing some decrease in the range of motion. On the right, ankle dorsiflexion is to 10 degrees. Straight leg raise bilaterally is 90 degrees. Internal and external rotation of the hips is within normal limits bilaterally. Abduction bilaterally is to 30 degrees passively.

Manual Muscle Testing: Strength of the lower extremities, including hip flexion, knee extension, and knee flexion, is 2/5; the patient is not able to move her extremity through the full range of motion. Hip flexion on the

Continued

CASE 2-20A—cont'd

right is at 1/5; the patient does elicit a muscle contraction but is not able to move the lower extremity against gravity.

Mobility: The patient transfers from her wheelchair to a mat with maximal assistance of her mother. It has been noted in the past that the patient was able to transfer from the wheelchair to the mat; however, she did require maximal assistance on this date. The patient is able to roll from supine to side-lying with minimal assistance. She transitions from a supine to sitting position with maximal assistance. She also transitions from sitting to standing with maximal assistance and with maximal assistance to remain standing.

Balance: The patient's balance was tested in a seated position. In short sitting, the patient is able to resist balance disturbances; however, she has some difficulty when trying to balance without the use of upper extremities for support. The patient particularly struggles with balance if an anterior balance disturbance is given. In long sitting, the patient is able to maintain the long-sit position with use of upper extremities for supports.

ASSESSMENT: The patient presents to physical therapy with decreased balance reactions, some decrease in range of motion of the lower extremities, and decrease in pelvic stabilization musculature, particularly on the left side. I believe this patient would benefit from a physical therapy program to adjust these issues. Goals for this patient include (1) that the patient's passive hip abduction will increase by 5 degrees for increased motion for daily activities; (2) that the patient will be able to maintain balance on a dynamic surface times 10 seconds without the use of upper extremities for increased balance; (3) that the patient's pelvic stability will be increased through activity such as tall kneeling and bridges, which will also help to improve her balance reaction; (4) that the patient will reach for rings while maintaining balance on a dynamic surface successfully on 8/10 trials.

PLAN: We will plan to see this patient two times a week for the summer programming utilization at dynamic surface to help encourage balance reactions. The patient may also be progressed into a home-exercise program for increased strengthening of the pelvic stabilizers. Thank you for this referral.

SERVICE CODE(S): _____

ICD-10-CM DX CODE(S): _____

(Answers to every other Case are located in Appendix D . The full answer key is only available in the TEACH Instructor Resources on Evolve.)

CASE 2-20B   *Physical Therapy Evaluation*

Terra presents to the Orthotics Department to be fitted with an ankle-foot orthotic. Report the orthotic fitting only.

LOCATION: Outpatient, Clinic

PATIENT: Terra Benson

REFERRING PHYSICIAN: Ronald Green, MD

PHYSICIAN: Mary Barneswell, MD

ORTHOTICS TECHNICIAN: Carl Enerson

DIAGNOSIS: Cerebral palsy with inversion tone, left ankle.

Terra was originally seen in our department 4 weeks ago on Tuesday, as per Dr. Barneswell's order for an AFO (ankle-foot orthosis). At that time, a negative impression of Terra's lower-left leg was obtained for the fabrication of the brace. Terra returned today to get fitted in her new AFO and appeared rather relaxed while casting, resulting in a neutral casting position. For optimal results, the brace is fabricated in 2 degrees of dorsiflexion and trimmed in a leaf-spring style posterior to the malleolus to afford a flexible brace. The foot portion of the brace terminates distal to her toes. The patient's leg was securely held in place with one proximal tibial Velcro strap. The patient's presenting footwear worked well in combination with the AFO. Overall fit was excellent.

The family is aware of the signs of skin irritation. Terra's improvement and function will be monitored through Dr. Barneswell. This fitting took 30 minutes. If any questions arise, please feel free to contact us at the Orthotics Department.

SERVICE CODE(S): _____

ICD-10-CM DX CODE(S): _____

(Answers to every other Case are located in Appendix D . The full answer key is only available in the TEACH Instructor Resources on Evolve.)

CASE 2-20C   *Physical Therapy Evaluation*

Dr. Green decides that Terra would benefit from a physical therapy program based on the initial assessment performed by Dr. Barneswell. Dr. Barneswell conducts a complete re-evaluation prior to the beginning of Terra's therapy program.

LOCATION: Outpatient, Clinic

PATIENT: Terra Benson

REFERRING PHYSICIAN: Ronald Green, MD

PHYSICIAN: Mary Barneswell, MD

SUBJECTIVE: Terra was referred for direct physical therapy on a twice-weekly basis to increase lower-extremity range of motion, and strength, and to increase weight-bearing tolerance, and for assisted transfer training. Programming should include therapeutic pool, if available. Terra recently underwent multiple orthopedic procedures at the Manytown Children's Hospital, including femoral derotation osteotomy on the left, bilateral rectus femoris lengthening, phenol injection, and two left hip adductor tendons. She returned to see Dr. Almaz last Monday to have a recheck appointment, at which time all restrictions were lifted, including weight-bearing. Referral was written

CASE 2-20C—cont'd

to begin physical therapy programming. Terra was accompanied today by her father, who lifted her from her manual wheelchair to the elevated mat for evaluation.

OBJECTIVE: Observation: Terra arrives seated in her manual wheelchair with her left hip in a position of internal rotation and adduction. Her right hip was in a neutral position. She stated that she has decreased endurance for lower-extremity weight bearing because her left hip begins to hurt after approximately 10 minutes of standing in her stander.

Lower-Extremity Passive Range of Motion:

JOINT	RIGHT	LEFT
Hip flexion	120 degrees	107 degrees
Hip abduction	25 degrees	16 degrees
Straight leg raising	90 degrees	85 degrees
Excessive dorsiflexion	20>	10 degrees

Lower Extremity Strength:

MUSCLE GROUP		
Quadriceps	F−/F+	F−
Hip abductors	P−	P−
Hip flexion	F−	F−
Hamstrings	F−	P+
Hip extensors	P−	P−

Tone in the lower extremities is increased. Mobility: Terra requires maximum assistance for standing pivot transfer from wheelchair to elevated mat. She requires a moderate assist to roll over from supine to prone and minimal assistance to roll from prone to supine. Her main means of mobility is by way of her power wheelchair. Gross Motor Skills: Terra is dependent on her power wheelchair for mobility. Her mom and dad lift her from her wheelchair instead of allowing her to use transfer with moderate to maximum assistance. Terra stands in her stander, but is no longer able to walk. Adaptive Equipment: She uses her power wheelchair at school and has a stander for home use.

ASSESSMENT: Impression: Patient's legs are very deconditioned as a result of her recent surgery and recovery. All restrictions are lifted, and she is ready to take responsibility for her own transfers with assist as needed. Strengths: (1) Interacts well with others in her environment; (2) motivated and cooperative. Problem list: (1) Left hip resting position of internal rotation and adduction; (2) she is not actively involved in her own transfers; (3) leg spasms causing her sitting posture to be asymmetrical; (4) decreased hip abduction on left leg to migrate into windswept position to her right. Goals: (1) To improve sitting balance: Terra will sustain erect sitting posture with upper- and lower-extremity support while seated on the bench or elevated mat; (2) improved lower-extremity passive range of motion: increased left hip flexion to 120 degrees and left hip abduction to 25 degrees; (3) increased lower-extremity strength by a half to a full muscle grade; (4) improved sliding board transfers with standby assistance from wheelchair to elevated mat or bed or standing pivot transfer with minimal to moderate assistance.

PLAN/RECOMMENDATION: (1) Terra is ready to begin a program of direct physical therapy on a twice-weekly basis for 3 to 4 months. A portion of that programming will occur in the therapeutic pool. (2) Plan of treatment for physical therapy program is listed under goals. (3) Patient will be seen in the gym during 1 session in the week and in the therapeutic pool for the other sessions to maximize her outcome. (4) Terra should place a towel roll between her knees when sitting in her wheelchair (to keep her hips in neutral alignment) to reduce her hip muscle spasms in her adductor muscle on the left. This will also promote body symmetry. (5) Her home exercise program should begin with standing in the stander on a daily basis for 10 to 30 minutes. She tolerated a 1-minute stand today and should increase her tolerance for standing gradually up to 30 minutes. Her home exercise program will be updated as needed. (6) Terra will return to the office for a recheck appointment in 4 months' time.

SERVICE CODE(S): _____

ICD-10-CM DX CODE(S): _____

(Answers to every other Case are located in Appendix D. The full answer key is only available in the TEACH Instructor Resources on Evolve.)

throughout the entire session. This is represented by codes 97032-97039.

Therapeutic Procedures (97110-97552) require direct patient contact and report services such as those performed to improve or develop strength, endurance, range of motion, and/or flexibility. Many of these services are exercises, neuromuscular re-education, water therapy, gait training, massage, and manipulation. There are also codes to report the services of fitting and training of orthotic or prosthetic devices.

Medical Nutrition Therapy

Medical Nutritional Therapy codes (97802-97804) are used to report medical nutritional therapy assessment or intervention services performed by a person other than a physician. The services are provided either individually or in a group. For example, a patient who the physician believes is not eating appropriately to maintain optimal health is referred to a dietitian for assessment and design of a more balanced eating plan. The dietitian's services are reported in increments of 15 minutes. If the dietitian spent 1 hour in an initial assessment with a patient, the services would be reported 97802 × 4, Medical nutritional therapy, initial assessment and intervention, individual, face-to-face with the patient, each 15 minutes.

Osteopathic and Chiropractic Manipulative Treatment

A doctor of osteopathy (DO) and a doctor of chiropractic (DC) are physicians who use alternative methods of treatment. Osteopathic Manipulative Treatment (OMT) codes (98925-98929) are used to report osteopathic manipulative treatment based on the number of body regions treated. Chiropractic Manipulative Treatment (CMT) codes (98940-98943) are used to report chiropractic manipulative treatment based on the number of spinal regions treated. Included in all these codes is a patient assessment and treatment. An E/M code is reported only if the physician provided a separate and distinct E/M service.

Special Services, Procedures, and Reports

This is the miscellaneous services section of the CPT for medical services. Codes 99000-99082 reflect services rendered at unusual hours of the day or on holidays, in unusual locations, for unusual supplies or materials, for preoperative and postoperative visits included in the surgical package (bundled), and for other miscellaneous services. These codes are used throughout the reporting of all medical services, such as 99070 for supplies and materials. There are also codes within this subsection that are not used often, for example, medical testimony, 99075. Take time to review all codes and descriptions within this often-used subsection of the CPT.

HCPCS Level II Modifiers

The Healthcare Procedural Coding System (HCPCS) is used with CPT codes and HCPCS Level II codes. The anatomical modifiers in this system are used to specify side, eyelid, thumb, finger/toe, and coronary artery.

-LT	Left side
-RT	Right side
-E1	Upper-left, eyelid
-E2	Lower-left, eyelid
-E3	Upper-right, eyelid
-E4	Lower-right, eyelid

-FA	Left hand, thumb
-F1	Left hand, second digit
-F2	Left hand, third digit
-F3	Left hand, fourth digit
-F4	Left hand, fifth digit
-F5	Right hand, thumb
-F6	Right hand, second digit
-F7	Right hand, third digit
-F8	Right hand, fourth digit
-F9	Right hand, fifth digit
-TA	Left foot, great toe
-T1	Left foot, second digit
-T2	Left foot, third digit
-T3	Left foot, fourth digit
-T4	Left foot, fifth digit
-T5	Right foot, great toe
-T6	Right foot, second digit
-T7	Right foot, third digit
-T8	Right foot, fourth digit
-T9	Right foot, fifth digit
-LC	Left circumflex, coronary artery
-LD	Left anterior descending coronary artery
-RC	Right coronary artery

Anatomical modifiers are not used with skin procedures, such as removal of skin tags from any area. The exception is with codes that indicate the skin of the feet, hands, fingers, legs, arms, and eyelids. A full list of HCPCS modifiers is located in the HCPCS Level II manual.

From the Trenches

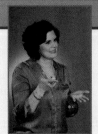

"The keys to success for a medical coder are the ability to anticipate and accept change and to always keep learning."

RACHEL E. BRIGGS
BA, CPC, CPMA, CENTC, CEMC

CASE 2-21A   *Office Procedure*

Sally Jones presented to Dr. Warner's office at the clinic for repair of a bilateral ingrown toenail of the great toe, which is a surgical procedure that can be performed in the physician's office using local anesthetic. Use HCPCS modifiers to indicate the digits repaired.

LOCATION: Outpatient, Clinic

PATIENT: Sally Jones

PHYSICIAN: Alma Naraquist, MD

SURGEON: Samuel Warner, MD

PREOPERATIVE DIAGNOSIS: Ingrown lateral borders, great toes, bilateral.

POSTOPERATIVE DIAGNOSIS: Ingrown lateral borders, great toes, bilateral.

SURGICAL PROCEDURE: Nail resection with chemical destruction and nail matrix lateral borders, great toes bilateral.

PROCEDURE: The patient's right and left feet were prepped and draped in the usual aseptic manner. The great toes were then anesthetized with 50/50 mixture of 2% lidocaine plain and 0.5% Marcaine plain with a quantity of 2.5 cc (cubic centimeters) into each

CASE 2-21A—cont'd

great toe. Treatment was first directed to the left great toe, where a mini-tourniquet was placed around the toe for hemostasis. The lateral border was then incised and excised in total. Phenol was then applied for 45 seconds, dry-swabbed, reapplied for 45 seconds, and dry-swabbed again. The area was then flushed with copious amounts of alcohol. The tourniquet was removed, and blood flow returned to normal. Sterile dressing with Neosporin cream was applied. Identical procedure then was performed on the right great toe lateral border. Following completion of both procedures, the dressings were taped in place. Stockinette was applied over the dressings, and surgical shoes were dispensed. The patient was given all verbal and written postoperative instructions. The patient is to use Extra-Strength Tylenol for pain. We will see the patient back in approximately 1 week's time for a checkup.

SERVICE CODE(S): _____

ICD-10-CM DX CODE(S): _____

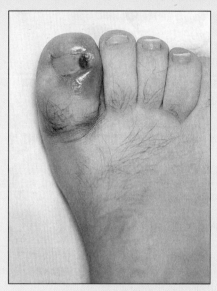

FIGURE 2–3 Ingrown toenail.

(Answers to every other Case are located in Appendix D . The full answer key is only available in the TEACH Instructor Resources on Evolve.)

CASE 2-21B   *Clinic Progress Note*

This is a patient of Dr. Naraquist's who comes in for a routine postoperative checkup during the postoperative period. A Z code would be reported for this follow-up examination, since the originally diagnosed condition of "ingrown toenail" no longer exists and the patient is still receiving services to consolidate the treatment. Reference the Index of the ICD-10-CM under the terms "Examination, follow-up, specified surgery NEC." Also, note that other "follow-up examination" codes are specific to chemotherapy, radiotherapy, etc.

LOCATION: Outpatient, Clinic

PATIENT: Sally Jones

PHYSICIAN: Alma Naraquist, MD

SURGEON: Samuel Warner, MD

The patient had phenol procedures performed to the lateral border on each great toe 6 days ago. She is doing well and presents without problems or complications.

EXAMINATION reveals a normal appearance from phenol procedure to the lateral border of each great toe. Mucus and granulation tissue was debrided from those margins.

She is encouraged to continue with soaks and return in 2 weeks for another postoperative check.

SERVICE CODE(S): _____

ICD-10-CM DX CODE(S): _____

(Answers to every other Case are located in Appendix D . The full answer key is only available in the TEACH Instructor Resources on Evolve.)

Audit the coding for the following reports.

Audit Report 2.1 Psychotherapy

This patient is seen by the psychiatrist, Fred Shongo, for supportive psychotherapy in the clinic.

LOCATION: Outpatient, Clinic

PATIENT: Joyce Epema

PRIMARY PHYSICIAN: Ronald Green, MD

CONSULTING PHYSICIAN: Fred Shongo, MD

There were brief periods of time when Joyce was grimacing in response to physical pain. She continues to hope that there will be a surgery or dramatic intervention with this pain. She made very clear it is episodic and sometimes is less severe.

We have addressed impulsive behaviors and especially irritability. It appears she is doing better with that at least by her report. Arrangement for follow-up will be made. I spent 20 minutes performing a psychiatric diagnostic evaluation of this patient.

DIAGNOSTIC IMPRESSION:
1. Major depression, mild, recurrent.
2. Impulse disorder, NOS.

One of the following codes is reported incorrectly for this case. Indicate the incorrect code.

PROFESSIONAL SERVICES: Psychotherapy, **90791**

ICD-10-CM DX: Depression, **F33.9**; Impulse disorder, **F63.9**

INCORRECT CODE: _____

Audit Report 2.2 Operative Report, Swan-Ganz

LOCATION: Inpatient, Hospital

PATIENT: Charles Carpenter

SURGEON: Leslie Alanda, MD

PREOPERATIVE DIAGNOSIS: Acute myocardial infarction, congestive heart failure with hypotension.

POSTOPERATIVE DIAGNOSIS: Same.

PROCEDURE PERFORMED: Insertion of Swan-Ganz catheter.

PROCEDURE: Consent was obtained from his sister. Right neck area was prepped. Sterile drapes were applied. Under sterile gowns and technique, right internal jugular vein was identified with 22-gauge needle from medial approach. 18-gauge catheter was inserted into the vein. A guide wire was passed through the vein. A 9-French introducer was inserted over the guide wire without difficulty. 7.5 French catheter was inserted. Right atrial pressures were 16, right ventricular pressure 34/10, pulmonary artery pressure 36/22 with a wedge pressure of 18. The patient tolerated the procedure well.

One or more codes should not have been reported or is missing for this case. Indicate the code(s) incorrectly reported or missing.

PROFESSIONAL SERVICES: Swan-Ganz catheter insertion, **93503**

ICD-10-CM DX: Acute myocardial infarction, **I21**; Congestive heart failure, **I50.9**; Hypotension, **I95.9**

INCORRECTLY REPORTED OR MISSING CODE(S): _____

Audit Report 2.3 Electroencephalogram

LOCATION: Outpatient, Hospital

PATIENT: Nolan Benson

PHYSICIAN: Timothy Pleasant, MD

FINDINGS: This is an 18-channel digital EEG recording performed on this 74-year-old male with a history of decreased mental status.

The background is characterized by diffuse slowing and disorganization consisting of medium-voltage theta rhythm at 4-6 Hz seen from all areas of the head. From anterior head areas, faster activity at beta range. Muscle artifacts and eye movements are noted and normal. EEG artifacts at 70 per minute were noted. Hyperventilation and photic stimulation were not performed at this time.

IMPRESSION: The EEG shows moderate encephalopathy process. Possible lesion cannot be ruled out at this time. Further studies are needed.

One of the following codes is reported incorrectly for this case. Indicate the incorrect code.

PROFESSIONAL SERVICES: Electroencephalography, **95816**

ICD-10-CM DX: Decreased mental status, **R41.82**; Abnormal EEG, **R94.01**

INCORRECT CODE: _____

CHAPTER 2—cont'd

Audit Report 2.4 Chart Note

LOCATION: Outpatient, Clinic

PATIENT: Ronald House

PHYSICIAN: Alma Naraquist, MD

AGE: 58

COVERAGE: Blue Cross Blue Shield

Patient presents for administration of a 3-dose schedule IM injection of Hepatitis B vaccine administered by Dr. Naraquist's nurse.

One or more of the following codes are reported incorrectly for this case. Indicate the incorrect code or codes.

SERVICE CODE(S): Evaluation and Management, **99211**; Unlisted vaccine/toxoid, **90749**; Immunization administration, **90471**

ICD-10-CM DX CODE(S):   Screening for other viral disease, **Z11.59**

INCORRECT/MISSING CODE(S): _____

Audit Report 2.5 Vascular Laboratory Report, Duplex Venous Examination

LOCATION: Outpatient, Hospital

PATIENT: Rebecca Stone

ORDERING PHSYCIAN: Ronald Green, MD

PHYSICIAN: James Noonar, MD

INDICATION: Edema, right extremities, right ankle fracture, rule out pulmonary embolism

The patient is a 65-year-old female with an ankle fracture. Since this has occurred, the patient has developed edema, and this is done to rule out pulmonary embolism.

Both legs were interrogated at the common femoral, superficial femoral, popliteal, and saphenous levels. The right leg could only be examined down to the knee. The left leg was examined below the knee as well. We examined for spontaneous flow, phasicity, augmentation, and compressibility. There is no evidence of thrombus.

CONCLUSION: This study is "negative," but the leg was not interrogated at the lower right leg, which would be the most concerned area. If the physician wishes, bandages could be removed and the technologist brought back for that.

There was no evidence of thrombophlebitis, but the study was not complete.

One or more of the following codes are reported incorrectly for this case. Indicate the incorrect code or codes.

SERVICE CODE(S):   Duplex scan of extremity veins, **93970**

ICD-10-CM DX CODE(S):   Localized edema, **R60.0**; Fracture of right lower leg, **S82.891A**; Other pulmonary embolism, **I26.99**

INCORRECT/MISSING CODE(S): _____

Audit Report 2.6 Photodynamic Therapy

LOCATION: Outpatient, Clinic

Dr. Barton will provide Tim Johnson with four photodynamic therapy exposures over the course of several weeks as a treatment for several Keratocanthomas on the skin of his back. Report todays session.

One or more of the following codes are reported incorrectly or missing for this case. Indicate the incorrect or missing code or codes.

SERVICE CODE(S):   Photodynamic therapy, **96567 × 4**

ICD-10-CM DX CODE(S):   Malignant neoplasm of skin of trunk, **C44.509**

INCORRECT/MISSING CODE(S): _____

(Auditing Review answers with rationales are only available in the TEACH Instructor Resources on Evolve.)

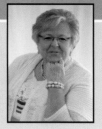
"If you are a detective at heart, you are going to be a great coder. A great coder can never call it good enough until they have exhausted every possible detail."

Radiology

http://evolve.elsevier.com/Buck/next

(Answers to every other Case are located in Appendix D, with the full answer key only available in the TEACH Instructor Resources on Evolve)
(Auditing Review answers with rationales are only available in the TEACH Instructor Resources on Evolve)

Radiology is the branch of medicine that uses radiant energy to diagnose and treat patients. The term originally referred to the use of x-rays to produce radiographs but is now commonly applied to all types of medical imaging. A physician who specializes in radiology is a **radiologist**. Radiologists can provide services to patients independent of or in conjunction with another physician of a different specialty. The Radiology section of the CPT manual is divided into the main subsections of Diagnostic Radiology, Diagnostic Ultrasound, Radiation Oncology, and Nuclear Medicine.

Positions and Placement

Terminology referring to planes of the body and positioning of the body is often used in the Radiology section. A **position** is how the patient is placed during the x-ray examination, and a **projection** is the path of the x-ray beam. **Figure 3-1** illustrates the major planes and the surfaces of the body that can be accessed by positioning the body.

Figure 3-2 shows proximal and distal directional body references that mean closest to (proximal) or farthest from (distal) the trunk of the body. These terms are relative, meaning they are used to describe the position of the part as compared with another part. Therefore, the term **proximal** describes a part as being closer to the body trunk than another part, and the term **distal** describes a part as being farther away from the body trunk than another part. The knee would be described as being proximal to the ankle, and it would also be described as being distal to the thigh or hip.

Figure 3-3 illustrates the **anteroposterior (AP)** (front to back) position, in which the patient has his or her front (anterior) closest to the x-ray machine, and the x-ray travels through the patient from the front to the back. In **Figure 3-4**, the **posteroanterior (PA)** position, the patient has his or her back (posterior) located closest to the machine, and the beam travels through the patient from back to front.

Lateral positions are side positions. When the patient's right side is closest to the film, it is called right lateral. When the patient's left side is closest to the film, it is called left lateral. **Figure 3-5** shows a left lateral position, and **Figure 3-6** shows a right lateral position. The use of these various positions allows the physician to view the body from a variety of angles.

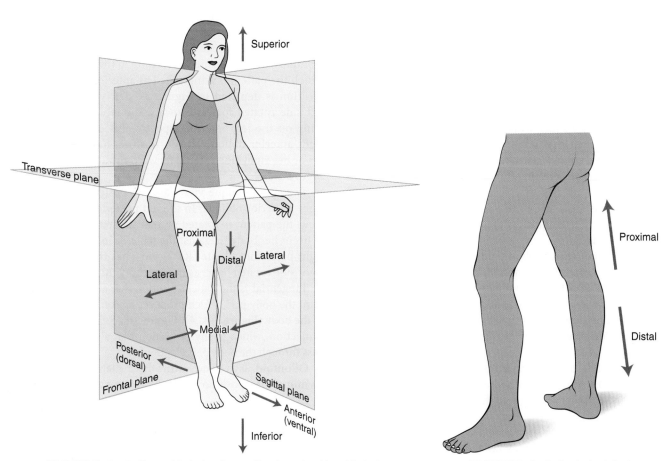

FIGURE 3–1 Planes of the body and terms of location and position of the body.

FIGURE 3–2 Proximal and distal.

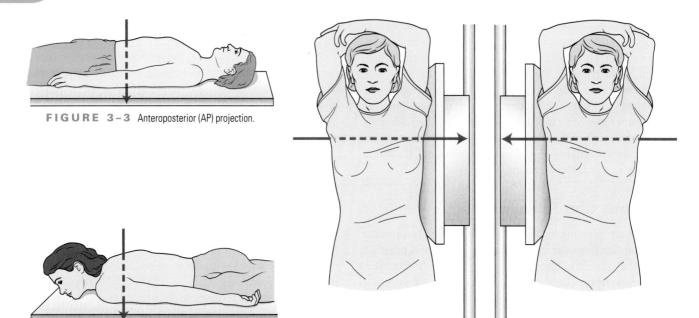

FIGURE 3-3   Anteroposterior (AP) projection.

FIGURE 3-4   Posteroanterior (PA) projection.

FIGURE 3-5   Left lateral position.

FIGURE 3-6   Right lateral position.

Dorsal, more commonly referred to as **supine,** means lying on the back (s<u>UP</u>ine means lying on the back with the face UP); **ventral,** more commonly referred to as **prone,** means lying on the stomach; and **lateral** means lying on the side.

Decubitus positions are recumbent positions; the x-ray beam is placed horizontally. Ventral decubitus (prone) is the act of lying on the stomach (**Figure 3-7, A**), and dorsal decubitus (supine) is the act of lying on the back (**Figure 3-7, B**). The term "decubitus," generally shortened to "decub," has a special meaning in radiology. The simple act of lying on one's back would be referred to as lying supine, but if a horizontal x-ray beam is used, the position becomes decubitus. The type of decubitus is determined by the body surface on which the patient is lying.

Recumbent means lying down. Thus, right lateral recumbent means the patient is lying on the right side (**Figure 3-7, C**), and left lateral recumbent means the patient is lying on the left side (**Figure 3-7, D**). In the ventral decubitus position, the patient is positioned prone, and the x-ray beam comes into the patient from the right side and exits on the left (**Figure 3-7, E**).

In the **left lateral decubitus** position, the patient is lying on the left side with the beam coming from the front and passing through to the back (anteroposterior) (**Figure 3-7, F**).

When the patient is positioned on his or her back (dorsal decubitus) and the x-ray beam comes into the left side of the patient, the positioning is dorsal decubitus, but the view obtained is a right lateral (because the right side is closest to the film) (**Figure 3-7, G**).

Oblique views refer to those obtained while the body is rotated; it is not in a full anteroposterior or posteroanterior position but is somewhat diagonal. Oblique views are termed according to the body surface on which the patient is lying. The left anterior oblique (LAO) position is depicted in **Figure 3-7, H,** with the patient's left side rotated forward toward the table. The patient is lying on the left anterior aspect of his or her body. The right anterior oblique (RAO) position has the patient on his or her right side rotated forward toward the table, as in **Figure 3-7, I**.

Two more oblique views are left posterior oblique and right posterior oblique. In the left posterior oblique (LPO) view, the patient is rotated so that the left posterior aspect of his or her body is against the table, as in **Figure 3-7, J**. The right posterior oblique (RPO) view has the patient on the right side rotated back, as in **Figure 3-7, K**.

Tangential is the patient position that allows the beam to skim the body part, which produces a profile of the structure of the body (**Figure 3-8, A**). **Figure 3-8, B** illustrates the **axial projection,** which is any projection that allows the beam to pass through the body part lengthwise.

Odontoid is a view with the patient's mouth open. **Swimmers** is a position in which the arms are over the head.

Component Coding

Coding radiology services often includes component coding. The following are components:

1. **Professional:** Describes the services of the physician/radiologist, including the supervision of the taking of the

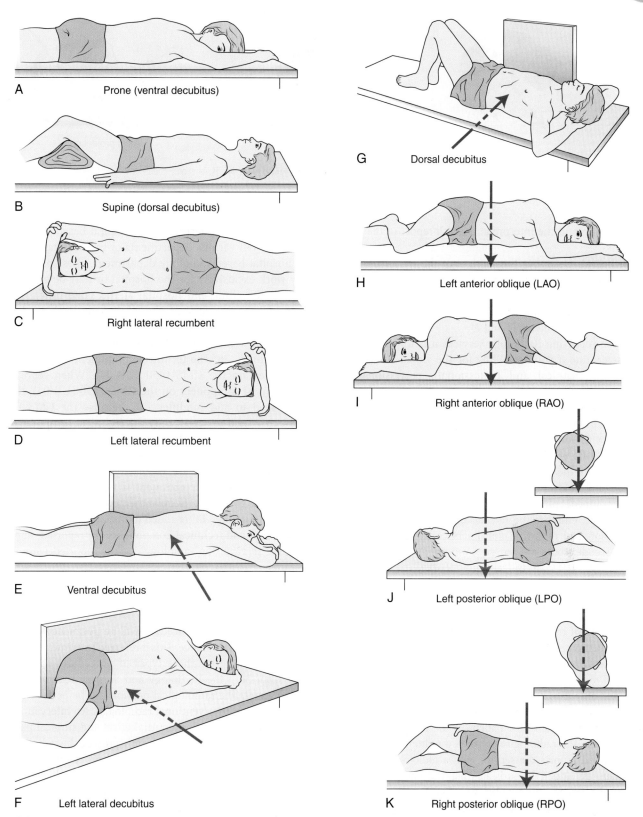

A Prone (ventral decubitus)

B Supine (dorsal decubitus)

C Right lateral recumbent

D Left lateral recumbent

E Ventral decubitus

F Left lateral decubitus

G Dorsal decubitus

H Left anterior oblique (LAO)

I Right anterior oblique (RAO)

J Left posterior oblique (LPO)

K Right posterior oblique (RPO)

FIGURE 3-7 Radiographic positions. **A,** Prone (ventral decubitus). **B,** Supine (dorsal decubitus). **C,** Right lateral recumbent. **D,** Left lateral recumbent. **E,** Ventral decubitus. **F,** Left lateral decubitus. **G,** Dorsal decubitus. **H,** Left anterior oblique (LAO). **I,** Right anterior oblique (RAO). **J,** Left posterior oblique (LPO). **K,** Right posterior oblique (RPO).

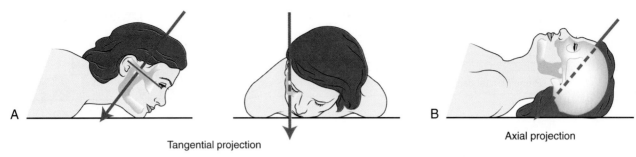

A

Tangential projection

B

Axial projection

FIGURE 3-8 Radiographic projections. **A,** Tangential projection. **B,** Axial projection.

x-ray film and the interpretation with report of the x-ray films.

2. **Technical:** Describes the services of the technologist, as well as the cost of the resources such as equipment, film, and usual supplies used to provide the service.

3. **Global:** Describes the combination of the professional and technical components (1 and 2).

When reporting Radiology services it is important that you determine if you are billing for the global component (both the technical and professional), professional, or technical only.

Global Component—When reporting both the professional (physician/radiologist) and technical portion (resources used such as equipment and supplies) of the service, report the CPT code without a modifier -26 or -TC, because this would inform the carrier that you are submitting for both the professional and technical portion of the service. For example, if the orthopedic physician owns the x-ray equipment located in his office, employs the technician, and also provides the supervision and report, a global service was provided, and the CPT code would not require a modifier -26 (professional component) or -TC (technical component).

Professional Component—When reporting the professional portion only of the service, it means that you are only reporting the physician/radiologist's supervision and interpretation with report and not the technical portion (cost of resources used such as equipment and supplies) of the service. When only the professional (physician) component is provided, report the CPT code with modifier -26 to indicate the physician provided only the professional portion of the service, not the entire service. For example, a radiologist from the local clinic analyzes x-rays taken of a patient at the hospital radiology department. The radiologist prepares a written report of the findings and reports the service with a radiology code with modifier -26 added to indicate that the equipment, film, technical services, and supplies were NOT provided by the physician preparing the report at the time of this service.

Two billing forms are used in the hospital setting: CMS-1500 for professional services provided by professional employees of the hospital and the CMS-1450 (UB-04) to report facility (hospital) services. At times the hospital will employ a radiologist to provide professional services, such

as mammography interpretation. Hospital-based physicians may also staff various departments of the hospital, such as the hospital-based radiology department. These physicians may work exclusively for the hospital or may be employed by both the clinic and hospital at the same time. When reporting the services of the physician portion of the service performed by a hospital-employed physician, you would report the professional service on the CMS-1500 with modifier -26. The technical component of the service is reported on the CMS-1450 (UB-04). When reporting the technical component on the CMS-1450 (UB-04), there is no need to add modifier -TC because the CMS-1450 (UB-04) is used to report only the technical component of the services.

At the clinic, both the professional (physician) and the technical components are reported on the CMS-1500. If only the professional component is reported, modifier -26 is added to the code. If only the technical component is provided, modifier -TC is added to the CPT code. If both the professional and technical components are reported, known as *global services,* the radiology code is reported without a modifier.

Interventional Radiology

Sometimes a surgical procedure will be performed with the use of radiologic guidance. This is referred to as interventional radiology. Billing for these types of procedures requires a code from both the Radiology and Surgery sections of the CPT manual. The radiological portion can be performed by a radiologist or interventional radiologist. An interventional radiologist can do both the radiological and surgical part of the procedure. A radiologist can only provide the radiological portion of the service, and the surgical procedure would be performed by the surgeon. The codes in the Radiology section describe the radiologic portion of the procedure only. When a procedure requiring the use of radiology is performed, the services are reported with a combination of CPT codes from the Surgery (for the procedure) and the Radiology sections (for the radiologic Supervision and Interpretation [RS&I]). The physician performing the procedure (such as biopsy, aspiration, injection, or placement of other materials) will report his portion of the procedure using a code from the Surgery section of the CPT manual. The physician performing the radiologic supervision and interpretation will report his service using the RS&I code. When a single physician performs both the procedure and the RS&I, he will report a combination of codes for each aspect of the procedure. For example, an ultrasound-guided fine needle aspiration biopsy is reported with 10005. In addition to performing the S&I, a permanently recorded image and report are required. The above rule regarding the use of a combination of codes does not apply to the Radiation Oncology procedures.

Contrast

Codes in the Radiology section describe only the radiology procedures, not the intra-articular (joint) injection or placement of other materials necessary to provide the service; therefore, these would be reported in addition to the radiology service. For example, contrast material that is injected during a radiographic procedure is reported separately. The phrase "with contrast" in the CPT manual means contrast that was injected. The supply of the injected contrast material is reported with a HCPCS Level II code, such as Q9952, Injection during MRI. If the procedure indicates that contrast was administered orally or rectally, the service is coded as "without contrast" because only intravascular contrast qualifies as "with contrast."

An **intra-articular** injection is one that is within a joint. An **intrathecal** injection is one that is placed through the theca (enclosing sheath) of the spinal cord into the subarachnoid space.

Contrast is typically administered in the following methods:

Does Not Qualify	Qualifies as with Contrast
• Oral: Mouth	• Intra-articular: Injected into a joint
• Rectal: Rectum	• Intravenously: Injected into a vein
	• Intrathecal: Injected into a subarachnoid/subdural space

Many **types** of contrast are often used with the various radiographic procedures. For example:

- Isovue → Nonionic CT
- Gadolinium → MRI
- Barium → Gastrointestinal
- Iodine → CT/IVP/arthrograms/angiograms

Facility Specifics

In the outpatient departments of the hospital, CPT codes for the radiologic examination are established by the facility *Chargemaster,* the computer software program used to process hospital billing. Many facilities have included modifiers programmed within the Chargemaster software. The modifiers automatically are placed on the insurance claim form without any intervention by coding staff.

The main difference in coding for the hospital facility in the outpatient setting is the use of ICD-10-PCS for the procedure codes.

Many facilities have specific policies designating which procedures performed within the facility will be assigned codes. Policies vary between the inpatient and outpatient setting within a hospital facility. These policies are usually reviewed annually because of the rapid changes in technology and the more invasive and complicated procedures that are being performed in the radiology department. For the purposes of this text, most of the invasive radiology procedures (entering the body) are performed in the hospital radiology department. Routine procedures, such as x-rays, CTs, and ultrasounds, are usually performed in the clinic outpatient setting.

Diagnostic Radiology

Codes 70010-76499, often used from the Radiology section, include both diagnostic radiology and diagnostic ultrasound. These codes describe diagnostic imaging, **computed axial tomography (CAT, CT), magnetic resonance imaging (MRI),** and magnetic resonance angiography (MRA). The codes are divided by x-ray, CAT/CT, MRI, and MRA

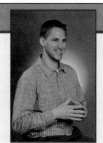

From the Trenches

"Coders have a great potential for growth and having a billing background will open doors to practice management and consulting positions."

MICHAEL HAAS
CPC, MBA

throughout the subsection. For example, subheading Spine and Pelvis (72020-72295) includes the following:

- Radiographic examination (x-rays) of the spine (72020-72120)
- CT of the spine (72125-72133)
- MRI of the spine (72141-72159)

If fewer than the total number of views specified in the code are taken, modifier -52 (reduced service) would be used to indicate to the third-party payer that less of the procedure was performed than described by the code unless a code already exists for the smaller number of views.

X-ray is a common diagnostic radiology service. The service can be provided on an outpatient or inpatient basis. Modifier -26 is used to indicate that only the professional component of the service was provided.

Hemodialysis Catheter Placement

A hemodialysis catheter is used to access the blood for hemodialysis. The catheter has two joined lines. One line is used to pull blood from the patient's blood system for cleaning, and the other line is used to return the cleaned blood back to the blood system. The catheter can be temporary or permanent. A temporary catheter is placed in the neck, chest, or groin by a nephrologist, general surgeon, or interventional radiologist. This type of catheter can stay in place for about 3 weeks. An x-ray will be taken to ensure that the catheter is in the correct location. Catheters are not ideal for permanent access. They can clog, become infected, or cause narrowing of the vessel into which the access catheter is placed. If the patient needs to start hemodialysis immediately, a catheter will suffice for several weeks while permanent access is developed. Catheters that will be needed for more than about 3 weeks are designed to be tunneled under the skin to increase comfort and reduce complications. A patient who needs dialysis for longer than 3 weeks will usually receive a permanent catheter. An x-ray is taken after placement to ensure that the catheter is in the correct location.

CASE 3-1   *Radiology Report, Chest*

Morris Lancer had a hemodialysis catheter placed. Report Dr. Monson's services for the follow-up x-ray performed to ensure correct placement of the catheter. For the purpose of a diagnosis, this is an "Encounter for dialysis catheter fitting and adjustment, extracorporeal." In hemodialysis, blood is removed from the body and circulated through an extracorporeal fluid circuit (outside the body), where it is cleansed of wastes and then returned to the patient.

LOCATION: Outpatient, Hospital

PATIENT: Morris Lancer

PHYSICIAN: Ronald Green, MD

RADIOLOGIST: Morton Monson, MD

EXAMINATION OF: Portable chest x-ray

CLINICAL SYMPTOMS: Follow-up placement of hemodialysis catheter

PORTABLE 15-DEGREE UPRIGHT AP (ANTERIOR POSTERIOR) CHEST X-RAY, 5:00 AM: An endotracheal tube ending is located well above the carina. An NG tube is present, the tip of which is not seen in our field of view but goes below level of the left hemidiaphragm. A central line from left subclavian ends in the right atrial contour. Cardiomegaly is noted. Confluent change is seen in all lung fields, sparing only the left apex. The finding has increased compared with 1 week previously, suggesting a fluid-overloaded failure pattern rather than pneumonia. Some atelectatic change is still seen at the right base. Partial collapse of left lung base is still present. These are stable findings. Effusions would not be seen on a 15-degree upright chest x-ray. No bony lesion of significance is seen.

IMPRESSION:

1. Support lines as mentioned.
2. Cardiomegaly with failure pattern. Failure pattern—increasing since yesterday morning's x-ray.

Partial collapsed right lower lobe and left lower lobe. Those are stable findings.

SERVICE CODE(S): _____

ICD-10-CM DX CODE(S): _____

(Answers to every other Case are located in Appendix D. The full answer key is only available in the TEACH Instructor Resources on Evolve.)

Types of Catheters

Many types of catheters are available, such as central venous catheters (for administration of fluids or medications), feeding tubes, or cardiac catheters (to obtain blood samples, intracardiac pressures, and for diagnostic purposes). Reference a medical dictionary under the term "catheter" to see all the various types of catheters. It is a common practice for an imaging service to be provided before and/or after a catheter placement.

CASE 3-2 *Radiology Report, Line Placement*

In the following case, Dr. Sanchez, general surgeon, placed a right internal jugular central venous catheter and has requested Dr. Monson to interpret the x-ray of the patient's chest to ensure that the catheter is correctly placed. Code Dr. Monson's service.

LOCATION: Outpatient, Hospital

PATIENT: George Barr

PHYSICIAN: Gary Sanchez, MD

RADIOLOGIST: Morton Monson, MD

EXAMINATION OF: Chest, single view

CLINICAL SYMPTOMS: Congestive heart failure

CHEST, SINGLE VIEW: FINDINGS: No previous examination is available for comparison. A right internal jugular central venous catheter is present. The distal tip of the catheter overlies the expected location of the superior vena cava. The heart size appears at the upper limits of normal. The pulmonary vasculature markings also appear at the upper limits of normal. Abnormal focal density is present within the retrocardiac region of the left lung base. Increased markings are present in the right infrahilar region as well. These densities could be related to either atelectasis or infiltrate. Blunting of the left costophrenic angle is consistent with a left-sided pleural effusion. Definite pneumothorax is not identified on this examination.

IMPRESSION:

1. Status post placement of right internal jugular central venous catheter as described above.
2. The heart size and pulmonary vasculature markings appear at the upper limits of normal.
3. Focal density is present within both lung bases, which could be related to either atelectasis or infiltrate. Documentation of radiographic clearing is recommended to exclude underlying lesions.
4. Small left-sided pleural effusion.

SERVICE CODE(S): _____

ICD-10-CM DX CODE(S): _____

(Answers to every other Case are located in Appendix D . The full answer key is only available in the TEACH Instructor Resources on Evolve.)

Nasogastric Tube

A nasogastric tube is placed through the nose and into the stomach. The tube is used to deliver nutrition to the patient. To ensure proper placement, an x-ray is taken after placement.

CASE 3-3 *Radiology Report, Abdomen*

Report Dr. Monson's professional service for an abdominal x-ray performed to check the placement of the tube. For the diagnoses for this patient, assign a Z code for the encounter for adjustment of a nonvascular catheter, followed by the presenting symptom of abdominal pain. Since this is a comparison study it is important to note that Dr. Monson also provided the previous study at 11:00 AM the same day.

LOCATION: Outpatient, Hospital (Observation Care)

PATIENT: Jody Cornwallace

PHYSICIAN: Ronald Green, MD

RADIOLOGIST: Morton Monson, MD

EXAMINATION OF: Abdomen

CLINICAL SYMPTOMS: Cor-Flo placement due to abdominal pain.

SINGLE VIEW OF ABDOMEN: Comparison is made with the previous study of 11:00 AM this day.

The nasogastric feeding tube is again identified. Its distal aspect lies at what appears to be the gastric antrum or possibly the first portion of the duodenum. This should be adequate for feeding the 3:00 PM study. The remainder of the abdomen is relatively unchanged.

CONCLUSION:

1. Interim repositioning of nasogastric feeding tube. Its distal aspect now lies at the gastric antrum or first portion of the duodenum. This should be adequate position for feeding.
2. The gastrointestinal air pattern is otherwise nonspecific.

SERVICE CODE(S): _____

ICD-10-CM DX CODE(S): _____

(Answers to every other Case are located in Appendix D . The full answer key is only available in the TEACH Instructor Resources on Evolve.)

The following cases will provide you an opportunity to code a variety of routine x-ray services.

CASE 3-4   *Radiology Report, Chest*

Report Dr. Monson's professional service.

LOCATION: Outpatient, Hospital

PATIENT: Lorenz Miller

PHYSICIAN: Ronald Green, MD

RADIOLOGIST: Morton Monson, MD

EXAMINATION OF: Chest

CLINICAL SYMPTOMS: Primary, malignant neoplasm of the hilus of the lung

TWO VIEWS, CHEST: Frontal and lateral views obtained of the chest. These are submitted on September 3 for interpretation. Comparison is made with a portable view of the chest, July 27. Blunting of the left posterior costophrenic sulcus suggests small pleural effusion on the left. Abnormal opacity, right perihilar/suprahilar region, is best seen on the frontal view. The patient has a history of lung cancer. Opacity was noted there previously. Previously noted bibasilar opacities appear essentially resolved. Oral contrast is noted within the abdomen.

IMPRESSION: Persistent opacity, right perihilar/suprahilar region, presumably reflecting the patient's clinical history of lung cancer. This was noted previously. Suspect small pleural effusion on the left. Basilar regions otherwise appear cleared since the prior study.

SERVICE CODE(S): _____

ICD-10-CM DX CODE(S): _____

(Answers to every other Case are located in Appendix D . The full answer key is only available in the TEACH Instructor Resources on Evolve.)

CASE 3-5   *Radiology Report, Femur*

Code the professional component of the service. Report HCPCS National Level II modifier to indicate the side of the body x-rayed.

LOCATION: Outpatient, Hospital

PATIENT: Simon Fields

PHYSICIAN: Leslie Alanda, MD

RADIOLOGIST: Morton Monson, MD

CLINICAL SYMPTOMS: Leg pain

EXAMINATION OF: Left femur

TWO VIEWS, LEFT FEMUR: This examination is compared with an AP (anterior posterior) view of the femur dated 3 months previously from a skeletal survey. Again seen is a mixed sclerotic and lytic lesion within the distal diaphysis of the left femur. This is not significantly changed since the previous examination dated 3 months previously. This is seen to involve the posterior aspect of the left femur. Finding is highly suspicious for the presence of metastatic disease. Vascular calcifications and surgical clips are noted to be present.

IMPRESSION: Mixed lytic and sclerotic lesion involving the distal left femur. This is highly suspicious for the presence of metastatic disease.

SERVICE CODE(S): _____

ICD-10-CM DX CODE(S): _____

(Answers to every other Case are located in Appendix D . The full answer key is only available in the TEACH Instructor Resources on Evolve.)

CASE 3-6   *Radiology Report, Knee*

Report the global service for this x-ray that was performed at the clinic where Dr. Monson supervised the technician and then interpreted the results and wrote a report of the findings. When reporting an ICD-10-CM code for a fracture, unless the skin is broken, code the fracture as "closed." If the documentation does not indicate whether the fracture is closed or open, report closed fracture. Distal means lower or farthest from the point of origin, and proximal means higher or nearest to the point of origin.

LOCATION: Outpatient, Clinic

PATIENT: Jason Glassheim

PHYSICIAN: Leslie Alanda, MD

RADIOLOGIST: Morton Monson, MD

EXAMINATION OF: Two views, left knee

CLINICAL SYMPTOMS: Fracture of the distal femur

TWO VIEWS, LEFT KNEE: A comminuted fracture involves the distal femur. This is incompletely demonstrated on this study. Medial angulation of the distal femoral shaft fragment appears to be present. Multiple fracture fragments are present over the fracture site. There is also mild anterior angulation of the distal femoral shaft and overriding at the fracture site with the proximal portion of the shaft anteriorly displaced by approximately ¼ to ⅓ shaft width.

IMPRESSION: Comminuted fracture, distal femur, incompletely demonstrated on these films.

SERVICE CODE(S): _____

ICD-10-CM DX CODE(S): _____

(Answers to every other Case are located in Appendix D . The full answer key is only available in the TEACH Instructor Resources on Evolve.)

CASE 3-7 *Radiology Report, Shoulder*

Report Dr. Monson's professional service for each of the x-rays of the right shoulder.

LOCATION: Outpatient, Hospital

PATIENT: Nelda Cavazos

PHYSICIAN: Mohomad Almaz, MD

RADIOLOGIST: Morton Monson, MD

EXAMINATION OF: Right shoulder

CLINICAL SYMPTOMS: Right shoulder pain

These films are from 15 days previously just now submitted for interpretation, having been with the orthopedist in the interval.

RIGHT SHOULDER: Two sets of films from 15 days previously performed at 11:20 am and another set performed at 1:00 pm. The three views are from 11:20 am and three from 1:00 pm on the same day, again, there is no change from 15 days prior. No fracturing is identified. Degenerative change is as described before.

IMPRESSION:

1. Degenerative change without fracture or dislocation.
2. Films are just now submitted for interpretation.

SERVICE CODE(S): _____

ICD-10-CM DX CODE(S): _____

(Answers to every other Case are located in Appendix D . The full answer key is only available in the TEACH Instructor Resources on Evolve.)

CASE 3-8 *KUB*

This patient underwent an outpatient surgical procedure for placement of a feeding tube for dysphagia resulting from a cerebrovascular accident 3 weeks ago. Report the professional component of the x-ray. For the diagnosis, report only the primary purpose for this encounter with a Z code, which in this case is adjustment of a nasogastric tube (nonvascular catheter).

LOCATION: Outpatient, Hospital

PATIENT: Sally Ozark

PHYSICIAN: Ronald Green, MD

RADIOLOGIST: Edward Riddle, MD

EXAMINATION OF: KUB (kidney, ureter, bladder), abdominal view

CLINICAL SYMPTOMS: Check Cor-Flo feeding tube placement

KUB, ONE FILM DONE PORTABLE SUPINE, 12:15 PM

No prior film. There is degenerative change in bony structures. Bowel gas pattern is nonspecific. Mainly we see stomach and colon gas. No distended bowel loops. Feeding tube extends from esophagus down into stomach and ends in the anticipated location of the second portion of the C-loop. That position could be used as a feeding tube. No organomegaly or significant calcification is seen on field of view.

IMPRESSION: This was performed to check feeding tube placement. It appears to end or have its tip in the anticipated location of the second portion of the C-loop.

SERVICE CODE(S): _____

ICD-10-CM DX CODE(S): _____

(Answers to every other Case are located in Appendix D . The full answer key is only available in the TEACH Instructor Resources on Evolve.)

Cine-Pharyngoesophagram

Cine-pharyngoesophagram, also called cineradiography or a video swallow, is a serial (moving picture) x-ray of the digestive tract. It allows dynamic (with motion) visualization of the swallowing function as well as strictures and other abnormalities.

CASE 3-9 *Video Swallow*

Dr. Monson is a clinic physician who reviews a video swallow (swallowing evaluation) that was performed at the local hospital outpatient department for a patient of Dr. Naraquist. Report Dr. Monson's service.

LOCATION: Outpatient, Hospital

PATIENT: Loren Zann

PHYSICIAN: Alma Naraquist, MD

RADIOLOGIST: Morton Monson, MD

EXAMINATION OF: Pharynx

CLINICAL SYMPTOMS: Dysphagia

VIDEO SWALLOW: FINDINGS: The patient's swallowing mechanism was examined using various liquid and solid barium consistencies. The patient demonstrated trace penetration on a single swallow with the nectar consistency barium by cup and also with the thin barium consistency by cup without and with chin tuck. No aspiration. Pooling of the liquid barium consistencies within the valleculae and piriform sinuses is seen.

SERVICE CODE(S): _____

ICD-10-CM DX CODE(S): _____

(Answers to every other Case are located in Appendix D . The full answer key is only available in the TEACH Instructor Resources on Evolve.)

CAT/CT Scans

Computerized axial tomography (CAT or CT) is a procedure by which selected planes of tissue are pinpointed through computer enhancement. The CAT is produced by means of a circular machine that takes pictures of the patient from many different angles. If needed, a three-dimensional image can be produced. The scan can be with or without contrast (remember that oral or rectal contrasts do not count as contrast). "Without" means there is no IV contrast. "With" means there is IV contrast. The scan can also be performed without contrast followed by with contrast, which means that the scan would be conducted first without contrast and then repeated again with contrast. The codes are usually divided based on the statement of with or without contrast and then the extent of the study. The codes are located in the index of the CPT manual under the term "CT Scan" and further subdivided by "Without and with Contrast," "Without Contrast," and "With Contrast." Locate "CT Scan" in the index of the CPT manual and note that these three divisions list the same or similar subterms, such as "Abdomen" in each division. The "Without and with Contrast" is when the CT scan is performed without contrast first and then repeated with contrast. The "Without Contrast" is the use of no intravenous contrast. The "With Contrast" is with the use of injected contrast.

A technician, under the supervision of a radiologist, performs the scan, and the radiologist interprets the results and writes a report. Do not report modifier -TC if the technical component is provided at the hospital because, as stated earlier, the CMS-1450 (UB-04) does not require the use of the technical modifier. If the radiologist performs only the professional component of the service, modifier -26 is added to the code.

From the Trenches

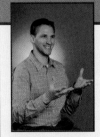

"Coding students should understand that becoming proficient coder takes patience and constant education."

MICHAEL HAAS
CPC, MBA

CASE 3-10   *CT Scan, Brain*

Report the radiologist's service for the following CT. For the diagnosis, report the presenting symptom as indicated "alteration of mental status." Because there are so many questionable diagnoses in this report that cannot be reported, the only definitive diagnosis is "alteration of mental status."

LOCATION: Outpatient, Hospital

PATIENT: John Doe

PHYSICIAN: Ronald Green, MD

RADIOLOGIST: Morton Monson, MD

EXAMINATION OF: Brain CT (computed tomography)

CLINICAL SYMPTOMS: Alteration of mental status

COMPUTED TOMOGRAPHIC EXAMINATION OF THE BRAIN was performed without contrast material. The study was performed in my absence and is presented for evaluation. There is movement in multiple images.

In image 11, there is questionable low density involving the superior surface of the left frontal lobe. Most probably, this is not real. Adjacent images do not show this low density; however, if the patient moved between images, there certainly would be misregistration.

I do believe there may be abnormal low density involving the base of the right frontal lobe. I believe this may represent encephalomalacia, most probably from an old injury of the right frontal lobe. There is a questionable, very small amount of similar low density within the left frontal lobe on image 11.

There are patchy areas of low density within the white matter of both hemispheres. These are symmetric. Most probably, they represent areas of gliosis of indeterminate etiology.

Bilaterally, several small areas of decreased density of the subcortical white matter of the insular regions are present that might be representative of previous ischemic change. I do not believe this is acute.

There is no hemorrhage. No mass. No indication of raised intracranial pressure.

IMPRESSION: Possible encephalomalacia at the base of the right frontal lobe, most probably from an old injury. Questionable encephalomalacia changes of left frontal lobe. Questionable low density (most probably not real) of the superior margin of the left temporal lobe. If this were real, it might be recent ischemic change. Possible small lacunar-type infarctions of the brain parenchyma are subjacent to each insular region. No hemorrhage.

SERVICE CODE(S): _____

ICD-10-CM DX CODE(S): _____

Reconstruction

A CT scan is a small slice (cross-sectional view) of a layer of the body. A **reconstruction** is when several of these cross-sectional views are put together (reconstructed) into a three-dimensional image. Reconstruction can be performed with CT scans, **MRIs,** or other **tomography** (body-section radiography). The reconstruction service is reported in addition to the radiographic procedure (CT, MRI, or other tomography). The reconstruction codes are located in the index of the CPT manual under CT Scan, 3-D Rendering and Magnetic Resonance Imaging, 3-D Rendering. The codes 76376 and 76377 are located within the "Other Procedures" subsection within the Radiology section. The two codes are differentiated by whether or not an independent workstation was required for the processing.

A **neuroradiologist** is a radiologist who specializes in radiographic procedures of the nervous system. Dr. Phillip Hart is a neuroradiologist employed by the hospital and is the head of the Radiology Department at the hospital. When radiographic service was provided in the hospital setting, thereby using the radiology equipment provided by the hospital, both the professional and technical portions of the radiology service were provided to the patient. The professional component is reported with modifier -26, and the technical portion of the service is reported with no modifier. You will be reporting services for Dr. Hart in the next three cases.

Congestive Heart Failure

Congestive heart failure (I50.9) is a condition in which the heart is unable to generate adequate output. When the heart has lost its ability to pump effectively, blood may back up into other organs, such as the liver or lungs. When the organs do not get a sufficient blood supply, the oxygen level is decreased, and the organ can be damaged and lose the ability to function properly.

Hypoxemia

Hypoxemia, also known as anoxia, is a deficiency in the level of oxygen in the arterial blood.

For the next three cases, 3-11A through 3-13A, the radiologist is employed by the clinic and is rendering services at the hospital. Assign the professional component only.

CASE 3-11   *CT Scan, Sinuses*

Report Dr. Hart's service.

LOCATION: Inpatient, Hospital

PATIENT: Cheryl West

PHYSICIAN: Ronald Green, MD

RADIOLOGIST: Phillip Hart, MD

CLINICAL SYMPTOMS: Intubated due to congestive heart failure, hypoxemia.

COMPUTED TOMOGRAPHIC EXAMINATION OF THE PARANASAL SINUSES was performed using thin, overlapping images in the axial plane. The patient's condition did not allow direct coronal images. Coronal reconstructions (3-D) were performed from the original data set and required an independent workstation.

Frontal, ethmoid, and sphenoid sinuses are virtually all filled with abnormal soft-tissue density. There is no bone erosion. The septations of the ethmoid complexes remain intact. Nasal cavity shows decreased aeration bilaterally.

Both maxillary sinuses show a considerable amount of abnormal soft-tissue density, but there is some aeration. There certainly could be fluid levels.

There is nasal intubation on the right.

IMPRESSION: Abnormal density almost filling all of the paranasal sinuses, as described above, without bone erosion. Certainly, this might be due to inflammation/infection; however, it is certainly not unusual for fluid to collect within paranasal sinuses when patients are intubated. The findings do need close clinical correlation.

SERVICE CODE(S): _____

ICD-10-CM DX CODE(S): _____

(Answers to every other Case are located in Appendix D . The full answer key is only available in the TEACH Instructor Resources on Evolve.)

CASE 3-12   *CT Scan, Sinuses*

Report Dr. Hart's service. Remember to also assign an ICD-10-CM Z code to report the "Dependence, on, ventilator."

LOCATION: Outpatient, Hospital

PATIENT: Lonny Barker

PHYSICIAN: Ronald Green, MD

RADIOLOGIST: Phillip Hart, MD

EXAMINATION OF: CT (computed tomography) of sinuses

CLINICAL SYMPTOMS: FUO (fever of unknown origin)

COMPUTED TOMOGRAPHIC EXAMINATION OF THE PARANASAL SINUSES was performed with intravenous contrast in the axial plane, computed for high-resolution bone algorithm. The patient is on a ventilator. Direct coronal images could not be obtained.

The left maxillary sinus is almost completely filled with abnormal soft-tissue density. The right maxillary sinus also shows a considerable amount of abnormal soft-tissue density, and there is a bubble appearance. I believe there is fluid within both sinuses.

Most of the ethmoid sinuses are filled with abnormal soft-tissue density. Septations of the ethmoid complexes are intact. Right sphenoid sinus shows some aeration. There are also mural nodulations of soft tissue within the left sphenoid sinus, but there might be a fluid level.

Both frontal sinuses are well aerated, but there is a rim of mucosal thickening of each frontal sinus, and there may be fluid within the left frontal sinus inferiorly.

IMPRESSION: All the paranasal sinuses show abnormalities as described above. Many of the air cells are filled with abnormal soft-tissue density. There is indication of fluid within at least the maxillary sinuses and perhaps the left sphenoid sinus. The findings can be consistent with a sinusitis condition; however, the patient is also on a ventilator. Patients with endotracheal intubation can have fluid in the sinuses without having a sinusitis condition.

SERVICE CODE(S): _____

ICD-10-CM DX CODE(S): _____

(Answers to every other Case are located in Appendix D . The full answer key is only available in the TEACH Instructor Resources on Evolve.)

CASE 3-13   *CT Scan, Chest*

Amyloidosis is a group of conditions in which a protein (amyloid) collects in the tissues and organs of the body to the point where the function is compromised. The following CT scan is of the chest of a patient with clinical symptoms of amyloidosis, and the scan is being performed to determine the extent of the disease. The elevated creatinine level, bilateral pleural effusions, adenopathy, degenerative osseous structures, and the lung opacity are all a part of the amyloidosis and therefore not reported separately. Report Dr. Hart's professional services.

LOCATION: Outpatient, Hospital

PATIENT: Jane Gallo

PHYSICIAN: Ronald Green, MD

RADIOLOGIST: Phillip Hart, MD

EXAMINATION OF: Diagnostic CT (computerized tomography) scan of the chest

CLINICAL SYMPTOMS: Amyloidosis

CT SCAN OF THE CHEST: Technique: Multiple computed axial tomograms were obtained from the thoracic inlet to ischial tuberosities following the administration of oral but not IV (intravenous) contrast. IV contrast was withheld secondary to the patient's elevated creatinine

status. Small bilateral pleural effusions/pleural thickening are seen, the left greater than the right. There is linear opacity in the right apex consistent with subsegmental volume loss or scarring. There is a very small area of nonspecific opacity in the posteromedial left lung base, which may be related to scarring, but it could also represent a small focal area of infiltrate or even volume averaging with the adjacent vessel. A short-term 3-month follow-up is suggested to document stability. The osseous structures demonstrate degenerative change. Evaluation for adenopathy is limited by a lack of IV contrast. Atherosclerotic change involves the aorta and its branches, including the coronary arteries. Small nonspecific pretracheal lymph nodes are present, none of which appear enlarged by CT criteria.

IMPRESSION:

1. Bilateral pleural effusions, left greater than right.
2. Study limited for evaluation of adenopathy due to lack of IV contrast.
3. Very tiny patchy, nonspecific opacity, left medial lung base. Short-term follow-up in 3 months is suggested.
4. Minimal linear opacity, right apex, is consistent with subsegmental volume loss or scarring.

SERVICE CODE(S): _____

ICD-10-CM DX CODE(S): _____

(Answers to every other Case are located in Appendix D . The full answer key is only available in the TEACH Instructor Resources on Evolve.)

In the previous three cases, the examinations were performed at the hospital and the radiologist is employed by the clinic. The clinic would bill the professional services, and the hospital would bill the technical component of the CT scan.

In cases where the radiologist is employed by the hospital, the hospital bill would include charges for both the professional component and the technical component of the CT scan. Now, back to reporting Dr. Monson's services.

CASE 3-14   *CT Scan, Abdomen and Pelvis*

The patient in this case also has amyloidosis. Dr. Monson, the clinic physician, provides the professional service for the CT scan that was performed at the hospital outpatient department. Code the professional component of the services rendered.

LOCATION: Outpatient, Hospital

PATIENT: Les Carlisle

PHYSICIAN: Ronald Green, MD

RADIOLOGIST: Morton Monson, MD

EXAMINATION OF: CT (computerized tomography) scan of abdomen and pelvis

CLINICAL SYMPTOMS: Amyloidosis

CT SCAN OF THE ABDOMEN AND PELVIS:

FINDINGS: Evaluation of visceral organs and adenopathy is limited by lack of IV (intravenous) contrast. The liver, spleen, adrenals, and kidneys have a normal noncontrasted CT appearance. Opacified portions of the bowel have a normal CT appearance. The pancreas demonstrates calcifications within the body and tail, as well as a larger calcification seen in the region of the head of the pancreas. Clinical correlation regarding possible previous pancreatitis is suggested. On this study, there is also questionable prominence of the head of the pancreas, but it is immediately adjacent to the duodenum and difficult to separate without IV contrast. Ultrasound may be helpful for evaluation of the pancreas, although the pancreas is not always well visualized with ultrasound. Vascular calcifications are seen in the aorta and its branches. Degenerative change is seen in the spine. The noncontrasted bladder has a normal CT appearance.

IMPRESSION:

1. Calcifications within the pancreas. Clinical correlation regarding possibility of prior pancreatitis is suggested.
2. Questionable prominence to the head of the pancreas is immediately adjacent to the bowel, and it is uncertain whether this represents volume averaging within the bowel. Please see above comments regarding ultrasound.
3. Atherosclerotic change involves the aorta and its branches.

SERVICE CODE(S): _____

ICD-10-CM DX CODE(S): _____

(Answers to every other Case are located in Appendix D . The full answer key is only available in the TEACH Instructor Resources on Evolve.)

CASE 3-15   *CT Scan, Chest*

Report Dr. Monson's service. The patient is status post mastectomy, which is reported with a Z code. Reference the Index of the ICD-10-CM under "Absence, breast, acquired" for the Tabular location of the code.

LOCATION: Outpatient, Hospital

PATIENT: Christina Saenz

PHYSICIAN: Gregory Dawson, MD

RADIOLOGIST: Morton Monson, MD

EXAMINATION OF: Chest diagnostic CT (computerized tomography)

CLINICAL SYMPTOMS: Shortness of breath

TECHNIQUE: The patient was scanned from the apices of the lungs through the adrenals following administration of intravenous contrast.

FINDINGS: This examination is compared with a prior chest CT scan dated July 11. The patient is status post left mastectomy. Postsurgical changes are similar in appearance to the prior examination. Definite axillary adenopathy is not seen on this examination. Definite mediastinal adenopathy is not seen. No hilar adenopathy is identified. There are bilateral pleural effusions present on this examination. The right is larger than the left. The right effusion is larger than what was seen previously, and the left effusion is new. The liver appears heterogeneous, which presumably relates to the phase of enhancement at which it was scanned. Multiple hypodensities are associated with the liver. These were evaluated on a recent abdomen CT with follow-up suggested on that CT. Please refer to that report. The adrenal glands demonstrate the presence of scattered fibrotic change. Also, hazy opacity is present within the right lower lung zone. This may relate to atelectasis or infiltrate. I would recommend progress studies to document clearing of the opacities as well as the pleural effusions to exclude underlying lesions.

IMPRESSION:

1. Postsurgical changes of the left hemithorax.
2. Bilateral pleural effusions, worsened since the prior examination.
3. Hazy opacity seen within the right lower lung zone, which may relate to atelectasis or infiltrate.
4. Additional scattered fibrotic change noted within the lungs.

SERVICE CODE(S): _____

ICD-10-CM DX CODE(S): _____

(Answers to every other Case are located in Appendix D . The full answer key is only available in the TEACH Instructor Resources on Evolve.)

CASE 3-16   *CT Scan, Chest, Abdomen, and Pelvis*

Report Dr. Monson's service.

LOCATION: Outpatient, Hospital

PATIENT: Thelma Olson

PHYSICIAN: Gregory Dawson, MD

RADIOLOGIST: Morton Monson, MD

EXAMINATION OF: CT (computerized tomography) of chest, abdomen, and pelvis

CLINICAL SYMPTOMS: Right lower-lobe mass, abdominal aortic aneurysm, increasing girth, and fatigue.

CT OF CHEST, ABDOMEN, AND PELVIS: Technique: CT of the chest, abdomen, and pelvis was performed with oral and IV (intravenous) contrast material with delayed images through the kidneys. No previous CTs for comparison.

FINDINGS: Chest: Moderate-sized right pleural effusion with associated compressive atelectasis. Patchy, somewhat rounded infiltrate in the right mid and lower lung, which is nonspecific and could represent a neoplastic or infectious process. There is a 6.8-cm (centimeter) bleb or bulla in the right lower lobe. Emphysematous changes in both lungs. No mediastinal, hilar, or axillary adenopathy. Coronary artery calcification. No left pleural effusion. No focal adrenal masses. Atheromatous changes in the thoracic aorta. Slight fibrosis or linear atelectasis left lower lobe. Bullous formation in the posterior aspect of the right upper lobe.

ABDOMEN AND PELVIS: Moderate amount of ascites in the abdomen and pelvis, most marked in the right paracolic gutter. Normal-appearing small bowel and large bowel. No focal hepatic lesions. No focal adrenal masses. There is a prominent retrocrural node (images 40 and 41), which measures upper limits of normal. No abdominal or pelvic adenopathy. No free air. Tiny low-density lesion in the midportion of the left kidney is too small to characterize. Infrarenal abdominal aortic aneurysm, which measures 3.5 cm in maximum AP (anterior posterior) diameter and extends for a length of 3 to 4 cm and does not include the aortic bifurcation. Atheromatous changes in the abdominal aorta. No bony destructive lesions.

SERVICE CODE(S): _____

ICD-10-CM DX CODE(S): _____

Discussion

This report is an excellent example of connecting the diagnoses to the service/procedure codes. A diagnostic CT (computerized tomography) scan of the chest (thorax) was performed because of the right lower-lobe mass; the CT of the abdomen was performed to assess the abdominal aortic aneurysm, and the pelvic scan was performed to assess the bowels and kidneys. Since these services were provided and are now going to be reported, diagnoses to support the submission of each service must be provided.

The Findings section of the report indicates the following (words from the report are highlighted):

Pleural effusion is the presence of fluid in pleural space that can cause atelectasis (incomplete expansion of the lung). In this case there is a moderate-sized pleural effusion of the right lung which is not identified as caused by another process; therefore, it is reported. Infiltrate into the right lung has occurred, but the physician indicates that this could be caused by a "neoplastic (like a neoplasm) or infectious process"; and since outpatient coders do not report these types of probable diagnoses, these statements are not considered when reporting the diagnoses for this case.

Presence of a "bleb or bulla" (both words mean the same thing—a distended space in the lung associated with emphysema) in right lower lobe, and "emphysematous" (of the nature of emphysema) changes in both lungs. It would seem that the patient has emphysema, but the physician did not state this directly, and as such emphysema is not coded.

"Coronary artery calcification." This is not the reason the services were rendered, so this would be an incidental finding, which could or could not be reported.

"Atheromatous changes in the abdominal aorta." Atheromatous describes the nature of atheroma, a gruel-type matter that fills a tumor. This is not a definitive diagnosis that can be reported.

"Slight fibrosis OR linear atelectasis left lower lobe." Stated as a differential (one OR the other) diagnosis, which outpatient coders do not report.

"Bullous formation in the posterior aspect of the right upper lobe." Bullous is derived from bulla, which means a distended space. This is not a diagnosis as much as it is a statement of what the lung area looks like (it is distended as in emphysema).

None of these statements is a definitive diagnosis, so the reason for the x-ray of the thorax remains most definitively as "mass of right lower lobe."

Now for the abdomen and pelvis CT scan results in terms of diagnoses. "Ascites" is an accumulation of fluid in the abdominal cavity and is the reason for the increased girth, as stated in the Clinical Symptoms section of the report.

"Tiny low-density lesion in the mid-portion of the kidney is too small to characterize." This is an incidental finding and will not be reported.

"Infrarenal (below or beneath the kidney) **abdominal aortic aneurysm."** This is the same as the entrance diagnosis and will be reported.

"Atheromatous changes in the thoracic aorta." Atheromatous is the nature of atheroma, which is a gruel-type matter that fills a tumor. This is not a definitive diagnosis that can be reported.

In the end, after analysis of the report there is only one diagnosis that will be reported in addition to the entrance diagnoses of right lower lobe mass and abdominal aortic aneurysm—ascites. The right lower lobe mass (which is not a neoplasm, but a mass) is reported, the abdominal aortic aneurysm is reported, and the ascites is reported. The fatigue may be reported but does not support any of the services provided, so it is an incidental diagnosis.

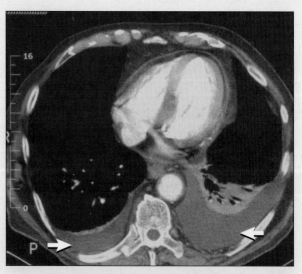

FIGURE 3–9 Pleural effusion.

CASE 3-17 *CT Scan, Abdomen*

This service is provided due to an abnormal radiological examination. You can begin your search for the correct diagnosis code in the Index of the ICD-10-CM under the term "Abnormal, diagnostic imaging" subtermed by the type of examination. Report Dr. Monson's service.

LOCATION: Outpatient, Hospital

PATIENT: Jamal Johnson

PHYSICIAN: Ronald Green, MD

RADIOLOGIST: Morton Monson, MD

EXAMINATION OF: CT (computerized tomography) of abdomen

CLINICAL SYMPTOMS: Previous abdomen radiography indicated abnormality

CT OF ABDOMEN: This study is performed on July 5, and comparisons were made with the prior study of January 1.

Images were obtained from the hemidiaphragm through the inferior pubic rami. Seven-mm (millimeter) 3-D reconstructions through the abdomen were performed with 10-mm 3-D reconstructions. Nonionic intravenous contrast was used for the patient's safety and convenience. Oral contrast was also administered.

The cardiac silhouette is enlarged. There is evidence of bilateral pleural effusions, increased when compared with the previous study, particularly on the right. Atelectasis involving portions of the right lung base is seen. Midline sternotomy is noted. There is evidence of previous left mastectomy. On the initial study, the liver is extremely heterogeneous. I believe this is most likely due to an arterial phase resulting from poor cardiac output. Delayed images reveal the liver to be somewhat less inhomogeneous. At least three distinct cystic areas involving the liver are seen, one along the anterior right lobe, which on today's study measures 2 × 1.7 cm (centimeter) and has densities of approximately 8 Hounsfield units. The area within the left lobe measures 1.8 × 1.7 cm and has densities that are −5, which are most likely averaging. A smaller cystic area within the right lobe is seen on image 19. This is really too small to measure well or characterize. These are basically similar compared with the previous study insofar as I can determine. Evidence is also seen of abdominal and pelvic ascites at this time. This was also seen previously. The volume is small. Fluid is seen along the presacral region in the sigmoid colon. There is also what appears to be fluid surrounding portions of the lower bowel loops. A small midline uterus is noted. It is difficult to see clearly the tissue planes along the fluid and uterus. I cannot really rule out some soft-tissue density within this region, which may or may not be associated with the uterus. These findings are very similar, however, compared with the previous study. The pancreas is somewhat difficult to assess and appears to be small and atrophic. The adrenal glands are not enlarged. The spleen is not grossly enlarged. There is satisfactory excretory function within the kidneys, with partially opacified bladder being present. There is heavy aortoiliac ASVD (arteriosclerotic vascular disease) without aneurysm. The remainder of the abdomen is basically stable and similar compared with the previous study.

CONCLUSION:

1. Status post midline sternotomy. There appears to be cardiac enlargement.
2. Bilateral pleural effusions, more prominent on the right, increased compared with the previous study. Atelectasis involving portions of the right lung base is also seen.
3. The initial study of the liver is quite inhomogeneous. I believe this is due to an arterial phase of the study resulting from the patient's apparent low cardiac output. The delayed images reveal the liver to be somewhat more homogeneous, although three apparent probable cystic areas are identified. These areas appear to be relatively stable and similar compared with the previous study. A small amount of abdominal ascites is also suggested. Fluid is seen within the pelvis, including the presacral region surrounding the sigmoid colon. These findings are relatively similar compared with the previous study. There are several low-lying bowel loops, which makes it difficult to assess whether there is fluid surrounding these bowel loops or some soft-tissue density. These findings, however, are basically unchanged compared with the previous study. The findings must be clinically correlated. An additional 6-month follow-up would be recommended to reassess again.
4. Aortoiliac ASVD without gross aneurysm. The remainder of the abdomen and pelvis is basically unchanged compared with the prior study.

SERVICE CODE(S): _____

ICD-10-CM DX CODE(S): _____

CASE 3-18 *CT Scan, Abdomen and Pelvis*

This service is provided due to an abnormal function study. You can begin your search for the correct diagnosis code in the Index of the ICD-10-CM under the term "Abnormal, function studies", subtermed by type of study. Report Dr. Monson's service.

LOCATION: Outpatient, Hospital

PATIENT: Amanda Longtree

PHYSICIAN: Larry Friendly, MD

RADIOLOGIST: Morton Monson, MD

EXAMINATION OF: CT (computerized tomography) of abdomen and pelvis

CLINICAL SYMPTOMS: Elevated liver function tests

CT OF ABDOMEN AND PELVIS: TECHNIQUE: 7-mm (millimeter) scans are obtained from the lung bases to the iliac crests and 10-mm scans from the iliac crests to the symphysis pubis. The study was done with oral and intravenous contrast.

Limited comparison with CT scan of the chest from July 11.

Scattered fibrotic changes are seen in the lower lung zones. A 1.6-cm (centimeter) hypodense lesion is noted along the anterior aspect of the upper liver on image 10. Hounsfield units are upper limits of that expected for a cyst. Characterization, however, is limited because this is seen on one cut only. An additional hypodense lesion is seen in the left lobe of the liver anteriorly on image 12. This has Hounsfield units consistent with a cyst. These lesions appear unchanged since the previous study. Two additional small hypodensities are seen in the right lobe of the liver, but they are too small to characterize further. The evaluation of the liver overall is somewhat limited because of the phase of the bolus. This appears to be early regarding vascular enhancement. It is therefore difficult to assess the density of the liver compared with the spleen, and I am unable to assess for the presence or absence of fatty infiltration. The pancreas is grossly unremarkable. Adrenal glands and kidneys are grossly unremarkable. A small soft-tissue density is seen in the pelvis bilaterally, likely reflecting patient's ovaries. Vascular calcifications are seen. There is hazy

Continued

CASE 3-18—*cont'd*

density seen in the presacral space, and there appears to be a small amount of fluid. This includes adjacent to the rectum.

IMPRESSION:

1. Two hypodense lesions are noted along the anterior aspect of the liver. One of these appears to be a cyst. The other lesion is difficult to characterize because of its small size, but it may also be a cyst. These lesions do not appear significantly changed from July 11. Two additional tiny hypodensities are seen in the liver. Suggest additional short-term follow-up in 3 to 4 months to document stability.

2. Unable to assess for the presence or absence of fatty infiltration of the liver because of the phase of enhancement.

SERVICE CODE(S): _____

ICD-10-CM DX CODE(S): _____

CT Guidance

The CT scan is also used for guidance for procedures, such as needle placement for biopsies, tissue ablation (destruction), radiation therapy, and vertebroplasty. Guidance or marking is reported separately from the procedure. See the index of the CPT manual entries under CT Scan, Guidance, for the location of the codes to report these guidance or marking services.

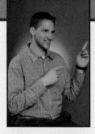

From the Trenches

"The most rewarding part of being a coder is collaborating with a team to solve problems."

MICHAEL HAAS
CPC, MBA

CASE 3-19 *CT-Guided Kidney Biopsy*

Dr. Riddle is an interventional radiologist who performed a CT-guided kidney biopsy. Report the biopsy and the guidance services provided by Dr. Riddle.

LOCATION: Outpatient, Hospital

PATIENT: Matt Barons

PHYSICIAN: Alma Naraquist, MD

RADIOLOGIST: Edward Riddle, MD

EXAMINATION OF: CT (computerized tomography)-guided kidney biopsy

CLINICAL SYMPTOMS: Severe chronic renal insufficiency and severe anemia

CT-GUIDED KIDNEY BIOPSY: HISTORY: This 70-year-old man presents with severe chronic renal insufficiency and severe anemia. The etiology of nephrotic syndrome and renal insufficiency is unknown.

FINDINGS: The procedure, risks, complications, and alternatives were explained to the patient and the patient's family. After questions and answers, they understand and agree to proceed.

The patient was prepped and draped in the standard fashion. With 1% Xylocaine with local anesthesia and conscious sedation with both Versed and fentanyl, the inferior third of the right lower pole kidney was selected with a van Sonnenberg needle. With a coaxial system, multiple 20-gauge core biopsies were obtained. Few glomeruli were evident. The tissue appeared very scarred and hyalinized. Then the middle third of the right kidney was selected, and similar results were obtained with the 20-gauge core biopsy. Then the inferior third of the left kidney was selected, this time with an 18-gauge ASAP needle. CT confirmed the position. Multiple core biopsies were obtained. Only one or two glomeruli were possibly evident but, similar to the other side of the tissue, appeared very scarred and hyalinized. At this point, we discussed the situation with the pathologist, and we agreed just to send the tissue out for further analysis.

Postprocedure CT scan through the retroperitoneal kidney region shows some mild bilateral retroperitoneal hemorrhage. The patient tolerated the procedure well, and we will follow up with him this afternoon and make some decisions as to whether or not he can be discharged to home or needs to stay in the hospital overnight.

IMPRESSION: Successful CT-guided core biopsies of the right kidney and left kidney as described above.

SERVICE CODE(S): _____

ICD-10-CM DX CODE(S): _____

Discussion

This service included CT scan guidance for biopsy needle placement, which is the first CPT code listed followed by the code for the bilateral (-50) kidney biopsy. Next, a follow-up (postprocedural) CT scan was performed, with -26 appended to indicate that only the professional portion of the service is being reported.

The diagnoses stated in the Clinical Symptoms section of the report (renal insufficiency and anemia) and the nephrotic syndrome found within the body of the report are reported. Nephrotic syndrome is a name for a group of diseases involving defective renal glomeruli that result in proteinuria (excess protein in urine) and lipiduria (excess lipids in urine).

CASE 3-20 *CT Scan, Brain*

CT scan provides excellent detail, as in the following case of brain hemorrhage and malignant neoplasm. Report Dr. Monson's service only.

LOCATION: Inpatient, Hospital

PATIENT: Daniel Quick

PHYSICIAN: Timothy Pleasant, MD

RADIOLOGIST: Morton Monson, MD

EXAMINATION OF: CT (computed tomography) of brain

CLINICAL SYMPTOMS: Brain hemorrhage and primary malignant parietal lobe neoplasm

COMPUTED TOMOGRAPHIC EXAMINATION OF THE BRAIN was performed without contrast material and is compared with 2 days previously.

In the interim, the patient has had surgical procedure for parietal removal of neoplasm and hemorrhage in the right frontoparietal region. Anterior portions of the lateral ventricles again are noted to be expanded, and these now contain a considerable amount of gas from the operative procedure. There is also linear gas more posteriorly in the right hemisphere, surrounding a fluid-filled cavity that I believe represents the posterior portion of the lateral ventricle. The gas appears to be external or along the margin of the ventricle.

There is blood within the posterior portions of the lateral ventricles. I do not believe there is evidence of significant raised intracranial pressure. There is a small amount of gas in the scalp at the surgical site.

IMPRESSION: Partial removal of neoplasm and tumor from the right hemisphere. Findings as described above. I do not believe there is increased intracranial pressure.

Small amount of gas in the scalp, which might represent postsurgical gas but might also represent a small dural leak if the dura was closed. It is recognized that this patient has had multiple surgical procedures, and there is most probably a significant amount of dural scarring.

SERVICE CODE(S): _____

ICD-10-CM DX CODE(S): _____

(Answers to every other Case are located in Appendix D. The full answer key is only available in the TEACH Instructor Resources on Evolve.)

Ultrasound

Diagnostic ultrasound is the use of high-frequency sound waves to image anatomic structures and to detect the cause of illness and disease. The physician uses it in the diagnosis process. Ultrasound moves at different speeds through tissue, depending on the density of the tissue. Forms and outlines of organs can be identified by ultrasound as the sound waves bounce back from the tissue (echo).

Codes for ultrasound procedures are found in three locations:

- Radiology section, Diagnostic Ultrasound subsection, 76506-76999, divided on the basis of the anatomic location of the procedure (e.g., chest, pelvis)
- Medicine section, Non-Invasive Vascular Diagnostic Studies subsection, 93880-93998, divided on the basis of the anatomic location of the procedure (cerebrovascular, extremity)
- Medicine section, Echocardiography (ultrasound of the heart and great arteries), 93303-93355

The ultrasound codes for heart and vessels are in the Medicine section; all other ultrasound codes are in the Radiology section.

Modes and Scans

The four different types of ultrasound listed in the CPT manual are A-mode, M-mode, B-scan, and real-time scan.

- **A-mode:** One-dimensional display reflecting the time it takes the sound wave to reach a structure and reflect back. This process maps the structure's outline. *A* stands for amplitude of sound return (echo).

- **M-mode:** One-dimensional display of the movement of structures. *M* stands for motion.
- **B-scan:** Two-dimensional display of the movement of tissues and organs. *B* stands for brightness. The sound waves bounce off tissue or organs and are projected onto a black-and-white television screen. Strong signals display as black, and weaker signals display as lighter shades of gray. B-scan is also called *gray-scale ultrasound*.
- **Real-time scan:** Two-dimensional display of both the structure and the motion of tissues and organs. The display indicates the size, shape, and movement of the tissue or organ.

These modes and scans are used to describe the codes throughout the Diagnostic Ultrasound subsection. Codes are often divided on the basis of the scan or mode that was used. The medical record will indicate the scan or mode used.

Several codes within the subsection include the use of Doppler ultrasound. **Doppler ultrasound** is the use of sound that can be transmitted only through solids or liquids. It is a specific version of ultrasonography, or ultrasound. Doppler ultrasound can be standard black-and-white or color. Color Doppler translates the standard black-and-white into colored images, and the code descriptions will specifically state "color-flow Doppler."

There is component coding in the subheading of Ultrasonic Guidance Procedures. The parenthetic information will refer you to the surgical procedure code. For example, code 76946 is for the radiologic supervision and interpretation of ultrasonic guidance for amniocentesis. The radiologist guides (76946) the insertion (59000) of a needle by the surgeon to withdraw fluid from the uterus. If one physician, such as an interventional radiologist, performs both parts of the procedure, report both codes for the one physician.

CASE 3-21   *Ultrasound, Right Lower Quadrant*

Report Dr. Monson's service. This ultrasound is looking for an inflamed appendix because the patient presents with symptoms of appendicitis; however, no appendix is visualized.

LOCATION: Outpatient, Hospital

PATIENT: Kathleen Lee

PHYSICIAN: Daniel G. Olanka, MD

RADIOLOGIST: Morton Monson, MD

RIGHT LOWER QUADRANT ULTRASOUND: Clinical information states right lower quadrant pain, chills, and fever. We are asked to look for an inflamed appendix. Right lower quadrant is imaged. There is bowel gas in that area. There is no fluid collection. There is no free fluid. There is no structure resembling the appendix.

IMPRESSION:

1. Normal ultrasound of right lower quadrant.
2. It must be remembered that failure to image an appendix does not exclude appendicitis.

SERVICE CODE(S): _____

ICD-10-CM DX CODE(S): _____

(Answers to every other Case are located in Appendix D . The full answer key is only available in the TEACH Instructor Resources on Evolve.)

CASE 3-22   *Ultrasound, Gallbladder*

Report Dr. Monson's service.

LOCATION: Outpatient, Hospital

PATIENT: Mary Lou Moe

PHYSICIAN: Larry Friendly, MD

RADIOLOGIST: Morton Monson, MD

EXAMINATION OF: Gallbladder ultrasound

CLINICAL SYMPTOMS: Abdominal pain

GALLBLADDER ULTRASOUND: Findings: A right pleural effusion is present. A normal gallbladder is not identified. In the region of the gallbladder fossa, there is an echogenic structure that does produce prominent posterior shadowing. This is not peristalsis, and there is adjacent peristalsis of bowel. Common bile duct is 7 mm (millimeter), which is upper normal.

IMPRESSION: Normal gallbladder is not identified. It is thought that there is a WES (wall echo shadow that occurs in patients with contracted gallbladders) sign consistent with a gallbladder packed with stones, but the differential diagnosis does include the absence of a gallbladder with echogenic bowel in the area. Clinical correlation is suggested.

SERVICE CODE(S): _____

ICD-10-CM DX CODE(S): _____

(Answers to every other Case are located in Appendix D . The full answer key is only available in the TEACH Instructor Resources on Evolve.)

CASE 3-23   *Ultrasound, Renal*

Report Dr. Monson's service.

LOCATION: Outpatient, Hospital

PATIENT: Jerry Alcester

PHYSICIAN: Alma Naraquist, MD

RADIOLOGIST: Morton Monson, MD

CLINICAL SYMPTOMS: Nephrotic syndrome

RENAL ULTRASOUND WITH ESTIMATION OF POSTVOID RESIDUAL URINARY BLADDER: No prior study. Right kidney is 11.6 × 6.6 × 5.3 cm (centimeter). It shows some cortical thinning appropriate for age. No cystic or solid mass or hydronephrosis is noted. No echogenic density to suggest calculus. Left kidney is 11.8 × 5.8 × 4.8 cm. No cystic or solid mass or hydronephrosis noted. Prevoid estimated volume is 68.2 ml (milliliter), postvoid urinary volume 7.94 ml. The prostate is enlarged, causing a bulge in the floor of the urinary bladder.

IMPRESSION:

1. Kidneys within normal limits.
2. Renal size normal bilaterally. No cystic or solid mass or hydronephrosis, right or left.
3. No significant urinary volume prevoid or postvoid.
4. Mild prostatic enlargement.

SERVICE CODE(S): _____

ICD-10-CM DX CODE(S): _____

(Answers to every other Case are located in Appendix D . The full answer key is only available in the TEACH Instructor Resources on Evolve.)

CASE 3-24 *Ultrasound, Gallbladder*

Report Dr. Monson's service.

LOCATION: Outpatient, Hospital

PATIENT: Billy Zack

PHYSICIAN: Ronald Green, MD

RADIOLOGIST: Edward Riddle, MD

EXAMINATION OF: Gallbladder sonogram

CLINICAL SYMPTOMS: Abdominal pain in the right upper quadrant

GALLBLADDER SONOGRAM: This examination is difficult because of patient body habitus and position as well as the patient being on a ventilator. The liver is markedly enlarged and extends into the left abdomen. Longest measurement shown is greater than 21 cm (centimeter). The gallbladder may demonstrate echogenic foci within it, which may be stones. No surrounding fluid is noted. No evidence of ductal dilatation is seen. The common hepatic duct and common bile duct measure 0.5 cm each.

SERVICE CODE(S): _____

ICD-10-CM DX CODE(S): _____

(Answers to every other Case are located in Appendix D . The full answer key is only available in the TEACH Instructor Resources on Evolve.)

CASE 3-25 *Ultrasound, Renal*

Report Dr. Monson's service.

LOCATION: Outpatient, Hospital

PATIENT: Pat Highland

PHYSICIAN: George Orbitz, MD

RADIOLOGIST: Morton Monson, MD

EXAMINATION OF: Renal sonogram

CLINICAL SYMPTOMS: Chronic cholecystitis; chronic renal failure

RENAL SONOGRAM: FINDINGS: The right kidney measures 9.0 × 4.1 × 4.1 cm (centimeter). The left kidney measures 9.8 × 4.4 × 4.6 cm. There is bilateral cortical thinning, consistent with the given history. Multiple cysts are seen bilaterally. On the right, the largest cyst measures 2.4 cm in maximum diameter. On the left, the largest cyst measures 1.4 cm in maximum diameter. The bladder volume after voiding is 16 cc (cubic centimeter). Incidental note of a large amount of ascites noted as well.

SERVICE CODE(S): _____

ICD-10-CM DX CODE(S): _____

(Answers to every other Case are located in Appendix D . The full answer key is only available in the TEACH Instructor Resources on Evolve.)

A radiological procedure is often performed because of an abnormal test, such as an abnormal blood chemistry or abnormal function test. You can locate the diagnosis in the Index in the ICD-10-CM under the main term "Findings, abnormal" and then subtermed by the test type. Take time now to review this important section of the Index and become familiar with the subterms located there.

CASE 3-26 *Ultrasound, Renal*

Increasing creatinine and BUN in the report represent a diagnosis of abnormal blood chemistry. Report Dr. Monson's service.

LOCATION: Outpatient, Hospital

PATIENT: Rosie O'Toole

PHYSICIAN: Ronald Green, MD

RADIOLOGIST: Morton Monson, MD

EXAMINATION OF: Renal ultrasound

CLINICAL SYMPTOMS: Increasing creatinine and BUN (blood urea nitrogen), low urine output

RENAL ULTRASOUND: The right kidney measures 10.7 cm (centimeter) long and 5 cm wide; AP (anterior posterior) height is 6.8 cm. There appears to be a calculus involving the upper pole with shadowing. This measures approximately 6 mm (millimeter). Gross hydronephrosis is not seen. The left kidney measures 11.8 × 5.9 × 5.6 cm, respectively. No gross hydronephrosis or calculus is seen. Visualization of both kidneys is somewhat limited because of the patient's body habitus. A Foley catheter is in place. The urinary bladder cannot be assessed.

CONCLUSION: Somewhat limited visualization because of the patient's body habitus. I do not think there is gross hydronephrosis or solid mass involving either kidney, other than what may be a small stone involving the upper pole of the right kidney, which measures 6 mm.

SERVICE CODE(S): _____

ICD-10-CM DX CODE(S): _____

(Answers to every other Case are located in Appendix D . The full answer key is only available in the TEACH Instructor Resources on Evolve.)

CASE 3-27 *Ultrasound, Retroperitoneal*

Report Dr. Monson's service.

LOCATION: Outpatient, Hospital

PATIENT: Shane Gustoworthy

PHYSICIAN: George Orbitz, MD

RADIOLOGIST: Morton Monson, MD

EXAMINATION OF: Renal ultrasound, limited

CLINICAL SYMPTOMS: Acute pyelonephritis

RETROPERITONEAL ULTRASOUND: FINDINGS: The right kidney measures approximately 10.8 cm (centimeter) in length and shows normal renal

echotexture with no evidence of focal scarring, hydronephrosis, calculi, or mass. Suboptimal visualization of the right kidney is due to overlying bowel gas. The left kidney measures approximately 10.1 cm in length and shows normal renal echotexture with no focal scarring, mass, hydronephrosis, or calculi. Cholelithiasis is incidentally noted. Suprapubic catheter is in place.

SERVICE CODE(S): _____

ICD-10-CM DX CODE(S): _____

(Answers to every other Case are located in Appendix D . The full answer key is only available in the TEACH Instructor Resources on Evolve.)

Ultrasound Guidance

Ultrasound is also used for guidance for such procedures as biopsy, aspiration, or injection. The guidance procedures are reported with CPT codes 76932-76965. The radiologist determines the location where the needle is to be inserted and the best route to the site, including the exact measurements to the site. The term "marking" is sometimes used in the reports, but marking is reported with a guidance code since there is no separate code for marking. Ultrasound can also be used during the placement of the needle, catheter, or device. The radiology code does not include the actual procedure, only the marking; guidance for the procedure itself would be reported separately. For example, in the following thoracentesis, the surgeon would report thoracentesis, the radiology physician would report the professional component of the ultrasound guidance for marking, and the facility (hospital) would report the thoracentesis code (32555) along with the technical component of the ultrasound guidance.

CASE 3-28 *Ultrasound, Right Lower Hemithorax—Marking*

Report Dr. Monson's professional service. Dr. Dawson's procedure report is not included in this text; therefore, the thoracentesis procedure code cannot be assigned.

LOCATION: Outpatient, Hospital

PATIENT: Danny Hopmann

PHYSICIAN: Gregory Dawson, MD

RADIOLOGIST: Morton Monson, MD

ULTRASOUND OF THE RIGHT LOWER HEMITHORAX:

HISTORY: Right pleural effusion marking for thoracentesis. Ultrasound guidance is provided to Dr. Dawson during thoracentesis. See his report for the details of the procedure.

FINDINGS: Limited ultrasound of the right lower hemithorax to mark for thoracentesis right-sided pleural effusion, which measures approximately 3.7 cm (centimeter) to the middle of the pocket of pleural fluid.

SERVICE CODE(S): _____

ICD 10 CM DX CODE(S): _____

(Answers to every other Case are located in Appendix D . The full answer key is only available in the TEACH Instructor Resources on Evolve.)

Radiation Oncology

Radiation Oncology deals with both professional and technical treatments using radiation to destroy tumors. The codes are divided on the basis of treatment. Professional and technical components are used extensively. The codes within this subheading include codes for the initial consultation through management of the patient throughout the course of treatment. When the initial consultation occurs, the code for the service would be an E/M code.

Clinical Treatment Planning

Clinical Treatment Planning reflects professional services by the physician. It includes interpretation of special testing, tumor localization, treatment volume determination, treatment time/dosage determination, choice of treatment modality (method), determination of the number and size of treatment ports, selection of appropriate treatment devices, and any other procedures necessary to develop an adequate course of treatment. A treatment plan is set up for all patients who require radiation therapy.

The three types of clinical treatment plans are simple, intermediate, and complex.

■ **Simple** planning requires that there is a single treatment area of interest that is encompassed by a single port or by simple parallel opposed ports with simple or no blocking (77261).

■ **Intermediate** planning requires that there are three or more converging ports, two separate treatment areas, multiple blocks, or special time/dose constraints (77262).

■ **Complex** planning requires that there is highly complex blocking, custom shielding blocks, tangential ports, special wedges or compensators, three or more separate treatment areas, rotational or special beam consideration, or a combination of therapeutic modalities (77263).

Simulation

Simulation aided field setting (77280-77299) is the service of determining treatment areas and placement of the ports for radiation treatment, but it does not include the administration of radiation. A simulation can be performed on a simulator designated for use only in simulations in a radiation therapy treatment unit or on a diagnostic x-ray machine. Codes are divided to indicate four levels of simulation-aided service:

■ **Simple** simulation of a single treatment area, with either a single port or parallel opposed ports and simple or no blocking (77280), also referred to as verification simulation.

■ **Intermediate** simulation of three or more converging ports, with two separate treatment areas and multiple blocks (77285).

■ **Complex** simulation of tangential ports, with three or more treatment areas, rotation or arc therapy, complex blocking, custom shielding blocks, brachytherapy source verification, hyperthermia probe verification, and any use of contrast material (77290).

■ **Three-dimensional** (#77295) computer-generated reconstruction of tumor volume and surrounding critical normal tissue structures based on direct CT scan and/ or MRI data in preparation for noncoplanar or coplanar therapy; this is a simulation that utilizes documented three-dimensional beam's-eye view volume dose displays of multiple or moving beams. Documentation of three-dimensional volume reconstruction and dose distribution is required (77295).

For most third-party payers, normal follow-up care is included for 3 months following completion of treatment that was reported using radiation oncology codes. You would not bill for the normal follow-up care that occurs within this 3-month period.

Medical Radiation Physics, Dosimetry, Treatment Devices, and Special Services codes (77295, 77300-77370) report the decision making of the physicians as to the type of treatment (modality), dose, and development of treatment devices (blocks, stents, bolus, etc.). It is common to have several dosimetry or device changes during a treatment course.

Dosimetry is the calculation of the radiation dose and placement. The number of calculations is reported on the basis of the level of treatment devices (simple, intermediate, and complex).

Radiation Treatment Delivery (77385-77587, 77401-77417, 77424-77425) is the technical component of the service or the actual delivery of the radiation. Radiation treatment is delivered in units called megaelectron volts (MeV). A megaelectron volt is a unit of energy. The radiation energy delivered by the machine is measured in megaelectron volts; the energy that is deposited in the patient's tissue is measured in rads (radiation-absorbed dose). The therapy dose in a cancer treatment would typically be in the thousands of rads.

To code Radiation Treatment Delivery services, you need to know the amount of radiation delivered and the number of the following:

■ Areas treated (single, two, three, or more)
■ Ports involved (single, three or more, tangential)
■ Blocks used (none, multiple, custom)

Radiation Treatment Management

Radiation Treatment Management (77427-77499) reports the professional component. The codes are used to report units of five treatments of radiation therapy. The notes under the heading Radiation Treatment Management state that clinical management is based on five fractions or treatment sessions, regardless of the actual time period in which the treatment is furnished. The services do not need to be furnished in consecutive days. Multiple fractions or treatment sessions consisting of two or more treatments on the same day may be reported separately, as long as there is a break in the therapy sessions. If the patient receives five treatments and then receives an additional one or two fractions, you do not report the additional fractions. Only if three or more fractions beyond the original five are delivered at the end of a course of treatment would you code using 77427 to indicate the additional treatment. If the complete course of treatment only includes one or two fractions, code 77431 would be reported in place of 77427.

Bundled into the Radiation Treatment Management codes are the following physician services:

■ Review of port films
■ Review of dosimetry, dose delivery, and treatment parameters
■ Review of patient treatment setup
■ Examination of the patient for medical evaluation and management (e.g., assessment of the patient's response to treatment, coordination of care and treatment, review of imaging and/or lab test results)

Proton Beam Treatment Delivery

The delivery of radiation treatment using a proton beam utilizes particles that are positively charged with electricity. The use of the proton beam is an alternative delivery method for radiation in which photon (electromagnetic) radiation traditionally would be used. The Proton Beam subheading (77520-77525) are divided according to whether there was simple, intermediate, or complex delivery.

Hyperthermia

Hyperthermia is an increase in body temperature; it is used as a treatment for cancer. The heat source can be ultrasound, microwave, or another means of increasing the temperature in an area. When the temperature of an area is increased, metabolism increases, which boosts the ability of the body to eradicate cancer cells. The location of the heat source can be external (to a depth of 4 cm or less), interstitial (within the tissues), or intracavitary (inside the body). External treatment would be application to the skin of a heat source such as ultrasound. Interstitial treatment is insertion of a probe that delivers heat directly to the treatment area.

Codes 77600-77615 are used to report external or interstitial treatment delivery.

Intracavitary treatment delivery requires insertion of a heat-producing probe into a body orifice, such as the rectum or vagina. Code 77620 is used to report intracavitary treatment and is the only code listed under Clinical Intracavitary Hyperthermia.

Clinical Brachytherapy

Clinical **brachytherapy** is the placement of radioactive material directly into or surrounding the site of the tumor, as illustrated in **Figure 3-10**. Placement may be **intracavitary** (within a body cavity) or **interstitial** (within the tissues), and material may be placed permanently or temporarily. The terms "source" and "ribbon" are used in the Clinical Brachytherapy codes (77750-77799). A **source** is a container holding a radioactive element that can be inserted directly into the body, where it delivers the radiation dose over time. Sources come in various forms, such as seeds or capsules, and are placed in a cavity (intracavitary) or permanently placed within the tissue (interstitial). **Ribbons** are seeds embedded on a tape. The ribbon is cut to the desired length to control the amount of radiation the patient receives. Ribbons are inserted temporarily into the tissue.

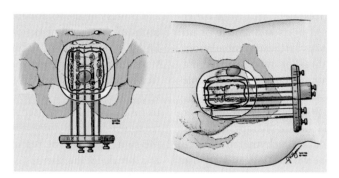

FIGURE 3-10 Proton beam therapy.

From the Trenches

"The coding field is exciting in that it is always challenging and always changing."

MICHAEL HAAS
CPC, MBA

CASE 3-29A   *Radiation Oncology Consultation Note*

Dr. Eagle is a radiation oncologist who specializes in the treatment of cancer and is employed by the clinic. Dr. Eagle is requested by Dr. Avila to consult on Garrison O'Grady, a patient with long-standing prostate cancer. Assign the code for Dr. Eagle's service.

LOCATION: Outpatient, Clinic

PATIENT: Garrison O'Grady

PHYSICIAN: Ira Avila, MD

RADIOLOGIST: James Eagle, MD

HISTORY: The patient is an 80-year-old male with a long-standing history of prostate cancer. He initially presented with right leg lymphedema and hematuria with an elevated PSA (prostate specific antigen). Biopsies of the prostate were performed last year, demonstrating adenocarcinoma with a Gleason's score of 10. He was found to have a pelvic mass with bone metastases as well as a right hydronephrosis. Nephrostomy tubes were placed at that time. He received a course of palliative radiotherapy to 4620 cGy (centigray) in 26 fractions to his pelvis, completed 9 months ago. Subsequently, he developed progressive right lower-extremity edema and initiation of left lower-extremity edema and scrotal edema. He received a second course of radiotherapy to the pelvis, receiving 4500 cGy in 25 fractions, completed 7 months ago. During the interim, the edema slowly increased involving both lower extremities and extending up to his waist. He has also developed a metastatic skin lesion involving the left flank. The patient has undergone several androgen blockade regimens consisting of Lupron, Casodex, and most recently ketoconazole and hydrocortisone. The patient reports that the metastatic skin lesion has increased in size and has become painful and associated with drainage. We have been asked to see the patient by Dr. Avila to render an opinion on the role of palliative radiotherapy for the symptoms of skin metastasis.

ALLERGIES: Allergic to environmental bee stings; otherwise, no known drug allergies.

PAST MEDICAL HISTORY: Significant for:

1. Essential hypertension.
2. Hyperlipidemia.
3. Osteoarthritis.
4. Paget's disease.
5. Locally advanced prostate cancer with metastases as outlined.

PAST SURGICAL HISTORY: Placement of a right nephrostomy tube.

PRESENT MEDICATIONS:

1. Coumadin 5 mg (milligram) q.d. (every day).
2. Dexamethasone 0.75 mg b.i.d. (twice a day).
3. Zaroxolyn 5 mg q.d.
4. Ketoconazole 200 mg t.i.d. (three times a day).
5. Hydrocortisone 20 mg q.a.m. (every morning) and 10 mg q.p.m. (every afternoon or evening).

SOCIAL HISTORY: The patient lives with his younger brother in Marshville, 20 miles east. They have much difficulty with travel arrangements and have requested that he stay at the local elder care unit during his course of radiotherapy. He does have one sister, who accompanies him today. The patient reports that he is essentially unable to ambulate because of the lower-extremity peripheral edema.

FAMILY HISTORY: The patient had a brother who was diagnosed with prostate cancer.

REVIEW OF SYSTEMS: Significant for progressive pain and drainage associated with his skin metastases involving the left flank. It is also significant for progressive lymphedema involving both lower extremities, right greater than left, which has made ambulation essentially impossible. It is negative for fevers, chills, sweats, anorexia, weight loss, difficulty swallowing, cough, hemoptysis, shortness of breath, chest pain, chest tightness, chest pressure, nausea, vomiting, diarrhea, constipation, or musculoskeletal pain. EENT is within normal limits. Neurologic responses are normal. Review of systems is otherwise negative.

EXAMINATION: The patient is an 80-year-old man who appears to be in no apparent distress. Pulse is 90 and respiratory rate is 18. Head is normocephalic and atraumatic. The auricular canals and tympanic membranes are clear and intact bilaterally. Eyes have EOMI (extraocular movement intact). PERRLA (pupils equal, round, reactive to light, and accommodation). Visual fields are full to confrontation. Sclerae are clear. Oral cavity is pink and moist without mucosal lesions. Dentition is in good repair. Lungs are clear to auscultation and percussion. Heart is regular without murmur. The left flank has a 13.5-cm (centimeter) wide lesion, which measures 5.5 cm in height and protrudes about 1.5 to 2 cm. The metastatic skin lesion is purplish and is mildly weeping throughout the consultation. A right nephrostomy tube is appreciated. There is pitting edema up through the ileal chest bilaterally and is significantly worse distally. Neurologically, he is oriented times three. Cranial nerves II through XII are intact. Gait is impossible, with the patient being wheelchair-bound.

IMPRESSION: Metastatic prostate cancer with symptomatic metastases to the left flank.

RECOMMENDATIONS: The patient is an 80-year-old man who presents with symptomatic skin metastases originating from his prostate cancer. I do believe he would benefit from palliative radiotherapy to the left flank for pain control as well as to decrease the drainage from the symptomatic skin metastases. The indications and goals of palliative radiotherapy have been discussed with the patient and his sister. Before initiating his palliative radiotherapy, the patient will require accommodations in the elder care unit. We contacted our social worker, who will facilitate living arrangements. Once the patient is able to become a resident within the elder care unit, he will then initiate his palliative radiotherapy. The patient and his family declined living arrangements here because of the difficulty with travel arrangements. All questions and concerns have been addressed.

Total time spent with the patient and his family today was 42 minutes.

We appreciate the opportunity to participate and to advise you in the care of your patient.

SERVICE CODE(S): _____

ICD-10-CM DX CODE(S): _____

Codes are divided on the basis of the number of sources or ribbons used in an application:

- Simple 1-4
- Intermediate 5-10
- Complex greater than 10

The Clinical Brachytherapy codes include the physician's work related to the patient's admission to the hospital as well as the daily hospital visits.

This patient is presenting for a consultation as stated in the last sentence of the History section of the report (Case 3-29A), "We have been asked to see the patient by Dr. Avila to render an opinion on the role of palliative radiotherapy for the symptoms of skin metastasis." The diagnosis for the secondary neoplasm of the skin (metastatic site) is listed first as per the directions in the *Official Guidelines for Coding and Reporting*. When the encounter is for the secondary site, the secondary site (skin metastasis) is listed first, and the primary site (neoplasm of the prostate) is listed second.

CASE 3-29B   *Radiation Oncology Treatment Planning Note*

Mr. O'Grady has been established at the elder care unit and is now ready to begin his palliative treatment. Palliative treatment is focused toward making the patient as comfortable as possible. The treatment is not intended to cure the condition but only to provide more comfort to a patient by relieving some of the pain. This is the clinical treatment planning of a complex level due to use of a custom-made Cerrobend block. Assign the code for Dr. Eagle's service.

LOCATION: Outpatient, Clinic

PATIENT: Garrison O'Grady

PHYSICIAN: Ira Avila, MD

RADIOLOGIST: James Eagle, MD

DIAGNOSIS: Stage IV (intravenous) metastatic adenocarcinoma of the prostate with symptomatic metastasis to the skin involving the left flank.

CLINICAL CONSIDERATIONS: The patient is an 80-year-old man with symptomatic skin metastasis to the left flank from this prostate cancer. The indications, goals, and side effects of palliative radiotherapy for the symptomatic skin metastases have been discussed in detail. The patient and his family appear to understand and have verbalized a desire to proceed with this option. Arrangements have been made for the patient to proceed with his radiotherapy while a resident at the elder care unit.

TECHNICAL CONSIDERATIONS: The patient is an 80-year-old man with symptomatic skin metastasis from his metastatic prostate cancer. The target volume will include the skin of the left flank for a total of 15 fractions. Normal tissues, which need to be considered, include the surrounding normal skin, kidney, spine, and small bowel.

The fractionation is 3750 cGy (centigray) in 15 fractions with an en face radiation treatment field at 100 SSD.

The palliative radiotherapy treatment field will be treated with 9 MEV electrons prescribed to the 90th percent Isodose line. A custom-made Cerrobend block (note this is the treatment device) will be designed for the electron field. Bolus will also be used to enhance the skin dose. He will require a complex simulation, at which time dose calculations will be performed to ensure that the prescribed dose will be delivered to the target volume. The patient will initiate his radiotherapy thereafter. All questions and concerns have been addressed. We appreciate the opportunity to participate in the care of your patient.

SERVICE CODE(S): _____

ICD-10-CM DX CODE(S): _____

(Answers to every other Case are located in Appendix D . The full answer key is only available in the TEACH Instructor Resources on Evolve.)

CASE 3-29C   *Radiation Oncology Simulation Note*

The simulation is now performed to calculate the amount of radiation that would be delivered during the treatment phase. The level of the simulation is indicated in the treatment-planning note in the previous report. The custom-made treatment block (treatment device) is reported with a separate CPT code. This is a complex simulation involving blocking. Assign the professional portion of this service.

LOCATION: Outpatient, Hospital

PATIENT: Garrison O'Grady

PHYSICIAN: Ira Avila, MD

RADIOLOGIST: James Eagle, MD

DIAGNOSIS: Stage IV (intravenous) symptomatic skin metastases involving the left flank originating from metastatic prostate cancer.

SIMULATION: After explaining to the patient the purpose of the simulation procedure, he was placed on the treatment table in the prone position. He was then placed in the treatment position.

THERAPEUTIC FIELD SETUP: An electron radiotherapy treatment field was clinically set at 100 SSD. A custom-made Cerrobend block (note this is the treatment device) will be constructed for the radiotherapy treatment field. We anticipate using 9-MeV (mega volt) electrons prescribed to the 90th percent Isodose line. Bolus will also be used to enhance the dose distribution to the skin. Dose calculations will be performed to ensure that the prescribed dose will be delivered to the target volume.

The entire simulation took approximately 40 minutes. The patient tolerated the procedure very well and was discharged in stable condition. We anticipate the patient initiating his radiotherapy later this week.

SERVICE CODE(S): _____

ICD-10-CM DX CODE(S): _____

Treatment Delivery

The physician writes one progress note for each week of treatment. Five fractions are delivered in a week, with one treatment a day for 5 days. The physician portion of the service is reported with 77427, once for each week with five fractions. The radiation oncology services are often provided in the hospital setting in an outpatient department, such as a radiation oncology department. The hospital outpatient coder then reports the services for the facility on the CMS-1450 (UB-04). The facility services are reported with different codes because the hospital is providing the physical location where the treatments are delivered and any additional service that may be required, such as in the following report, where port films are taken. The port films are x-rays that are taken to ensure the correct positioning of the treatment portals for the patient who is receiving external beam radiation therapy. Port films charges are for the technical component only, with no professional component provided or reported. The hospital would report the port image(s) (77417), in addition to the radiation therapy treatment delivery, on a per-session basis.

CASE 3-29D *Radiation Oncology Progress Note—Week 1, 5 Days*

This is the first week of treatment delivery. Report the code for the professional portion of this service.

LOCATION: Outpatient, Hospital

PATIENT: Garrison O'Grady

PHYSICIAN: Ira Avila, MD

RADIOLOGIST: James Eagle, MD

HISTORY: The patient is an 80-year-old man with stage IV (intravenous) prostate cancer with symptomatic skin metastases involving the left flank. He has received 1250 cGy (centigray) in 5 fractions to his left flank. He has had a significant reduction in the metastatic lesion; however, he has also had a reaction from the tape required for his dressing. He denies any change in his energy level or changes in his bowel habits.

PHYSICAL EXAMINATION: Pulse is 84. Respiratory rate is 18. The neck is supple without adenopathy. Lungs are clear.

Heart is regular without murmur. There is a palpable mass within the left flank that measures 12 3 5 cm (centimeters), which protrudes less than at his consultation. There is a suggestion of necrosis with drainage from his tumor.

BEAM REVIEW: The patient's treatment position is as initially planned. The dose calculations have been reviewed and indicate the correct setting for all treatments.

PORT FILMS: The patient has been seen clinically with the setup being accepted.

DISPOSITION: The patient will continue with his radiation treatments as prescribed. He will continue with his dressings consisting of Telfa gauze and ABD (Adriamycin, bleomycin, dacarbazine) dressing with the use of a tape. We will initiate the use of a tape prep to protect his skin during his treatment process. We will continue to monitor for further radiation side effects and treat as indicated.

SERVICE CODE(S): _____

ICD-10-CM DX CODE(S): _____

(Answers to every other Case are located in Appendix D . The full answer key is only available in the TEACH Instructor Resources on Evolve.)

CASE 3-29E *Radiation Oncology Progress Note—Week 2, 5 Days*

This is the second week of treatment delivery. Report the code for the professional portion of this service.

LOCATION: Outpatient, Hospital

PATIENT: Garrison O'Grady

PHYSICIAN: Ira Avila, MD

RADIOLOGIST: James Eagle, MD

HISTORY: The patient is an 80-year-old man with a stage IV prostate cancer with symptomatic skin metastases involving the left flank. He has initiated a course of palliative radiotherapy and is receiving 25 Gy (gray) in 10 fractions. He continues to have drainage from tumor necrosis. He has also had a skin reaction from the tape required for his dressings. He denies any changes in his energy level or change in his bowel or bladder habits.

EXAM: Pulse 80. Respiratory rate is 18. The neck is supple without adenopathy. Lungs are clear to auscultation. Heart is regular without murmur. A palpable mass remains within the left flank, measuring 11 3 4.5, which protrudes much less than last week. There continues to be necrosis from the central portion of his tumor, which also has diminished from last week.

BEAM REVIEW: The patient's treatment position is as initially planned. The dose calculations have been reviewed and indicate the correct settings for all treatments.

PORT FILMS: The patient has been seen clinically with the setup being accepted.

DISPOSITION: The patient will continue with his radiation treatments as prescribed. He will continue with his dressings on a daily basis using Telfa gauze and an ABD (Adriamycin, bleomycin, dacarbazine) dressing with the use of tape. The skin will be prepped before application of the gauze and tape. We will monitor for radiation side effects and treat as indicated.

SERVICE CODE(S): _____

ICD-10-CM DX CODE(S): _____

(Answers to every other Case are located in Appendix D . The full answer key is only available in the TEACH Instructor Resources on Evolve.)

Nuclear Medicine

Nuclear medicine deals with the placement of radionuclides within the body and the monitoring of emissions from the radioactive elements.

There are two subsections in Nuclear Medicine: Diagnostic (78012-78999) and Therapeutic (79005-79999). The services listed do not include the radium or other radioelement. You would assign a HCPCS National Level II supply code to report the radium or radioelement. The Diagnostic Nuclear Medicine subsection is divided by organ system (i.e., Endocrine, Gastrointestinal, etc.). The codes report imaging, such as the organ system gastrointestinal, subdivided into, for example, liver and salivary gland imaging. There are usually several imagings or studies that can be performed; for example, there are three codes for salivary gland:

78230	Salivary gland imaging
78231	Salivary gland imaging, with serial images
78232	Salivary gland function study

For the imaging procedure, a radiotracer (radioactive isotope) is injected, and the salivary gland is imaged with a gamma camera (a special camera used to take images of the radiotracers). In the serial imaging procedure, several (a series of) images are taken, and then the patient is given a substance that stimulates the salivary gland (such as a lemon candy) and images are again taken. The function study includes a radioactive substance being placed under the tongue, which stimulates the salivary glands, and images then are taken of the salivary glands to assess the function.

The therapeutic services (79005-79999) contain codes for various treatments in which radiopharmaceuticals are needed to treat lesions and thyroid malfunctions.

Intracavitary and interstitial radioactivity colloid therapies (79200, 79300) are sources that are placed into the body at the site of the tumor, and over time the source emits radiation. An advantage of this method of treatment is that the source gives a high dose of radiation to the tumor and much lower dose to the surrounding areas.

Intravascular and intra-articular therapy involves the placement of radiopharmaceuticals directly into a vessel (intravascular) or a joint (intra-articular). After placement, the radiopharmaceutical destroys the lesion.

Nuclear medicine procedures are located in the index of the CPT manual under Nuclear Medicine.

CASE 3-30   *Diagnostic Pulmonary Function Study*

To locate the correct CPT code, reference "Pulmonary Perfusion Imaging, Nuclear Medicine" in the CPT Index. Assign the professional code for this service.

LOCATION: Outpatient, Hospital

PATIENT: Mary Blue

PHYSICIAN: Ronald Green, MD

RADIOLOGIST: Morton Monson, MD

EXAMINATION OF: Lungs

CLINICAL SYMPTOMS: Hypoxemia, shortness of breath

VENTILATION-PERFUSION SCAN OF LUNGS: DOSE: The patient received 2.0 millicuries of technetium-99m DTPA (diethylene-triamine penta-acetic acid) by aerosol and 6.0 millicuries of technetium-99m labeled MAA (macroaggregated albumin) intravenously.

FINDINGS: This examination is interpreted in conjunction with a chest radiograph dated last month. Overall perfusion appears better than ventilation. The ventilation is very patchy and inhomogeneous. Because of the inhomogeneity, this study is indeterminate for the possibility of pulmonary embolus. There is an apparent triple match present within the right lung base. This also makes the study indeterminate for the possibility of pulmonary embolus. A few scattered matched perfusion defects are seen. Definite unmatched perfusion defects are not seen on this examination.

IMPRESSION: Because of the inhomogeneous ventilation and the triple match within the right lung base, this study is indeterminate for the possibility of pulmonary embolus.

SERVICE CODE(S): _____

ICD-10-CM DX CODE(S): _____

(Answers to every other Case are located in Appendix D . The full answer key is only available in the TEACH Instructor Resources on Evolve.)

CASE 3-31 *Ventilation-Perfusion Lung Scan*

Assign Dr. Monson's service code.

LOCATION: Outpatient, Hospital

PATIENT: Hilda Torgerson

PHYSICIAN: Marvin Elhard, MD

RADIOLOGIST: Morton Monson, MD

EXAMINATION OF: Ventilation-perfusion lung scan

CLINICAL SYMPTOMS: Right chest pain

VENTILATION-PERFUSION LUNG SCAN

DOSE: The patient received 2.0 millicuries of technetium-99m DTPA (diethylene-triamine penta-acetic acid) by aerosol and 6.0 millicuries of technetium-99m labeled MAA (macroaggregated albumin) intravenously.

FINDINGS: This examination is interpreted in conjunction with a chest radiograph, which is dated last year. Evaluation of ventilation and perfusion images demonstrates the presence of small, scattered, matched ventilation and perfusion defects within both lungs. A moderately large perfusion defect is present within the right lung base. This matches on ventilation and perfusion images. A focal opacity is present within this area on the chest radiograph. The findings constitute a triple match, and the study is therefore indeterminate for pulmonary embolus. Definite perfusion mismatches are not seen on this examination.

IMPRESSION: Triple match identified within the right lower lung zone. The study is therefore indeterminate for the possibility of pulmonary embolus. Definite mismatch is not identified.

SERVICE CODE(S): _____

ICD-10-CM DX CODE(S): _____

(Answers to every other Case are located in Appendix D . The full answer key is only available in the TEACH Instructor Resources on Evolve.)

Interventional Radiology

Component or combination coding means that a code from the Radiology section, as well as a code from one of the other sections of the CPT manual, must be used to fully describe the procedure. For example, an interventional radiologist may inject contrast material; place stents, catheters, or guidewires; or perform any number of procedures that could also be performed by two separate physicians—a radiologist and a surgeon. Interventional radiologists perform both the radiology and surgical portions of the procedure. Many times, before radiology procedures can be performed, a contrast material is used to make organs or vessels stand out more clearly on the radiographic image. When this contrast material is injected, a CPT code from the Surgery section must be used to indicate the injection service. For example, if the interventional radiologist performed a placement of percutaneous interstitial markers for radiation therapy guidance (32553) with ultrasonic guidance (76942). If the intervention radiologist performs both portions of the

service, both codes would be reported. If, however, a surgeon performed the placement procedure and a radiologist performed the ultrasonic guidance portion of the service, each would report his or her portion of the service. Remember to append modifier -26 to the CPT code when reporting only the professional component of the radiology services.

Central Venous Access Procedures

Locate the Central Venous Access Procedures codes 36555 and 36566 in the CPT manual. Codes 36555 and 36556 are for **temporary** nontunneled catheters (5-7 days). A tunneled catheter is one that is burrowed into the skin at a distance from the vascular access site. Codes 36557-36561 are for tunneled catheters, but 36557 and 36558 are **level with the skin** with a button-type access. This access is like a PICC (peripherally inserted central catheter) line that is used for direct access for long-term antibiotic IV therapy. Note that 36557 and 36558 are for "without subcutaneous port or pump" and 36560 and 36561 are for "with subcutaneous port."

CASE 3-32 *Radiology Report, Hemodialysis Catheter Placement*

Code the professional interventional radiology services provided by Dr. Riddle.

LOCATION: Outpatient, Hospital

PATIENT: Harry Sportsmann

PERSONAL PHYSICIAN: George Orbitz, MD

RADIOLOGIST: Edward Riddle, MD

EXAMINATION OF: Placement of tunneled hemodialysis catheter

CLINICAL SYMPTOMS: Chronic renal failure

PLACEMENT OF AN ANGIODYNAMICS MORE-FLOW HEMODIALYSIS CATHETER: The patient is a 54-year-old man with a history of renal

failure. Placement of a tunneled hemodialysis catheter was requested by Dr. Orbitz.

Prior to the start of the study, the procedure was explained to the patient, including the risks, complications, and alternatives. The patient understood and consented to the exam.

The patient was prepped and draped in the usual sterile fashion. An Ioban II (antimicrobial film) was placed on the skin.

Using sterile technique under ultrasound guidance following administration of local anesthesia (1% lidocaine), a 21-gauge micropuncture needle was advanced into the right internal jugular vein in the lower neck region. Using a microvena kit, a 0.18 stainless steel wire was used to measure the distance from the junction of the right atrium/superior vena cava to the skin site, and

Continued

CASE 3-32—cont'd

the appropriate-sized catheter was obtained. A 5-French straight catheter was advanced into the internal jugular vein. The catheter was then placed to flush.

A small skin incision was placed in the upper chest region. Following administration of local anesthesia (1% lidocaine), a tunnel was obtained between the two skin incisions. A vascular sheath was then placed through the tunnel, and the More-Flow was then advanced through the peel-away sheath. The 5-French straight catheter then was removed over an extra-stiff wire, and a peel-away sheath was placed into the right internal jugular vein. The dilator and wire were then removed, and the end of the peel-away sheath was crimped to avoid blood loss with the patient holding his breath. The tip of the catheter then was advanced through the peel-away sheath with the tip at the proximal right atrium. The peel-away sheath was removed, and the catheter was adjusted to obtain a smooth transition. The

cuff of the catheter was approximately 1 to 2 cm (centimeters) from the incision site. A single 2-0 Prolene suture was then placed at the catheter insertion site, and two sutures were placed at the lower-neck incision site. No obvious bleeding was seen. Contrast was infused through both ports, which revealed adequate placement. Ultrasound shows the tip of the catheter terminating in the right atrium.

The patient tolerated the procedure well. The patient denied pain and shortness of breath at termination of the study.

IMPRESSION: Placement of a 14.5-French AngioDynamics More-Flow hemodialysis catheter through the internal jugular vein as described above.

SERVICE CODE(S): _____

ICD-10-CM DX CODE(S): _____

CASE 3-33   *Gastrojejunostomy Catheter Placement*

Report Dr. Riddle's services only. In this case, a gastrojejunostomy catheter is placed (the service) for nutritional support of this patient who has nutritional deficiency (the diagnosis). This service includes the percutaneous insertion of the gastrostomy tube and radiologic guidance. Pay close attention to the notes that follow the gastrostomy tube initial placement codes.

LOCATION: Outpatient, Hospital

PATIENT: Brian Neilson

PERSONAL PHYSICIAN: Leslie Alanda, MD

RADIOLOGIST: Edward Riddle, MD

EXAMINATION OF: Placement of gastrojejunostomy catheter

CLINICAL SYMPTOMS: Nutritional support due to nutritional deficiency

PLACEMENT OF GASTROJEJUNOSTOMY CATHETER: The patient is a 63-year-old man with extensive medical history including intracranial hemorrhage. Placement of a percutaneous gastrojejunostomy catheter was requested by Dr. Alanda for nutritional support.

Before start of the study, the procedure was explained to the patient's wife, including the risks, complications, and alternatives. The patient's wife understood and consented to the exam.

The patient was prepped and draped in the usual sterile fashion. Using ultrasound guidance, the edge of the liver was localized. Through a previously placed nasogastric tube, the stomach was distended with air.

Using fluoroscopic guidance following administration of local anesthesia (1% lidocaine), gastropexy was performed using four Medi-Tech T-tacks at the mid to distal aspect of the stomach.

Using multiple wires and catheters, an extra stiff guidewire was ultimately placed with the tip in the proximal jejunum. Following multiple dilatations, a no. 14 French Shetty gastrojejunostomy was placed with the tip in the proximal jejunum. A small amount of contrast was administered, which revealed adequate placement. No evidence of extravasation or other significant abnormalities was seen.

The patient tolerated the procedure well. No evidence of bleeding was seen at the termination of the study.

IMPRESSION: Placement of a No. 14-French Shetty gastrojejunostomy catheter with the tip in the proximal jejunum as described above.

SERVICE CODE(S): _____

ICD-10-CM DX CODE(S): _____

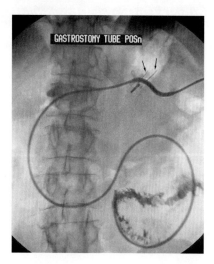

FIGURE 3-11 Gastrojejunostomy.

CASE 3-34   *Gastrojejunostomy Catheter Placement*

There will be a code from the Surgery section to report the gastrostomy tube inserted percutaneously (with the addition of the modifier that indicates a discontinued procedure). The Impression section of the report indicates that the procedure was discontinued. Report Dr. Riddle's professional services.

LOCATION: Outpatient, Hospital

PATIENT: Malcolm Fox

PHYSICIAN: Ronald Green, MD

RADIOLOGIST: Edward Riddle, MD

EXAMINATION OF: Attempted placement of gastrojejunostomy catheter

CLINICAL SYMPTOMS: Abdominal pain and malnutrition

ATTEMPTED PLACEMENT OF GASTROJEJUNOSTOMY CATHETER: The patient is an 86-year-old man with an extensive medical history that includes abdominal pain and malnutrition. Placement of a gastrojejunostomy catheter was requested by Dr. Green.

Before start of the study, the procedure was explained to the patient's daughter, including the risks, complications, and alternatives. The patient's daughter understood and consented to the procedure.

The patient was prepped and draped in the usual sterile fashion. The patient was also sedated.

The gastrojejunostomy catheter could not be safely placed percutaneously because of the patient's anatomy. There is marked dilatation of what is thought to represent small bowel, which is displacing the stomach superiorly. If distension of the small bowel is relieved, percutaneous placement may be possible at a later date.

IMPRESSION: Percutaneous gastrojejunostomy catheter could not be placed because of the patient's anatomy, as described above.

SERVICE CODE(S): _____

ICD-10-CM DX CODE(S): _____

(Answers to every other Case are located in Appendix D . The full answer key is only available in the TEACH Instructor Resources on Evolve.)

CASE 3-35   *Gastrojejunostomy Catheter Placement*

This service involves not only the percutaneous insertion of a gastrostomy tube by Dr. Riddle, but also x-ray guidance performed by Dr. Riddle. Because Dr. Riddle is an interventional radiologist, he has expertise in performing both the percutaneous insertion of the gastrostomy tube and the radiological guidance for the placement. Report Dr. Riddle's services. Pay attention to the notes that follow the gastrostomy tube initial placement codes and descriptions in the CPT manual to report the following services correctly.

LOCATION: Inpatient, Hospital

PATIENT: Jane Wellington

PERSONAL PHYSICIAN: Ronald Green, MD

RADIOLOGIST: Edward Riddle, MD

EXAMINATION OF: Placement of a gastrojejunostomy catheter

CLINICAL SYMPTOMS: CVA (stroke/cardiovascular accident)

PERCUTANEOUS GASTROJEJUNOSTOMY PLACEMENT: The patient is a 60-year-old woman with a history of a stroke and ARDS (acute or adult respiratory distress syndrome) on a ventilator. Placement of a gastrojejunostomy catheter for nutritional support was requested by Dr. Green.

Before start of the study, the procedure was explained to the patient's husband on the phone, including the risks, complications, and alternatives. The patient's husband understood and consented to the procedure.

The patient was prepped and draped in the usual sterile fashion. Using ultrasound guidance, the edge of the liver was localized. Through a previously placed nasogastric tube, the stomach was distended with air.

Using fluoroscopic guidance following administration of local anesthesia (1% lidocaine), gastropexy was performed using four Medi-Tech T-tacks at the mid to distal aspect of the stomach.

Using multiple wires and catheters, an extra-stiff guidewire was ultimately placed with the tip in the proximal jejunum. Following multiple dilatations, a 14-French Shetty gastrojejunostomy was placed with the tip in the proximal jejunum. A small amount of contrast was administered, which revealed adequate placement. There is no evidence of extravasation or other significant abnormalities.

The patient tolerated the procedure well. No evidence of bleeding was seen at termination of the study.

IMPRESSION: Placement of a 14-French Shetty gastrojejunostomy catheter with the tip in the proximal jejunum as described above.

SERVICE CODE(S): _____

ICD-10-CM DX CODE(S): _____

(Answers to every other Case are located in Appendix D . The full answer key is only available in the TEACH Instructor Resources on Evolve.)

CHAPTER 3   *Auditing Review*

Audit the coding for the following reports.

Audit Report 3.1 Interventional Radiology Services
Report the interventional radiology services of Dr. Riddle.

LOCATION: Outpatient, Hospital

PATIENT: Micah Alberta

PHYSICIAN: Ronald Green, MD

SURGEON/RADIOLOGIST: Edward Riddle, MD

CLINICAL SYMPTOMS: Chronic renal failure

PLACEMENT OF A TUNNELED 14.5-FRENCH ANGIODYNAMIC HEMODIALYSIS CATHETER: The patient is a 37-year-old male with history of renal failure. Placement of tunneled hemodialysis catheter was requested by Dr. Green.

Prior to the start of the study, the procedure was explained to the patient including the risk, complications, and alternatives. The patient understood and consented to the examination.

The patient was prepped and draped in the usual sterile fashion. An Ioban II (antimicrobial film) was placed on the skin.

Using sterile technique under ultrasound guidance following administration of local anesthesia (1% lidocaine), a 21-gauge micropuncture needle was advanced into the right internal jugular vein in the lower neck region. Utilizing the microvena kit, a 0.18 stainless-steel wire was utilized to measure the distance from the junction of the right atrium/superior vena cava to the skin site and the catheter was cut to size. A 5-French straight catheter was advanced into the internal jugular vein. The catheter was then placed to flush.

A small skin incision was made in the upper chest region. Following administration of local anesthesia (1% lidocaine), a tunnel was obtained between the two skin incisions. A vascular sheath was then placed through the tunnel, and the catheter was then advanced through the peel-away sheath.

The 5-French straight catheter was then removed over a Rosen wire and a 10-French peel-away sheath was placed into the right internal jugular vein. The dilator and wire were then removed, and the end of the peel-away sheath was crimped to avoid blood loss with the patient holding his breath. The tip of the catheter was then advanced through the peel-away sheath with the tip at the junction of the right atrium/superior vena cava. The peel-away sheath was then removed and the catheter was adjusted to obtain a smooth transition. The cuff of the catheter was approximately 1 to 2 cm from the incision site. There was no evidence of bleeding.

Contrast was infused through the single port, which revealed adequate placement.

Post-placement chest x-ray did not reveal pneumothorax.

The patient tolerated the procedure well. The patient denied pain and shortness of breath at termination of the study.

IMPRESSION: Placement of a tunneled 14.5-French angiodynamic hemodialysis catheter through the right internal jugular vein as described above.

One of the following codes is reported incorrectly for this case. Indicate the incorrect code.

PROFESSIONAL SERVICES: Catheterization, **36558**; Fluoroscopy Guidance, **77001-26**

ICD-10-CM DX: Chronic renal failure, NOS, **N18.9**

INCORRECT CODE: _____

Audit Report 3.2 Emergency Brain CT Scan

LOCATION: Inpatient, Hospital

PATIENT: Annabelle Castaneda

PHYSICIAN: Ronald Green, MD

RADIOLOGIST: Morton Monson, MD

EXAMINATION OF: Emergency brain CT

CLINICAL SYMPTOMS: Hematoma, meninges of brain

COMPUTED TOMOGRAPHIC EXAMINATION OF THE BRAIN was performed without contrast material as an emergency procedure. The patient has had multiple CT examinations, the most recent being last month. She also has had multiple MR examinations, the most recent being 6 months ago. The patient is known to have a large extradural neoplasm adjacent to the right hemisphere. She has had several operative procedures for this neoplasm. Although the neoplasm is thought to be a meningioma, it is obviously aggressive in that it has recurred so frequently.

The most recent brain examination was on March 18th of last year. Apparently that study again showed a solid contrast-enhancing mass (with low-density portions) in relation to the front frontoparietal junction. Significant encephalomalacia of the right frontal lobe is again noted.

On today's CT examination, I believe there has been acute or subacute hemorrhage into the neoplasm of the meninges. The hemorrhage has decompressed into the ventricular system with resultant blood in the posterior portions of both lateral ventricles. I believe there is some swelling of the right hemisphere. However, the patient had previously had much of the right frontal lobe removed. Presently, there is no shift of midline structures from right to left. Left lateral ventricle is larger than normal. Although it has previously been larger than normal, today's examination shows increased enlargement of the frontal and temporal horns. Therefore, there might be some obstruction, although it certainly might not be acute. Cerebral sulci of the left hemisphere can be visualized, as are basal cisterns. Overall, I do not feel that there is significant raised intracranial pressure.

One of the following codes is reported incorrectly for this case. Indicate the incorrect code.

PROFESSIONAL SERVICES: Brain CT scan, **70470-26**

ICD-10-CM DX: Hemorrhagic meninges, **I60.8**; Meninges neoplasm, **D49.7**

INCORRECT CODE: _____

CHAPTER 3—cont'd

Audit Report 3.3 Radiology, Ultrasound

LOCATION: Outpatient, Hospital

PATIENT: Julia Olivia

ORDERING PHYSICIAN: Ronald Green, MD

RADIOLOGIST: Morton Monson, MD

PELVIC TRANSABDOMINAL SONOGRAM AND ABDOMEN COMPLETE SONOGRAM

HISTORY: Chronic abdominal pain

PELVIC AND TRANSABDOMINAL STUDY: The uterus measures 7.1 × 4.7 × 3.3 cm. The endometrial stripe measures 0.6 cm in thickness. The right ovary measures 1.8 × 2.5 × 2.1 cm and the left ovary measures 2.5 × 1.2 × 2.3 cm. No obvious mass is noted in the adnexal regions, although there is a hypoechoic focus adjacent to the right ovary that does not demonstrate flow within it and may be due to small amount of free fluid surrounding it or is perhaps a prominent fallopian tube. Since transvaginal images were not submitted, this is incompletely evaluated.

ABDOMINAL SONOGRAM: The aorta is of normal caliber. The pancreatic head and body are normal. The liver is normal. The gallbladder demonstrates dependent echoes with no evidence of shadowing stones. There is no wall thickening. No ductal dilatation. The common hepatic and common bile duct measure 0.2 and 0.3 cm, respectively. No free fluid in Morison's pouch. The right kidney is normal in length at 8.8 cm and the left kidney measures 9.6 cm in length. No evidence of hydronephrosis bilaterally.

One of the following codes is reported incorrectly for this case. Indicate the incorrect code.

PROFESSIONAL SERVICES: Pelvic ultrasound, **76856-26**; Abdomen ultrasound, **76700-26**

ICD-10-CM DX: Abdominal pain, **R10.84**

INCORRECT CODE: _____

Audit Report 3.4 CT Scan, Abdomen and Pelvis

LOCATION: Outpatient, Hospital

PATIENT: Steve Hart

PHYSICIAN: Ronald Green, MD

RADIOLOGIST: Morton Monson, MD

EXAMINATION OF: CT scan of abdomen and pelvis

CLINICAL SYMPTOMS: Pelvic abscess, previous colon surgery

CT SCAN OF THE ABDOMEN WITHOUT IV CONTRAST: Axial images obtained with oral contrast only, previously given. Compared to 4/13. Atelectatic changes are noted in both lung bases, more pronounced on the left. Underlying left basilar pneumonia could not be excluded. Small left pleural effusion is seen and stable in size from prior study, if not minimally smaller. Previous laminectomy changes of the lumbar spine are present regarding these organs. Gallbladder is distended, a new finding. No layering sludge or gallstones are appreciated, however. No bile duct dilatation is seen. No free air is present. No ascites is noted, either. Bowel is less distended on the current study than seen on prior exam.

CT SCAN OF THE PELVIS WITHOUT IV CONTRAST: Axial images obtained with oral contrast only. Compared to 4/13. Ostomy site is again noted. Findings of pelvic abscesses are again seen with residual wall

thickening around the abscesses noted. These have not significantly changed in size. The smaller, more superficial pocket seen on the left now demonstrates a small amount of air within it. Again noted is presacral soft tissue thickening, which may be inflammatory given the abscesses. Surgical changes are noted here within the pelvis. Tumor cannot be completely excluded.

IMPRESSION:

1. Bibasilar atelectatic changes, more pronounced on the left.
2. Minimal change in left pleural effusion.
3. Gallbladder distention with no radiopaque stones or biliary duct dilation seen.
4. Residual abscess collections noted in the pelvis with minimal change since 4/13.
5. Continued presacral soft tissue thickening. Inflammatory versus tumor.

One or more of the following codes are reported incorrectly or missing for this case. Indicate the incorrect or missing code or codes.

SERVICE CODE(S): Computed tomography, **74177**

ICD-10-CM DX CODE(S): Peritoneal abscess, **K65.1**

INCORRECT/MISSING CODE(S): _____

Audit Report 3.5 CT Scan, Chest, Abdomen, and Pelvis

LOCATION: Outpatient, Hospital

PATIENT: Amy Larson

PHYSICIAN: Gregory Dawson, MD

RADIOLOGIST: Morton Monson, MD

EXAMINATION OF: CT of chest, abdomen, and pelvis

CLINICAL SYMPTOMS: Shortness of breath, nodule of lung, and level 1 trauma due to motor vehicle collision.

CT OF CHEST, ABDOMEN AND PELVIS: Technique: CT of the chest, abdomen, and pelvis was performed with oral and IV contrast material. No previous CTs for comparison.

FINDINGS: Chest: Small lymph nodes are noted within both axillae, but none are pathologically sized. However, there is lymphadenopathy within the mediastinum with nodes seen within the pretracheal, precarinal, paratracheal, and prevascular regions. The largest node is seen in the right paratracheal region and has a diameter of approximately 1.3 cm in short axis diameter. There are other nodules of approximately 1 cm in size. Bilateral pleural effusions are noted with presumed compressive atelectasis. There is some

Continued

opacification in the left hilar region with air bronchograms seen within it, which could be due to atelectasis, although other etiology is possible. Aortic atherosclerotic change with mural thrombus is noted. There is some focal opacity seen, especially in the right lung with air bronchograms within it. Again, this is presumed to be due to some atelectasis. Posterolaterally within the left lung base there is also a pleural based opacity, again of uncertain significance. Multiple other right lung pleural based opacities are noted. This could be loculated pleural fluid collection, although other etiology, including a nodule, is not even excluded in this scenario. The adrenal glands are within limits as to size. The kidneys are small. A lesion within the spleen is not entirely excluded in this setting. Increased mural thrombus is noted within the aorta at the take-off of the celiac and SMA. On the lung window, there is diffuse increase in the density of the lungs, which is seen within lungs, which are fully expanded. Again seen are the numerous bilateral pleural based opacities as described previously. Nodular density seen is consistent with a subcentimeter calcified granuloma.

ABDOMEN AND PELVIS: Mild diffuse fatty infiltration of the liver with no focal hepatic or splenic lesions. There are several lower right rib fractures. NG tube with tip in the proximal stomach. Negative adrenal glands, kidneys, gallbladder. Mild diffuse atrophy of the pancreas. Aortoiliac calcification. The abdominal aorta is of normal caliber. Foley catheter is within the bladder. No free air, free fluid, or adenopathy within the abdomen or pelvis. No fractures are seen involving the spine or pelvis.

One or more of the following codes are reported incorrectly or missing for this case. Indicate the incorrect or missing code or codes.

SERVICE CODE(S):   Computed tomography, **71270, 74178**

ICD-10-CM DX CODE(S):   Pleural effusion, **J90;** Shortness of breath, **R06.02**

INCORRECT/MISSING CODE(S): _____

Audit Report 3.6 Ultrasound, Abdomen

LOCATION: Outpatient, Hospital

PATIENT: Delores Flats

PHYSICIAN: Larry Friendly, MD

RADIOLOGIST: Morton Monson, MD

EXAMINATION OF: Abdomen ultrasound

CLINICAL SYMPTOMS: Nausea and vomiting; abdominal pain. Rule out cholelithiasis.

ABDOMINAL ULTRASOUND: FINDINGS: The liver is normal in size and echo texture with no focal masses. Large shadowing stone in the gallbladder lumen with gallbladder wall thickening and pericholecystic

fluid. No bile duct dilatation. Survey view of the right kidney shows mild to moderate amount of free fluid in the right lower quadrant. The appendix itself is not identified.

One or more of the following codes are reported incorrectly for this case. Indicate the incorrect code or codes.

SERVICE CODE(S): Ultrasound, **76700**

ICD-10-CM DX CODE(S): Nausea with vomiting, **R11.2;** Abdominal pain, **R10.9**

INCORRECT/MISSING CODE(S): _____

(Auditing Review answers with rationales are only available in the TEACH Instructor Resources on Evolve.)

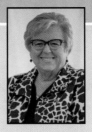

"As a coder, being a member of the health care team means that we do our part by reporting the services provided with the greatest integrity and attention to specificity."

Pathology and Laboratory

http://evolve.elsevier.com/Buck/next

(Answers to every other Case are located in Appendix D, with the full answer key only available in the TEACH Instructor Resources on Evolve)
(Auditing Review answers with rationales are only available in the TEACH Instructor Resources on Evolve)

Types of Services

The codes in the Pathology and Laboratory section of the CPT manual cover a wide variety of services. The following are the types of services most commonly used:

Organ- or Disease-Oriented Panels (80047-80081)

Therapeutic Drug Assays (80150-80299)

Urinalysis (81000-81099)

Chemistry (82009-84999)

Hematology and Coagulation (85002-85999)

Immunology (86000-86849)

Superbill/Requisition Form

Tests are often requested by means of a **superbill** or requisition form as illustrated in **Figure 4-1**. Note on the superbill/requisition form that the area under the "Code" column would contain the CPT laboratory code, but for the purposes of this text, the codes have been deleted and you will be removing Figure 4-1 from the text and placing the codes on the form as you work through this chapter. When you are finished with the chapter, you will use the requisition form to complete several coding cases. In the office, the physician would place a check mark in the blank column to the left of the "Code" column, as illustrated in **Figure 4-2** (see "Test ordered by physician"). The physician would complete the requisition form, or the nursing staff would complete the requisition form per the physician's direction. The requisition form contains areas for the date and time the test was ordered, the priority of the test, whether the order is for a recurring test that will be conducted several times during the stated time, and any special instructions the physician wants to convey to the laboratory staff regarding the test(s). There is a space to indicate whether the collection of the specimen was conducted in the office or in the laboratory. An example of a physician collecting the specimen would be when the physician performs a spinal tap to aspirate spinal fluid for examination. The fluid then would be sent to the laboratory with a requisition form indicating that the fluid was obtained by the physician in the office, along with directions from the physician for the specific laboratory test(s) requested. The aspiration service performed by the physician is reported separately. An example of the laboratory personnel collecting the specimen would be when the patient takes the General Laboratory Test Requisition to the laboratory where the technician performs the test(s) ordered by the physician. The requisition form is developed by the medical facility to reflect the organization's most commonly requested laboratory tests. There are also spaces on the requisition form to request tests not listed on the form. The requisition form also has a location for the written indication or diagnosis along with the diagnosis code.

The services in the Pathology and Laboratory section of the CPT manual include **the laboratory test only. The collection of the specimen is coded separately.** For example, if a patient had a technician in a clinic laboratory withdraw blood by means of a venipuncture, and the blood sample was then analyzed in the laboratory, 36415 is reported for the venipuncture in addition to a code to report the test performed on the blood.

Indicators are written physician orders to the laboratory that set standards. When a test is found to be positive, the physician would want further information about the condition by means of additional laboratory tests. For example, if a routine urinalysis is performed, a culture is performed if a positive bacteria result is found. If a culture is performed to identify the organism, a sensitivity test is performed if the bacteria are of a certain type or count (as predetermined by the medical facility) to warrant the additional laboratory studies. Some indicators are also located on the requisition form. For example, on Figure 4-1 under the Immunology (Blood) section, the ASO screen (Antistreptolysin O, a blood test which measures antibodies produced to fight streptococcal bacteria) has an indicator specifying that another test is to be performed if the screening test is positive.

From the Trenches

"Anyone can do this job, it just takes dedication and a willingness to keep learning."

CHRISTINA CIATTI
CPC, CPC-I, CPB

Order Date: _____   Order Time: _____

PRIORITY (Routine unless otherwise specified)
☐ ASAP   ☐ STAT   All tests: ☐ Yes   ☐ No
If No, Specify Tests: _____

☐ **RECURRING ORDER** (not to exceed 12 months)
Frequency: _____   Start Date: _____   End Date: _____

SPECIAL INSTRUCTIONS

FOR PHYSICIAN OFFICE COLLECTION ONLY:
Collected: Date: _____   Time: _____   By: _____

FOR LAB COLLECTION ONLY:
Collected: Date: _____   Time: _____   By: _____

General Laboratory Requisition

Code	CHEMISTRY	DX
	Albumin/Serum	
	Alkaline phosphatase	
	ALT/SGPT	
	Amylase	
	Arterial Blood Gas	
	AST/SGOT	
	Bilirubin, direct	
	Bilirubin, total	
	BUN, Quant	
	Calcium, total	
	Carbon dioxide (CO_2)	
	CEA	
	Chloride, blood	
	Cholesterol, serum	
	CK (creatine kinase)	
	Creatinine, blood	
	FSH	
	Ferritin	
	Folic Acid (Folate), blood	
	GGT	
	Glucose, blood non-reag	
	Glycated Hgb (Hgb A1C)	
	HCG-Qualitative	
	HCG-Quantitative	
	HDL Cholesterol	
-90	Immun. Electrophoresis	
	Iron	
	Iron Binding Capacity	
NC	% saturation requires iron & IBC to be ordered	
	LDH (lactate dehydrogenase)	
	LH (luteinizing hormone)	
	Magnesium	
	Phosphorus, blood	
	Potassium, blood	
	Prolactin, blood	
	Protein, total	
-90	Protein Electrophoresis, serum	
	PSA, total	
	Sodium, serum	
	T4, free (thyroxine)	
	TSH	
	Triglycerides	
	Uric Acid, blood	
	Vitamin B12	
	CALCULATIONS	
NC	LDL requires Chol & HDL to be ordered	
NC	CHOL/HDL requires Chol & HDL to be ordered	

Code	TOXICOLOGY/ THERAPEUTIC DRUGS	DX
	Last Dose:	
	Carbamazepine	
	Digoxin	
	Lithium	
	Phenobarbital	
	Phenytoin (Dilantin)	
	Salicylate	
	Valproic Acid	
	Theophylline	

Code	IMMUNOLOGY (Blood)	DX
	ANA (FANA) Screen	
	if ANA positive, 86039 titer	
	performed, if titer >1:160	
	cascade performed (anti-ds DNA, ENA I & ENA II)	
	Anti-ds DNA	
	ENA I (Sm, RNP)	
	ENA II (SSA, SSB)	
	ASO screen (ASO titer if screen positive 86060)	
	Rheumatoid factor (qual)	
	RPR (Syphilis Serology), quant	
	Cold Agglutinin titer	
	Hep B surface antigen	
-90	Hep B surface antigen OB (PHL)	
-90	HIV	
	Mono test	
	Rubella Antibody	

Code	PANELS	DX
	Electrolytes CO_2, Cl, K, Na	
	Bas Met, cal ion	
	Bas Met, cal tot	
	Comprehensive metabolic Alb, Bili tot, Ca tot, Cl, Creat, Glu, Alk phos, K, Prot tot, Na, AST, ALT, BUN, CO_2	
	Hepatic Function Alb, Bili tot and dir, Alk phos, AST, ALT, Prot tot	
	Lipid Chol tot, HDL, Trig., calc, LDL, Chol/HDL ratio	
	Gen health, Comp met, CBC, TSH	

Code	HEMATOLOGY	DX
	Hemogram	
	WBC, auto WBC diff	
	Hemogram micro exam, WBC diff	
	Hemogram micro exam, w/o diff	
	Hemogram manual WBC diff, buffy	
	Hematocrit	
	Hemoglobin	
	Platelet count, auto	
	Reticulocyte count, manual	
	Sedimentation Rate, auto	
	WBC, automated	
	CBC, with diff Hgb, Hct, RBC, WBC, Platelet	
	CBC, w/o diff Hgb, Hct, RBC, WBC, Platelet	

Code	COAGULATION	DX
☐ Coumadin ☐ Heparin		
	APTT	
	Prothrombin time	
	Bleeding time	

Code	OFFICE TESTING	DX
	UA, Dipstick in Office	

Code	URINE/STOOL	DX
	UA, Routine	
	UA SAVE (for possible urine culture if requested)	
	UA with microscopic	
	Urinalysis, Dipstick, Lab	
	Occult Blood	
	Urine HCG	
	Diabetic urine cascade	

Code	TIMED URINE	DX
	Hours:	
	Creatinine Clearance	
	Calcium, Urine, Quant.	
	Uric acid	

Code	BODY FLUID	DX
	Fluid Source:	
	Cell Count w/o Diff	
	Protein	
	Glucose	
	Semen Analysis	
	Semen Analysis, Comp	

Code	IMMUNOHEMATOLOGY	DX
	Blood type ABO, Rh(D)	
	Weak D performed if Rh negative	
	Antibody Screen	
	Identification, if positive, titer if indicated	
	Direct Coombs additional testing if positive	

WRITE-IN TESTS	DX	Lab Use

Medical Necessity Statement: Tests ordered on Medicare patients must follow CMS rules regarding medical necessity and FDA approval guidelines and must include diagnosis, symptoms, or reason for testing as indicated on the medical record. For any patient of any payor (including Medicare and Medicaid) that has a medical necessity requirement, order only those tests which are medically necessary for the diagnosis and treatment of the patient.

DX	CODE	WRITTEN INDICATION/DIAGNOSIS (Match Diagnosis # to Test)
1		
2		
3		
4		

LAB USE ONLY	
Arterial Puncture	
Venipuncture	
Venipuncture MC/MA	
Handling Fee	
Urine Volume Measurement	
-90 PKU	

Chart #: _____   Date: _____
Name: _____   M/F
DOB: _____
Physician: _____

Medicare #: _____   Medicaid #: _____
☐ No ABN needed   ☐ Patient refused to sign ABN
Nursing Home Part A Medicare: ☐ Yes ☐ No
Worker's Comp: ☐ Yes ☐ No
Company Account: _____

FIGURE 4–1 General Laboratory Requisition Form.

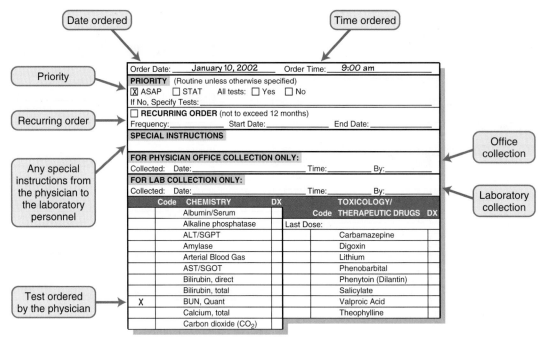

FIGURE 4–2 A physician would complete the form by placing a check mark in the blank column.

Organ- or Disease-Oriented Panels

The codes in the Organ- or Disease-Oriented Panels are grouped according to the usual laboratory work ordered by a physician for the diagnosis of, or screening for, various diseases or conditions. Groups of tests may be performed together, depending on the situation or disease. For example, during the first obstetric visit, the patient commonly has baseline laboratory tests performed to ensure that appropriate antepartum care can be given. CPT code 80055 describes an obstetric **panel** that would typically be used for the first obstetric visit. **To assign a panel code, each test listed in the panel description must be performed.** Additional tests are coded and billed separately. The development of panels saves the facility from having to bill for each test separately, and it is often more economical for the patient.

List each laboratory test separately unless the tests are part of a panel. You cannot report modifier -52 (reduced service) with a panel. For example, if all the tests in the obstetric panel were performed except the syphilis test, you could not report 80055 (Obstetrical Panel) with modifier -52. You would instead list separately each of the tests that were performed with the corresponding CPT code.

Figure 4-3 illustrates the panel codes from the General Laboratory Test Requisition form. The types of codes on the form are based on the requirements of the medical facility. Not all panels are present on the requisition form. Following each panel entry on the requisition form is a list of abbreviations for the tests included in that panel.

Now enter the panel codes onto the General Laboratory Test Requisition form in the blank to the left of the panel test name in the "Panels" section of the requisition form on Figure 4-1. When you have completed all of the activities in this chapter, the superbill/requisition form will have all the necessary codes and will be ready to use in several coding activities from that point on in your coding assignments.

Code	PANELS	DX
	Electrolytes CO_2, Cl, K, Na	
	Bas Met, cal ion	
	Bas Met, cal tot	
	Comprehensive metabolic Alb, Bili tot, Ca tot, Cl, Creat, Glu, Alk phos, K, Prot tot, Na, AST, ALT, BUN, CO_2	
	Hepatic Function Alb, Bili tot and dir, Alk phos, AST, ALT, Prot tot	
	Lipid Chol tot, HDL, Trig., calc, LDL, Chol/HDL ratio	
	Gen health, Comp met, CBC, TSH	

FIGURE 4–3 Panel codes.

CASE 4-1

Identify the panel code and the meaning of the abbreviations by referring to the code description in the CPT manual. For example:

Code: 80051 Electrolyte

CO₂ — carbon dioxide
Cl — chloride

K — potassium
Na — sodium

4-1A Basic Metabolic Panel (Calcium, Total)

The basic metabolic panel that specifies "calcium, ionized" is 80047 and has one code in the panel that is different from the basic metabolic panel with a "calcium total" (80048). What is that one code in 80047 that is different?

Code: _____

Ca tot _____

CO₂ _____
Cl _____
Creat _____
Glu _____
K _____
Na _____
BUN _____

4-1B Comprehensive Metabolic Panel
Code: _____

Alb _____
Bili tot _____
Ca tot _____
CO₂ _____
Cl _____
Creat _____

Glu _____
alk phos _____
K _____
Prot tot _____
Na _____
AST _____
ALT _____
BUN _____

4-1C Hepatic Function Panel
Code: _____

Prot tot _____
Alb _____

Bili tot, dir (There are two separate tests represented here.)
_____
alk phos _____
AST _____
ALT _____

4-1D Lipid Panel
Code: _____

Chol tot _____

HDL _____
Trig _____

4-1E General Health Panel
Code: _____

Comp met _____

CBC _____
TSH _____

(Answers to every other Case are located in Appendix D . The full answer key is only available in the TEACH Instructor Resources on Evolve.)

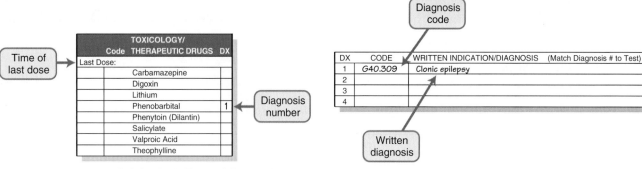

FIGURE 4-4 Toxicology for the Therapeutic Drugs section.

FIGURE 4-5 Diagnosis.

Therapeutic Drug Assays

Figure 4-4 illustrates the Toxicology for Therapeutic Drugs section from the General Laboratory Test Requisition form. Note the location of the diagnosis number that is placed in the "DX" column. The DX is numbered on the requisition form in order to identify the specific diagnosis code and written diagnosis statement correlating to the performed test. (Although some providers may allow submission for more diagnoses on one laboratory requisition form, a maximum of four diagnoses lines are shown on the General Laboratory Requisition template in this text.) For example, if a patient were prescribed phenobarbital for a clonic seizure disorder, the patient's blood ideally would contain a level of phenobarbital within the therapeutic drug range of 15 to 40 µg per milliliter (toxic range is about 40-100 µg per milliliter). Periodically, the physician would have the phenobarbital level of the patient's blood assessed to ensure that the level was within the therapeutic range. The physician or the assistant would complete the requisition form by placing the written diagnosis on the form, as illustrated in **Figure 4-5,** and placing number 1 after "Phenobarbital" in the "DX" column (as illustrated in **Figure 4-4**) to indicate that the therapeutic drug assay was being performed because of the diagnosis of clonic epilepsy. Sometimes the physician or the assistant would also enter the diagnosis code, and in other instances the medical coder would assign the diagnosis code based on the written description. The code is placed on the line that indicates the diagnosis. For example, if the physician indicated that diagnosis as clonic epilepsy:

Referenced in the Index under the term "Epilepsy, myoclonus, myoclonic—*see* Epilepsy, generalized, idiopathic." That entry directs the coder to G40.309.

CASE 4-2A *Therapeutic Drug Assays and Drug Monitoring*

Code the following drug assays that can be located in the Therapeutic Drug Assays subsection of the CPT manual (80150-80299):

CODE	DRUG	USED TO TREAT
1 _____	Carbamazepine, total	Seizures, neuralgia, depressive disorders, alcohol withdrawal, psychotic disorders
2 _____	Digoxin; total	Congestive heart failure, atrial fibrillation and flutter, tachycardia
3 _____	Lithium	Bipolar disorder, cluster headaches, premenstrual syndrome, alcoholism, dyskinesia, hyperthyroidism, mental disorders
4 _____	Phenobarbital	Seizures, hyperbilirubinemia
5 _____	Phenytoin, total (Dilantin)	Seizures, neuralgia, Bell's palsy, dysrhythmias, neuropathy pain
6 _____	Salicylate	Inflammation, pain (aspirin)
7 _____	Valproic acid (dipropylacetic acid); total	Seizures, migraines
8 _____	Theophylline	Bronchospasm

Enter the Therapeutic Drug Assay codes onto the requisition form (Figure 4-1).

(Answers to every other Case are located in Appendix D . The full answer key is only available in the TEACH Instructor Resources on Evolve.)

CASE 4-2B   *Drug Monitoring (Serum)*

The following are drug-monitoring tests ordered on a variety of patients with the report generated in the laboratory and sent to the ordering physician. The > symbol means "greater than," and the < symbol means "less than." This patient's acetaminophen level is 275, which the laboratory staff has flagged as abnormally high. The "Toxic" column indicates that for acetaminophen, any value greater than 250 (>250) is dangerous. This patient is 25 pg/ml (picogram/milliliter) higher than the top end of normal and would be contacted by the physician to adjust the amount of acetaminophen being taken. Code each of the following:

				NORMAL	TOXIC
9 _____	Acetaminophen* (UA)	275	H	10-20 pg/ml	>250
10 _____	Salicylate (serum)	50	L	100-250 pg/ml	>300
11 _____	Tobramycin (serum)	8		5-10 pg/ml	>10
12 _____	Phenobarbital (serum)	60	H	15-40 pg/ml	>80
13 _____	Gentamicin (serum)	6		5-10 pg/ml	>10
14 _____	Aminophylline (serum) (another name for theophylline)	2	L	10-20 pg/ml	>20

*Some laboratory reports will draw the physician's attention to abnormal values with an asterisk.

(Answers to every other Case are located in Appendix D . The full answer key is only available in the TEACH Instructor Resources on Evolve.)

It is important that the diagnosis and laboratory test correlate to ensure accurate reporting and reimbursement for services provided to the patient.

The drugs are listed by their generic or chemical names, not their brand names. For example, 80162 is for the generic drug Digoxin; total sold under the brand names of Lanoxin, Purodigin, etc. A current copy of *Physician's Desk Reference* for drug reference will be helpful as you report drug assays.

Urinalysis, Molecular Pathology, and Chemistry

Many types of tests are located under the Urinalysis, Molecular Pathology, and Chemistry subsections of the CPT manual. **Urinalysis** codes are for nonspecific tests performed on urine. Chemistry codes are used to report specific tests performed on material from any source (e.g., urine, blood, breath, feces, sputum). For example, a urinalysis using a dipstick (81000-81003) would report the presence and quantity of the following constituents: **bilirubin, glucose, hemoglobin, ketones, leukocytes,** nitrite, pH protein, **specific gravity,** and **urobilinogen.** Any number of these constituents may be analyzed and reported using one code from the range 81000-81003. If the physician ordered an analysis of the urine specifically to determine the presence of urobilinogen (reduced bilirubin) and the exact amount of urobilinogen present (quantitative analysis), you would choose a code from the Chemistry subsection (84580). When assigning codes from the Urinalysis or Chemistry subsection, you need to know:

1. The identification of specific tests
2. Whether the test is automated (done by machine) or nonautomated (done manually)
3. The number of tests performed
4. The identification of combination codes for similar types of tests
5. Whether the results are qualitative (type) or quantitative (amount)
6. The methodology used for testing

Urine/Stool

Figure 4-6 illustrates the "Urine/Stool" analysis that the medical facility routinely performs. As you read the paragraphs below that refer to these analyses, place the code numbers on Figure 4-1 next to the correct test name.

A nonautomated urinalysis is performed when a dipstick or tablet **reagent** (a substance that changes color when exposed to another substance) is exposed to urine (81000-81003). The stick or reagent changes color, and that color is compared with a color chart that indicates the various levels of constituents in the sample.

The sample may then be analyzed for any number of constituents in one reading (bilirubin, glucose, hemoglobin, ketones, leukocytes, nitrite, pH, protein, specific gravity, and/or urobilinogen). A manual (a comparison performed

Code	URINE/STOOL	DX
	UA, Routine	
	UA SAVE (for possible urine culture if requested)	
	UA with microscopic	
	Urinalysis, Dipstick, Lab	
	Occult Blood	
	Urine HCG	
	Diabetic urine cascade	

FIGURE 4-6 Urine/stool analysis.

by a person without the aid of a machine—nonautomated) urinalysis is reported with 81000 (with microscopy) or 81002 (without microscopy). An automated urinalysis (using a machine) is reported with 81001 (with microscopy) or 81003 (without microscopy).

The "UA, Routine" on the General Laboratory Test Requisition form is an 81003 (automated without microscope) and would represent the most commonly ordered urinalysis. The "Diabetic urine cascade" under "Urine/Stool" on the form is also 81003 and is placed on the form developed by the medical facility because the physicians in the facility often refer to laboratory tests by that name. The "UA with microscopic" on the form is reported with 81001 (automated with microscope). The "Urinalysis, Dipstick, Lab" is 81002 (nonautomated without microscope). Be certain to read the full description of these codes in the CPT manual as you are placing the codes on the requisition form displayed in Figure 4-1.

The **Occult Blood** is an analysis of a stool sample to detect the presence of blood. Usually the patient takes a kit home and takes three stool samples. The kit is then returned to a laboratory for analysis. Multiple samples improve the accuracy of the test. The test is reported with 82270 for three consecutive collected specimens that are analyzed with a single determination. This test is sometimes called a stool guaiac ("gwy-ack") or FOB (fecal occult blood). Guaiac is the resin of a tree used as a reagent in tests for the presence of blood. Code 82270 reports only the presence or absence of blood in the stool sample (qualitative) and does not report the exact amount of blood present (quantitative). When the physician obtains a diagnostic stool sample during the DRE (digital rectal exam), the laboratory CPT code is 82272.

The urine pregnancy test is reported with 81025 and is located on the form as "Urine HCG" in the Urine/Stool section of the report. HCG stands for human chorionic gonadotropin and is the hormone that the reagent or strip reacts to and the presence of which indicates a positive pregnancy test.

Timed Urine

Timed urine tests are illustrated in **Figure 4-7.** The "Creatinine Clearance" is reported with 82575 and is a kidney function test. The assessment is conducted on a urine sample that is taken over a period of time—usually 24 hours—and calculates the creatinine expelled over that period. In a 24-hour sample, the patient would discard the first urine passed of the day and then collect and refrigerate every urine passed during the next 24-hour period. The "Calcium, Urine, Quant" is a 24-hour sample of urine that is analyzed to determine the amount of calcium expelled over a 24-hour period and is reported with 82340. The "Uric acid" is reported with 84560 and is also a 24-hour urine sample that is analyzed for uric acid. Increased

FIGURE 4–7 Timed urine tests.

levels of uric acid are indicative of gout or increased risk for kidney stones.

Enter the codes above onto the requisition form in Figure 4-1.

Molecular Pathology

The Molecular Pathology codes are divided into Tier 1 and Tier 2 codes. Tier 1 codes (81161, 81200-81383) report services for molecular assays that are more commonly performed. For example, 81162 is an assay to determine the presence of a breast cancer gene—BRCA1 and BRCA2 (*DNA repair associated*). There are many conditions in which a genetic predisposition can be predicted, such as cystic fibrosis and colon cancer. Tier 2 codes 81400-81408, or unlisted molecular pathology procedure code, 81479 involve less commonly performed analyses and are arranged by the required level of technical resources and the level of physician or other qualified health professional interpretation.

Chemistry

The Chemistry codes can appear to be the most challenging codes in all of the CPT because of the technical language used in the code descriptions. So let's start at the very beginning on this subsection so you can see that it is not really difficult if you adhere to a few simple steps. The tests in the Chemistry subsection can be from any source (i.e., blood, urine, serum, plasma) unless the code descriptions specifically indicate the source. Therefore, if no source is indicated in the code description, the code covers a sample from any source. An example of codes with a specified source in the code description include 80320-80322 for alcohol drug testing by means of any specimen except breath, since code 82075 is reported for a breath alcohol test. Codes 80329-80331 are used to report acetaminophen (Tylenol) as a non-opioid analgesic from any source.

The tests are listed alphabetically in the Chemistry subsection, although several parenthetical notes are included there which provide direction in order to facilitate location of tests for certain substances, such as acetaminophen, alcohol, or amphetamine, which are located under the Definitive Drug Testing subheading and not in the

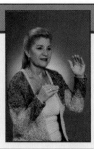

From the Trenches

"The most rewarding part of being a medical coder is making sure that the provider is reimbursed for all services that are provided."

CHRISTINA CIATTI
CPC, CPC-I, CPB

CASE 4-3   *Chemistry Tests*

Enter a code for each Chemistry test listed by first referencing the index of the CPT manual and then from the main portion of the CPT manual, choosing the correct code to place in the blank to the left of the chemistry test stated.

1 _____ Albumin, serum	26 _____ 90 Immunofixation electrophoresis, serum
2 _____ Alkaline phosphatase	*(The medical facility sends the sample to an*
3 _____ ALT/SGPT	*outside laboratory for analysis, indicated by*
4 _____ Amylase	*modifier -90.)*
5 _____ Arterial blood gas	27 _____ Iron
6 _____ AST/SGOT	28 _____ Iron-binding capacity
7 _____ Bilirubin, direct	NC % saturated requires iron and IBC to be
8 _____ Bilirubin, total	ordered
9 _____ BUN, quant	29 _____ LDH (lactate dehydrogenase)
10 _____ Calcium, total	30 _____ LH (luteinizing hormone)
11 _____ Carbon dioxide (CO_2)	31 _____ Magnesium
12 _____ CEA	32 _____ Phosphorus, blood
13 _____ Chloride, blood	33 _____ Potassium, blood
14 _____ Cholesterol, serum	34 _____ Prolactin, blood
15 _____ CK (creatine kinase)	35 _____ Protein, total, serum
16 _____ Creatinine, blood	36 _____ 90 Protein Electrophoresis, serum
17 _____ FSH	*(The medical facility sends the sample to an outside*
18 _____ Ferritin	*laboratory for analysis indicated by modifier -90.)*
19 _____ Folic acid (Folate), blood	37 _____ PSA, total
20 _____ GGT	38 _____ Sodium, serum
21 _____ Glucose, blood, non-reagent	39 _____ T4, free (thyroxine)
22 _____ Glycated Hgb (Hgb A1C)	40 _____ TSH
23 _____ hCG—Qualitative	41 _____ Triglycerides
24 _____ hCG—Quantitative	42 _____ Uric acid, blood
25 _____ HDL Cholesterol	43 _____ Vitamin B$_{12}$

Place the codes onto the requisition form in Figure 4-1.

Code the following clinical chemistry (blood, serum, plasma) tests. Serum is the clear portion of any body fluid. For example, blood serum is the clear liquid that separates from the blood when blood is allowed to clot completely.

Continued

CASE 4-3—cont'd

	06/06	HIGH/LOW	NORMAL
44 Insulin, fasting, plasma _____ (total)	2	L	5-25 μ/ml
45 Iron, serum _____	21	WNL	75-175 μ/dl
46 Iron-binding capacity _____	602	H	20-410 μ/dl
	02/27		NORMAL
47 Vitamin A, serum _____	10	L	20-80 μg/dl
48 Vitamin B$_{12}$ _____	150	L	180-900 pg/ml
	04/30/XX		NORMAL
49 Creatinine _____ (CK) serum			
Male	0.6	H	0.2-0.5 mg/dl
50 Bilirubin, serum			
Direct _____	0.3	WNL	0.1-0.4 mg/dl
51 Bilirubin, serum			
Total _____	0.6	WNL	0.3-1.1 mg/dl
	12/24/XX		NORMAL
52 Thyroxine-binding globulin _____			
TBG _____	22	WNL	15.0-34.0 g/ml
	07/02/XX		NORMAL
53 Prolactin, serum _____			
Male _____	18	H	1.0-15.0 mg/dl

(Answers to every other Case are located in Appendix D . The full answer key is only available in the TEACH Instructor Resources on Evolve.)

Chemistry subsection. Each test may be found in the CPT Index, either by locating the specific substance name or under the term, "Pathology and Laboratory", and then locating the specific substance name. For instance, the test for chromium can be found under the term, "chromium", or under the term, "Pathology and Laboratory, Chemistry", and then under "chromium", with the same directive to reference code 82495. The cross-referencing system in the CPT index is especially useful when locating chemistry tests, which are often stated in abbreviation form. For example, for BUN, you are directed by the notes in the CPT index under the entry (BUN) to *See* Blood Urea Nitrogen; Urea Nitrogen.

Calculations

The "Calculations" section of the report located at the bottom of the Chemistry section (**Figure 4-8**) contains spaces for the physician to indicate that the technician is to calculate the LDL (low-density lipoprotein) and/or the HDL (high-density lipoprotein). This calculation does not have a separate code because it is not reported separately.

Chromatography

Chromatography is the measurement of a substance while the substance is moving (mobile phase) and while not moving (stationary phase or sorbent). Knowing about the mobile and stationary phases is important to the coder because each phase is reported separately. (For example, 82542 reports quantitative chromatography for a single analyte, with single mobile and stationary phase. If multiple analytes with a single stationary and mobile phase are performed, you would report with 82542.) The chemistry codes for chromatography are 82542, 84999. The CPT index lists these specialized tests under "Chromatography."

Order Date: _____ Order Time: _____

PRIORITY (Routine unless otherwise specified)
☐ ASAP ☐ STAT All tests: ☐ Yes ☐ No
If No, Specify Tests: _____
☐ **RECURRING ORDER** (not to exceed 12 months)
Frequency: _____ Start Date: _____ End Date: _____
SPECIAL INSTRUCTIONS

FOR PHYSICIAN OFFICE COLLECTION ONLY:
Collected: Date: _____ Time: _____ By: _____
FOR LAB COLLECTION ONLY:
Collected: Date: _____ Time: _____ By: _____

General Laboratory Requisition

Code	CHEMISTRY	DX
	Albumin/Serum	
	Alkaline phosphatase	
	ALT/SGPT	
	Amylase	
	Arterial Blood Gas	
	AST/SGOT	
	Bilirubin, direct	
	Bilirubin, total	
	BUN, Quant	
	Calcium, total	
	Carbon dioxide (CO_2)	
	CEA	
	Chloride, blood	
	Cholesterol, serum	
	CK (creatine kinase)	
	Creatinine, blood	
	FSH	
	Ferritin	
	Folic Acid (Folate), blood	
	GGT	
	Glucose, blood non-reag	
	Glycated Hgb (Hgb A1C)	
	HCG-Qualitative	
	HCG-Quantitative	
	HDL Cholesterol	
-90	Immun. Electro. Phoresis	
	Iron	
	Iron Binding Capacity	
NC	% saturation requires iron & IBC to be ordered	
	LDH (lactate dehydrogenase)	
	LH (luteinizing hormone)	
	Magnesium	
	Phosphorus, blood	
	Potassium, blood	
	Prolactin, blood	
	Protein, total	
-90	Protein Electrophoresis, serum	
	PSA, total	
	Sodium, serum	
	T4, free (thyroxine)	
	TSH	
	Triglycerides	
	Uric Acid, blood	
	Vitamin B12	
	CALCULATIONS	
NC	LDL requires Chol & HDL to be ordered	
NC	CHOL/HDL requires Chol & HDL to be ordered	

TOXICOLOGY/
Code	THERAPEUTIC DRUGS	DX
Last Dose:		
	Carbamazepine	
	Digoxin	
	Lithium	
	Phenobarbital	
	Phenytoin (Dilantin)	
	Salicylate	
	Valproic Acid	
	Theophylline	

Code	IMMUNOLOGY (Blood)	DX
	ANA (FANA) Screen	
	if ANA positive, 86039 titer	
	performed, if titer >1:160	
	cascade performed (anti-ds DNA, ENA I & ENA II)	
	Anti-ds DNA	
	ENA I (Sm, RNP)	
	ENA II (SSA, SSB)	
	ASO screen (ASO titer if screen positive 86060)	
	Rheumatoid factor (qual)	
	RPR (Syphilis Serology), quant	
	Cold Agglutinin titer	
	Hep B surface antigen	
-90	Hep B surface antigen OB (PHL)	
-90	HIV	
	Mono test	
	Rubella Antibody	

Code	PANELS	DX
	Electrolytes CO_2, Cl, K, Na	
	Bas Met, cal ion	
	Bas Met, cal tot	
	Comprehensive metabolic	
	Alb, Bili tot, Ca tot, Cl, Creat,	
	Glu, Alk phos, K, Prot tot,	
	Na, AST, ALT, BUN, CO_2	
	Hepatic Function	
	Alb, Bili tot and dir, Alk phos,	
	AST, ALT, Prot tot	
	Lipid Chol tot, HDL, Trig.,	
	calc, LDL, Chol/HDL ratio	
	Gen health, Comp met,	
	CBC, TSH	

Code	HEMATOLOGY	DX
	Hemogram	
	WBC, auto WBC diff	
	Hemogram micro exam, WBC diff	
	Hemogram micro exam, w/o diff	
	Hemogram manual WBC diff, buffy	
	Hematocrit	
	Hemoglobin	
	Platelet count, auto	
	Reticulocyte count, manual	
	Sedimentation Rate, auto	
	WBC, automated	
	CBC, with diff	
	Hgb, Hct, RBC, WBC, Platelet	
	CBC, w/o diff	
	Hgb, Hct, RBC, WBC, Platelet	

Code	COAGULATION	DX
☐ Coumadin ☐ Heparin		
	APTT	
	Prothrombin time	
	Bleeding time	

Code	OFFICE TESTING	DX
	UA, Dipstick in Office	

Code	URINE/STOOL	DX
	UA, Routine	
	UA SAVE (for possible urine culture if requested)	
	UA with microscopic	
	Urinalysis, Dipstick, Lab	
	Occult Blood	
	Urine HCG	
	Diabetic urine cascade	

Code	TIMED URINE	DX
Hours:		
	Creatinine Clearance	
	Calcium, Urine, Quant.	
	Uric acid	

Code	BODY FLUID	DX
Fluid Source:		
	Cell Count w/ Diff	
	Protein	
	Glucose	
	Semen Analysis	
	Semen Analysis, Comp	

Code	IMMUNOHEMATOLOGY	DX
	Blood type ABO, Rh(D)	
	Weak D performed if Rh negative	
	Antibody Screen	
	Identification, if positive, titer if indicated	
	Direct Coombs	
	additional testing if positive	

WRITE-IN TESTS	DX	Lab Use

Medical Necessity Statement: Tests ordered on Medicare patients must follow CMS rules regarding medical necessity and FDA approval guidelines and must include diagnosis, symptoms, or reason for testing as indicated on the medical record. For any patient of any payor (including Medicare and Medicaid) that has a medical necessity requirement, order only those tests which are medically necessary for the diagnosis and treatment of the patient.

DX	CODE	WRITTEN INDICATION/DIAGNOSIS	(Match Diagnosis # to Test)
1			
2			
3			
4			

LAB USE ONLY	
Arterial Puncture	
Venipuncture	
Venipuncture MC/MA	
Handling Fee	
Urine Volume Measurement	
-90 PKU	

Chart #: _____ Date: _____
Name: _____ M/F _____
DOB: _____
Physician: _____

Medicare #: _____ Medicaid #: _____
☐ No ABN needed   ☐ Patient refused to sign ABN
Nursing Home Part A Medicare: ☐ Yes ☐ No
Worker's Comp: ☐ Yes ☐ No
Company Account: _____

FIGURE 4–8 Calculation section.

Hematology and Coagulation

The Hematology and Coagulation subsection of the CPT manual contains codes based on the various blood-drawing methods and tests. The method used to do the test is often what determines code assignment. A common laboratory test is a **hemogram,** which is a graphic picture of the various blood constituencies. A **differential** is an actual count of the amount or number of the constituency. For example, a leukocyte (white blood cell [WBC]) differential would include the following constituencies:

Myelocytes
Band neutrophils
Segmented neutrophils
Lymphocytes
Monocytes
Eosinophils
Basophils

A physician would order a WBC and the patient would arrive at the laboratory, where a technician would draw a specimen by venipuncture, finger stick, or heel stick for an infant. The blood would be analyzed and a report of the findings sent to the ordering physician. For example, a physician who ordered a WBC for a patient received the following laboratory information in the laboratory report:

WBC	01/03/02		Normal
Myelocytes	2	H	0%
Band neutrophils	2	L	3%-5%
Segmented neutrophils	50	L	54%-62%
Lymphocytes	27	WNL	25%-33%
Monocytes	5	WNL	3%-7%
Eosinophils	4	H	1%-3%
Basophils	2	H	0%-1%

Note that the "Normal" ranges for each component of the WBC are displayed and represent the limits for a normal test result. Also, for each constituent above the "Normal" limit, an "H" is entered to indicate "high." For each constituent below "Normal," an "L" is entered to indicate "low" to enable the physician to locate quickly the constituents that vary from normal. WNL indicates "within normal limits." Although each medical facility has its own format for laboratory test results, the informational components displayed would be similar to these.

Laboratory Use Only

The codes in the Pathology and Laboratory section represent only the test performed, not the drawing of the sample. Note on **Figure 4-9** the section titled "Lab Use Only" in the lower-right corner of the form. The technician would place a check mark next to "Arterial Puncture" if the blood were drawn by means of an arterial puncture (36600) or by "Venipuncture" if a venipuncture (36415) were performed. Also note that there is a space to check off a handling fee if the sample is sent to an outside laboratory for analysis (99000). A urine volume measurement is reported with 81050. The PKU is a phenylketonuria, which is a urine and blood test performed in neonates to detect the presence of phenylketonuria, a genetic disease that if left untreated leads to brain damage (84030).

Figure 4-10 illustrates the Hematology codes on the General Laboratory Test Requisition form representing commonly requested hematology procedures in a general outpatient setting. An automated hemogram with an automated WBC differential count is reported with 85004. When an automated blood count (hemogram) with an automated differential count of the leukocytes (WBC) is not sufficient, the physician may order a manual microscopic review of the blood. Manual microscopic review of the blood is usually performed in one of three ways:

1. Manual differential WBC with a microscopy (85007)
2. Microscopic examination without manual differential (85008)
3. Manual differential WBC count with buffy coat (a special study performed when the leukocyte count is so low that the standard evaluation cannot be performed) (85009)

A complete CBC (complete blood count) is a hemogram that includes the RBC (red blood count), WBC (white blood count), HGB (hemoglobin), HCT (hematocrit), PLT (platelet or thrombocyte count), and indices (which includes MCHC, mean corpuscular hemoglobin; MCV, mean corpuscular volume; and RDW, red cell distribution width). There are two types of complete CBCs: 85025, which includes an automated differential WBC, and 85027, which does not include an automated differential WBC count.

Note that the hemogram codes in the 85032-85049 range are counts of certain constituents (i.e., red blood cells or reticulocyte) divided based on whether the test was manual or automated.

Order Date: _____	Order Time: _____

PRIORITY (Routine unless otherwise specified)
☐ ASAP ☐ STAT All tests: ☐ Yes ☐ No
If No, Specify Tests: _____

☐ **RECURRING ORDER** (not to exceed 12 months)
Frequency: _____ Start Date: _____ End Date: _____

SPECIAL INSTRUCTIONS

FOR PHYSICIAN OFFICE COLLECTION ONLY:
Collected: Date: _____ Time: _____ By: _____

FOR LAB COLLECTION ONLY:
Collected: Date: _____ Time: _____ By: _____

General Laboratory Requisition

Code	CHEMISTRY	DX
	Albumin/Serum	
	Alkaline phosphatase	
	ALT/SGPT	
	Amylase	
	Arterial Blood Gas	
	AST/SGOT	
	Bilirubin, direct	
	Bilirubin, total	
	BUN, Quant	
	Calcium, total	
	Carbon dioxide (CO_2)	
	CEA	
	Chloride, blood	
	Cholesterol, serum	
	CK (creatine kinase)	
	Creatinine, blood	
	FSH	
	Ferritin	
	Folic Acid (Folate), blood	
	GGT	
	Glucose, blood non-reag	
	Glycated Hgb (Hgb A1C)	
	HCG-Qualitative	
	HCG-Quantitative	
	HDL Cholesterol	
-90	Immun. Electrophoresis	
	Iron	
	Iron Binding Capacity	
NC	% saturation requires iron & IBC to be ordered	
	LDH (lactate dehydrogenase)	
	LH (luteinizing hormone)	
	Magnesium	
	Phosphorus, blood	
	Potassium, blood	
	Prolactin, blood	
	Protein, total	
-90	Protein Electrophoresis, serum	
	PSA, total	
	Sodium, serum	
	T4, free (thyroxine)	
	TSH	
	Triglycerides	
	Uric Acid, blood	
	Vitamin B12	
	CALCULATIONS	
NC	LDL requires Chol & HDL to be ordered	
NC	CHOL/HDL requires Chol & HDL to be ordered	

Code	TOXICOLOGY/ THERAPEUTIC DRUGS	DX
Last Dose:		
	Carbamazepine	
	Digoxin	
	Lithium	
	Phenobarbital	
	Phenytoin (Dilantin)	
	Salicylate	
	Valproic Acid	
	Theophylline	

Code	IMMUNOLOGY (Blood)	DX
	ANA (FANA) Screen	
	if ANA positive, 86039 titer	
	performed, if titer >1:160	
	cascade performed (anti-	
	ds DNA, ENA I & ENA II)	
	Anti-ds DNA	
	ENA I (Sm, RNP)	
	ENA II (SSA, SSB)	
	ASO screen (ASO titer if	
	screen positive 86060)	
	Rheumatoid factor (qual)	
	RPR (Syphilis Serology), quant	
	Cold Agglutinin titer	
	Hep B surface antigen	
-90	Hep B surface antigen OB (PHL)	
-90	HIV	
	Mono test	
	Rubella Antibody	

Code	PANELS	DX
	Electrolytes CO_2, Cl, K, Na	
	Bas Met, cal ion	
	Bas Met, cal tot	
	Comprehensive metabolic	
	Alb, Bili tot, Ca tot, Cl, Creat,	
	Glu, Alk phos, K, Prot tot,	
	Na, AST, ALT, BUN, CO_2	
	Hepatic Function	
	Alb, Bili tot and dir, Alk phos,	
	AST, ALT, Prot tot	
	Lipid Chol tot, HDL, Trig.,	
	calc, LDL, Chol/HDL ratio	
	Gen health, Comp met,	
	CBC, TSH	

Code	HEMATOLOGY	DX
	Hemogram WBC, auto WBC diff	
	Hemogram micro exam, WBC diff	
	Hemogram micro exam, w/o diff	
	Hemogram manual WBC diff, buffy	
	Hematocrit	
	Hemoglobin	
	Platelet count, auto	
	Reticulocyte count, manual	
	Sedimentation Rate, auto	
	WBC, automated	
	CBC, with diff Hgb, Hct, RBC, WBC, Platelet	
	CBC, w/o diff Hgb, Hct, RBC, WBC, Platelet	

Code	COAGULATION	DX
☐ Coumadin ☐ Heparin		
	APTT	
	Prothrombin time	
	Bleeding time	

Code	OFFICE TESTING	DX
	UA, Dipstick in Office	

Code	URINE/STOOL	DX
	UA, Routine	
	UA SAVE (for possible urine culture if requested)	
	UA with microscopic	
	Urinalysis, Dipstick, Lab	
	Occult Blood	
	Urine HCG	
	Diabetic urine cascade	

Code	TIMED URINE	DX
Hours:		
	Creatinine Clearance	
	Calcium, Urine, Quant.	
	Uric acid	

Code	BODY FLUID	DX
Fluid Source:		
	Cell Count w/o Diff	
	Protein	
	Glucose	
	Semen Analysis	
	Semen Analysis, Comp	

Code	IMMUNOHEMATOLOGY	DX
	Blood type ABO, Rh(D)	
	Weak D performed if Rh negative	
	Antibody Screen	
	Identification, if positive, titer if indicated	
	Direct Coombs additional testing if positive	

WRITE-IN TESTS	DX	Lab Use

Medical Necessity Statement: Tests ordered on Medicare patients must follow CMS rules regarding medical necessity and FDA approval guidelines and must include diagnosis, symptoms, or reason for testing as indicated on the medical record. For any patient of any payor (including Medicare and Medicaid) that has a medical necessity requirement, order only those tests which are medically necessary for the diagnosis and treatment of the patient.

DX	CODE	WRITTEN INDICATION/DIAGNOSIS (Match Diagnosis # to Test)
1		
2		
3		
4		

LAB USE ONLY	
Arterial Puncture	
Venipuncture	
Venipuncture MC/MA	
Handling Fee	
Urine Volume Measurement	
-90 PKU	

Chart #: _____	Date: _____
Name: _____	M/F
DOB: _____	
Physician: _____	

Medicare #: _____ Medicaid #: _____
☐ No ABN needed ☐ Patient refused to sign ABN
Nursing Home Part A Medicare: ☐ Yes ☐ No
Worker's Comp: ☐ Yes ☐ No
Company Account: _____

FIGURE 4–9 Lab Use Only section.

Code	HEMATOLOGY	DX
	Hemogram WBC, auto WBC diff	
	Hemogram micro exam, WBC diff	
	Hemogram micro exam, w/o diff	
	Hemogram manual WBC diff, buffy	
	Hematocrit	
	Hemoglobin	
	Platelet count, auto	
	Reticulocyte count, manual	
	Sedimentation Rate, auto	
	WBC, automated	
	CBC, with diff Hgb, Hct, RBC, WBC, Platelet	
	CBC, w/o diff Hgb, Hct, RBC, WBC, Platelet	

FIGURE 4-10 Hematology codes.

CASE 4-4   *Hematology*

Fill in the hemogram code of each of the counts indicated on the Hematology section of the form as follows:

1 _____ Hemogram
         blood count, auto WBC diff

2 _____ Hemogram
         microexam, manual WBC diff

3 _____ Hemogram
         smear, microexam, w/o diff

4 _____ Hemogram
         manual WBC diff, buffy

5 _____ Hematocrit

6 _____ Hemoglobin

7 _____ Platelet count, auto

8 _____ Reticulocyte count, manual

9 _____ Sedimentation rate, auto

10 _____ WBC, automated

11 _____ CBC, with auto diff
          Hgb, Hct, RBC, WBC, Platelet

12 _____ CBC, w/o diff
          Hgb, Hct, RBC, WBC, Platelet

Enter the codes from the above activity onto the requisition form in Figure 4-1.

The following laboratory tests were conducted on a variety of patients on January 21. The test performed appears in the left column, the results under the 01/21 column, an indication of an abnormal result in the "Rate" column, and the normal results for that test in the "Normal" column. Assign codes to the tests:

LABORATORY TEST	01/21	RATE	NORMAL
13 Coombs test* Direct _____	N	N	Negative
14 Coombs test _____ Indirect, qual _____	P	P	Negative
15 Hematocrit (Hct) Male† _____	62	H	40-54 ml/dl
16 Hematocrit (Hct) Newborn† _____	30	L	49-54 ml/dl
17 Hemoglobin (Hgb) Female† _____	6	L	12.0-16.0 g/dl

CASE 4-4—cont'd

18 Hemoglobin, fetal _____ chemical			
_____ fetal qual	2	H	<1.0% of total
19 Hemoglobin A$_2$ quan _____	2	WNL	1.5%-3.0% of total
20 Hemoglobin, plasma _____	4	WNL	0-5.0 mg/dl
21 Methemoglobin _____ qual			
_____ quan	16	L	30-130 mg/dl
22 Sedimentation rate (ESR)			
Wintrobe test, Male _____ non-automated	4	WNL	0-5 mm/hr
_____ automated			

*Coombs test is also known as antierythrocyte antibodies (anti-RBC). **Direct Coombs** measures the presence of the anti-RBC antibodies that are bound to the surface of circulating RBCs. **Indirect Coombs** measures the "free" antibodies that are not bound to the surface of the circulating RBCs. The test is used to detect autoimmune anemia. As such, the negative test result (N) indicates the normal test result, and a positive test result (P) indicates an abnormal test result.

†Relates to laboratory value only and has nothing to do with code choice.

CASE 4-4—cont'd

Code the following laboratory results:

LABORATORY TEST	01/21	RATE	NORMAL
23 Alkaline phosphatase, leukocyte _____	58	WNL	14-100
24 Leukocytes, differential, manual _____			
Myelocytes	2	H	0%
Band neutrophils	4	WNL	3%-5%
Segmented neutrophils	58	WNL	54%-62%
Lymphocytes	27	WNL	25%-33%
Monocytes	5	WNL	3%-7%
Eosinophils	4	H	1%-3%
Basophils	2	H	0%-1%
25 Platelets, automated _____	150,000	WNL	150,000-350,000/mm³
26 Reticulocytes, manual _____	33,000	WNL	25,000-75,000/mm³ (0.5%-15% of erythrocytes)

(Answers to every other Case are located in Appendix D . The full answer key is only available in the TEACH Instructor Resources on Evolve.)

Coagulation

Many blood coagulation tests are located in the Hematology and Coagulation subsection. The codes are divided based on the particular factor being tested. Great care must be taken to ensure that the correct factor has been reported based on the information in the medical record.

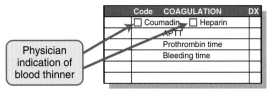

FIGURE 4–11 Coagulation section.

The **Coagulation** codes are reported for services to patients who take blood thinners. For example, Coumadin and heparin are prescribed to patients with conditions such as blood clots or heart attack. As illustrated in **Figure 4-11**, the Coagulation section has a place for the physician to indicate whether the patient is currently taking Coumadin or heparin. The coagulation test is performed for that specific medication. The three assessments under the Coagulation section of the form are:

■ APTT is an activated partial thromboplastin time, most often referred to as a PTT or partial thromboplastin time, and is used to assess coagulation. You can locate this test in the index of the CPT manual under the entry "Thromboplastin, Partial Time."

CASE 4-5 *Coagulation*

Enter the codes for the following coagulation tests:

1 _____ PTT
2 _____ Prothrombin time
3 _____ Bleeding time

Record the codes for these coagulation tests on the requisition form in Figure 4-1.

Code the following tests, some of which are not on the requisition form:

COAGULATION TESTS	02/09	RATE	NORMAL
4 Bleeding time (template) _____	2.32	L	2.75-8.0 min
5 Coagulation time (glass tube) _____	10	WNL	5-15 min
6 D-dimer, semiquant (Fibrin Degradation) _____	0.2	WNL	<0.5 µg/ml
7 Factor VIII and other coagulation factors _____ (related antigen)	20	L	50%-150% of normal
8 Fibrin split products (Thrombo-Welco test) _____ (paracoagulation)	8	L	>10 µg/dl
9 Fibrinogen, activity _____	300	WNL	200-400 mg/dl
10 Partial thromboplastin time (PTT) _____	29	H	20-15s
11 Prothrombin time (PT) _____	13	WNL	12.0-14.0s

(Answers to every other Case are located in Appendix D . The full answer key is only available in the TEACH Instructor Resources on Evolve.)

■ A prothrombin time is a one-stage coagulation assessment using an automated device and is also used with patients who are on anticoagulation medications. You can locate the prothrombin time in the index of the CPT manual under the entry "Prothrombin Time."

■ The bleeding time is measured by nicking the patient's vein and recording the amount of time it takes to stop the bleeding. This measures the platelet function or the coagulation of the blood. The physician then adjusts the patient's medication based on the bleeding times or coagulation assessments. You can locate the bleeding time assessments in the index of the CPT manual under the entry "Bleeding Time."

Immunohematology

As illustrated in **Figure 4-12,** the Immunohematology section of the requisition form indicates four tests that are commonly requested:
■ Blood typing is identification of the patient's blood group as O, A, B, or AB. In addition, this test also indicates if there is an Rh factor present. You can locate this test in the index of the CPT manual under the entry "Blood Typing, ABO Only."

■ Weak D is an Rh typing that determines whether the blood is positive or negative. You can locate this test in the index of the CPT manual under the entry "Blood Typing, Rh(D)."
■ Antibody screen is a test to detect a certain antibody that affects red blood cells, the presence of which may present difficulties during childbirth or blood transfusion. You can locate this test in the index of the CPT manual under the entry "Antibody, Red Blood Cell."
■ Direct Coombs or a direct antiglobulin test (DAT) is used to identify the makeup of the surface of the red blood cell. The test is used to detect various types of anemia and other red blood cell conditions. You can locate the test in the CPT index under the entry "Coombs Test."

Code	IMMUNOHEMATOLOGY	DX
	Blood type ABO, Rh(D) Weak D performed if Rh negative	
	Antibody Screen Identification, if positive, titer if indicated	
	Direct Coombs additional testing if positive	

FIGURE 4-12 Immunohematology section.

CASE 4-6   *Immunohematology*

Enter the codes for the following tests:

1 _____ Blood type ABO, serologic
2 _____ Rh(D), serologic Weak D performed if Rh negative

3 _____ Antibody screen identification, if positive, titer if indicated
4 _____ Direct Coombs, additional testing if positive

(Answers to every other Case are located in Appendix D . The full answer key is only available in the TEACH Instructor Resources on Evolve.)

Immunology

Figure 4-13 illustrates the **Immunology (Blood)** codes that deal with the identification of conditions of the immune system caused by the action of antibodies (e.g., hypersensitivity, allergic reactions, immunity, and alterations of body tissue). The tests on the form are as follows:

- ANA (FANA) screen, an antinuclear antibodies titer or a fluorescent antinuclear antibody, is a screen of the antibodies of the cell nucleus and is used as a diagnostic test for autoimmune disease, such as scleroderma or lupus. Note that an indicator is stated on the requisition form that if the ANA screen is positive, an 86039 ANA titer should be performed. If the titer is less than 1:160, another indicator, an anti-ds DNA, ENA I, and ENA II are to be performed, which are further analyses. You can locate these antibody tests in the index of the CPT manual under "Antinuclear Antibodies."

- Anti-ds DNA or deoxyribonucleic acid (DNA) antibody is a test that identifies the presence of certain

antibodies that are not infectious, such as smooth-muscle antibody or mitochondrial antibody. The "D.S." means double strand. This test is not a titer (a report on the level of the antibody) but rather a report of the presence or absence of the antibody. It is reported with 86255.

- ENA I, or extractable nuclear antigen, is an assessment of a number of antibodies that are listed in the parenthetical information of this code. The "Sm" and "RNP" are types of antibodies, but other types of antibodies may be reported with this code as listed in the code description. Each of the antibodies is indicative of certain conditions; for example, RNP is the ribonucleic protein, and the presence of this antibody is used in the diagnosis of lupus and scleroderma as well as other autoimmune diseases. This code has "×2" following it because each antibody assessment is reported separately. The physician orders the assessments (Sm and RNP) by placing a check next to ENA I. The next entry of ENA II is a second group of antigens—SSA, SSB; the physician places a check mark in the ENA II column to order assessment of these two antigens. You can locate this test in the index of the CPT manual under "Nuclear Antigen, Antibody."

- ASO stands for "antistreptolysin O" and is a laboratory test used to measure antibodies produced to fight streptococcal bacteria. This test is routinely performed for patients with infectious mononucleosis or rheumatoid arthritis. There are two different ASO tests, one a screen (qualitative or presence of) and one a titer (quantitative or count). Also on the requisition form is an indicator stating that if the screen is positive, the laboratory technician is to conduct a titer on the sample. You can locate this test in the index of the CPT manual under "Antistreptolysin O."

- Rheumatoid factor is often referred to as RF and is an immunoglobulin found in the blood of patients with rheumatoid arthritis. There is a screen code and a titer code. The RF test on the form is a qualitative test (presence of). You can locate this test in the index of the CPT manual under "Rheumatoid Factor."

Code	IMMUNOLOGY (Blood)	DX
	ANA (FANA) Screen if ANA positive, 86039 titer performed, if titer >1:160 cascade performed (anti-ds DNA, ENA I & ENA II)	
	Anti-ds DNA	
	ENA I (Sm, RNP)	
	ENA II (SSA, SSB)	
	ASO screen (ASO titer if screen positive 86060)	
	Rheumatoid factor (qual)	
	RPR (Syphilis Serology), quant	
	Cold Agglutinin titer	
	Hep B surface antigen	
-90	Hep B surface antigen OB (PHL)	NC
-90	HIV	NC
	Mono test	
	Rubella Antibody	

FIGURE 4–13 Immunology (Blood) codes.

■ RPR is a rapid plasma reagin and is a syphilis test. There is a qualitative and a quantitative code. The test on the form is a quantitative test. You can locate this test in the index of the CPT under "Syphilis Test."

■ Cold agglutinin is a test to assess for IgM (immuno-globulin M), which is the first immunoglobulin produced in an immune response. The presence of IgM may indicate *Mycoplasma pneumoniae*, anemia, or other conditions. There are codes for both a screen and titer. Screen is to separate from, and titer is an amount of one substance necessary to react with another substance. You can locate this test in the index of the CPT under "Cold Agglutinin."

■ Hep B surface antigen identifies the presence of HBsAg, which is a lipoprotein that covers the surface of the virus that causes hepatitis B. There are two codes for hepatitis B surface antigen—one for the screening to identify the presence of HBsAg and a neutralization test, which is a further test performed when the hepatitis B surface antigen test is repeatedly positive; the neutralization test can rule out false-positives. You can locate this test in the index of the CPT under "Hepatitis Antigen, B surface."

■ Hep B surface antigen OB is the same test as above, except that in the medical facility represented by the General Laboratory Test Requisition form, the test for the pregnant patient is sent to an outside laboratory and, as such, modifier -90 is placed after the CPT code

and NC (no charge) is indicated because the laboratory doing the analysis will submit the bill for the test directly to the third-party payer.

■ HIV is a test for the human immunodeficiency virus. There are codes for HIV-1, HIV-2, or a combination code for HIV-1 and HIV-2 in one test. HIV-2 is a strain of HIV that originated in primates (monkeys). There is also a code for confirmation of HIV (86689). The code on the requisition form is for HIV-1. You can locate this test in the index of the CPT under "HIV, Antibody."

■ Mono test is a test for mononucleosis or heterophile antibody screen. There are many codes that can be used to report "mono tests." For example, 86663 reports an Epstein-Barr, which tests for exposure to the virus and is called an early antigen test (EA). 86664 reports a test that is more extensive and assesses at the cellular level for the presence of the virus. 86665 reports a viral capsid antigen test (VCA) that is more efficient and is often reported. 86308 is a screening test that is very inexpensive and efficient and is most often reported for Epstein-Barr virus screen. On the requisition form in this text, the "mono test" is reported with 86308.

■ Rubella Antibody is a titer for German measles, and it evaluates the level of antibodies in the patient's blood. You can locate this test in the index of the CPT under "Antibody, Rubella."

CASE 4-7   *Immunology*

Enter the codes for the following Immunology tests:

1 _____ ANA (FANA) Screen	9 _____ Hep B surface antigen
2 _____ Anti-D.S. (double stranded) DNA	10 _____ Hep B surface antigen OB, NC sent to outside
3 _____ ENA I (Sm, RNP)	lab—Mod 90
4 _____ ENA II (SS-A, SS-B)	11 _____ HIV-1, NC sent to outside lab—Mod 90
5 _____ ASO screen	12 _____ Mono test*
6 _____ Rheumatoid factor (qual)	13 _____ Rubella Antibody
7 _____ RPR (Syphilis Serology), quant	
8 _____ Cold Agglutinin titer	

*Mono = Epstein-Barr virus.

(Answers to every other Case are located in Appendix D . The full answer key is only available in the TEACH Instructor Resources on Evolve.)

Body Fluid

The Body Fluid section of the requisition form illustrated in **Figure 4-14** has a selection of commonly performed laboratory tests that are performed on a variety of body fluids.

■ Cell count w/Diff is a cell count performed on miscellaneous body fluids, such as cerebrospinal fluid,

pleural fluid, peritoneal fluid, or joint fluid. For example, cerebrospinal fluid can be analyzed for the presence of various bacteria (bacterial meningitis), such as *S. pneumoniae*, *E. coli*, or *N. meningitidis*. The differential represented by the "w/Diff" is a study performed in addition to the basic cell count. The differential examination includes counting types of cells present in

Code	BODY FLUID	DX
Fluid Source:		
	Cell Count w/o Diff	
	Protein	
	Glucose	
	Semen Analysis	
	Semen Analysis, Comp	

FIGURE 4–14 Body Fluid section.

the sample. You can locate this test in the index of the CPT under "Cell Count, Body Fluid."

■ The term "protein" represents a prostate specific antigen (PSA) test and is used to diagnose prostate cancer and to monitor recurrent prostate cancer. There are three different PSA tests, one for a complex PSA, one for total serum, and one for free PSA. The one on the requisition form is for a free PSA. You can locate this test in the index of the CPT under "Prostate Specific Antigen."

■ Glucose is found in many bodily fluids other than blood; for example, urine, and higher or lower levels than normal can indicate a disease condition. You can locate this test in the index of the CPT under "Glucose, Body Fluid."

■ Semen Analysis is the analysis of the presence and/or motility of sperm that may include the Huhner test, which is an analysis of the sperm after intercourse. The sperm is removed from the vaginal area by means of a swab for analysis. You can locate this test in the index of the CPT under "Semen Analysis."

■ Semen Analysis, Comp is a complete semen analysis that includes the volume, count, motility, and differential. This test can also be located in the index in the same location as the previous semen analysis.

CASE 4-8   *Body Fluid*

Enter the codes for the following Body Fluid tests:

1 _____ Cell Count w/Diff
2 _____ Protein, total
3 _____ Glucose (not blood)
4 _____ Semen Analysis (presence and/or motility post coital)

5 _____ Semen Analysis, Comp (volume, count, motility, and differential)

Enter the CPT codes for the Body Fluid tests on the requisition form in Figure 4-1.

(Answers to every other Case are located in Appendix D . The full answer key is only available in the TEACH Instructor Resources on Evolve.)

Office Testing

Each medical facility will have tests that the physician performs in the office rather than having the patient go to the laboratory for the test. In the medical facility represented on the General Laboratory Test Requisition form, the physicians in the practice commonly have their nursing staff perform routine in-office urinalysis (UA) by means of a dipstick (nonautomated) as illustrated in **Figure 4-15.** Place the correct code for this service on the requisition form.

Code	OFFICE TESTING	DX
	UA, Dipstick in Office	

FIGURE 4–15 Office testing.

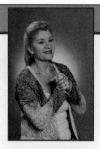

From the Trenches

"Medical coding is a challenging, rewarding profession knowing that coders not only help the Provider, but also the Patient."

CHRISTINA CIATTI
CPC, CPC-I, CPB

CASE 4-9 *Office Testing*

Enter the code for the urinalysis.

1 _____ UA, Dipstick in Office

There is no microscopic analysis with this office test. You can locate this test in the index of the CPT under "Urinalysis, Routine."

Enter the code on the requisition form in Figure 4-1.

(Answers to every other Case are located in Appendix D . The full answer key is only available in the TEACH Instructor Resources on Evolve.)

Other Laboratory and Pathology Services

In addition to the most commonly used laboratory codes, which are often placed on a superbill/requisition form similar to the one you just coded, are the following:

Drug Assay (80305-80377)
Evocative/Suppression Testing (80400-80439)
Transfusion Medicine (86850-86999)
Microbiology (87003-87999)
Anatomic Pathology (88000-88099)
Pathology Clinical Consultations (80503-80506)
Molecular Pathology (81161-81479)
Multianalyte Assays with Algorithmic Analyses (81490-81599)
Cytopathology (88104-88199)
Cytogenetic Studies (88230-88299)
Surgical Pathology (88300-88399)
Transcutaneous Procedures (88720-88749)
Other Procedures (89049-89240)
Reproductive Medicine Procedures (89250-89398)
Proprietary Laboratory Analyses (0001U-0520U)

Presumptive Drug Class Screening

The screening of drug classes (80305-80307) is divided based on method performed. Codes 80305-80307 include drugs that may be easily detected either by direct optical observation devices, such as dipsticks, cups, cards, or cartridges, or instrumental testing procedures, which include chemistry analyzers using immunoassay or enzyme assay.

Code 80305 reports single or multiple drug class procedures from Drug Class Test using direct optical observation and is reported only once per date of service. CPT 80306 reports single drug class screenings that use instrumented testing procedures and is only reported once per date of service.

Code 80307 is reported for presumptive screening of any number of drug classes using chemical analyzers and chromatography, and is reported once per date of service.

Diagnoses Coding in Drug Test and Drug Abuse

In the Index of ICD-10-CM, locate the term "Test(s)." Next, locate the subterm "blood-alcohol" and "blood-drug," and note that you are referred to Z04.89. When referencing the Tabular, the description of the code indicates "blood-alcohol tests" or "blood-drug tests." Therefore, if a patient presents for a test to assess the presence or absence of either a drug or alcohol, the service is reported with Z04.89.

Return to the term "Test(s)" in the Index. Review all of the subterms under this heading and see that this is a good location for directions to many commonly reported diagnoses when coding laboratory services. For example, pregnancy tests, tuberculin (Mantoux), paternity, and fertility tests.

If blood is drawn to assess the level of a therapeutic drug, such as when a patient takes Heparin (blood thinner), the diagnosis is reported Z51.81. This is found in the Index under "Encounter, therapeutic drug level monitoring, Z51.81."

If the laboratory test is performed as a confirmation, the patient is already known to have a more definitive diagnosis and it is that diagnosis that would be reported, not a Z code for screening for the presence of a substance or condition. For example, if the patient had a drug screen to check for the presence of cocaine, the diagnosis code for the screening service would be Z04.89. Upon return for a confirmation of the initial test, which is standard procedure, the diagnosis would be reported as F14.10, nondependent cocaine abuse. Turn to the term "Abuse" in the Index, and review the

subterms listed there. You must **never** code directly from the Index and must *always* reference the Tabular before assigning a code. Using the Index is only half of the coding process, but it is the first step to locating the codes in the Tabular.

Many laboratory procedures are for conditions that are known or suspected. For example, if a patient presents to the laboratory for an insulin tolerance panel for suspected insulin deficiency, the diagnosis code would be E27.40 (Deficiency, corticoadrenal). This is another good example of why you must know your medical terminology (corticoadrenal), since there is no entry for insulin.

CASE 4-10 *Presumptive Drug Class Screening*

1. Martin Morison is a 17-year-old high school student sent to the laboratory for a routine drug screen conducted by chromatography that included multiple drugs.

SERVICE CODE(S): _____

ICD-10-CM DX CODE(S): _____

2. A drug screen is conducted for cocaine, read by direct observation.

SERVICE CODE(S): _____

ICD-10-CM DX CODE(S): _____

3. Alice Harnes, a nurse at the local hospital, is brought in to the laboratory for a drug screening that includes amphetamine, cocaine, and barbiturates. Using instrument assisted direct observation.

SERVICE CODE(S): _____

ICD-10-CM DX CODE(S): _____

(Answers to every other Case are located in Appendix D . The full answer key is only available in the TEACH Instructor Resources on Evolve.)

Evocative/Suppression Testing

Evocative/Suppression testing is performed to determine measurements of the effect of evocative or suppressive agents on chemical constituents. For example, code 80400 is reported when a patient undergoes testing to determine whether adrenocorticotropic hormone is being stimulated for production in the body. The physician may suspect that the patient suffers from adrenal gland insufficiency.

Note that following each of the code descriptions is a statement of the services that must have been provided for the code to be applicable. For example, the requirement to report 80400 ACTH stimulation panel is "Cortisol (82533 × 2)" or two cortisol tests as described in 82533. You will have to read the description for code 82533 to ensure that it is the correct test before you can report 80400.

CASE 4-11 *Evocative/Suppression Testing*

1. Mary Hopewell has low blood pressure of undetermined etiology and is sent by her primary care physician to the laboratory in the clinic for an insulin tolerance panel that included five cortisol and five glucose assessments for what is suspected to be a deficiency in her adrenocorticotropic hormone (corticoadrenal deficiency).

SERVICE CODE(S): _____

ICD-10-CM DX CODE(S): _____

2. Joe Franklin is sent to the laboratory by his family physician to receive a complete pituitary panel (Evocative/Suppression test) for his suspected malignant tumor of the pituitary gland resulting in visual field impairment and headaches.

SERVICE CODE(S): _____

ICD-10-CM DX CODE(S): _____

(Answers to every other Case are located in Appendix D . The full answer key is only available in the TEACH Instructor Resources on Evolve.)

Transfusion Medicine

The Transfusion Medicine subsection deals with tests performed on blood or blood products. Tests include screening for antibodies, Coombs testing, autologous blood collection and processing, blood typing, compatibility testing, and preparation of and treatments performed on blood and blood products.

CASE 4-12   *Transfusion Medicine*

1. Jessi Welter presented to the laboratory for blood typing for a paternity test, which identified his ABO (three main blood types), Rh (rhesus factor), and MN antigens.

SERVICE CODE(S): _____

ICD-10-CM DX CODE(S): _____

2. The blood bank technician prepares 6 units of blood for freezing.

SERVICE CODE(S): _____

ICD-10-CM DX CODE(S): _____

Microbiology

Microbiology deals with the study of microorganisms. Cultures for the identification of organisms as well as the identification of sensitivities of the organism to antibiotics (called culture and sensitivity) are found in this subsection. Culture codes must be reviewed carefully because some codes are used to indicate screening only to detect the presence of an organism; some codes indicate the identification of specific organisms; and others indicate additional sensitivity testing to determine which antibiotic would be best for treatment of the specified bacteria. You should report all tests performed on the basis of whether they are quantitative or qualitative and/or a sensitivity study.

CASE 4-13   *Microbiology*

1. Sally Jane Newman is brought to the laboratory by her father for a urinalysis for a bacterial culture that includes a quantitative colony count. Her pediatrician indicates a diagnosis of dysuria.

SERVICE CODE(S): _____

ICD-10-CM DX CODE(S): _____

2. Rachel Bose has symptoms of dysuria, vaginal discharge, and odor. She is sent to the laboratory by her obstetrician for a *Chlamydia* culture. According to physician documentation, the test was positive for *Chlamydia trachomatis*.

SERVICE CODE(S): _____

ICD-10-CM DX CODE(S): _____

(Answers to every other Case are located in Appendix D. The full answer key is only available in the TEACH Instructor Resources on Evolve.)

Anatomic Pathology

Anatomic Pathology deals with examination of the body fluids or tissues in postmortem examination. Postmortem examination involves the completion of gross microscopic and limited autopsies. The codes in this section report the physician's service only and are divided according to the extent of the examination. This subsection also contains codes for forensic examination and coroners' cases.

CASE 4-14   *Anatomic Pathology*

1. Grey Lonewolf performs an autopsy on a 13-year-old female who died in an automobile accident. The autopsy includes both gross and microscopic examinations and includes the brain and spinal cord.

SERVICE CODE(S): _____

2. The county coroner performs a forensic examination on an 18-year-old male who sustained fatal knife wounds to the chest during an altercation.

SERVICE CODE(S): _____

(Answers to every other Case are located in Appendix D. The full answer key is only available in the TEACH Instructor Resources on Evolve.)

Pathology Clinical Consultations

A clinical pathologist, on request from a primary care physician, will perform a consultation to render additional medical interpretation regarding test results. For example, a primary care physician reviews laboratory test results and requests a clinical pathologist to review, interpret, and prepare a written report on the findings.

These consultation codes (80503-80506) can be based on either the level of medical decision making (MDM) or the total time spent on the date of consultation. When submitted to a third-party payer, the submission is accompanied by a written report.

If reporting based on MDM, determine whether the level was straightforward (80503), moderate (80504), or high (80505), but also based on two out of the three MDM elements.

If assigning these codes based instead on time, then total time spent on the date of consultation must be documented for all activities personally performed by the consultant in the report, but not including activities usually performed by clinical staff. Report 80503 for 5-20 minutes of total time, 80504 for 21-40 minutes of total time, and 80505 for 41-60 minutes of total time. Each additional 30 minutes after the initial 60 minutes of total time should be reported with 80506 as an add-on code to 80505 only.

These are not the only pathology consultation codes in the Pathology and Laboratory section of the CPT manual. There are also consultation codes toward the end of the section in the Surgical Pathology subsection, codes 88321-88334. These consultation codes are used to report the services of a pathologist who reviews and gives an opinion or advice concerning pathology slides, specimens, material, or records that were prepared elsewhere or for pathology consultation during surgery.

CASE 4-15 *Pathology Clinical Consultations*

1. Dr. Green's patient, Lonnie Glenn, was currently in the hospital when Dr. Green asked Dr. Lonewolf to consult with him on Lonnie's therapeutic drug levels. Dr. Lonewolf indicated that he provided a limited consultation.

   SERVICE CODE(S): _____

   ICD-10-CM DX CODE(S): _____

2. Dr. Alanda sent three slides to Dr. Lonewolf, asking him to review the slides that were prepared at the patient's hometown clinic's laboratory. Dr. Lonewolf reviews the slides and prepares a written report that is sent to Dr. Alanda. The patient has malignant primary prostate cancer.

   SERVICE CODE(S): _____

   ICD-10-CM DX CODE(S): _____

3. Dr. Green requests that Dr. Lonewolf provide a surgical pathology consultation during a surgical procedure for a female patient with malignant primary breast cancer.

   SERVICE CODE(S): _____

   ICD-10-CM DX CODE(S): _____

(Answers to every other Case are located in Appendix D . The full answer key is only available in the TEACH Instructor Resources on Evolve.)

Cytopathology and Cytogenetic Studies

The Cytopathology subsection deals with laboratory work performed to determine whether cellular changes are present. For example, a common **cytopathology** procedure is the Papanicolaou smear (Pap smear). Cytopathology may also be performed on fluids that have been aspirated from a site to identify cellular changes. Cytogenetic studies include tests performed for genetic and chromosomal studies.

CASE 4-16 *Cytopathology and Cytogenetic Studies*

1. A bone marrow sample is received in the laboratory with a request for a culture for a suspected generalized neoplastic disease in a patient with severe anemia.

   SERVICE CODE(S): _____

   ICD-10-CM DX CODE(S): _____

2. A chromosome analysis for amniotic fluid cells was performed due to abnormal amniotic fluid results. The test included cell counts for 10 colonies and banding.

   SERVICE CODE(S): _____

   ICD-10-CM DX CODE(S): _____

(Answers to every other Case are located in Appendix D . The full answer key is only available in the TEACH Instructor Resources on Evolve.)

Surgical Pathology

A pathology department, usually located in a hospital, medical school, or outside medical laboratory facility, would analyze tissue removed from a patient during a surgical procedure, and that facility would report the analysis with codes from 88300-88309, Surgical Pathology. The clinic or other medical facility can send the tissue to an outside laboratory for analysis, reimburse the outside facility for the service, and then bill the third-party payer for reimbursement using modifier -90 to indicate that the service was actually provided by an outside laboratory. Pathology codes describe the evaluation of specimens to determine the pathology of disease processes. When choosing the correct code for pathology, you must identify the source of the specimen and the reason for the surgical procedure. The Surgical Pathology subsection contains codes that are divided into six levels (Levels I through VI) based on the specimen examined and the level of work required by the pathologist. Pathology testing is done on all tissue removed from the body. The surgical pathology classification level is determined by the complexity of the pathologic examination.

The 88300-88309 surgical pathology examination codes contain a technical and professional component. Let's look at four examples of settings and how the reporting of the examination would be handled:

1. The pathologist is an employee of the hospital, and the pathological examination of the surgical specimen was performed in the hospital's pathology laboratory. The hospital would report the professional employee (professional component) and the facility expenses of establishing and maintaining a laboratory (technical component). The professional component would be reported on the CMS1500 with modifier -26. The technical component would be reported on the CMS1450 with no modifier because the CMS1450 is only used to report the technical portion of services.

2. The pathologist is an employee of the clinic, and the pathologist went to the hospital and used the hospital facilities to perform the examination of the surgical specimen. The clinic would report the professional component on the CMS-1500 with modifier -26 to indicate that only the physician portion of the service was being reported. The hospital would report the technical portion of the service on the CMS-1500 with no modifier.

3. The pathologist is an employee of the clinic and performed the surgical specimen examination at a clinic-based pathology laboratory. Using the CMS-1500, the clinic would report the specimen examination code once, with no modifier to indicate that both the professional and technical portion of the service was provided.

4. The pathologist is an employee of the hospital and performed the surgical specimen examination at a clinic-based pathology laboratory. The hospital would report the professional component on the CMS-1500, and the clinic would report the technical component on a CMS-1500 with modifier -TC (technical component) to indicate that only the technical component of the service was provided.

As you can see from the above examples, who employs the professional and the location in which the services are provided are essential to correctly reporting the surgical pathology examination. For the purposes of this text, you will not be required to report the components of the surgical pathology examination codes (88300-88309).

Usually the coder does not add modifier -26 to codes 88300-88309 because the clinic or hospital software system automatically generates the necessary modifier to indicate where and by whom the service was provided. So, again, for this text and for the 88300-88309 codes only, you do not need to consider whether the service is technical, professional, or global (both technical and professional).

Level I pathology code 88300 identifies specimens that normally do not need to be viewed under a microscope for pathologic diagnosis (e.g., a tooth)—those for which the probability of disease or malignancy is minimal.

Level II pathology code 88302 deals with tissues that are usually considered normal tissue and have been removed, not because of the probability of the presence of disease or malignancy, but for some other reason (e.g., a fallopian tube for sterilization, foreskin of a newborn).

Level III pathology code 88304 is assigned for specimens with a low probability of disease or malignancy. For example, a gallbladder may be neoplastic (benign or malignant), but when the gallbladder is removed for cholecystitis (inflammation of the gallbladder), it is usually inflamed from chronic disease and not because of cancerous changes.

Level IV pathology code 88305 carries a higher probability of malignancy or decision making for disease pathology. For example, a uterus is removed because of a diagnosis of prolapse. There is a possibility that the uterus is malignant or there are other causes of disease pathology.

Level V pathology code 88307 classifies more complex pathology evaluations (e.g., examination of a uterus that was removed for reasons other than prolapse or neoplasm).

Level VI pathology code 88309 includes examination of neoplastic tissue or very involved specimens, such as a total resection of a colon.

The remaining codes at the end of the subsection classify specialized procedures, utilization of stains, consultations performed, preparations used, and/or instrumentation needed to complete testing. These types of procedures can be reported in addition to the examination of the specimen(s).

Throughout the remainder of this text, you will be presented with operative reports and the corresponding pathology reports to which you will assign the surgical pathology codes.

Specimens

A specimen is a sample of tissue, blood, or urine that requires individual examination and pathologic diagnosis. In order to identify separate specimens from a patient, the surgeon must submit each specimen for individual examination based on the surgical report. Documentation should indicate each separate container that is individually marked or by a physical mark on each specimen in order to distinguish the specimens if multiple specimens are submitted together. Having separate containers or more than one tissue does not constitute having separate specimens. The tissue may have required several excisions or would not fit into one cassette. When there is no identification for separate specimens, only one unit of pathology service is reported.

For example, if liver tissue is received for pathologic examination comprising of multiple specimens for individual and separate attention, and individual examination and pathologic diagnosis, each specimen's gross and microscopic examination performed is considered a single unit of service. The appropriate surgical pathology (88300-88309) code would be reported.

Other Procedures

Other Procedures include miscellaneous testing on body fluids, the use of special instrumentation, and testing performed on oocyte and sperm.

CASE 4-17 *Surgical Pathology Report*

The following pathology report is a gastrointestinal pathology report from Chapter 7 of this text. Assign a CPT and an ICD-10-CM code to the pathologist's service:

LOCATION: Outpatient, Hospital
PATIENT: Jatin Al-Assad
SURGEON: Larry Friendly, MD
PATHOLOGIST: Morton Monson, MD
CLINICAL HISTORY: Polyp
TISSUE RECEIVED: Five separate colon polyps in five separate cassettes
GROSS DESCRIPTION: Each specimen is labeled with the patient's name and "colon polyp A-E." Specimen labeled "A from rectum" consists of colon mucosa and is 0.2 cm (centimeters) in dimension. Specimen labeled "B from sigmoid colon" consists of colon mucosa and is 4 mm (millimeters) in dimension. Specimen labeled "C from ascending colon" consists of colon mucosa and is 3mm in size. Specimen labeled "D from descending colon" consists of colon mucosa and is 0.9 cm in dimension. Specimen labeled "E from splenic flexure" consists of colon mucosa and is .5 cm in size.

MICROSCOPIC DESCRIPTION: Sections of each of the five separate polyps show surface epithelium and underlying glands lined by a serrated feathery surface epithelium.

DIAGNOSIS: Colon polyp A: Hyperplastic polyp
Colon polyp B: Hyperplastic polyp
Colon polyp C: Hyperplastic polyp
Colon polyp D: Hyperplastic polyp
Colon polyp E: Hyperplastic polyp

SERVICE CODE(S): _____
ICD-10-CM DX CODE(S): _____

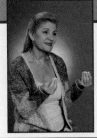

From the Trenches

"All coders should be encouraged to keep advancing in the field. There will always be a job out there that can utilize their knowledge and experience."

CHRISTINA CIATTI
CPC, CPC-I, CPB

CASE 4-18 *Other Procedures*

Report only the collection of the specimens, not the analysis.

1. Dr. Friendly performs a cell count on cerebrospinal fluid.
SERVICE CODE(S): _____

2. Dr. Friendly performs a nasal smear to determine the level of eosinophils.
SERVICE CODE(S): _____

CASE 4-19 *Pathology and Laboratory Section Review*

Now that you have reviewed the Pathology and Laboratory section of the CPT manual, it is time to combine the code laboratory tests from across the section. Code the following patient services and diagnoses.

Laboratory for a 60-year-old male patient with a chief complaint of heartburn with reflux (GERD):

SERVICE CODE(S)

1. *Helicobacter pylori* antibody _____

ICD-10-CM DX CODE(S): _____

Laboratory tests for a 50-year-old female patient with genital herpes simplex infection:

SERVICE CODE(S)

2. Tzanck smear with Wright stain (a special stain) _____
3. Viral culture _____
4. Herpes antibody testing _____

ICD-10-CM DX CODE(S): _____

Laboratory tests for a 24-year-old female with HIV (human immunodeficiency virus) screening due to high-risk lifestyle. (Both the **screening** for a specified viral disease and the **problem** with lifestyle are reported with Z codes.):

SERVICE CODE(S)

5. Western blot _____
6. Complete automated CBC _____
7. ANA _____

Continued

CASE 4-19—cont'd

ICD-10-CM DX CODE(S): _____

Laboratory tests for a 16-year-old male patient with diabetes for confirmation of ketoacidosis:

	SERVICE CODE(S)
8. Plasma glucose	_____
9. Ketones, qualitative	_____
10. Electrolytes panel	_____
11. Arterial blood gases	_____

ICD-10-CM DX CODE(S): _____

Laboratory tests for a 62-year-old female with hyperlipidemia:

	SERVICE CODE(S)
12. Total cholesterol	_____
13. HDL cholesterol	_____

ICD-10-CM DX CODE(S): _____

Laboratory tests for a 46-year-old man with impotence (organic):

	SERVICE CODE(S)
14. CBC	_____
15. Thyroid (TSH)	_____
16. Prolactin	_____
17. Free testosterone	_____

ICD-10-CM DX CODE(S): _____

Laboratory tests for a 26-year-old female with chronic myelocytic leukemia:

	SERVICE CODE(S)
18. CBC	_____
19. Automated platelet count, including electrolytes	_____
20. Calcium, total	_____
21. Magnesium	_____
22. Uric acid/blood	_____
23. Prothrombin time	_____
24. Partial thromboplastin time	_____

ICD-10-CM DX CODE(S): _____

Laboratory tests for a 6-year-old female with familial polycythemia:

	SERVICE CODE(S)
25. BUN	_____
26. Creatinine	_____
27. CBC	_____
28. Blood smear	_____

ICD-10-CM DX CODE(S): _____

Laboratory tests for a patient with suspected type I diabetes mellitus: Symptoms include weight loss and polydipsia. There is also a strong family history of type I diabetes. (There are three diagnoses to report here: weight loss, polydipsia, and family history of diabetes.)

	SERVICE CODE(S)
29. Blood glucose	_____

ICD-10-CM DX CODE(S): _____

Laboratory tests for a morbidly obese 39-year-old female who has been experiencing excessive thirst:

	SERVICE CODE(S)
30. Blood glucose	_____

ICD-10-CM DX CODE(S): _____

	SERVICE CODE(S)
31. Lipid panel	_____

ICD-10-CM DX CODE(S): _____

Laboratory tests for an 86-year-old male with endocarditis:

	SERVICE CODE(S)
32. Sedimentation rate (automated)	_____
33. CBC	_____

ICD-10-CM DX CODE(S): _____

Laboratory tests for a 21-year-old female with endometriosis of uterus:

	SERVICE CODE(S)
34. BUN	_____
35. Urinalysis (automated)	_____

ICD-10-CM DX CODE(S): _____

Laboratory tests for a 73-year-old male with Bell's palsy:

	SERVICE CODE(S)
36. CBC	_____
37. Sedimentation rate (automated)	_____
38. Glucose	_____
39. Urea nitrogen, urine	_____
40. BUN	_____
41. Hepatic function enzymes panel	_____
42. Creatinine	_____

ICD-10-CM DX CODE(S): _____

	SERVICE CODE(S)
43. Bone Marrow Biopsy	_____
Pathology Exam	
Bone Smear	_____

PREOPERATIVE DIAGNOSIS: Amyloidosis.

POSTOPERATIVE DIAGNOSIS: Amyloidosis.

The patient was sterilized and anesthetized by standard procedure. One bone marrow core biopsy was obtained from the left posterior iliac crest with moderate to severe discomfort. At the end of the procedure, the patient did not have any discomfort. There were no obvious complications.

Pathology report on the specimen: _____

Smear interpretation: _____

ICD-10-CM DX CODE(S): _____

Order Date: _____ Order Time: _____

PRIORITY (Routine unless otherwise specified)
[X] ASAP [ ] STAT   All tests: [ ] Yes [ ] No
If No, Specify Tests: _____

[ ] **RECURRING ORDER** (not to exceed 12 months)
Frequency: _____ Start Date: _____ End Date: _____

SPECIAL INSTRUCTIONS

FOR PHYSICIAN OFFICE COLLECTION ONLY:
Collected: Date: _____ Time: _____ By: _____

FOR LAB COLLECTION ONLY:
Collected: Date: _____ Time: _____ By: _____

General Laboratory Requisition

Code	CHEMISTRY	DX
	Albumin/Serum	
	Alkaline phosphatase	
	ALT/SGPT	
	Amylase	
	Arterial Blood Gas	
	AST/SGOT	
	Bilirubin, direct	
X	Bilirubin, total	
	BUN, Quant	
	Calcium, total	
	Carbon dioxide (CO_2)	
	CEA	
	Chloride, blood	
	Cholesterol, serum	
	CK (creatine kinase)	
	Creatinine, blood	
	FSH	
	Ferritin	
	Folic Acid (Folate), blood	
	GGT	
	Glucose, blood non-reag	
	Glycated Hgb (Hgb A1C)	
	HCG-Qualitative	
	HCG-Quantitative	
	HDL Cholesterol	
-90	Immun. Electrophoresis	
	Iron	
	Iron Binding Capacity	
NC	% saturation requires	
	iron & IBC to be ordered	
	LDH (lactate dehydrogenase)	
	LH (luteinizing hormone)	
	Magnesium	
	Phosphorus, blood	
	Potassium, blood	
	Prolactin, blood	
	Protein, total	
-90	Protein Electrophoresis, serum	
	PSA, total	
	Sodium, serum	
	T4, free (thyroxine)	
	TSH	
	Triglycerides	
	Uric Acid, blood	
	Vitamin B12	
	CALCULATIONS	
NC	LDL requires Chol & HDL	
	to be ordered	
NC	CHOL/HDL requires Chol	
	& HDL to be ordered	

Code	TOXICOLOGY/ THERAPEUTIC DRUGS	DX
Last Dose:		
	Carbamazepine	
	Digoxin	
	Lithium	
	Phenobarbital	
	Phenytoin (Dilantin)	
	Salicylate	
	Valproic Acid	
	Theophylline	

Code	IMMUNOLOGY (Blood)	DX
	ANA (FANA) Screen	
	if ANA positive, 86039 titer	
	performed, if titer >1:160	
	cascade performed (anti-	
	ds DNA, ENA I & ENA II)	
	Anti-ds DNA	
	ENA I (Sm, RNP)	
	ENA II (SSA, SSB)	
	ASO screen (ASO titer if	
	screen positive 86060)	
	Rheumatoid factor (qual)	
	RPR (Syphilis Serology), quant	
	Cold Agglutinin titer	
	Hep B surface antigen	
-90	Hep B surface antigen	
	OB (PHL)	
-90	HIV	
	Mono test	
	Rubella Antibody	

Code	PANELS	DX
	Electrolytes CO_2, Cl, K, Na	
	Bas Met, cal ion	
	Bas Met, cal tot	
X	Comprehensive metabolic / Alb, Bili tot, Ca tot, Cl, Creat, Glu, Alk phos, K, Prot tot, Na, AST, ALT, BUN, CO_2	
	Hepatic Function / Alb, Bili tot and dir, Alk phos, AST, ALT, Prot tot	
	Lipid Chol tot, HDL, Trig., calc LDL, Chol/HDL ratio	
	Gen health, Comp met, CBC, TSH	

Code	HEMATOLOGY	DX
	Hemogram	
	WBC, auto WBC diff	
	Hemogram	
	micro exam, WBC diff	
	Hemogram	
	micro exam, w/o diff	
	Hemogram	
	manual WBC diff, buffy	
	Hematocrit	
	Hemoglobin	
	Platelet count, auto	
	Reticulocyte count, manual	
	Sedimentation Rate, auto	
	WBC, automated	
	CBC, with diff	
	Hgb, Hct, RBC, WBC, Platelet	
	CBC, w/o diff	
	Hgb, Hct, RBC, WBC, Platelet	

Code	COAGULATION	DX
[ ] Coumadin [ ] Heparin		
	APTT	
	Prothrombin time	
	Bleeding time	

Code	OFFICE TESTING	DX
	UA, Dipstick in Office	

Code	URINE/STOOL	DX
	UA, Routine	
	UA SAVE (for possible	
	urine culture if requested)	
	UA with microscopic	
	Urinalysis, Dipstick, Lab	
	Occult Blood	
	Urine HCG	
	Diabetic urine cascade	

Code	TIMED URINE	DX
Hours:		
	Creatinine Clearance	
	Calcium, Urine, Quant.	
	Uric acid	

Code	BODY FLUID	DX
Fluid Source:		
	Cell Count w/o Diff	
	Protein	
	Glucose	
	Semen Analysis	
	Semen Analysis, Comp	

Code	IMMUNOHEMATOLOGY	DX
	Blood type ABO, Rh(D)	
	Weak D performed if	
	Rh negative	
	Antibody Screen	
	Identification, if positive,	
	titer if indicated	
	Direct Coombs	
	additional testing if	
	positive	

WRITE-IN TESTS	DX	Lab Use

Medical Necessity Statement: Tests ordered on Medicare patients must follow CMS rules regarding medical necessity and FDA approval guidelines and must include diagnosis, symptoms, or reason for testing as indicated on the medical record. For any payor (including Medicare and Medicaid) that has a medical necessity requirement, order only those tests which are medically necessary for the diagnosis and treatment of the patient.

DX	CODE	WRITTEN INDICATION/DIAGNOSIS (Match Diagnosis # to Test)
1		Idiopathic renal stone recurrent
2		
3		
4		

LAB USE ONLY	
Arterial Puncture	
Venipuncture	
Venipuncture MC/MA	
Handling Fee	
Urine Volume Measurement	
-90 PKU	

Chart #: _____1384B_____ Date: __01/10/02__
Name: _____Mary Brown_____ M (F)
DOB: _____06/07/40_____
Physician: ___Ronald Green, MD___

Medicare #: _____ Medicaid #: _____
[X] No ABN needed   [ ] Patient refused to sign ABN
Nursing Home Part A Medicare: [ ] Yes [ ] No
Worker's Comp: [ ] Yes [ ] No
Company Account: _____

44.

SERVICE CODE(S): _____

ICD-10-CM DX CODE(S): _____

Order Date: _____ Order Time: _____

PRIORITY (Routine unless otherwise specified)
[X] ASAP □ STAT All tests: □ Yes □ No
If No, Specify Tests: _____
□ **RECURRING ORDER** (not to exceed 12 months)
Frequency: _____ Start Date: _____ End Date: _____

SPECIAL INSTRUCTIONS

FOR PHYSICIAN OFFICE COLLECTION ONLY:
Collected: Date: _____ Time: _____ By: _____

FOR LAB COLLECTION ONLY:
Collected: Date: _____ Time: _____ By: _____

General Laboratory Requisition

Code	CHEMISTRY	DX
	Albumin/Serum	
	Alkaline phosphatase	
	ALT/SGPT	
	Amylase	
	Arterial Blood Gas	
	AST/SGOT	
	Bilirubin, direct	
	Bilirubin, total	
	BUN, Quant	
	Calcium, total	
	Carbon dioxide (CO_2)	
	CEA	
	Chloride, blood	
	Cholesterol, serum	
	CK (creatine kinase)	
	Creatinine, blood	
	FSH	
	Ferritin	
	Folic Acid (Folate), blood	
	GGT	
	Glucose, blood non-reag	
	Glycated Hgb (Hgb A1C)	
	HCG-Qualitative	
	HCG-Quantitative	
	HDL Cholesterol	
-90	Immun. Electrophoresis	
	Iron	
	Iron Binding Capacity	
NC	% saturation requires iron & IBC to be ordered	
	LDH (lactate dehydrogenase)	
	LH (luteinizing hormone)	
	Magnesium	
	Phosphorus, blood	
	Potassium, blood	
	Prolactin, blood	
	Protein, total	
-90	Protein Electrophoresis, serum	
	PSA, total	
	Sodium, serum	
	T4, free (thyroxine)	
	TSH	
	Triglycerides	
	Uric Acid, blood	
	Vitamin B12	
	CALCULATIONS	
NC	LDL requires Chol & HDL to be ordered	
NC	CHOL/HDL requires Chol & HDL to be ordered	

Code	TOXICOLOGY/ THERAPEUTIC DRUGS	DX
	Last Dose:	
	Carbamazepine	
	Digoxin	
	Lithium	
	Phenobarbital	
	Phenytoin (Dilantin)	
	Salicylate	
	Valproic Acid	
	Theophylline	

Code	IMMUNOLOGY (Blood)	DX
	ANA (FANA) Screen	
	if ANA positive, 86039 titer performed, if titer >1:160 cascade performed (anti-ds DNA, ENA I & ENA II)	
	Anti-ds DNA	
	ENA I (Sm, RNP)	
	ENA II (SSA, SSB)	
	ASO screen (ASO titer if screen positive 86060)	
	Rheumatoid factor (qual)	
	RPR (Syphilis Serology), quant	
	Cold Agglutinin titer	
	Hep B surface antigen	
-90	Hep B surface antigen OB (PHL)	
-90	HIV	
	Mono test	
	Rubella Antibody	

Code	PANELS	DX
	Electrolytes CO_2, Cl, K, Na	
	Bas Met, cal ion	
	Bas Met, cal tot	
	Comprehensive metabolic	
	Alb, Bili tot, Ca tot, Cl, Creat, Glu, Alk phos, K, Prot tot, Na, AST, ALT, BUN, CO_2	
	Hepatic Function	
	Alb, Bili tot and dir, Alk phos, AST, ALT, Prot tot	
	Lipid Chol tot, HDL, Trig., calc, LDL, Chol/HDL ratio	
	Gen health, Comp met, CBC, TSH	

Code	HEMATOLOGY	DX
	Hemogram	
	WBC, auto WBC diff	
	Hemogram micro exam, WBC diff	
	Hemogram micro exam, w/o diff	
	Hemogram manual WBC diff, buffy	
	Hematocrit	
	Hemoglobin	
X	Platelet count, auto	
	Reticulocyte count, manual	
	Sedimentation Rate, auto	
	WBC, automated	
	CBC, with diff	
	Hgb, Hct, RBC, WBC, Platelet	
	CBC, w/o diff	
	Hgb, Hct, RBC, WBC, Platelet	

Code	COAGULATION	DX
	□ Coumadin □ Heparin	
	APTT	
X	Prothrombin time	
X	Bleeding time	

Code	OFFICE TESTING	DX
	UA, Dipstick in Office	

Code	URINE/STOOL	DX
	UA, Routine	
	UA SAVE (for possible urine culture if requested)	
	UA with microscopic	
	Urinalysis, Dipstick, Lab	
	Occult Blood	
	Urine HCG	
	Diabetic urine cascade	

Code	TIMED URINE	DX
	Hours:	
	Creatinine Clearance	
	Calcium, Urine, Quant.	
	Uric acid	

Code	BODY FLUID	DX
	Fluid Source:	
	Cell Count w/o Diff	
	Protein	
	Glucose	
	Semen Analysis	
	Semen Analysis, Comp	

Code	IMMUNOHEMATOLOGY	DX
	Blood type ABO, Rh(D)	
	Weak D performed if Rh negative	
	Antibody Screen	
	Identification, if positive, titer if indicated	
	Direct Coombs additional testing if positive	

WRITE-IN TESTS	DX	Lab Use

Medical Necessity Statement: Tests ordered on Medicare patients must follow CMS rules regarding medical necessity and FDA approval guidelines and must include diagnosis, symptoms, or reason for testing as indicated on the medical record. For any patient of any payor (including Medicare and Medicaid) that has a medical necessity requirement, order only those tests which are medically necessary for the diagnosis and treatment of the patient.

DX	CODE	WRITTEN INDICATION/DIAGNOSIS (Match Diagnosis # to Test)
1		Thrombocytopenia
2		
3		
4		

LAB USE ONLY	
Arterial Puncture	
Venipuncture	
Venipuncture MC/MA	
Handling Fee	
Urine Volume Measurement	
-90 PKU	

Chart #: _8214J_   Date: _01/10/02_

Name: _Scott Jubelio_   Ⓜ F

DOB: _08/01/64_

Physician: _Ronald Green, MD_

Medicare #: _____ Medicaid #: _____

[X] No ABN needed   □ Patient refused to sign ABN

Nursing Home Part A Medicare: □ Yes □ No

Worker's Comp: □ Yes □ No

Company Account: _____

45.

SERVICE CODE(S): _____

ICD-10-CM DX CODE(S): _____

Order Date: _____ Order Time: _____

PRIORITY (Routine unless otherwise specified)
[X] ASAP   [ ] STAT   All tests: [ ] Yes [ ] No
If No, Specify Tests: _____

[ ] **RECURRING ORDER** (not to exceed 12 months)
Frequency: _____ Start Date: _____ End Date: _____

SPECIAL INSTRUCTIONS

FOR PHYSICIAN OFFICE COLLECTION ONLY:
Collected: Date: _____ Time: _____ By: _____

FOR LAB COLLECTION ONLY:
Collected: Date: _____ Time: _____ By: _____

General Laboratory Requisition

Code	CHEMISTRY	DX		Code	TOXICOLOGY/ THERAPEUTIC DRUGS	DX
	Albumin/Serum				Last Dose:	
	Alkaline phosphatase					
	ALT/SGPT				Carbamazepine	
	Amylase				Digoxin	
	Arterial Blood Gas				Lithium	
	AST/SGOT				Phenobarbital	
	Bilirubin, direct				Phenytoin (Dilantin)	
	Bilirubin, total				Salicylate	
	BUN, Quant				Valproic Acid	
	Calcium, total				Theophylline	
	Carbon dioxide (CO_2)			Code	IMMUNOLOGY (Blood)	DX
	CEA				ANA (FANA) Screen	
	Chloride, blood				if ANA positive, 86039 titer	
	Cholesterol, serum				performed, if titer >1:160	
	CK (creatine kinase)				cascade performed (anti-	
	Creatinine, blood				ds DNA, ENA I & ENA II)	
	FSH				Anti-ds DNA	
	Ferritin				ENA I (Sm, RNP)	
	Folic Acid (Folate), blood				ENA II (SSA, SSB)	
	GGT				ASO screen (ASO titer if	
	Glucose, blood non-reag				screen positive 86060)	
	Glycated Hgb (Hgb A1C)				Rheumatoid factor (qual)	
	HCG-Qualitative				RPR (Syphilis Serology), quant	
	HCG-Quantitative				Cold Agglutinin titer	
	HDL Cholesterol				Hep B surface antigen	
-90	Immun. Electrophoresis			-90	Hep B surface antigen	
	Iron				OB (PHL)	
	Iron Binding Capacity			-90	HIV	
NC	% saturation requires				Mono test	
	iron & IBC to be ordered				Rubella Antibody	
	LDH (lactate dehydrogenase)					
	LH (luteinizing hormone)					
	Magnesium			Code	PANELS	DX
	Phosphorus, blood				Electrolytes CO_2, Cl, K, Na	
	Potassium, blood				Bas Met, cal ion	
	Prolactin, blood				Bas Met, cal tot	
	Protein, total				Comprehensive metabolic	
-90	Protein Electrophoresis, serum				Alb, Bili tot, Ca tot, Cl, Creat,	
	PSA, total				Glu, Alk phos, K, Prot tot,	
	Sodium, serum				Na, AST, ALT, BUN, CO_2	
X	T4, free (thyroxine)				Hepatic Function	
X	TSH				Alb, Bili tot and dir, Alk phos,	
	Triglycerides				AST, ALT, Prot tot	
	Uric Acid, blood				Lipid Chol tot, HDL, Trig.,	
	Vitamin B12				calc LDL, Chol/HDL ratio	
	CALCULATIONS				Gen health, Comp met,	
NC	LDL requires Chol & HDL				CBC, TSH	
	to be ordered					
NC	CHOL/HDL requires Chol					
	& HDL to be ordered					

Code	HEMATOLOGY	DX
	Hemogram	
	WBC, auto WBC diff	
	Hemogram	
	micro exam, WBC diff	
	Hemogram	
	micro exam, w/o diff	
	Hemogram	
	manual WBC diff, buffy	
	Hematocrit	
	Hemoglobin	
	Platelet count, auto	
	Reticulocyte count, manual	
X	Sedimentation Rate, auto	
	WBC, automated	
	CBC, with diff	
	Hgb, Hct, RBC, WBC, Platelet	
	CBC, w/o diff	
	Hgb, Hct, RBC, WBC, Platelet	

Code	COAGULATION	DX
[ ] Coumadin [ ] Heparin		
	APTT	
	Prothrombin time	
	Bleeding time	

Code	OFFICE TESTING	DX
	UA, Dipstick in Office	

Code	URINE/STOOL	DX
	UA, Routine	
	UA SAVE (for possible	
	urine culture if requested)	
	UA with microscopic	
	Urinalysis, Dipstick, Lab	
	Occult Blood	
	Urine HCG	
	Diabetic urine cascade	

Code	TIMED URINE	DX
Hours:		
	Creatinine Clearance	
	Calcium, Urine, Quant.	
	Uric acid	

Code	BODY FLUID	DX
Fluid Source:		
	Cell Count w/o Diff	
	Protein	
	Glucose	
	Semen Analysis	
	Semen Analysis, Comp	

Code	IMMUNOHEMATOLOGY	DX
	Blood type ABO, Rh(D)	
	Weak D performed if	
	Rh negative	
	Antibody Screen	
	Identification, if positive,	
	titer if indicated	
	Direct Coombs	
	additional testing if	
	positive	

WRITE-IN TESTS		DX	Lab Use

Medical Necessity Statement: Tests ordered on Medicare patients must follow CMS rules regarding medical necessity and FDA approval guidelines and must include diagnosis, symptoms, or reason for testing as indicated on the medical record. For any patient of any payor (including Medicare and Medicaid) that has a medical necessity requirement, order only those tests which are medically necessary for the diagnosis and treatment of the patient.

DX	CODE	WRITTEN INDICATION/DIAGNOSIS (Match Diagnosis # to Test)
1		Hyperthyroidism
2		
3		
4		

LAB USE ONLY	
Arterial Puncture	
Venipuncture	
Venipuncture MC/MA	
Handling Fee	
Urine Volume Measurement	
-90 PKU	

Chart #: __1496B__ Date: __01/10/02__
Name: __Larry Blaine__ (M)/F
DOB: __11/03/74__
Physician: __Alma Naraquist, MD__

Medicare #: _____ Medicaid #: _____
[X] No ABN needed [ ] Patient refused to sign ABN
Nursing Home Part A Medicare: [ ] Yes [ ] No
Worker's Comp: [ ] Yes [ ] No
Company Account: _____

46.

SERVICE CODE(S): _____

ICD-10-CM DX CODE(S): _____

Order Date: _____ Order Time: _____

General Laboratory Requisition

PRIORITY (Routine unless otherwise specified)
[X] ASAP [ ] STAT All tests: [ ] Yes [ ] No
If No, Specify Tests: _____

[ ] **RECURRING ORDER** (not to exceed 12 months)
Frequency: _____ Start Date: _____ End Date: _____

SPECIAL INSTRUCTIONS

FOR PHYSICIAN OFFICE COLLECTION ONLY:
Collected: Date: _____ Time: _____ By: _____

FOR LAB COLLECTION ONLY:
Collected: Date: _____ Time: _____ By: _____

Code	CHEMISTRY	DX
	Albumin/Serum	
X	Alkaline phosphatase	
	ALT/SGPT	
	Amylase	
	Arterial Blood Gas	
	AST/SGOT	
	Bilirubin, direct	
	Bilirubin, total	
	BUN, Quant	
	Calcium, total	
	Carbon dioxide (CO_2)	
	CEA	
	Chloride, blood	
	Cholesterol, serum	
	CK (creatine kinase)	
	Creatinine, blood	
	FSH	
	Ferritin	
	Folic Acid (Folate), blood	
	GGT	
	Glucose, blood non-reag	
	Glycated Hgb (Hgb A1C)	
	HCG-Qualitative	
	HCG-Quantitative	
	HDL Cholesterol	
-90	Immun. Electrophoresis	
	Iron	
	Iron Binding Capacity	
NC	% saturation requires	
	iron & IBC to be ordered	
	LDH (lactate dehydrogenase)	
	LH (luteinizing hormone)	
	Magnesium	
X	Phosphorus, blood	
	Potassium, blood	
	Prolactin, blood	
	Protein, total	
-90	Protein Electrophoresis, serum	
	PSA, total	
	Sodium, serum	
	T4, free (thyroxine)	
X	TSH	
	Triglycerides	
	Uric Acid, blood	
	Vitamin B12	
	CALCULATIONS	
NC	LDL requires Chol & HDL	
	to be ordered	
NC	CHOL/HDL requires Chol	
	& HDL to be ordered	

Code	TOXICOLOGY/ THERAPEUTIC DRUGS	DX
	Last Dose:	
	Carbamazepine	
	Digoxin	
	Lithium	
	Phenobarbital	
	Phenytoin (Dilantin)	
	Salicylate	
	Valproic Acid	
	Theophylline	

Code	IMMUNOLOGY (Blood)	DX
	ANA (FANA) Screen	
	if ANA positive, 86039 titer	
	performed, if titer >1:160	
	cascade performed (anti-	
	ds DNA, ENA I & ENA II)	
	Anti-ds DNA	
	ENA I (Sm, RNP)	
	ENA II (SSA, SSB)	
	ASO screen (ASO titer if	
	screen positive 86060)	
	Rheumatoid factor (qual)	
	RPR (Syphilis Serology), quant	
	Cold Agglutinin titer	
	Hep B surface antigen	
-90	Hep B surface antigen	
	OB (PHL)	
-90	HIV	
	Mono test	
	Rubella Antibody	

Code	PANELS	DX
	Electrolytes CO_2, Cl, K, Na	
	Bas Met, cal ion	
	Bas Met, cal tot	
	Comprehensive metabolic	
	Alb, Bili tot, Ca tot, Cl, Creat,	
	Glu, Alk phos, K, Prot tot,	
	Na, AST, ALT, BUN, CO_2	
	Hepatic Function	
	Alb, Bili tot and dir, Alk phos,	
	AST, ALT, Prot tot	
	Lipid Chol tot, HDL, Trig.,	
	calc, LDL, Chol/HDL ratio	
	Gen health, Comp met,	
	CBC, TSH	

	Code	HEMATOLOGY	DX
		Hemogram	
		WBC, auto WBC diff	
		Hemogram	
		micro exam, WBC diff	
		Hemogram	
		micro exam, w/o diff	
X		Hemogram	
		manual WBC diff, buffy	
		Hematocrit	
		Hemoglobin	
		Platelet count, auto	
		Reticulocyte count, manual	
X		Sedimentation Rate, auto	
		WBC, automated	
		CBC, with diff	
		Hgb, Hct, RBC, WBC, Platelet	
		CBC, w/o diff	
		Hgb, Hct, RBC, WBC, Platelet	

	Code	COAGULATION	DX
		[ ] Coumadin [ ] Heparin	
		APTT	
		Prothrombin time	
		Bleeding time	

	Code	OFFICE TESTING	DX
		UA, Dipstick in Office	

X	Code	URINE/STOOL	DX
X		UA, Routine	
		UA SAVE (for possible	
		urine culture if requested)	
		UA with microscopic	
		Urinalysis, Dipstick, Lab	
		Occult Blood	
		Urine HCG	
		Diabetic urine cascade	

	Code	TIMED URINE	DX
		Hours:	
		Creatinine Clearance	
		Calcium, Urine, Quant.	
		Uric acid	

	Code	BODY FLUID	DX
		Fluid Source:	
		Cell Count w/o Diff	
		Protein	
		Glucose	
		Semen Analysis	
		Semen Analysis, Comp	

	Code	IMMUNOHEMATOLOGY	DX
		Blood type ABO, Rh(D)	
		Weak D performed if	
		Rh negative	
		Antibody Screen	
		Identification, if positive,	
		titer if indicated	
		Direct Coombs	
		additional testing if	
		positive	

WRITE-IN TESTS	DX	Lab Use

Medical Necessity Statement: Tests ordered on Medicare patients must follow CMS rules regarding medical necessity and FDA approval guidelines and must include diagnosis, symptoms, or reason for testing as indicated on the medical record. For any patient of any payor (including Medicare and Medicaid) that has a medical necessity requirement, order only those tests which are medically necessary for the diagnosis and treatment of the patient.

DX	CODE	WRITTEN INDICATION/DIAGNOSIS (Match Diagnosis # to Test)
1		Osteoporosis
2		
3		
4		

LAB USE ONLY	
Arterial Puncture	
Venipuncture	
Venipuncture MC/MA	
Handling Fee	
Urine Volume Measurement	
-90 PKU	

Chart #: __4920C__   Date: __01/10/02__
Name: __Alma Covett__   M (F)
DOB: __06/09/40__
Physician: __Leslie Alanda, MD__

Medicare #: _____ Medicaid #: _____
[X] No ABN needed   [ ] Patient refused to sign ABN
Nursing Home Part A Medicare: [ ] Yes [ ] No
Worker's Comp: [ ] Yes [ ] No
Company Account: _____

47.

SERVICE CODE(S): _____

ICD-10-CM DX CODE(S): _____

Order Date: _____   Order Time: _____

PRIORITY (Routine unless otherwise specified)

[X] ASAP   [ ] STAT   All tests: [ ] Yes   [ ] No

If No, Specify Tests: _____

[ ] **RECURRING ORDER** (not to exceed 12 months)

Frequency: _____ Start Date: _____ End Date: _____

SPECIAL INSTRUCTIONS

FOR PHYSICIAN OFFICE COLLECTION ONLY:

Collected: Date: _____ Time: _____ By: _____

FOR LAB COLLECTION ONLY:

Collected: Date: _____ Time: _____ By: _____

General Laboratory Requisition

Code	CHEMISTRY	DX
	Albumin/Serum	
	Alkaline phosphatase	
	ALT/SGPT	
	Amylase	
	Arterial Blood Gas	
	AST/SGOT	
	Bilirubin, direct	
	Bilirubin, total	
	BUN, Quant	
	Calcium, total	
	Carbon dioxide (CO_2)	
	CEA	
	Chloride, blood	
	Cholesterol, serum	
	CK (creatine kinase)	
	Creatinine, blood	
	FSH	
	Ferritin	
	Folic Acid (Folate), blood	
	GGT	
	Glucose, blood non-reag	
	Glycated Hgb (Hgb A1C)	
	HCG-Qualitative	X
	HCG-Quantitative	
	HDL Cholesterol	
-90	Immun. Electrophoresis	
	Iron	
	Iron Binding Capacity	
NC	% saturation requires	
	iron & IBC to be ordered	
	LDH (lactate dehydrogenase)	
	LH (luteinizing hormone)	
	Magnesium	
	Phosphorus, blood	
	Potassium, blood	
	Prolactin, blood	
	Protein, total	
-90	Protein Electrophoresis, serum	
	PSA, total	
	Sodium, serum	
	T4, free (thyroxine)	
	TSH	
	Triglycerides	
	Uric Acid, blood	
	Vitamin B12	
	CALCULATIONS	
NC	LDL requires Chol & HDL	
	to be ordered	
NC	CHOL/HDL requires Chol	
	& HDL to be ordered	

Code	TOXICOLOGY/ THERAPEUTIC DRUGS	DX
	Last Dose:	
	Carbamazepine	
	Digoxin	
	Lithium	
	Phenobarbital	
	Phenytoin (Dilantin)	
	Salicylate	
	Valproic Acid	
	Theophylline	

Code	IMMUNOLOGY (Blood)	DX
	ANA (FANA) Screen	
	if ANA positive, 86039 titer	
	performed, if titer >1:160	
	cascade performed (anti-	
	ds DNA, ENA I & ENA II)	
	Anti-ds DNA	
	ENA I (Sm, RNP)	
	ENA II (SSA, SSB)	
	ASO screen (ASO titer if	
	screen positive 86060)	
	Rheumatoid factor (qual)	
	RPR (Syphilis Serology), quant	
	Cold Agglutinin titer	
	Hep B surface antigen	
-90	Hep B surface antigen	
	OB (PHL)	
-90	HIV	
	Mono test	
	Rubella Antibody	

Code	PANELS	DX
	Electrolytes CO_2, Cl, K, Na	
	Bas Met, cal ion	
	Bas Met, cal tot	
	Comprehensive metabolic	
	Alb, Bili tot, Ca tot, Cl, Creat,	
	Glu, Alk phos, K, Prot tot,	
	Na, AST, ALT, BUN, CO_2	
	Hepatic Function	
	Alb, Bili tot and dir, Alk phos,	
	AST, ALT, Prot tot	
	Lipid Chol tot, HDL, Trig.,	X
	calc, LDL, Chol/HDL ratio	
	Gen health, Comp met,	
	CBC, TSH	

Code	HEMATOLOGY	DX
	Hemogram	
	WBC, auto WBC diff	
	Hemogram	
	micro exam, WBC diff	
	Hemogram	
	micro exam, w/o diff	
	Hemogram	
	manual WBC diff, buffy	
	Hematocrit	
	Hemoglobin	
	Platelet count, auto	
	Reticulocyte count, manual	
	Sedimentation Rate, auto	
	WBC, automated	
	CBC, with diff	
	Hgb, Hct, RBC, WBC, Platelet	
	CBC, w/o diff	
	Hgb, Hct, RBC, WBC, Platelet	

Code	COAGULATION	DX
[ ] Coumadin [ ] Heparin		
	APTT	
	Prothrombin time	
	Bleeding time	

Code	OFFICE TESTING	DX
	UA, Dipstick in Office	

Code	URINE/STOOL	DX
	UA, Routine	
	UA SAVE (for possible	
	urine culture if requested)	
	UA with microscopic	
	Urinalysis, Dipstick, Lab	
	Occult Blood	
	Urine HCG	
	Diabetic urine cascade	

Code	TIMED URINE	DX
	Hours:	
	Creatinine Clearance	
	Calcium, Urine, Quant.	
	Uric acid	

Code	BODY FLUID	DX
	Fluid Source:	
	Cell Count w/o Diff	
	Protein	
	Glucose	
	Semen Analysis	
	Semen Analysis, Comp	

Code	IMMUNOHEMATOLOGY	DX
	Blood type ABO, Rh(D)	
	Weak D performed if	
	Rh negative	
	Antibody Screen	
	Identification, if positive,	
	titer if indicated	
	Direct Coombs	
	additional testing if	
	positive	

WRITE-IN TESTS	DX	Lab Use

Medical Necessity Statement: Tests ordered on Medicare patients must follow CMS rules regarding medical necessity and FDA approval guidelines and must include diagnosis, symptoms, or reason for testing as indicated on the medical record. For any patient of any payor (including Medicare and Medicaid) that has a medical necessity requirement, order only those tests which are medically necessary for the diagnosis and treatment of the patient.

DX	CODE	WRITTEN INDICATION/DIAGNOSIS (Match Diagnosis # to Test)
1		Meniere's Disease
2		
3		
4		

LAB USE ONLY		
	Arterial Puncture	
	Venipuncture	
	Venipuncture MC/MA	
	Handling Fee	
	Urine Volume Measurement	
-90	PKU	

Chart #: ___2346B___ Date: ___01/10/02___

Name: ___Peter Bartlett___ (M) F

DOB: ___04/04/47___

Physician: ___Ronald Green, MD___

Medicare #: _____ Medicaid #: _____

[X] No ABN needed   [ ] Patient refused to sign ABN

Nursing Home Part A Medicare: [ ] Yes [ ] No

Worker's Comp: [ ] Yes [ ] No

Company Account: _____

48.

SERVICE CODE(S): _____

ICD-10-CM DX CODE(S): _____

Order Date: _____ Order Time: _____

| **PRIORITY** (Routine unless otherwise specified) |
| [X] ASAP [ ] STAT All tests: [ ] Yes [ ] No |
| If No, Specify Tests: _____ |
| [ ] RECURRING ORDER (not to exceed 12 months) |
| Frequency: _____ Start Date: _____ End Date: _____ |
| **SPECIAL INSTRUCTIONS** |
| **FOR PHYSICIAN OFFICE COLLECTION ONLY:** |
| Collected: Date: _____ Time: _____ By: _____ |
| **FOR LAB COLLECTION ONLY:** |
| Collected: Date: _____ Time: _____ By: _____ |

General Laboratory Requisition

CHEMISTRY

Code	CHEMISTRY	DX
	Albumin/Serum	
	Alkaline phosphatase	
	ALT/SGPT	
	Amylase	
	Arterial Blood Gas	
	AST/SGOT	
	Bilirubin, direct	
	Bilirubin, total	
	BUN, Quant	
	Calcium, total	
	Carbon dioxide (CO_2)	
	CEA	
	Chloride, blood	
	Cholesterol, serum	
	CK (creatine kinase)	
	Creatinine, blood	
	FSH	
	Ferritin	
	Folic Acid (Folate), blood	
	GGT	
	Glucose, blood non-reag	
	Glycated Hgb (Hgb A1C)	
	HCG-Qualitative	
	HCG-Quantitative	
	HDL Cholesterol	
-90	Immun. Electrophoresis	
	Iron	
	Iron Binding Capacity	
NC	% saturation requires	
	iron & IBC to be ordered	
	LDH (lactate dehydrogenase)	
	LH (luteinizing hormone)	
	Magnesium	
	Phosphorus, blood	
	Potassium, blood	
	Prolactin, blood	
	Protein, total	
-90	Protein Electrophoresis, serum	
X	PSA, total	
	Sodium, serum	
	T4, free (thyroxine)	
	TSH	
	Triglycerides	
	Uric Acid, blood	
	Vitamin B12	
	CALCULATIONS	
NC	LDL requires Chol & HDL	
	to be ordered	
NC	CHOL/HDL requires Chol	
	& HDL to be ordered	

TOXICOLOGY/THERAPEUTIC DRUGS

Last Dose:

Code	THERAPEUTIC DRUGS	DX
	Carbamazepine	
	Digoxin	
	Lithium	
	Phenobarbital	
	Phenytoin (Dilantin)	
	Salicylate	
	Valproic Acid	
	Theophylline	

IMMUNOLOGY (Blood)

Code	IMMUNOLOGY (Blood)	DX
	ANA (FANA) Screen	
	if ANA positive, 86039 titer	
	performed, if titer >1:160	
	cascade performed (anti-ds DNA, ENA I & ENA II)	
	Anti-ds DNA	
	ENA I (Sm, RNP)	
	ENA II (SSA, SSB)	
	ASO screen (ASO titer if screen positive 86060)	
	Rheumatoid factor (qual)	
	RPR (Syphilis Serology), quant	
	Cold Agglutinin titer	
	Hep B surface antigen	
-90	Hep B surface antigen OB (PHL)	
-90	HIV	
	Mono test	
	Rubella Antibody	

PANELS

Code	PANELS	DX
	Electrolytes CO_2, Cl, K, Na	
	Bas Met, cal ion	
	Bas Met, cal tot	
	Comprehensive metabolic	
	Alb, Bili tot, Ca tot, Cl, Creat,	
	Glu, Alk phos, K, Prot tot,	
	Na, AST, ALT, BUN, CO_2	
	Hepatic Function	
	Alb, Bili tot and dir, Alk phos,	
	AST, ALT, Prot tot	
	Lipid Chol tot, HDL, Trig.,	
	calc, LDL, Chol/HDL ratio	
	Gen health, Comp met,	
	CBC, TSH	

HEMATOLOGY

Code	HEMATOLOGY	DX
	Hemogram	
	WBC, auto WBC diff	
	Hemogram micro exam, WBC diff	
X	Hemogram micro exam, w/o diff	
	Hemogram manual WBC diff, buffy	
	Hematocrit	
	Hemoglobin	
	Platelet count, auto	
	Reticulocyte count, manual	
	Sedimentation Rate, auto	
	WBC, automated	
	CBC, with diff	
	Hgb, Hct, RBC, WBC, Platelet	
	CBC, w/o diff	
	Hgb, Hct, RBC, WBC, Platelet	

COAGULATION

Code	COAGULATION	DX
	[ ] Coumadin [ ] Heparin	
	APTT	
	Prothrombin time	
	Bleeding time	

OFFICE TESTING

Code	OFFICE TESTING	DX
	UA, Dipstick in Office	

URINE/STOOL

Code	URINE/STOOL	DX
	UA, Routine	
	UA SAVE (for possible urine culture if requested)	
	UA with microscopic	
	Urinalysis, Dipstick, Lab	
	Occult Blood	
	Urine HCG	
	Diabetic urine cascade	

TIMED URINE

Hours:

Code	TIMED URINE	DX
	Creatinine Clearance	
	Calcium, Urine, Quant.	
	Uric acid	

BODY FLUID

Fluid Source:

Code	BODY FLUID	DX
	Cell Count w/o Diff	
	Protein	
	Glucose	
	Semen Analysis	
	Semen Analysis, Comp	

IMMUNOHEMATOLOGY

Code	IMMUNOHEMATOLOGY	DX
	Blood type ABO, Rh(D)	
	Weak D performed if Rh negative	
	Antibody Screen	
	Identification, if positive, titer if indicated	
	Direct Coombs additional testing if positive	

WRITE-IN TESTS

WRITE-IN TESTS	DX	Lab Use

Medical Necessity Statement: Tests ordered on Medicare patients must follow CMS rules regarding medical necessity and FDA approval guidelines and must include diagnosis, symptoms, or reason for testing as indicated on the medical record. For any patient of any payor (including Medicare and Medicaid) that has a medical necessity requirement, order only those tests which are medically necessary for the diagnosis and treatment of the patient.

DX	CODE	WRITTEN INDICATION/DIAGNOSIS (Match Diagnosis # to Test)
1		Prostatitis, acute
2		
3		
4		

LAB USE ONLY

LAB USE ONLY
Arterial Puncture
Venipuncture
Venipuncture MC/MA
Handling Fee
Urine Volume Measurement
-90 PKU

Chart #: 6498B

Name: Loren Brown Ⓜ/F

DOB: 01/30/56

Physician: Ronald Green, MD

Date: 01/10/02

Medicare #: _____ Medicaid #: _____

[X] No ABN needed [ ] Patient refused to sign ABN

Nursing Home Part A Medicare: [ ] Yes [ ] No

Worker's Comp: [ ] Yes [ ] No

Company Account: _____

49.

SERVICE CODE(S): _____

ICD-10-CM DX CODE(S): _____

Order Date: _____ Order Time: _____

PRIORITY (Routine unless otherwise specified)
[X] ASAP [ ] STAT All tests: [ ] Yes [ ] No
If No, Specify Tests: _____

[ ] **RECURRING ORDER** (not to exceed 12 months)
Frequency: _____ Start Date: _____ End Date: _____

SPECIAL INSTRUCTIONS

FOR PHYSICIAN OFFICE COLLECTION ONLY:
Collected: Date: _____ Time: _____ By: _____

FOR LAB COLLECTION ONLY:
Collected: Date: _____ Time: _____ By: _____

General Laboratory Requisition

Code	CHEMISTRY	DX		Code	TOXICOLOGY/ THERAPEUTIC DRUGS	DX
	Albumin/Serum				Last Dose:	
	Alkaline phosphatase					
	ALT/SGPT				Carbamazepine	
	Amylase				Digoxin	
	Arterial Blood Gas				Lithium	
	AST/SGOT				Phenobarbital	
	Bilirubin, direct				Phenytoin (Dilantin)	
	Bilirubin, total				Salicylate	
	BUN, Quant				Valproic Acid	
	Calcium, total				Theophylline	
	Carbon dioxide (CO_2)			Code	IMMUNOLOGY (Blood)	DX
	CEA				ANA (FANA) Screen	
	Chloride, blood				if ANA positive, 86039 titer	
	Cholesterol, serum				performed, if titer >1:160	
	CK (creatine kinase)				cascade performed (anti-	
	Creatinine, blood				ds DNA, ENA I & ENA II)	
X	FSH				Anti-ds DNA	
	Ferritin				ENA I (Sm, RNP)	
	Folic Acid (Folate), blood				ENA II (SSA, SSB)	
	GGT				ASO screen (ASO titer if	
	Glucose, blood non-reag				screen positive 86060)	
	Glycated Hgb (Hgb A1C)				Rheumatoid factor (qual)	
	HCG-Qualitative				RPR (Syphilis Serology), quant	
	HCG-Quantitative				Cold Agglutinin titer	
	HDL Cholesterol				Hep B surface antigen	
	-90 Immun. Electrophoresis				-90 Hep B surface antigen	
	Iron				OB (PHL)	
	Iron Binding Capacity				-90 HIV	
NC	% saturation requires				Mono test	
	iron & IBC to be ordered				Rubella Antibody	
	LDH (lactate dehydrogenase)					
X	LH (luteinizing hormone)					
	Magnesium			Code	PANELS	DX
	Phosphorus, blood				Electrolytes CO_2, Cl, K, Na	
	Potassium, blood				Bas Met, cal ion	
	Prolactin, blood				Bas Met, cal tot	
	Protein, total				Comprehensive metabolic	
	-90 Protein Electrophoresis, serum				Alb, Bili tot, Ca tot, Cl, Creat,	
	PSA, total				Glu, Alk phos, K, Prot tot,	
	Sodium, serum				Na, AST, ALT, BUN, CO_2	
X	T4, free (thyroxine)				Hepatic Function	
X	TSH				Alb, Bili tot and dir, Alk phos,	
	Triglycerides				AST, ALT, Prot tot	
	Uric Acid, blood				Lipid Chol tot, HDL, Trig.,	
	Vitamin B12				calc, LDL, Chol/HDL ratio	
	CALCULATIONS				Gen health, Comp met,	
NC	LDL requires Chol & HDL				CBC, TSH	
	to be ordered					
NC	CHOL/HDL requires Chol					
	& HDL to be ordered					

Code	HEMATOLOGY	DX
	Hemogram	
	WBC, auto WBC diff	
	Hemogram	
	micro exam, WBC diff	
	Hemogram	
	micro exam, w/o diff	
	Hemogram	
	manual WBC diff, buffy	
	Hematocrit	
	Hemoglobin	
	Platelet count, auto	
	Reticulocyte count, manual	
	Sedimentation Rate, auto	
	WBC, automated	
	CBC, with diff	
	Hgb, Hct, RBC, WBC, Platelet	
	CBC, w/o diff	
	Hgb, Hct, RBC, WBC, Platelet	

Code	COAGULATION	DX
[ ] Coumadin [ ] Heparin		
	APTT	
	Prothrombin time	
	Bleeding time	

Code	OFFICE TESTING	DX
	UA, Dipstick in Office	

Code	URINE/STOOL	DX
	UA, Routine	
	UA SAVE (for possible	
	urine culture if requested)	
	UA with microscopic	
	Urinalysis, Dipstick, Lab	
	Occult Blood	
	Urine HCG	
	Diabetic urine cascade	

Code	TIMED URINE	DX
	Hours:	
	Creatinine Clearance	
	Calcium, Urine, Quant.	
	Uric acid	

Code	BODY FLUID	DX
	Fluid Source:	
	Cell Count w/o Diff	
	Protein	
	Glucose	
	Semen Analysis	
	Semen Analysis, Comp	

Code	IMMUNOHEMATOLOGY	DX
	Blood type ABO, Rh(D)	
	Weak D performed if	
	Rh negative	
	Antibody Screen	
	Identification, if positive,	
	titer if indicated	
	Direct Coombs	
	additional testing if	
	positive	

WRITE-IN TESTS		DX	Lab Use

Medical Necessity Statement: Tests ordered on Medicare patients must follow CMS rules regarding medical necessity and FDA approval guidelines and must include diagnosis, symptoms, or reason for testing as indicated on the medical record. For any patient of any payor (including Medicare and Medicaid) that has a medical necessity requirement, order only those tests which are medically necessary for the diagnosis and treatment of the patient.

DX	CODE	WRITTEN INDICATION/DIAGNOSIS (Match Diagnosis # to Test)
1		Hyperprolactinemia
2		
3		
4		

LAB USE ONLY
Arterial Puncture
Venipuncture
Venipuncture MC/MA
Handling Fee
Urine Volume Measurement
-90 PKU

Chart #: __6241E__   Date: __01/10/02__
Name: __Manly Edwards__   (M)/F
DOB: __07/04/33__
Physician: __Ronald Green, MD__

Medicare #: _____ Medicaid #: _____
[X] No ABN needed [ ] Patient refused to sign ABN
Nursing Home Part A Medicare: [ ] Yes [ ] No
Worker's Comp: [ ] Yes [ ] No
Company Account: _____

50.

SERVICE CODE(S): _____

ICD-10-CM DX CODE(S): _____

Order Date: _____   Order Time: _____

PRIORITY (Routine unless otherwise specified)
[X] ASAP   [ ] STAT   All tests: [ ] Yes   [ ] No
If No, Specify Tests: _____

[ ] **RECURRING ORDER** (not to exceed 12 months)
Frequency: _____   Start Date: _____   End Date: _____

SPECIAL INSTRUCTIONS

FOR PHYSICIAN OFFICE COLLECTION ONLY:
Collected: Date: _____ Time: _____ By: _____

FOR LAB COLLECTION ONLY:
Collected: Date: _____ Time: _____ By: _____

General Laboratory Requisition

CHEMISTRY

Code	CHEMISTRY	DX
	Albumin/Serum	
	Alkaline phosphatase	
	ALT/SGPT	
	Amylase	
	Arterial Blood Gas	
	AST/SGOT	
	Bilirubin, direct	
	Bilirubin, total	
X	BUN, Quant	
	Calcium, total	
	Carbon dioxide (CO_2)	
	CEA	
	Chloride, blood	
	Cholesterol, serum	
	CK (creatine kinase)	
X	Creatinine, blood	
	FSH	
	Ferritin	
	Folic Acid (Folate), blood	
	GGT	
	Glucose, blood non-reag	
	Glycated Hgb (Hgb A1C)	
	HCG-Qualitative	
	HCG-Quantitative	
	HDL Cholesterol	
-90	Immun. Electrophoresis	
	Iron	
	Iron Binding Capacity	
NC	% saturation requires iron & IBC to be ordered	
	LDH (lactate dehydrogenase)	
	LH (luteinizing hormone)	
	Magnesium	
	Phosphorus, blood	
	Potassium, blood	
	Prolactin, blood	
	Protein, total	
-90	Protein Electrophoresis, serum	
	PSA, total	
	Sodium, serum	
	T4, free (thyroxine)	
	TSH	
	Triglycerides	
	Uric Acid, blood	
	Vitamin B12	
	CALCULATIONS	
NC	LDL requires Chol & HDL to be ordered	
NC	CHOL/HDL requires Chol & HDL to be ordered	

TOXICOLOGY/THERAPEUTIC DRUGS

Last Dose: _____

Code	THERAPEUTIC DRUGS	DX
	Carbamazepine	
	Digoxin	
	Lithium	
	Phenobarbital	
	Phenytoin (Dilantin)	
	Salicylate	
	Valproic Acid	
	Theophylline	

IMMUNOLOGY (Blood)

Code	IMMUNOLOGY (Blood)	DX
	ANA (FANA) Screen if ANA positive, 86039 titer performed, if titer >1:160 cascade performed (anti-ds DNA, ENA I & ENA II)	
	Anti-ds DNA	
	ENA I (Sm, RNP)	
	ENA II (SSA, SSB)	
	ASO screen (ASO titer if screen positive 86060)	
	Rheumatoid factor (qual)	
	RPR (Syphilis Serology), quant	
	Cold Agglutinin titer	
	Hep B surface antigen	
-90	Hep B surface antigen OB (PHL)	
-90	HIV	
	Mono test	
	Rubella Antibody	

PANELS

Code	PANELS	DX
	Electrolytes CO_2, Cl, K, Na	
	Bas Met, cal ion	
	Bas Met, cal tot	
	Comprehensive metabolic Alb, Bili tot, Ca tot, Cl, Creat, Glu, Alk phos, K, Prot tot, Na, AST, ALT, BUN, CO_2	
	Hepatic Function Alb, Bili tot and dir, Alk phos, AST, ALT, Prot tot	
	Lipid Chol tot, HDL, Trig., calc, LDL, Chol/HDL ratio	
	Gen health, Comp met, CBC, TSH	

HEMATOLOGY

Code	HEMATOLOGY	DX
	Hemogram	
	WBC, auto WBC diff	
	Hemogram micro exam, WBC diff	
	Hemogram micro exam, w/o diff	
	Hemogram manual WBC diff, buffy	
	Hematocrit	
	Hemoglobin	
	Platelet count, auto	
	Reticulocyte count, manual	
	Sedimentation Rate, auto	
	WBC, automated	
	CBC, with diff Hgb, Hct, RBC, WBC, Platelet	
	CBC, w/o diff Hgb, Hct, RBC, WBC, Platelet	

COAGULATION

Code	COAGULATION	DX
	[ ] Coumadin [ ] Heparin	
	APTT	
	Prothrombin time	
	Bleeding time	

OFFICE TESTING

Code	OFFICE TESTING	DX
	UA, Dipstick in Office	

URINE/STOOL

Code	URINE/STOOL	DX
	UA, Routine	
	UA SAVE (for possible urine culture if requested)	
	UA with microscopic	
	Urinalysis, Dipstick, Lab	
	Occult Blood	
	Urine HCG	
	Diabetic urine cascade	

TIMED URINE

Hours: _____

Code	TIMED URINE	DX
	Creatinine Clearance	
	Calcium, Urine, Quant.	
	Uric acid	

BODY FLUID

Fluid Source: _____

Code	BODY FLUID	DX
	Cell Count w/o Diff	
	Protein	
	Glucose	
	Semen Analysis	
	Semen Analysis, Comp	

IMMUNOHEMATOLOGY

Code	IMMUNOHEMATOLOGY	DX
	Blood type ABO, Rh(D)	
	Weak D performed if Rh negative	
	Antibody Screen	
	Identification, if positive, titer if indicated	
	Direct Coombs additional testing if positive	

WRITE-IN TESTS	DX	Lab Use

Medical Necessity Statement: Tests ordered on Medicare patients must follow CMS rules regarding medical necessity and FDA approval guidelines and must include diagnosis, symptoms, or reason for testing as indicated on the medical record. For any patient of any payor (including Medicare and Medicaid) that has a medical necessity requirement, order only those tests which are medically necessary for the diagnosis and treatment of the patient.

DX	CODE	WRITTEN INDICATION/DIAGNOSIS (Match Diagnosis # to Test)
1		Chronic renal failure
2		
3		
4		

LAB USE ONLY	
Arterial Puncture	
Venipuncture	
Venipuncture MC/MA	
Handling Fee	
Urine Volume Measurement	
-90 PKU	

Chart #: _____5899C_____   Date: _01/10/02_
Name: _Randy Chalette_   (M)/F
DOB: _06/30/74_
Physician: _Leslie Alanda, MD_

Medicare #: _____   Medicaid #: _____
[X] No ABN needed   [ ] Patient refused to sign ABN
Nursing Home Part A Medicare: [ ] Yes   [ ] No
Worker's Comp: [ ] Yes   [ ] No
Company Account: _____

51.

SERVICE CODE(S): _____

ICD-10-CM DX CODE(S): _____

CHAPTER 4   *Auditing Review*

Audit the coding for the following reports.

Audit Report 4.1 Laboratory Workup

A 65-year-old female with ESRD, hypertension, diabetes mellitus type 2, and atrial fibrillation on Coumadin presents to the lab for the following:

Comprehensive metabolic panel _____

Magnesium _____

Prothrombin time (PT) _____

UA (Automated with microscope)

One or more of the following codes are reported incorrectly for this case. Indicate the incorrect code or codes.

PROFESSIONAL SERVICES: Comprehensive metabolic panel, **80053**; Creatinine, **82565**; Magnesium, **83735**; Prothrombin time, **85610**; Urinalysis, **81003**

ICD-10-CM DX: Hypertensive kidney disease, **I12.0**; End-stage renal disease, **N18.6**; Diabetes, **E11.9**; Atrial fibrillation, **I48.91**; Long-term drug therapy, **Z79.01**

INCORRECT CODE(S): _____

Audit Report 4.2 Laboratory Workup

A patient with acquired hemolytic anemia reports to the lab for the following blood work:

Ferritin _____

Iron _____

Hemoglobin _____

One of the following codes was incorrectly reported for this case. Indicate the incorrect code.

PROFESSIONAL SERVICES: Ferritin, **82728**; Iron, **83540**; Hemoglobin, **83051**

ICD-10-CM DX: Anemia, **D59.9**

INCORRECT CODE: _____

Audit Report 4.3 Pathology Report

LOCATION: Inpatient, Hospital

PATIENT: Martin Glass

SURGEON: Ira Avila, MD

ATTENDING PHYSICIAN: Ira Avila, MD

PATHOLOGIST: Grey Lonewolf, MD

CLINICAL HISTORY: Adenoma, prostate, and nodules and prostate

TISSUES RECEIVED:

FA. LT pelvic lymph nodes (FS). A. LT pelvic lymph nodes (FS). FB. RT pelvic lymph nodes (FS).

B. RT pelvic lymph nodes (FS). C. Prostate.

GROSS DESCRIPTION: Received in a container labeled "left pelvic nodes" are multiple tan and red lymph nodes up to 2.5 cm.

INTRAOPERATIVE FROZEN SECTION DIAGNOSIS: As per Dr. Lonewolf: Left pelvic lymph nodes: Negative for tumor.

The lymph nodes are submitted as A.

Received in a container labeled "right pelvic lymph nodes" are multiple tan and red lymph nodes up to 2.5 cm.

INTRAOPERATIVE FROZEN SECTION DIAGNOSIS: As per Dr. Lonewolf: Right pelvic lymph nodes: Negative for tumor.

The lymph nodes are submitted as B.

Received in a container labeled "prostate" is a prostate measuring 5.8 × 5.5 × 4 cm in greatest dimension and weighing 65 g. The surface has a tan to gray-purple appearance and diffuse multinodularity. The seminal vesicles are identified and show no abnormalities. The specimen is step sectioned and demonstrates a varied pattern with multiple foci of yellow infiltrative solid areas amongst the gray-tan moist cut surface. The right seminal vesicle is submitted as C1 and C2. The left seminal vesicle is submitted as C3 and C4. The right portion of the specimen from posterior to anterior is submitted as C5 to C13 and C37 to C40. The left portion is submitted as C14 to C24 and the midline is submitted as C25 to C32. The apex is submitted as C33 to C36.

MICROSCOPIC DESCRIPTION: The lymph nodes of the left pelvic region are negative for tumor and show sinus histiocytosis.

The lymph nodes of the right pelvic region are negative for tumor and show sinus histiocytosis.

The prostate demonstrates multiple areas of glands that vary in size and configuration and are lined by cells that are slightly enlarged with vesicular nuclei. The cells are relatively uniform and show intraglandular papillations and foci of hyperplasia. The seminal vesicles show normal morphology. Rare small foci demonstrate closely crowded glands that contain enlarged cells with vesicular nuclei showing prominent nucleoli. The cytoplasm varies in amounts. Large numbers of the glands are cystically dilated and lined by flattened epithelium. Foci of squamous metaplasia are present in rare glands.

DIAGNOSIS: Lymph nodes, left pelvic: Negative for tumor; sinus histiocytosis.

Lymph nodes, right pelvic: Negative for tumor; sinus histiocytosis.

Continued

CHAPTER 4—*cont'd*

Prostate, total prostatectomy: Adenocarcinoma, well differentiated, Gleason's grade 2 + 2 = 4, occasional foci; adenomatous hyperplasia; prostatic intraepithelial neoplasia, high grade, extensive.

COMMENT: The surgical margins of resection appear free of tumor. Case reviewed with Dr. Avila.

One of the following codes is reported incorrectly for this case. Indicate the incorrect code.

PROFESSIONAL SERVICES: Surgical pathology, **88309-26**; Surgical pathology, **88305-26**; Pathology surgical consultation, first tissue block, **88331**; Pathology surgical consultation, additional tissue block, **88332**

ICD-10-CM DX: Prostate neoplasm, **C61**

INCORRECT CODE: _____

Audit Report 4.4 Immunohematology

One or more of the following codes are reported incorrectly for this case. Indicate the incorrect code or codes.

86156	Cold agglutinin; titer
86277	Growth hormone, human, antibody
86480	Tuberculosis, intradermal
86592	Syphilis test; quantitative

INCORRECT/MISSING CODE(S): _____

Audit Report 4.5 Body Fluids

One or more of the following codes are reported incorrectly for this case. Indicate the incorrect code or codes.

84160	Protein, serum, total
82947	Glucose
89300	Semen Analysis, Complete
85004	Cell Count w/Diff

INCORRECT/MISSING CODE(S): _____

Audit Report 4.6 Transfusion Medicine

One or more of the following codes are reported incorrectly for this case. Indicate the incorrect code or codes.

1. Delores, a laboratory technician, performs splitting of blood products, 1 unit.

SERVICE CODE(S):   Irradiation of blood product, **86945**

2. Jessica, a laboratory technician, performs screening of RBC antibodies, serum technique.

SERVICE CODE(S):   RBC antibody identification, **86870**

INCORRECT/MISSING CODE(S): _____

(Auditing Review answers with rationales are only available in the TEACH Instructor Resources on Evolve.)

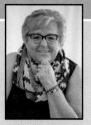

"Endlessly fascinating! That is what coding is. It can capture you for a lifetime and keep you interested in what is next. That's a great career."

Integumentary System

http://evolve.elsevier.com/Buck/next

(Answers to every other Case are located in Appendix D, with the full answer key only available in the TEACH Instructor Resources on Evolve)
(Auditing Review answers with rationales are only available in the TEACH Instructor Resources on Evolve)

Debridement

Debridement cleans surface areas and removes necrotic tissue. Codes in this category describe services of debridement based on depth, body surface, and condition. The first debridement codes (11000 and 11001) are assigned to report debridement of eczematous or infected skin. The dead tissue may have to be cut away with a scalpel or scissors or washed with saline solution. Code 11000 is used to report debridement of 10% of the body surface or less, and add-on code 11001 is used to report each additional 10%. Codes 11004-11006 are used to report debridement of the skin, subcutaneous tissue, muscle, and fascia for necrotizing soft-tissue infection, which is a very serious condition. These codes are divided by location. Codes 11010-11012 are used to report debridement associated with open fracture and are divided by the extent (depth) of debridement. Codes 11042-11047 are used to report debridement not associated with fracture or infected/eczematous or necrotizing tissue. These codes are divided by the extent (depth) of debridement involved and the square centimeters debrided.

CASE 5-1   *Operative Report, Excision Fat Necrosis*

This patient is in a 90-day postoperative global period. Assign codes for the surgeon's service.

LOCATION: Inpatient, Hospital

PATIENT: Terri Morgan

SURGEON: Gary Sanchez, MD

INDICATION FOR PROCEDURE: This patient has had extensive fat necrosis of the lower abdominal wound following a panniculectomy that I performed 24 days ago.

PREOPERATIVE DIAGNOSIS: Fat necrosis, lower abdominal wound

POSTOPERATIVE DIAGNOSIS: Fat necrosis, lower abdominal wound

SURGICAL FINDINGS: This is an area of about 10 × 6 cm (centimeter) diameter fat necrosis in the center of the wound and fat necrosis laterally in the wounds in a sulcus that was buried underneath the upper abdominal flap. The measurement of the wound from side to side was 50 cm in its total dimensions, and it was 6 cm proximally in its greatest width.

PROCEDURE PERFORMED: Excision of fat necrosis

ANESTHESIA: General endotracheal

ESTIMATED BLOOD LOSS: 25 cc

DESCRIPTION OF PROCEDURE: Under satisfactory general endotracheal anesthesia, the patient's abdomen was prepped with Betadine scrub and solution and draped in the routine sterile fashion. The dead fat was excised from the central portion of the wound, leaving the wound with about 6 mm (millimeter) width. We noted there was some dead fat in both lateral aspects of the wounds, which we excised, and there was an undermined area laterally in both aspects of the wound, which we opened up and curetted out at its base but remaining within the subcutaneous level. We also sharply removed the dead fat from these areas. Totally, 60 sq. cm. of subcutaneous tissue was debrided. We applied Silvadene cream and ABD (Adriamycin, bleomycin, dacarbazine) pads for dressing. Estimated blood loss was 25 cc. The patient tolerated the procedure well and left the area in good condition.

Pathology Report Later Indicated: Fat necrosis

SERVICE CODE(S): _____

ICD-10-CM DX CODE(S): _____

CASE 5-1— *cont'd*

Discussion

A panniculectomy, which is a major surgical procedure in which excess skin and subcutaneous tissue are removed, includes a 90-day postoperative period within the global surgical package. As a result of the previous panniculectomy, the patient developed "fat necrosis" and was returned to the OR (operating room) for excision. A postoperative complication that requires a return to the operating room is not considered "routine" postoperative care. Modifier -78 indicates a return to the operating room within the global period by the same physician who originally performed the surgical procedure. The third-party payer would decide if this debridement would be paid separately or included within the initial surgical package.

Fat necrosis (**Figure 5-1**) is a condition in which neutral fats in the cells of adipose (fatty) tissue are split and produce chalky white areas. In this surgical procedure, the physician removes the areas of necrosis by first using a scalpel or a dermatome (an instrument that slices layers of skin off) and removes the superficial necrotic areas. The epidermal layer is then excised to remove any areas of epidermal necrosis to the level of healthy tissue. This is a skin and subcutaneous tissue debridement.

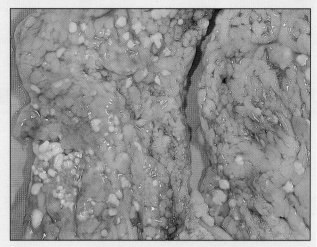

FIGURE 5-1 Fat necrosis.

(Answers to every other Case are located in Appendix D . The full answer key is only available in the TEACH Instructor Resources on Evolve.)

CASE 5-2A   *Operative Report, Debridement*

The debridement in this case is performed to a deeper level than the debridement performed in 5-1A. In 5-1A, the depth was to the subcutaneous level; but in 5-2A the operative report indicates the debridement was to the level of bone, with cultures taken from the necrotic area.

LOCATION: Inpatient, Hospital

PATIENT: Arnold Rolf

SURGEON: Gary Sanchez, MD

INDICATIONS FOR THIS PROCEDURE: This patient has had an apparent full-thickness loss of an area of previous surgery overlying the medial aspect of the left lower tibia. The patient sustained a compound tibial fracture 2 months previously, and this was immediately plated by Dr. Almaz. The patient subsequently developed a full-thickness loss in this area, and I saw him last week in an attempt to try to dry this area out and possibly salvage any tissue overlying the plate. When he was seen in the office, I felt he probably had a full-thickness loss and scheduled him for debridement. The patient was not set up at this time for soleus muscle flap, although that has been discussed as the possible definitive management, although it is slightly low for a soleus muscle flap. The only other alternative is a free flap.

PREOPERATIVE DIAGNOSIS: Full-thickness tissue loss, left lower extremity, medial aspect of lower third of leg. (This is an ulcer.)

POSTOPERATIVE DIAGNOSIS: Full-thickness tissue loss, left lower extremity, medial aspect of lower third of leg.

PROCEDURE PERFORMED: Debridement of soft tissue of left lower extremity, and culture and sensitivity of two deep soft-tissue sites and two bone sites, with the fourth bone site being from the medullary cavity.

ANESTHESIA: General endotracheal

SURGICAL FINDINGS: A 3-cm (centimeter)-diameter, full-thickness skin loss overlying a previously plated fracture.

Lying on top of the plate and overlying two of the plate holes was a liquefactive (conversion to liquid) necrotic area. In one of the holes for the plate, there was some cloudy drainage of which we obtained a culture and sensitivity. We also obtained culture and sensitivity of another deep soft-tissue site and the other hole in the tibia in conjunction with the plate. There were actually loose bone particles in this area. We debrided 20 sq. cm. of bone.

PROCEDURE: The patient's left leg was prepped with Betadine scrub and solution and draped in a routine sterile fashion. We lifted up the eschar (slough produced by a heat burn) with sharp dissection and noted there was liquefactive necrosis underneath the eschar and actually lying on top of the plate. We took some of the tissue from underneath the eschar on its deep surface and placed this for culture and sensitivity, labeling it "deep tissue with eschar, left lower extremity." Number two was also labeled "deep tissue over plate." Specimen number three was labeled "culture and sensitivity of bone and tissue." Number four was labeled "bone from medullary cavity, left tibia." After we obtained these cultures, we placed Xeroform on the wound and put a 4 × 4 over this. We wrapped it with a Kerlix roll and replaced the splint that the patient had arrived with. Estimated blood loss was zero. The patient seemed to tolerate the procedure well and left the operating room in good condition.

Pathology Report Later Indicated: Non-pressure ulcer with bone necrosis

SERVICE CODE(S): _____

ICD-10-CM DX CODE(S): _____

CASE 5-2A—cont'd

Discussion

Fracture care has a 90-day global period. This patient is within a 90-day global period with Dr. Almaz; but since the surgeon in this case is different, the -78 modifier is not needed to report Dr. Sanchez's surgery.

(Answers to every other Case are located in Appendix D . The full answer key is only available in the TEACH Instructor Resources on Evolve.)

CASE 5-2B   *Radiology Report, Leg*

Report the professional service only.

LOCATION: Inpatient, Hospital

PATIENT: Arnold Rolf

SURGEON: Gary Sanchez, MD

RADIOLOGIST: Morton Monson, MD

EXAMINATION OF: Left lower extremity ultrasound

CLINICAL SYMPTOMS: Extremity pain

LEFT LOWER EXTREMITY ULTRASOUND: HISTORY: History of fracture

FINDINGS: Ultrasound examination with compression of the deep venous system of the left lower extremity is negative for DVT (deep vein thrombosis). The left popliteal, greater saphenous, and femoral veins are patent and negative for thrombus. Unable to evaluate the calf veins.

SERVICE CODE(S): _____

ICD-10-CM DX CODE(S): _____

Discussion

This report is an excellent example of how the outpatient coder must only report the diagnostic statements made within the one report that is being coded. In this case, you know that the patient is in for debridement of an ulcer on his lower leg; however, the radiology report indicates the diagnosis under the Clinical Symptoms section of the report is "extremity pain." It is this pain in the leg that is reported as the reason for the radiology service by way of the diagnosis code.

(Answers to every other Case are located in Appendix D . The full answer key is only available in the TEACH Instructor Resources on Evolve.)

Skin Biopsy and Skin Tags

A skin biopsy is a procedure where a sample of skin or lesion is removed and reported with codes from 11102-11107. There are several different biopsy techniques, such as tangential (shave), punch, and incisional. A single biopsy is reported with a code, and each additional biopsy is reported with an add-on code. For example, if a patient comes in with 3 lesions and punch biopsies were performed, codes reported would be 11104 and 11105 x 2. If simple closure was required, it would be included in the codes. When different biopsy techniques are performed on the lesions, report the code for the first lesion and the add-on code(s) for each additional lesion [i.e., punch (11105), shave (11103), incisional (11107)].

Skin tags are **benign lesions** (**Figure 5-2**) that can appear anywhere but most often appear on the neck or trunk, especially in older people. Skin tags are removed by a variety of methods, such as scissors, blades, ligatures, electrosurgery, or chemicals, as illustrated in **Figure 5-3.** Whatever method of removal is used, simple closure is included in the skin tag codes, as is any local anesthesia used. Codes 11200 and 11201 are used to report skin tag removal and are based on the first 15 lesions and then on each additional 10 lesions or part thereof after the first 15.

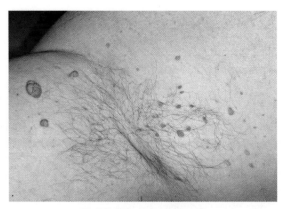

FIGURE 5–2 Skin tags.

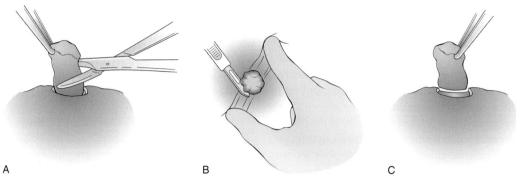

FIGURE 5−3 **A,** Scissors removal. **B,** Shaving of a lesion with a scalpel. **C,** Removal with tweezers.

From the Trenches

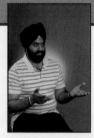

"Hard work always pays off and keeping yourself in the game is the key to success."

KHUSHWINDER SINGH
MHA, CPC, CPMA, CRC, CPCO

CASE 5-3A   *Operative Report, Skin Biopsy*

LOCATION: Outpatient, Hospital

PATIENT: Stephanie Dvorak

SURGEON: Gary Sanchez, MD

PREOPERATIVE DIAGNOSIS: Nevus of the chest

POSTOPERATIVE DIAGNOSIS: Nevus of the chest

PROCEDURE PERFORMED: Punch biopsy

ANESTHESIA: 1% Lidocaine with 1:100,000 epinephrine

PROCEDURE: The risks and benefits of the procedure were discussed, and the patient consented to the procedure. Using for local anesthesia,

a 6-mm punch biopsy was obtained for the left upper chest. Biopsy submitted to pathology. Biopsy site was closed with a top layer of 4.0 nylon. The skin sutures need to be removed in 10 to 14 days. Dressing was applied and wound care instructions were explained.

Pathology Report Later Indicated: Compound nevus

SERVICE CODE(S): _____

ICD-10-CM DX CODE(S): _____

CASE 5-3B   *Operative Report, Skin Tags*

LOCATION: Outpatient, Hospital

PATIENT: DiAnn Hopke

SURGEON: Gary Sanchez, MD

PREOPERATIVE DIAGNOSIS: Fibroepithelial skin tags of the neck

POSTOPERATIVE DIAGNOSIS: Fibroepithelial skin tags of the neck

PROCEDURE PERFORMED: Excision of multiple (10) skin tags of neck

ANESTHESIA: General endotracheal, supplementing with 1% Xylocaine with 1:100,000 epinephrine, approximately 5 cc

SURGICAL FINDINGS: Fibroepithelial skin tags of the neck.

PROCEDURE: The neck was prepped with Betadine scrub and solution and draped in a routine sterile fashion. Skin tags were removed by electrocautery. The bases of the skin tag were cauterized where appropriate. Antibiotic ointment and Band-Aids were applied. The multiple skin tags were submitted for permanent sections (biopsy section that takes several days to prepare, as compared to frozen section, which is immediately examined). The patient tolerated the procedure well and left the area in good condition.

Pathology Report Later Indicated: Benign skin tags (10)

SERVICE CODE(S): _____

ICD-10-CM DX CODE(S): _____

Discussion

The diagnosis is stated in the Postoperative Diagnosis section of the report as skin tags, and the ICD-10-CM Index directs the coder to L91.8 under the entry "Tag, skin." The code description for L91.8 does not include the term "skin tag." This is an excellent example of how the coder must trust the Index of the ICD-10-CM to include terms that may not be in the Tabular.

Lesion Excision

Codes 11400-11646 are used to report the **excision** of malignant and benign lesions based on the **site, number,** and **size** and whether the lesion is **malignant** or **benign.** To calculate the size of the lesion, both the lesion (at the greatest dimension) and the margin (at its narrowest dimension) must be known. The margin is the healthy skin that is taken from around the lesion to ensure that the entire lesion is removed. See the illustration in **Figure 5-4.** Take the measurements from the operative report because the lesion may shrink when placed in the fluids in which it is preserved until it is examined by the pathologist. The pathology report should be used to identify the size of the lesion only if no other record of the size can be documented. Based on the above information, let's determine the excised diameter of a lesion. For example, a benign lesion of the arm that measures 1.0 cm at the widest point and is removed with a 0.5-cm margin at the narrowest point is reported as a 2.0-cm lesion (11402).

The operative report must not be coded until the pathology report on the specimen has been prepared. The pathologist is a physician, and the diagnosis stated on the report prepared by the pathologist should be reported. For example, a surgeon removes a skin lesion and the operative report indicates a postoperative diagnosis of "skin lesion," but the pathology report indicates "malignant melanoma." The coder would report the diagnosis as malignant melanoma because it is the most definitive diagnosis. If the specimen indicated "skin lesion" and the pathology report indicated "neoplasm of uncertain behavior," the neoplasm of uncertain behavior would be reported.

Do not code directly from the Neoplasm Table in the Index. Always locate the neoplasm morphology within the Index for instructions on how to use the Neoplasm Table, and then reference the Tabular.

The malignant lesion codes (11600-11646) are the same whether the lesion is malignant melanoma or basal cell carcinoma.

Read the notes that precede codes 11400 and 11600 before coding the reports that follow.

Keratosis

Keratosis is a callus or horny growth. For the purposes of reporting the CPT code, an excision of a keratosis is excision of a benign lesion.

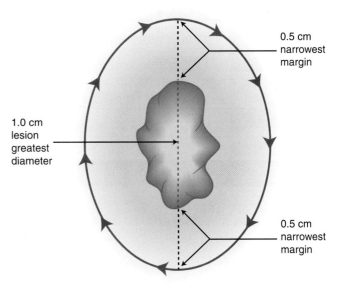

FIGURE 5-4 Calculating the size of a lesion.

CASE 5-4A   *Operative Report, Lesions*

LOCATION: Outpatient, Hospital

PATIENT: Tom Boll

SURGEON: Gary Sanchez, MD

PREOPERATIVE DIAGNOSIS: Lesions, left lower extremity

POSTOPERATIVE DIAGNOSIS: Undetermined lesion, left lower extremity, most likely benign with clear margins.

SURGICAL FINDINGS: There was a 2-cm (centimeter) diameter, raised erythematous lesion with a central pore of keratin. (This is keratosis.) Frozen section showed clear margins. Although it essentially looked benign, there is some question of well-differentiated squamous cell carcinoma, and this is reserved as a possible diagnosis.

SURGICAL PROCEDURE: Excision of lesion, left lower extremity

ANESTHESIA: Spinal

DESCRIPTION OF PROCEDURE: Under satisfactory spinal anesthesia, the patient's left leg was prepped with Betadine scrub and solution and draped in a routine sterile fashion. The lesion was excised with a 1-cm margin laterally and with a 2-cm margin proximally and distally tagging the superomedial aspect with a silk suture. Dissection was carried down to the deep layer of fascia, and bleeding was electrocoagulated. One 2-0 Monocryl suture was used subcuticularly to take tension off the wound, and then the skin was closed with interrupted vertical mattress sutures of 3-0 Prolene. We submitted the specimen for frozen section, and the frozen-section diagnosis was probably benign with the possibility of well-differentiated squamous cell carcinoma. The pathology report leaned in favor of this being a benign lesion; however, we went well around the lesion. I returned to the operating room, rescrubbed, and regloved and placed a Xeroform dressing, Kerlix fluffs over the wound, and Kerlix fluffs around the malleoli on the heels, wrapping the foot and leg from the foot to the knee with a Kerlix roll times two, Kling times two, and two Sof-Rol. The patient tolerated the procedure well and left the operating room in good condition.

Pathology Report Later Indicated: See report 5-4B.

SERVICE CODE(S): _____

ICD-10-CM DX CODE(S): _____

CASE 5-4A—cont'd

Discussion

Note that in this case the pathologist had been in the operating room and had taken a frozen section. The frozen section was examined by the pathologist immediately to determine if there was cancer in the specimen. The pathologist made the determination that the specimen was benign, and as such the surgeon returned to the operating room to close the wound. Although the frozen section is not as accurate as a permanent section, it provides a preliminary pathological diagnosis. The pathologist would also conduct a permanent section on the specimen, and the final pathological diagnosis would be made.

CASE 5-4B   *Pathology Report*

Assign codes for the pathologist only. Note that within this report the pathologist went to the operating room and provided an immediate consultation (frozen section). The heading "Intraoperative Frozen Section Diagnosis" is the indication for this service. Locate directions to this code in the index of the CPT under "Pathology, Surgical, Consultation, Intraoperative." The frozen section is reported in addition to the pathological examination permanent section of the specimen.

LOCATION: Outpatient, Hospital

PATIENT: Tom Boll

SURGEON: Gary Sanchez, MD

PATHOLOGIST: Grey Lonewolf, MD

CLINICAL HISTORY: A 2-cm (centimeter) lesion, left leg

SPECIMEN RECEIVED: Lesion, left leg with FS (frozen section)

GROSS DESCRIPTION:

The specimen is labeled with the patient's name and "lesion left leg," which consists of a 4 3 2 3 0.8-cm skin ellipse with a central nodular area, 1.5 cm in diameter with scale crust. A suture identifies the superior medial ellipse, which is identified with black ink. The inferior/lateral ellipse is identified with green ink, the superior margin with red ink, and the inferior margin with blue ink. Representative sections are frozen and processed in cassettes.

INTRAOPERATIVE FROZEN SECTION DIAGNOSES per Dr. Lonewolf. Lesion left leg, excision: Margins benign, defer to permanent sections.

Sections of skin show mild hyperkeratosis with pseudoepitheliomatous hyperplasia with central scale crust and underlying epidermal cysts. There are mild chronic inflammatory infiltrates. Margins are benign.

DIAGNOSIS: Skin lesion, left leg, excision: Skin showing mild hyperkeratosis with central scale crust, pseudoepitheliomatous hyperplasia, epidermal cysts, and mild chronic inflammation; margins are benign.

SERVICE CODE(S): _____

ICD-10-CM DX CODE(S): _____

Discussion

Note that even though the Diagnosis section of the report started off with "skin lesion," the diagnosis was hyperkeratosis later in the section, which is the highest level of specificity of the lesion and must be coded as such.

CASE 5-5   *Operative Report, Lesions*

This service is being provided to remove two chest lesions in a patient with a personal history of a malignant breast neoplasm. In addition to the code to report the current chest lesions, the history is reported with a Z code. Locate directions to the Z code by referencing "History, personal" in the Index, subtermed by type of history. Report only Dr. Sanchez's service and the surgery codes for the facility. Do not assign codes for the pathologist's service.

LOCATION: Outpatient, Hospital

PATIENT: Bernice Pries

SURGEON: Gary Sanchez, MD

PREOPERATIVE DIAGNOSIS: Lesions, chest, times two

POSTOPERATIVE DIAGNOSIS: Lesions, chest, times two

PROCEDURE PERFORMED: Removal of two lesions, chest, in previous total mastectomy site

HISTORY: This patient had a segmental mastectomy due to malignancy and then subsequently had radiotherapy in the past. She developed a recurrent breast cancer, and I did a total mastectomy. She now has two areas that are very hard; these are likely fat necrosis, but we are not sure. It is elected to remove them.

When I first saw her in the office, it was the most medial aspect of her incision that was hard, but I felt a new area right along the incision and a little more lateral toward the axilla, and she wanted that removed too. I marked both these areas in the same-day holding room with the patient's husband and the nurse present.

PROCEDURE: The patient was given an anesthetic. She was prepped and draped in a supine fashion. We started with the medial lesion. We

Continued

CASE 5-5—cont'd

made an incision and then developed superior flaps and inferior flaps. We removed this lesion going right down to the muscle, but did not include the muscle. The first lesion measured approximately 1.7 cm (centimeter), and the second lesion measured 2.0 cm. We obtained excellent hemostasis. I did the same with the smaller lesion that was on the lateral aspect. These both appeared to be fat necrosis. We did frozen sections, and they both appeared to be benign lesions. We obtained excellent hemostasis and brought the subcutaneous tissues together with Vicryl. We closed the skin with subcuticular Vicryl also. We could not apply Steri-Strips because of her allergy to tape. That is why we used subcuticular Vicryl instead of my usual subcuticular Prolene with Steri-Strips. The patient tolerated this well and went to the recovery room in good condition.

Pathology Report Later Indicated: Benign lesions

SERVICE CODE(S): _____

ICD-10-CM DX CODE(S): _____

(Answers to every other Case are located in Appendix D . The full answer key is only available in the TEACH Instructor Resources on Evolve.)

CASE 5-6 *Operative Report, Lipoma*

LOCATION: Outpatient, Hospital

PATIENT: Florence DeFrang

SURGEON: Gary Sanchez, MD

PREOPERATIVE DIAGNOSIS: Lesion, left lower neck anterior

POSTOPERATIVE DIAGNOSIS: Lesion, left lower neck anterior

PROCEDURE PERFORMED: Removal of lipoma

HISTORY: This patient has a small lipoma of her anterior lower neck. I tried removing it with EMLA cream (local anesthetic cream) in the ambulatory patient care center, but she completely lost it and it was impossible to do; so I elected to bring her to the operating room and do this with IV (intravenous) sedation.

DESCRIPTION OF PROCEDURE: The patient was prepped and draped in the supine position. We made a skin incision along Langer's lines. We removed the lesion in toto (means in total), and the lesion measured 0.8 cm (centimeter), including margins. We obtained excellent hemostasis with cautery and then brought the subcutaneous tissue together with 3-0 Vicryl, and the skin was closed with a 5-0 Vicryl in a subcuticular fashion. Steri-Strips, gauze, and tape were applied. The patient tolerated the procedure well and went to the recovery room in excellent condition.

Pathology Report Later Indicated: Benign lipoma

SERVICE CODE(S): _____

ICD-10-CM DX CODE(S): _____

(Answers to every other Case are located in Appendix D . The full answer key is only available in the TEACH Instructor Resources on Evolve.)

CASE 5-7 *Operative Report, Nevus*

LOCATION: Outpatient, Hospital

PATIENT: Beverly Weik

SURGEON: Gary Sanchez, MD

INDICATIONS FOR PROCEDURE: This patient has a giant congenital nevus of the anterior aspect of the midline of the neck, which has a 4% to 20% chance of development of malignant melanoma at some time in the patient's life.

PREOPERATIVE DIAGNOSIS: Giant congenital nevus (compound nevus), neck

POSTOPERATIVE DIAGNOSIS: Giant congenital nevus (compound nevus), neck

PROCEDURE PERFORMED: Excision of giant congenital nevus of the neck

SURGICAL FINDINGS: A 4 × 1.5-cm (centimeter) diameter irregular, oval-shaped giant congenital nevus of the neck

ANESTHESIA: General endotracheal with 3 cc (cubic centimeter) of 1% Xylocaine with 1:100,000 epinephrine

COMPLICATIONS: None

DRAINS: None

SPONGE AND NEEDLE COUNTS: Correct

PROCEDURE: The patient's neck was prepped with Betadine scrub and solution and draped in the routine sterile fashion. Anesthesia was administered in the concentration and amount mentioned above. The lesion was then excised elliptically with a margin of a few millimeters around it. Bleeding was electrocoagulated. The wound was closed with subcuticular 4-0 Monocryl, and $1/2$-inch Steri-Strips were applied. A soft cervical collar was not available, and we will attempt to use a firm cervical collar for the immobilization of the neck. Otherwise, the patient tolerated the procedure well and left the operating room in good condition.

Pathology Report Later Indicated: Benign giant nevus. (This is a benign skin lesion.)

SERVICE CODE(S): _____

ICD-10-CM DX CODE(S): _____

(Answers to every other Case are located in Appendix D . The full answer key is only available in the TEACH Instructor Resources on Evolve.)

CASE 5-8 *Operative Report, Epithelioma*

LOCATION: Outpatient, Hospital

PATIENT: Larry Harris

SURGEON: Gary Sanchez, MD

PREOPERATIVE DIAGNOSIS: Inclusion cyst, left eyebrow

POSTOPERATIVE DIAGNOSIS: Calcifying epithelioma (benign skin lesion) of Malherbe, left eyebrow, middle aspect

SURGICAL FINDINGS: A 0.7-cm (centimeter)-diameter ruptured calcifying epithelioma of Malherbe

SURGICAL PROCEDURE: Excision of calcifying epithelioma of Malherbe

ANESTHESIA: General endotracheal anesthesia plus 1 cc of 1% Xylocaine with 1:100,000 epinephrine

ESTIMATED BLOOD LOSS: Negligible

DESCRIPTION OF PROCEDURE: The patient's left eyebrow was prepped with Betadine scrub and solution and draped in a routine sterile fashion. We injected 1 cc of 1% Xylocaine with 1:100,000 epinephrine around it and waited about 5 minutes. We made an incision in the axis of the eyebrow and entered the capsule of the epithelioma. We were then able to dissect the capsule out completely along with the contents of the sac. There were no contents of the sac or sac left within the wound. We closed the wound with two plain sutures of 5-0 Prolene and a horizontal mattress suture of 5-0 Prolene. Surgical and an ophthalmic antibiotic ointment were applied. The patient tolerated the procedure well and left the operating room in good condition.

Pathology Report Later Indicated: Benign lesion

SERVICE CODE(S): _____

ICD-10-CM DX CODE(S): _____

(Answers to every other Case are located in Appendix D . The full answer key is only available in the TEACH Instructor Resources on Evolve.)

CASE 5-9 *Operative Report, Keratosis Excision*

LOCATION: Outpatient, Hospital

PATIENT: Glen Croaker

SURGEON: Gary Sanchez, MD

PREOPERATIVE DIAGNOSIS: Bowen's disease, right cheek

POSTOPERATIVE DIAGNOSIS: Actinic keratosis, right cheek, by frozen section

PROCEDURE PERFORMED: Excision of keratosis, right cheek (1.5-cm [centimeter] diameter)

ANESTHESIA: Ten cc of 1% Xylocaine with 1:800,000 epinephrine with MAC anesthesia

ESTIMATED BLOOD LOSS: Negligible

COMPLICATIONS: None

SURGICAL FINDINGS: A 1.5-cm-diameter raised pink lesion with keratosis on surface, morphologically resembling Bowen's disease

DESCRIPTION OF PROCEDURE: The patient's face was prepped with Betadine scrub and solution and draped in a routine sterile fashion. A margin of about 0.5 cm was taken around the specimen, and we submitted this for frozen section, tagging the inferior aspect with a silk suture. It was the pathologist's opinion this was bowenoid keratosis, and the pathologist felt that we were sufficiently around this to forego any further surgery. The lesion had been closed with interrupted subcuticular 4-0 Vicryl and interrupted 5-0 Prolene. Xeroform and a 4 × 4 were applied for dressing. The patient tolerated the procedure well and left the area in good condition.

Pathology Report Later Indicated: Actinic keratosis, benign. (This is a benign skin lesion.)

SERVICE CODE(S): _____

ICD-10-CM DX CODE(S): _____

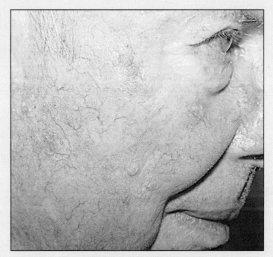

FIGURE 5–5 Actinic keratosis.

(Answers to every other Case are located in Appendix D . The full answer key is only available in the TEACH Instructor Resources on Evolve.)

CASE 5-10   *Operative Report, Wide Excision, Melanoma*

This patient had a lesion that was excised 9 days ago by Dr. Sanchez. After the original excision the lesion was determined to be malignant and the pathology exam revealed that the margins were involved. The lesion needs to be re-excised to assure complete removal. For more information on re-excision, go to the CPT manual and read the instructions preceding code 11600. Assign codes for both the physician and facility.

LOCATION: Outpatient, Hospital

PATIENT: Roger Ulland

SURGEON: Gary Sanchez, MD

PREOPERATIVE DIAGNOSIS: Malignant melanoma, left shoulder (2 cm [centimeter])

POSTOPERATIVE DIAGNOSIS: Malignant melanoma, left shoulder (2 cm)

PROCEDURE PERFORMED: Wide excision of malignant melanoma, posterior aspect of left shoulder

ANESTHESIA: General endotracheal with supplementary 1% Xylocaine with 1:100,000 epinephrine, approximately 10 cc

ESTIMATED BLOOD LOSS: Negligible

PROCEDURE: The shoulder was prepped with Betadine scrub and solution and draped in the routine sterile fashion. A margin of about 3 cm laterally and medially around the healed incision site was taken, tapering to a 4 to 5 cm proximally and distally. The incision was carried down to the base of the dermis. Bleeding was electrocoagulated, and the wound was closed in layers with subcuticular 2-0 Monocryl and some twists and pulley sutures of 2-0 Monocryl in the center of the wound, where the most tension was. Kerlix fluffs and a sling were applied followed by an external Ace bandage. The patient tolerated the procedure well and left the area in good condition.

Pathology Report Later Indicated: Malignant melanoma. (This is a primary, malignant neoplasm of the skin.)

SERVICE CODE(S): _____

ICD-10-CM DX CODE(S): _____

(Answers to every other Case are located in Appendix D . The full answer key is only available in the TEACH Instructor Resources on Evolve.)

CASE 5-11   *Operative Report, Squamous Cell Carcinoma*

LOCATION: Outpatient, Hospital

PATIENT: Kyle Pearce

SURGEON: Gary Sanchez, MD

PREOPERATIVE DIAGNOSIS: Nonhealing ulcer with eschar of the left temple

POSTOPERATIVE DIAGNOSIS: Squamous cell carcinoma of the left temple

SURGICAL FINDINGS: A 2-cm (centimeter)-diameter nonhealing ulcer of the left temporal region with an eschar overlying it

SURGICAL PROCEDURE: Excision of squamous cell carcinoma of the left temple

ANESTHESIA: Standby with 6.5 cc (cubic centimeter) of 1% Xylocaine with 1:800,000 epinephrine

ESTIMATED BLOOD LOSS: Negligible

COMPLICATIONS: None

SPONGE AND NEEDLE COUNTS: Correct

DESCRIPTION OF PROCEDURE: The patient's face was prepped with Betadine scrub and solution and draped in a routine sterile fashion. A margin of 1 cm on each side of the lesion laterally and medially was outlined with 1-cm margins proximally and distally. We incised this elliptically down to the orbicularis oculi and the frontalis muscle. Bleeding was electrocoagulated. We tagged the medial end with a silk suture. This was submitted for frozen section, and there did not appear to be any residual squamous cell located within the lesion; the lesion was also widely clear on frozen section. We returned to the operating room, and after some undermining, we closed the wound with interrupted vertical mattress sutures of 3-0 Prolene. Xeroform and 4 × 4 dressing were applied. The patient tolerated the procedure well and left the operating room in good condition.

Pathology Report Later Indicated: Primary squamous cell carcinoma. (This is a primary, malignant neoplasm of the skin of temple.)

SERVICE CODE(S): _____

ICD-10-CM DX CODE(S): _____

(Answers to every other Case are located in Appendix D . The full answer key is only available in the TEACH Instructor Resources on Evolve.)

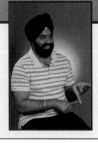

From the Trenches

"Proper coding and clinic documentation can be rewarding because it improves the quality of life for our patients."

KHUSHWINDER SINGH
MHA, CPC, CPMA, CRC, CPCO

CASE 5-12   *Operative Report, Wide Excision, Malignant Melanoma*

In this report there is a wide excision due to the location and extent of the lesion. In order to affect repair afterwards, the surgeon "undermined the skin after the manner of a subcutaneous facelift and brought the skin up . . . " However, note that the closure was only of the skin, there was no layered closure. If there had been a layered closure indicated in the report, an intermediate repair would also have been reported, but since there is only skin closure, there is no additional repair reported.

LOCATION: Outpatient, Hospital

PATIENT: Terry Uebe

SURGEON: Gary Sanchez, MD

PREOPERATIVE DIAGNOSIS: Malignant melanoma, left preauricular area. See clinic chart for depth of melanoma.

POSTOPERATIVE DIAGNOSIS: Malignant melanoma with clear margins on preauricular area

PROCEDURE PERFORMED: Wide excision of malignant melanoma, left preauricular area

ANESTHESIA: General endotracheal with supplementary 1% Xylocaine with 1:800,000 epinephrine

ESTIMATED BLOOD LOSS: Approximately 25 cc (cubic centimeter)

PROCEDURE: The patient's left face and ear were prepped with Betadine scrub and solution and draped in a routine sterile fashion. The 0.8-cm (centimeter) lesion was excised to include the crus of the left ear in the dissection because this was the only method to provide at least 2 cm of width around the excision site. We were able to get about 2.5 cm on the anterior excision site and at least 3 cm proximally and distally. We submitted the specimen, tagged the superior aspect with a silk suture, cauterized the bleeding, and then using separate instrument and gloves, we undermined the skin after the manner of a subcutaneous facelift and brought the skin up, suturing it to the more posterior edge with interrupted 3-0 Prolene. We dressed the wound with Xeroform, Kerlix fluffs, and a Kerlix roll plus Kling. The patient tolerated the procedure well and left the operating table in good condition.

Pathology Report Later Indicated: Malignant melanoma of ear

SERVICE CODE(S): _____

ICD-10-CM DX CODE(S): _____

(Answers to every other Case are located in Appendix D . The full answer key is only available in the TEACH Instructor Resources on Evolve.)

Nails

The Nails codes (11719-11765) are reported for the trimming of fingernails and toenails, debridement of nails, removal of nails, drainage of hematomas, biopsies of nails, repair of nails, reconstruction of nails, and excision of cysts of the nails. Code 11719 is used to report trimming of nails that are not defective. This is a minimal service, and the code covers trimming one fingernail/toenail or many fingernails/toenails. Code 11720 is a more complex service that reports the debridement of nail(s) by any method, up to five nails and includes the use of tools to accomplish the service, cleaning materials/solutions, and files. Supplies used for nail services are included in the codes and not reported separately.

Codes 11730-11732 report avulsion of the nail plate, which is removal of the nail plate, leaving the root so the nail will grow back. After injection with local anesthetic, the nail is lifted away from the nail bed and all or a portion of the nail is removed.

The nail treatment codes do not require the use of modifier -51 because the codes indicate the number of nails included in the code. Units are used to report the service of multiple nails. For example, when reporting the removal of 3 nails, 11730 is used to report the first nail, and 11732 × 2 reports the second and third nails. Modifiers may be added, depending on the payer. Some payers will require the use of -RT and -LT to indicate right or left, and others, such as Medicare, will require the use of the HCPCS modifiers F1-F9 and FA to report the fingers; T1-T9 and TA are used to report the toenails as illustrated in **Figures 5-6** and **5-7.**

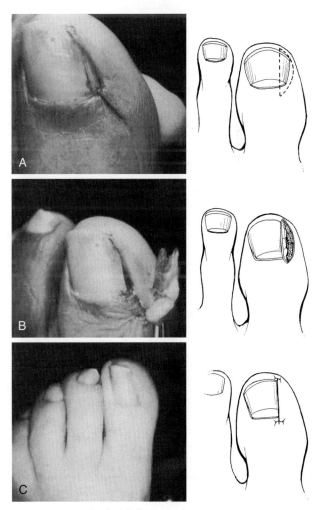

FIGURE 5-6 Onychectomy.

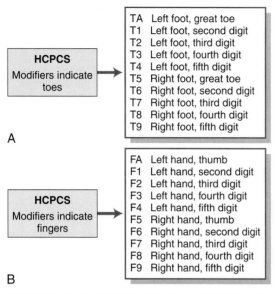

A common condition that is treated by physicians and reported with the Nail subheading code is onychocryptosis (ingrown toenail). This is a painful condition in which the nail grows down and into the soft tissue of the nail fold and often leads to infection. Treatment for severe cases is a partial permanent **onychectomy** (removal of the nail plate and root). The toe is anesthetized, and a portion of the nail plate is removed (11750). The nail will not grow back where the base has been removed. The local anesthetic and supplies necessary to remove the nail are included in the nail codes and are not reported separately.

FIGURE 5−7 A, HCPCS modifiers for toes. **B,** HCPCS modifiers for fingers.

CASE 5-13   *Clinic Progress Note*

Violet Berg presents to Dr. Warner's office with a chronic ingrown toenail. Use HCPCS modifiers when reporting the service. Report the physician's service only.

LOCATION: Outpatient, Clinic

PATIENT: Violet Berg

FAMILY PHYSICIAN: Leslie Alanda, MD

PODIATRIST: Samuel Warner, MD

This 14-year-old girl presents with her mom with a chronic ingrown lateral border, right great toenail. She has had the nail removed times two by Dr. Alanda, and it continues to come back. I would recommend that we do a more permanent-type procedure. She is not allergic to anything. She does get exercise-induced asthma. She is on Claritin and cold medications as needed. She has been dealing with this on and off for the last 3 years. She has actually had trouble with both great toenails. The only one sore today, though, is the right lateral border. She is quite nervous and anxious.

OBJECTIVE EVALUATION: Vascular status: Pulses are palpable, dorsalis pedis and posterior tibial. There is no ankle edema, swelling, or erythema. Feet are warm to touch. Dermatologic: She has paronychia, the lateral border of the right great toenail. Dr. Alanda mentioned in a note that it was the left great toenail, but the mother states that it was this toe times two. It is locally cellulitic. No signs of ascending cellulitis, paronychia, or pus formation. It is inflamed.

ASSESSMENT: Chronic ingrown lateral border, right great toenail with cellulitis (onychocryptosis)

PLAN:

1. I would recommend that we locally anesthetize the right great toe, prep and drape, and remove the lateral border in an attempt

at permanent treatment to prevent regrowth. Consent was obtained.

2. We did locally anesthetize the right great toe. She was quite nervous during this but did tolerate it very well. We did prep and drape the right great toe in the standard sterile fashion. I did give her an additional 2 cc (cubic centimeter) of 1% lidocaine and 0.5% Marcaine plain. Tourniquet was applied to the base of the right great toe. The lateral border of the right great toenail was avulsed. All nail spiculization and necrotic debris were removed as encountered. Phenol was applied to the nail bed and matrix tissues for the appropriate length of time and curetted aggressively between applications. Tourniquet was removed, and normal vascular status returned to the right great toe. Alcohol was used to wash the toe. Bacitracin ointment and a dry sterile dressing were applied. The patient tolerated the procedure and anesthesia well.

The patient was given written and verbal instructions on wound care regarding t.i.d. (three times a day). Epsom salt soaks for 5 to 10 minutes, two drops of Cortisporin otic solution, and cover with a dry sterile dressing or Band-Aid. I would recommend that she avoid tight-fitting shoes, take Tylenol as needed for pain, and we will see her back in 7 to 10 days for a postoperative check or sooner if any problems arise.

SERVICE CODE(S): _____

ICD-10-CM DX CODE(S): _____

(Answers to every other Case are located in Appendix D . The full answer key is only available in the TEACH Instructor Resources on Evolve.)

Repair (Closure)

There are three types of wounds and three levels of repair or closure: simple, intermediate, and complex. A simple wound involves the **epidermis, dermis,** and/or **subcutaneous** tissue. A simple repair (one-layer) (12001-12021) is required to close a simple wound. Understanding what the definition of a simple repair is will provide useful knowledge because often you will have to report a closure that is more than a simple closure. A simple repair (closure) is bundled into excision codes, and if the wound required a closure that was more than a one-layer repair (simple), the closure may be reported separately. For example, if an excision of a lesion that would usually require a simple closure required an intermediate closure, you would report the excision and the closure separately. An intermediate wound involves one or more layers of the subcutaneous tissue and superficial fascia. Fascia is the sheet of tissue that covers other tissue, such as the muscles. An **intermediate repair** (12031-12057) requires more than a single-layer closure in which the physician repairs deeper layers of tissue with dissolving stitches and then closes the epidermis, often with different type (number) of suture. If the documentation in the medical record indicates that a simple wound is extensively debrided (cleaned), an intermediate repair is reported. A **complex repair** (13100-13160), such as revision, debridement, extensive undermining, stents, or retention sutures, requires complicated wound closure and more than layered closure.

After reading the medical documentation and making a decision about the **complexity** of the repair as simple, intermediate, or complex, the next step is to code correctly the repair and closure based on the location of the wound. The codes in the CPT manual are grouped together by complexity, which you already have learned about, and then by **location.** For example, 12001 reports superficial wounds of the scalp, neck, axillae, external genitalia, trunk, and/or extremities (including the hands and feet), and 12011 reports superficial repair of wounds of the face, ears, eyelids, nose, lips, and/or mucous membranes.

The codes are then further divided based on the **length** of the repair. The CPT measurements are in the metric system, so at first it is difficult to imagine the length of these measurements. An inch equals 2.54 cm. Physicians usually report the measurements using the metric system, but if they do not, you must convert the measurements to metric in order to select the correct code. If the physician stated that the wound was 5 inches long, you would multiply 5 inches by 2.54 as a means of converting the measurement to 12.7 cm.

Repairs of the same complexity and location are added together and reported with one code. For example, two superficial (complexity) wounds are repaired. One 2.1-cm (length) wound is located on the arm (location), and another is 2.3 cm (length) and is on the neck (location). The wounds are of the same complexity and grouped in the same locations as referred to in code description 12001

(neck and extremities). Add the two wounds together (4.4 cm) and report with 12002, which is assigned to repairs of scalp, neck, axillae, external genitalia, trunk and/or extremities totaling 2.6 to 7.5 cm. If the wounds are of different complexities or location, you cannot add the lengths together but must instead report them separately. When reporting multiple wounds, place the most complex repair first and follow with the subsequent repair codes with modifier -59 added.

If the wound is grossly contaminated and requires extensive debridement, a separate debridement procedure may be coded (11000-11047 for extensive debridement). A debridement code can also be reported when the skin is broken and contaminated with an open fracture repair.

Do not report the following wound repair services separately:

- Simple **ligation** (tying) of vessels is considered part of the wound repair and is not listed separately.
- Simple **exploration** of surrounding tissue, nerves, vessels, and tendons is considered part of the wound repair process and is not listed separately.
- Normal **debridement** (cleaning and removing skin or tissue from the wound until normal, healthy tissue is exposed) is not listed separately.

There are substances, much like super-strength household glue, that are used to glue the edges of wounds together. Dermabond is one of these special skin glues that the physician places in the wound, pulls the edges together, and then places a bandage over the area. HCPCS code G0168 is used to report skin closure for Medicare patients, and other third-party payers use the simple repair codes to report these skin closures using adhesives based on the location and length of the repair.

Read the notes preceding the Repair (Closure) codes to ensure that you understand wound repair before coding the cases that follow.

External causes are reported with codes in the V01-Y99 range and the External Cause Index is referenced to locate these codes.

External Cause codes are never used as a principal diagnosis. Rather, External Cause codes are used to clarify the cause of an injury or adverse effect. External Cause code terms describe the external circumstances under which an accident, injury, or act of violence occurred. The main terms in this section usually represent the type of accident or violence (e.g., assault, collision), with the specific agent or other circumstance listed below the main term. You must be sure to read all the information under a term in the External Cause code index, then locate the code in the External code section of Volume 1, Tabular.

In the outpatient setting, especially the emergency department, it is up to each facility to determine if external cause codes are to be reported, as recording external cause codes is not yet mandatory.

CASE 5-14 *Operative Report, Laceration*

While returning from a concert, Virgil Rhone fell asleep (there is an external cause code for this) at the wheel and lost control of his automobile. His car slid into a ditch and struck a tree. He sustained lacerations on both ears. Assign an External Cause code to indicate how the accident happened.

LOCATION: Outpatient, Hospital Emergency Department

PATIENT: Virgil Rhone

SURGEON: Paul Sutton, MD

PREOPERATIVE DIAGNOSIS: Right and left ear lacerations

POSTOPERATIVE DIAGNOSIS: Right and left ear lacerations

PROCEDURE PERFORMED: Cleaning and suturing of right and left ear lacerations

ANESTHESIA: 1% Xylocaine

INDICATIONS FOR PROCEDURE: The patient is a 45-year-old white male who was involved in a motor vehicle accident. The patient sustained bilateral ear lacerations, and he is now undergoing repair.

PROCEDURE: The patient was prepped and draped in the usual manner. Xylocaine was used as local anesthesia. The right ear was cleaned, and a 5.2-cm (centimeter) laceration was sutured with interrupted 5-0 nylon sutures. Next the left ear was cleaned, and a 4.8-cm laceration was sutured with interrupted 5-0 nylon sutures. The patient tolerated the procedure well.

SERVICE CODE(S): _____

ICD-10-CM DX CODE(S): _____

(Answers to every other Case are located in Appendix D . The full answer key is only available in the TEACH Instructor Resources on Evolve.)

CASE 5-15 *Operative Report, Laceration*

Don Ehlers was a passenger in Virgil Rhone's car and sustained a laceration of the lip. Report an External Cause code in addition to the diagnosis code.

LOCATION: Outpatient, Hospital, Emergency Department

PATIENT: Don Ehlers

SURGEON: Paul Sutton, MD

PREOPERATIVE DIAGNOSIS: Laceration, left lip

POSTOPERATIVE DIAGNOSIS: Laceration, left lip

PROCEDURE PERFORMED: Complex repair of laceration

OPERATIVE NOTE: The 6-cm (centimeter) area of the laceration was inspected carefully and irrigated to remove all debris (pieces of glass and other debris). The laceration extends from the outside of the mouth, not through the lip itself, but below the lip into the mouth region. By turning the lip inside out, we were able to place some chromic sutures of 3-0 on the inside. The outside was then closed using 5-0 nylon in an interrupted fashion. The patient tolerated the procedure well and was discharged from the emergency room in stable condition.

SERVICE CODE(S): _____

ICD-10-CM DX CODE(S): _____

(Answers to every other Case are located in Appendix D . The full answer key is only available in the TEACH Instructor Resources on Evolve.)

Modifier -59

Modifier -59 is used to indicate that services usually bundled into one Procedural Service payment were provided as separate services. The description of the modifier is as follows:

Under certain circumstances, the physician may need to indicate that a procedure or service was distinct or independent from other services performed on the same day. Modifier -59 is used to identify procedures/services that are not normally reported together, but are appropriate under the circumstances. This may represent a different session or patient encounter, different procedure or surgery, different site or organ system, separate incision/excision, separate lesion, or separate injury (or area of injury in extensive injuries) not ordinarily encountered or performed on the same day by the same physician. However, when another already established modifier is appropriate, it should be used rather than modifier -59. Only if no more descriptive modifier is available and the use of modifier -59 best explains the circumstances should modifier -59 be used.

As the code description notes, modifier -59 is used to identify the following:

■ Different session or patient encounter
■ Different procedure or surgery
■ Different site or organ system
■ Separate incision/excision
■ Separate lesion
■ Separate injury or area of injury in extensive injuries

Modifier -59 is reported with codes from all sections of the CPT manual except E/M and anesthesia codes. Medicare has lists of codes that cannot be reported together; they are called edits. These edits have been established to ensure that providers do not report services that are included in the bundle for a given code. For example, you would not report a standard preoperative visit related to a major surgical procedure and report separately the surgery and follow-up care. All three services—preoperative, intraoperative, and postoperative—are packaged together in one major surgical CPT code. The use of modifier -59 indicates that the service was not a part of the primary service but, indeed, was a distinct service.

Modifier -59 distinguishes a procedure performed on the same day as another procedure that normally would not be reported separately (e.g., a biopsy of one lesion on the right leg and an excision of another lesion on the same leg).

Although this resource does not follow specific payer coding guidelines, it is important to note that CMS has created four HCPCS modifiers, collectively referred to as modifiers -X{EPSU}, which identify subsets of modifier -59 (Distinct Procedural Services):

XE: Separate Encounter
XP: Separate Practitioner
XS: Separate Structure/Organ
XU: Unusual Non-overlapping service

CMS will continue to recognize modifier -59, but may selectively require the use of one of these more specific modifiers, as determined by their National Correct Coding Initiative (NCCI) edits that will identify which -X{EPSU} modifier would be payable rather than the -59 modifier.

Only modifier -59 will be included in the answers found in this text, and the CMS HCPCS modifiers will not by utilized.

CASE 5-16   *Operative Report, Excision Histiocytic Tumor*

The following case involves the excision of a lesion that requires more than a simple closure. In addition, there are multiple procedures conducted during the same operative session.
Assign the codes for the surgeon only.

LOCATION: Inpatient, Hospital

PATIENT: Erik Moti

SURGEON: Gary Sanchez, MD

PREOPERATIVE DIAGNOSIS: Residual plexiform fibrous histiocytic tumor of the left costovertebral angle area

POSTOPERATIVE DIAGNOSIS: Residual plexiform fibrous histiocytic tumor of left costovertebral angle area

PROCEDURE PERFORMED: Excision of plexiform fibrous histiocytic tumor of left costovertebral angle and evacuation of hematoma, left costovertebral angle

ANESTHESIA: General endotracheal with approximately 20 cc (cubic centimeter) of tumescent solution prepared by adding to 1 L of Ringer's lactate, 25 cc 2% Xylocaine, 1 cc of 1:100,000 epinephrine, and 3 cc of 8.4% sodium bicarbonate.

ESTIMATED BLOOD LOSS: Negligible

SURGICAL FINDINGS: There was a 50-cc hematoma beginning to organize in the area of the left costovertebral angle in the subcutaneous space on top of the latissimus dorsi muscle.

DESCRIPTION OF PROCEDURE: The patient was intubated and turned in the prone position. The area of the left costovertebral angle was prepped with Betadine scrub and solution and draped in a routine sterile fashion. An incision was made 2 cm (centimeter) and carried down to the fascia of the muscle, where a hematoma was entered and drained. The skin portion of that lesion was removed, and the fascia and a portion of the muscle of the latissimus dorsi were removed secondarily. The lesion measured 2.9 cm at the widest point. Bleeding was electrocoagulated, and a no. 7 Jackson-Pratt drain was inserted in the depth of the wound. The wound was closed with interrupted 0 Monocryl for the deep fascia layer and subcuticular 4-0 Monocryl using a few vertical mattress sutures of 3-0 Monocryl. Steri-Strips and Kerlix fluffs plus Elastoplast were applied. The patient tolerated the procedure well and left the operating room in good condition.

Pathology Report Later Indicated: Benign lesion of the soft tissue of the costovertebral angle area

SERVICE CODE(S): _____

ICD-10-CM DX CODE(S): _____

Discussion

The costovertebral angle is located in the back. It is the space on either side of the vertebral column between the last rib and the lumbar vertebrae.

(Answers to every other Case are located in Appendix D . The full answer key is only available in the TEACH Instructor Resources on Evolve.)

CASE 5-17   *Operative Report, Umbilicoplasty*

This case is of a complex repair in which the surgeon repaired an area of scarring by removal of the scarred area. The surgeon also removed a mass and then closed the area. The repair is the most resource-intensive procedure.

LOCATION: Outpatient, Hospital

PATIENT: Teresa Wiley

SURGEON: Gary Sanchez, MD

PREOPERATIVE DIAGNOSIS: Scarring and retraction of umbilicus, status post partial slough of umbilical skin

POSTOPERATIVE DIAGNOSIS: Scarring and retraction of umbilicus, status post partial slough of umbilical skin

SURGICAL FINDINGS:

1. There was a remnant of buried 1-cm (centimeter) diameter umbilical skin still attached to the umbilical stalk and some granulation tissue and scar tissue located within the depth of the umbilical wound.
2. Fat necrosis, left inguinal area.

Continued

CASE 5-17—cont'd

SURGICAL PROCEDURES:

1. Excision of fat necrosis, left inguinal region
2. Umbilicoplasty utilizing a 3-cm diameter flap that was 5 mm (millimeter) wide

ANESTHESIA: General endotracheal. Supplementary local approximately 6 cc of 1% Xylocaine with 1:100,000 epinephrine.

DESCRIPTION OF PROCEDURE: The patient's abdomen was prepped with Betadine scrub and solution and draped in a routine sterile fashion. Several cc of 1% Xylocaine with 1:100,000 epinephrine was injected into the scar laterally, overlying the mass in the inguinal area. This mass measured about 1 cm in diameter. We excised the scar over the mass and came down on the mass, which had the appearance of fat necrosis and measured 2.9 cm at the greatest width. This was excised, and all the palpably firm tissue was removed. We cauterized the bleeding and closed the subcutaneous layer with 3-0 Vicryl and the subdermal layer with interrupted 3-0 Vicryl using 4-0 Prolene for the skin. A plain 4 × 4 was applied. The umbilicus was approached by excision of the scar for about 2 cm above the previous umbilical site beginning at the 12 o'clock position and also 2 cm below the 6 o'clock position. I incised the apparent scar tissue circumferentially and came down on a mass of apparent granulation tissue and fat necrosis, which I excised, trimming this off the umbilical stalk. Attached to the umbilical stalk was a nubbin of about 1 cm of umbilicus in a semicircular shape that was 5 mm wide and 3 cm from one side of the flap to the other. This flap was then sutured with half-mattress sutures to the 12 and 6 o'clock positions also, suturing it back to the original site with a subdermal half-mattress suture of 3-0 Monocryl, following closure of the donor areas with interrupted 3-0 Prolene, and the completion of the closure of the outer ring of the bilateral flaps with interrupted 3-0 Prolene. Dressing consisted of a glycerin-soaked cotton ball and a 4 × 4. We did put some Nitro paste in the depth of the wound. The patient tolerated the procedure well and left the operating room in good condition.

Pathology Report Later Indicated: Necrotic, fatty mass; benign tissue

SERVICE CODE(S): _____

ICD-10-CM DX CODE(S): _____

Discussion

The scarring and retraction of the umbilicus required excision and revision; this is reported with a complex wound repair code. The fat necrosis in the inguinal area was excised and is reported with a benign lesion excision code. The umbilical scar revision is the more complex procedure and is sequenced first followed by the inguinal lesion (fat necrosis) excision code. Did you remember to use the multiple procedure modifier to indicate that both procedures took place during the same operative session?

(Answers to every other Case are located in Appendix D. The full answer key is only available in the TEACH Instructor Resources on Evolve.)

CASE 5-18   *Operative Report, Scar Revision, Dermabrasion*

LOCATION: Outpatient, Hospital

PATIENT: Daniel Vaa

SURGEON: Gary Sanchez, MD

PREOPERATIVE DIAGNOSIS: Unsightly widened scar of anterior chest wall

POSTOPERATIVE DIAGNOSIS: Unsightly widened scar of anterior chest wall

PROCEDURES PERFORMED:

1. Dermabrasion
2. Scar revision

ANESTHESIA: General endotracheal with approximately 7 cc of 1% Xylocaine and 1:100,000 epinephrine

ESTIMATED BLOOD LOSS: Less than 25 cc

COMPLICATIONS: None

SPONGE AND NEEDLE COUNTS: Correct

INDICATION: This patient has a widened scar with large suture marks as a result of resection of a dermatofibrosarcoma protuberans about 2 years ago.

SURGICAL FINDINGS: A 27-cm-long unsightly scar of left anterior chest wall with suture marks and widening of the scar. The scar is in the shape of a triangle with its base pointing medially and the apex pointing toward the coronoid process.

DESCRIPTION OF PROCEDURE: The patient's chest was prepped with Betadine scrub and solution and draped in a routine sterile fashion. The scar was injected with 7 cc of 1% Xylocaine and 1:100,000 epinephrine and dermabraded. It was excised to include parts of the suture marks. This was excised down to fat, but some residual scarring remained. This was left in to help provide support and blood supply. We closed the wound with subcuticular 3-0 Monocryl and interrupted twists of 5-0 Prolene. The dressing consisted of thymol iodide powder and 4 × 4s. The patient tolerated the procedure well and left the area in good condition.

SERVICE CODE(S): _____

ICD-10-CM DX CODE(S): _____

CASE 5-18—cont'd

Discussion

The complex repair codes 13100-13160 contain an interesting format that you need to understand to report the codes correctly. Turn to this code range in the CPT manual. With the text open to the code range, note that code 13100 is for a complex repair on the trunk that measures 1.1 cm to 2.5 cm and that 13101 is for a complex repair on the trunk that measures 2.6 cm to 7.5 cm. The add-on code 13102 is to be reported for each additional 5 cm or less after the first 7.5 cm.

In this case you had a 27-cm scar that was repaired. Code 13100 is only reported for repairs between 1.1 cm and 2.5 cm, and per the note in the CPT manual the add-on code 13102 is only reported in conjunction with

13101, not 13100. The first 7.5 cm are reported with 13101, because that is the maximum length you can report for the primary code. The remaining 19.5 cm are reported with the add-on code 13102, which is only used with 13101. Also note that the add-on code is for each additional 5 cm **or less.** You would report the 27-cm scar repair with the following codes:

- 13101 for the first 7.5 cm — **7.5** cm (Primary code.)
- 13102 for the next additional 5 cm — **5** cm (Add-on code.)
- 13102 for the next additional 5 cm — **5** cm (Add-on code.)
- 13102 for the next additional 5 cm — **5** cm (Add-on code.)
- 13102 for the remaining 4.5 cm — **4.5** cm (Add-on code.)

(Answers to every other Case are located in Appendix D . The full answer key is only available in the TEACH Instructor Resources on Evolve.)

CASE 5-19   *Operative Report, Dermabrasion*

LOCATION: Outpatient, Hospital

PATIENT: Florence DeFrang

SURGEON: Gary Sanchez, MD

PREOPERATIVE DIAGNOSIS: Scar of neck

POSTOPERATIVE DIAGNOSIS: Scar of neck

PROCEDURE PERFORMED: Dermabrasion of neck scar with revision of complex scar of neck (closure of complex wound)

ANESTHESIA: 7 cc (cubic centimeter) of 1% Xylocaine with 1:100,000 epinephrine

ESTIMATED BLOOD LOSS: Negligible

DESCRIPTION OF PROCEDURE: The patient's neck was prepped with Betadine scrub and solution and draped in a routine sterile fashion.

Dermabrasion was carried out with a hand engine, using one of the larger burs, and then we injected with 7 cc of 1% Xylocaine with 1:100,000 epinephrine. The scar measured 14 cm (centimeter) in length by about 1.5 cm in width with a 1.5-cm Y-extension. The scar was dermabraded, as noted, and then excised. Bleeding was electrocoagulated, and the wound was closed with subcuticular 3-0 and 4-0 Monocryl and interrupted twists of 5-0 Prolene using one horizontal mattress suture of 5-0 Prolene in the Y-portion of the scar. Thymol iodide powder was applied with Kerlix fluffs and a soft cervical collar was applied. The patient tolerated the procedure well and left the operating room in good condition.

SERVICE CODE(S): _____

ICD-10-CM DX CODE(S): _____

(Answers to every other Case are located in Appendix D . The full answer key is only available in the TEACH Instructor Resources on Evolve.)

CASE 5-20   *Operative Report, Scar Revision*

LOCATION: Outpatient, Hospital

PATIENT: Kim Plante

SURGEON: Gary Sanchez, MD

PREOPERATIVE DIAGNOSIS: Foreign body granuloma of the nose and scar of dorsum of nose

POSTOPERATIVE DIAGNOSIS: Foreign body granuloma of the nose and scar of dorsum of nose

SURGICAL FINDINGS: There was about a 1.5-cm (centimeter) transverse scar located at about the level of the supratarsal fold, and beneath this there was extensive foreign body reaction extending beneath the procerus muscles over the nasal bone extending, in fact, down into the nasal bone in the nasal frontal angle area. There was extensive involvement of the subcutaneous tissue and the tissue extending all the way down to the nasal bone as mentioned.

PROCEDURE PERFORMED:

1. A 1.5-cm complex scar revision, dorsum of the nose
2. Excision of extensive (2.5 cm) foreign body granuloma of the nose involving the procerus and nasalis muscles

ANESTHESIA: General endotracheal with approximately 2 cc of 1% Xylocaine with 1:100,000 epinephrine

ESTIMATED BLOOD LOSS: Negligible

COMPLICATIONS: None

SPONGE AND NEEDLE COUNT: Correct

DESCRIPTION OF PROCEDURE: The patient's face was prepped with Betadine scrub and solution and draped in a routine sterile fashion. The scar was dermabraded and then we excised it. In the subcutaneous tissue, we came down on a foreign body granulomatous reaction that contained what appeared to be a mixture in the previous

Continued

CASE 5-20—cont'd

foreign body (glue). We excised this on top of the musculature, but some of the foreign body extended down below the musculature of the procerus muscles and obviously had separated the muscles at the midline. It (the glue) appeared that this had been injected underneath the muscles and went from the bridge of the nose at about the level of the canthi bilaterally up to the nasal frontal angle. This chronic inflammatory and granulomatous process was involved over about a 2.5 × 2.5-cm area of the nose. After removal of this, considerable dead space remained, and we cauterized the bleeding. I reapproximated the procerus muscles with 5-0 Monocryl, put subcuticular 5-0 Monocryl to close the dead space partially, but needed to use horizontal mattress sutures of 6-0 Prolene to complete closure of the dead space in the subcutaneous area. I did not think a subcuticular suture would be helpful in obtaining the type of closure

that we wanted, and therefore the horizontal mattress sutures were used. We then better apposed the skin edges with interrupted 7-0 Prolene using a combination of twists and plain sutures. I applied Surgicel and antibiotic ointment. A portion of the specimen was submitted for frozen section and showed foreign body granulomatous reaction, which in fact had multiple sites of what appeared to be the previously injected glue surrounded by intense foreign body reaction. Interestingly, there were some muscle fibers present on the specimen. The patient tolerated the procedure well and left the operating room in good condition.

SERVICE CODE(S): _____

ICD-10-CM DX CODE(S): _____

(Answers to every other Case are located in Appendix D . The full answer key is only available in the TEACH Instructor Resources on Evolve.)

Adjacent Tissue Transfers or Rearrangements

Adjacent **tissue transfers** are procedures in which a segment of skin is moved from one area to an adjacent area. One side of the moved skin (flap) is left attached to the blood supply to keep the area viable. The flap is then sutured into place. The procedures are often termed V-plasty, W-plasty, Z-plasty, rotation flaps, or advancement flaps.

Adjacent tissue transfers (14000-14350) are reported according to the size of the **recipient site** measured in square centimeters. Simple repair of the donor site is included in the tissue transfer code and is not reported separately. Complex closure or grafting of the donor site is reported separately. To code transfers, you need to know the location of the defect, the size of the defect, and any donor area.

Unlike the repair codes where lesion excisions performed at the time of the repair are reported separately, when a lesion is excised at the site of the repair and then repaired by adjacent tissue transfer, the lesion excision is included in the tissue transfer code and not reported separately.

CASE 5-21   *Operative Report, Wide Excision, Basal Cell Carcinoma*

LOCATION: Outpatient, Hospital

PATIENT: Karen Rhodes

SURGEON: Gary Sanchez, MD

PREOPERATIVE DIAGNOSIS: Left leg lateral lesion

POSTOPERATIVE DIAGNOSIS: Basal cell carcinoma, left calf

PROCEDURE PERFORMED: Excision of the left leg basal cell carcinoma

SURGICAL FINDINGS: A 1 × 1-cm lesion, morphologically resembling a basal cell carcinoma

ANESTHESIA: General endotracheal; 30 mL of Marcaine was infiltrated into the wound prior to making the incision.

DESCRIPTION OF PROCEDURE: The patient was brought to the operating room, and the left leg was dressed. An elliptical incision taking a 0.5-cm margin was made around the previous basal cell carcinoma, and dissection was carried down to subcutaneous tissue. After this, hemostasis was obtained with electrocautery, and the wound was closed with mattress sutures of 4-0 nylon. This was sterilely dressed. The patient tolerated the procedure well and was returned to the recovery room in good condition. Sponge and needle counts were correct.

Pathology Report Later Indicated: Basal cell carcinoma.

SERVICE CODE(S): _____

ICD-10-CM DX CODE(S): _____

(Answers to every other Case are located in Appendix D . The full answer key is only available in the TEACH Instructor Resources on Evolve.)

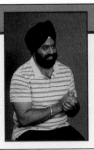

From the Trenches

"The key to success in the medical coding field is getting certifications in difference specialities and keeping abreast of all newer guidelines."

KHUSHWINDER SINGH

MHA, CPC, CPMA, CRC, CPCO

CASE 5-22A   *Operative Report, Wide Excision, Basal Cell Carcinoma*

Assign the pathology codes in Case 5-22B.

LOCATION: Outpatient, Hospital

PATIENT: Irene Reep

SURGEON: Gary Sanchez, MD

PREOPERATIVE DIAGNOSIS: Basal cell carcinoma, left alar crease

POSTOPERATIVE DIAGNOSIS: Basal cell carcinoma, left alar crease

SURGICAL FINDINGS: A 7-mm (millimeter)-diameter raised lesion, morphologically resembling a cystic basal cell carcinoma, located in the left alar crease.

INTRAOPERATIVE FROZEN SECTION: Grey Lonewolf, MD

SURGICAL PROCEDURE: Wide excision of basal cell carcinoma, left alar crease with reconstruction of the defect by a 4 × 2.5-cm nasolabial flap.

ANESTHESIA: General endotracheal with 13 cc of 1% Xylocaine with 1:100,000 epinephrine.

ESTIMATED BLOOD LOSS: 25 cc (cubic centimeter)

DESCRIPTION OF PROCEDURE: The patient's face was prepped with Betadine scrub and solution and draped in a routine sterile fashion. We initially outlined a margin of 5 mm around the lesion, excising it down to nasal musculature and the facial musculature lateral to the nasolabial (nose/lip) line. The margins were 1 cm on the proximal distal ends. The superior part was tagged with a silk suture. After excision of this lesion and once the inferior part was taken all the way down to the mucosa, we submitted it for frozen section, and there was involvement in both lateral and medial margins and some of the inferior margin. Also the deep margin was involved. I returned to the operating room and took another 5 mm of skin around this in continuity with the underlying musculature, going all the way down to the pyriform fossa and going all the way down to the mucosa of the nasal cavity. More laterally, we included some of the superficial musculature of the cheek and then obtained hemostasis. We cauterized the bleeding, following which a 4 × 2.5-cm (centimeter) nasolabial flap was developed from the cheek and rotated into the defect, insetting it with mostly interrupted horizontal mattress sutures of 4-0 Prolene. The wound was dressed with Surgicel and glycerin-soaked cotton with a few dry cotton balls on top and taped over this. The estimated blood loss was approximately 25 cc. As stated above, we did a second frozen section, which showed clear margins on all specimens. One margin was very close; however, I felt that grossly we had no tumor involvement in the margin in question.

Pathology Report Later Indicated: See 5-22B.

SERVICE CODE(S): _____

ICD-10-CM DX CODE(S): _____

Discussion

You need to identify the location, size, and repair to correctly code this service. According to the Surgical Procedure section of the report and substantiated within the body of the report are these three items:

SURGICAL PROCEDURE: Wide excision of basal cell carcinoma, left alar crease (**location** is beside the nose in this case) with reconstruction of the defect by 4 × 2.5-cm (**size** is 4 × 2.5 cm = 10 sq cm) nasolabial flap (**repair** type is a skin flap or an "adjacent tissue transfer").

In the index of the CPT manual you can locate the code for this transfer under "Skin Graft and Flap, Tissue Transfer." These codes are divided based on the location, such as trunk, arm, hands, etc., and total square centimeters.

Figure 5-8 illustrates basal cell carcinoma of the nose.

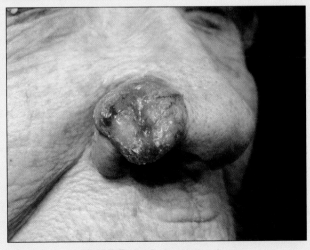

FIGURE 5-8 Basal cell carcinoma.

(Answers to every other Case are located in Appendix D. The full answer key is only available in the TEACH Instructor Resources on Evolve.)

CASE 5-22B   *Pathology Report*

LOCATION: Outpatient, Hospital

PATIENT: Irene Reep

SURGEON: Gary Sanchez, MD

PATHOLOGIST: Grey Lonewolf, MD

CLINICAL HISTORY: A 7-mm (millimeter) lesion, left alar crease

SPECIMEN RECEIVED:

A. Lesion, left alar crease with FS (frozen section)
B. Re-excision of same lesion with FS

GROSS DESCRIPTION:

A. The specimen is labeled with the patient's name and "lesion, left alar crease," which consists of a 2 × 2 × 1.5-cm (centimeter) nodule. The superior aspect is tagged, which is also identified with black ink, the inferior aspect with green, the right (medial) aspect with red, and the left (lateral) aspect with blue ink. Frozen sections are processed in cassettes A1-4; the remaining tissue is in cassette A5.

INTRAOPERATIVE FROZEN-SECTION DIAGNOSIS per Dr. Lonewolf: Left alar crease skin lesion: Basal cell carcinoma involving margins.

B. The specimen is labeled with the patient's name and "re-excision left alar crease lesion, tagged superior," which consists of a 3.5 × 2.8 × 1.0-cm roughly spherical skin segment with a central biopsy cavity. The superior aspect is identified with black ink, inferior aspect with green ink, right (medial) aspect with red ink, and left (lateral)

aspect with blue ink. The specimen is serially sectioned and frozen. The frozen sections are processed in cassettes B1-9.

INTRAOPERATIVE FROZEN-SECTION DIAGNOSIS: Per Dr. Lonewolf: Re-excision left alar crease lesion: Focal residual basal carcinoma; margins benign.

MICROSCOPIC DESCRIPTION:

A. Permanent sections confirm the frozen-section diagnosis showing basal cell carcinoma involving the surgical margins. The tumor is characterized by downward growth of irregular nests of basaloid cells showing palisading of the peripheral cell layer. Tumor is associated with a reactive fibrous stoma.
B. Sections show skin with underlying subcutaneous adipose tissue with admixed skeletal muscle and focal hyaline cartilage. There is focal residual basal cell carcinoma similar in appearance to that described above in A. All margins are benign.

DIAGNOSIS:

A. Skin lesion, left alar crease excision: Basal cell carcinoma, involving margins.
B. Re-excision left alar crease excision: Focal residual basal cell carcinoma, margins benign.

SERVICE CODE(S): _____

ICD-10-CM DX CODE(S): _____

Discussion

Based on the pathology report, the pathologist provided three services:

- First frozen section
- Second frozen section
- One microscopic examination

An intraoperative consultation includes the pathologist's opinion provided during surgery. If the pathologist was present in the operating room and provided an opinion and only a gross examination (using the eyes only), the service would be reported with 88329. If the pathologist was present at surgery, provided a gross examination, and took a frozen section (specimen

that is immediately frozen in cold liquid or environment), the service would be reported with 88331 for the first specimen and 88332 for each additional specimen. This report indicates that the pathologist was present in the operating room, provided a gross examination, and took two frozen sections.

In addition to the codes to report the intraoperative consultations, a microscopic examination (in the report labeled Microscopic Description) was conducted on both specimens (A&B). The microscopic description is reported with the correct level code from the 88300-88309 range. Since there were two microscopic examinations indicated in the report, then 88305 is reported × 2.

(Answers to every other Case are located in Appendix D. The full answer key is only available in the TEACH Instructor Resources on Evolve.)

Skin Grafts

A free **skin graft** is a piece of skin that is either of a split-thickness autograft (epidermis and part of the dermis) or a full-thickness autograft (epidermis and all the dermis). These grafts are completely freed from the donor site and are placed over the recipient site without a connection left between the graft and the donor site. As with adjacent tissue transfers, the free skin grafts are reported by the site, size, and type of repair to the **recipient** site.

The **recipient** site is specified within the code descriptions as the location, such as trunk, arms, or legs.

CPT includes the Lund-Browder Diagram and Classification Method Table **(Figure 5-9)**, which is used specifically to estimate the extent, depth, and percentage of burns. Lund-Browder takes into consideration the age of the patient, with adjustments made in the percentages of the head and legs according to patient age.

The **types** of grafts are varied and specified within the codes as pinch, split, or full-thickness autograft. A pinch graft is a small, split-thickness repair; a split graft is a repair that involves the epidermis and some of the dermis; and a full-thickness graft is a repair that involves the epidermis and all of the dermis. Often a split-thickness skin graft is documented in the patient record as STSG and a full-thickness skin graft as FTSG.

The **donor** site is the place from which the tissue for the graft is taken. If the donor site for the graft requires repair by

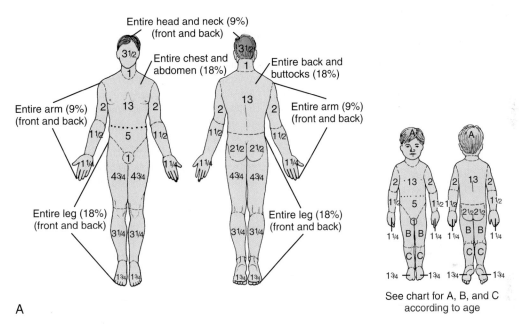

AGE	Birth–1 yr	1–4 yr	5–9 yr	10–14 yr	15 yr	Adult
Head	19	17	13	11	9	7
Neck	2					
Ant trunk	13					
Post trunk	13					
R buttock	2½					
L buttock	2½					
Genitalia	1					
R U arm	4					
L U arm	4					
R L arm	3					
L L arm	3					
R hand	2½	6½	8	8½	9	9½
L hand	2½	6½	8	8½	9	9½
R thigh	5½	5	5½	6	6½	7
L thigh	5½	5	5½	6	6½	7
R leg	5					
L leg	5					
R foot	3½					
L foot	3½					

B　　　　　　　　BODY AREA

FIGURE 5–9 Example of Lund-Browder Classification Method.

grafting, an additional graft code is reported. Simple repair (closure) of the donor site is included in the graft code, and as such, simple repairs are not reported separately.

A temporary graft may be placed on the recipient site, such as a bilaminate (artificial skin). Autografts are grafts taken from the patient's body, allografts are taken from other persons (alive or cadaver), and xenografts are taken from other species (such as pigs).

Surgical preparation of the recipient site prepares the area to receive the graft and includes removal of scar tissue or lesions. If surgical preparation of a site is required, it is reported separately with codes 15002-15005.

CASE 5-23   *Operative Report, Split-Thickness Autograft*

The diagnosis in this report is that of a nonhealing wound, which can be located by first referencing the ICD-10-CM Index under the main term "Complication[s]," followed by the subterms "postprocedural," "specified NEC," "skin and subcutaneous tissue." Reference the ICD-10-CM Index under the main term "Wound," followed by the subterms "open," "nonhealing surgical." The service is a split graft, which is a free skin graft.

LOCATION: Inpatient, Hospital

PATIENT: Roger Ulland

SURGEON: Gary Sanchez, MD

PREOPERATIVE DIAGNOSIS: Nonhealing wound of left lower quadrant of abdomen **(site)**

POSTOPERATIVE DIAGNOSIS: Nonhealing wound of left lower quadrant of abdomen

SURGICAL PROCEDURE: Split-thickness skin graft from the right thigh to the left lower quadrant of the abdomen measuring 2.5 × 2.5 cm (centimeter)

INDICATION: This patient has a nonhealing wound of a previously skin-grafted site of the lower abdomen.

SURGICAL FINDINGS: A 2.5 × 2.5-cm **(size)** nonhealing wound of the right lower abdomen with exuberant granulation tissue.

ANESTHESIA: Standby with about 6 cc of 1% Xylocaine with 1:800,000 epinephrine.

COMPLICATIONS: None

SPONGE AND NEEDLE COUNT: Correct

DESCRIPTION OF PROCEDURE: The patient's right thigh and abdomen were prepped with Betadine scrub and solution and draped in a routine sterile fashion. The right thigh was anesthetized with 1% Xylocaine with 1:800,000 epinephrine (6 cc), and Shur-Clens was applied. The skin graft was taken with a Goulian Weck blade with an 8-thousands-of-an-inch-thick shim on the blade. This was sewed to the defect with a running 5-0 Vicryl. A dressing of Xeroform glycerin-soaked cotton and a Kerlix fluff were then applied using Elastoplast to hold the dressing in place. The donor site was covered with scarlet red and an ABD (Adriamycin, bleomycin, dacarbazine) pad. The patient tolerated the procedure well and left the area in good condition.

SERVICE CODE(S): _____

ICD-10-CM DX CODE(S): _____

(Answers to every other Case are located in Appendix D . The full answer key is only available in the TEACH Instructor Resources on Evolve.)

CASE 5-24A   *Operative Report, Muscle Flap*

The procedure that Dr. Sanchez is performing involves deeper tissue than what is reported with the Free Skin Graft codes. In this case, the repair is of the muscle (muscle flap) and of the skin (skin graft), and both procedures are reported.

LOCATION: Inpatient, Hospital

PATIENT: Josh Peterson

SURGEON: Gary Sanchez, MD

PREOPERATIVE DIAGNOSIS: Ulcer, left lower extremity, with exposed tibia and exposed plate

POSTOPERATIVE DIAGNOSIS: Ulcer, left lower extremity, with exposed tibia and exposed plate

PROCEDURES PERFORMED:

1. Soleus muscle flap
2. Split-thickness skin graft 2.5 × 2.5 cm (centimeter) from the left thigh to the left lower extremity

ANESTHESIA: General endotracheal

ESTIMATED BLOOD LOSS: 130 cc (cubic centimeter)

DRAINS: One no. 10 Jackson-Pratt

SURGICAL FINDINGS: There was an open wound extending from the lower third of the tibia up into the middle third of the leg with an exposed plate, but tissue loss of the lower third of the leg was evident. Dr. Almaz, orthopedics, had previously inserted antibiotic beads.

PROCEDURE: An incision was made 2.5 cm medial to the tibial border. We developed a bilobed flap and identified the separation of the soleus muscle and the gastrocnemius medial head following incision of the deep fascia. I dissected the soleus muscle free distally as far as possible and then cut it distally at the Achilles tendon insertion, transposing it through a tunnel of the bilobed flap and covering the area of soft-tissue loss by using bolsters that were tied in place with 0 Prolene. This effectively covered the open area, and then we closed the remainder of the area with 0 Prolene, closing the donor area also with 0 Prolene. We put Nitro paste along the edges where there

CASE 5-24A—cont'd

was some skin blanching and put a no. 10 Jackson-Pratt drain in the distal end of the wound, bringing it out through a separate stab wound incision. A split-thickness skin graft of about 2.5 × 2.5 cm was taken from the left thigh, meshed with 1:1.5 mesher, and applied to the defect area measuring 2.5 × 2.5 cm with 2-0 Prolene sutures and staples. We dressed the wound with Xeroform, Kerlix fluffs, Kerlix roll, Kling, and Sof-Rol, and then a cast

was applied by the orthopedic technician. The donor site was dressed with scarlet red and an ABD (Adriamycin, bleomycin, dacarbazine) pad. The patient tolerated the procedure well and left the area in good condition.

SERVICE CODE(S): _____

ICD-10-CM DX CODE(S): _____

(Answers to every other Case are located in Appendix D . The full answer key is only available in the TEACH Instructor Resources on Evolve.)

CASE 5-24B   *Radiology Report, Ultrasound, Lower Extremity*

The diagnosis on this report is an ulcer of the skin of the lower leg, which requires an L97.2-- code and aftercare for a fracture of the leg, which requires an S82.9---. In ICD-10-CM, the Z code for aftercare is not reported for aftercare for injuries (I.C.21.7.). Assign the acute injury code with the 7th character "D". Assign codes for the professional portion of a vascular study of the veins of the leg.

LOCATION: Inpatient, Hospital

PATIENT: Josh Peterson

SURGEON: Gary Sanchez, MD

RADIOLOGIST: Morton Monson, MD

EXAMINATION OF: Left lower extremity ultrasound

CLINICAL SYMPTOMS: Ulcer, lower extremity, calf

LEFT LOWER EXTREMITY ULTRASOUND: History of traumatic fracture

FINDINGS: Ultrasound examination of the deep venous system of the left lower extremity is negative for DVT (deep vein thrombosis). The left popliteal, greater saphenous, and femoral veins are patent and negative for thrombus. Unable to evaluate the calf veins due to existing cast.

SERVICE CODE(S): _____

ICD-10-CM DX CODE(S): _____

(Answers to every other Case are located in Appendix D . The full answer key is only available in the TEACH Instructor Resources on Evolve.)

CASE 5-25   *Operative Report, Full-Thickness Skin Graft*

Avulsion is ripping or tearing apart. When referencing the Index under the terms "Avulsion, skin and subcutaneous tissue", the coder is directed to "see Wound, open, by site".

LOCATION: Outpatient, Hospital

PATIENT: Brenda Payne

SURGEON: Gary Sanchez, MD

INDICATION: This patient had an avulsion injury of the dorsum of the left thumb.

PREOPERATIVE DIAGNOSIS: Partial-thickness avulsion, dorsum of left thumb **(location)**

POSTOPERATIVE DIAGNOSIS: Partial-thickness avulsion, dorsum of left thumb

SURGICAL FINDINGS: There is about a 4 × 2.5-cm (centimeter) **(size)** area of avulsion of the skin of the dorsum of left thumb extending from about the base of the nail to the metacarpophalangeal joint.

PROCEDURE PERFORMED: Full-thickness skin graft **(type of repair)**

ANESTHESIA: General

COMPLICATIONS: None

SPONGE AND NEEDLE COUNT: Correct

DESCRIPTION OF PROCEDURE: The arm and hand were prepped with Betadine scrub and solution and draped in a routine sterile fashion. The left groin was also prepped with Betadine scrub and solution and draped in a routine sterile fashion. The area of the left thumb was inspected, and a full-thickness graft was taken from the left groin and applied to the defect of the left thumb using a tie-over dressing of Xeroform and glycerin-soaked cotton balls. The donor site area was closed with subcuticular 3-0 Monocryl. The remainder of the hand dressing was Kerlix fluffs, Kerlix roll, Kling, Sof-Rol, and a short-arm fiberglass cast. The donor site was covered with Xeroform and 4 × 4. The patient tolerated the procedure well and left the area in good condition.

SERVICE CODE(S): _____

ICD-10-CM DX CODE(S): _____

(Answers to every other Case are located in Appendix D . The full answer key is only available in the TEACH Instructor Resources on Evolve.)

CASE 5-26 *Operative Report, Muscle Flap*

LOCATION: Outpatient, Hospital

PATIENT: Janet Larae

SURGEON: Gary Sanchez, MD

PREOPERATIVE DIAGNOSIS: Open wound, left lower extremity, with exposed tibia and exposed plate

POSTOPERATIVE DIAGNOSIS: Open wound, left lower extremity, with exposed tibia and exposed plate. (This is an ulcer.)

PROCEDURES PERFORMED:

1. Soleus muscle flap (muscle flap 15733-15738)
2. Split-thickness skin graft 5.0 × 5.0 cm (centimeter) from the left thigh to the left lower extremity (split autograft 15100-15121)

ANESTHESIA: General endotracheal

ESTIMATED BLOOD LOSS: 80 cc (cubic centimeter)

DRAINS: One no. 1 Jackson-Pratt

SURGICAL FINDINGS: There was an open wound extending from the lower third of the tibia up into the middle third of the leg with an exposed plate, but tissue loss of the lower third of the leg was evident.

PROCEDURE: An incision was made 5.0 cm medial to the tibial border. We developed a bilobed flap and identified the separation of the soleus muscle and the gastrocnemius medial head following incision of the deep fascia. The soleus muscle was freed distally as far as possible and then cut distally at the Achilles tendon insertion. The bilobed flap was found covering the area of soft-tissue loss by using bolsters that were tied in place with 0 Prolene. The open area was covered, and then we closed the remainder of the area, closing the donor area also with 0 Prolene. We put Nitro paste along the edges where there was some skin blanching and put a no. 1 Jackson-Pratt drain in the distal end of the wound, bringing it out through a separate stab wound incision. A split-thickness skin graft of about 5.0 × 5.0 cm was taken from the left thigh, meshed with a mesher, and applied to the defect with 2-0 Prolene, sutures, and staples. We dressed the wound with Xeroform, Kerlix fluffs, Kerlix roll, Kling, and a Sof-Rol, and then the orthopedic technician applied a cast. The donor site was dressed with scarlet red and an ABD (Adriamycin, bleomycin, dacarbazine) pad. The patient tolerated the procedure well and left the area in good condition.

SERVICE CODE(S): _____

ICD-10-CM DX CODE(S): _____

(Answers to every other Case are located in Appendix D . The full answer key is only available in the TEACH Instructor Resources on Evolve.)

Other Procedures

The next three reports will provide you with an opportunity to code a variety of services.

CASE 5-27 *Operative Report, Composite Graft*

LOCATION: Outpatient, Hospital

PATIENT: Doreen Anderson

SURGEON: Gary Sanchez, MD

PREOPERATIVE DIAGNOSIS: Lentigo maligna, right side of nose overlying alar cartilage

POSTOPERATIVE DIAGNOSIS: Lentigo maligna, right side of nose overlying alar cartilage

PROCEDURE PERFORMED: Excision, lentigo maligna alar of the right side of nose with repair by composite graft **(type)** from the right ear

SURGICAL FINDINGS: There is about a 5-mm (millimeter) raised scar along the nostril rim

ANESTHESIA: General endotracheal with 6 cc (cubic centimeter) of 1% Xylocaine and 1:800,000 epinephrine

ESTIMATED BLOOD LOSS: Negligible

DESCRIPTION OF PROCEDURE: The patient's face and right ear were prepped with Betadine scrub and solution and draped in a routine sterile fashion. Both sites (i.e., the ear and nose) were injected with 1% Xylocaine and 1:800,000 epinephrine, and a through-and-through excision was accomplished of the right alar lesion with a margin of 1 cm (centimeter) from the farthest edge of the scar. This was excised in the form of a triangle and, after obtaining hemostasis, I took a composite graft from the right ear with a no. 11 knife blade measuring about 2 cm in its maximal width. The cartilage was trimmed somewhat in this area. Then I sutured the vestibular lining in with interrupted 4-0 Monocryl using interrupted 5-0 Prolene for the external sutures. A dressing of Xeroform was rolled up and placed in the nose. It was placed in the right nostril and then a Xeroform and 4 × 4 were placed over it externally. The right ear had been repaired with interrupted 3-0 Prolene. Surgicel and a Band-Aid were applied to the right ear. The patient tolerated the procedure well and left the operating room in good condition.

Pathology Report Later Indicated: Carcinoma in situ

SERVICE CODE(S): _____

ICD-10-CM DX CODE(S): _____

(Answers to every other Case are located in Appendix D . The full answer key is only available in the TEACH Instructor Resources on Evolve.)

CASE 5-28   *Operative Report, Abdominoplasty*

LOCATION: Inpatient, Hospital

PATIENT: Harriet Bergh

SURGEON: Gary Sanchez, MD

INDICATIONS FOR PROCEDURE: This patient has a nonhealing vertical wound below the umbilicus for which we have attempted conservative management with failure of conservative management. This wound probably will not heal without removal of the large panniculus that the patient has. Complications were discussed with the patient, including hematoma, infection, pulmonary embolus, fat necrosis, skin necrosis, urinary tract infection, and atelectasis.

PREOPERATIVE DIAGNOSIS: Massive abdominal panniculus (localized fat)

POSTOPERATIVE DIAGNOSIS: Massive abdominal panniculus

SURGICAL FINDINGS: Massive abdominal panniculus weighing a total of 8.99 kg (kilogram)

SURGICAL PROCEDURE: Abdominoplasty (skin only) with relocation of the umbilicus

ANESTHESIA: General endotracheal

ESTIMATED BLOOD LOSS: 200 cc (cubic centimeter)

FLUIDS: Three liters of Ringer's lactate

DRAINS: Four no. 10 Jackson-Pratts

DESCRIPTION OF PROCEDURE: A lower abdominal incision was marked out, and 400 cc of tumescent solution was infiltrated along the suture lines in the abdomen. Tumescent solution was prepared by adding 25 cc of 2% Xylocaine, 1 cc of 1:100,000 epinephrine, and 3 cc of sodium bicarbonate to 1 L of Ringer's lactate. The umbilicus was circumscribed and cut down to the abdominal wall, undermining the skin at the supra-areolar fascial level on the abdominal wall, up to the costal margin. We then plexed the table, pulled the areas of resection down, and resected them by halving each side. We obtained a total of 8.99 kg from both sides, and after appropriate trimming, we closed the superficial layer with interrupted 0 Monocryl using subcuticular 0 Monocryl for the skin closure and staples. We then located the umbilicus by palpation underneath the abdominal wall. We had inserted four Jackson-Pratt drains and brought them out through separate stab wound incisions. After location of the abdominal wall, along the iliac crest, we made a 15-mm (millimeter) incision transversely over the proposed site of the umbilicus and brought it out in the skin, suturing to the skin with 3-0 Prolene. We did not suture it to the fascia because of the scarring around the umbilicus, and we inserted Xeroform in that using a dressing of ABD (Adriamycin, bleomycin, dacarbazine) pads, Sof-Rol, and a plaster cast, on which we placed a 10-pound sandbag. Estimated blood loss was 200 cc. The patient tolerated the procedure well and left the operating room in good condition.

Pathology Report Later Indicated: Benign skin and fat

SERVICE CODE(S): _____

ICD-10-CM DX CODE(S): _____

(Answers to every other Case are located in Appendix D . The full answer key is only available in the TEACH Instructor Resources on Evolve.)

CASE 5-29   *Operative Report, Post Skin Graft*

This is a return to the operating room (during the postoperative period of the initial procedure) by the same surgeon who originally performed a full-thickness graft 5 days before. This report describes the service of a dressing change and a diagnosis of admission for a change of surgical dressing.

The ICD-10-CM aftercare codes are not reported for injuries. Assign the acute care code with the 7th character "D" for subsequent care (ICD-10-CM Official Guidelines for Coding and Reporting I.C. 21.7.).

LOCATION: Outpatient, Hospital

PATIENT: Helen Mittag

SURGEON: Gary Sanchez, MD

INDICATION: This patient had a thin, full-thickness graft from the groin applied to the dorsum of the right index finger 5 days ago after being burned by a bonfire. We are going to change her dressing under anesthesia to prevent any dislodgment of the graft secondary to movement.

PREOPERATIVE DIAGNOSIS: Status post full-thickness skin graft, right groin to dorsum of right index finger overlying the proximal phalanx.

POSTOPERATIVE DIAGNOSIS: Status post full-thickness skin graft, right groin to dorsum of right index finger overlying the proximal phalanx

SURGICAL FINDINGS:

1. A 2.5 × 1.5-cm (centimeter) intact full-thickness graft of the dorsum of the right index finger overlying the proximal phalanx.
2. Healed groin wound except for one 2-mm (millimeter) area of maceration of the skin in the center of the area. There was also a small amount of rash in the medial aspect of the groin.

PROCEDURE PERFORMED: Dressing change

ANESTHESIA: General

COMPLICATIONS: None

SPONGE AND NEEDLE COUNT: Correct

DESCRIPTION OF PROCEDURE: Under satisfactory LMA anesthesia, the cast was removed and the dressing was removed. We removed the dressing down to the tie over portion of it and then draped it in a routine sterile fashion. The Monocryl sutures were cut near their origins, and the tie-over dressing was removed. The skin graft measuring about 2.5 × 1.5 cm was intact. There was a bit of serosanguineous drainage from one edge, and we took a culture and sensitivity of this. A dressing was reapplied using Xeroform immediately

Continued

CASE 5-29—cont'd

on top of the graft, followed by glycerin-soaked cotton ball, a 3-inch Kling, Kerlix roll, Kerlix fluffs at the base and the palm, and a 3-inch Kling for the outside of the dressing. For support and for immobilization, we taped the index and middle fingers to minimize motion in the fingers. A cast was not reapplied. The twists and single horizontal mattress suture in the groin were removed with a no. 11 knife blade, and a dry dressing was applied. There

was one small 2-mm (millimeter) area of maceration of the center of the wound. The patient tolerated the procedure well and left the operating room in good condition.

SERVICE CODE(S): _____

ICD-10-CM DX CODE(S): _____

(Answers to every other Case are located in Appendix D . The full answer key is only available in the TEACH Instructor Resources on Evolve.)

Pressure Ulcers

A pressure ulcer is a decubitus ulcer or a bedsore found on areas of the body that have bony projections, such as the hips, ankle projections, heels, and the area above the tailbone. Pressure on these areas causes decreased blood flow, and sores form. With continued pressure, the sores ulcerate, and deeper layers of tissue, such as fascia, muscle, and bone, may be affected. Ulcers are identified by stages—1, 2, 3, and 4.

Although a pressure ulcer can be seen, the depth to which the ulceration has penetrated cannot be seen. The ulcer may involve only superficial skin or may affect deeper layers. (Gangrene and/or osteomyelitis are possible complications.) The treatment for a pressure ulcer (15920-15999) is excision of the ulcerated area to the depth of unaffected tissue, fascia, or muscle. If a free skin graft is used to close the ulcer, that closure would be reported separately.

CASE 5-30 *Operative Report, Debridement*

LOCATION: Inpatient, Hospital

PATIENT: Mabel Rud

SURGEON: Gary Sanchez, MD

PREOPERATIVE DIAGNOSIS:

1. Left ischial pressure ulcer
2. Osteomyelitis, left ischium

POSTOPERATIVE DIAGNOSIS:

1. Left ischial pressure ulcer
2. Osteomyelitis, left ischium

PROCEDURE PERFORMED: Debridement, left ischial ulcer, with ostectomy of the ischial tuberosity and primary closure

INDICATION: The patient had a recurrent left ischial ulcer secondary to osteomyelitis and shearing forces.

ESTIMATED BLOOD LOSS: 100 cc (cubic centimeter)

DRAINS: One no. 10 Jackson-Pratt

DESCRIPTION OF PROCEDURE: Under satisfactory general endotracheal anesthesia, the patient was turned in the prone position and draped in a routine sterile fashion. She had been prepped with Betadine scrubbing solution. We excised the ulcer elliptically and dissected down to the ischial tuberosity, which was covered with granulation tissue, and we removed this as a unit with the osteotome. We took a piece of bone from deep in the ischial tuberosity and submitted it for culture and sensitivity. Bleeding was electrocoagulated, and we placed a no. 10 Jackson-Pratt in the wound, bringing it out through a separate stab wound incision laterally. I closed the wound by advancing the posterior thigh musculature to suture it to the gluteus maximus muscle with 0 Monocryl. The remainder of the wound was closed with no. 2 Prolene. We cauterized the granulation tissue on top of a 1.5-cm (centimeter) superficial sacral ulcer and then dressed the wound with Xeroform, Kerlix, and Elastoplast. The patient tolerated the procedure well and left the area in good condition.

SERVICE CODE(S): _____

ICD-10-CM DX CODE(S): _____

(Answers to every other Case are located in Appendix D . The full answer key is only available in the TEACH Instructor Resources on Evolve.)

Breast Procedures

To report **mastectomy** procedures correctly, it is necessary to determine the extent of the procedure, that is, whether pectoral muscles, axillary lymph nodes, or internal mammary lymph nodes were also removed. The mastectomy codes are for unilateral procedures and are reported with either the -RT (right) or -LT (left) modifiers; bilateral procedures are reported with use of modifier -50 (bilateral procedures).

Breast biopsies can be performed by means of an incision made into the lesion in which a small portion of the lesion is taken out, or by **excisional biopsy** in which the entire lesion is removed. The lesion may be marked preoperatively. Percutaneous breast biopsies are reported with 19081-19086 based on the guidance method. A location device (clip, metallic pellet, wire, needle, radioactive seed) placed without a biopsy is reported with 19281-19288 based on the guidance method.

There are multiple codes for mastectomies (19300-19307). You should carefully review the operative report to confirm whether pectoral muscles, axillary lymph nodes, or internal mammary lymph nodes were also removed. This information will be necessary to determine the correct mastectomy code.

CASE 5-31A   *Operative Report, Breast Biopsy*

Use the HCPCS modifier that identifies the left side.

LOCATION: Inpatient, Hospital

PATIENT: Marina Wild

SURGEON: Gary Sanchez, MD

PREOPERATIVE DIAGNOSIS: Left breast mass

POSTOPERATIVE DIAGNOSIS: Left breast mass

PROCEDURE PERFORMED: Biopsy, left breast mass

ANESTHESIA: General anesthesia

INDICATIONS: This is a 42-year-old female with a previous history of breast biopsy laterally in the left axillary tail **(previous location)** area. She has some scar tissue present in this area, and just lateral and superior to the tail of Spence in the axilla **(current location),** she has a firm area, which is worrisome to the patient. She has had a normal workup for breast mass.

DESCRIPTION OF PROCEDURE: She was taken to the operating room and laid supine on the operating room table, anesthetized, and put to sleep. The left axilla, tail of breast, was prepped and draped in the usual fashion. We utilized a slightly oblique and transverse incision overlying the firm area and dissected down through the subcutaneous tissue with a combination of blunt and sharp dissection, tying off bleeding with silk suture material. The area represented breast tissue, and we grasped and elevated it with an Allis clamp and cored out a large area of tissue. The residual cavity had no palpable masses, and the area was closed. The dermal layer was closed with interrupted

chromic, and skin edges were closed with interrupted nylon. Dressings were applied. She tolerated this well. Dr. Monson was present for the entire case.

Pathology Report Indicated: See Report 5-31B.

SERVICE CODE(S): _____

ICD-10-CM DX CODE(S): _____

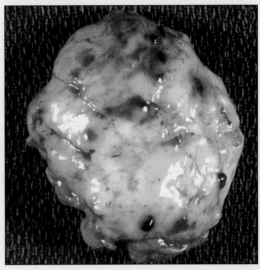

FIGURE 5–10 Breast biopsy.

(Answers to every other Case are located in Appendix D . The full answer key is only available in the TEACH Instructor Resources on Evolve.)

CASE 5-31B   *Pathology Report*

Assign codes for the physician service only.

LOCATION: Inpatient, Hospital

PATIENT: Marina Wild

SURGEON: Gary Sanchez, MD

PATHOLOGIST: Morton Monson, MD

CLINICAL HISTORY: Breast lump

TISSUE RECEIVED: OR (operating room) Consult

LEFT BREAST BIOPSY: Axillary tail area

GROSS DESCRIPTION: The specimen is labeled with the patient's name and "left breast lump," which consists of two yellow fatty tissues, one of which is 5 × 3.5 × 2.5 cm (centimeter) and the other 4 × 3 × 1.5 cm. Cut surfaces reveal largely yellow adipose tissue throughout. The specimen is

serially sectioned and processed in toto in 25 cassettes with the smaller specimen in cassettes 1-9 and the larger specimen in cassettes 10-25.

INTRAOPERATIVE FROZEN SECTION DIAGNOSIS per Dr. Monson: Left breast biopsy, axillary tail area: Grossly benign, defer to permanent sections.

MICROSCOPIC DESCRIPTION: Sections show predominantly mature adipose tissue with intersecting bands of fibrous tissue. Sections from the smaller tissue segment show a focus of benign ducts. Sections of the large tissue section show a few benign lymph nodes with mild fatty change.

DIAGNOSIS: Left breast biopsy, axillary area: Adipose tissue with a single focus of benign ducts and nine benign axillary lymph nodes.

SERVICE CODE(S): _____

ICD-10-CM DX CODE(S): _____

(Answers to every other Case are located in Appendix D . The full answer key is only available in the TEACH Instructor Resources on Evolve.)

CASE 5-31C   *Progress Note*

This service is reported with Z codes to report aftercare that involved the removal of dressing in a follow-up situation. The patient has no current symptoms or illness. Assign codes for the physician service only.

LOCATION: Outpatient, Clinic

PATIENT: Marina Wild

SURGEON: Gary Sanchez, MD

The patient comes in for a postoperative check after biopsy of a left breast mass. The biopsy specimen showed adipose tissue with a single focus of benign ducts and nine benign axillary lymph nodes. It was in

the tail of Spence where the biopsy occurred. She has been doing well since her surgery. She complains of some pain and numbness, but this is improving. She takes Tylenol for the pain; no narcotics.

PHYSICAL EXAMINATION: The wound is clean and dry. No cellulitis. No evidence of a seroma. Stitches were removed. No Steri-Strips were applied.

IMPRESSION: Routine postoperative check

PLAN: Return to clinic p.r.n. (as needed)

SERVICE CODE(S): _____

ICD-10-CM DX CODE(S): _____

(Answers to every other Case are located in Appendix D . The full answer key is only available in the TEACH Instructor Resources on Evolve.)

From the Trenches

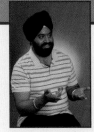

"Getting auditing certification and adding specialities will help enhance a coder's career."

KHUSHWINDER SINGH
MHA, CPC, CPMA, CRC, CPCO

CASE 5-32A   *Operative Report, Breast Mass*

LOCATION: Outpatient, Hospital

PATIENT: Donna Senne

SURGEON: Gary Sanchez, MD

PREOPERATIVE DIAGNOSIS: Right breast mass

POSTOPERATIVE DIAGNOSIS: Right breast mass

OPERATIVE NOTE: With the patient under general anesthesia, the right breast was prepped and draped in a sterile manner. A standard breast line incision was made over the palpated mass. Sharp dissection was carried down to the mass. The mass was grasped with an Allis clamp and then was excised from the surrounding breast tissue. Hemostasis

was maintained with electrocautery, and then the breast tissue was reapproximated using 2 and 3-0 chromic. The skin was closed using 4-0 Vicryl in a subcuticular fashion. Steri-Strips were applied at the conclusion of the procedure. The patient tolerated the procedure well and was returned to the recovery area in stable condition. At the end of the procedure, all sponges and instruments were accounted for.

Pathology Report Later Indicated: See Report 5-32B.

SERVICE CODE(S): _____

ICD-10-CM DX CODE(S): _____

(Answers to every other Case are located in Appendix D . The full answer key is only available in the TEACH Instructor Resources on Evolve.)

CASE 5-32B *Pathology Report*

Assign codes for the pathologist.

LOCATION: Outpatient, Hospital

PATIENT: Donna Senne

SURGEON: Gary Sanchez, MD

PATHOLOGIST: Grey Lonewolf, MD

CLINICAL HISTORY: Right abnormal mammogram

SPECIMEN RECEIVED: Right breast biopsy

GROSS DESCRIPTION: The specimen is labeled with the patient's name and "right breast biopsy" and consists of a biopsy of white-tan lobulated tissue with adipose at the periphery, 4.7 × 3.5 × 2.0 cm (centimeter). Surgical margins are inked black. Cut sections show a white-tan, moderately firm, lobulated, somewhat glistening lesion, 3.5 × 2.8 × 1.6 cm. The lesion shows solid white-tan tissue throughout. Representative sections are submitted in six cassettes.

MICROSCOPIC DESCRIPTION: Sections show a well-circumscribed lesion showing a mildly cellular stroma consisting of spindled cells showing no cell atypia or mitotic activity. There is proliferation of variably sized glands with focal leaflike processes protruding into cystic spaces. Many of the ducts are collapsed into slitlike spaces. The epithelial elements consist of luminal epithelial cells and a myoepithelial layer.

DIAGNOSIS: Right breast biopsy: Benign fibroadenoma

SERVICE CODE(S): _____

ICD-10-CM DX CODE(S): _____

(Answers to every other Case are located in Appendix D . The full answer key is only available in the TEACH Instructor Resources on Evolve.)

CASE 5-33A *Operative Report, Breast Biopsy with Needle Localization*

This patient presents for the removal of a breast lesion that was previously marked prior to surgery with a radiological marker. Microcalcification of the breast is fibrosis of the breast.

LOCATION: Outpatient, Hospital

PATIENT: Marilyn Agnes

SURGEON: Gary Sanchez, MD

PREOPERATIVE DIAGNOSIS: Right breast microcalcification by mammogram

POSTOPERATIVE DIAGNOSIS: Right breast microcalcification by mammogram

PROCEDURE PERFORMED: Right breast biopsy with needle localization

ANESTHESIA: 1% Xylocaine local; 16 cc (cubic centimeter) was used. The patient also received IV (intravenous) sedation.

INDICATIONS FOR SURGERY: The patient is a 77-year-old white female who had undergone mammography. The patient was found to have microcalcifications in her right breast. The patient was taken to the operating room for biopsy.

DESCRIPTION OF PROCEDURE: The patient had previously undergone needle localization on the right breast microcalcification. She was brought back to the operating room. The patient was then prepped and draped in the usual manner. One percent Xylocaine was used as local anesthesia; a total of 16 cc was used. The patient also received IV sedation. An incision was made over the guidewire. The guidewire and surrounding breast tissue were incised and sent to pathology. Hemostasis was obtained using Bovie cautery. The operative area was thoroughly irrigated. The incision was then closed with figure-of-eight 2-0 chromic sutures for the deep and superficial layers. The skin was closed with 4-0 Vicryl subcuticular stitch, and Steri-Strips were applied. The patient tolerated the operation and returned to recovery in stable condition.

Pathology Report Later Indicated: See Report 5-33B.

SERVICE CODE(S): _____

ICD-10-CM DX CODE(S): _____

(Answers to every other Case are located in Appendix D . The full answer key is only available in the TEACH Instructor Resources on Evolve.)

CASE 5-33B *Pathology Report*

Assign codes for the pathologist.

LOCATION: Outpatient, Hospital

PATIENT: Marilyn Agnes

SURGEON: Gary Sanchez, MD

PATHOLOGIST: Grey Lonewolf, MD

CLINICAL HISTORY: Right breast microcalcification

SPECIMEN RECEIVED: Right breast biopsy after wire localization

GROSS DESCRIPTION: Submitted in formalin and labeled with the patient's name and "right breast biopsy after wire localization" is a piece of lobulated yellow fatty tissue measuring 6.5 × 4 × 1.5 cm (centimeter) with an intact localizing wire. First, serial sections are submitted in cassettes 1-3, and sections from the region of the wire tip are submitted in cassettes 4-7. No gross lesion is identified. No gross lesions are identified in the remainder of the specimen, and representative sections are submitted in cassettes 8-12.

MICROSCOPIC DESCRIPTION: The slides show multiple sections of breast parenchyma featuring prominent adipose tissue replacement. A focus of mild fibrosis with coarse microcalcifications is present on slide 4, corresponding to the abnormality seen on accompanying specimen mammogram.

DIAGNOSIS: Breast, right, biopsy:

1. Focal fibrosis with coarse microcalcifications, corresponding to the abnormality seen on accompanying specimen mammogram.
2. Adipose tissue replacement of breast parenchyma.

SERVICE CODE(S): _____

ICD-10-CM DX CODE(S): _____

(Answers to every other Case are located in Appendix D . The full answer key is only available in the TEACH Instructor Resources on Evolve.)

CASE 5-34 *Operative Report, Segmental Mastectomy with Sentinel Node Injection*

Glory Nisley had cancer of the right breast, and in this operative report, Dr. Sanchez performed a segmental mastectomy that removed a portion of her breast. Additionally, the surgeon injected dye into the patient, and when the dye reached the lymph nodes, the node appeared blue, which is "a hot node." The hot node was sampled and sent to the pathology lab for analysis. This injection procedure would be used when a lymphadenectomy (removal of the lymph node) is performed to ensure that all of the positive nodes are removed. The sentinel node injection procedure is reported separately. Do not report the frozen sections, as this would be reported by the pathologist. Assign the codes for the physician for the surgical procedure.

LOCATION: Outpatient, Hospital

PATIENT: Glory Nisley

SURGEON: Gary Sanchez, MD

PREOPERATIVE DIAGNOSIS: Cancer of right breast

POSTOPERATIVE DIAGNOSIS: Cancer of right breast

PROCEDURE PERFORMED: Segmental mastectomy with frozen-section margins, sentinel node biopsy times two, limited axillary dissection

ANESTHESIA: General

PROCEDURE: The patient was given a general anesthetic. I used 3 cc of isosulfan blue, and I injected just lateral to the cavity. I massaged for 5 minutes. Her right arm was free draped, and she was prepped and draped in this position. We marked 2 cm (centimeter) on every margin superior, inferior, medially, and laterally. We then developed our superior flap and went down to the chest wall. We developed the inferior flap and went down to chest wall. We then removed this segmental mastectomy going from medial to lateral. We oriented it with silk suture for pathological assessment. The frozen section margins came back negative. We then made an incision in the right axilla. We went down to the clavipectoral fascia and opened it up. We identified a very hot node that was blue. The counts are well documented in the chart. We sent another node, which was right against the first sentinel node. Both these nodes were blue. Once we got the second node out, our background was negligible. We sent both of these out for frozen section. We did a tissue to make sure that we did not have a false-negative result. After waiting, we found that the sentinel node biopsies times two were also benign. We then put a medium Hemovac drain in both sites and sutured the drains in place with silk sutures. We brought the subcutaneous tissue together with Vicryl. Staples were placed in the skin. Telfa, toppers, and gauze were applied. The patient tolerated the procedure well and went to the recovery room in good condition.

Pathology Report Later Indicated: Primary carcinoma of breast tissue

SERVICE CODE(S): _____

ICD-10-CM DX CODE(S): _____

(Answers to every other Case are located in Appendix D . The full answer key is only available in the TEACH Instructor Resources on Evolve.)

CASE 5-35A   *Preoperative Consultation*

This is an E/M service at which a decision for surgery was made, which might require the use of modifier -57 on the E/M code. You report not only the diagnosis of breast mass but also the history of malignant breast neoplasm.

LOCATION: Outpatient, Clinic

PATIENT: Ann Rose

PHYSICIAN: Ronald Green, MD

CONSULTANT: Gary Sanchez

Mrs. Rose is a lady who in 1990 had a left modified radical mastectomy for breast cancer. She apparently had at least five lymph nodes positive at that time and underwent chemotherapy, and she has been symptom-free since then. She states that earlier in October, she noticed that there was a lump present in her right breast, which had not been there before. She only examines herself intermittently, and she says probably once about every 6 to 8 weeks. There has been no pain, no nipple discharge, and no history of trauma. She has had a partial evaluation by Dr. Green, who has requested this consultation, including a bone scan and chest x-ray for the possibility of metastatic disease. The patient is otherwise doing well. She apparently lost her husband 8 years ago. He died of cancer, and she is concerned because her daughter's mother-in-law also has cancer at the present time and apparently not doing well.

PHYSICAL EXAMINATION shows a lady who is very bright and oriented. Cervical and supraclavicular examination shows a soft lymph node in the posterior triangle of the left neck. There are no carotid bruits. The mastectomy site on the left has healed reasonably well. There is no evidence of any lymphadenopathy, and there is no evidence of recurrence. On the right side, in the 2 o'clock position, approximately 7 cm (centimeter) from the areola, there is a firm to hard mass that is approximately 2 cm in diameter. It is mobile within the breast tissue and not fixed to either the skin or the deeper structures. There is no evidence of any axillary node involvement. Periareolar area is normal.

Examination of the mammograms suggests a 2- to 2.5-cm lesion in the area of the palpable mass, and this is certainly suspicious for malignancy.

I went over in detail with the patient and her daughters the various options for her, but the patient basically wants to proceed with the biopsy of the area. Then, if it is malignant, she wants a mastectomy done at the same time. We did go through the risks of the procedure, and she is aware of these. I also reviewed in detail the other options, which would include lumpectomy with radiation therapy and chemotherapy, simple mastectomy with radiation, and axillary dissection, etc. After going through these, she says that she really is not inclined to proceed with anything other than the biopsy and breast resection, a modified radical, as indicated at the time of surgery, and she only wants to undergo one anesthetic. She apparently had significant problems with the biopsy the last time, and she does not want to proceed with this at this time. Consequently, we will be proceeding with the procedure. Because she is taking aspirin, even though it is only 80 mg (milligram) a day, we will stop that today, and we will do the biopsy and probably mastectomy next week because I do feel this is most likely malignant.

Total time spent with patient today was 35 minutes.

SERVICE CODE(S): _____

ICD-10-CM DX CODE(S): _____

(Answers to every other Case are located in Appendix D . The full answer key is only available in the TEACH Instructor Resources on Evolve.)

CASE 5-35B   *Operative Report, Modified Radical Mastectomy*

Assign codes for the surgeon only.

LOCATION: Inpatient, Hospital

PATIENT: Ann Rose

PHYSICIAN: Ronald Green, MD

SURGEON: Gary Sanchez, MD

PREOPERATIVE DIAGNOSIS: Lump in the right breast, upper, inner quadrant

POSTOPERATIVE DIAGNOSIS: Infiltrating intraductal carcinoma of the right breast

PROCEDURES PERFORMED: Right breast biopsy followed by a modified radical mastectomy with level II axillary dissection

This lady, in 1990, had a left mastectomy for breast cancer. This was done in Manytown, and she does not remember the surgeon's name. However, she presented with a mass in the right breast, and in further discussions had decided that, should this turn out to be a malignancy, then she wanted immediate mastectomy. She was not interested in breast reconstruction, nor was she interested in any other form of therapy such as lumpectomy. Risks have been explained in detail to her and her daughter.

Under general anesthesia, the right breast was prepped and draped, and then an incision was made parallel to a skin crease approximately 5 cm (centimeter) away from the areola at the 2 o'clock position. Because of the clinical characteristics, there was high probability of malignancy, and the incision was placed in such a way that we could do the mastectomy as necessary with minimal risk. The skin incision was made, and then the lump itself was removed without difficulty. Electrocautery was not used because of the concern for interference with the histology. Once the lesion was removed, however, small bleeders were controlled with electrocautery. The skin was then closed with a subcuticular 4-0 Vicryl. At this time, the specimen was reviewed by pathology, and they confirmed the presence of probably a grade 2 infiltrating intraductal carcinoma.

The patient's drapes were removed, and then the right breast and axilla were prepped and draped secondarily. All surgeons also changed. Once this was completed, then a standard right modified radical mastectomy was completed to incorporate the incision from the biopsy site. The upper flap was able to be developed and not enter the biopsy site. The vessels were either suture ligated for the larger penetrating vessels or ligated and/or cauterized for the small flaps. Once the upper flap was developed, then the lower flap was developed in such a way that there would be an adequate amount of skin for closure. The axillary dissection was performed by initially dissecting along the pectoralis major and minor muscles, and the dissection stopped just at the pectoralis minor border. However, there was one lymph node that was more palpable up in probably a level III area, and because of this palpable nature, this was removed as an isolated

Continued

CASE 5-35B—cont'd

node and marked for the pathologist. The majority of the dissection of the axilla was completed with blunt and then sharp dissection, but the larger lymphatics were ligated with 3-0 Vicryl. The arteries were ligated with 3-0 Vicryl as well. The intercostal brachial nerves were identified and preserved with the exception of one small branch, which went through a fairly dense area but was thought to be lymph nodes, and consequently this small branch was sacrificed. At completion of this procedure, the breast was then removed from the chest wall using electrocautery and, as noted above, the larger vessels being suture-ligated with 3-0 Vicryl. After the breast was removed, the entire area was irrigated. There were no further bleedings that required any intervention other than mild cautery. At this point, no. 10 Jackson-Pratts were placed, one into the axilla, and one into the subcuticular tissue through two separate

stab wounds in the inferior flap. The skin was then approximated by using 2-0 Vicryl to approximate the deeper fatty tissue and then subcuticular 4-0 Vicryl for the skin. Half-inch Steri-Strips were then applied. The drains were sutured in place using 3-0 nylon, and then the dressing was applied around these.

Total blood loss was less than 100 ml (milliliter). The patient tolerated the procedure well. Further care will depend on the pathology in this area.

Pathology Report Later Indicated: See Report 5-35C.

SERVICE CODE(S): _____

ICD-10-CM DX CODE(S): _____

(Answers to every other Case are located in Appendix D . The full answer key is only available in the TEACH Instructor Resources on Evolve.)

CASE 5-35C   *Pathology Report*

LOCATION: Inpatient, Hospital

PATIENT: Ann Rose

PHYSICIAN: Ronald Green, MD

SURGEON: Gary Sanchez, MD

PATHOGIST: Morton Monson, MD

CLINICAL HISTORY:

1. Lesion, right breast, upper inner quadrant
2. Suture at superior apical
3. Apical node (separate), just anterior axillary

TISSUE RECEIVED:

A. RT breast BX (FS)
A. RT breast BX (PS)
B. RT breast suture in apex
C. Apical node, right axilla

GROSS DESCRIPTION:

A. The specimen is labeled with the patient's name and "mass right breast" and consists of a piece of yellow and white fibrofatty tissue, 3.8 × 2.5 × 2 cm (centimeter). Sectioning reveals a white solid mass measuring 2 × 1.8 × 1.4 cm with spiculated border.

INTRAOPERATIVE FROZEN SECTION DIAGNOSIS: As per Dr. Monson: Infiltrating ductal carcinoma.

B. The specimen is labeled with the patient's name and "right breast" and consists of the product of a right modified radical

mastectomy with skin ellipse measuring 23 × 12 cm with centrally placed everted nipple. Biopsy site is noted in the upper medial portion. Biopsy cavity reveals hemorrhagic tan tissue. No distinct evidence of residual neoplasm is seen. Representative section of nipple is placed in cassette labeled B1. Representative sections of biopsy site are placed in cassettes labeled B2 through B8. The remainder of the breast parenchyma is composed primarily of fat with occasional fibrous strands. Random representative sections of breast are placed in cassettes labeled B9 through B10. Sections of axillary tail reveal multiple lymph nodes ranging from 1 cm down to 0.3 cm.

C. The specimen is labeled with the patient's name and "apical node right axilla" and consists of a 0.5-cm diameter apparent lymph node.

MICROSCOPIC DESCRIPTION:

A. Sections of breast showing an infiltrating neoplasm consisting of sheets, cords, and nests of cells infiltrating the desmoplastic stroma. Cells are enlarged and have increased nuclear-cytoplasmic ratio.
B. Lymph nodes were negative for malignancy with normal cells throughout.

SERVICE CODE(S): _____

ICD-10-CM DX CODE(S): _____

(Answers to every other Case are located in Appendix D . The full answer key is only available in the TEACH Instructor Resources on Evolve.)

CASE 5-35D   *Discharge Summary*

LOCATION: Inpatient, Hospital

PATIENT: Ann Rose

PHYSICIAN: Ronald Green, MD

SURGEON: Gary Sanchez, MD

REASON FOR HOSPITALIZATION: Right breast mass

BRIEF HISTORY: This patient had left mastectomy for breast cancer in 1990. She was now found to have a right breast mass and decided that should this turn out to be a malignancy she wanted an immediate mastectomy.

HOSPITAL COURSE: The patient underwent a right breast biopsy with frozen section showing infiltrating ductal carcinoma. At that time, a right modified radical mastectomy was performed. The patient tolerated the

CASE 5-35D—cont'd

procedure well and was transferred to the floor with two Jackson-Pratt drains in place. The patient's pain was controlled after surgery quite nicely. On postoperative day one, the patient was voiding without difficulty and tolerating her diet. She remained afebrile. Her wound did not show any signs of infection or drainage throughout her hospital course. The remainder of the patient's hospital course was uneventful, and she went home with her axillary Jackson-Pratt drain in place. Pathology on the specimen did reveal infiltrating ductal carcinoma grade 2 of 3 on her right breast. Six of six axillary nodes did not show any evidence of malignancy. One separate axillary node also did not show evidence of malignancy.

FOLLOW-UP: The patient was scheduled to return to the clinic in three to four days for follow-up and drain removal.

DISCHARGE INSTRUCTIONS:

1. Activity as tolerated
2. Diet as tolerated

DISCHARGE MEDICATIONS:

1. Lotensin 10 mg (milligram) 1 p.o. (by mouth) q.d. (every day).
2. Metoprolol 25 mg 1 p.o. b.i.d. (twice a day).
3. Tylenol no. 3, 1-2 p.o. q.4-6h. (every 4 to 6 hours) as needed for pain. The patient was sent home with 25.

PRINCIPAL DIAGNOSIS: Infiltrating ductal carcinoma grade 2 of 3, right breast, upper inner quadrant. Six of six axillary lymph nodes were negative. Now status post right modified radical mastectomy.

PRINCIPAL PROCEDURE: Right breast biopsy followed by a modified radical mastectomy with level II axillary dissection.

CONDITION ON DISCHARGE: Stable

SERVICE CODE(S): _____

ICD-10-CM DX CODE(S): _____

(Answers to every other Case are located in Appendix D . The full answer key is only available in the TEACH Instructor Resources on Evolve.)

CASE 5-35E   *Progress Note*

This is a postoperative visit. The reason for the service is a follow up after surgery. A history of cancer code is not reported since the patient is still being followed for cancer, with her current referral to the oncologist.

LOCATION: Outpatient, Clinic

PATIENT: Ann Rose

PHYSICIAN: Ronald Green, MD

SURGEON: Gary Sanchez, MD

Mrs. Rose is now several weeks after her right modified mastectomy for invasive carcinoma of the breast. She had previous carcinoma of the breast and mastectomy in 1990. The patient states that she just had a fullness under her arms. She has noticed no problems with arm motion other than just a little bit of stiffening when she raises it above her head. She has no swelling of the arm.

PHYSICAL EXAMINATION: She is alert and oriented. Her chest is clear. The mastectomy site is healing well. There is a fold of fatty tissue in the posterior axillary area that is still a little edematous, and there is a mild amount of edema on the inferior flap on the medial aspect. Other than this, there is no sign of infection or fluid collections. The patient can move her arm relatively well. She is able to put the arm and hand up above her head.

The area is healing well. We did go over the issue regarding the swelling in these areas. She does not want anything done with respect to the fat fold in the area. I did caution her regarding the area of the swelling that if it gets worse or if there are any changes in the skin color, etc. Otherwise, I will see her in about a month's time for follow-up, and she is going to be seeing the surgical oncologist in the near future regarding any further therapy.

SERVICE CODE(S): _____

ICD-10-CM DX CODE(S): _____

(Answers to every other Case are located in Appendix D . The full answer key is only available in the TEACH Instructor Resources on Evolve.)

CASE 5-36   *Operative Report, Breast Reduction*

Linda Halaas has been admitted to the hospital for a bilateral breast reduction. The admission for breast reduction is the first listed code and is reported with a Z code. The additional diagnoses are those conditions that support the reason the breast reduction is being performed. Report the services provided to her by Dr. Erickson, the clinic's plastic surgeon.

LOCATION: Inpatient, Hospital

PATIENT: Linda Halaas

SURGEON: Mark Erickson, MD

PREOPERATIVE DIAGNOSIS:

1. Bilateral mammary hypertrophy and hyperplasia
2. Bilateral mammary ptosis

POSTOPERATIVE DIAGNOSIS:

1. Bilateral mammary hypertrophy and hyperplasia
2. Bilateral mammary ptosis

PROCEDURE PERFORMED: Bilateral breast reduction using inferior pedicle technique.

1. 615 g (gram) resected from the right side
2. 609 g from the left side

ANESTHESIA: General endotracheal with 225 cc (cubic centimeter) of tumescent solution on the right side and 200 cc of tumescent solution on the left side. Tumescent solution was prepared by adding to 1 L of Ringer's lactate, 25 cc of 2% Xylocaine, 1 cc of 1:100,000 epinephrine, and 3 cc of 8.4% sodium bicarbonate.

Continued

CASE 5-36—cont'd

ESTIMATED BLOOD LOSS: 75 cc

DRAINS: None

SPONGE AND NEEDLE COUNTS: Correct

COMPLICATIONS: None

SURGICAL FINDINGS: Predominantly fatty breasts with fibrocystic disease obvious throughout both breasts, particularly around the periareolar area

DESCRIPTION OF PROCEDURE: The patient's chest was prepped with Betadine scrub and solution and draped in a routine sterile fashion. In accordance with the preoperatively marked new nipple site at 22 cm (centimeter) from the sternal notch and 12.5 cm from the midsternal line, we marked out an inferior pedicle breast pattern using the 45-mm (millimeter) cookie cutter marker for the new areolar size and the new areolar window. We marked the 12, 6, 9, and 3 o'clock positions at these points, and then we resumed our marking of the inferior pedicle, making the vertical limb 5 cm long. After marking of the inferior pedicle pattern, de-epithelialization of the right side was carried out, leaving about a 1.5-cm cuff of the de-epithelialized tissue above the areola. Deep dissection started at the 12 o'clock position and came toward the 3 o'clock position between the upper end of the vertical limb and the lateral edge of the medial flap. We began to bevel away from the vertical limb, starting at the caudal edge of the medial flap and connecting with the inframammary incision. An incision was then made on the caudal edge of the medial flap to connect to the apex of the triangle with the inframammary incision, and we carried this down the pectoralis major fascia, resecting the medial triangle at that level. Bleeding was electrocoagulated using the insulated forceps for the cautery directly. At the edge of the pedicle, we used a no. 22 knife blade to incise down to pectoralis major fascia. Deep dissection was then started at the 12 o'clock position and came toward the 9 o'clock position coming between the upper and the vertical limb and the medial edge of the lateral flap. We began to bevel away from the vertical limb, starting at the caudal edge of the lateral flap, and we made our incision near the vertical limb with a no. 22 knife blade down to the pectoralis major fascia, connecting it at the inframammary level and the incision on the caudal edge of the lateral flap at the pectoralis major fascia. The incision on the caudal edge of the lateral flap was made in such a manner as to leave 1.5 mm of thickness on the flap and to include the tail of Spence in the resection. Hemostasis was achieved, and then we divided the lateral and medial flaps completely from the upper end of the vertical limb but did not extend this down to the pectoralis major fascia. The skin was dissected away from the superior triangular area, and then we resected the superior triangle by connecting our lateral and medial flap incisions between the respective vertical limbs with a periareolar window incision superiorly. After appropriate resection and trimming, we obtained a final weight of 615 g (gram) on the right side. The estimated amount was 750 g. I then separated the dermis from the skin inferiorly, and at the midpoint of the vertical limb, I inset the lateral and medial flaps with a horizontal half mattress suture of 0 Prolene. The points marked at the 3, 6, 9, and 12 o'clock positions were inset with subcuticular 3-0 Monocryl, and then the vertical limb was closed with an interrupted 3-0 Monocryl using subcuticular 3-0 Monocryl also for the inframammary limb. Where better apposition of the skin edges and eversion were needed, we used skin staples, particularly in the area of the areola. The circulation was excellent in the nipple areolar complex, and there was no apparent ischemia of either flap. The left breast was then approached in a similar manner, but we made the pedicle about 9 cm wide instead of 8 cm wide as on the right side. We had instilled 225 cc of tumescent solution in the right side, and we instilled 200 cc of tumescent solution in the left side through junctional incisions. I then de-epithelialized the vertical stalk and left a 1.5-cm cuff of de-epithelialized tissue above. Deep dissection was started at the 12 o'clock position and came, with the cautery, toward the 9 o'clock between the upper end of the vertical limb and the medial flap, beveling away from the vertical limb starting at the caudal edge of the medial flap and connecting with the inframammary incision, and an incision on the caudal edge of the medial flap was made in such a manner as to leave 1.5 cm of thickness on the flap. After resection of the medial triangle, a lateral triangle resection was started at the 12 o'clock position and came toward the 3 o'clock position, coming between the upper end of the vertical limb and the lateral flap. I then resected the lateral triangle by connecting with the lateral flap in such a manner as to leave 1.5 cm of thickness of the flap and to include the tail of Spence in the resection. The superior triangle was then resected, and hemostasis was obtained using the cautery. A no. 22 knife blade was used to make the incision near the vertical pedicle, and following separation of the dermis inferiorly of the vertical pedicle, I inset the lateral and medial flaps with a horizontal mattress suture of 0 Prolene. A running subcuticular suture was used for the inframammary area, and a few interrupted sutures of 3-0 Monocryl were used for the areolar inset and the vertical limb. Skin staples were used to appose the edges better, and the dressing consisted of Xeroform, Kerlix fluffs, a support bra, and an external Ace bandage. Estimated blood loss was 75 cc. The patient seemed to tolerate the procedure well and left the operating room in good condition.

Pathology Report Later Indicated: Benign breast tissue

SERVICE CODE(S): _____

ICD-10-CM DX CODE(S): _____

(Answers to every other Case are located in Appendix D . The full answer key is only available in the TEACH Instructor Resources on Evolve.)

CASE 5-37   *Operative Report, Breast Augmentation*

The reason for this service is for admission for breast augmentation. Remember to use the bilateral modifier on this service as a breast augmentation code reports the procedure on only one breast. Report the surgeon's service.

LOCATION: Inpatient, Hospital

PATIENT: Sheila Lynch

SURGEON: Mark Erickson, MD

INDICATIONS FOR PROCEDURE: The patient has bilateral mammary hypoplasia following childbirth and wants to have an increase in breast volume just to fill out her clothes.

PREOPERATIVE DIAGNOSIS: Bilateral mammary hypoplasia

POSTOPERATIVE DIAGNOSIS: Bilateral mammary hypoplasia

PROCEDURE PERFORMED: Bilateral breast augmentation using McGhan style 468, 195-205 cc (cubic centimeter) implant inflated to 205 cc. Lot number was 441693. The left side had a number designation of 4488. The right had 4489.

ANESTHESIA: General endotracheal plus 5 cc of 1% Xylocaine with 1:100,000 epinephrine and 250 cc total of tumescent solution prepared by adding 25 cc of 2% Xylocaine, 1 cc of 1:100,00 epinephrine, and 3 cc of 8.4% sodium bicarbonate to 1 L of Ringer's lactate.

ESTIMATED BLOOD LOSS: Negligible

DESCRIPTION OF PROCEDURE: The patient's chest was prepped with Betadine scrub and solution and draped in a routine sterile fashion. Incision was made over the sixth rib and carried down through the subcutaneous tissue and fascia to the pectoralis muscle origin, which we incised along the rib, elevating it off of the rib and taking care not to dissect down on the rib or traumatize rib. We injected 150 cc of tumescent solution on the right side in the subpectoral space and used balloon dissection to further elevate the pectoralis muscle rapidly. Dissection was completed by sharp and blunt medially and inferiorly to detach the pectoralis insertion fibers. After detachment of those fibers, we inserted a balloon dissector and inflated to about 300 cc. We then went to the left side and made an incision over the sixth rib and dissected using the balloon dissector with some difficulty inserting 200-cc sizer. We left the balloon dissector in. We did insert the mammary sizer at this time. We left the balloon dissector in, went to the left side, made an incision over the sixth rib after injection of 1% Xylocaine and 1:100,000 epinephrine, carried down to the pectoralis fascia, incising the pectoralis major muscle, entering the subpectoral space where we injected 100 cc of tumescent solution, and then used the balloon dissector to elevate the pectoralis off the chest wall. We completed our pocket dissection, sharp and blunt dissection, and left the balloon dissector in place. We then went to the right side and removed the balloon dissector with some difficulty inserting a 200-cc sizer. The pocket was somewhat asymmetrical at this time, and we did further blunt dissection to enlarge the pocket. We went to the left side and removed our balloon dissector, completing the pocket dissection with very little bleeding. We inserted an inflatable saline implant, McGhan style 468, which we inflated to a total of 5 cc in the submuscular, subpectoral pocket. The muscle was closed with interrupted 3-0 Ethibond, the fascial layer was closed with interrupted 4-0 Vicryl, and a subcuticular Vicryl was used to complete the closure with a few twists of 6-0 Prolene. Steri-Strips were applied. On the right side, the pocket was clipped and completed to achieve symmetry, and after removal of the expander, we inserted the partially inflated McGhan style 468 with all the air removed, and after insertion of the pocket, we completed the filling to 205 cc. This brought the right breast implant into better asymmetry with the left side. Then we closed the muscle pocket with interrupted 3-0 Ethibond using interrupted 4-0 Vicryl for the fascial layer and subcuticular 4-0 Vicryl followed by a few twists of 6-0 Prolene. Steri-Strips were applied. Dressing consisted of the Steri-Strips, Kerlix fluffs, Kerlix roll, Kling, and an Ace bandage. Estimated blood loss was negligible. The patient tolerated the procedure well and left the operating room in good condition.

SERVICE CODE(S): _____

ICD-10-CM DX CODE(S): _____

(Answers to every other Case are located in Appendix D . The full answer key is only available in the TEACH Instructor Resources on Evolve.)

CASE 5-38   *Operative Report, Removal of Tissue Expander*

The reason for this service is a complication of a breast prosthetic, which was a tissue expander that was previously implanted and now is leaking. A tissue expander is placed status post mastectomy to stretch the skin and can be a sac of fluid or air, or a plastic insert. The stretched skin can be harvested for skin grafting or as in this case, placed to expand the skin to allow for a breast implant at a later date. When the implant malfunctions, such as the one in this case that is leaking, it is considered a mechanical complication.

ICD-10-CM: Reference the Index of the ICD-10-CM, under the main term "Complication" followed by subterms, "breast implant [prosthetic], mechanical leakage," to be directed to the correct code.

LOCATION: Outpatient, Hospital

PATIENT: Donna Polanski

SURGEON: Gary Sanchez, MD

PREOPERATIVE DIAGNOSIS: Status post tissue expansion, left breast, with 500-cc (cubic centimeter) tissue expander

POSTOPERATIVE DIAGNOSIS: Status post tissue expansion, left breast, with 500-cc tissue expander

SURGICAL FINDINGS: There was some exudate on the breast implant. There was a small amount of serosanguineous fluid within the pocket that appeared to be old. The capsule was very thin, and it was felt that it was indicated to leave this capsule intact.

Continued

CASE 5-38—cont'd

SURGICAL PROCEDURE: Removal of tissue expander, left breast, with reinsertion of 440-cc inflatable McGhan implant. See details and appropriate labeling for model number.

ANESTHESIA: General endotracheal; approximately 3 cc of 1% Xylocaine with 1:100,000 epinephrine were used for the incision line.

ESTIMATED BLOOD LOSS: Negligible

DESCRIPTION OF PROCEDURE: The patient was prepped with Betadine scrub and solution and draped in a routine sterile fashion. The Betadine was removed from the incision site, and the scar was outlined with a fine marker. We injected 3 cc of 1% Xylocaine with 1:100,000 epinephrine along the suture line and excised the scar down to the capsule of the breast, which was opened with the cutting cautery set at 30. I noted that there was some exudate within the capsule, and culture and sensitivity of this were obtained. The cavity itself contained a small amount of serosanguineous fluid, perhaps 5 cc or so, and this was thought to be old and nonintroduced. We irrigated the pocket with about 250 cc of Ringer's lactate, and then

I inspected the anterior aspect of the expander. There was some leakage upon rather extreme pressure from around the injection site, but this was minimal, and it was only produced with extreme pressure. The breast implant, which was a 440-460 McGhan inflatable textured anatomic-type implant, was inflated to 300 cc, and the air was removed from the implant. It was inserted in the pocket, and the complete inflation of the implant was then carried out, inflating it to 440 cc. The expander tube was then removed, and the capsule itself was closed with interrupted 2-0 Ethibond, following which the subcuticular layer was done with interrupted 4-0 Monocryl. One twist of 6-0 Prolene was placed in the lateral aspect of the incision, and Steri-Strips were applied. Kerlix fluffs and a support bra were applied. The patient tolerated the procedure well and left the area in good condition.

SERVICE CODE(S): _____

ICD-10-CM DX CODE(S): _____

(Answers to every other Case are located in Appendix D . The full answer key is only available in the TEACH Instructor Resources on Evolve.)

CHAPTER 5   *Auditing Review*

Audit the coding for the following reports.

Audit Report 5.1 Operative Report, Biopsy

LOCATION: Inpatient, Hospital

PATIENT: Arvid Comer

SURGEON: Mohomad Almaz, MD

ATTENDING PHYSICIAN: Mohomad Almaz, MD

PREOPERATIVE DIAGNOSIS: Cellulitis of the right hip

POSTOPERATIVE DIAGNOSIS: Cellulitis of the right hip

OPERATIVE PROCEDURE: Biopsy of the right hip cellulitis

ANESTHESIA: 1% Xylocaine

INDICATIONS FOR PROCEDURE: The patient is a 73-year-old Caucasian male who is critically ill. The patient has developed cellulitis of his right hip, and a biopsy was needed for diagnostic purposes for culture.

DESCRIPTION OF PROCEDURE: The patient was prepped with Betadine solution. One percent Xylocaine was used as local. An elliptical incision was used to excise a segment of skin. The segment of skin was divided for microbiology examination and also pathologic examination. The specimens were sent. Hemostasis was obtained using pressure. The incision was then approximated with 3-0 nylon suture. Dressing was applied. The patient tolerated the procedure.

One of the following codes is reported incorrectly for this case. Indicate the incorrect code.

PROFESSIONAL SERVICES: Hip biopsy, **27040**

ICD-10-CM DX: Lower limb cellulitis, **L03.115**

INCORRECT CODE: _____

Audit Report 5.2 Operative Report, Debridement

LOCATION: Inpatient, Hospital

PATIENT: Paul O'Reilly

SURGEON: Mark Erickson, MD

PREOPERATIVE DIAGNOSIS: Multiple wounds of left leg and left thigh.

POSTOPERATIVE DIAGNOSIS: Multiple wounds of left leg and left thigh (four wounds).

SURGICAL FINDINGS:

1. 20 × 10 cm open wound of the medial aspect of the left leg that is clean.
2. 20 × 7 cm left lower leg lateral wound that is clean.
3. 24 × 11 left lateral thigh wound that is clean with exposed fascia.
4. 13 × 1.5 cm wound of the left anterior thigh with gangrenous fat within the wound.

PROCEDURE PERFORMED:

1. Debridement of wound left anterior aspect, left thigh.
2. Split-thickness skin graft from the right thigh to the medial aspect of the left leg measuring 20 × 10 cm.
3. Split-thickness skin graft from the right thigh to the lateral aspect of the left lower leg measuring 20 × 7 cm.
4. A split-thickness skin graft from the right thigh to the left lateral thigh measuring 24 × 11 cm.
5. Split-thickness skin graft from the right thigh to the left anterior thigh measuring 13 × 1.5 cm.

ESTIMATED BLOOD LOSS: Negligible.

ANESTHESIA: General endotracheal anesthesia.

DESCRIPTION OF PROCEDURE: The legs were prepped with Betadine scrub and solution, draped in a routine sterile fashion. The anterior left thigh wound was debrided and split-thickness skin grafts measuring 10,000th to 11,000th of an inch thick were taken from the right thigh, meshed with the 3:1 ratio mesher, and applied to all of the defects mentioned above of the left leg in the measurements noted. They were stapled to the wounds, mostly on the edges, and dressings then consisted of Xeroform, Kerlix fluffs, Kerlix roll, Kling and an Ace bandage. Estimated blood loss was negligible. Scarlet red was applied to the donor site. The patient tolerated the procedure well and left the area in good condition.

One of the codes is not reported for this case. Indicate the missing code.

PROFESSIONAL SERVICES: Split-thickness graft to left thigh and left leg, **15100, 15101 × 6**; Preparation of left anterior thigh for split-thickness graft, **15002-51**.

ICD-10-CM DX: Open wound left leg, **S81.802A**; Open wound of left thigh, **S71.102A**.

MISSING CODE: _____

Audit Report 5.3 Operative Report, Carcinoma Lower Lip

LOCATION: Inpatient, Hospital

PATIENT: Larry Montiff

SURGEON: Mark Erickson, MD

PREOPERATIVE DIAGNOSES:

1. Squamous cell carcinoma, left lower lip.
2. Submental and submandibular area mass.

POSTOPERATIVE DIAGNOSES: Same.

PROCEDURE PERFORMED:

1. Excision of squamous cell carcinoma in skin of the left lower lip, 3.25 cm.
2. Suprahyoid neck dissection.
3. Bilateral advancement flap closure of surgical defect, 16 square cm.

ANESTHESIA: Local with IV sedation.

ESTIMATED BLOOD LOSS: Less than 25 cc.

INDICATIONS: A 70-year-old male with a mass on the submental and submandibular areas. He has a recurrent squamous cell carcinoma with palpable mass in the submental area and patient is now here for definitive review and surgery.

Continued

CHAPTER 5—*cont'd*

DESCRIPTION OF PROCEDURE: After consent was obtained, the patient was taken to the operating room and placed on the operating room table in the supine position. After an adequate level of IV sedation was obtained, the patient's lower face and neck were prepped with Betadine and then draped in a sterile manner. The incision was outlined in the lower lip area down to the mental crease area. An incision was also marked on the upper neck in the medial aspect just above the hyoid bone. The incision was extended also to the left submandibular area. The area was then infiltrated with I cc of Xylocaine with 1:100,000 units of epinephrine.

Attention was first focused on the lip. Utilizing sharp dissection, full-thickness excision was accomplished to include mucosa and skin. Three-mm margins on each side were utilized. Frozen section reported squamous cell carcinoma, completely excised with negative margins. At the time that frozen section was being done, the neck was addressed. Sharp dissection was carried down to the skin and subcutaneous tissue. Superior and inferior subplatysmal flaps were elevated. The lymphoid tissue in the suprahyoid area extending from the submental area to the left proximal submandibular area was then dissected and removed along with the masses. Dissection was carried down to the digastric muscle fascia. Hemostasis was achieved with silk ties and bipolar cautery. That area was sprayed with HemaSeal and then the wound was closed with the deeper tissue approximated with

interrupted 4-0 Vicryl suture and the skin approximated with skin staples. Bacitracin ointment and a dressing were applied.

Attention was then refocused on the lip. Bilateral advancement flaps were developed again by extending the incision along the mental crease line. The mucosa was left intact. The flaps were approximated with interrupted 4-0 Vicryl suture; 4-0 Vicryl suture was then utilized in interrupted mattress closure fashion to close the mucocutaneous area of the lower lip, as well as the mucosa. The skin was approximated with interrupted closure of 6-0 nylon. Bacitracin ointment was then applied. The patient tolerated the procedure well. There was no break in technique. The patient was awakened and taken to the postanesthesia care unit in good condition.

One of the following codes is reported incorrectly for this case. Indicate the incorrect code.

PROFESSIONAL SERVICES: Suprahyoid neck dissection, **38700**; Bilateral advancement flaps, **14060-51**; Excision of left lower lip lesion, **11644-51**

ICD-10-CM DX: Neck mass, **R22.1**; Squamous cell carcinoma of the skin of the lip, **C44.02**

INCORRECT CODE: _____

Audit Report 5.4 Operative Report, Debridement

LOCATION: Inpatient, Hospital

PATIENT: Arnie Holmes

PREOPERATIVE DIAGNOSIS: Right heel ulcer

POSTOPERATIVE DIAGNOSIS: Right heel ulcer with *Staphylococcus aureus* infection

SURGEON: Gary Sanchez, MD

PROCEDURE PERFORMED: Debridement of right heel ulcer down to the bone

INDICATIONS FOR THIS PROCEDURE: Mr. Holmes is a 58-year-old male who has a large heel ulcer, measuring at least 7 cm × 3.5 cm in a curvilinear ovoid shape. This needs to be sharply debrided. There is a lot of necrotic tissue here. We need to see how deep this goes. We also need to obtain cultures. We need to determine for sure if he also has osteo. If he does have other ongoing infection (this is reportable), this will require antibiotic therapy. Cultures will be obtained of the deep tissues as well. The procedure and the risks were all discussed with the patient and his wife preoperatively. They understand, and their questions were answered. I also met with them in the preop holding room, and they had no new questions.

PROCEDURE: The more proximal aspect of this wound on the plantar aspect of the heel went deep, basically down to the bone. This was all sharply debrided back. We cleared some of the tissue overlying the bones there. The tissues were basically all necrotic down to there. We sent this off as a specimen. The remainder of the heel ulcer was not as deep. We sharply debrided the eschar off of it. We sharply debrided all of the edges of the wound. The tissues appeared to be viable there. I am somewhat concerned about how much deeper tissue of the foot and surrounding areas is necrotic. We appear to have some area of viability there. Hemostasis was achieved. We washed it out with a liter of antibiotic solution of Bacitracin and Kanamycin using an Ortholav system. The wound was packed open with wet-to-dry dressings. The patient tolerated the procedure well.

Pathology Report Later Indicated: *Staphylococcus aureus*

One or more of the following codes are reported incorrectly for this case. Indicate the incorrect code or codes.

SERVICE CODE(S):   Bone debridement, **11044, 11047**

ICD-10-CM DX CODE(S):   Pressure ulcer with muscle necrosis, right heel, **L97.413**

INCORRECT/MISSING CODE(S): _____

Audit Report 5.5 Operative Report, Malignant Melanoma

LOCATION: Outpatient, Hospital

PATIENT: Jane Love

SURGEON: Gary Sanchez, MD

PREOPERATIVE DIAGNOSIS: Large lipoma of the lower abdomen

POSTOPERATIVE DIAGNOSIS: Malignant melanoma, lower abdomen

PROCEDURE PERFORMED: Radical excision of large mass of the lower abdomen, which measured 9 cm × 12 cm

ANESTHESIA: General anesthesia

INDICATION: The patient has a mass in the lower back. This is becoming quite bothersome to her. We discussed treatment options of observation versus surgical excision. She wishes to have this excised. We discussed the procedure as well as the risk involved. She understands and wishes to proceed.

CHAPTER 5—cont'd

PROCEDURE: The patient was brought to the operating room and placed in the supine position on the operating table and received general anesthetic. She was prepped and draped in sterile fashion. The area of the mass was identified and marked out. This was an ovoid lesion measuring 9 × 12 cm. This was basically between the iliac crest and lower abdomen. An incision line down the central aspect of this in a transverse fashion was infiltrated with 0.5% Marcaine. After waiting a couple of minutes, an incision was made. Dissection was carried down into the subcutaneous tissues. We then sharply circumferentially dissected out a large lipomatous mass. This was quite large. This was sent to pathology and came back as malignant melanoma. To minimize scarring, we did not go all the way to the end with our skin incision; however, we were able to retract this up and dissect out the lipomatous mass from under it. This was taken out all the way down to the fascia. This was then removed in total. There did not appear to be any masses there. Hemostasis was achieved. This left a 12.5 cm open wound and the subcutaneous tissues were closed with layered sutures of 3-0 Vicryl. The skin was closed with 4-0 Vicryl in running subcuticular fashion. Steri-Strips and sterile dressings, multiple Fluffs and ABDs,

and then an Ace wrap were applied. The Ace wrap went around a few times across the lower abdomen and pelvic region as well as across the iliac structures to help provide pressure to the area and to decrease the chance of developing seromas or hematomas. The patient tolerated the procedure well and went to the recovery room in stable condition.

I met with the patient's mother postoperatively and discussed the diagnosis. Discharge instructions were discussed with the patient and her mother. I discussed a referral to oncology for further treatment. Their questions were answered.

Pathology Report Later Indicated: Malignant melanoma

One or more of the following codes are reported incorrectly for this case. Indicate the incorrect code or codes.

SERVICE CODE(S):   Excision malignant lesion, **11606**

ICD-10-CM DX CODE(S):   Malignant neoplasm of skin of trunk, **C44.509**

INCORRECT/MISSING CODE(S): _____

Audit Report 5.6 Operative Report, Laceration

LOCATION: Hospital Emergency Department

PATIENT: Brad Nelson

SURGEON: Paul Sutton, MD

PREOPERATIVE DIAGNOSIS: Complex eyebrow laceration, 2.8 cm.

POSTOPERATIVE DIAGNOSIS: Complex eyebrow laceration, 2.8 cm.

PROCEDURE PERFORMED: Cleaning and suturing of laceration.

ANESTHESIA: 1% Lidocaine with epinephrine.

INDICATIONS FOR PROCEDURE: The patient is a 12-year-old male who fell off a four-wheeler while driving it. The patient sustained a complex eyebrow laceration, and he is now undergoing repair.

PROCEDURE: The area was anesthetized with 1% Lidocaine with epinephrine. We then irrigated the area thoroughly. The wound was then scrubbed with Betadine. The entire skin area was prepped with the

same Betadine solution. Sterile dressings were placed around the wound. The wound was then closed in 2 layers, the first layer with interrupted 4-0 Vicryl suture. The skin was then closed with 5-0 interrupted nylon suture in the area of the eyebrow. The rest of the incision in both directions was closed with interrupted 6-0 nylon suture. This was a complex laceration. The wound was then covered with Bacitracin. The patient was then discharged home with a prescription for Keflex. He has had a recent tetanus shot, so this will not be necessary. He is instructed to follow up in 1 week to have the sutures removed.

One or more of the following codes are reported incorrectly for this case. Indicate the incorrect code or codes.

SERVICE CODE(S):   Complex repair, **13152** _____

ICD-10-CM DX CODE(S):   Periocular laceration, **S01.119** _____

INCORRECT/MISSING CODE(S): _____

(Auditing Review answers with rationales are only available in the TEACH Instructor Resources on Evolve.)

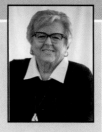

"Coders are a special group of people. They tend to be the investigative, intelligent, interested, and caring. They strive to always do their very best."

Cardiovascular System

http://evolve.elsevier.com/Buck/next

(Answers to every other Case are located in Appendix D, with the full answer key only available in the TEACH Instructor Resources on Evolve)
(Auditing Review answers with rationales are only available in the TEACH Instructor Resources on Evolve)

A cardiologist is a physician who specializes in diseases of the heart and vessels. A cardiothoracic surgeon is a physician who specializes in surgical procedures of the heart and chest. A variety of physicians frequently use the codes, as you will see as you code the services and procedures within this chapter. Examples of procedures include valve repair, beating heart surgery, aortic dissections, and excision of tumors of the chest wall.

When coding cardiovascular services, the coder will commonly use codes from the Evaluation/Management, Surgery, Medicine, and Radiology sections of the CPT manual.

The more common cardiovascular presenting problems are chest pain, hypertension, edema, murmur, mitral valve prolapse, palpitations, congestive heart failure, acute ischemia, abnormal stress tests, arrhythmias, congenital heart disease, syncope (fainting), hyperlipidemia, and claudication.

Evaluation and Management Services

Often the E/M services provided to a patient with a cardiac condition are very complex and extensive. The history and physical examination of the patient with a suspected cardiovascular condition are of critical importance to proper medical management of the patient. The physician has training, skills, knowledge, and experience that cannot be replaced by a laboratory test; rather, the tests assist the physician in the diagnosis process. Through the history and physical examination, the physician gathers a wide range of information necessary to diagnose the patient. For example, the symptom of chest pain, which is a cardinal manifestation of cardiac disease, could be caused by conditions of the aorta, pulmonary **artery,** bronchopulmonary tree, pleura, mediastinum, esophagus, diaphragm, tissues of the neck or thoracic wall (including the skin, thoracic muscles, cervicodorsal spine, costochondral junctions, breasts, sensory nerves, or spinal cord), stomach, duodenum, pancreas, or gallbladder. There are many potential causes for just one of the symptoms of cardiac disease.

Consultations are a frequent cardiologist service. Cardiology consultations can be provided to the inpatient or outpatient, and the choice of the correct E/M code for the consultation is based on documentation of key components and contributing factors. The cardiology consultation often produces lengthy, complex medical reports.

Arteriosclerosis

Arteriosclerosis is a chronic disease of the arterial system that results in thickened and hardened walls of the vessels resulting in loss of the artery elasticity. Gradually, the arterial lumen narrows. This results in increased blood pressure because the heart has to pump harder to force the blood through the artery, weakening of the arterial walls that then become more susceptible to rupture, and insufficient perfusion to the tissues of the body. **Atherosclerosis** is a form of arteriosclerosis in which deposits of fat and fibrin (insoluble protein) accumulate on the vessel walls. These accumulations are atheromas. When referencing the Index under the main term "Atherosclerosis," the coder is directed to "*see* Arteriosclerosis." Under the main term "Arteriosclerosis, arteriosclerotic" the coder is directed to **I70.90.** In the Tabular, the code description indicates "Atherosclerosis" that is not further specified. There are more specific diagnosis codes available for assignment based on the location of the disease, such as aorta (I70.0), renal artery (I70.1), extremities (I70.209), bypass graft of extremities (I70.309), of other specified arteries (I70.8), or generalized or unspecified atherosclerosis (I70.90).

One commonly diagnosed condition is atherosclerosis of the coronary artery. To assign a code to this condition, you start by referencing "Arteriosclerosis, coronary" in the Index. You are then directed to I25.10. The code includes arteriosclerotic heart disease (ASHD), atherosclerotic heart disease, and coronary artery sclerosis.

The assignment of additional characters is based on the location of the atherosclerosis and other factors, such as with or without angina pectoris (heart pain). For example, the following more common diagnoses are reported with six-character codes:

- "Of native coronary artery" indicates the atherosclerosis is within an original artery of the heart (I25.119).
- "Of autologous biological bypass graft" indicates that the atherosclerosis is within a vein graft that was taken from within the patient (I25.729).
- "Of nonautologous biological bypass graft" indicates the atherosclerosis is within a vessel grafted from a source other than the patient (I25.739).
- "Of artery bypass graft" indicates the atherosclerosis is within the internal mammary artery that was grafted from within the patient (I25.799).
- "Of unspecified type of bypass graft" is for reporting atherosclerosis of a bypass graft, but the origin of the graft is not otherwise specified (I25.810).

Review the subterms listed under the main term "Arteriosclerosis, arteriosclerotic" in the Index to become familiar with the entries located there and then review the codes you are directed to from the Index.

You will be coding other cardiovascular E/M services throughout this chapter.

CASE 6-1   *Cardiothoracic Surgery Consultation*

Time to put your cardiology coding knowledge to work by coding an E/M service provided by a cardiologist. A decision to perform surgery was made during this E/M visit, so remember to use the modifier that will indicate it.

LOCATION: Inpatient, Hospital

PATIENT: Manuel Lopez

PHYSICIAN: David Barton, MD

REASON FOR CONSULTATION: Atherosclerotic heart disease

HISTORY OF PRESENT ILLNESS: This 62-year-old Hispanic male was being considered for knee replacement and in his preoperative workup underwent a stress test, which did not show any ischemia; however, because of angioplasty 6 months ago, the patient was considered a candidate for angiography.

CARDIAC RISK FACTORS: Risk factors include a remote history of cigarette smoking, hypertension, previous coronary stent, dyslipidemia, and adult-onset diabetes mellitus.

MEDICAL HISTORY: Previous operations include the following:

1. Rotator cuff surgery in December of last year
2. Right coronary artery stent 6 months ago after right coronary artery occlusion with myocardial infarction

CURRENT MEDICATIONS:

1. Lotrel, 5/20 mg (milligram), 1 p.o. (by mouth) daily
2. Atenolol, 50 mg p.o. daily
3. Protonix, 40 mg, 1 to 2 daily
4. Lipitor, 10 mg daily
5. Hydrocodone as needed for knee pain
6. Nitroglycerin sublingual, 4/10 of 1 mg as needed.
7. Zoloft, 150 mg daily
8. Celebrex, 200 mg p.o. b.i.d. (twice a day)
9. 1 adult aspirin daily
10. Isosorbide, 30 mg p.o. daily
11. Glucosamine and chondroitin sulfate, 1 tablet b.i.d.
12. Actos, 40 mg p.o. daily
13. Magnesium, 400 mg p.o. t.i.d. (three times a day)

FAMILY HISTORY: Positive for coronary disease

SOCIAL HISTORY: The patient is married and lives with his wife in Manytown. He drinks minimally and stopped smoking years ago.

REVIEW OF SYSTEMS: Review of systems is significant for bilateral knee osteoarthritis. Echocardiogram done last year showed normal ventricular size with concentric hypertrophy and apical area of aneurysm.

PHYSICAL EXAMINATION: On examination, the patient is a 272-pound, 6-foot Hispanic male in no apparent distress, supine after his cardiac catheterization. Jugular venous pressure is normal. Carotids were 2+, equal, and quiet. The CHEST is clear and equal. The HEART has a regular rhythm with a rate of 70 without murmur, gallop, or rubs. The ABDOMEN is soft and obese without organomegaly. The upper and lower EXTREMITIES show no cyanosis, clubbing, or edema. Pulses are intact peripherally. The patient is grossly and neurologically intact. The chest x-ray shows normal cardiothoracic ratio. LUNG fields are clear.

The ECG (electrocardiogram) shows normal sinus rhythm with anterolateral ST (sinus tachycardia) segment and T-wave changes.

LABORATORY STUDIES: The laboratory shows sodium of 135, BUN (blood urea nitrogen) of 24, glucose of 115. The lipids are within satisfactory limits. The protime is 12.7 and PTT (partial thromboplastin time) is 31.6. White blood cell count is low at 3.5. Hemoglobin is 13.6, and platelets are 176,000.

Cardiac catheterization by Dr. Elhart 6 months ago showed good left ventricular contractility with, perhaps, some anterior early relaxation. The dominant right coronary artery had a 70% lesion at the posterior descending proximally. The left main was narrowed 40% distally. The left-to-right and right-to-left fill. The diagonal branch was diseased but small. The left circumflex was narrowed at two obtuse marginal branches at 70% to 90% proximally, respectively.

IMPRESSION: Three-vessel atherosclerotic heart disease in a 62-year-old Hispanic male with adult-onset diabetes mellitus, normal left ventricular function, and need for knee replacement.

DISPOSITION: The patient will be retained in the hospital and will undergo coronary vascularization tomorrow. Operation, complications including blood transfusion, risks, and alternatives were discussed with the patient and his family.

SERVICE CODE(S): _____

ICD-10-CM DX CODE(S): _____

(Answers to every other Case are located in Appendix D . The full answer key is only available in the TEACH Instructor Resources on Evolve.)

Coronary Artery Bypass Grafts

The Surgery section, Cardiovascular System subsection, codes are divided into Heart/Pericardium (33016-33999) and Arteries/Veins (34001-37799). In the Arteries and Veins subheading, you will find many of the same types of procedures that are found in the Heart and Pericardium subheading, except the Arteries and Veins are for procedures on noncoronary vessels elsewhere in the body.

When coronary arteries clog with plaque (arteriosclerotic coronary artery disease [ASCAD]), the flow of blood is lessened. **Figure 6-1** is a drawing that was placed in the patient's medical record by the cardiologist to indicate the blockage of the patient's heart vessels. Note that the figure

indicates the percentage of blockage of the involved vessels. For example, the right coronary artery (RCA) is 100% blocked by plaque. **Figure 6-2** illustrates an artery on fluoroscopy that is blocked with plaque. The heart muscle may begin to function below normal levels—reversible ischemia. If the heart muscle is denied adequate blood flow for an extended period, the muscle may die—irreversible ischemia.

A coronary artery bypass graft (CABG) bypasses the clogged area(s) of the vessels to improve blood flow. There are three types of coronary artery bypass grafts:

1. CABG with venous graft only (33510-33516)
2. CABG with venous and arterial grafts (33517-33530)
3. CABG with arterial graft only (33533-33536)

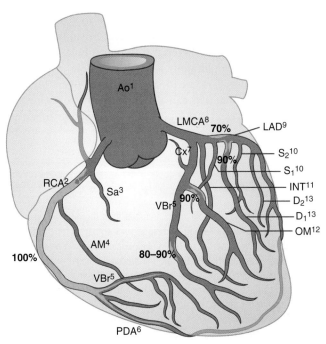

FIGURE 6–1 The percentages indicate the amount of blockage of the patient's heart vessels. The right coronary artery (RCA) is 100% blocked by plaque.

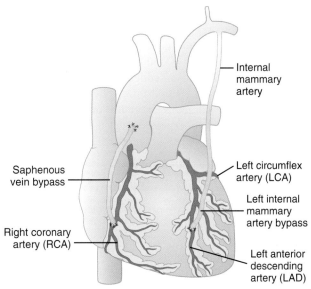

FIGURE 6–3 Coronary artery bypass.

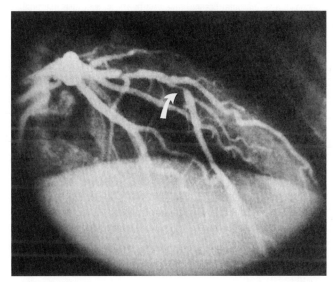

FIGURE 6–2 RAO cranial view showing the second LAD lesion (arrow).

The heart has two main coronary arteries—the left (left main) and right (right coronary artery). The left main (LM) artery divides into the left anterior descending (LAD) and left circumflex (LCA) arteries **(Figure 6-3)**. The right coronary artery (RCA) supplies the right ventricle and continues down the back of the heart (posterior aspect), where it is called the posterior descending artery (PDA). The coronary artery can be bypassed with an artery using the internal mammary artery, gastroepiploic artery, epigastric artery, radial artery, and arterial grafts from other areas. Note in Figure 6-3 that

the internal mammary artery (originates from the subclavian artery) is attached to the subclavian artery on one end, and the distal end is detached from its origin and reattached to the coronary artery to bypass the area of damage. Other times, the surgeon removes a portion of a **vein** and uses it for a graft, such as a right or left saphenous vein that is removed and used for a bypass graft. The procurement of the artery or vein is included in the CABG code and would not be reported separately. If an upper-extremity **artery,** such as the radial artery, is harvested for grafting, however, the harvesting service can be reported with add-on code 35600 (Harvest of upper extremity artery, one segment for coronary artery bypass procedure) or harvesting of an upper-extremity **vein** can be reported separately with add-on code 35500 (Harvest of upper-extremity vein, one segment for lower extremity or coronary artery bypass procedure).

Codes are selected based on the type (venous or arterial) of graft (harvested) and the number of grafts placed on the coronary artery (recipient). The number of grafts is determined by counting the number of distal anastomoses where the bypass graft is sutured to the diseased artery. For example, RCA and LAD receive two saphenous vein grafts. The type of graft is venous (harvested), and there were two grafts: one placed on the right coronary artery and one placed on the left anterior descending artery (recipients). The physician will often refer to the harvested and recipient, so you will need to know these terms to interpret the service provided correctly.

A CABG with venous and arterial grafts (33517-33530) is never used alone but only with the arterial graft codes (33533-33536). You can use the arterial graft codes alone (33533-33545) and the venous codes alone (33510-33516), but you can never report the Combined Arterial-Venous Grafting for Coronary Bypass codes alone. A helpful hint is to write "combination AV only" next to the codes

33517-33530 in your CPT manual as a reminder that these codes are used to report the venous graft(s) only when a combined arterial-venous graft is performed. Note that the codes from range 33517-33530 have a plus sign in front of them that indicates add-on codes and are never reported alone.

Cardiovascular surgeons often use artificial materials, such as Gore-Tex, to repair damaged areas of vessels. This artificial material is less susceptible to rejection and calcification than human tissue and can be readily available. The surgeon uses this material to repair a hole in a vessel as a seamstress would apply a patch to a hole in a pair of jeans. The material is cut to size and sewn over the hole. These artificial materials can also be formed into a tube and inserted into a vessel as a support for weakened or collapsed vessel walls.

CASE 6-2 *Coronary Artery Bypass*

Code the following CABG. Be certain to identify the number, location, and type of grafts.

LOCATION: Inpatient, Hospital

PATIENT: Manuel Lopez

SURGEON: David Barton, MD

PREOPERATIVE DIAGNOSIS: Atherosclerotic heart disease

POSTOPERATIVE DIAGNOSIS: Same

PROCEDURE PERFORMED: Coronary artery bypass grafts × 4 with left internal mammary artery to left anterior descending bypass and sequential saphenous vein bypass from the aorta to the first and second obtuse marginal branch of the left circumflex with an ongoing graft to the posterior descending coronary artery.

ANESTHESIA: General

INDICATIONS: This 62-year-old Hispanic male with a history of degenerative knee disease was considered a candidate for orthopedic surgical management; however, preoperatively he underwent stress testing, which was equivocal but prompted angiography, which showed severe three-vessel disease with normal ventricular function.

FINDINGS AT SURGERY: The vein was a 4-mm (millimeter)-diameter vessel of good quality and was used in reverse fashion. The left internal mammary artery was a 1.5-mm-diameter vessel of good quality. The left anterior descending was a 2-mm-diameter vessel of good quality. The first and second obtuse marginal branches were both 2 mm in diameter and of good quality. The posterior descending was, likewise, 2 mm in diameter and of good quality. All the grafts were appropriate prior to closure and were placed distal to palpable disease.

DESCRIPTION OF PROCEDURE: The patient was brought to the operating room and placed in the supine position. With the patient under general intubation anesthesia, the anterior chest, abdomen, and legs were prepped and draped in the usual manner. A segment of the greater saphenous vein was harvested from the left thigh using the endoscopic vein-harvesting technique and prepared for grafting. The pericardium was incised sharply and a pericardial well created. The patient was systemically heparinized and placed on single right atrial-to-aortic cardiopulmonary bypass with a stump in the main pulmonary artery for cardiac decompression. The patient was cooled to 26° C and, on fibrillation, aortic cross-clamp was applied and potassium-rich cold crystalline cardioplegic solution was administered through the aortic root with satisfactory cardiac arrest. Subsequent doses were given down the vein graft as the anastomosis was completed and also via the coronary sinus in a retrograde fashion. The end of the greater saphenous vein was then anastomosed to the proximal third of the posterior descending coronary artery using 7-0 Prolene. The graft was brought to the patient's left and then anastomosed side to side to the second obtuse marginal branch, followed by the first obtuse marginal branch, all with 7-0 continuous Prolene. The left internal mammary artery was then brought down to the midportion of the left anterior descending and anastomosed thereto with 8-0 continuous Prolene. The aortic cross-clamp was removed after 62 minutes with spontaneous cardioversion to a normal sinus rhythm. The patient was then warmed to 37° C esophageal temperature, during which time the vein graft was trimmed to size and anastomosed to the ascending aorta using 5-0 continuous Prolene technique. The patient was weaned from cardiopulmonary bypass without difficulty using no inotropes after 99 minutes. The patient was decannulated, protamine was given, and hemostasis was obtained. Temporary pacer wires were placed from the right atrium and right ventricles. The chest was drained with two Argyle chest tubes and closed in layers in the usual fashion. The leg was closed similarly. Sterile compression dressings were applied. The patient returned to the surgical intensive care unit in satisfactory condition. Sponge and needle counts were correct × 2.

SERVICE CODE(S): _____

ICD-10-CM DX CODE(S): _____

(Answers to every other Case are located in Appendix D . The full answer key is only available in the TEACH Instructor Resources on Evolve.)

From the Trenches

"The most rewarding part about being a medical coder is having the opportunity to learn something new everyday."

TANECKA POE
CCS, CPC, COC

Pacemaker

A pacemaker is an electrical device that is inserted into the body to shock the heart electrically into regular rhythm. The two parts of a pacemaker are the battery and electrode. The electrode is the device that emits the electrical charge. The electrode is also called the lead and is a flexible, thin tube. The battery is also called a pulse generator. Some generators are programmable and have a wide range of programming options. The pulse generator is placed into a pocket either under the clavicle, as illustrated in **Figure 6-4,** or under the muscle of the abdomen below the rib cage.

Either an epicardial or transvenous approach can be used to implant the electrode portion of the pacemaker. The epicardial approach involves opening the chest to the view of the surgeon and the device being placed on the heart. The transvenous approach is most commonly used because it is the least traumatic to the patient and involves inserting a needle with a wire attached (guidewire) into a vein. The guidewire then directs the placement of the electrode into the heart while the surgeon views the progression using a fluoroscope. The electrode is then attached to the pulse generator.

The pacemaker can be a single- or dual-chamber unit. A single-chamber pacemaker uses one pulse generator and one electrode, which is placed in either the atrium or the ventricle. A dual-chamber pacemaker uses a pulse generator and two electrodes—one placed in the atrium and the other placed in the ventricle.

Pacemakers can be permanent or temporary. A temporary pacemaker can be used when the heart needs only short-term pacing support. For example, when a patient is waiting for placement of a permanent pacemaker or a patient is experiencing postsurgical cardiac instability. After the pacemaker is placed, the physician will test the device to ensure that it is operating correctly. The pacemaker implantation report will include a statement such as "thresholds were obtained and were adequate." The testing and setting are included in the implantation service and are not reported separately. Special or extensive pacing, if noted in the report as being above the usual service, can be reported separately.

An **implantable defibrillator** is an implantable electronic device that has both the pulse generator and the electrodes, but it is capable of more functions than the pacemaker. The device senses irregularities in the heart rhythm and emits electrical charges to regulate the heart rhythm and pace the heart to correct heart rhythm. The device can be programmed to sense a wide variety of heart irregularities and then further programmed to emit various electrical charges in response. The device is used for antitachycardia (stops rapid heartbeat) pacing, low-energy cardioversion (restoration of normal heartbeat), or defibrillating shocks to treat tachycardia or fibrillation (quivering).

A single-chamber implantable defibrillator has a lead or leads inserted into a **single** chamber; a dual-chamber implantable defibrillator has leads inserted into **both** the atrium and ventricle. These electrode(s) may be placed through a vein (transvenous), on the heart surface (epicardial), or under the skin (subcutaneous). The number of leads used does not indicate a single- or dual-chamber implantable defibrillator because when a single chamber is being paced, multiple leads into that single chamber may be used. It is the number of **chambers** into which the leads are placed, not the number of leads used, that impacts code choice.

During insertion, electrophysiologic testing of an implantable defibrillator and electrical analysis of a pacemaker would often be conducted as a part of the insertion or reinsertion procedure. This testing and analysis would be reported separately using Medicine section codes 93264, 93279-93285. Perioperative testing is also reported separately with Medicine section codes 93286 and 93287. Remember to use modifier -26 if you are reporting only the professional component (physician) of the electrical analysis.

When a pacemaker or implantable defibrillator battery is changed, it is actually the pulse generator that is replaced. As a part of the usual 90-day surgical package that accompanies the implantation service, follow-up visits would be considered part of the global service by the third-party payer and therefore not reimbursed.

Removal of only the pulse generator without insertion of a new pulse generator is reported with 33233 or 33241. If the pulse generator is replaced without insertion or replacement of transvenous electrode(s), both the removal and insertion of another pulse generator is reported with only one code. 33227-33229 (permanent pacemaker) or 33262-33264 (implantable defibrillator), depending on the lead system number already in place. Removal and replacement of a permanent pacemaker pulse generator and transvenous electrode(s) is reported with 33233 in addition to 33234 or 33235 and 33206-33208. Removal and replacement of an implantable defibrillator pulse generator and subcutaneous or transvenous electrode(s) are reported with 33241 in addition to 33243 or 33244, 33249, 33270 or 33272.

Sick Sinus Syndrome

Sick sinus syndrome is a group of abnormal heartbeats (arrhythmias). The exact cause of this syndrome is

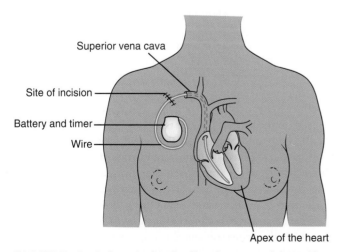

Superior vena cava

Site of incision

Battery and timer

Wire

Apex of the heart

FIGURE 6-4 Pacemaker insertion. The pulse generator is inserted into the upper chest area.

CASE 6-3   *Cardiology Follow-Up Note*

With the information you just learned about pacemakers, code the following E/M services to a patient who, after several tests, will have a pacemaker implanted.

LOCATION: Outpatient, Clinic

PATIENT: Herbert Gillford

PHYSICIAN: Marvin Elhart, MD

DIAGNOSES:

1. Symptomatic sick sinus syndrome
2. Dementia
3. Dilated cardiomyopathy with previous history of congestive heart failure

MEDICATIONS: Tylenol; Lasix 40 mg (milligram) as needed; Vasotec 5 mg once daily; Colace; aspirin: Ambien; and Arthrotec.

I evaluated this patient approximately 2 years ago. He was seen by Dr. Pleasant again last year on referral from Dr. Green because of episodes of falling down. The episodes are significant to the point that he had a hip fracture. Apparently, he was transferred to a nursing home in his hometown.

The history from the patient is almost useless because he does not recollect any symptoms and he says he feels fine and has no shortness of breath or falling down. The patient has been diagnosed with dementia previously. We tried to contact his relative, but we got the answering machine.

We reviewed the previous notations from Dr. Green and Dr. Pleasant and myself. Predominantly the problem is that the patient has had repeated falls and has been diagnosed with sinus bradycardia with first-degree AV (arteriovenous) block and bundle-branch block; a Holter monitor read by myself recently revealed predominantly atrial block.

EXAMINATION today reveals an elderly man in a wheelchair in no acute distress. His blood pressure was 124/68 with a heart rate of 60. Lungs did not reveal any rales. Cardiovascular examination reveals distant heart tones with normal S1 (first heart sound) and S2 (second heart sound) with a holosystolic murmur, grade 1/6, over the mitral area. Abdomen was obese. Extremities: No edema.

ECG (electrocardiogram) in the office reveals him to be in sinus bradycardia with a rate of 49 with first-degree AV block and left bundle-branch block. The Holter monitor revealed him to be predominantly in atrial fibrillation; his minimum rate was 49 and maximum 114 with an average of 74. At that time, the notation did show that he was taking Lanoxin, which apparently he is not taking at this time.

An echocardiogram also read by myself revealed the patient to have dilated cardiomyopathy with severe LV (left ventricle) dysfunction with mild aortic insufficiency and significant mitral insufficiency.

IMPRESSION AND RECOMMENDATIONS: Symptomatic sick sinus syndrome with evidence of paroxysmal atrial fibrillation. It is very difficult to assess this patient symptom-wise because he does not have a lot of insight into his symptoms. He has been diagnosed with dementia. It seems to me that there is enough evidence that this patient's falling down episodes might be related to his rhythm because that is the most common finding. The only solution to this problem would be implantation of a dual-chamber pacemaker.

We attempted to contact his family to discuss this and to obtain a consent, but we did not get an answer. We will contact the family again and discuss with them the recommendations. If they consent to it and agree to proceed, we will bring him in for implantation of a dual-chamber pacemaker. Total time spent with the patient today was 45 minutes.

SERVICE CODE(S): _____

ICD-10-CM DX CODE(S): _____

(Answers to every other Case are located in Appendix D . The full answer key is only available in the TEACH Instructor Resources on Evolve.)

---

unknown, but it is thought to be caused by a malfunction of the sinus node, which is the heart's natural pacemaker. It can result in many arrhythmias, including tachycardia (fast heart rate), bradycardia (slow heart rate), sinus arrest, sinus node exit block, and sinus bradycardia. These arrhythmias are not reported separately because they are symptoms of the syndrome. Rather, the syndrome is reported. You can locate direction to the code in the Index by referencing "Syndrome, sick, sinus."

In reports 6-5B and 6-5C, you will be coding the pacemaker implantation for the patient in report 6-3A, but you must learn a few more terms before you code the implantation service. Let us begin with echocardiography services.

Echocardiography

Cardiomyopathy (CMP) is a disease of the heart muscle. The exact cause(s) of cardiomyopathy are not known, and the symptoms of the disease are similar to those displayed in patients with myocarditis (infections of the heart muscle caused by virus, bacteria, or parasites), toxic effects of various drugs, **myocardial** infarction, various cardiac disorders (pericarditis, congestive heart disease, or stenosis), and various other conditions. As a part of the diagnostic process, the physician may order an electrocardiogram, chest x-rays, Doppler and echocardiography, radionuclide studies, cardiac catheterization, or blood tests.

Echocardiography obtains ultrasonic signals from the heart and coronary arteries with a two-dimensional image and/or Doppler ultrasound. **Transthoracic echocardiography** is a noninvasive procedure in which a transducer (transmitter) is placed on the skin and sound waves go through the structure of the body and bounce off the heart. From the frequency with which the waves return from the internal structures and bounce back to the transducer, the physician can determine the position and motion of the heart walls and internal structures of the heart and neighboring tissue.

Transesophageal echocardiography (TEE) is a procedure in which the transesophageal echography probe transducer is placed into the mouth and advanced into the esophagus, allowing a posterior view of the heart, as illustrated in **Figure 6-5**. Varieties of TEEs are reported with codes

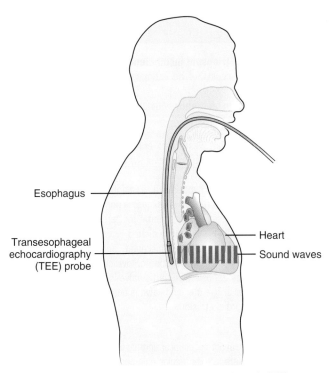

Esophagus

Transesophageal
echocardiography
(TEE) probe

Heart

Sound waves

FIGURE 6–5 Transesophageal echocardiography (TEE).

93312-93318. The codes are divided into those done for congenital cardiac conditions (93315-93317) and those done for noncongenital cardiac conditions (93312-93314). The stand-alone codes 93312 and 93315 are for the full service, and the indented codes are for components of the service. For example, 93313 is used to report the placement of the transesophageal probe only. Code 93318 is used to report a TEE for monitoring purposes. These monitoring functions are not limited to monitoring of the heart but also include monitoring of numerous organs, such as the lungs and mediastinum. These monitoring services are not the usual diagnostic service but instead are urgent services that are required for a critically ill or injured patient. Code 93355 is reported exclusively for guidance of a transcatheter intracardiac or great vessel intervention, such as a transcatheter aortic valve replacement or paravalvular regurgitation repair. It is an all-inclusive code; therefore, no additional codes are reported for color flow, Doppler, 3D, or administration of ultrasound contrast. (In Case 6-14A, you will be coding a TEE service prior to a cardioversion.)

Doppler echocardiography is a technique that records the flow of blood through the cardiovascular system by tracking the movement of the red blood cells by ultrasound. The pulsed-wave or continuous-wave Doppler produces a video recording or strip chart detailing the force with which the blood passes through the cardiovascular system and the direction of the blood. A **color-flow Doppler** is similar to the pulsed-wave or continuous Doppler, but in addition to the color flow is a two-dimensional color display. The color makes identification of blood flow easier. Code 93306 is a complete transthoracic echocardiography that includes M-mode, when performed, and spectral and color-flow Doppler. A limited transthoracic echocardiography, without spectral and color-flow Doppler, is reported with 93307. Note that you cannot report 93320 (complete Doppler), 93321 (limited Doppler), or color-flow velocity mapping (93325) with 93307.

Valve Insufficiencies

Insufficiency of a heart valve means the valve does not close properly, which may lead to hypertrophy (enlargement) of the heart because blood will pool in the chambers. Rheumatic heart disease is a result of rheumatic fever, which is a febrile (fever) disease caused by a *streptococcal* infection and results in valvular deformities. The ICD-10-CM divides codes for nonrheumatic valvular insufficiencies from valvular insufficiencies that are a result of (sequela) rheumatic heart disease. Category I34 is for **nonrheumatic** or **other specified** causes. This code is also assigned for **unspecified** causes when only one valve is involved. The documentation is often aortic stenosis (I35.0) of unknown cause. When there are multiple valves involved in the diagnosis *or* the documentation specifies rheumatic, refer to I05 to I08. For example, a commonly documented diagnosis is aortic and mitral valve regurgitation (not specified as rheumatic), which is reported with I08.0. When both **mitral** and **aortic** valves are involved, the ICD-10-CM presumes an etiology (cause) of rheumatic heart disease, and the physician does not need to document rheumatic heart disease. Also, when the diagnosis involves the **tricuspid valve,** the etiology also is presumed to be rheumatic heart disease if multiple heart valves are involved.

CASE 6-4 *Echocardiogram*

The patient presented to Dr. Elhart with complaints of chest discomfort. A 2-D Doppler and color-flow Doppler were performed at the local hospital in the outpatient cardiology department, and Dr. Elhart monitored the echocardiography.

LOCATION: Outpatient, Hospital

PATIENT: Herbert Gillford

PHYSICIAN: Marvin Elhart, MD

STUDY: The study is 2-D and a color-flow Doppler echocardiography.

INDICATION FOR STUDY: Sinus bradycardia

Chamber dimension by M-mode:

1. The left atrial diameter is 62 mm (millimeter), which is consistent with moderate atrial enlargement.
2. The aortic root is 39 mm.
3. Left ventricular diastolic diameter is 75 mm; systolic diameter is 65 mm.
4. Shortening fraction is 13%.
5. Ejection fraction is estimated at 26%.
6. Wall thickness is 7 mm.

DOPPLER:

1. Mild aortic insufficiency. The peak velocity across the aortic valve was estimated at 2 m/second. There is no evidence of significant aortic stenosis.
2. There is eccentric jet of mitral insufficiency. The E-velocity is estimated at 1.1 m/second, and that certainly corresponds with severe mitral insufficiency. There did not appear to be any significant mitral stenosis, even though the opening was decreased due to low cardiac output state.

3. There is moderate **tricuspid insufficiency.** The RV (right ventricle) systolic pressure could not be estimated because of incomplete spectral envelopes.
4. Mild **pulmonary insufficiency** without stenosis.

2-D ECHO (ECHOCARDIOGRAM):

1. Mild to moderate left ventricular enlargement. The overall left ventricular systolic function is severely depressed, and ejection fraction is estimated at 15% to 20%.
2. There is severe global hypokinesia. The inferoposterior segment appears to be akinetic. The wall thickness is normal.
3. Right ventricle, right atrium, and aortic root are within the normal limits. The left atrium is moderately dilated.
4. The mitral valve is minimally thickened, and the excursion is decreased and most likely is due to low cardiac output state rather than mitral stenosis. The aortic valve is fibrocalcific without significant stenosis. The tricuspid valve is unremarkable.
5. There is no pericardial effusion.

CONCLUSION:

1. This is a markedly abnormal echocardiogram that reveals the presence of mild to moderate left ventricular enlargement with severe global left ventricular systolic dysfunction due to valvular insufficiency.
2. Mild **aortic insufficiency.**
3. Severe **mitral insufficiency.**

RECOMMENDATIONS:

1. I would suggest aggressive medical therapy with the use of ACE inhibitors, diuresis, and possible ACE inhibitors. SBE (subacute bacterial endocarditis) prophylaxis.

SERVICE CODE(S): _____

ICD-10-CM DX CODE(S): _____

Discussion

This patient was referred for the symptom of sinus bradycardia (R00.1); but there are more definitive diagnoses available based on the test results. In the Conclusion section of the report, the physician indicates "left ventricular enlargement with severe global left ventricular systolic dysfunction due to valvular insufficiency." The ventricular enlargement and dysfunction are "due to" another more specific condition (valves are not functioning properly) and therefore neither the enlargement nor the dysfunction are reported separately. The physician indicated both **aortic** and **mitral** insufficiency and, in the Doppler section of the report, he indicated **tricuspid** and **pulmonary** insufficiency. No specific cause for these conditions was specified, so each of the conditions must be reported.

There are two codes required to report these diagnoses. In the Index of the ICD-10-CM, reference the main term "Insufficiency" and subterms "**mitral, with, aortic** valve disease", which is coded to I08.0; however, "**tricuspid** [valve] disease" is also documented. A combination code describing combined rheumatic disorders of mitral, aortic, and tricuspid valves is assigned. Although documentation does not indicate that the multiple valve diseases are rheumatic in nature, the "Includes" note under category I08 states that this category also includes multiple valve diseases that are unspecified, therefore, I08.3 is assigned. In the "Doppler" section of the report, the physician indicates that the patient also has **tricuspid** and **pulmonary** insufficiencies. The pulmonary valve insufficiency is reported with I08.8.

(Answers to every other Case are located in Appendix D . The full answer key is only available in the TEACH Instructor Resources on Evolve.)

Holter

Another commonly used cardiac diagnostic tool is the Holter monitor, which is a portable electrocardiography device that is worn by the patient, usually for 24 hours but up to 48 hours. The monitor records the electrical function of the heart and allows the physician to analyze the data to diagnose various cardiac conditions.

The sequence of events is important to know before you code the Holter monitor service. When the patient's physician evaluates the patient and determines that the patient requires the monitoring of cardiac function by means of a Holter monitor, the physician orders the monitoring, and at a later time the patient presents to the cardiology laboratory to be fitted with a monitor. The technician, under the supervision of the cardiologist, outfits the patient with the monitor, and the patient leaves the department wearing the monitor for a specified period of time (usually 24 to 48 hours for a Holter). The patient returns to the cardiology department, and the technician removes the monitor. The cardiologist interprets tracing of the Holter and writes a report of findings that is sent to the physician who ordered the monitoring. In the meantime, after the monitoring has been performed, but before the results are returned and reviewed by the physician, the coder reports the services. This sequence is important in identifying the diagnosis for which the services were provided. The coder does not wait for the results of the various tests to be returned before reporting the services for reimbursement. The coder does, however, wait for the test to be conducted prior to submitting for reimbursement. The physician's diagnosis will be used to report the services for the Holter monitoring in the following report. After the physician reads the report, he or she may change the diagnosis of the patient to reflect the test results, but only the physician can make the determination of the diagnosis. Perhaps the physician ordered several tests and the interpretation as to the diagnosis varied. It is the ordering physician's responsibility to assess all test results and make the conclusion as to the final diagnosis. When coding the various reports in this text, you will be seeing the report results. However, you would usually only know that the test had been requested and performed, not the results.

CASE 6-5A   *Holter Report*

Code the following Holter service, assuming the test had been ordered and performed. Report the global service. For the diagnosis, you would use the information presented in the "Indication" section of the report, because that would be the reason the physician ordered the test.

LOCATION: Outpatient, Clinic

PATIENT: Herbert Gillford

PHYSICIAN: Dr. Marvin Elhart

INDICATION: Patient with atrial fibrillation on Lanoxin. Patient has known cardiomyopathy.

BASELINE DATA: An 86-year-old man with congestive heart failure who is taking Elavil, Vasotec, Lanoxin, and Lasix.

The patient was monitored for 24 hours during which time the analysis was performed.

INTERPRETATION:

1. The predominant rhythm is atrial fibrillation. The average ventricular rate is 74 beats per minute, minimum 49 beats per minute, and maximum 114 beats per minute.
2. A total of 4948 ventricular ectopic beats were detected. There were four forms. There were 146 couplets with 1 triplet and 5 runs of bigeminy. There were two runs of ventricular tachycardia, the longest for 5 beats at a rate of 150 beats per minute. No ventricular fibrillation was noted.
3. There were no prolonged pauses.

CONCLUSION:

1. Predominant rhythm is atrial fibrillation with well-controlled ventricular rate.
2. There are no prolonged pauses.
3. Asymptomatic, nonsustained, ventricular tachycardia.

SERVICE CODE(S): _____

ICD-10-CM DX CODE(S): _____

(Answers to every other Case are located in Appendix D . The full answer key is only available in the TEACH Instructor Resources on Evolve.)

CASE 6-5B   *Radiology Report, Preimplantation*

Code the preimplantation services.

LOCATION: Outpatient, Hospital

PATIENT: Herbert Gillford

PHYSICIAN: Dr. Marvin Elhart

RADIOLOGIST: Dr. Morton Monson

EXAMINATION OF: Chest

CLINICAL SYMPTOMS: Sick sinus syndrome

CHEST, TWO VIEWS, FRONTAL AND LATERAL, 11:00 AM: Comparison is made to films taken 3 years ago. There is cardiomegaly. Overt failure is not identified. There is only a moderate degree of inspiration. Osseous structures show old compression deformity of the lower thoracic spine. Calcification is identified within a tortuous aorta. The portion of the abdomen that was seen is unremarkable.

IMPRESSION:

1. Sick sinus syndrome.
2. Cardiomegaly. There is a poor inspiration effort, but overt failure is not suggested grossly at this time.
3. Progress studies should be obtained as considered clinically warranted.

SERVICE CODE(S): _____

ICD-10-CM DX CODE(S): _____

(Answers to every other Case are located in Appendix D . The full answer key is only available in the TEACH Instructor Resources on Evolve.)

CASE 6-5C *Operative Report, Pacemaker Implantation*

LOCATION: Outpatient, Hospital

PATIENT: Herbert Gillford

SURGEON: Marvin Elhart, MD

PROCEDURE PERFORMED: Dual-chamber pacemaker implantation

INDICATION: Bradyarrhythmia

BRIEF HISTORY: This patient has been experiencing recurrent syncope. He was evaluated in the last year or so. Because of the presence of first-degree AV (atrioventricular) block and sinus bradycardia, the cause for his syncope is his bradyarrhythmia; for that reason, a dual-chamber pacemaker implantation was recommended after discussion with his cousin, who consented to the procedure. The cousin was informed of all potential complications, including infection, hematoma, pneumothorax, hemothorax, myocardial infarction, and even death. He agreed to proceed.

PROCEDURE: The patient was brought to the cardiac catheterization laboratory. He was placed on the catheterization table, where he was prepped and draped in the usual fashion. The procedure was extremely difficult to perform as a result of the patient's agitation despite adequate sedation. With reasonable hemostasis, the pacemaker pocket was performed in the left infraclavicular area after anesthetizing the area with 0.5 cc (cubic centimeter) of Xylocaine. Hemostasis was secured with cautery. The patient had excessive venous oozing from Valsalva and straining, and that was controlled with pressure. A single stick was performed because of the patient's agitation. Using a 9-French peel-away sheath, we introduced an atrial and a ventricular lead and placed them in an excellent position.

Thresholds were obtained adequately. The leads were sutured using 0 silk over their sleeves and secured. The pulse generator was connected. The pacemaker pocket was flushed with antibiotic solution. The pacemaker and leads were placed in the pocket and the pocket closed in two layers.

COMPLICATION: None

EQUIPMENT USED: Pulse generator was Medtronic model 60 Thera DRI, serial B28H. The ventricular lead was Medtronic serial L420V, model 4524 Link. The atrial lead was Medtronic 24-58, serial 326V.

The following parameters were obtained after implantation: Pacing threshold in the atrium was excellent at 0.5 msec and 0.5 V, and impedance was 445 ohms and sensing 2.1 mV. In the ventricle, 0.5 msec and 0.3 V with R wave of 19.9 mV and impedance 668 (device evaluation).

The following parameters were left at implantation: DDDR with lower rate limit of 70 and an upper rate limit of 120. The amplitude was 3.5 V in the atrium at 0.4 msec with a sensitivity of 0.5 mV. The ventricle was 3.5 V and 0.4 msec at 2.8-mV sensitivity (device evaluation).

CONCLUSION: Successful implantation of dual-chamber pacemaker without immediate complications.

PLAN: Patient to return to recovery unit and to be discharged late this evening to the nursing home with routine postpacemaker care.

SERVICE CODE(S): _____

ICD-10-CM DX CODE(S): _____

(Answers to every other Case are located in Appendix D . The full answer key is only available in the TEACH Instructor Resources on Evolve.)

CASE 6-5D *Radiology Report, Postimplantation*

Two diagnoses are reported with this postimplantation service. The first listed diagnosis is a Z code that indicates "Status, post, pacemaker, cardiac." The Z code is listed first, as that is the reason for the service (checking on the placement of the pacemaker). The bradycardia is also reported, but sequenced after the Z code.

LOCATION: Outpatient, Hospital

PATIENT: Herbert Gillford

PHYSICIAN: Dr. Marvin Elhart

RADIOLOGIST: Dr. Morton Monson

EXAMINATION OF: Chest

CLINICAL SYMPTOMS: Status post pacemaker placement, bradycardia

CHEST, SINGLE VIEW, FRONTAL: FINDINGS: This examination is compared with an examination performed earlier on the same day at 11:00 AM. Since the previous examination, there has been interval placement of a pacemaker. One of the leads overlies the expected location of the right ventricle. The proximal lead overlies the expected location of the right atrium near the junction with the superior vena cava. Cardiomegaly is present on this examination. This is unchanged when compared with the previous examination. The pulmonary vascular markings appear within normal limits. The examination otherwise appears unchanged compared with the previous examination. Definite pneumothorax is not identified on this examination.

SERVICE CODE(S): _____

ICD-10-CM DX CODE(S): _____

(Answers to every other Case are located in Appendix D . The full answer key is only available in the TEACH Instructor Resources on Evolve.)

Preimplantation, Implantation, and Postimplantation

A chest x-ray is performed prior to the pacemaker implantation. The pacemaker is implanted, and another chest x-ray is performed after the implantation to ensure proper pacemaker placement.

Stress Tests

A cardiovascular **stress test** is a special type of echocardiogram that compares the electrical system of the heart at rest and under exertion. The test is used by the physician to diagnose various diseases, such as coronary artery disease (atherosclerosis), coronary ischemia (dead or dying heart muscle), and arrhythmias (irregular heartbeats). The technician administers the stress test under the direct supervision of the physician. Usually the test is conducted while the patient is exercised on a treadmill or bicycle and continuous recordings are made of the electrical activity of the heart. Electrodes are attached to the chest of the patient, as is a blood pressure monitor. The patient begins to exercise at a low speed. The speed is increased at set intervals until the patient's maximal or submaximal heart rate is reached and sustained. Three services are bundled into the complete stress test procedure as described in 93015:

- Supervision
- Tracing
- Interpretation with written report

Codes in the range 93016-93018 are used when only a component of the test is provided:

- Supervision only without interpretation and report (93016)
- Tracing only (93017)
- Interpretation and report only (93018)

In order to report the correct code selection, place of service must be considered. If a physician performs continuous monitoring, supervises the stress test, interprets the data, and compiles a report in an office or physician clinic setting, the entire service would be coded as 93015 without any modifier to show that the global service is being reported to include both the professional and technical components. This will indicate that the physician not only provided the service but also owns the equipment and only one entity will be submitting a charge. Often the stress test is performed in a hospital setting, which will require that the physician and facility each report their distinct component codes without appending any modifiers, since specific codes are provided that describe their respective services. When the physician provides supervision of the stress test but without the interpretation and report, only 93016 would be reported. Code 93018 would be reported when the physician provides the interpretation and report. When the physician reports either 93016 or 93018, the facility would report the technical component for the stress test tracing with code 93017.

Sometimes, as the result of physical limitations, a patient is unable to exercise on a treadmill or bicycle. In these instances, the patient can be administered a drug, such as Persantine, adenosine, Cardiolite, or dobutamine to mimic the stress to the heart that would be brought about by exercise by dilating the vessels. These agents are administered in the outpatient setting at the hospital, and the hospital would report the cost of the pharmacologic agent, not the physician. Where tests are performed and who performed each of the components will have an effect on how the services are coded. For instance, if the test was administered at the local hospital and the physician did the supervision only, he would report the supervision component with 93016. The hospital would report the tracing portion of the service with 93017. If the outpatient facility employed a physician to do the supervision and interpretation and a technician to do the tracing, 93015 would be reported for the complete stress test service.

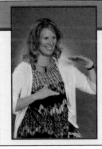

From the Trenches

"A medical coder must always have patience and be willing to accept change."

TANECKA POE
CCS, CPC, COC

CASE 6-6A   *Adenosine Cardiolite Stress Test*

The stress test was conducted at the cardiology laboratory at the local hospital with the clinic physician supervising the test and interpreting the results.

LOCATION: Outpatient, Hospital

PATIENT: Eleanor Montgomery

PHYSICIAN: Marvin Elhart, MD

INDICATIONS: Atherosclerotic heart disease with prior myocardial infarction, evaluate for potential ischemia

Electrocardiogram at rest in the exercise lead position reveals the presence of normal sinus rhythm with a somewhat atypical left bundle-branch block with related repolarization abnormalities. Subsequently the patient was injected with 140 μg (microgram) per kilogram per minute of IV (intravenous) Adenoscan over a 6-minute period. At the 3-minute mark, Cardiolite was injected. At the 10-minute mark, the patient was brought for Cardiolite imaging. The patient had a little chest pain and chest tightness during this test that resolved by the end of the Adenoscan infusion. At no point did any diagnostic ST (sinus tachycardia) abnormalities develop beyond baseline.

No ectopy was seen other than one PVC (premature ventricular contraction).

The pulses ranged in the 60s to 70s during this test. Systolic blood pressures ranged in the 130s to 160s during this test.

CONCLUSION:

1. The patient did have some chest discomfort during this test, which could potentially represent an anginal equivalent.
2. By facility criteria, there was no evidence of any induction of ischemia.

SERVICE CODE(S): _____

ICD-10-CM DX CODE(S): _____

(Answers to every other Case are located in Appendix D . The full answer key is only available in the TEACH Instructor Resources on Evolve.)

Myocardial Perfusion Scan

Depending on the results of the exercise stress test, the physician may recommend an additional test, such as a **myocardial perfusion scan** or stress thallium scan. A myocardial perfusion scan or myocardial perfusion imaging is a radiology procedure performed to assess the amount of blood that is reaching the heart muscle, areas of blocked arteries, or the effectiveness of a coronary artery bypass or **angioplasty.** This may be performed at rest and/or during stress. After an exercise stress test, the patient is injected with a radioactive tracer, such as adenosine or dipyridamole, and a specially equipped camera (gamma camera) is used to take a picture of the heart shortly after injection of the substance. The camera is attached to a computer, which displays the images. The tracer then circulates through the body and collects in the heart, at which time another image of the heart is taken that reveals areas where there are insufficient amounts of blood, which indicates dead or dying heart tissue. Myocardial perfusion scans are usually reported with codes from the Radiology section, Cardiovascular System subsection (78414-78499). Codes 78451-78454 and 78472-78492 are reported in addition to the appropriate stress testing code from range 93015-93018.

Ejection fraction is the percentage of blood pumped with each contraction of the heart and is related to the chamber volume. When the ejection fraction is low, the amount of blood pumped on each contraction is low. This test is included in the myocardial perfusion scan (78451-78454).

CASE 6-6B   *Radiology Report, Perfusion Scan*

LOCATION: Outpatient, Hospital

PATIENT: Eleanor Montgomery

PHYSICIAN: Dr. Marvin Elhart

EXAMINATION OF: Stress and rest myocardial perfusion scan with ejection fraction quantifications

INDICATIONS: Arteriosclerosis, coronary vessel

CLINICAL SYMPTOMS: Postmyocardial infarction, 20xx, angiography, 20xx

STRESS AND REST MYOCARDIAL PERFUSION SCAN: TECHNIQUE: Yesterday 31.4 mCi (millicurie) of technetium-99 m sestamibi was administered following stress with adenosine. Today, 24.4 mCi of technetium-99 m sestamibi was administered at rest. SPECT (single photon emission computed tomography) imaging was performed.

FINDINGS: There is minimal thinning of the cardiac apex on the stress images that shows some reversibility at rest. There is also a mild defect involving the inferolateral portion of the left ventricle extending from the periapical portion of the mid-left ventricle. This also shows reversibility in the inferior portion of the left ventricle. Ejection fraction about 35%.

IMPRESSION: Mild myocardial perfusion defects involving the apex and the periapical inferolateral portion of the left ventricle, which show reversibility on rest image. Diagnosis is coronary arteriosclerosis.

SERVICE CODE(S): _____

ICD-10-CM DX CODE(S): _____

(Answers to every other Case are located in Appendix D . The full answer key is only available in the TEACH Instructor Resources on Evolve.)

In the information preceding Case 6-4 of this chapter, you learned about coding a Doppler, and you once again have an opportunity to test your skills by coding the following report.

CASE 6-6C *Echo Doppler Report*

The patient's chest pains may or may not be related to the aortic and mitral insufficiency, so the chest pain would be reported in addition to the insufficiencies.

LOCATION: Outpatient, Hospital

PATIENT: Eleanor Montgomery

PHYSICIAN: Marvin Elhart, MD

INDICATION: Chest pain; evaluate heart function.

M-Mode, 2-D echo, and Doppler studies with color-flow analysis were performed. Findings are as follows:

1. CHAMBER SIZES: The left ventricle appears to be mildly enlarged on the 2-D images and mildly concentrically hypertrophied except for the septum, which is relatively thin compared with the rest of the left ventricle. The left atrium appears to be mildly enlarged and normal in thickness. The right ventricle and right atrium appear to be of normal size and thickness.
2. WALL MOTION (This is pulsed wave): All cardiac chambers contract normally except for the left ventricular interventricular septum;

anterior wall appears to be hypokinetic with moderate impairment of LVEF, visually on the order of about 35% or so.
3. The AORTIC ROOT is normal in size.
4. There is no pericardial effusion.
5. VALVES: The aortic valve and mitral valve leaflets are nonspecifically fibrocalcific. The tricuspid valve and pulmonic valve appear normal. No cardiac valves appear to prolapse.
6. DOPPLER WITH COLOR-FLOW INTERROGATION reveals mild aortic insufficiency. There also appears to be moderate mitral insufficiency. No other valvular, stenotic, or regurgitation lesions are seen.

CONCLUSION: The present echo Doppler study reveals mild aortic insufficiency along with moderate mitral insufficiency. The left ventricle and left atrium appear to be moderately enlarged. (The hypertrophy is a result of the insufficiency.) There appears to be left ventricular septal and anterior-wall hypokinesis along with moderate impairment of LVEF in the order of about 35% or so. Please see above report for details.

SERVICE CODE(S): _____

ICD-10-CM DX CODE(S): _____

(Answers to every other Case are located in Appendix D . The full answer key is only available in the TEACH Instructor Resources on Evolve.)

CASE 6-7A *Cardiology Consultation*

In Case 6-7, Eleanor Montgomery presents a year after the services you coded in Case 6-6 with the chief complaint of chest tightness. She is initially seen by Dr. James Noonar, Cardiology, at the request of her internal medicine physician, Dr. Naraquist.

LOCATION: Outpatient, Clinic

PATIENT: Eleanor Montgomery

CARDIOLOGIST: James Noonar, MD

I have been asked by Dr. Naraquist to render an opinion regarding the patient's chest tightness. She has a history of chest discomfort that led to an angiogram that showed mild atherosclerotic heart disease, nothing critical enough to warrant any intervention, and thereafter she had a normal Cardiolite stress test. Over the years, she has had rare episodes of chest discomfort. Lately, however, she has had in the last several weeks three bouts of chest discomfort—all relieved with nitroglycerin sprays × 2 each time. She indicates that she is not doing anything in particular when the episodes occur. She became concerned about this. She had no associated diaphoresis, shortness of breath, or any lightheadedness, but these were retrosternal chest pressures radiating toward the back, all promptly relieved with the two nitroglycerin sprays done serially.

Her ECG (electrocardiogram) in my office today shows normal sinus rhythm with left bundle-branch block with related repolarization abnormalities. This left bundle-branch block is a little more

prominent in terms of the QRSs (Q-wave, R-wave, S-wave) being slightly wider, but she did have a left bundle-branch block even back in December.

The patient has history of ALLERGY TO PENICILLIN AND SULFA DRUGS.

MEDICAL HISTORY includes the above as well as history of cancer of the uterus that has not recurred after having had TAH-BSO (total abdominal hysterectomy-bilateral salpingo-oophorectomy) with incidental appendectomy.

She has not had any other surgeries. There is also a history of right-wrist Colles fracture.

FAMILY HISTORY is negative for myocardial infarction and is otherwise noncontributory.

SOCIAL HISTORY: Nonsmoker. No history of alcohol abuse. No illegal drug use.

REVIEW OF SYSTEMS: Noncontributory except for above. General: No recent fevers, chills, or rigors. Weight has been stable. Neurologic: No strokelike or TIA (transient ischemic attack)-like symptoms. Endocrine: No diabetes mellitus or thyroid dysfunction noted. Hematologic: No anemia. Respiratory: No cough or hemoptysis. Cardiac: As per above with no PND (paroxysmal nocturnal dyspnea), orthopnea, or pedal edema. No syncope or presyncope. No bright red blood per rectum, melena, hemoptysis, or hematemesis. Musculoskeletal: No arthritis complaints. Psychiatric: No depression. Integumentary: No rashes.

Continued

CASE 6-7A—cont'd   *Cardiology Consultation*

CARDIAC RISK FACTORS include the following:

1. Postmenopausal state
2. History of aortic insufficiency
3. History of remote MI

MEDICATIONS:

1. Detrol
2. Meclizine
3. Premarin
4. Vitamin B_{12}
5. Omega vitamins
6. Folic acid as per above

PHYSICAL EXAMINATION: Patient is a well-developed female, age-appropriate for appearance, alert and oriented × 3. No apparent distress. Vital signs are stable. Afebrile. Blood pressure is 144/80. Pulse is 77 and regular. Weight is 152 pounds. Height is 5 feet 5 inches. HEENT (head, ears, eyes, nose, throat) examination is benign with head atraumatic and normocephalic. Oropharynx, teeth, and gums appear normal. Neck is supple without any significant jugular venous distention. No carotid bruits. No lymphadenopathy. No thyromegaly. Lungs are clear to auscultation. Cardiac examination: S1 (first heart sound) and S2 (second heart sound) are normal with a I-II/VI left sternal border soft systolic murmur. No other murmurs, gallops, clicks, or rubs are noted. The apical impulse is not palpable. No lifts, thrills, or heaves are noted. Abdominal examination: soft, nontender

abdomen. Normoactive bowel sounds. No organomegaly or palpable masses. Back without CVAT and no spinal percussion tenderness. All four extremities are without clubbing, cyanosis, or edema. Peripheral pulses are normal throughout. No femoral bruits are present. Skin is without rashes. No xanthomas or xanthelasmas are seen. Neurologic exam is grossly normal.

Old clinic notes indicate that this patient has had a history of a remote MI; however, she did have a normal cardiac stress test 5 years ago.

IMPRESSION AND RECOMMENDATIONS: This woman presents to me because of intermittent episodes of chest tightness. Of interest, she had an unremarkable angiogram back in 19xx or so. At this juncture, with her having this chest discomfort and having a possible heart murmur on exam, with a history of aortic insufficiency documented on echocardiogram a number of years ago, I will set her up for a Cardiolite stress test with an echocardiogram and return to clinic. If okay with her primary care physician, I will check screening lab results as ordered for further evaluation of this patient with a chest pain syndrome. I want to be sure that it is definitely not ischemia in someone who also has a history of atherosclerotic heart disease and a history of aortic insufficiency.

Thank you again for this consultation.

SERVICE CODE(S): _____

ICD-10-CM DX CODE(S): _____

(Answers to every other Case are located in Appendix D . The full answer key is only available in the TEACH Instructor Resources on Evolve.)

Review of Previous History

If the physician reviews a recent history (ROS and PFSH) and then references this review in the current history, this reference qualifies the current history for the same level as the previously documented level if the date and location of the information are specified. For example, when the documentation from Case 6-7A, 10/14/XX is referenced, the ROS and PFSH are of a comprehensive level. This previous service qualifies the current service for a comprehensive level of ROS and PFSH. The physician must reference the specific date and service along with a statement of "changes included" or "no changes noted" for this review of documentation to qualify for the history portion of the current service.

CASE 6-7B   *Hospital Service*

After Eleanor's cardiology consultation with Dr. Noonar, she was scheduled for a stress test. Dr. Noonar reviewed the results of the stress test and made arrangements to admit Eleanor to the hospital for further examination. Code the services provided to her.

LOCATION: Hospital, Inpatient

PATIENT: Eleanor Montgomery

CARDIOLOGIST: James Noonar, MD

HISTORY: The patient is being admitted for an angiogram because of positive Cardiolite stress test for ischemia last week. At the present interview, she had no ongoing complaints. I did a full review at the clinic, and as part of the workup, because of her chest-tightness problems, a Cardiolite stress test was performed that unfortunately showed some evidence of ischemia. That is why she is being admitted. For full details of her medical history, social history, family history, review of systems, and so on, all of which have not changed since our last visit, please refer to the previous history dated August 10. Her cardiac risk factors and her medications are also summarized in that note.

PHYSICAL EXAMINATION: No changes since 10/14/xx with no stigmata of congestive heart failure. Normal heart tones except for a 1-2/6 left sternal

border soft systolic murmur noted. She has no peripheral edema. LUNGS are clear. (Note: Your review of the medical record of 10/14/xx [those in report 6-7A], indicates that a comprehensive level of history was done.)

Recent echo Doppler study showed mild aortic insufficiency with moderate mitral insufficiency.

IMPRESSION/RECOMMENDATIONS: Patient is a woman with a history of intermittent chest tightness problems who recently had a Cardiolite stress test that was positive for ischemia. She also has a heart murmur on exam, and recent echocardiogram showed mild aortic insufficiency and moderate MR (mitral regurgitation). Thus, at this point, I will set her up for a diagnostic cardiac cath and a view of her valvular heart disease when we do this cardiac cath. We will do this bilaterally. Further notes will follow pending the clinical course on this patient who has also had, on further review of systems, some fatigue problems. In view of her valvular disease, when we do the cardiac cath, we will do the cardiac cath bilaterally.

SERVICE CODE(S): _____

ICD-10-CM DX CODE(S): _____

CASE 6-7C *Radiology Report, Chest*

LOCATION: Inpatient, Hospital

PATIENT: Eleanor Montgomery

CARDIOLOGIST: James Noonar, MD

RADIOLOGIST: Morton Monson, MD

EXAMINATION OF: Chest, two views, frontal and lateral

CLINICAL SYMPTOMS: Positive cardiac stress test; chest pain

CHEST, TWO X-RAYS: Findings: No previous examination is available for comparison at this time. The heart size and pulmonary vascular markings appear within normal limits. There are atherosclerotic changes of the thoracic aorta. No focal infiltrates are seen within the lungs. No pleural effusions are seen. Hypertrophic changes are present within the thoracic spine.

IMPRESSION:
1. ASCVD (arteriosclerotic cardiovascular disease)
2. No evidence for congestive failure or infiltrate

SERVICE CODE(S): _____

ICD-10-CM DX CODE(S): _____

(Answers to every other Case are located in Appendix D . The full answer key is only available in the TEACH Instructor Resources on Evolve.)

CASE 6-7D *Cardiothoracic Surgical Consultation*

LOCATION: Inpatient, Hospital

PATIENT: Eleanor Montgomery

CARDIOTHORACIC SURGEON: David Barton, MD

CARDIOLOGIST: James Noonar, MD

PRIMARY CARE PHYSICIAN: Alanda Naraquist, MD

REASON FOR CONSULTATION: Atherosclerotic heart disease and mitral insufficiency

HISTORY OF PRESENT ILLNESS: I have been asked by Dr. Noonar to render an opinion regarding the patient's ASHD (arteriosclerotic heart disease). Patient has a known history of atherosclerotic heart disease and has noted increasing symptoms of fatigability and intermittent chest pain over the past several months. She apparently did suffer a myocardial infarction in approximately 19xx. She remembers being given streptokinase at that time. She did have a coronary angiogram in 19xx that revealed mild atherosclerotic heart disease. A Cardiolite stress test in 19xx was normal by report. In the past several months, she has noted some increasing fatigability. She also has noticed some complaints of intermittent chest pain. She was given nitro spray to be used as needed and has used it approximately once per week for the past month or so according to her husband. The chest pain she has is retrosternal and occasionally radiates into the upper portion of the chest. She denies any accompanying shortness of breath, nausea, vomiting, or palpitations. The pain is relieved with nitroglycerin or rest. She also states that sometimes the pain is relieved with antacids. Today she underwent cardiac catheterization and coronary angiography revealing moderate atherosclerotic heart disease, preserved left ventricular systolic function, and moderate mitral insufficiency. Specifically, coronary angiography revealed a 50% stenosis of an obtuse marginal branch and a 70% stenosis of the left anterior descending artery. Distal to the stenosis, the LAD (left anterior descending coronary artery) was quite small. There was also a 75% stenosis in the extreme apical portion of the left anterior descending artery. The distal right coronary artery has a 60% stenosis. There is 3+ mitral insufficiency. A recent Cardiolite stress test revealed mild perfusion defects involving the apex and the periapical inferolateral wall. Patient ejection fraction was calculated to be 41%. Cardiothoracic surgery was consulted to discuss the option of surgical revascularization and possibly mitral valve repair or replacement.

MEDICAL HISTORY:

1. Atherosclerotic heart disease as described above
2. History of uterine cancer
3. Arthritis

She specifically denies any known history of diabetes mellitus, cerebrovascular accident, hepatitis, tuberculosis, asthma, or seizures.

SURGICAL HISTORY:

1. Total abdominal hysterectomy with bilateral salpingo-oophorectomy
2. Appendectomy

MEDICATIONS ON ADMISSION:

1. Detrol 1.25 mg (milligram) p.o. (by mouth) q.d. (every day)
2. Meclizine 12.5 mg p.o. q.d.
3. Premarin 1.25 mg p.o. q.d.
4. Aspirin 325 mg p.o.
5. Vitamin B_{12}
6. Omega-3
7. Folic acid
8. Nitro spray as described above

ALLERGIES: Penicillin and sulfa, which cause swelling and rashes. She also states that she is allergic to smoke, grapes, and oranges. The allergy to the grapes and oranges, however, appears to be a side effect (bloating and gas).

FAMILY HISTORY: Unremarkable for atherosclerotic heart disease according to the patient.

SOCIAL HISTORY: The patient is married and lives with her husband. He also has atherosclerotic heart disease and apparently had a stroke recently. She does not smoke cigarettes or drink alcohol.

REVIEW OF SYSTEMS: GENERAL: The patient denies any fever, chills, weight loss, or night sweats. CARDIAC: Essentially as that described in the history of present illness. RESPIRATORY: Unremarkable for any hemoptysis, productive cough, or wheezing. GASTROINTESTINAL: Remarkable only

Continued

CASE 6-7D—cont'd   *Cardiothoracic Surgical Consultation*

for symptoms of GE reflux. She denies any jaundice, abdominal pain, or change in bowel habits. GENITOURINARY: Remarkable for intermittent incontinence. She denies any hematuria or dysuria. MUSCULOSKELETAL: Remarkable only for arthritic symptoms in her hands and fingers. She denies any muscle pain or joint swelling other than in her fingers. NEUROLOGIC: The patient denies any severe migraines or seizures of focal weakness. SKIN: Unremarkable for any new rashes or lesions. ENDOCRINE: Unremarkable for any polydipsia, polyuria, or temperature intolerance. HEMATOLOGIC: Unremarkable for any history of anemia or bleeding tendencies.

PHYSICAL EXAMINATION: The patient is a well-developed, well-nourished, thin, white female appearing her stated age in no acute distress. Blood pressure 140/80; pulse 74 and regular; respirations 14. HEENT (head, ears, eyes, nose, throat): The patient is normocephalic. Pupils were equal, round, and reactive to light. Nose and throat exams were grossly unremarkable. The patient wears eyeglasses. The tympanic membranes were not examined. NECK: Supple without palpable adenopathy or thyromegaly. I could not detect any carotid bruits. There was no jugular venous distention with the patient sitting at 45 degrees. Auscultation of the CHEST reveals essentially clear breath sounds bilaterally. CARDIAC exam reveals a regular rhythm with a 1/6 systolic murmur heard best along the left sternal border. The murmur does not radiate. ABDOMEN: Soft abdominal organomegaly. GENITOURINARY/RECTAL: Deferred. The patient has a Foley catheter in place. Examination of the EXTREMITIES revealed palpable radial and femoral pulses. The left dorsalis pedis and posterior tibial pulse are faintly palpable. I could not detect any pedal pulses on the right foot. There is no significant peripheral cyanosis or edema. There are several superficial venous varicosities over both lower extremities. NEUROLOGIC: The patient is alert and oriented × 4. Gait was not tested. Strength was grossly normal in the upper extremities.

LABORATORY DATA: White blood cell count was 5600; hemoglobin 13.6; hematocrit 39.7; platelet count 244,000. Pro-time was 10.5; INR 0.8; PTT (partial thromboplastin time) 25.2. Total cholesterol was 212 with an HDL (high-density lipoprotein) fraction of 68 and an LDL (low-density lipoprotein)

fraction of 92. Sodium was 137, potassium 4.3, BUN (blood urea nitrogen) 16, creatinine 1.3, and glucose 78.

A 12-lead ECG (electrocardiogram) revealed a normal sinus rhythm with left bundle-branch block. Rate was 69.

IMPRESSION: The patient is a woman with a known history of atherosclerotic heart disease who has noticed increased fatigability and intermittent chest pain over the past several months. She has used nitroglycerin spray intermittently but only about once a week according to her and her husband. She is on no other cardiac medications. The results of the heart catheterization, Cardiolite stress test, and echocardiogram were reviewed with the physician. The prognosis as well as the risks and benefits of more aggressive medical therapy versus surgical revascularization and possible mitral valve surgery were discussed at length. Patient questions concerning her options for therapy were answered. I explained that because she had really been on minimal, if any, medical therapy that this certainly was an option. I explained that if she did not want to try a more aggressive medical therapy, surgery would be the next step. I also explained that if she wanted to try medical therapy and she experienced significant improvement in her symptoms, we could certainly try medical therapy for the time being. If, however, she did have breakthrough angina or developed symptoms of congestive heart failure, I think surgery would be her only other option. The patient appeared to understand the above findings and after a short discussion expressed the desire to proceed with a more aggressive medical therapy. I discussed the above findings with Dr. Noonar and Dr. Naraquist.

PLAN: The patient will be started on a more aggressive medical therapy. Dr. Naraquist will handle that. If she does not notice any improvement or experiences increasing symptoms, I think surgery should be strongly reconsidered.

Total time spent today was 65 minutes.

SERVICE CODE(S): _____

ICD-10-CM DX CODE(S): _____

(Answers to every other Case are located in Appendix D . The full answer key is only available in the TEACH Instructor Resources on Evolve.)

CASE 6-7E   *Radiology Report, Chest*

LOCATION: Inpatient, Hospital

PATIENT: Eleanor Montgomery

CARDIOLOGIST: James Noonar, MD

RADIOLOGIST: Morton Monson, MD

EXAMINATION OF: Chest

CLINICAL SYMPTOMS: Rales, left lung, cough

PA (POSTERIOR/ANTERIOR) & LATERAL CHEST, 11:05 AM: FINDINGS: Study is compared with the study of 11/01/xx at 8:40 AM. Cardiac

silhouette and pulmonary vasculature are within normal limits. No focal infiltrate or pleural effusion is identified. The aorta is tortuous with atherosclerotic change. Degenerative change involves the dorsal spine.

IMPRESSION: Stable chest

SERVICE CODE(S): _____

ICD-10-CM DX CODE(S): _____

(Answers to every other Case are located in Appendix D . The full answer key is only available in the TEACH Instructor Resources on Evolve.)

CASE 6-8   *Echo Doppler Report*

In January, the patient returns to the hospital outpatient department for another echocardiography. Code the physician portion of the service that was provided in the cardiology laboratory of the hospital.

LOCATION: Outpatient, Hospital

PATIENT: Eleanor Montgomery

PRIMARY CARE PHYSICIAN: Alanda Naraquist, MD

CARDIOLOGIST: James Noonar, MD

INDICATIONS: Evaluation of mitral regurgitation

M-Mode, 2-D, and Doppler studies with color-flow analysis were performed, and the findings are as follows:

1. CHAMBER SIZES: The left ventricle on the 2-D image is mildly enlarged and mildly concentrically hypertrophied. The LA (left atrium) appears to be mildly enlarged and on the 2-D images is normal in thickness. The right ventricle and right atrium appear to be of normal size and thickness.
2. WALL MOTION: All cardiac chambers contract normally, except for the left ventricle, which displays interventricular septal and anterior lateral wall mild hypokinesis. There also appears to be a double kick on relaxation consistent with right bundle-branch block type of conduction. The overall LVEF by visual estimation is on the order of about 35% to 40% at best.
3. The aortic root is of normal size.
4. There is no pericardial effusion.
5. VALVES: The aortic valve and mitral valve leaflets are nonspecifically mildly fibrocalcific. The tricuspid valve and pulmonic valve appear to be grossly normal. No cardiac valves appear to prolapse.
6. Doppler with color-flow interrogation reveals mild mitral insufficiency, mild aortic insufficiency, and trace tricuspid insufficiency. No other valvular stenotic or regurgitant lesions are seen.

CONCLUSION: The present echo Doppler study reveals mild enlargement of the left ventricle and left atrium, along with some LVH (left ventricular hypertrophy). There also appears to be mild aortic insufficiency, mild mitral insufficiency, and trace tricuspid insufficiency. There appear to be regional wall motion abnormalities as discussed above, with an EF (ejection fraction) of around 35% to 40% at best. Please see above report for details.

ADDENDUM: Doppler interrogation of mitral valve inflow reveals a prominent A-wave suggestive of decreased left ventricular compliance for which I apologize for not mentioning above.

SERVICE CODE(S): _____

ICD-10-CM DX CODE(S): _____

(Answers to every other Case are located in Appendix D . The full answer key is only available in the TEACH Instructor Resources on Evolve.)

CASE 6-9   *Cardiology Consultation*

In February, the patient was again admitted through the emergency room for atrial fibrillation. Her primary care physician requested a cardiology consultation. Code the cardiology consultation services. The patient has atrial fibrillation, anemia, and a heart murmur; additionally, a code is needed to report that this anemia is a complication of a surgical procedure.

LOCATION: Inpatient, Hospital

PATIENT: Eleanor Montgomery

CARDIOLOGIST: James Noonar, MD

REASON FOR ADMISSION: Rapid paroxysmal atrial fibrillation

HISTORY: I am being asked by Dr. Naraquist to render an opinion regarding this patient's paroxysmal atrial fibrillation. The patient was recently discharged after having bypass by Dr. Barton. During the admission she had some paroxysmal atrial fibrillation. She was discharged home yesterday and then, at about 3:00 in the morning today, she awoke with palpitations and a feeling of rapid heart rate. She saw her doctor, Dr. Naraquist, who found her to be in rapid atrial fibrillation. Apparently she was given verapamil and adenosine. I do not have those records at the time of this dictation, but by the time she arrived here she was in normal sinus rhythm with PACs (premature atrial contractions) occasionally, and that is what her rhythm is right now on telemetry (normal sinus rhythm with occasional PACs). She has not had any further atrial fibrillation. Lab results that have come back already include a digoxin level at 0.79 g/ml (gram/milliliter) with TSH (thyroid stimulating hormone) of 2.62, free T_4 (thyroxine) 1.0, BUN (blood urea nitrogen) 14, sodium 135, potassium 4.3, chloride 102, glucose 140, creatinine 1.4, calcium 8.2, albumin 2.5, alkaline phosphatase 102, bilirubin total 0.3, SGOT (serum glutamic oxaloacetic transaminase [AST]) 23, total protein 5.4, and CO_2 (carbon dioxide) 24.7.

On presentation, she showed a white blood cell count of 7170 with hemoglobin 8.6, hematocrit 26.2, and a normal platelet count and normal MCV (mean corpuscular volume). Recent hemoglobin around the time of her discharge earlier this week showed 8.6.

The patient at the present interview has no ongoing complaints.

Of interest, the patient had atrial fibrillation briefly during her hospitalization post bypass, which converted to sinus rhythm after getting some IV (intravenous) digitalis at that time.

MEDICAL HISTORY: Includes the above as well as prior myocardial infarction in 20xx; then in 20xx she had endometrial cancer treatment with TAH-BSO (total abdominal hysterectomy-bilateral salpingo-oophorectomy) without any recurrence of that cancer and had apparently 29 or so radiation therapy treatments, after which there were no recurrences of that cancer. She is status post remote appendectomy.

Continued

CASE 6-9—cont'd

ALLERGIES: Penicillin and sulfa

MEDICATIONS:

1. Detrol
2. Premarin
3. Vitamin B_{12}
4. Omega
5. Folic acid
6. Enteric-coated aspirin
7. Propranolol
8. Dyazide
9. Digoxin
10. KCl

The medications list said Lopressor 25 mg (milligram) b.i.d. (twice a day), but I just started that here. She was on propranolol 10 mg b.i.d. prior to this admission at the time of her recent discharge.

SOCIAL HISTORY: Nonsmoker, nondrinker. No history of alcohol abuse. No illegal drug use. Married.

FAMILY HISTORY: Patient has two sisters and two brothers who have myocardial infarctions in their later years. The rest of the family history is noncontributory.

REVIEW OF SYSTEMS: Noncontributory except for above. GENERAL: Since her bypass, she has not had any reports of fever, chills, or rigors. Weight has been stable. NEUROLOGIC: No stroke-like or TIA (transient ischemic attack)-like symptoms. ENDOCRINE: No diabetes mellitus or thyroid dysfunction noted. HEMATOLOGIC: Anemic since bypass, with hemoglobin as low as in the 7s post bypass that was 8.6 by the time of discharge without transfusion apparently given. RESPIRATORY: No cough or hemoptysis. CARDIAC: As per above with no PND (paroxysmal nocturnal dyspnea), orthopnea, or pedal edema. No syncope or presyncope was noted. No angina that she recognized as similar to the angina that she used to have before her bypass. She has a little chest wall pain from her bypass. That is about it, and she feels that she is healing well. GI (gastrointestinal): No nausea, vomiting, bloody stools, or black stools were noted. GU (genitourinary): No reports of any dysuria or hematuria, but she has some occasional urinary frequency for which she takes the Detrol, and that is chronic for her. MUSCULOSKELETAL: No complaints of any arthritis other than her left wrist chronically bothering her where she has an old fracture site that did not heal well.

CARDIAC RISK FACTORS: Include her recent bypass and two prior myocardial infarctions and family history of myocardial infarction and history of hypercholesterolemia; otherwise, negative.

PHYSICAL EXAMINATION: Well-developed, older female, age-appropriate for appearance, alert and oriented × 3, in no apparent distress. VITAL SIGNS stable; afebrile; blood pressure, 138/70; pulse, 74, occasionally irregular consistent with PACs and otherwise regular; respirations 14 and normal. HEENT (head, ears, eyes, nose, throat): Grossly benign with head atraumatic, normocephalic. Pharynx, teeth, and gums appear normal. NECK: Supple without any significant jugular venous distention. Carotids are normal in upstroke and volume. I do not appreciate any carotid bruits, but I can hear heart tones in her right neck. LUNGS: Clear to auscultation and percussion. CARDIAC: S1 (first heart sound) and S2 (second heart sound) normal with a 2/6 apical soft systolic murmur. Apical impulse is not palpable. No lifts, thrills, or heaves. ABDOMEN: Soft, nontender. Normoactive bowel sounds. No organomegaly, no palpable masses. BACK: Without CVA (stroke/cardiovascular accident) tenderness, no spinal percussion tenderness. EXTREMITIES: Without clubbing, cyanosis, or edema; both upper and lower extremities. Peripheral pulses are normal throughout, except for trace pedal pulses bilaterally. No femoral bruits. SKIN: Without rashes, no xanthomas, no xanthelasma. NEUROLOGIC: Grossly normal.

Chest-wall wound from recent bypass as well as epigastric drain site and saphenous vein strip site from her left thigh area all appear to be healing well without any stigmata of infection or dehiscence.

Admission ECG (electrocardiogram) pending.

IMPRESSION/RECOMMENDATIONS: The patient is an older woman with a history of prior myocardial infarction, followed by the development of worsening angina recently that led to bypass recently. During that hospitalization, she had some brief paroxysmal atrial fibrillation after just being discharged home yesterday afternoon. At 3:00 in the morning today, she had rapid atrial fibrillation and was seen by her local physician; she apparently received some verapamil and adenosine, and by the time she arrived here, she was back in sinus rhythm with occasional PACs, which is her current status. She appears otherwise stable and looks well otherwise. I am not convinced there is anything active going on that we need to make any changes for except that she is on such a low dose of propranolol, which I will change to Lopressor 25 mg b.i.d. (twice a day), and that will be better for atrial fibrillation prophylaxis than the low-dose propranolol. I will keep her on telemetry, and as long as she remains otherwise stable, I would recommend this patient up for discharge home tomorrow.

ADDENDUM: The patient is anemic. Her hemoglobin is only 8.6, and this is postsurgical because of blood loss with surgery as per prior records. I think ideally keeping her hemoglobin over 10 mg percent would help her and also help prophylaxis against recurrent atrial fibrillation. In this patient with recent bypass who now has a heart murmur on exam, that might be just a flow murmur due to her anemia. We will get her tanked up with some blood, get her hemoglobin over 10 gm and if she continues to have a heart murmur, I recommend an Echo. Thus, I will give her 2 units of packed cells.

Today the patient does have, in her right forearm area, a mildly cellulitic area that looks like it is an IV site infection from a prior IV placement in this patient with a history of penicillin and sulfa allergy. For this, I will empirically start her on Cipro 500 mg p.o. (by mouth) b.i.d. for 10 days.

SERVICE CODE(S): _____

ICD-10-CM DX CODE(S): _____

(Answers to every other Case are located in Appendix D . The full answer key is only available in the TEACH Instructor Resources on Evolve.)

Cardiac Catheterization

Invasive cardiology is an area of medicine in which the physician not only diagnoses the cardiac condition but also performs the cardiac procedures that involve entry into the heart and circulatory system. For example, the cardiologist would perform cardiac catheterization, coronary angioplasty, and electrophysiologic studies of the heart.

Cardiac catheterization is an invasive procedure in which the physician percutaneously inserts a catheter into a vein and manipulates the catheter into the heart or coronary vessel (**Figure 6-6**). A fine-gauge needle is inserted into an artery, such as the right subclavian artery, internal jugular, femoral, external jugular, or brachial vessel. A guidewire, followed by a catheter, is then inserted into the artery. The surgeon manipulates the catheter into position by means of fluoroscopy (viewing on a monitor).

The three parts to a cardiac catheterization service are **placement** of the catheter, **injection** of dye into the vessel, and **imaging** of the vessel. Historically, each component of a cardiac catheterization was reported with a code; however, now all three components are included in most of the catheterization codes. For example, a left heart catheterization code 93452 now includes the catheterization, injection, and imaging in one code. The supervision and interpretation are also included in these combination codes.

Once the catheter is positioned into the left coronary artery, and the catheter is repositioned into another vessel, for example, the left ventricle, the repositioning is included in the introduction. If, however, both the left coronary artery and left ventricle were injected and imaged, each injection (2) and each imaging service (2) would be reported separately.

The cardiac catheterization is often accompanied by placement of a **stent** or angioplasty. **Angioplasty** is repair of a vessel. Percutaneous transluminal coronary angioplasty (PTCA) is a procedure in which the physician makes an incision into a vessel and inserts a catheter. The catheter is manipulated into the vessel that is blocked with plaque.

A second catheter with a balloon at the tip is threaded into the blocked area. The balloon is then inflated, pushing the plaque against the vessel wall (**Figure 6-7**). Angioplasty is done to improve the caliber of the vessel and thereby increase the blood flow. Angioplasty is reported with 92920 for a single

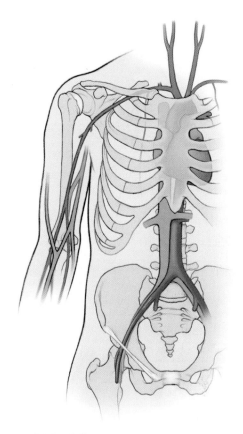

FIGURE 6–6 Cardiac catheterization.

major coronary artery or branch and add-on code 92921 for each additional branch of a major coronary artery.

Stenting, illustrated in **Figures 6-8** and **6-9,** is reinforcing a weakened area in a vessel, in addition to forcing open and holding in place that area of a vessel that is occluded. For example, if it was discovered on cardiac catheterization that the patient's coronary vessel was obstructed with atherosclerosis, the physician could widen the area and place a stent into the vessel to keep the vessel open, thereby increasing blood flow through the damaged area. The placement of the stent using the percutaneous transcatheter approach (by means of the catheter) is reported with 92928 for a single major coronary artery or branch and add-on code 92929 for each additional branch of a major coronary artery.

The terminology used in the cardiology services often refers not only to the location of the vessels but also the procedures,

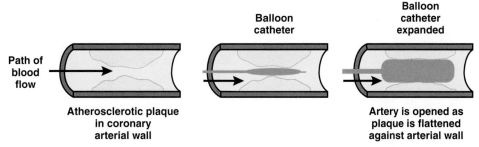

Path of blood flow

Atherosclerotic plaque in coronary arterial wall

Balloon catheter

Balloon catheter expanded

Artery is opened as plaque is flattened against arterial wall

FIGURE 6–7 Balloon-tipped catheter with the balloon inflated is used to push back plaque against the wall of the vessel.

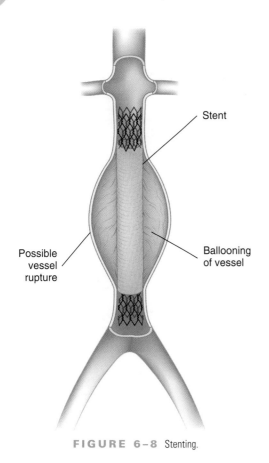

FIGURE 6–8 Stenting.

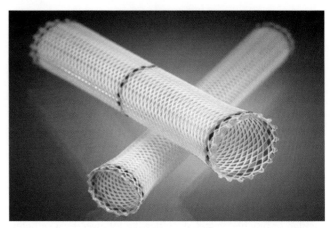

FIGURE 6–9 Stent.

for example, the LAD (left anterior descending artery) and RCA (right coronary artery). A good medical dictionary and/or abbreviation text is a necessity as you begin to code from the various catheterization, angioplasty, and stenting records.

In this report, the catheter was placed, then two injections and two images were performed in different vessels. Point III indicates an angiography; this requires an injection of contrast and an imaging. Point IV (intravenous) indicates a ventriculography; this requires an injection of contrast and an imaging. The initial introduction of the catheter includes repositioning—in this case from the left coronary artery to the left ventricle (separate vessels).

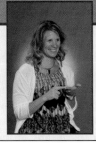

From the Trenches

"A coder should consider getting certified because most places require certification and it show that you really care about the quality of your coding."

TANECKA POE
CCS, CPC, COC

CASE 6-10A   *Emergency and Outpatient Record*

The following reports are for a 50-year-old white male who is seen in the emergency department of the local hospital. The patient was first seen in the emergency department by the physician on staff. The emergency department physician then turned the case over to Dr. Elhart, the cardiologist from the local clinic who was on call. Dr. Elhart admitted the patient to the hospital. Code the emergency outpatient services provided to the patient by Dr. Sutton.

LOCATION: Outpatient, Hospital

PATIENT: Kenneth Peters

PHYSICIAN: Paul Sutton, MD

SUBJECTIVE: This is a 50-year-old white male who has a history of hypertension. He has no other significant ongoing medical problems and takes no other medications. He is on aspirin and nifedipine. He has no known allergies. He presents acutely to the emergency room today with a history of suddenly developing substernal chest pressure radiating to his jaw that started about 1 hour prior to his arrival. He had diaphoresis and some nausea associated with this. He had no significant dyspnea, however. Other than his history of hypertension and remote smoking history when he quit smoking about 23 years ago, he has no significant risk factors for coronary artery disease.

REVIEW OF SYSTEMS: CONSTITUTIONAL: No fevers, sweats, or chills. GASTROINTESTINAL: No vomiting or diarrhea. GU (genitourinary): No urgency, frequency, or dysuria. RESPIRATORY: No cough or significant shortness of breath. CARDIOVASCULAR: Chest pain as outlined above. No history of peripheral edema.

CASE 6-10A—cont'd

OBJECTIVE: He is afebrile (99) and stable. VITAL SIGNS: There is no evidence of diaphoresis or dyspnea at this time. His HEENT (head, ears, eyes, nose, throat) exam is grossly unremarkable. NECK: Supple. There is no thyromegaly or adenopathy. HEART: S1 (first heart sound) and S2 (second heart sound), no S3 (third heart sound) or S4 (fourth heart sound). The rhythm is regular. No murmur. LUNG sounds are clear. ABDOMEN: Bowel sounds are present and active. No organomegaly, masses, or hernias are noted. Generally, soft and nontender. There is no evidence of a pulsatile mass, and his femoral pulses are equal bilaterally. EXTREMITIES: All are negative for cyanosis or edema.

His ECG (electrocardiogram) revealed a sinus rhythm with obvious inferior ST (sinus tachycardia) elevation changes. He had taken aspirin at home prior to his arrival here. He was started on IV (intravenous) nitroglycerin at 5 μg/min (microgram/minute). He was started on nasal-prong oxygen and given two sublingual nitroglycerin sprays, all of which did afford some improvement. He was given a bolus with 5000 units of IV heparin and started on 1000 units per hour heparin drip. The remainder of a cardiac panel was ordered and is pending at this time.

ASSESSMENT: Acute myocardial ischemic event

PLAN: The case was discussed with Dr. Elhart, who was on call for Cardiology. He arrived to evaluate further and assume care, and the patient was admitted and transferred to the cath lab.

SERVICE CODE(S): _____

ICD-10-CM DX CODE(S): _____

(Answers to every other Case are located in Appendix D . The full answer key is only available in the TEACH Instructor Resources on Evolve.)

CASE 6-10B *Radiology Report, Chest*

Even though you know from the previous report that this patient had an acute myocardial ischemic event, you can only code the diagnostic statement made on this one report, which is chest pain.

LOCATION: Outpatient, Hospital
PATIENT: Kenneth Peters
PHYSICIAN: Paul Sutton, MD
RADIOLOGIST: Morton Monson, MD
EXAMINATION OF: Chest
CLINICAL SYMPTOMS: Chest pain
ONE-VIEW CHEST, 9/22/xx, 4:15 PM: A portable AP (anterior posterior) supine view was obtained of the chest. No previous examinations were available for comparison. Cardiac size is within normal limits. Pulmonary vascularity is grossly unremarkable. No focal pulmonary infiltrates are seen. There is no evidence of pulmonary edema.

IMPRESSION:

1. Portable AP view of the chest shows no evidence of pulmonary edema or focal pulmonary infiltrates.
2. Scattered degenerative/hypertrophic changes are noted in the dorsal spine.

SERVICE CODE(S): _____

ICD-10-CM DX CODE(S): _____

(Answers to every other Case are located in Appendix D . The full answer key is only available in the TEACH Instructor Resources on Evolve.)

CASE 6-10C *Hospital Admission*

The angina is a symptom of myocardial infarction and is not reported separately.

LOCATION: Inpatient, Hospital
PATIENT: Kenneth Peters
PHYSICIAN: Marvin Elhart, MD
REASON FOR ADMISSION: Acute inferior-wall MI and unstable angina
HISTORY: This 50-year-old man came to the emergency room with acute inferior-wall MI with ongoing unstable angina. He has ST (sinus tachycardia) elevation in the inferior leads, reciprocal lateral changes in leads 1 and L. He has never had any prior MI. His chest pain began about 1 hour ago when he was sitting around at his home without any activities going on, and this suddenly developed retrosternally associated with some diaphoresis, but nothing else was going on otherwise. He came to the emergency room, where oxygen and sublingual nitroglycerin were administered. Right now, his chest discomfort is down to about 2/10 in intensity. He has no other ongoing complaints.

MEDICAL HISTORY: Notable for recurrent diagnosis of hypertension made by Dr. Naraquist. He was started on some medication, but I do not have the name of the medication at this admission. Otherwise, he has not been on any medications. No known drug allergies; no prior operations.

His medical history is notable for the above problem and is otherwise totally unremarkable except for the fact that he was born with retinitis pigmentosa and is on Social Security disability for that because of tunnel vision that is related to his retinitis pigmentosa and his recent documentation of hypertension. That is about it in his health history; this man has otherwise been healthy.

Continued

CASE 6-10C—cont'd

SOCIAL HISTORY: Former five- to six-packs-a-year smoker. He quit smoking more than 23 years ago. No history of alcohol abuse. No illegal drug use is noted.

FAMILY HISTORY: Negative for MI and otherwise noncontributory

REVIEW OF SYSTEMS: Noncontributory except for above. In general, no recent fevers, chills, or rigors. Weight has been stable. NEUROLOGIC: No history of any strokelike or TIA (transient ischemic attack)-like symptoms. ENDOCRINOLOGIC: No diabetes mellitus or thyroid dysfunction is noted. HEMATOLOGIC: No anemia. PSYCHIATRIC: No depression. RESPIRATORY: No cough or hemoptysis. CARDIAC: As per above with no PND (paroxysmal nocturnal dyspnea), orthopnea, or pedal edema. No syncope or presyncope. No palpitations. GI (gastrointestinal): No nausea, vomiting, bloody stools, or black stools. GU (genitourinary): No dysuria or hematuria. MUSCULOSKELETAL: No arthritis.

CARDIAC RISK FACTORS: Scant remote cigarette use and recent documentation of hypertension. Otherwise negative.

PHYSICAL EXAMINATION: Man with no known drug allergies. Well-developed, middle-aged man who is alert, and oriented × 3, complaining of mild chest discomfort. Age is appropriate for appearance. Medium build. VITAL SIGNS: Stable. He is afebrile. Blood pressure is 130/74. Pulse is 63 and regular. Respirations are 20. HEENT (head, ears, eyes, nose, throat) EXAMINATION: Benign with head atraumatic and normocephalic. Pharynx, teeth, and gums appear normal. NECK: Supple without any significant jugular venous distention. Carotids are normal in upstroke and volume. No carotid bruits. No thyromegaly. LUNGS: Clear to auscultation and percussion. CARDIAC EXAMINATION: S1 (first heart sound) and S2 (second heart sound) normal. No audible murmurs, gallops, clicks, or rubs. Apical impulse is not palpable. No lifts, thrills, or heaves. ABDOMINAL EXAM: Soft, nontender abdomen. Normoactive bowel sounds. No organomegaly, no palpable masses. No abdominal bruits. BACK: Without CVA (stroke/cardiovascular accident) tenderness, no spinal percussion tenderness. EXTREMITIES: Without clubbing, cyanosis, or edema. Peripheral pulses are normal throughout. No femoral bruits. SKIN: Without rashes, no xanthomas, no xanthelasmas. NEUROLOGIC EXAM: Grossly normal.

In discussion with the patient, I advised him about the risks and benefits of cardiac catheterization with potential acute intervention with angioplasty and stenting versus thrombolytic therapy. He and I both agree that there is an edge to going right to the cath lab as we can get our cath mobilized right away. We will bring him stat to the cath lab and do an emergency angiogram and, if need be, go ahead and do angioplasty and stenting, all depending, of course, on the results of our cardiac cath. Further notes will follow pending upcoming clinical course in the cath lab.

SERVICE CODE(S): _____

ICD-10-CM DX CODE(S): _____

(Answers to every other Case are located in Appendix D . The full answer key is only available in the TEACH Instructor Resources on Evolve.)

CASE 6-10D   *Cardiac Catheterization Report*

LOCATION: Inpatient, Hospital

PATIENT: Kenneth Peters

SURGEON: Marvin Elhart, MD

PROCEDURES PERFORMED: Left-sided heart catheterization, selective coronary arteriography, left ventriculography

INDICATION: Ongoing unstable angina with acute inferior-wall MI. See the present records for further details.

PROCEDURE NOTE: Please refer to the procedure note in the enclosed cardiac catheterization log sheet. This procedure is done through the modified Seldinger technique via the right femoral approach without any complications. At the end of the case, the right femoral arterial sheath was left in place, and the decision was made to intervene with angioplasty and stenting. See the upcoming angioplasty and stenting reports for details. The patient suffered no complications from the angiogram.

RESULTS: Results are as follows.

I. HEMODYNAMICS: Hemodynamics are listed fully on separate sheets within this report. Please refer to those separate sheets for details.

II. FLUOROSCOPY: Fluoroscopy reveals no valvular calcifications. No coronary artery calcifications are noted.

III. ANGIOGRAPHY:

    A. LEFT MAIN CORONARY ARTERY: The left main coronary artery is normal.

    B. LEFT ANTERIOR DESCENDING CORONARY ARTERY: The anterior descending coronary artery at its midportion has a 75% focal stenosis followed by a 50% focal stenosis in its midportion. The remainder of the LAD (left anterior descending coronary artery) system is normal.

    C. LEFT CIRCUMFLEX ARTERY: The left circumflex artery is an anatomically dominant vessel. The left circumflex artery is stump-occluded at its midportion. Just before this midportion stump occlusion, the left circumflex artery gives rise to its major marginal branch. This major marginal branch has a 95% focal stenosis proximally. The rest of the left circumflex system appears normal.

    D. RIGHT CORONARY ARTERY: The right coronary artery is an anatomically nondominant, small 2-mm-caliber vessel. The right coronary artery is diffusely diseased at its proximal through early midsection over about a 20-mm (millimeter) length with up to 95% luminal compromise. The rest of this RCA (right coronary artery) system is normal.

IV. VENTRICULOGRAPHY:

    A. QUALITATIVE: The left ventricle displays normal contractility except there is slight localized inferior hypokinesis near the apex. No mitral valve prolapse or mitral regurgitation is seen on normal sinus rhythm beats.

    B. QUANTITATIVE: The calculated left ventricular ejection fraction is 65%.

CASE 6-10D—cont'd

Note that the coronary artery lesions described above are atherosclerotic in nature.

CONCLUSION:

1. Severe three-vessel atherosclerotic heart disease with the culprit for his MI being a stump-occluded dominant circumflex.
2. Well-preserved left ventricular function with only slight inferior-wall localized hypokinesis.
3. Angiographically normal cardiac output.
4. See report above for details.

RECOMMENDATIONS: Angioplasty and stenting of the patient's culprit for the MI being his stump-occluded circumflex. While we are at this procedure, if this goes smoothly, I will go ahead and angioplasty and consider stenting his circumflex marginal and also angioplasty his RCA system and LAD system.

SERVICE CODE(S): _____

ICD-10-CM DX CODE(S): _____

(Answers to every other Case are located in Appendix D . The full answer key is only available in the TEACH Instructor Resources on Evolve.)

In this report the catheter was placed, then two injections and two images were performed in different vessels. Point III indicates an angiography; this requires injection and imaging codes. Point IV (intravenous) indicates a ventriculography; this requires an injection of contrast and an imaging. The initial introduction of the catheter includes repositioning — in this case from the left coronary artery to the left ventricle (separate vessels).

CASE 6-10E   *PTCA/Stenting Report*

Use appropriate HCPCS modifiers to indicate stenting locations.

LOCATION: Inpatient, Hospital

PATIENT: Kenneth Peters

SURGEON: Marvin Elhart, MD

PROCEDURE PERFORMED: Percutaneous transluminal coronary angioplasty/stenting of the left circumflex, and LAD (left anterior descending coronary artery), with angioplasty of the RCA (right coronary artery).

INDICATION: Culprit circumflex occlusion with this patient having severe disease in these other vessels as mentioned. See the present records for further details on this patient with an acute inferior-wall MI and arteriosclerosis of the coronary artery.

PROCEDURE NOTE: Please refer to the procedure log in the enclosed cardiac catheterization log sheet. This procedure is done through the modified Seldinger technique via the right femoral approach without any complications. At the end of the procedure, the right femoral arterial sheath was left in place and the patient was brought to the ICU (intensive care unit) for monitoring purposes. He suffered no complications from this procedure. Note that ReoPro was given during this procedure per the ReoPro protocol. Results are as follows.

A. PREANGIOPLASTY ANGIOGRAPHY of the right and left coronary systems is well described in the earlier cath report. See that earlier cath report for details.

B. POSTANGIOPLASTY AND STENTING ANGIOGRAPHY of the left coronary system shows the former 75% mid-LAD lesion has been reduced to 9% luminal residual post-PTCA (percutaneous transluminal coronary angioplasty)/stenting. The former 100% stump-occluded circumflex itself has been reduced to 0% luminal residual post PTCA/stenting. The remainder of the left coronary system is otherwise unchanged compared with prior to angioplasty and stenting. The LAD still has a residual midportion 50% lesion that I left alone at this time.

The RCA system, which was nondominant and small in caliber, had the former 95% diffuse proximal and midportion disease angioplastied successfully to 20% to 30% smooth luminal residual post PTCA.

Note that there was good TIMI grade 3 filling seen into the entire right and left coronary systems postprocedure. The patient was free of chest pain after the procedure.

CONCLUSION: Successful multivessel angioplasty and stenting, with angioplasty and stenting done of an occluded circumflex as well as angioplasty and stenting done of the diseased LAD and circumflex marginal and angioplasty of the RCA. This multivessel angioplasty and stenting procedure was highly successful. The patient was brought to the ICU for monitoring purposes, chest pain-free, after the procedure.

SERVICE CODE(S): _____

ICD-10-CM DX CODE(S): _____

(Answers to every other Case are located in Appendix D . The full answer key is only available in the TEACH Instructor Resources on Evolve.)

CASE 6-11A   *Hospital Admission*

This 63-year-old male presents to the ED with the chief complaint of palpitations and is seen by his cardiologist, Dr. Elhart. He had been discharged from the same hospital the day before this visit. He is again admitted into the hospital by Dr. Elhart where a history and physical, blood workup, electrocardiography, and chest x-ray are done. Code the services provided to this patient.

LOCATION: Inpatient, Hospital

PATIENT: Randall Meyers

PHYSICIAN: Marvin Elhart, MD

HISTORY: The patient is 63 years old and complaining of palpitations. Although initially he mentioned that he has had these symptoms for the last week or two, with the help of his brother, he clarified that he has been having this for 1 or 2 years, although infrequent. It has occurred more often in the last week or two. Last Saturday he was hospitalized for palpitations. He felt his heart beating fast and hard and also had some shooting pains in the left arm and a burning sensation in the left chest. He states that x-rays and ECGs (electrocardiograms) were done. He apparently had low sodium, potassium, and magnesium levels that were replaced. He was told that he had an "irregular heartbeat." He also has a history of irregular heartbeat according to his records.

He was discharged on Wednesday. Wednesday night, however, he returned to the hospital because he again experienced fast heartbeats. He was just discharged yesterday. He comes in today because this morning he had another episode when he felt his heart was beating fast. He states that it was about 100 beats per minute. He tells me that when he was in the hospital during the second hospitalization, he was found to have a heart rate of 120. This was during the night. He also had what sounds like a 2-second pause within that time. He also had a CT (computerized tomography) scan done of his head and an EEG (electroencephalogram). He is uncertain exactly why this was done. He did not state that he had any strokelike problems. He is scheduled to have an echocardiogram Tuesday in the hospital. At this time he does not complain of palpitations and has no shortness of breath or chest pains.

MEDICAL HISTORY: History of palpitations for 1 to 2 years. There has been some question in his old medical records about whether he has had atrial fibrillation in the past. History of open-heart surgery at age 16 for what sounds like aortic coarctation. (His brother knows that since then he has been able "always to feel his heart beating"). History of TURP and bladder spasms, appendectomy, and hypertension.

SOCIAL HISTORY: He is married. He does not smoke; he quit 7 years ago. Prior to that, he smoked one-half pack per day since his teenage years. Alcohol: He drinks about three whiskies a day. He states that he waters these down; however, he initially stated he did not drink, and his brother helped to clarify this history.

REVIEW OF SYSTEMS: Patient denies any history of migraines or seizures. EENT: Negative. CARDIAC: Per HPI. No PND (paroxysmal nocturnal dyspnea) or orthopnea. RESPIRATORY: No chronic cough or hemoptysis. GI (gastrointestinal): No melena or hematochezia. No vomiting or diarrhea. GU (genitourinary): History of TURP. He has no problems with his stream now. EXTREMITIES: Negative. No clubbing. NEUROLOGIC: Normal.

MEDICATIONS: Cardura, K-Dur, Prinivil, amitriptyline, phenazopyridine, over-the-counter Pepcid, Cipro, and magnesium tablets.

ALLERGIES: None to drugs known.

PHYSICAL EXAMINATION: Sixty-three-year-old in no acute distress. VITAL SIGNS: Blood pressure, 167/80. Pulse 88. Respirations 20. Temperature 36.5° C (Celsius). HEENT (head, ears, eyes, nose, throat): Head, normocephalic. Eyes are clear. TMs (tympanic membranes) are normal. PERL. EOMs (extraocular movements) intact. Nose without congestions or discharge. Oral pharynx without inflammation or exudate. NECK: Supple, no lymphadenopathy or thyromegaly. No JVD (jugular vein distention). HEART: Tones regular. S1 (first heart sound), S2 (second heart sound), no murmur appreciated. LUNGS: Clear bilaterally with good air entry. ABDOMEN: Soft, nontender. No guarding or rebound. No hepatosplenomegaly. GU: Negative. EXTREMITIES: All without cyanosis or edema.

CHEST X-RAY: PA (posterior/anterior) and lateral show no acute pulmonary disease. Radiology report pending. ECG showed sinus tachycardia, poor R-wave progression V1 through V4. Appreciate no ischemic changes.

CBC (complete blood count) was unremarkable. Electrolytes, BUN (blood urea nitrogen), and creatinine within normal limits. Glucose 114.

ASSESSMENT: Palpitations

PLAN: An echo will be performed and also a Holter monitor will be set up. Patient is comfortable with these recommendations.

SERVICE CODE(S): _____

ICD-10-CM DX CODE(S): _____

(Answers to every other Case are located in Appendix D . The full answer key is only available in the TEACH Instructor Resources on Evolve.)

CASE 6-11B   *General Chemistry*

The services in Cases 6-11B, 6-11C, 6-11D, and 6-11E were performed as part of the ED services. The diagnosis for 6-11B, 6-11C, and 6-11D is palpitations.

LOCATION: Inpatient, Hospital

PATIENT: Randall Meyers

PHYSICIAN: Marvin Elhart, MD

TIME:	REF RANGE	UNITS		+0905
BUN	7-22	mg/dl		12
Sodium	135-145	mmol/L		135
Potassium	3.6-5.5	mmol/L		5.2
Chloride	98-109	mmol/L		100
Carbon dioxide	23-33	mmol/L		29.3
Timed glucose	70-110	mg/dl	H	114
Creatinine	0.5-1.2	mg/dl		0.9
Calcium (total)	8.4-10.6	mg/dl		9.1

SERVICE CODE(S): _____

ICD-10-CM DX CODE(S): _____

(Answers to every other Case are located in Appendix D . The full answer key is only available in the TEACH Instructor Resources on Evolve.)

CASE 6-11C *Hematology*

There are two services to be coded in 6-11C—an automated blood cell count with manual differential and an automated differential.

LOCATION: Inpatient, Hospital

PATIENT: Randall Meyers

PHYSICIAN: Marvin Elhart, MD

AUTOMATED BLOOD COUNT WITH MANUAL DIFFERENTIAL

DATE: TIME:	REF RANGE	02/10/XX UNITS	+0905
WBC	3.6-11.0	K/UL	6.23
RBC	4.40-5.90	M/UL	4.82
HGB	13.0-18.0	g/dl	14.5
HCT	40-52	%	42.2
MCV	80-100	FL	87.6
MCH	26-34	PG	30.1
MCHC	32-36	g/dl	34.4
RDW	37-50	FL	42.3
PLT	150-440	K/UL	296
MPV	8.0-13.0	FL	9.8

AUTO WBC DIFFERENTIAL

DATE:	REF RANGE	02/10/XX UNITS		+0905
Neutrophil	54-74	%		70.5
Lymphocyte	22-42	%	L	18.6
Monocyte	2-8	%	H	9.3
Eosinophil	0-6	%		1.1
Basophil	0-2	%		0.5
Neutrophil	1.5-8.5	K/UL		4.39
Lymphocyte	1.1-3.5	K/UL		1.16
Monocyte	0.2-0.8	K/UL		0.58
Eosinophil	0.0-0.6	K/UL		0.07
Basophil	0.0-0.2	K/UL		0.03

SERVICE CODE(S): _____

ICD-10-CM DX CODE(S): _____

(Answers to every other Case are located in Appendix D . The full answer key is only available in the TEACH Instructor Resources on Evolve.)

CASE 6-11D *Electrocardiography*

The physician you are coding for, Dr. Naraquist, did the interpretation with a report for the following electrocardiography. Note that there is a code for the tracing only and a code for the interpretation with report only as well as a code for the complete service, which includes the tracing and the interpretation with the report.

LOCATION: Inpatient, Hospital

PATIENT: Randall Meyers

PHYSICIAN: Marvin Elhart, MD

Age: 63-year-old male

Clinical Presentation: Palpitation

Time: 7:42:02

Previous ECG (electrocardiogram): 23 December, 12:20:04 (8 years ago)

133	Sinus tachycardia, rate 104	Normal P axis, rate >=100
99	Late translation	QRS negative in V5 and V6
195	Borderline low voltage in QMART Artifact in leads (s_ II, III, aVF)	6 frontal leads <0.6mV

SERVICE CODE(S): _____

ICD-10-CM DX CODE(S): _____

(Answers to every other Case are located in Appendix D . The full answer key is only available in the TEACH Instructor Resources on Evolve.)

CASE 6-11E *Radiology Report, Chest*

LOCATION: Inpatient, Hospital

PATIENT: Randall Meyers

PHYSICIAN: Marvin Elhart, MD

RADIOLOGIST: Morton Monson, MD

EXAMINATION OF: Chest, two views

CLINICAL SYMPTOMS: Palpitations

CHEST, TWO VIEWS: Comparison is made to a previous examination dated 12-24.

FINDINGS: The heart size and pulmonary vascular markings appear within normal limits. There is new focal density present within the right lung base, which may reflect either atelectasis or infiltrate. Please correlate this clinically. There is radiographic evidence of COPD (chronic obstructive pulmonary disease). Rib changes are seen on the left, suggesting previous thoracotomy.

IMPRESSION:

1. Chronic obstructive pulmonary disease
2. Focal density is present within the right lung base, which may represent either atelectasis or infiltrate.

SERVICE CODE(S): _____

ICD-10-CM DX CODE(S): _____

(Answers to every other Case are located in Appendix D . The full answer key is only available in the TEACH Instructor Resources on Evolve.)

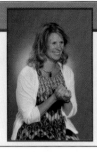

From the Trenches

"Medical coding is not just using what the doctor puts as the diagnosis. All documentation needs to support the code."

TANECKA POE
CCS, CPC, COC

CASE 6-12A   *Hospital Admission*

The patient in Case 6-11 was subsequently discharged to home. Twenty-three days after the discharge, the 63-year-old male patient was again admitted to the hospital by Dr. Elhart with a chief complaint of chest pain.

LOCATION: Inpatient, Hospital

PATIENT: Randall Meyers

PHYSICIAN: Marvin Elhart, MD

REASON FOR ADMISSION: Chest pain

HISTORY IS AS FOLLOWS: This 63-year-old man came to my service for admission and a Cardiolite stress test. Even before we started, he started having chest pain and became bradycardic after a sublingual nitroglycerin spray, and he had to be given atropine. His heart rate was down to about 40. After the atropine, the heart rate returned to normal. Blood pressure was briefly down to the 90s and high 80s systolic, but then after a fluid bolus, it returned to normal. The chest pain, which was retrosternal chest pressure, slowly ameliorated, although it is still about 1 to 2/10, and I decided to cancel the Cardiolite stress test and admit him to the ICU (intensive care unit).

He has had a history the last several months of exertional and resting chest pains, which he describes as burning in intensity, and also has had pounding in his chest occasionally. This man had an echocardiogram showing borderline concentric LVH (left ventricular hypertrophy) with mild aortic insufficiency and mild aortic stenosis with a negative non-Cardiolite stress test about 1 year ago. At the present interview, when I had him admitted, he was still having mild chest pain. He was admitted to ICU at the time that I initially had him admitted and was started on IV (intravenous) nitroglycerin.

His MEDICAL HISTORY is notable for multiple cystoscopies for urethral stricture, prostatitis, aortic coarctation that was repaired as a child, what sounds like paroxysmal atrial fibrillation, history of hypertension and history of SIADH (syndrome of inappropriate secretion of anti-diuretic hormone) in the past, and gastroesophageal reflux disease.

SOCIAL HISTORY reveals him to be married with no children. He was a former smoker, about 50 to 60 pack years.

He quit smoking about 6 to 7 years ago. No history of alcohol abuse. No illegal drug use.

FAMILY HISTORY: Negative for a mycocardial infarction otherwise, noncontributory.

REVIEW OF SYSTEMS: Noncontributory except for above with no PND (paroxysmal nocturnal dyspnea), orthopnea, pedal edema, and no syncope or presyncope. No bright red blood per rectum, melena, hemoptysis, or hematemesis.

CARDIAC RISK FACTORS: History of essential hypertension and tobacco use, and all other systems are otherwise negative.

ALLERGIES: None known, although on Floxin he gets nausea and vomiting.

CHRONIC MEDICATIONS FOR THIS MAN HAVE INCLUDED AS PER NURSING ADMISSION NOTES:

1. Cardura
2. Hydrochlorothiazide
3. Atenolol
4. Magnesium
5. KCl
6. Amitriptyline

EXAMINATION AT PRESENT: Well-developed, elderly man, age-appropriate for appearance, fully oriented, comfortable and in apparent distress, somewhat vague historian, but fully oriented × 3 and alert. Vital signs are stable. Afebrile. Blood pressure at present now is 120/70; pulse 70 and regular; respirations 22 and normal; weight 172 pounds; height 5 feet 10 inches. HEENT (head, ears, eyes, nose, throat): Grossly benign. Fundi not examined. NECK: Supple without any significant jugular venous distention. Carotids are normal in upstroke and volume. No carotid bruits. No thyromegaly. LUNGS: clear. CARDIAC: S1 (first heart sound) and S2 (second heart sound) normal with 1/6 apical to left sternal border soft systolic murmur. No other murmurs heard. No gallops, clicks, or rubs. Apical pulse is not palpable. No lifts, thrills, or heaves. ABDOMEN: Soft, nontender abdomen. Normoactive bowels sounds. No organomegaly; no palpable masses. BACK: Without CVA (stroke/cardiovascular accident) clubbing, cyanosis, or edema. Peripheral pulses are normal throughout. No femoral bruits. SKIN: Without rashes; no xanthomas; no xanthelasmas. NEUROLOGIC: Grossly normal.

ADMISSION LABORATORY AND ECG (electrocardiogram): Pending, except an ECG done at the time we were going to do the Cardiolite stress test showed no evidence of any ischemia or infarction and was otherwise unremarkable. Palpation of the chest wall shows no evidence of any tenderness, and the abdominal examination is totally benign with no evidence of abdominal tenderness.

OVERALL IMPRESSIONS AND RECOMMENDATIONS are that this man with recent chest pains, which is difficult to sort out, was scheduled for Cardiolite stress today. Before we even hooked him up, he was having burning chest pain. He had no significant ECG changes, but because of that and the fact that he became hypotensive after sublingual nitroglycerin for which we had to start IV fluids and IV atropine, my feeling is that the best decision is to place him in the ICU, cancel his Cardiolite stress test, and schedule him for a cardiac catheterization. The patient agrees with

CASE 6-12A—*cont'd*

this strategy. By the way, he had chest pain, which I did not mention off and on all last night as well. With this story, we really must consider that he has unstable angina and rule out myocardial infarction. He is scheduled for a cardiac catheterization today. I think there is no reason now to do a Cardiolite stress test because we are going to do a cardiac catheterization. The cardiac catheterization will be scheduled later today. Further notes to follow pending his clinical course.

ADDENDUM: Please note that the H and P (history and physical) was dictated somewhat late as I already had an admission thereafter

and could not dictate this until now; but after I did this dictation, we subsequently brought him down to the cardiac catheterization laboratory and found normal coronary arteries! Therefore, I will undertake a noncardiac workup for chest pain and do an upper GI (gastrointestinal) in the morning. I am going to ask Dr. Noonar to consult on this patient.

SERVICE CODE(S): _____

ICD-10-CM DX CODE(S): _____

(Answers to every other Case are located in Appendix D . The full answer key is only available in the TEACH Instructor Resources on Evolve.)

CASE 6-12B   *Cardiology Consultation*

The patient was discharged and now presents for a consultation.

LOCATION: Outpatient, Clinic

PATIENT: Randall Meyers

ATTENDING PHYSICIAN: Marvin Elhart, MD

CONSULTANT: James Noonar, MD

REASON FOR CONSULTATION: The patient has been referred for an opinion on the problem of chest pain.

HISTORY IS AS FOLLOWS: He is a somewhat vague historian, a nice man who is 63 years of age and has noticed in the last several months intermittent exertional and resting chest pains during which he feels his chest burning. He also has had palpitations. A recent 24-hour Holter monitor showed some nonsustained PSVT (paroxysmal supraventricular tachycardia) for which he tried to increase his atenolol to 100 mg (milligram) a day, but that slowed his pulse down to the 40s and he went back to his usual 50 mg of atenolol per day and still is having palpitation problems. On the Holter monitor, there is also a suggestion of some ischemia on the monitored ECG (electrocardiogram). Echocardiogram was done in May that also showed borderline concentric left ventricular hypertrophy with mild aortic insufficiency and aortic stenosis. He had a negative non-Cardiolite stress test about one year ago. Back then he was not having any chest pain per se he tells me. Note that the patient has never had a myocardial infarction. He is presently on Cardura 2 mg daily; hydrochlorothiazide a half tablet daily; atenolol 50 mg daily; magnesium 64 mg, two tablets b.i.d. (twice a day); KCI (potassium chloride) 20 mEq (milliequivalent) b.i.d.; amitriptyline 10 mg q.h.s. (each bedtime). He has no known true drug allergies, although when he is taking Floxin he has nausea and vomiting.

MEDICAL HISTORY is notable for the above. Additionally:

1. He has had multiple cystoscopes for urethral stricture.
2. Prostatitis.
3. Repair of aortic coarctation as a child.
4. History in the past of what sounds like paroxysmal atrial fibrillation.
5. History of hypertension.
6. History of hyponatremia believed in the past to be due to SIADH (syndrome of inappropriate secretion of anti-diuretic hormone).
7. He also has had a history suggestive of gastroesophageal reflux disease.

SOCIAL HISTORY: He is married with no children, a former smoker, about 50 to 60 packs per year. He quit smoking 6 to 7 years ago. No history of alcohol use or abuse. No illegal drug use.

FAMILY HISTORY: Negative for myocardial infarction and otherwise noncontributory.

REVIEW OF SYSTEMS: Noncontributory except for above with no PND (paroxysmal nocturnal dyspnea), orthopnea, or pedal edema; no syncope or presyncope, no bright red blood per rectum, melena, hemoptysis, or hematemesis.

CARDIAC RISK FACTORS: History of essential hypertension and tobacco use; all organ systems are otherwise negative.

ALLERGIES: He has no known true drug allergies, although when taking Floxin he gets nausea and vomiting.

PRESENT MEDICATIONS include:

1. Cardura 2 mg daily
2. Hydrochlorothiazide, $^1/_2$ tablet daily
3. Atenolol 50 mg daily
4. Magnesium 64 mg, 2 tablets t.i.d. (three times a day)
5. KCI 20 mEq b.i.d.
6. Amitriptyline 10 mg q.h.s.

PHYSICAL EXAMINATION: Well-developed older man, age-appropriate for appearance. Fully oriented, comfortable, and in no apparent distress. Vital signs are stable. Afebrile. Blood pressure is 130/74. Pulse is 72 and regular. Respirations are 20 and normal. Weight is 172 pounds. Height: 5 feet 10 inches. HEENT (head, ears, eyes, nose, throat) examination is grossly benign. Fundi are not examined. Neck is supple without any significant jugular venous distention. Carotids are normal in upstroke and volume; no carotid bruits; no thyromegaly. Lungs are clear. Cardiac examination: S1 (first heart sound) and 2 (second heart sound) are normal with a I/VI apical to left sternal border soft systolic murmur. No other murmurs are heard; no gallops, clicks, or rubs. Apical impulse is not palpable. No lifts, thrills, or heaves. Abdominal examination reveals a soft, nontender abdomen with normoactive bowel sounds. There is no organomegaly. There are no palpable masses. Back reveals no CVAT and no spinal percussion tenderness. Extremities are without clubbing, cyanosis, or edema. Peripheral pulses are normal throughout. No femoral bruits. Skin without rashes. No xanthomas. No xanthelasmas. Neurologic examination is grossly normal.

Continued

CASE 6-12B—cont'd

ECG today: Normal sinus rhythm with right bundle-branch block with diffuse ST-T abnormalities.

My IMPRESSION/RECOMMENDATIONS for this patient with a history of some recent chest pain problems are somewhat difficult to sort out given that he has a history suggestive of gastroesophageal reflux disease. It sounds to me that, with his cardiac risk factors, he is developing angina, and at this point I would suggest the following:

1. An ECG.
2. Set up a Cardiolite stress test in the morning.
3. Given his slight heart murmur and mild aortic insufficiency, he is given SBE (subacute bacterial endocarditis) prophylaxis card.

ADDENDUM: The patient has a history of a coarctation in the aorta repaired many years ago. When I check his radial pulses both in the left and right arm and check that against his femoral pulses in the right and left legs, I see no timing delay in his femorals. Because there is no timing delay between radial and femoral pulses, there is no clinical evidence of any significant recurrent coarctation.

I will make further comments about what to do next for this man who also has had some nonsustained PSVT (paroxysmal supraventricular tachycardia) seen on a recent 24-hour Holter monitor that did not tolerate higher doses of a beta-blocker. Right now, though, I want to see how he does on a stress test and then make a decision about whether he needs to have an angiogram. I suspect his Cardiolite stress test will be positive. His clinical story and recent 24-hour Holter monitor did suggest some ischemic problems potentially. Further notes will follow pending the clinical course. Thank you for the consultation.

SERVICE CODE(S): _____

ICD-10-CM DX CODE(S): _____

(Answers to every other Case are located in Appendix D . The full answer key is only available in the TEACH Instructor Resources on Evolve.)

CASE 6-12C *Radiology Report, Chest*

LOCATION: Outpatient, Hospital

PATIENT: Randall Meyers

ATTENDING PHYSICIAN: Marvin Elhart, MD

RADIOLOGIST: Morton Monson, MD

EXAMINATION OF: Chest

CLINICAL SYMPTOMS: Chest pain, precatheterization

CHEST, SINGLE VIEW: COMPARISON: Comparison is made to a previous examination dated 1 year ago.

FINDINGS: The heart size appears at the upper limits of normal. The pulmonary vascular markings appear within normal limits. This examination is somewhat rotated. This accentuates the right paratracheal markings. Definite focal infiltrates are not seen within the lungs. No pleural effusions are seen.

IMPRESSION: No evidence for infiltrate or congestive failure.

SERVICE CODE(S): _____

ICD-10-CM DX CODE(S): _____

(Answers to every other Case are located in Appendix D . The full answer key is only available in the TEACH Instructor Resources on Evolve.)

CASE 6-12D *Cardiac Catheterization Report*

LOCATION: Outpatient, Hospital

PATIENT: Randall Meyers

ATTENDING PHYSICIAN: Marvin Elhart, MD

SURGEON: Marvin Elhart, MD

PROCEDURES PERFORMED: Left-sided heart catheterization, selective coronary angiography, left ventriculography

INDICATION: Clinical unstable angina. See the present hospital records for further details.

PROCEDURE NOTE: Refer to the procedure log in the enclosed cardiac catheterization log sheet. Note that this procedure was done via the modified Seldinger technique via the right femoral approach without any complications. At the end of the case, sheaths were removed and good hemostasis was achieved. The patient suffered no complications from this procedure.

RESULTS:

I. HEMODYNAMICS: Hemodynamics are listed fully on separate sheets within this report and are normal.

II. FLUOROSCOPY: Fluoroscopy reveals no valvular calcifications. No coronary artery calcifications are noted.

III. ANGIOGRAPHY (This is the injection and interpretation of the arteries):
   A. LEFT MAIN CORONARY ARTERY: Normal
   B. LEFT ANTERIOR DESCENDING CORONARY ARTERY and its branches are normal.
   C. LEFT CIRCUMFLEX ARTERY: Normal.
   D. There is a ramus intermedius branch. This ramus intermedius branch is normal.
   E. RIGHT CORONARY ARTERY: The right coronary artery is an anatomically dominant vessel. The right coronary artery and its branches are normal.

IV. VENTRICULOGRAPHY (This is the injection and interpretation of the ventricle, a different [separate] vessel):
   A. QUALIFICATIONS: The left ventricle displays normal contractility. No regional wall motion abnormalities are identified. No mitral valve prolapse or mitral regurgitation is seen.
   B. QUANTITATIVE: The calculated left ventricular ejection fraction is pending at the time of this dictation but by visual estimation is normal.

CASE 6-12D—cont'd

CONCLUSION:

1. Normal coronary arteries
2. Normal left ventricular systolic function
3. Angiographically normal cardiac output
4. See report above for details

RECOMMENDATIONS: Noncardiac workup of chest pain. The patient has no underlying coronary artery disease seen at this time, and even though he clinically had unstable angina in retrospect with his normal angiogram study, one must consider pursuing a noncardiac workup of chest pain.

SERVICE CODE(S): _____

ICD-10-CM DX CODE(S): _____

(Answers to every other Case are located in Appendix D . The full answer key is only available in the TEACH Instructor Resources on Evolve.)

CASE 6-12E   *Radiology Report, GI*

Immediately after the cardiac catheterization, the following x-ray was taken.

LOCATION: Outpatient, Hospital

PATIENT: Randall Meyers

ATTENDING PHYSICIAN: Marvin Elhart, MD

RADIOLOGIST: Morton Monson, MD

EXAMINATION OF: Upper GI (gastrointestinal)

CLINICAL SYMPTOMS: Chest pain

UPPER GI: CLINICAL HISTORY: Chest pain

FINDINGS: A biphasic examination of the upper gastrointestinal tract was performed. The esophagus, stomach, and duodenum appear morphologically normal. There is no evidence of ulceration. During the course of the examination, multiple episodes of gastroesophageal reflux were noted. This reflux is considered of mild to moderate degree. Definite hiatal hernia was not seen.

IMPRESSION:

1. Mild to moderate gastroesophageal reflux
2. No evidence of ulceration

SERVICE CODE(S): _____

ICD-10-CM DX CODE(S): _____

(Answers to every other Case are located in Appendix D . The full answer key is only available in the TEACH Instructor Resources on Evolve.)

Miscellaneous Reports

Cardioversion

Cardioversion is electrical stimulation of the heart to achieve normal heart rhythm. The procedure can be performed as an emergency procedure or a planned procedure to correct an abnormal heart rhythm. There are two approaches used for cardioversion—an internal procedure (92961, the heart is exposed and paddles are placed directly on the heart) and an external procedure (92960, the paddles are placed directly on the chest).

CASE 6-13   *Cardioversion*

The patient had a diagnosis of atrial fibrillation and atrial flutter, and Dr. Noonar has recommended cardioversion to correct the abnormal rhythm.

LOCATION: Outpatient, Hospital

PATIENT: Karen Blackwell

PHYSICIAN: James Noonar, MD

PROCEDURE PERFORMED: Cardioversion

INDICATIONS: Atrial fibrillation and atrial flutter

DESCRIPTION OF PROCEDURE: Informed consent was obtained. After adequate sedation and while the patient's heart rate, blood pressure, and O_2 (oxygen) saturation were being monitored, cardioversion was done successfully using 300 synchronized joules with which the patient converted to sinus bradycardia; however, she had frequent PACs (premature atrial contractions).

RECOMMENDATIONS: We will load the patient up with 1 g (gram) of procainamide in an attempt to maintain her sinus mechanism.

SERVICE CODE(S): _____

ICD-10-CM DX CODE(S): _____

(Answers to every other Case are located in Appendix D . The full answer key is only available in the TEACH Instructor Resources on Evolve.)

CASE 6-14 *Transesophageal Echocardiogram Report*

LOCATION: Outpatient, Hospital

PATIENT: Mary South

PHYSICIAN: David Barton, MD

RADIOLOGY: Morton Monson, MD

PROCEDURE: Transesophageal echocardiogram

INDICATION: To evaluate the patient for the presence of atrial thrombi prior to cardioversion

DESCRIPTION OF PROCEDURE: Informed consent was obtained. The patient was premedicated with intravenous Versed and fentanyl. (Note: These drugs indicate conscious sedation.) The throat was anesthetized with Hurricane spray. After adequate sedation and local anesthesia were obtained, the transesophageal echocardiogram was performed in the usual manner.

FINDINGS:

CARDIAC CHAMBER: The left atrium was dilated. The left atrial appendage was dilated. There was no evidence of atrial thrombi. The left ventricle was normal sized. There was moderate diffuse hypokinesis. The overall left ventricular systolic function was moderately reduced with an

ejection fraction of about 30%, markedly better than her echocardiogram from a couple of days ago. The right atrium and right ventricle were markedly dilated. The aortic root was normal sized.

VALVES: The mitral valve was mildly thickened but opened normally. There was mild aortic sclerosis without stenosis. The tricuspid valve was grossly normal. The pulmonic valve was also normal.

DOPPLER AND COLOR DOPPLER INTERROGATION revealed the presence of moderate mitral insufficiency and what appeared to be also moderate tricuspid insufficiency.

CONCLUSION:

1. No evidence of atrial thrombi
2. Dilated left atrium
3. Dilated right atrium and right ventricle
4. Moderate mitral and what appears to be (?) moderate tricuspid insufficiency

SERVICE CODE(S): _____

ICD-10-CM DX CODE(S): _____

CASE 6-15 *Operative Report, Thromboendarterectomy*

LOCATION: Outpatient, Hospital

PATIENT: Mary Heidorn

SURGEON: Gary Sanchez, MD

PREOPERATIVE DIAGNOSIS: Right carotid stenosis

POSTOPERATIVE DIAGNOSIS: Right carotid stenosis

PROCEDURE PERFORMED: Right carotid thromboendarterectomy

This patient was monitored with EEG (electroencephalogram). There were some depressions when we clamped, but this returned to normal after re-establishing circulation.

ANESTHESIA: General

DESCRIPTION OF PROCEDURE: Under general anesthesia, the patient's right side of the neck was prepped and draped in the usual manner. An incision was made across the medial border of the sternocleidomastoid. The platysma was divided. The common carotid artery was localized. We then put a

LigaLoop around it, and then we isolated the external and internal carotid arteries and placed LigaLoops around them. We saw the hypoglossal nerve. We put the retractors in and retracted on the upper end of the wound, and then we gave the patient heparin and proceeded with the arteriotomy.

After placing clamps on the internal, common, and external carotid arteries, the arteriotomy was done. This was a severe stenosing atherosclerotic plaque. This was removed. We then sutured the artery up with a 5-0 Prolene at the distal and then at the proximal and meeting in the middle, producing back bleeding, and then we closed the artery. The wound was then closed in layers after placing a Hemovac in the wound. The wound was approximated with 2-0 chromic, 2-0 plain, and surgical staples on skin. A dressing was applied. The patient was discharged to recovery.

SERVICE CODE(S): _____

ICD-10-CM DX CODE(S): _____

CASE 6-16A *Radiology Report, Venogram*

This patient has chronic renal failure, and the nephrologist is going to create a fistula (channel between two structures) between a vein and an artery to be used for hemodialysis. Prior to the surgery, a venogram is performed to ensure the vessels are adequate for the fistula creation. The hospital provides the technician and equipment and Dr. Monson provides the supervision, interpretation, and report of the radiology service.

LOCATION: Outpatient, Hospital

PATIENT: Maggie Sodium

PHYSICIAN: George Orbitz, MD

RADIOLOGIST: Morton Monson, MD

EXAMINATION OF: Limited venogram of left upper extremity

CLINICAL SYMPTOMS: CRF, intraoperative evaluation of veins of the left forearm

LIMITED VENOGRAM OF LEFT UPPER EXTREMITY

Injection of a vein in the region of the wrist was performed, and there was visualization of the veins predominantly at and above the antecubital region. There is no evidence of thrombus within the veins, and there is no evidence of extravasation. The veins are adequate for an AV fistula; surgery will be scheduled.

SERVICE CODE(S): _____

ICD-10-CM DX CODE(S): _____

CASE 6-16B   *Operative Report, Arteriovenous Fistula*

LOCATION: Outpatient, Hospital

PATIENT: Maggie Sodium

SURGEON: George Orbitz, MD

PREOPERATIVE DIAGNOSIS: Chronic renal failure

POSTOPERATIVE DIAGNOSIS: Chronic renal failure

PROCEDURE PERFORMED: Placement of primary arteriovenous fistula, left wrist

ANESTHESIA: General

PROCEDURE: With the patient under general anesthesia, the arm was marked for the vein. There was a fairly large cephalic vein at the wrist on the left, but we are not certain as to whether there was a continuous vein going up the arm. We then prepped and draped the arm. We first made a small incision about midway up the forearm over an area where we could no longer palpate the vein. After marking this incision and freeing up the vein in this location, we could see that there was an adequate vein going up to just below the elbow. With this in mind, we then made an extended incision at the wrist and were able to mobilize the cephalic vein toward the radial artery. We were also able to free the radial artery. We took down some tributaries of the vein with 4-0 silk ligatures and then in a similar fashion took down tributaries of the artery. Once we had both vessels well immobilized, we brought them together with vascular loops, gave the patient 5000 units of heparin, and then performed a primary anastomosis between the artery and vein using 6-0 Prolene. With completion of the anastomosis, there was excellent flow with a palpable thrill. We ligated three tributary branches of vein to increase the flow up the arm. We passed a Fogarty catheter all the way up the arm and then gently pulled it back with the balloon partially inflated to dilate the vein. This showed that we had a patent vein all the way up the arm and that we were able to dilate the vein back down to the anastomosis. This Fogarty catheter was introduced through the distal venous segment, which was then ligated using 2-0 silk. On completion of the procedure, the patient had an intact vascular anastomosis with good flow documented to the hand in both the radial and ulnar arteries. The patient had a palpable thrill going up the lower portion of the arm. The incisions were then closed using an inner layer of 3-0 chromic and a skin layer of 4-0 nylon. Sterile dressings were applied. The patient tolerated the procedure well and was discharged from the operating room in stable condition.

SERVICE CODE(S): _____

ICD-10-CM DX CODE(S): _____

(Answers to every other Case are located in Appendix D . The full answer key is only available in the TEACH Instructor Resources on Evolve.)

CASE 6-17   *Operative Report, Arteriovenous Fistula*

LOCATION: Inpatient, Hospital

PATIENT: Samuel Mortonson

SURGEON: Gary Sanchez, MD

PREOPERATIVE DIAGNOSIS: End-stage renal disease

POSTOPERATIVE DIAGNOSIS: End-stage renal disease

OPERATIVE PROCEDURE: Primary arteriovenous fistula, right radiocephalic

INDICATION: This 48-year-old man has end-stage renal disease and is on hemodialysis. He has fair-sized cephalic vein clinically. I discussed the primary AV (arteriovenous) fistula between the radial artery and cephalic vein. I had previously discussed this procedure with him. I said that we should try to get this to work first. Sometimes, though, veins do not dilate up nicely, depending on how many times they have been "poked" for IV (intravenous) access and blood draws. He has been in the hospital a number of times, and so they have had some access to this but overall clinically it looks pretty good.

PROCEDURE: The patient was brought to the operating theater and placed in a supine position on the operating room table. After receiving some IV sedation, he was prepped and draped in a sterile fashion. His cephalic vein was marked out, as was his radial artery. An incision line was marked halfway between these two. This was longitudinal. It was infiltrated with 0.5% Marcaine with epinephrine, which was left to set for a couple of minutes. An incision was then made. We dissected out the cephalic vein first. This was done sharply. We were able to get around the circumferential. A couple of small side branches were ligated with 4-0 silks and transected. We were able to dissect up a good segment of the cephalic vein and then dissected out the radial artery. This was also done sharply. We were able to dissect down to it and dissect it sharply in a circumferential manner. This had a fair amount of calcifications within it. Two tiny side branches were taken down with 4-0 silks and transected. We then put a right-angle clamp on the distal aspect of the cephalic vein. It was transected. We ligated this with 2-0 Vicryl and attached a Titus needle onto the end of the cephalic vein. This dilated nicely and flushed out easily. We then occluded the radial artery proximally and distally with mini vessel loops in a Potts loop fashion. Arteriotomy was made. Bleeding was still coming distally. This was controlled then with a small profunda clamp. This worked well. We then irrigated it out with a heparinized saline both proximally and distally for heparinization and spatulated the end of the vein and cut it to length. We then performed an end-to-side anastomosis using Gore-Tex CV-7 suture. Prior to placing the last couple of bites, we back-bled and forward-bled and flushed everything out with heparinized saline. We then placed the last couple of suture bites and secured the suture line. We opened up the vein and then the proximal radial artery. We let the flow initially go through this and into the vein. We then opened up the distal radial artery. A light thrill was present. Pulses were heard with the Doppler of the radial artery on the wrist distally

Continued

CASE 6-17—cont'd

to our anastomosis as well as on the ulnar artery. The palmar arch also had good flow both proximally and distally. There was distal artery flow and good capsular refill in all fingers. There was good long diastolic flow through the cephalic vein up the forearm. A light thrill was present over the area. A good bruit was also audible with a sterile stethoscope. Hemostasis was present. We closed the subcutaneous tissue with 3-0 Vicryl in interrupted fashion. The skin was closed with 4-0 Vicryl in a running subcuticular fashion. Sterile dressings of Telfa and Tegaderm were applied. The patient tolerated the procedure well and went to the recovery room in stable condition.

SERVICE CODE(S): _____

ICD-10-CM DX CODE(S): _____

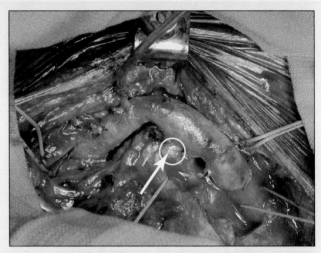

FIGURE 6-10 Arteriovenous fistula.

(Answers to every other Case are located in Appendix D . The full answer key is only available in the TEACH Instructor Resources on Evolve.)

CASE 6-18A   *Operative Report, Abdominal Aortic Aneurysm*

LOCATION: Inpatient, Hospital

PATIENT: Tom Hoff

SURGEON: Gary Sanchez, MD

PREOPERATIVE DIAGNOSIS: Ruptured abdominal aortic aneurysm

POSTOPERATIVE DIAGNOSIS: Ruptured abdominal aortic aneurysm. Anemia due to acute blood loss

OPERATIVE PROCEDURE: Repair of ruptured abdominal aortic aneurysm with a 20 × 10 bifurcated aortobifemoral graft

ANESTHESIA: General

INDICATIONS FOR SURGERY: The patient is a 36-year-old male who came to the emergency room with severe back and abdominal pain. The patient was found to have a ruptured abdominal aortic aneurysm, and he was taken immediately to the operating room for surgery.

DESCRIPTION OF OPERATION: The patient was taken to the operating room with a ruptured abdominal aortic aneurysm. A midline abdominal incision was made. The abdomen was entered. The patient's entire right side and middle part of his abdomen were full of blood. Attempts were made, and finally control was obtained by clamping the aorta at the level of the diaphragm. The aneurysm was then opened, and there was aneurysmal wall on the anterior surface. It had completely blown out. After searching, we were able to find the neck of the aneurysm and the aorta. A clamp was placed on this level, and the clamp at the hilum was released. The distal iliac arteries were also aneurysmal, and these were located with some difficulty. After these were packed off, the proximal aneurysmal aorta was partially transected, leaving the posterior wall intact. A 20 × 10-mm (millimeter) bifurcated Dacron graft was then sewn end to end to the aorta using a running 3-0 Prolene suture. The vascular clamp then was placed on the graft, and the clamp on the aorta was then released. There was some bleeding on the left lateral aspect of the anastomosis, and this was controlled with 3-0 Prolene sutures. After this, the anastomosis was tight. The distal iliac artery openings were then oversewn. It was difficult to ascertain the openings in the distal iliac arteries because of the aneurysmal dilatation. Before this was done, the bleeding from the iliac arteries was controlled by dissecting both femoral arteries

and clamping the femoral arteries to decrease the backflow. The iliac arteries were oversewn from the inside; at least this attempt was made. The right and left limbs were then tunneled into each groin area. An end-to-side anastomosis was then done on each femoral artery. Just prior to completion of the left femoral anastomosis, the clamp on the aortic graft was released to allow flow to go through the left limb of the graft. When this occurred, there was extreme backflow of blood into the abdomen through the iliac arteries. We did not sew the opening closed. After multiple attempts to try to control this, we were unable to do so and again a large amount of blood loss was obtained because of this bleeding. Therefore, we packed the artery off and opened up the abdomen initially from the left groin into the abdomen lying out the iliac artery. When this was done, we then ligated the iliac artery with 0 silk sutures. After we completed this, the anastomosis was completed on the left side and blood was allowed to flow in the left femoral artery. The right anastomosis was completed and then blood was allowed to flow into this artery. The patient's blood pressure was initially below 50, but blood pressure was finally over 100. The estimated blood loss was unable to be obtained because of the huge amount of blood loss sustained during the operation. The patient received 5351 cc (cubic centimeter) of Cellsaver, 24,000 cc of crystalloid, 500 cc of albumin, 6978 cc of RBCs (red blood cells), 245 cc of platelets, 1051 cc of fresh frozen plasma, and 6000 cc of lactated Ringer's. The patient's incisions were partially closed, and the abdominal wound was left open. Steri-Drapes were placed within the abdominal wall, and then towels were placed over the Steri-Drapes, followed by Jackson-Pratt drains, and then followed by adhesive loban drapes. This would allow for expansion of the abdomen because of the edema that occurred during surgery. Also, the right colon appeared to have a large amount of ecchymosis in this area, and there is some question as to whether or not this will be survivable. The patient put out less than 100 cc of urine during the entire operation, which lasted over 5 hours. The patient was taken back to the intensive care unit in critical condition.

SERVICE CODE(S): _____

ICD-10-CM DX CODE(S): _____

CASE 6-18B *Pathology Report*

LOCATION: Inpatient, Hospital

PATIENT: Tom Hoff

SURGEON: Gary Sanchez, MD

PATHOLOGIST: Grey Lonewolf, MD

CLINICAL HISTORY: Leaking abdominal aortic aneurysm, ruptured

SPECIMEN RECEIVED: Abdominal aortic plaque and clot

GROSS DESCRIPTION: The specimen is labeled with the patient's name and "abdominal aortic plaque and clot," which consists of multiple pink-tan laminated fibrin thrombus fragments up to 6 cm (centimeter) in greatest dimension. Admixed are numerous fragments of dark red blood clots up to 7 cm in greatest dimension. A few tan-yellow atherosclerotic plaque segments up to 2.5 cm in greatest dimension were seen, with representative sections in five cassettes.

MICROSCOPIC DIAGNOSIS: Fibrohyalinized tissue with severe atherosclerosis and plaque hemorrhage with laminated fibrin thrombus and blood clot consistent with abdominal aortic aneurysm.

SERVICE CODE(S): _____

ICD-10-CM DX CODE(S): _____

(Answers to every other Case are located in Appendix D . The full answer key is only available in the TEACH Instructor Resources on Evolve.)

CASE 6-19 *Operative Report, Femoral Artery Laceration*

You will be coding the services of both the surgeon and the assistant surgeon in the following case. The diagnosis code for this service will be the complication, which was an accidental puncture or laceration that occurred during the initial stenting procedure.

LOCATION: Inpatient, Hospital

PATIENT: Nora Hycliff

ATTENDING PHYSCIAN: Ronald Green, MD

SURGEON: Gary Sanchez, MD

ASSISTANT SURGEON: Terry Moltz, MD

PREOPERATIVE DIAGNOSIS:

1. Retroperitoneal bleed
2. Right femoral artery laceration

POSTOPERATIVE DIAGNOSIS:

1. Retroperitoneal bleed
2. Right femoral artery laceration

PROCEDURE PERFORMED: Repair of femoral artery laceration

INDICATIONS: This is a 57-year-old female who underwent a heart catheterization/stenting today. This actually had been performed through a left femoral artery; however, the procedure started with an attempt on the right. They had to take a few sticks apparently to get into the right femoral artery. They were able to cannulate it, though, and were able to pass a guidewire a short distance. They were unable to pass it any farther. This was removed. They subsequently then went over to the left groin and performed their procedure. Actually, I had been called to see her regarding a stenosis of the left common femoral artery. She had a pulseless left foot; however, decreasing to a 4-French catheter, there was no flow by the catheter noted on angiography. The catheter was then subsequently removed and was closed with a VasoSeal. She had a pulse in the anterior tibial artery on the left and seemed to have at times weak pulse in the posterior tibial on the right. She was subsequently transferred up to the medical ICU (intensive care unit). I checked on her shortly thereafter. She was awake, alert, and doing okay. We could not identify any pulses in the left foot but could on the right foot. Arterial Doppler study also could not find any pulses in the foot. I therefore contacted interventional radiology about performing a left leg angiogram. They were going to do this within the hour. Subsequently, she apparently became hypotensive, and she was managed for this by Dr. Noonar and then by Dr. Green.

When she came down to interventional radiology, she was rather hypotensive. She then had a CT (computed tomography) scan ordered by Dr. Green and was brought there. I was notified that she was going to the scanner. I went to see her. She was noted to have a large retroperitoneal bleed on the right side. I thought this was most likely coming from her right femoral stick.

I met with the patient's husband. I discussed the patient's diagnosis and my recommendations of a right femoral artery exploration and possibly a left femoral artery exploration to re-establish flow in the left foot as necessary.

PROCEDURE: The patient was brought to the operating room as a class 1. She went right back to room 9 and had a cardiac arrest at this point. She became pulseless. We started chest compressions. She had, of course, already been intubated. Code was managed by anesthesia. We kept giving her IV (intravenous) boluses of fluids. We were able to get her pressure back. We then quickly prepped and draped her. Even while I was scrubbing in, she had another episode of pulseless electrical activity. They were able to get her pulse back again. We then prepped and draped in a sterile fashion. A vertical incision was made in the right groin. Dissection was carried down through the subcutaneous tissues. I tried to come in high on this to be sure that we could get in proximally to the lesion. We came down on the external oblique and cleaned this all off down to the artery. It was at this point that some bleeding occurred. We could see that there was a laceration in the anterior wall of the common femoral artery; however, we did not really have the artery very cleaned out at this point, nor could I get proximal control. We tried to get proximal control above this, but with the bleeding and the patient being obese, we just could not get control. We then extended the incision in hockey-stick fashion up the right side. We carried this down to the fascia. We divided this and entered the retroperitoneal space. There was a huge amount of sanguineous fluid but no clot in this. Again, because of the body habitus, we still could not get down to really good control in the external iliac. I was able, though, to control it somewhat with a finger. Dr. Moltz then came in to provide surgical assistance. I was then able to take 5-0 Prolene stitch to oversew the laceration. This was on the

Continued

CASE 6-19—cont'd

anterior wall of the common femoral artery. We were able to fix this with a figure-of-eight ligature. This had been bleeding rather profusely. I am not sure whether the wire had caught on something as it came out or if it had been kind of tangentially lacerated with the needle, but there was a hole of approximately 3 to maybe even 4 mm (millimeter). With this controlled, visualization was much better in the groin. She had a couple of other bleeding points from our dissection that were controlled with either Prolene ligatures or through Vicryl ligatures. A small branch had been avulsed off the common femoral vein. Again, this was a small branch. The soft tissue site was ligated with 3-0 Vicryl. A small hole in the vein was ligated with and repaired with a 6-0 Prolene suture. We packed Gelfoam and thrombin in these areas. We then reinspected the wound after a little while. Again, we continued to achieve hemostasis in the soft tissues with either 3-0 Vicryl ligatures or cautery. She had a lot of soft-tissue areas that were just oozing. The patient had received multiple units of blood and had also received FFP (fresh frozen platelets) as well as platelets. She was going into DIC (disseminated intravascular coagulation). With packing of the wound, though, things actually seemed to settle down and seemed to be rather hemostatic overall. We placed a no. 10 flat Jackson-Pratt drain and brought this out through a separate stab wound. This was attached to the skin with 2-0 silk. We closed the retroperitoneal exposure site and the fascia overlying it with 2-0 Vicryl suture. The ilioinguinal ligament also had been partially divided in a vertical fashion prior to this. This was also repaired with interrupted sutures of 2-0 Vicryl in a figure-of-eight fashion. We then closed the subcutaneous tissues in three layers of interrupted 2-0 Vicryl. The skin was closed with staples. Sterile dressings were applied. We had checked for pulses in the feet during the procedure. Pulses were present, but she had excellent capillary refill. She had good flow through her femorals on both sides. Distally to our anastomotic repair, she had a good pulse and also good flow through Doppler with good diastolic waves. I could even feel a thrill in the artery. On the left side, she had a good Doppler flow again with long diastolic waves. Her feet and toes showed very good capillary refill and were pink. The patient was in no condition at this time to undergo an exploration of her left femoral artery to see what we could do to improve the flow in her left foot. She may develop an occlusion here, but again she is going into DIC. She has had multiple units of blood. She has had two codes of PEA (pulseless electrical activity). I have been trying to keep her pressure just up to diastolic of 90. The amount of fluid was huge. We are taking the risk of potentially having a limb loss, but I think at this time we are going to have to do everything we can just to get her to survive all of this. She was then transferred to the surgical ICU in critical and unstable condition.

SERVICE CODE(S): _____

ICD-10-CM DX CODE(S): _____

(Answers to every other Case are located in Appendix D . The full answer key is only available in the TEACH Instructor Resources on Evolve.)

CHAPTER 6 *Auditing Review*

Audit the coding for the following reports.

Audit Report 6.1 Echocardiogram Report

LOCATION: Inpatient, Hospital

PATIENT: Marilyn Aschoff

ATTENDING PHYSICIAN: David Barton, MD

RADIOLOGIST: Morton Monson, MD

INDICATION: Shortness of breath and atrial fibrillation

FINDINGS by means of 2-D and M-mode echocardiography:

CARDIAC CHAMBERS: The left atrium was mildly dilated and measured 4.4 cm. There was no evidence of atrial thrombi. The aortic root dimensions were within normal limits. The left ventricle was normal in size. There was mild concentric left ventricular hypertrophy. There was severe diffuse hypokinesis. The apex was kinetic. The overall ejection fraction was about 15%-20%. The right atrium was mildly dilated. The right ventricle was normal in size.

VALVES: The mitral valve has mild fibrocalcific changes, but more so the posterior leaflet, with mitral annulus calcification. The mitral valve excursion was adequate. There was aortic sclerosis, without significant stenosis. The tricuspid valve was grossly normal. The pulmonic valve was not well visualized.

DOPPLER AND COLOR DOPPLER INTERROGATION reveals the presence of severe mitral and tricuspid insufficiency. The calculated right ventricular systolic pressure was 42 mmHg.

CONCLUSION:

1. Severe left ventricular dysfunction.
2. Severe mitral and tricuspid insufficiency.
3. Mild to moderate pulmonary hypertension.

RECOMMENDATIONS:

1. Digitalization.
2. Afterload reducing agents.
3. Diuretics.
4. If this patient is labile, then bilateral heart catheterization should be considered. Although the LV function is severely reduced, part of that could be due to the fact that she has been tachycardic for a long period of time, i.e., can be tachycardia induced.

One of the codes is not reported for this case. Indicate the missing code.

PROFESSIONAL SERVICES: Echocardiography, **93306-26**

ICD-10-CM DX: Ventricular dysfunction, **I51.9**; Mitral valve insufficiency with tricuspid insufficiency, **I08.1**

MISSING CODE: _____

Audit Report 6.2 Cardiac Catheterization Report

LOCATION: Inpatient, Hospital

PATIENT: Marilyn Aschoff

SURGEON: David Barton, MD

ATTENDING PHYSICIAN: David Barton, MD

PROCEDURES PERFORMED: Left heart catheterization, selective coronary angiography, and left ventriculography

INDICATION: Chest pain in spite of being on IV nitroglycerin

DESCRIPTION OF PROCEDURE: Please see the computer report. Please note that the procedure was done using the right radial artery approach.

COMPLICATIONS: None

RESULTS:

1. HEMODYNAMICS: The left ventricular pressure before the LV gram was 8 with an LVEDP of 10. After the LV gram, the left ventricular pressure was 126/68 with an LVEDP of 14. The aortic pressure on pullback was 126/68. There was no significant gradient across the aortic valve.
2. LEFT VENTRICULOGRAPHY showed that the left ventricle is normal in size. There are no significant segmental wall motion abnormalities. The overall left ventricular systolic function is excellent with an ejection fraction of better than 70%.
3. SELECTIVE CORONARY ANGIOGRAPHY:
   A. RIGHT CORONARY ARTERY was a large dominant artery that has no significant obstructive disease.
   B. LEFT MAIN CORONARY ARTERY is a short artery that is free of significant obstructive disease.
   C. LEFT CIRCUMFLEX ARTERY was a medium to large-size, nondominant artery that appeared to have no significant obstructive disease. The proximal lesion that was seen on the previous angiogram back in March was no longer visible. Multiple views were taken; however, none of the views revealed any significant atherosclerotic disease.
   D. LEFT ANTERIOR DESCENDING CORONARY ARTERY is a large-size artery proximally, but a small-to medium-size artery in the mid to distal portion. The left anterior descending artery has only mild surface irregularities in the mid to distal portion.

CONCLUSION: Normal overall left ventricular systolic function. There is no evidence of any significant atherosclerotic heart disease whatsoever.

RECOMMENDATION: Due to the discrepancy I am seeing between this angiogram and the angiogram back in March of this year that showed moderate proximal left circumflex artery stenosis, I would proceed with intracoronary ultrasound to make sure that we are not missing anything angiographically.

One or more codes should not have been reported for this case. Indicate the code(s) incorrectly reported.

PROFESSIONAL SERVICES: Left heart catheterization, **93458-26;** Catheterization injection, **93565**

ICD-10-CM DX: Chest pain, **R07.9**

INCORRECTLY REPORTED CODE(S): _____

Continued

Audit Report 6.3 Angioplasty/Stenting Report

LOCATION: Inpatient, Hospital

PATIENT: Marilyn Aschoff

SURGEON: David Barton, MD

ATTENDING PHYSICIAN: David Barton, MD

PROCEDURE PERFORMED: Angioplasty/stenting of 70% ostial right coronary artery stenosis

INDICATION: Chronic ischemic heart disease

DESCRIPTION OF PROCEDURE: Please see the computer report. Please note that we started first by dilating the ostium using a 2.5 × 15 mm cutting balloon. After that, we deployed a 3.0 × 8 mm BX Velocity stent. The stent was then post-dilated using a 3.225 × 8 mm PowerSail up to 24 atmospheres.

COMPLICATIONS: None

RESULTS: Successful angioplasty/stent of 70% ostial right coronary artery stenosis with no residual stenosis at the end of the procedure.

One of the following codes is reported incorrectly for this case. Indicate the incorrect code.

PROFESSIONAL SERVICES: Coronary artery stent insertion, **92921-LC**

ICD-10-CM DX: Coronary arteriosclerosis, **I25.10;** Ischemic heart disease, **I25.9**

INCORRECT CODE: _____

Audit Report 6.4 Coronary Artery Bypass

LOCATION: Inpatient, Hospital

PATIENT: Michael Phelps

SURGEON: David Barton, MD

PREOPERATIVE DIAGNOSIS: Atherosclerotic heart disease

POSTOPERATIVE DIAGNOSIS: Same

PROCEDURE PERFORMED: Coronary artery bypass graft from the left internal mammary artery to left anterior descending bypass and sequential saphenous vein bypass grafts from the aorta to the first and then to the third obtuse marginal branches of the left circumflex.

ANESTHESIA: General

INDICATIONS: This 57-year-old male patient with progressive angina was noted on cardiac catheterization to have distal left main disease as well as high-grade proximal dominant left circumflex disease.

FINDINGS AT SURGERY: Revealed a greater saphenous vein conduit, which was 3.5 mm in diameter, was of good quality, and was used in reverse fashion. The left internal mammary artery was a 1-mm diameter vessel and was of good quality with excellent flow. The left anterior descending artery was 2 mm in diameter and was of good quality. The first and third obtuse marginal branches were both 2 mm in diameter and were of good quality. All grafts were probed and patent prior to closure.

DESCRIPTION OF PROCEDURE: The patient was brought to the operating room and placed in the supine position. Under general intubation anesthesia, the anterior chest, abdomen, and legs were prepped and draped in the usual manner. A segment of greater saphenous vein was harvested from the right leg using the endoscope. A segment of greater saphenous vein was harvested from the left thigh using the endoscope and prepared for grafting. The sternum was opened in the usual fashion, and the left internal mammary artery was taken down and prepared for grafting. The pericardium was incised sharply, and a pericardial well was created. The patient was systemically heparinized and placed on single right atrial to aortic cardiopulmonary bypass with a pump in the main pulmonary artery for cardiac decompression. The patient was cooled to 26 degrees, and upon fibrillation the aortic cross-clamp was applied and potassium-rich cold crystalline cardioplegic solution was administered through the aortic root with satisfactory cardiac arrest. Subsequent doses were given via the coronary sinus in a retrograde fashion. The end of the greater saphenous vein was anastomosed to the aorta and then the first obtuse marginal branch. The end of the other greater saphenous vein was then anastomosed to the third obtuse marginal branch with 7-0 Prolene. The left internal mammary artery was then brought down to the midportion of the left anterior descending artery and then anastomosed with 8-0 continuous Prolene. The aortic cross-clamp was removed after 56 minutes with spontaneous cardioversion to normal sinus rhythm. The patient was then warmed to 37 degrees esophageal temperature and weaned from cardiopulmonary bypass without difficulty after 78 minutes. The patient was decannulated, protamine was given, and hemostasis obtained. Temporary pacer wires were placed in the right atrium and right ventricle. The chest was drained with two Argyle chest tubes and closed in layers in the usual fashion. The leg was closed similarly. Sterile compression dressings were applied, and the patient returned to the surgical intensive care unit in satisfactory condition. Sponge count and needle count was correct × 2.

One or more of the following codes are reported incorrectly for this case. Indicate the incorrect code or codes.

SERVICE CODE(S): Coronary artery bypass graft, **33533;** Harvest of extremity artery, **35601-51;** CABG with venous graft, **33518;** Endoscopic harvest of vein(s) for CABG, **33508-51**

ICD-10-CM DX CODE(S): Atherosclerosis of native coronary artery, **I25.10**

INCORRECT/MISSING CODE(S): _____

CHAPTER 6—cont'd

Audit Report 6.5 Adenosine Cardiolite Stress Test

LOCATION: Outpatient, Hospital

PATIENT: Matt Arman

PHYSICIAN: Marvin Elhart, MD

INDICATIONS: The patient is status post heart catheterization and stent placement × 3 and now has recurring chest pain.

IDENTIFICATION: 61-year-old male, 5′ 8″, 210 pounds.

The patient underwent stress test according to Bruce protocol with Myoview injection.

HEMODYNAMIC RESPONSE: Heart rate at rest was 68 and at peak exercise was 132. Blood pressure at rest was 138/78 and at peak was 168/78.

During the stress test, the patient had no chest pain. The test was stopped due to fatigue. At baseline, the patient had a normal sinus rhythm with no ST segment changes. At peak exercise, the patient had no ST segment changes noted.

The patient exercised for a total of 10 minutes, achieving 11.3 METS.

CONCLUSION:

1. Excellent exercise tolerance.
2. Good hemodynamic response to exercise.
3. This EKG stress test is not suggestive for significant obstructive disease. No chest pain clinically. The Myoview part of the stress test will be reported separately.

One or more of the following codes are reported incorrectly for this case. Indicate the incorrect code or codes.

SERVICE CODE(S):   Cardiovascular stress test, **93015-26**

ICD-10-CM DX CODE(S):   Chest pain, **R07.9**

INCORRECT/MISSING CODE(S):   _____

Audit Report 6.6 Echo Doppler Report

LOCATION: Outpatient, Hospital

PATIENT: Allison Gunderson

PRIMARY CARE PHYSICIAN: Alanda Naraquist, MD

CARDIOLOGIST: James Noonar, MD

INDICATION: Congestive heart failure

A 2-D echocardiographic study with color-flow interrogation, spectral Doppler, and M-mode measurements was performed.

2-D AND M-MODE MEASUREMENTS:

1. Aortic root 3.8 cm.
2. Aortic valve excursion not measured.
3. Left atrium 5.2 cm.
4. Right ventricle not measured.
5. Left ventricle end-diastole 4.7 cm.
6. Left ventricle end-systole 4.2 cm.
7. Fractional shortening 0.10.
8. Ejection fraction 23%.
9. Interventricular septum 1.1 cm.
10. Left ventricular posterior wall 1.1 cm.

DOPPLER MEASUREMENTS:

1. Aortic valve peak velocity 3.19 m/sec.
2. Aortic valve peak gradient 41 mmHg.
3. Aortic valve mean gradient 30 mmHg.
4. Aortic valve area 0.82 cm #2 by continuity equation.
5. Severe aortic stenosis by continuity equation.
6. Trace mitral regurgitation.
7. Trace tricuspid regurgitation.

2-D ECHOCARDIOGRAPHIC REPORT:

1. Technically adequate study.
2. Normal left ventricular cavitary dimensions, end-diastole and end-systole. Mild left ventricular concentric hypertrophy. Moderate LV systolic dysfunction. Dyskinetic LV wall motion consistent with atrial fibrillation.
3. Mildly dilated aortic root.
4. Severely calcified, thickened, fibrotic aortic valve with markedly restricted opening and markedly reduced leaflet excursion. Severe aortic stenosis by continuity equation with aortic valve area of 0.82 cm #2, aortic valve peak velocity 3.2 m/s, peak gradient 41 mmHg, and mean gradient 30 mmHg. Fibrocalcific disease of the aortic valve root and annulus.
5. Mildly thickened, calcified mitral valve leaflets with good opening and adequate excursion. Mitral annular calcification. Normal subvalvular chordae tendineae apparatus. No prolapse, flail, redundancy, or myxomatous changes of mitral valve leaflets.
6. Dilated left atrial cavitary dimensions.
7. Top normal right-sided chamber dimensions and function. Normal morphologic appearance of the tricuspid valve.
8. Trace mitral insufficiency. Trace tricuspid insufficiency.
9. No significant pericardial effusion, intracardiac mass, or thrombus. No intracavitary spontaneous echo contrast. No valvular vegetations or left ventricular apical mural thrombus detected. Intact interatrial and interventricular septum. No PFO by color-flow Doppler.

IMPRESSION: Normal LV cavitary dimensions. Mild concentric left ventricular hypertrophy. Moderate LV systolic dysfunction. Left ventricular dyskinesis secondary to conductive arrhythmia, atrial fibrillation. Ejection fraction 23%. Moderate global hypokinesis with dyskinetic wall motion secondary to atrial fibrillation. Mildly dilated aortic root. Highly calcified, thickened, restricted aortic valve leaflet opening and markedly diminished leaflet excursion. Severe aortic valvular stenosis with aortic valve area of 0.82 cm #2 by continuity equation, aortic valve peak velocity 3.2 m/s, peak gradient 41 mmHg, mean gradient 30 mmHg. Trace MR. Trace tricuspid insufficiency. Mitral annular calcification. Left atrial enlargement. (The preceding findings are indicative of congestive heart failure.)

One or more of the following codes are reported incorrectly for this case. Indicate the incorrect code or codes.

SERVICE CODE(S):   Transthoracic echocardiography, **93306;** Pulsed Doppler echocardiography, **93320;** Color flow velocity mapping Doppler echocardiography, **93325**

ICD-10-CM DX CODE(S):   Heart failure, **I50.9**

INCORRECT/MISSING CODE(S):   _____

(Auditing Review answers with rationales are only available in the TEACH Instructor Resources on Evolve.)

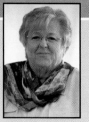

"Coding is the financial support of the health care system. The skill of coding will always be an important part of health care. Learn your craft well, practice it carefully, and always demonstrate integrity."

Digestive System, Hemic/Lymphatic System, and Mediastinum/Diaphragm

http://evolve.elsevier.com/Buck/next

(Answers to every other Case are located in Appendix D, with the full answer key only available in the TEACH Instructor Resources on Evolve)
(Auditing Review answers with rationales are only available in the TEACH Instructor Resources on Evolve)

Digestive System

Digestive system (40490-49999) complaints are common and are treated by a wide variety of physicians. The **gastrointestinal** tract includes the items indicated in **Figure 7-1.** Common gastrointestinal symptoms are abdominal pain, nausea, vomiting, difficulty swallowing, heartburn, indigestion, bleeding, diarrhea, and constipation. Common conditions are stomatitis, peptic ulcer, gastroesophageal reflux, hemorrhoids, diverticulitis, bowel obstruction, gastritis, appendicitis, and colorectal cancer.

Conditions of the liver, gallbladder, and bile ducts are part of the gastrointestinal system; common signs or symptoms include jaundice, ascites (fluid in the abdominal cavity), and abnormal liver function tests. Common conditions of the liver are cirrhosis, hepatitis, and hyperbilirubinemia; of the gallbladder, gallstones and cholecystitis; of the pancreas, pancreatitis and carcinomas.

A physician who specializes in the diagnoses and treatment of the digestive system is a **gastroenterologist.** These specialists provide operative services using various approaches, such as rectal, endoscopic, laparoscopic, and open surgical procedures. The approach will be a determining factor in the code you choose.

General surgeons often use digestive system codes because they perform many of the abdominal procedures. For example, a gastroenterologist would diagnose a patient with appendicitis, and the general surgeon would remove the appendix. The gastroenterologist usually does the endoscopic procedures (through the mouth or the anus) and diagnoses gastrointestinal system conditions; if the conditions require surgery, the general surgeon would do the laparoscopic (through the abdomen) or open (incisional) procedures.

Not all of the codes in the Digestive System subsection are for procedures that you consider as being in the gastrointestinal system; for example, the Abdomen, Peritoneum, and Omentum (49000-49999), in which you will find codes such as those for laparotomy (49000-49010), subdiaphragmatic and retroperitoneal abscess drainage (49020-49062), and **laparoscopy** (49320-49329), just to name a few. When an abdominal laparoscopic procedure is performed for diagnostic purposes and no procedure is conducted, you would report the diagnostic procedure with a Digestive section code. For

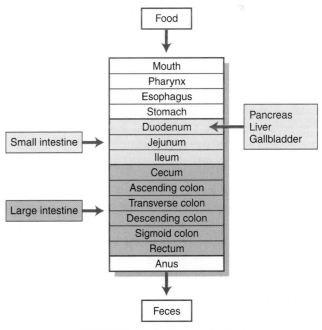

FIGURE 7-1 Gastrointestinal tract.

example, the surgeon performs a diagnostic laparoscopy (49320) for the purpose of examining the adrenal gland. The surgeon removes a portion of the adrenal gland, and the procedure becomes a surgical laparoscopy (60650). Read the notes above 60650, and you will find that the note refers you to 49320 if the laparoscopy was diagnostic.

The Introduction, Revision, Removal subcategory (49400-49465) contains codes for insertion, revision, replacement, or removal of air, contrast, **catheter,** or shunt into the abdomen (peritoneal/intraperitoneal cavity). For example, placement (insertion) of a dialysis catheter for peritoneal **hemodialysis** would be reported with 49421.

E/M Services

Report 7-1A is a surgical consultation for a patient with a bowel obstruction. A bowel obstruction is a blockage of the small or large intestine. Postoperative adhesions are the most common cause of bowel obstruction of the small intestine, with hernias and neoplasms also being common. Cancer is the most common cause of large intestine obstruction; volvulus (twisting of intestine) and diverticulitis are also common. Clinical presentations would often be abdominal pain, nausea, vomiting, or bloating. Clinical findings include blood in the stool, fever (especially if the bowel is perforated), absence of bowel sounds or a tinkling sound, and abdominal tenderness. No laboratory tests are available that can be used to indicate bowel obstruction. X-ray, contrast studies, and CT scan are the main tests that the physician would use to assist in the diagnostic process.

If the diagnosis is obstructed bowel, a general surgeon would usually perform an open surgical procedure, and nearly all complete obstructions require surgery. After an abdominal surgery, although uncommon, the anastomosis can leak and allow air and bowel contents into the abdominal cavity, possibly placing the patient in an emergency situation requiring immediate attention.

Intestinal Obstruction

Obstruction of the intestinal tract can occur in a variety of ways. **Intussusception** (K56.1) is the prolapse of part of the intestine into another adjacent part of the intestine.

Intussusception may be enteric (ileoileal, jejunoileal, jejunojejunal), colic (colocolic), or intracolic (ileocecal, ileocolic). See **Figure 7-2.** Usually this causes strangulation of the blood supply (causing ischemic colon, gangrene) and is most common in infants. **Paralytic ileus** (K56.0) is the loss of the peristaltic action of the intestine. Usually this occurs after intestinal trauma or a gastrointestinal surgical procedure (complication code K91.89) and can occur in the large and small intestines. **Volvulus** (K56.2) is the twisting of a segment of the intestine (also known as torsion) and is most common in the large intestine of the elderly. See **Figure 7-3. Impaction** of the intestine can occur through fecal material impacted in the colon (K56.41), gallstone obstruction of the intestine (K56.3),

or other types of obstruction (K56.49) such as enterolith. Other specified types of intestinal obstructions, such as intestinal or peritoneal adhesions, occur after an operation or an infection (K56.5-). Unspecified intestinal obstruction (K56.609) is assigned to those obstructions where there is no clear indication of the type of obstruction.

External Procedures

External procedures are those that can be performed in the area of the rectum, such as drainage of rectal abscess or hemorrhoidectomy. These external procedures performed with an **anoscope,** as illustrated in **Figure 7-4,** are reported with endoscopy codes. The anoscope codes are located in the Endoscopy subcategory (46600-46615) of the Anus category. The stand-alone code 46600 states "Anoscopy;..." and is then followed by the indented codes based on the procedure performed, such as biopsy, foreign body removal, or control of bleeding. Note that there is a distinction made for the method of removal of tumors (46610-46611); 46612 is for removal of multiple tumors, polyps, or lesions using hot biopsy forceps, cautery, or snare. This means that if one tumor was removed with cautery, you would code 46610, and if multiple tumors were removed, you would code with 46612. It would not be appropriate to list the single tumor removal code with modifier -51 on the second code (i.e., 46610 and 46610-51); rather, you must list only 46612 to report the multiple removal.

A **fistula** (K60.3X) is an abnormal channel that connects two places that would ordinarily not be connected, for example, an anal fistula in which a channel leads from the anal canal into the tissue surrounding the channel. The channel then becomes clogged with fecal material, and often an abscess (K61.0) will form at the end of the channel. The channel can be closed with sutures or excised. Codes to report the excision of anal fistula are in the Excision subcategory (46200-46320). If a diagnostic anoscopy were performed (46600) as well as the surgical excision of a fistula, each would be coded separately with modifier -51 added to the exploration anoscope. This is because the anoscopy is performed by using a scope and the removal of the fistula is by surgical excision. If both a fistula and an abscess are present, each is reported separately. Packing placed into an abscessed area is not reported separately.

Some gastroenterologists perform these anal procedures, or a general surgeon may be called in to perform the procedure at the request of the gastroenterologist or other physician who diagnosed the condition. Most gastroenterologists perform the procedures that use an endoscope and refer the open abdominal procedures to a general surgeon. Smaller facilities have no gastrointestinal specialists, and these procedures are performed by general surgeons.

If an abscess is simply lanced and drained, report the services with an incision code (46020-46083).

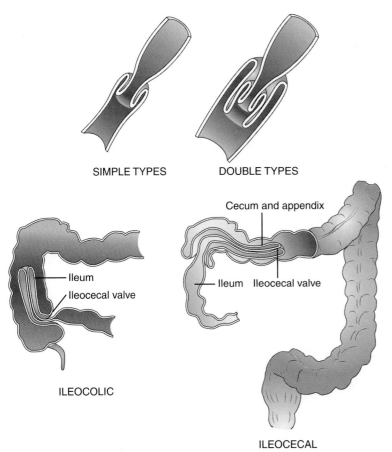

SIMPLE TYPES   DOUBLE TYPES

Cecum and appendix

Ileum
Ileocecal valve

ILEOCOLIC

Ileum   Ileocecal valve

ILEOCECAL

FIGURE 7–2 Types of intussusception.

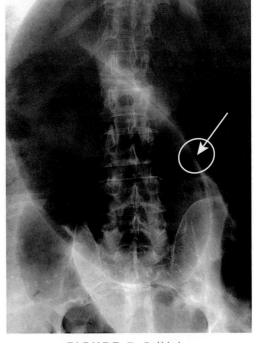

FIGURE 7–3 Volvulus.

CASE 7-1   *Inpatient Consultation*

The patient had a gastrointestinal operation 4 weeks ago, but the report does not clearly indicate that the current obstruction is due to the surgical procedure; therefore, a "complication of surgery" code would not be appropriate in this case.

LOCATION: Inpatient, Hospital

PATIENT: Martin Newwell

PHYSICIAN: Alma Naraquist, MD

CONSULTANT: Daniel Olanka, MD

HISTORY OF PRESENT ILLNESS: This patient was operated on by Dr. Sanchez approximately 4 weeks ago for a misdiagnosis of appendicitis. He underwent ileocecal resection. He has had a variety of problems in the postoperative period, including renal failure, respiratory failure, tracheostomy, etc. He is currently under the care of Dr. Naraquist and is off the ventilator and breathing through the tracheostomy. He has been intermittently fed through small-bowel Cor-Flo tube, but this has the appearance of a bowel obstruction. Dr. Naraquist has asked me to evaluate the patient for his possible bowel obstruction. The family has also requested that another surgeon get involved in his care, and so I have been tagged to review his case.

PHYSICAL EXAMINATION: On examination, the patient is resting comfortably in bed. He does have a tracheostomy in place. He is alert and does respond. The chest is clear to auscultation. There is a catheter in place for dialysis, although the patient is not currently on dialysis. The abdomen is markedly distended. It is tympanitic. Tinkling bowel sounds are heard. There are no rashes. The midline scar is well healed. There is no particular focal tenderness, and no hernias are appreciated.

Review of the patient's films shows marked dilatation of the small bowel. Review of the CT (computerized tomography) scan shows marked dilatation of the small bowel with what appears to be a transition zone in the distal ileum. The colon is deflated.

DISCUSSION: By physical examination, this patient has chronic bowel obstruction, at least partial in nature. Certainly his x-rays support that there is a major problem intra-abdominally. My recommendation would be that the patient should be considered for re-exploration for bowel obstruction. I do not know whether the problem is at the anastomosis or near the anastomosis. I think patient would benefit from some total parenteral nutrition (TPN) and aggressive hydration over the next few days, and then we will plan to take him to the operating room next week.

SERVICE CODE(S): _____

ICD-10-CM DX CODE(S): _____

(Answers to every other Case are located in Appendix D . The full answer key is only available in the TEACH Instructor Resources on Evolve.)

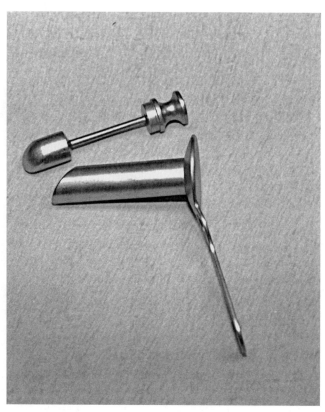

FIGURE 7-4 Anoscope.

CASE 7-2 | *Operative Report, Anal Fistula*

LOCATION: Inpatient, Hospital

PATIENT: Russell Cornwall

SURGEON: Larry P. Friendly, MD

PREOPERATIVE DIAGNOSIS: Anal fistula

POSTOPERATIVE DIAGNOSIS: Anal fistula

TITLE OF PROCEDURE:

1. Fistulotomy.
2. Anoscopy.

ANESTHESIA: General

INDICATIONS: The patient is a 46-year-old male with fever of unknown origin whom I had seen several months ago with perianal fistula. Since that time, he has had decreased drainage but still has pain and fevers. He presents today for elective fistulotomy, and he understands the risk of bleeding and infection and the possible risk of damage to the sphincter muscle, and he wishes to proceed with procedure.

The patient was brought to the operating room, placed under spinal anesthesia, placed in the jackknife position, and prepped and draped sterilely. Digital rectal examination was first performed, and there were no masses. Anoscopy was then performed, and there was no internal anal fistulous opening. At the 4 o'clock position, we could feel this hard, indurated mass that drained purulent material. We then opened this with a no. 15 blade and debrided a necrotic capsule from this area. We then cauterized the base, injected it with 30 cc of 0.5% Sensorcaine with epinephrine solution, and packed it with 4 × 4 gauze. The patient tolerated this well and was taken to the postanesthesia recovery room in stable condition.

SERVICE CODE(S): _____

ICD-10-CM DX CODE(S): _____

(Answers to every other Case are located in Appendix D . The full answer key is only available in the TEACH Instructor Resources on Evolve.)

CASE 7-3 | *Operative Report, Intersphincteric Abscess*

LOCATION: Inpatient, Hospital

PATIENT: Mortica Kellogg

PHYSICIAN: Ronald Green, MD

SURGEON: Larry P. Friendly, MD

PREOPERATIVE DIAGNOSIS: Rectal pain

POSTOPERATIVE DIAGNOSIS: Intersphincteric abscess

OPERATIVE PROCEDURE: Examination under anesthesia and drainage of perirectal abscess

OPERATIVE NOTE: The patient was placed under general anesthesia and was placed in the lithotomy position. The rectal area was prepped and draped in a sterile manner. Examination of the external anus showed no

CASE 7-3—cont'd

evidence of a fissure or obvious perirectal abscess. I palpated around the anus carefully and could not really appreciate any pathology. We then proceeded to dilate the anus to three fingers and introduced the bivalve speculum. While carefully inspecting the inner lining of the anus in the lithotomy position proximally at the 6 or 7 o'clock location, we encountered a fluctuant feeling area, which with mild pressure from the finger ruptured and drained purulent material. This was cultured. We were then in a small abscess cavity, which appeared to be in an intersphincteric location in between the subcutaneous and the deep sphincters. This was completely drained and then irrigated with some saline. We then packed the area with gauze. The patient tolerated the procedure well and was discharged to the recovery room in stable condition.

SERVICE CODE(S): _____

ICD-10-CM DX CODE(S): _____

(Answers to every other Case are located in Appendix D . The full answer key is only available in the TEACH Instructor Resources on Evolve.)

CASE 7-4   *Operative Report, Perirectal Fistulectomies*

In this case a fistula is removed with no mention of an abscess.

LOCATION: Inpatient, Hospital

PATIENT: George Papenfuss

SURGEON: Larry Friendly, MD

PREOPERATIVE DIAGNOSIS: Perirectal fistulas

POSTOPERATIVE DIAGNOSIS: Perirectal fistulas

PROCEDURE PERFORMED: Perirectal fistulectomies

ANESTHESIA: General anesthetic.

INDICATIONS FOR SURGERY: The patient is a 61-year-old white male who had draining perirectal fistulas, which had been incised and drained in the past. The patient is now being admitted for incision of these fistulas.

DESCRIPTION OF PROCEDURE: The patient was placed in a jackknife position. He was prepped and draped in the usual manner. The patient was given a general anesthetic. The fistulous tracts were in the 2 and 11 o'clock positions. The fistulous tracts were excised; one had an abscessed pocket, which was excised in its entirety. The tracts continued over the 12 o'clock midline position over into about the 2 o'clock position. All these tracts were combined into one large incision, and all the inflammatory tissue was excised sharply. The rectum was also dilated up and examined. No evidence of any tract could be seen draining directly into the rectum at this time, and no induration was seen. The inflammatory tissue present on the outer skin area was completely excised. The operative area was thoroughly irrigated. Hemostasis was obtained using Bovie cautery. The wounds were left open, and dressings were applied. The patient tolerated the operation and returned to recovery in stable condition.

SERVICE CODE(S): _____

ICD-10-CM DX CODE(S): _____

(Answers to every other Case are located in Appendix D . The full answer key is only available in the TEACH Instructor Resources on Evolve.)

Hemorrhoids

Hemorrhoids (piles) are caused by increased pressure on the hemorrhoid veins, such as constipation, straining during heavy lifting, lesions, or pregnancy. This pressure causes the hemorrhoid vein to bulge (like a varicose vein), causing anal bleeding, itching, and/or pain. See **Figure 7-5**. Hemorrhoids are graded, similar to how ulcers are graded.

- Grade I hemorrhoids project into the anal canal but do not protrude outside of the anus.
- Grade II hemorrhoids protrude (external) from the anus on straining, but return upon cessation of straining.
- Grade III hemorrhoids protrude upon straining and only return if manually reduced (returned to normal position).
- Grade IV hemorrhoids permanently protrude.

The complexity of the procedure depends on the type of hemorrhoid and the complexity of repair.

A common term when speaking of hemorrhoids is thrombosed, which means one containing clotted blood.

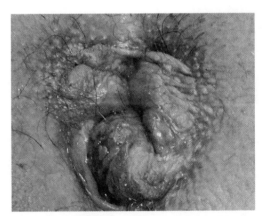

FIGURE 7–5 Hemorrhoids.

The diagnosis code for hemorrhoids is K64.-.

A fourth character indicates with or without complications, and a fifth character indicates bleeding, prolapsed, strangulated, or ulcerated.

If the hemorrhoid occurs during pregnancy, O22.4-, Other venous complications, is used to report the diagnosis.

CASE 7-5 *Operative Report, Hemorrhoidectomy*

LOCATION: Outpatient, Hospital

PATIENT: Pricilla Stephanopolis

PHYSICIAN: Gary Sanchez, MD

SURGEON: Ronald Ripple, MD

PREOPERATIVE DIAGNOSIS: Symptomatic internal hemorrhoid, grade II

POSTOPERATIVE DIAGNOSIS: Symptomatic internal hemorrhoid, grade II

PROCEDURE PERFORMED: Hemorrhoidectomy (excision of single internal hemorrhoid). This is the largest and the only bleeding hemorrhoid.

ANESTHESIA: General endotracheal anesthesia plus 30 cc (cubic centimeter) of 0.5% Marcaine with epinephrine

The patient, on examination under anesthesia, had other smaller, Grade I hemorrhoids that were higher up in the anal canal, but the decision was made not to excise these because they were not bleeding.

PROCEDURE IN DETAIL: After good general endotracheal anesthesia, the patient was carefully placed in the prone position. After this, a total of 30 cc of Marcaine was infiltrated into the area around the hemorrhoid. The hemorrhoid was grasped with an Allis clamp, and a straight clamp was placed across the base. A running stitch was then placed below the clamp for hemostasis. Next the hemorrhoid was excised above the clamp, and a running stitch going in the opposite direction was then looped over the straight clamp. The straight clamp was removed, and the looped stitch was then tightened up. Another layer of suture was then run down the length of the excised hemorrhoid. Hemostasis was obtained with this maneuver. No other large thrombosed or extruding hemorrhoids were noted. After this, Vaseline gauze was placed over the wound. ABD (Adriamycin, bleomycin, dacarbazine) dressing and knit mesh pants were placed on the patient to hold the dressing in place. She was returned to the recovery room in good condition.

SERVICE CODE(S): _____

ICD-10-CM DX CODE(S): _____

(Answers to every other Case are located in Appendix D . The full answer key is only available in the TEACH Instructor Resources on Evolve.)

Catheters

Intraperitoneal catheters are inserted into the abdomen (peritoneal cavity) for the purposes of drainage. The choice of catheter depends on the purpose for which the catheter is being placed and the physician's preference.

Reports often refer to the catheters by brand name, such as Tenkhoff, Foley, and Swan neck. Catheters are inserted on either a permanent or a temporary basis. The approach for placement can be closed (percutaneous) or open. The closed placement requires a puncture wound made on the abdomen with the catheter threaded through the incision and into the abdominal cavity. During an open procedure, the surgeon may place a drain, securing the catheter in place outside of the abdomen. The drain placement is bundled into the procedure and not reported separately.

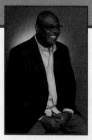

From the Trenches

"A successful coder is one who isn't afraid to inquire when he/she is unsure. There is a correct answer out there and guessing isn't part of the equation."

ROLANDO RUSSELL

MBA, RHIA, CPC, CPAR

CASE 7-6 *Operative Report*

LOCATION: Inpatient, Hospital

PATIENT: Gladys Hanson

SURGEON: Gary Sanchez, MD

PREOPERATIVE DIAGNOSIS: End-stage renal disease

POSTOPERATIVE DIAGNOSIS: End-stage renal disease

PROCEDURE PERFORMED: Placement of a tunneled peritoneal dialysis catheter

INDICATION: This 23-year-old female has end-stage renal disease and is going to need permanent dialysis. She elected peritoneal dialysis. Please see clinic consultation for further details of the discussion of procedure and risks involved.

PROCEDURE: The patient was brought to the operating theater and placed in the supine position on the operating room table. After receiving a general anesthetic, she was prepped and draped in a sterile fashion. An incision line that was infraumbilical and vertical was infiltrated with

CASE 7-6—cont'd

0.5% Marcaine. An incision was then made and carried down through the subcutaneous tissues down to the anterior fascia. The anterior fascia was grasped and divided sharply. The peritoneum was also divided sharply. The peritoneal cavity was entered. A peritoneal dialysis catheter was then inserted using a Bozeman catheter into the pelvis. The patient had been placed in a Trendelenburg position. We then were able to place the catheter with ease. We placed a 2-0 Vicryl in a pursestring fashion through the peritoneum. This was also attached to the cuff in adjacent spots. This was then secured. Interrupted sutures of 2-0 Vicryl were then used to close the fascia. The sutures in the cuff were also placed through the cuff to help secure this in place. It was then tunneled out to the left side. The cuff was buried in the subcutaneous tissues. The subcutaneous tissues and vertical midline incision were closed with

interrupted sutures of 3-0 Vicryl around and over the catheter. The skin was closed with 4-0 Vicryl in a running subcuticular fashion. Steri-Strips and a sterile dressing were applied. The catheter-retaining device was used at the exit site to help secure it in place. We had also flushed this intermittently with heparinized saline during the procedure at various steps and then let the drain back out at all times as well as at the end of the procedure. This flushed well and irrigated well. The patient tolerated the procedure well and went to the recovery room in stable condition. No family was present to meet with postoperatively to discuss the results.

SERVICE CODE(S): _____

ICD-10-CM DX CODE(S): _____

(Answers to every other Case are located in Appendix D . The full answer key is only available in the TEACH Instructor Resources on Evolve.)

Endoscopy Procedures

Procedures are often performed by means of an endoscope and laparoscopy. The surgical approach determines the code. For example, if the patient has a lesion on the outside of the intestine, the physician would open the abdomen (open procedure) or use a laparoscopy (tube inserted through the abdominal wall) to excise the lesion. Codes for the open procedure are located in the Intestine, Excision category (44100-44160). Codes for the laparoscopic approach are located in the Intestine, Laparoscopy category. If the lesion was inside the intestine and the surgeon used an endoscope inserted through the anus to remove the lesion, you would report the service with a code from Intestines, Endoscopy (44360-44408). There are endoscopic, laparoscopic, and open approaches in many of the subheadings of the Digestive System subsection.

The **endoscopic** procedure uses an existing orifice (opening), a **laparoscopic** procedure uses a small incision, and an **open** procedure uses a larger incision.

There are endoscopic and laparoscopic codes for the gastrointestinal tract, such as the esophagus, stomach, intestines, and anus as well as abdomen, peritoneum, and omentum.

Remember to code to the full extent of the procedure, which is the point at which the procedure terminates. For example, if the procedure begins with an endoscope being placed into the mouth, through the esophagus, and terminating in the stomach, the full extent is the stomach. Although the operative report will state the procedure performed in the identifiers of the report, such as "Procedure Performed," you must always read the full operative report to ensure the full extent is reported. For example, the Procedure Performed identifier may state esophagogastroscopy (full extent is the stomach), but upon reading the report, you may find that the duodenum was referenced, making the procedure an esophagogastroduodenoscopy (full extent is the duodenum).

Use the correct approach and code to the fullest extent of the procedure.

Gastritis and Duodenitis

Gastritis is a severe inflammation of the stomach. **Acute gastritis** (K29.0-) is usually superficial erosions of the surface epithelium brought about by drugs, chemicals, or *Helicobacter pylori* bacteria. **Atrophic gastritis** (K29.4-) is a chronic inflammation of the stomach that results in destruction of the cells of the mucous lining of the stomach. **Duodenitis** (K29.8-) is a severe inflammation of the duodenum.

Ulcer

Ulcer is an erosive area or a break. The term "peptic" pertains to pepsin or to digestion. A peptic ulcer occurs on the mucosal lining of the stomach (K25) or duodenum (K26) and results in the submucosal areas being exposed to the gastric secretions. The site may be unspecified (K27) in the medical record. Additional code would be reported to identify alcohol abuse and dependence (F10.-)

Hernia

Hernias of the groin are the most common type of hernia, accounting for 80% of all hernias. There are two major types of inguinal hernias (K40.9-): indirect (oblique) and direct. **Indirect inguinal hernias** result when the intestines emerge through the abdominal wall in an indirect fashion through the inguinal canal. **Direct inguinal hernias** penetrate through the abdominal wall in a direct fashion. **Femoral hernias** occur at the femoral ring where the femoral vessels enter the thigh.

A common type of hernia is a hiatal or esophageal hernia, also referred to as a sliding hernia or diaphragmatic hernia.

When the diaphragmatic hernia is mentioned with obstruction, report the diagnosis with K44.0; when it is without obstruction, report the diagnosis with K44.9.

Rectal Procedures

Rectal endoscopic procedures are:

- Proctosigmoidoscopy: Endoscopic examination of the rectum (proct/o = rectum) and the sigmoid colon (45300-45327)
- Sigmoidoscopy: Endoscopic examination of the sigmoid colon and may include the descending colon (45330-45350)
- Colonoscopy: Endoscopic examination of the colon (from rectum to cecum, which is the uppermost portion of the large intestine and may include the lower portion of the small intestine, ileum) (45378-45392)

The codes are divided based on the extent and the purpose of the procedure. Note that the stand-alone codes 45300, 45330, and 45378 each have a list of indented codes

---

CASE 7-7   *Operative Report, Esophagogastroduodenoscopy*

LOCATION: Outpatient, Hospital

PATIENT: David Amron

PHYSICIAN: Larry Friendly, MD

PREOPERATIVE DIAGNOSIS: Upper gastrointestinal bleeding

POSTOPERATIVE DIAGNOSIS: Mild gastritis, mild duodenitis, a 5-mm (millimeter) gastric ulcer, not actively bleeding; biopsies obtained for *Helicobacter pylori;* also hiatal hernia

INDICATION: A 70-year-old white man who has chronic renal failure secondary to amyloidosis presents with 1 week of coffee-ground emesis. He smokes two to three packs per day and has two to three melenic stools per day. We do not have any results of laboratory tests. He was just admitted. We suspect upper gastrointestinal bleeding. He has not been on any NSAIDs (nonsteroidal antiinflammatory drugs). He has never had an ulcer. He has no other gastrointestinal symptoms.

PROCEDURE PERFORMED: Esophagogastroduodenoscopy

PREOPERATIVE MEDICATION: Demerol 50 mg (milligram) IV (intravenous); Versed 4 mg IV

FINDINGS: The flexible Pentax video pediatric endoscope was passed without difficulty into the oropharynx. The gastroesophageal junction was seen at 40 cm (centimeter). Inspection of the esophagus revealed no erythema, ulceration, exudate, friability, or other mucosal abnormalities. From 40 to 43 cm, there was a 3-cm hiatal hernia. Along the lower border of the hernia sac, there was a 5 × 2-mm ulceration. It was not actively bleeding. Photograph was obtained. The stomach proper was entered. Coffee-ground material was present, but no fresh blood. Endoscope was advanced to the second duodenum. Inspection of the second duodenum revealed no abnormalities. The first duodenum and duodenal bulb revealed some mild patchy erythema and no ulceration. The antrum revealed patchy erythema but no ulceration. Retroflexion revealed the previously described minimal ulcer and hiatal hernia. Nothing was seen in the fundus or cardia. Biopsies were obtained of the antrum to rule out *H. pylori*. The patient tolerated the procedure well.

IMPRESSION: Some old blood present, no active bleeding. A 5-mm gastric ulcer along the inferior border of the 3-mm hiatal hernia, not bleeding. Mild gastritis and mild duodenitis are present. Biopsies obtained for *Helicobacter pylori*.

PLAN: Will observe patient for 24 hours and possibly discharge, follow hemoglobins. At this point, it does not appear that the patient has amyloid of the gastrointestinal tract.

SERVICE CODE(S): _____

ICD-10-CM DX CODE(S): _____

(Answers to every other Case are located in Appendix D . The full answer key is only available in the TEACH Instructor Resources on Evolve.)

based on the purpose (such as biopsy, foreign body removal, ablation, control of bleeding, etc.).

As specified in the CPT guidelines, as well as in the Colonoscopy Decision Tree, if the patient was fully prepared for the colonoscopy and the colonoscope could not be advanced to the splenic flexor, report the procedure as a flexible sigmoidoscopy with code 45330. If the patient was undergoing a screening or diagnostic procedure and the colonoscope was advanced beyond the splenic flexor but not to the cecum due to extenuating circumstances, report the procedure with CPT code 45378 and append modifier -53, Discontinued Procedure. If a therapeutic colonoscopy was begun but the colonoscope could be advanced beyond the splenic flexure but not to the cecum, report the appropriate therapeutic procedure code and append modifier -52, Reduced Service. These extenuating circumstances could indicate that the patient's vital signs became unstable or the bowel preparation for the surgery was not sufficient to continue the procedure. Some payers, including Medicare, require modifier -53 to be reported whenever a procedure cannot be completed. Diagnosis code, Z43.09 (Surgical procedure not carried out due to contraindication), should be reported as a secondary code.

Polyps

A polyp is a growth on a pedicle (stem) that bleeds easily and may become malignant. In the Index, the codes for a diagnosis of polyp(s) are located under the main term "Polyp, polypus" subtermed by location, such as nose (J33.9), labia (N84.3), and gum (K06.8). These codes are then referenced in the Tabular for further information regarding code assignment. A polyp is not a neoplasm; rather, it is an abnormal growth of normal cells. Sometimes the term "hyperplastic" is used in the pathology report of a polyp specimen. The term means that there is an increase in the number of normal cells.

CASE 7-8A *Operative Report, Colon Polypectomy*

Report the services for the following case. When reporting the diagnosis for the operative procedure, reference the pathology report located in 7-8B.

LOCATION: Outpatient, Hospital

PATIENT: Jatin Al-Assad

SURGEON: Larry Friendly, MD

SCOPE USED: Pentax video colonoscope

MEDICATIONS GIVEN: Fentanyl 75 μg (microgram) and Versed 3 mg (milligram) IV (intravenous) prior to the procedure

PREOPERATIVE DIAGNOSIS: Polyp on sigmoidoscopy

POSTOPERATIVE DIAGNOSIS: Colon polyps

PROCEDURE PERFORMED: Colonoscopy with removal of polyps

INDICATION: The patient is a 48-year-old male who presented for screening sigmoidoscopy on January 15. He was found to have several adenomatous polyps in the sigmoid colon and rectum. This procedure is being done to remove those polyps and any other polyps in the more proximal colon.

FINDINGS: About five polyps were seen, three pedunculated and two sessile. These were snared. The remainder of the colon and rectum were normal.

DESCRIPTION OF TECHNIQUE: After informed consent was obtained, the patient was prepared for colonoscopy. He was placed in the left lateral decubitus position. A digital rectal examination was performed and was unremarkable. The lubricated Pentax video colonoscope was then guided digitally into the rectum and advanced to the cecum. The scope was withdrawn and the mucosa inspected. The cecum, ascending colon, transverse colon, and descending colon were normal. Through the sigmoid colon and rectum, five polyps were seen. The largest measured about 1 cm (centimeter) in diameter. Three were pedunculated. These were snared. Two others were smaller and sessile. The distal rectum was normal. The scope was withdrawn. The patient tolerated the procedure well and was discharged ambulatory with a driver.

RECOMMENDATIONS: Follow-up colonoscopy in 2 years due to the relatively large number of polyps seen on this examination in a relatively young man.

Pathology Report Later Indicated: See Report 7-8B.

SERVICE CODE(S): _____

ICD-10-CM DX CODE(S): _____

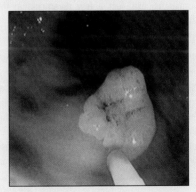

FIGURE 7-6 Polypectomy.

(Answers to every other Case are located in Appendix D . The full answer key is only available in the TEACH Instructor Resources on Evolve.)

CASE 7-8B   *Pathology Report*

LOCATION: Outpatient, Hospital

PATIENT: Jatin Al-Assad

SURGEON: Larry Friendly, MD

PATHOLOGIST: Morton Monson, MD

CLINICAL HISTORY: Polyp

TISSUE RECEIVED: Colon polyp

GROSS DESCRIPTION: The specimen is labeled with the patient's name and "colon polyps" and consists of five polypoid segments of colon mucosa up to 0.9 cm (centimeter) in greatest dimension. The two larger polyps are submitted in cassette 1 and the three smaller polyps in cassette 2. The specimen is submitted in toto in two cassettes.

MICROSCOPIC DESCRIPTION: Sections reveal five polyps showing surface epithelium and underlying glands lined by a serrated feathery surface epithelium.

DIAGNOSIS: Colon, polypectomy: hyperplastic polyps (five)

SERVICE CODE(S): _____

ICD-10-CM DX CODE(S): _____

(Answers to every other Case are located in Appendix D . The full answer key is only available in the TEACH Instructor Resources on Evolve.)

Abnormal Findings

When a patient has an abnormal finding as the preoperative diagnosis, reference "Abnormal" in the Index of the ICD-10-CM. In the following case, the patient presents for a sigmoidoscopy because of abnormal findings on x-ray. This would be a common reason for the patient to have an endoscopic procedure of the lower gastrointestinal tract. Also, if the patient has a family history or personal history of gastrointestinal lesions, the physician will recommend a screening endoscopic procedure.

As you read the reports, if there are terms you do not understand, you should take the time now to look them up in a medical dictionary. Your medical terminology skills will improve quickly and greatly if you make a practice of doing this.

Coder's Rule: Never pass by a medical term that you do not understand.

CASE 7-9   *Operative Report, Sigmoidoscopy*

LOCATION: Outpatient, Hospital

PATIENT: James Acheson

SURGEON: Larry Friendly, MD

PREOPERATIVE DIAGNOSIS: Abnormal findings on x-ray; GI (gastrointestinal) tract

POSTOPERATIVE DIAGNOSIS: Normal flexible sigmoidoscopy; no volvulus. Normal mucosa, just a few diverticula in the descending sigmoid colon

PROCEDURE PERFORMED: Flexible sigmoidoscopy

INDICATION: The patient is a 19-year-old white male who apparently had a perforated appendix with abscess. He had a cecectomy and has had a complicated hospital course with renal failure and sepsis. He has been getting tube feedings, which have been poorly tolerated. His CT (computerized tomography) scan showed dilated bowel in the midabdomen and pelvis and also a loop in the sigmoid colon, which is abnormal, thought to be possibly a volvulus or inflammatory infectious process in that area. The procedure is indicated to determine whether obstruction is present.

PREOPERATIVE MEDICATION: None

FINDINGS: The Pentax video sigmoidoscope was inserted without difficulty to 60 cm (centimeter). Careful inspection in the mid-descending (this is the colon), distal descending, sigmoid, and rectum revealed no erythema, ulceration, exudate, friability, or other mucosal abnormalities. There were a few diverticula present. The mucosa was normal. No volvulus were noted. No diverticulitis and no obstructing lesion were seen. The patient tolerated the procedure well.

IMPRESSION: Normal flexible sigmoidoscopy to 60 cm. No obstruction or volvulus was noted. The mucosa was normal.

DISCUSSION/PLAN: The patient needs to have a small bowel obstruction ruled out. We have recommended small bowel series.

SERVICE CODE(S): _____

ICD-10-CM DX CODE(S): _____

(Answers to every other Case are located in Appendix D . The full answer key is only available in the TEACH Instructor Resources on Evolve.)

CASE 7-10A   *Operative Report, Sigmoidoscopy*

LOCATION: Outpatient, Hospital

PATIENT: Jason Bell

SURGEON: Larry Friendly, MD

SCOPE USED: Pentax video sigmoidoscope

MEDICATIONS GIVEN: None

PREOPERATIVE DIAGNOSIS: Screen

POSTOPERATIVE DIAGNOSIS: Sigmoid and rectal polyps

INDICATION: The patient is a 51-year-old man who presents for screening sigmoidoscopy. He is asymptomatic. There is no family history of colon cancer or polyps.

FINDINGS: Four polyps were seen on this examination scattered between the rectum and proximal sigmoid colon. The largest measured about 1 cm (centimeter) in diameter.

The others were diminutive, about 4 or 5 mm (millimeter) in diameter. Biopsies were taken of two of these polyps.

DESCRIPTION OF TECHNIQUE: After informed consent was obtained, the patient was prepared for a sigmoidoscopy. He was placed in the left lateral decubitus position and given no medication. A digital rectal examination was performed and was unremarkable. The lubricated Pentax video sigmoidoscope was guided digitally into the rectum and advanced to 60 cm. Four polyps were seen to range from 4 to 10 mm in diameter between the sigmoid colon and the proximal rectum. Biopsies were taken of two of these. They appeared to be adenomas. There were no diverticula. The distal rectum was normal. The scope was withdrawn. The patient tolerated the procedure well and was discharged ambulatory.

RECOMMENDATIONS: Review polyp biopsies. These appear to be adenomas, and the patient will be scheduled for colonoscopy for polypectomy.

Pathology Report Later Indicated: See Report 7-10B.

SERVICE CODE(S): _____

ICD-10-CM DX CODE(S): _____

(Answers to every other Case are located in Appendix D . The full answer key is only available in the TEACH Instructor Resources on Evolve.)

CASE 7-10B   *Pathology Report*

LOCATION: Outpatient, Hospital

PATIENT: Jason Bell

SURGEON: Larry Friendly, MD

PATHOLOGIST: Morton Monson, MD

CLINICAL HISTORY: Screening for colon polyps

SPECIMEN RECEIVED: Colon polyps biopsy

GROSS DESCRIPTION: Received in a container labeled "colon polyps biopsy" are two frozen fragments of tan tissue measuring 0.1 to 0.4 cm (centimeter) in greatest dimension. The specimen is totally submitted.

MICROSCOPIC DESCRIPTION: The colon biopsy demonstrates a polyp showing adenomatous and villous epithelial features within the glandular and surface epithelium. The glands vary in size and configuration and are separated by an intact lamina propria. The cells are enlarged with elongated hyperchromatic nuclei. Pseudostratification and crowding are evident.

DIAGNOSIS: Colon and rectum biopsy, mucosal: tubulovillous adenoma (this is a benign neoplasm).

SERVICE CODE(S): _____

ICD-10-CM DX CODE(S): _____

(Answers to every other Case are located in Appendix D . The full answer key is only available in the TEACH Instructor Resources on Evolve.)

Abdominal Pain

Abdominal pain is a common complaint with many possible causes. The physician must rely on his or her expert clinical skills in obtaining a thorough history and examination that will lead to the correct diagnosis and correct treatment. The history would include assessment of the onset (chronic or acute), progression, location, type, and associated signs and symptoms, such as vomiting or change in bowel habits.

CASE 7-11A   *Operative Report, Colonoscopy*

Dr. Friendly performs a colonoscopy on a patient with a history of diarrhea for the past month.

LOCATION: Inpatient, Hospital

PATIENT: Gloria Hathorne

PRIMARY PHYSICIAN: Ronald Green, MD

SURGEON: Larry Friendly, MD

PROCEDURE PERFORMED: Colonoscopy with biopsies

PREPROCEDURE DIAGNOSIS: Abdominal pain, anemia

POSTPROCEDURE DIAGNOSIS: Ulcerative circumferential mass in the ascending colon consistent with either adenocarcinoma or lymphoma

PREOPERATIVE MEDICATION: Demerol 50 mg (milligram) IV (intravenous); Versed 2 mg IV

INDICATION: This is a very pleasant 40-year-old white female who I referred for evaluation of anemia and lower abdominal pain. The patient has had bilateral lower abdominal pain for 4 weeks. She has also developed diarrhea in the last few months. She had a gastric lymphoma 1 year ago that was treated with chemotherapy, and I believe also radiation. Her pain has disappeared, but her hemoglobin is 8.7. The patient had a CT (computerized tomography) scan that showed thickening in the ascending colon and cecum.

PROCEDURE: The Pentax video colonoscope was inserted without difficulty to the cecum. The ileocecal valve was identified. The appendiceal orifice was seen. The cecum was normal; however, just above the cecum in the proximal ascending colon was a large circumferential mass with ulceration and friability. Biopsies were obtained and a photograph obtained. Inspection in the remainder of the ascending colon, hepatic flexure, transverse colon, splenic flexure, descending colon, sigmoid colon, and rectum revealed no erythema, ulceration, exudate, friability, or other mucosal abnormalities. The patient tolerated the procedure well.

IMPRESSION: Large circumferential mass in the proximal ascending colon consistent with adenocarcinoma of the colon versus lymphoma

PLAN: Will await biopsy results, test accordingly, and do esophagogastroduodenoscopy.

Pathology Report Later Indicated: Adenocarcinoma, ascending colon

SERVICE CODE(S): _____

ICD-10-CM DX CODE(S): _____

(Answers to every other Case are located in Appendix D . The full answer key is only available in the TEACH Instructor Resources on Evolve.)

CASE 7-11B   *Surgical Consultation*

Dr. Sanchez serves as a consultant to assess the feasibility of undergoing resection of the colon the next day.

LOCATION: Inpatient, Hospital

PATIENT: Gloria Hathorne

PRIMARY PHYSICIAN: Ronald Green, MD

CONSULTANT: Gary Sanchez, MD

HISTORY OF PRESENT ILLNESS: The patient is a 40-year-old white female who has been having difficulty with diarrhea for the past month. The patient was recently admitted to the hospital because of abdominal pain and this diarrhea problem. The patient has a history of gastric lymphoma 2 years ago that was treated with chemotherapy and radiation therapy. The patient underwent evaluation for abdominal pain. Dr. Friendly did an upper endoscopy that showed radiation gastritis in the stomach area, and colonoscopy revealed an ascending colon lesion. Biopsies taken by Dr. Friendly showed an adenocarcinoma. The patient is now being seen for consideration of resection of her right colon for adenocarcinoma of the ascending colon.

PAST MEDICAL HISTORY:

OPERATIONS:

1. Open cholecystectomy
2. Total abdominal hysterectomy
3. Coronary artery bypass graft

ILLNESSES:

1. Diabetes mellitus
2. Hypertension
3. History of lymphoma

MEDICATIONS:

1. Advil
2. Compazine
3. Furosemide
4. Insulin
5. Lorazepam
6. Paxil
7. Remeron
8. Ultram
9. Zestril
10. Aciphex
11. Iron

ALLERGIES: None known.

REVIEW OF SYSTEMS: The patient does not smoke or drink. Neuro: The patient denies any history of seizure disorder, headaches, or dizziness. Cardiac: No history of myocardial infarction or congenital heart disease. The patient has hypertension and had heart bypass surgery in 1998. Pulmonary: No history of asthma, hay fever, or pneumonia. No history of hemoptysis. GI (gastrointestinal): See history of present illness. GU (genitourinary): The patient denies any urgency, frequency, or dysuria. GYN (gynecology): Gravida 1, para (to bring forth) 1, AB 0. Status TAH-BSO (total abdominal hysterectomy-bilateral salpingo-oophorectomy). Hematologic: The patient has received blood transfusions recently during this hospitalization. She has not noted any rectal bleeding. However, the patient does have bleeding from her colon cancer.

EXAMINATION: Mrs. Hathorne is a 40-year-old white female who is oriented to time, place, and person. Chest: Lungs are clear. No rales or rhonchi are heard. Heart: Regular rhythm. No murmur.

CASE 7-11B—cont'd

Abdomen: Normal bowel sounds. No masses or hepatosplenomegaly. The patient's abdomen is nontender at this time. She has a right subcostal incision scar and lower abdominal incision scar from her previous surgeries.

IMPRESSION:

1. Ascending colon adenocarcinoma
2. Status post lymphoma treatment 2 years ago
3. Hypertension
4. Diabetes mellitus
5. Pacemaker

PLAN: The patient has been counseled for resection of her colon cancer. She has agreed to the operation. All her questions about the surgery were answered. The patient will undergo a bowel prep tonight and surgery tomorrow.

Thank you for the consultation.

SERVICE CODE(S): _____

ICD-10-CM DX CODE(S): _____

(Answers to every other Case are located in Appendix D . The full answer key is only available in the TEACH Instructor Resources on Evolve.)

A **hemicolectomy** is a partial resection of about half the colon. See **Figure 7-7**. The designations of right and left indicate the location of the resection as either the left or right half of the colon from the middle of the transverse segment to the rectum. This procedure is performed for a variety of reasons, such as cancer or Crohn's disease (inflamed, ulcerated, thickened, and sometimes obstructed intestine). The colon is then joined with the ileum. Great care is taken to ensure that the anastomosis (joining of the two ends of the intestine) is secure so that it does not leak into the abdominal cavity.

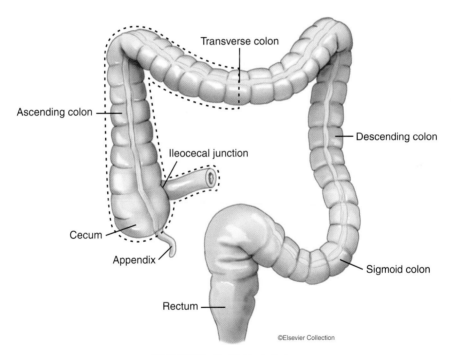

©Elsevier Collection

FIGURE 7-7 Hemicolectomy.

From the Trenches

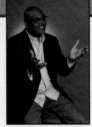

"Working in medical coding has many benefits, including being able to work remotely, as well as having the opportunity to work as an independent contractor."

ROLANDO RUSSELL
MBA, RHIA, CPC, CPAR

CASE 7-11C   *Operative Report, Hemicolectomy*

Some time later, the patient is taken to the operating room for a hemicolectomy by Dr. Sanchez. When assigning the diagnoses codes to this report, be certain to use the pathology report for the most definitive diagnosis. This report is an example of how code selection using only the surgical report can lead to incorrect or incomplete coding. According to the surgical report, you would only report the ascending colon adenocarcinoma, but upon referencing the pathology report, you will see that there is metastasis from the primary site to the mesentery, the secondary site.

LOCATION: Inpatient, Hospital

PATIENT: Gloria Hathorne

PRIMARY PHYSICIAN: Ronald Green, MD

SURGEON: Gary Sanchez, MD

PREOPERATIVE DIAGNOSIS: Adenocarcinoma of the ascending colon

POSTOPERATIVE DIAGNOSIS: Perforated adenocarcinoma of the ascending colon with attachment to the lateral abdominal wall

PROCEDURE PERFORMED: Right hemicolectomy with anastomosis

ANESTHESIA: General

INDICATIONS FOR SURGERY: Mrs. Hathorne is a 40-year-old white female who is having difficulties with her bowels. The patient was found to have an adenocarcinoma of the ascending colon that was proven by biopsy. The patient is taken to the operating room after a bowel prep yesterday for surgery.

PROCEDURE: The patient was prepped and draped in the usual manner. A midline abdominal incision was made. The patient has had previous surgeries, which included an appendectomy, hysterectomy, cholecystectomy, and radiation treatment to her abdomen for lymphoma. The patient had adhesions from her multiple previous surgeries and radiation therapy. These adhesions were taken down sharply using the Bovie cautery and Metzenbaum scissors. After this was done, the right colon was elevated using the Bovie cautery to divide the peritoneum on the right lateral gutter. The colon was then brought up into the operative area. The small bowel ileum was adherent down into the pelvis from her previous surgeries. These were taken down using Metzenbaum scissors and then allowed the small bowel to be freed up into the incision area. The dissection was carried

to the transverse colon in about the midpoint of the transverse colon. A Penrose drain was then placed around the transverse colon and also one around the ileum.

During the dissection of the cancer from the lateral abdominal wall, the cancer was firmly adherent to the abdominal wall. When this was finally freed up, there was an opening in the colon, which appeared to be a perforation of the area of cancer, which had been sealed by the lateral abdominal wall. No gross evidence of any tumor on the abdominal wall was seen. The opening in the colon was closed with a 2-0 silk suture. Next the mesentery was scored using the Bovie cautery. The mesentery was clamped and divided using Kelly clamps and tied with interrupted 2-0 silk sutures. After this was completed, the bowel clamp was placed on the proximal ileum and also on the distal colon. Kocher clamps were placed on the specimen side of the ileum and the colon. The colon and ileum were then transected, and the specimen was sent to pathology. An end-to-end anastomosis was then done. A two-layer closure was done. Interrupted 3-0 silk sutures were placed on either end of the anastomosis, and the posterior layer was then placed. All sutures were placed before they were tied. After this was completed, the inner layer was then run using a running 3-0 Vicryl suture using a locking stitch for the posterior layer and a running stitch on the anterior layer. After this was completed, the bowel clamps were removed. The anterior outer layer was then placed using interrupted 3-0 silk sutures. There was an excellent anastomosis following this procedure. The opening in the mesentery was closed with a running 2-0 Vicryl suture. The operative area was thoroughly irrigated. There were a few small bleeders that were found after the irrigation, and these were controlled by 2-0 silk ties or Bovie cautery. An additional adhesion was taken down of the omentum attached to the pelvis down into the pelvic gutter, and this was freed. After all the adhesions were taken down (don't be tempted to code the adhesions separately), the operative area again was thoroughly irrigated. The bowel was returned to the abdomen. The anastomosis was again checked and was excellent. The abdominal incision was then closed with a running no. 1 looped PDS suture for the fascia and the peritoneum in a single-layer closure. The subcutaneous tissues were then thoroughly irrigated, and the skin was closed with skin clips. The patient tolerated the operation and returned to recovery in stable condition.

Pathology Report Later Indicated: See Report 7-11D.

SERVICE CODE(S): _____

ICD-10-CM DX CODE(S): _____

(Answers to every other Case are located in Appendix D . The full answer key is only available in the TEACH Instructor Resources on Evolve.)

CASE 7-11D   *Pathology Report*

LOCATION: Inpatient, Hospital

PATIENT: Gloria Hathorne

PRIMARY PHYSICIAN: Ronald Green, MD

SURGEON: Gary Sanchez, MD

PATHOLOGIST: Morton Monson, MD

CLINICAL HISTORY: Ascending colon adenocarcinoma

SPECIMEN RECEIVED: Right colon

GROSS DESCRIPTION:

The specimen is labeled with the patient's name and "right ascending colon" and consists of a right hemicolectomy specimen including 4 cm (centimeter) of distal ileum including ileocecal valve with attached cecum and approximately 10 cm of colon. Also attached is mesentery. The appendix is absent. Approximately 5 cm from the ileocecal valve, a constricting lesion is noted grossly, which puckers the serosal surface. Cut section reveals a somewhat excavating circumferential mass measuring approximately 3 cm

CASE 7-11D—cont'd

in length that consists of gritty tan tissue. On cut section, it appears that the above-described lesion penetrates the full thickness of the bowel wall on the mesenteric side. Multiple small lymph nodes are found in the mesenteric fat and are placed in cassettes labeled 8-15.

MICROSCOPIC DESCRIPTION:

Sections of proximal and distal resection margins show no evidence of neoplasm. Sections of the previously described neoplasm consist of an excavating tumor consisting of small glandular strictures with abundant mucin production. The tumor infiltrates to the full thickness of the wall to the mesenteric fat. Several small foci of tumor are noted in the mesenteric fat. Sections of 11 lymph nodes show no evidence of neoplasm.

DIAGNOSIS:

Right hemicolectomy:

1. Moderately differentiated infiltrating adenocarcinoma with full-thickness penetration and multiple small discrete mesenteric metastatic nodules.
2. Twelve mesenteric lymph nodes showing no evidence of neoplasm.
3. Proximal and distal resection margins negative for tumor.

COMMENT: Although no tumor is seen in microscopically recognizable lymph nodes, several small tumor nodules are present in the mesenteric fat.

SERVICE CODE(S): _____

ICD-10-CM DX CODE(S): _____

(Answers to every other Case are located in Appendix D . The full answer key is only available in the TEACH Instructor Resources on Evolve.)

CASE 7-12A   *Hospital Inpatient Service*

In this next case, you will have the opportunity to code an extensive case (7-12A to 7-12H) for a patient initially admitted for nausea, vomiting, and diarrhea. The patient was in the hospital for 6 days and had multiple and varied services.

LOCATION: Inpatient, Hospital

PATIENT: Maynard Peters

ATTENDING PHYSICIAN: George Orbitz, MD

Patient is being admitted primarily because of intractable nausea, vomiting, and diarrhea.

The patient is a 32-year-old white gentleman who was diagnosed as having type 1 diabetes mellitus at 12 years of age. His diabetes has been complicated by diabetic retinopathy/blindness with multiple eye laser treatments; diabetic vascular neuropathy/autonomic neuropathy manifested by significant gastroparesis and erectile dysfunction; and diabetic nephropathy. He has had a kidney and pancreas transplant performed in May 20xx and January 20xx, respectively. According to the patient, he has not had any episodes of rejection of either organ per repeated biopsies.

History started around 1 to 2 weeks prior to admission, when the patient started to have intermittent episodes of diarrhea, which have been attributed to some irritable bowel syndrome component. During the course of his evaluation in the clinic and in the hospital, the patient was noted to have a significant cytomegalovirus infection, for which he was placed on ganciclovir intravenous treatment.

In the ensuing days, the patient continued to have persistent nausea, vomiting, and diarrhea. He has been coordinating his care with Dr. Jayco as well as with the transplant center in Denver. It is believed his diarrhea and other gastrointestinal symptoms stem primarily from either the cytomegalovirus infection and/or the intravenous ganciclovir treatment per se, thereby necessitating that his dose of ganciclovir be reduced to every 24 hours instead of every 12 hours as he had been taking. This dosage adjustment was done fairly recently, within the past 2 days.

The patient was seen by Dr. Jayco in the clinic on Monday and was advised to go to the emergency room, where he was given 2 L of intravenous fluids. After coming home, the patient relates that he continued to have persistent diarrhea, and this time he has had vague epigastric abdominal discomfort, nonradiating, not related to meals or change in position or bowel movements. On examination, he did not really have a surgical abdomen, as there is no evidence of rebound or guarding. Furthermore, his bowel sounds seem to be normal. A KUB (kidney, ureter, bladder) was performed, however, which did show evidence of air fluid levels, which would be suggestive of small bowel obstruction. Please note that the serum potassium is 5.4.

At this time, the plan is to admit the patient to the medical floor. We will check his daily weights and his inputs and outputs, and we will give him IV (intravenous) fluids, mainly 0.9% normal saline infusing at a rate of 150 to 200 ml (milliliter) per hour. I will continue the same medications, including rapamycin, Prograf, and ganciclovir every 24 hours as he has been taking. We will ask Dr. Olanka from gastroenterology to evaluate the patient in the morning to see if he has any recommendations. With absence of significant distention of the abdomen, I do not feel compelled to place a nasogastric tube at this time. Again, it is possible that these gastrointestinal symptoms may stem primarily from a long-standing history of diabetic autonomic neuropathy/gastroparesis plus/minus ganciclovir treatment per se plus/minus cytomegalovirus infection. In the morning, Dr. Jayco will assume care from the nephrology standpoint, and he will be coordinating with the Denver transplant coordinators.

PAST MEDICAL/SURGICAL HISTORY:

1. Type 1 insulin-dependent diabetes mellitus
   A. Diabetic retinopathy with multiple laser surgeries; status post vitrectomy right eye ×2, left eye ×1
   B. Diabetic vascular neuropathy, erectile dysfunction
   C. Diabetic autonomic neuropathy, gastroparesis, gastroesophageal reflux disease, chronic nausea, and vomiting (?)
   D. Diabetic nephropathy, history of hemodialysis requirement
2. Status post toenail surgery, right and left
3. Status post angiography, February 2001, showing minimal atherosclerotic disease with normal LV (left ventricle) function and some LV dilatation
4. Hyperlipidemia

Continued

CASE 7-12A—cont'd

5. Chronic mild metabolic acidosis most likely relating to chronic renal insufficiency/pancreas transplant draining into the bladder
6. Depression
7. Asthma
8. Hypertension secondary to diabetic nephropathy/chronic renal insufficiency/renal failure

SOCIAL HISTORY: He is married and has two children. He is on disability, I believe. He denies any current or previous history of alcohol, tobacco, or intravenous or recreational drugs.

FAMILY HISTORY: Positive for heart disease. Negative for hypertension, diabetes, stroke, cancer, kidney disease, bleeding disorder, or dyscrasia. A cousin has had spina bifida, heart disease, and seizures. Mother was diagnosed as having Crohn's disease.

CURRENT MEDICATIONS:

1. Rapamycin 2 mg (milligram) q.d. (every day).
2. Prograf 2 mg b.i.d. (twice a day).
3. Lipitor 10 mg q.h.s. (each bedtime).
4. Aspirin 81 mg q.d.
5. Sodium bicarbonate 650 per tab, 2 tabs q.i.d. (four times a day).
6. Zoloft 100 mg q.d.
7. Ganciclovir IV q.24h. (recently adjusted from 12h dosing; see note above).

ALLERGIES: ACE inhibitors apparently cause some swelling. Penicillin and sulfa medications cause rash.

LABORATORY TESTS: Sodium 135, potassium 5.4, chloride 98, CO_2 (carbon dioxide) 21, BUN (blood urea nitrogen) and creatinine are 28/3.1, glucose 135, calcium 8.8. Hemogram shows an H&H (hematocrit and hemoglobin) of 12.5/37, WBC (white blood count) 8.6, and platelets 319. There is a slight left shift as neutrophils are 89.8%.

REVIEW OF SYSTEMS: CONSTITUTIONAL: No fever or chills. Positive weight loss. He appears to be fairly nourished. No night sweats. SKIN: No skin lesions. No active dermatosis. EYES: No eye discharge. No eye itching. Positive diabetic retinopathy/legally blind. ENT: No ear discharge. No hearing difficulty. No pharyngeal hyperemia, congestion, or exudate. LYMPH NODES: No lymphadenopathy in the neck, axillae, or groin. NEUROLOGIC: No headaches. No gait instability. No falls. No seizures. PSYCHIATRIC: No behavioral changes. NECK: No thyromegaly. RESPIRATORY: No cough. No colds. No hemoptysis. No shortness of breath. CARDIOVASCULAR: No chest pain. No palpitations. No orthopnea. No paroxysmal nocturnal dyspnea. GASTROINTESTINAL: Positive anorexia. Positive nausea. Positive vomiting. No dysphagia. No odynophagia. No constipation. Positive diarrhea. Positive abdominal pain. No fecal incontinence. Positive history of irritable bowel syndrome is questionable. No hematemesis. No hematochezia. No melena. GENITOURINARY: No urgency. No frequency. No dysuria. No hematuria. No urinary incontinence. No nocturia. No penile discharge. No penile lesion. Positive history of erectile dysfunction related to diabetic vascular neuropathy. MUSCULOSKELETAL: No joint pains. No muscle pain/weaknesses. HEMATOLOGIC: No bleeding tendencies. No purpura. No petechia. No ecchymosis. ENDOCRINOLOGIC: No heat/cold intolerance.

PHYSICAL EXAMINATION: Vital signs are stable. Blood pressure 120s/80s. Heart rate in the 80s to 90s. Respirations 20. He is afebrile. Normocephalic and atraumatic. Pink palpebral conjunctivae, anicteric sclerae. No nasal or aural discharge. Moist tongue and buccal mucosa. No pharyngeal hyperemia, congestion, or exudates. Supple neck. No lymphadenopathy. Symmetric chest expansion. No retractions. Positive rhonchi. No crackles or wheezes. S1 (first heart sound) and S2 (second heart sound) are distinct. No S3 (third heart sound) or S4 (fourth heart sound). Regular rate and rhythm. Abdomen: Positive bowel sounds, soft. No rebound. No guarding. Positive direct tenderness over the epigastrium only on deep palpation but not on light palpation. No abdominal bruits appreciated during this examination. Renal allograft appears to be nontender without any bruits appreciated. No edema. No arthritic changes noted on both upper and lower extremities. Pulses are fair.

ASSESSMENT/PLAN: Impression for this patient is as follows:

1. Nausea, vomiting, and diarrhea, questionable etiology.
   A. Gastroenteritis unlikely because of the chronic nature of his symptomatology.
   B. Medications, namely ganciclovir. Questionable Prograf. Will need to discuss with transplant coordinators. Will check Prograf levels. Agree with decreasing ganciclovir to every 24-hour dosing.
   C. Diabetic autonomic neuropathy/gastroparesis/irritable bowel syndrome, questionable.
   D. Cytomegalovirus infection per se.

At this time, plan is to hydrate the patient with IV fluids, namely, 0.9% normal saline. We will continue to monitor his chemistries, labs, etc.

Because of the air fluid levels on the KUB, which suggest a small bowel obstruction, I am going to ask Dr. Olanka from gastroenterology to give us his opinion regarding this patient. Please note this patient does not have any evidence of ileus or hypokalemia.

2. Chronic renal failure, hypertensive, (latest creatinine clearance is 43 ml [milliliter]/min with a creatinine of 1.8, total volume of 2000 ml, and 1.36 g proteinuria performed last month), status post kidney, pancreas transplant with no previous episodes of rejection. Will check urinary amylase because this patient's pancreas is allegedly draining into the urinary bladder. If urinary amylase is slow, this may suggest rejection. Please note that this patient's creatinine has been in the 2.8 to 3.1 range over the past several weeks to months. His baseline creatinine is in the 1.4 to 1.6 range.

Aggressive IV fluid hydration as noted above.

3. Hyperlipidemia. Continue Lipitor 10 mg at q.h.s.
   A. Questionable mild atherosclerotic heart disease (see past medical/surgical history). Continue aspirin 81 mg q.d.
   B. Mild chronic metabolic acidosis related to pancreatic drainage into the urinary bladder. Continue bicarbonate supplements.
   C. Depression. Continue Zoloft 100 mg q.d.

PLAN: As dictated above. Dr. Jayco will take over in the morning and will reassume care. Dr. Olanka of gastroenterology will evaluate the patient in the morning.

I have spent a total of 90 minutes evaluating and reviewing this patient's medical records and formulating a treatment strategy. An additional 40 minutes was spent discussing the case in great detail with the patient and his family.

SERVICE CODE(S): _____

ICD-10-CM DX CODE(S): _____

CASE 7-12A—cont'd

Discussion

There are so many diagnoses to consider in this report. When deciding which diagnosis to report, consider why the patient initially presented for care. In an inpatient setting, all of the diagnoses would be reported, but in the outpatient setting, those conditions that prompted the encounter and demonstrate medical necessity are reported. Under the Assessment/Plan section of the report, the first-listed statement is the nausea, vomiting, and diarrhea, which must be reported as it was the primary reason for the patient presenting for care. There is a combination code for the nausea with vomiting and another code for the diarrhea. The hypertensive renal failure could be reported, as indicated in point 2 of the Assessment/Plan section of the report, and most coders would definitely report that. The diabetes with the diabetic retinopathy and neuropathy could be reported. The history of transplants (kidney, Z94.0 and pancreas, Z94.83) also has major impact on the care of this patient, so that also could be reported.

(Answers to every other Case are located in Appendix D . The full answer key is only available in the TEACH Instructor Resources on Evolve.)

CASE 7-12B *Infectious Disease Consultation*

On this report, the order of the diagnoses has changed. The physician lists as the first point under the Impression section the diarrhea and vomiting. There is no mention of the nausea on this report. In points 2 and 3, the kidney and pancreas transplants are noted, with indication that the patient's immune system is depressed due to the transplants. When people undergo organ transplants, the patient is given immunosuppressants to decrease the likelihood of rejection of the transplanted organ. The transplant status should be reported using Z codes. You can find direction to the correct Z code by locating "Transplant" in the Index.

LOCATION: Inpatient, Hospital

PATIENT: Maynard Peters

PHYSICIAN: Gordon Jayco, MD

CONSULTANT: Lou Lin, MD

REASON FOR REFERRAL: Diarrhea in an immunocompromised host.

IMPRESSION:

1. Two-week duration of diarrhea, vomiting, night sweats, and chills, progressing on ganciclovir.
2. Immune compromise secondary to transplantation.
3. Renal transplant with apparently a living related donor in May 20xx with a pancreatic cadaver transplant in December 20xx with drainage to the bladder in a patient who apparently is CMV (cytomegalovirus) positive and has not had any opportunistic infections or complications. Now on an immunosuppressive regimen of sirolimus and FK-506.
   For approximately 2 months after each transplant, the patient received a course of ganciclovir and a month or two ago completed 2 to 3 months of oral acyclovir for apparent herpes of the eye.
4. Hyperlipidemia
5. Diabetes mellitus type 1 with complications of retinopathy, vasculopathy, autonomic neuropathy, gastroparesis, and neuropathy
6. Chronic renal failure with a creatinine clearance of 43 in December, status posttransplant as above
7. Hematuria, etiology unclear
8. Depression
9. Asthma
10. Hypertension
11. Coronary artery disease with an angiogram done in January 20xx when he had minimal coronary disease

RECOMMENDATIONS:

1. I think it is important that we try to make a diagnosis to see whether this is an infectious etiology versus a partial small bowel obstruction. He will need a colonoscopy and upper endoscopy. Certainly, if lesions are found, biopsy should be obtained for specific viral studies.
2. *C. difficile (Clostridium difficile)* toxin should be obtained.
3. Stool cultures and white blood cell stains should be obtained.
4. CMV titer of either a CMV P-65 or a quantitative CMV titer should be obtained.
5. CT (computerized tomography) scan
6. Consideration of surgical consultation as well

HISTORY OF PRESENT ILLNESS: This 32-year-old gentleman is status post renal transplant and pancreatic transplant in May 20xx and January 20xx for underlying diabetic nephropathy. His transplant has been uneventful. He has been on sirolimus and FK-506. First, he has had a chronic history of constipation followed by diarrhea for years, which he usually takes Imodium, which stops his diarrhea. About 2 weeks ago, he developed increasing diarrhea that was not responsive to Imodium with vomiting, night sweats, and chills. He was treated with acyclovir for a week and it had no effect. Apparently, he had a CMV titer that was positive at the transplant center in Denver and then was started on IV (intravenous) ganciclovir. Despite that, he continues to get worse with worsening diarrhea and cramps.

When seen in the emergency room, he was hydrated. He continues to have relapses with dehydration. Subsequently, he was admitted to the hospital for hydration as well as diagnosis. Because of this, an infectious disease consultation was obtained.

FAMILY HISTORY: Father died at age 39 of cardiac problems. Mother died at 76 and had recently been diagnosed with Crohn's disease. A cousin has spina bifida, heart disease, and seizures of unknown origin.

PAST MEDICAL HISTORY: He has had diabetes mellitus now for 19 years, on insulin. It has been complicated by retinopathy requiring multiple laser treatments. He is essentially blind. He had vasculopathy, autonomic neuropathy, gastroparesis, neuropathy, and nephropathy that eventually required the transplant. He also had a long history of irritable bowel syndrome, hyperlipidemia, depression, asthma, and hypertension. He has coronary artery disease. He had an angiogram in January 20xx that showed minimal disease. He had his transplant in May 20xx, which was apparently a living donor from his wife, and a pancreatic cadaver transplant in January 20xx, with

Continued

CASE 7-12B—cont'd

drainage to the bladder. Apparently, he has not had any opportunistic infections. He was treated with prophylactic ganciclovir for 2 months, approximately after the kidney transplant and then again for about 2 months after the pancreatic transplant. About 2 months ago, he completed 2 to 3 months of acyclovir for what sounds like herpes of the eye.

MEDICATIONS: Besides the antirejection medications sirolimus and FK-506, he is on atorvastatin, an aspirin a day, Prevacid, and Zoloft.

ALLERGIES: ACE inhibitors cause swelling. Penicillin and sulfa cause manifestation of rash.

REVIEW OF SYSTEMS: Complete, negative except he has had a little bit of dyspnea related to this illness. He had some dysuria yesterday. Although he had some chronic low back pain and some chronic arthralgias, predominantly hip and shoulders, it seems to have become worse in the last week or two. OPHTHALMOLOGIC: Negative. OTOLARYNGOLOGIC: Negative. CARDIOVASCULAR: Negative. RESPIRATORY: Negative. GU (genitourinary): Negative. MUSCULOSKELETAL INTEGUMENTARY: Negative. NEUROLOGIC: Negative. PSYCHIATRIC: Negative. ENDOCRINE: Negative. HEMATOLOGIC: Negative. LYMPHATIC: Negative.

TRAVEL: No recent travel, hunting, or fishing.

ANIMAL EXPOSURE: He does have animal exposure to cats, dogs, and horses. He does not have any direct care of these.

SOCIAL HISTORY: He is married and has two children. No tobacco use. No alcohol use.

PHYSICAL EXAMINATION: He is alert. His T-max is 37.2. Pulse is 110. Respiratory rate is 22. Blood pressure is 126/75. HEENT (head, ears, eyes, nose, throat): Head, nontraumatic. The tympanic membranes are clear bilaterally. The conjunctivae are clear. Red reflex is seen. Pupils are irregular, probably related to prior surgery. He has evidence of the fundus with multiple laser treatments. The nasal membranes are clear. The pharynx is clear. Moist mucous membranes. I do not hear a carotid bruit. NECK is supple. There is no cervical adenopathy. No thyroid tenderness. There is no supraclavicular adenopathy. Chest is symmetrical. PULMONARY exam is clear. There are no secondary muscles of respiration and no axillary or epitrochlear adenopathy. ABDOMEN: He is distended. I can hear tinkling bowel sounds. There is no tenderness with deep palpation. No rebound. There is no groin adenopathy. INTEGUMENTARY: No other rashes or eruptions.

LABORATORY DATA: He has a white count of 8.6, hemoglobin of 21.5, and platelet count of 319. Urinalysis showed 10-15 RBCs (red blood cells). Sodium was 135, potassium 5.4. BUN (blood urea nitrogen) was 38. Creatinine was 3.1. His glucose was 135. Blood cultures: He had urine cultures, stool, and cultures done 2 months ago. Apparently, no pathogen has been identified.

I have discussed the case with Dr. Jayco, and we will implement the interventions.

SERVICE CODE(S): _____

ICD-10-CM DX CODE(S): _____

(Answers to every other Case are located in Appendix D . The full answer key is only available in the TEACH Instructor Resources on Evolve.)

Cytomegalovirus

Cytomegalovirus (CMV) is a herpes virus that infects humans, monkeys, and rodents. CMV is also known as salivary gland virus. The virus produces unique large cells.

Transmission is associated with close contact, not only sexual contact. It does not produce genital symptoms, but rather produces nonspecific and often mild clinical symptoms, such as colitis.

CASE 7-12C   *Operative Report, Colonoscopy*

LOCATION: Inpatient, Hospital

PATIENT: Maynard Peters

ATTENDING PHYSICIAN: Gordon Jayco, MD

SURGEON: Daniel Olanka, MD

PROCEDURE: Colonoscopy with multiple biopsies

PREOPERATIVE DIAGNOSIS: Rule out cytomegalovirus colitis

POSTOPERATIVE DIAGNOSIS: Mild patchy erythema in the descending, sigmoid, and rectum, nonspecific, not characteristic of colitis

INDICATION: This is a 32-year-old white man with pancreatic and kidney transplant secondary to diabetes who presents with 1 week of diarrhea, abdominal cramping, and nausea and vomiting. He was treated with ganciclovir at the transplant center in Denver for presumed CMV enteritis based on rising CMV serology. He was not seen, however, by anyone. He presents now dehydrated and with creatinine of 3.1. The procedure is indicated to rule out CMV (cytomegalovirus) colitis.

PREOPERATIVE MEDICATION: Demerol 50 mg (milligram) IV (intravenous); Versed 4 mg IV

FINDINGS: The Pentax video colonoscope was inserted easily into the cecum. Ileocecal valve was identified. The appendiceal orifice was seen. The terminal ileum was entered a distance of 5 cm (centimeter). No lesions were seen. Inspection of the cecum, ascending colon, hepatic flexure, transverse colon, and splenic flexure revealed no erythema, ulceration, exudate, or friability in the mucosa. Biopsies were obtained in the right colon of normal mucosa. The distal distending, sigmoid, and rectum revealed patchy erythema without ulceration, no friability, and really no loss of vascular pattern. There was erythematous area, nonspecific. Biopsies were obtained of these areas also. The patient tolerated the procedure well.

IMPRESSION: Nonspecific mild erythema in the distal descending, sigmoid, and rectum, not characteristic of CMV colitis. Biopsies of terminal ileum were benign as per pathology. Normal colon otherwise.

PLAN: Esophagogastroduodenoscopy.

SERVICE CODE(S): _____

ICD-10-CM DX CODE(S): _____

(Answers to every other Case are located in Appendix D . The full answer key is only available in the TEACH Instructor Resources on Evolve.)

CASE 7-12D   *Operative Report, Esophagogastroduodenoscopy*

In this report, the diagnosis changed to gastritis.

LOCATION: Inpatient, Hospital

PATIENT: Maynard Peters

ATTENDING PHYSICIAN: Gordon Jayco, MD

SURGEON: Daniel Olanka, MD

OPERATIVE PROCEDURE: Esophagogastroduodenoscopy

PREOPERATIVE DIAGNOSIS: Rule out cytomegalovirus gastritis

POSTOPERATIVE DIAGNOSIS: Mild gastritis, nonspecific; biopsied

INDICATION: A 32-year-old white male with diabetes who had kidney and pancreatic transplant, presents with 1 week of nausea, vomiting, and diarrhea. He was treated for a presumptive CMV (cytomegalovirus) enteritis elsewhere with ganciclovir, and he continues to be ill. We just performed colonoscopy, which showed nonspecific erythema in the distal descending sigmoid and rectum.

PREOPERATIVE MEDICATION: As per colonoscopy.

FINDINGS: The flexible Pentax video pediatric endoscope was passed without difficulty into the oropharynx. The gastroesophageal junction was seen at 42 cm (centimeter). Inspection of the esophagus revealed no erythema, ulceration, exudate, friability, varices, or other mucosal abnormalities. The stomach proper was entered, and the endoscope advanced to the second duodenum. Inspection of the second duodenum, first duodenum, duodenal bulb, and pylorus revealed no abnormalities. Retroflexion revealed no lesions of the cardia or fundus. Inspection of the body revealed no abnormalities. The antrum revealed some patchy and linear erythema; no friability. There were some coffee-ground specks present. Biopsies were obtained, and photograph was obtained. The patient tolerated the procedure well.

IMPRESSION: Mild gastritis, biopsied.

PLAN: We placed a nasogastric tube for this patient because he is having severe vomiting of large amounts of liquids. Will treat the patient conservatively and hydrate him and see how he does, and then we will review the biopsy.

Pathology Report Later Indicated: Gastritis.

SERVICE CODE(S): _____

ICD-10-CM DX CODE(S): _____

(Answers to every other Case are located in Appendix D . The full answer key is only available in the TEACH Instructor Resources on Evolve.)

CASE 7-12E   *KUB*

The report references that this KUB is done prior to barium study. A barium study is a study in which barium is used as a contrast medium.

LOCATION: Inpatient, Hospital

PATIENT: Maynard Peters

PRIMARY PHYSICIAN: Gordon Jayco, MD

RADIOLOGIST: Morton Monson, MD

EXAMINATION OF: KUB (kidney, ureter, bladder)

CLINICAL SYMPTOMS: Nausea, vomiting, and diarrhea in a patient with kidney and pancreas transplants.

KUB DONE PRIOR TO BARIUM STUDY: There is no prior study for comparison. No bony lesion is appreciated. There are surgical clips over the right side of vertebral body L5 (fifth lumbar vertebra) and the right side of the sacrum. That is presumably either transplanted kidney or transplanted pancreas site. There are vascular or surgical clips over the left sacroiliac joint, midportion, and that is again either the site of the transplanted kidney or site of the pancreas transplant presumably. Bowel gas pattern is nonspecific. No distended bowel loops are seen. There is bowel gas from stomach to rectum. No enlargement of liver or spleen. No significant calcification seen. Entirety of pelvis not imaged on film.

IMPRESSION:

1. History of kidney and pancreas transplants
2. Nonspecific bowel gas pattern
3. Surgical clips, low abdomen/upper pelvis
4. No bony lesion seen

SERVICE CODE(S): _____

ICD-10-CM DX CODE(S): _____

(Answers to every other Case are located in Appendix D . The full answer key is only available in the TEACH Instructor Resources on Evolve.)

CASE 7-12F   *KUB*

Two days after the initial KUB, the patient was returned to the radiology department for a recheck.

LOCATION: Inpatient, Hospital

PATIENT: Maynard Peters

ATTENDING PHYSICIAN: Gordon Jayco, MD

RADIOLOGIST: Morton Monson, MD

EXAMINATION OF: KUB (kidney, ureter, bladder)

CLINICAL SYMPTOMS: Barium recheck in patient with diarrhea, vomiting in a patient with a history of kidney and pancreas transplant.

KUB, 8 AM: FINDINGS: There is barium throughout the decompressed colon to the level of the rectum. Gaseous distention of a few loops of small bowel that are of normal caliber in the midabdomen. NG tube with tip in the distal stomach. Surgical clips projected over the left aspect of the pelvis.

SERVICE CODE(S): _____

ICD-10-CM DX CODE(S): _____

(Answers to every other Case are located in Appendix D . The full answer key is only available in the TEACH Instructor Resources on Evolve.)

CASE 7-12G   *KUB*

The next day, the patient was returned to the radiology department for "barium in the belly," which refers to the previous day's results that indicated there was heavy barium residue in the colon. This residue would prevent clarity on visualization. Dr. Jayco wants the patient to have a CT scan.

LOCATION: Inpatient, Hospital

PATIENT: Maynard Peters

ATTENDING PHYSICIAN: Gordon Jayco, MD

RADIOLOGIST: Morton Monson, MD

EXAMINATION OF: KUB (kidney, ureter, bladder)

CLINICAL SYMPTOMS: Barium in belly in patient with diarrhea, vomiting in a patient with a history of kidney and pancreas transplant.

KUB: This is performed pre-CT (computerized tomography) to determine whether barium has cleared adequately to obtain a CT. This is 8:45 AM.

Comparison is made with previous study performed yesterday. Heavy barium is again seen within portions of the descending and sigmoid colon. This is decreased compared with the previous study; however, the heavy barium still would create a significant artifact. I would recommend that CT be rescheduled for perhaps tomorrow or Monday to ensure that this heavy barium is no longer present. The gastrointestinal air pattern is relatively nonspecific.

CONCLUSION: Residual heavy barium seen within portions of the transverse, descending, and sigmoid colon. It is decreased compared with the previous study, and yet still a significant amount is present, which I believe would create significant artifact on the CT scan that is planned. I would recommend delaying it until this barium has cleared.

SERVICE CODE(S): _____

ICD-10-CM DX CODE(S): _____

(Answers to every other Case are located in Appendix D . The full answer key is only available in the TEACH Instructor Resources on Evolve.)

CASE 7-12H   *Discharge Summary*

LOCATION: Inpatient, Hospital

PATIENT: Maynard Peters

ATTENDING PHYSICIAN: Gordon Jayco, MD

FINAL DIAGNOSES:

1. Small-bowel obstruction, etiology to be determined
2. Dehydration, secondary to no. 1
3. Acute renal failure, secondary to no. 1, recovering

4. Status post kidney transplant
5. Status post pancreas transplant
6. Diabetes mellitus type 1
7. Immunocompromised state, secondary to transplantation, hyperlipidemia
8. History of asthma
9. Minimal history of coronary artery disease
10. Metabolic acidosis and electrolyte imbalance, secondary to acute renal failure

CASE 7-12H—*cont'd*

HOSPITAL COURSE: This patient was admitted for dehydration, electrolyte imbalance, and acute renal failure superimposed on his living, unrelated-donor kidney transplant and pancreas transplant. The kidney was significantly involved, and the pancreas was not affected. They were on the mend during his hospital course. He received electrolyte repletion. He had both ends scoped and was believed not to have CMV (cytomegalovirus) colitis, for which he was being empirically treated. *C. difficile (Clostridium difficile)* was negative, and there was no other obvious explanation for his problem except that we suspected a partial small-bowel obstruction on admission. This did not resolve. It actually got worse, and the situation was severe enough for us to proceed with our evacuation plan, which was devised on Friday; that is, if he did not continue to get better, we would transfer him to the primary transplant center for further evaluation. There was an area in the middle of the small bowel that was abnormal and that we could not visualize well, and we were trying to get a CT (computerized tomography) scan done, but his barium was not cleaning out properly. In any case, that will be resolved at the transplant center.

Time spent preparing and reviewing his chart was 30 minutes.

SERVICE CODE(S): _____

ICD-10-CM DX CODE(S): _____

(Answers to every other Case are located in Appendix D . The full answer key is only available in the TEACH Instructor Resources on Evolve.)

Laparoscopic Procedures

Laparoscopic procedures are those in which a scope is inserted into the abdomen by way of small incisions, as illustrated in **Figure 7-8.** Trocar ports are introduced. The port is a sharp-ended hollow tube that is inserted into the abdomen and serves as an entry point for the scope. The surgeon will place additional trocar ports as needed to view the internal structures from the correct angle and to insert instruments as needed. The number of ports has no influence on the code choice. The physician then performs the procedure by means of manipulation of the instruments inserted through the ports. Many abdominal procedures can be accomplished using this less invasive method that reduces the recovery time for the patient and is less painful because the incision size is reduced. These procedures are often done in an ambulatory surgery center, that is, at the hospital, clinic, or free-standing surgical center. The patients seen in these centers are outpatients, even if the center is part of a hospital. The physician reports his or her services, and the hospital reports the facility service.

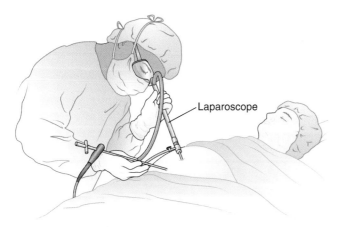

FIGURE 7 – 8 Laparoscopic procedure.

Closed Procedures Converted to Open Procedures

An operative procedure that began as a closed procedure (a procedure being performed by means of scope) that was **converted** to an open procedure (operation completed through an incision) is reported with codes from category Z53.3. Also note that Z53.09 is available for assignment for surgical or other procedures **not carried out** because of contraindications. Contraindication means literally "against indication" that would be recommended by the **physician.** Z53.1 is a surgical procedure not carried out because of the **patient's** decision. Z53.8 is assigned for procedures not carried out for other reasons. The Z code is sequenced last.

CASE 7-13   *Operative Report, Appendectomy*

In this report, note that there was a complication (see highlighted area on the report) in which a small serosal tear was created by one of the surgical instruments (Kitner). This is reported with two codes, one for the complication (K91.--) and one for the location of the complication (the tear/injury). Begin the code assignment process for the location of the complication in the Index of the ICD-10-CM under the main term "Injury" and subterm by location of the injury. You will be directed to the Tabular to assign the code. Never code directly from the Index.

LOCATION: Outpatient, Hospital

PATIENT: Samantha Young

PHYSICIAN: Larry Friendly, MD

PREOPERATIVE DIAGNOSIS: Colitis, terminal ileitis, and possible appendicitis.

POSTOPERATIVE DIAGNOSIS: Acute appendicitis. No evidence of abscess or peritonitis. No pus in the abdomen.

PROCEDURE PERFORMED: Laparoscopic abdominal exploration, laparoscopic mobilization of the cecum converted to open appendectomy.

SPECIMEN: Appendix

COMPLICATIONS: A small serosal tear in the terminal ileum was a retraction injury. This was repaired during the open part of the case with 3-0 silk.

ESTIMATED BLOOD LOSS: Less than 100 cc (cubic centimeter)

ANESTHESIA: General endotracheal with 30 cc of Marcaine local augmentation.

PROCEDURE IN DETAIL: After good general endotracheal anesthesia, the patient was prepped and draped in the usual sterile fashion. A Foley and NG (nasogastric) tube were both placed to decompress the stomach and also the bladder. A small infraumbilical incision was made, and under direct vision the fascia was nicked. The Veress needle was placed in the fascia, and the abdomen was insufflated to 16 Torr. After this, the fascial incision was lengthened, and a no. 10 trocar was placed. The camera was placed through this, and the abdomen was inspected. The cecum was quite inflamed. The base of the appendix was noted. The appendix itself was stuck down to the cecum. The area of terminal ileum just adjacent to the cecum was inflamed. The cecum was mobilized, and the peritoneal reflection was taken down. This was done with hot scissors. Care was taken not to injure bowel. The ovary was inspected and was normal. The appendix was felt to be quite friable, and there was a small serosal tear created in the ileum with the Kitner while mobilizing the cecum (this represents a complication during surgery). We were unable to determine laparoscopically whether this is just a serosal tear, and additionally the tissue was so friable that we were not confident that we would be able to close the stump of the appendix with an endoscopic stapler. Therefore, the decision was made to open the abdomen. This was done with appendiceal incision. A Rocky-Davis incision was made after anesthetizing the area with Marcaine. The external oblique and transversus abdominis fascia was incised, and a muscle-sparing technique was applied. The peritoneum was entered, and the cecum was brought up into the wound. The base of the appendix was identified, and it was so friable that we could not simply tie off the base of the appendix and amputate the appendix distally. It was necessary to close the cecum where the appendix was attached and to divide the appendix off the cecum. This was done with running 3-0 Vicryl. After this, some imbricating 3-0 silk stitches were placed. Attention was then turned to the serosal injury. This indeed turned out to be just serosa. This was on the terminal ileum. The serosal injury was repaired with interrupted 3-0 silk. Next the abdomen was irrigated and pneumoperitoneum was sucked out. The pneumoperitoneum was released. The two ports, the no. 10 port and the no. 5 subport, were removed. The camera port was also removed. This was done prior to opening the abdomen. All the fascial stitches were used to close the umbilical port and also the left no. 10 port sites. The appendiceal wound was closed in layers with the peritoneum, and two layers of fascia were closed separately. The skin was closed with 4-0 Vicryl. Steri-Strips and sterile dressings were applied. The patient tolerated the procedure well, and sponge and needle counts were correct. She was extubated in the operating room and returned to the recovery room in good condition.

Pathology Report Later Indicated: Acute Appendicitis

SERVICE CODE(S): _____

ICD-10-CM DX CODE(S): _____

(Answers to every other Case are located in Appendix D . The full answer key is only available in the TEACH Instructor Resources on Evolve.)

Cholecystectomy

Removal of the gallbladder, **cholecystectomy,** is a procedure performed for diseased or malfunctioning gallbladder conditions. The procedure can be performed either open (47600-47620) or laparoscopic (47562-47570, **Figures 7-9** and **7-10**). The CPT codes are divided based on the method (open/laparoscopic) and the extent of the procedure (with or without exploration of the common bile duct, repairs, removal of portion of bile duct or intestine). The preferred method continues to be the open cholecystectomy due to a higher complication rate from hemorrhage or bile leakage following laparoscopic procedures. One benefit of the laparoscopic procedure is that the hospital stay is an average of 4 days compared with the more invasive open procedure with a hospital stay of 7 days.

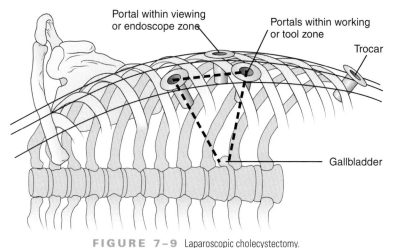

FIGURE 7–9 Laparoscopic cholecystectomy.

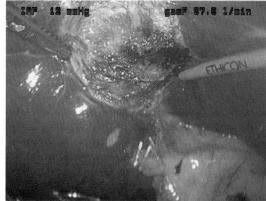

FIGURE 7–10 Laparoscopic cholecystectomy.

CASE 7-14 *Operative Report, Cholecystectomy*

The patient in this case presents with biliary dyskinesia (gallbladder dysfunction). The gallbladder of a patient with biliary dyskinesia appears normal on ultrasound scan, but when the gallbladder is stimulated to contract with food or with the stimulating hormone CCK, the gallbladder does not contract properly. Another diagnostic tool often used is the HIDA scan, which is a special type of isotope scan used to visualize the gallbladder emptying (ejection fraction). The patient in the following case has an abnormal CCK and HIDA scan and is having the gallbladder removed.

LOCATION: Outpatient, Hospital

PATIENT: Karen Daniels

PHYSICIAN: Larry Friendly, MD

PREOPERATIVE DIAGNOSIS: Biliary dyskinesia

POSTOPERATIVE DIAGNOSIS: Biliary dyskinesia

PROCEDURE PERFORMED: Laparoscopic cholecystectomy

ANESTHESIA: General

INDICATION: The patient is a 39-year-old female who presents with an abnormal CCK HIDA (hydroxy iminodiacetic acid [imaging test]) scan. She presents today for elective laparoscopic cholecystectomy. She understands the risks of bleeding, infection, possible damage to the biliary system, and possible conversion to open procedure, and she wishes to proceed.

PROCEDURE: The patient was brought to the operating table and placed under general anesthesia. Foley catheter and orogastric tubes were inserted, and she was prepped and draped sterilely. A supraumbilical skin incision was made with a no. 11 blade, and dissection was carried down through subcutaneous tissues. Bluntly, midline fascia was grasped with a Kocher clamp, and 0 Vicryl sutures were placed on either side of the midline fascia. The Veress needle was then inserted into the abdominal cavity; drop test confirmed placement within the peritoneal space. The abdomen was insufflated with carbon dioxide, and a 10-mm (millimeter) trocar port and laparoscope were introduced, showing no damage to the underlying viscera. Under direct vision, three additional trocar ports were placed, one upper midline 10 mm, two right upper quadrant 5 mm. The gallbladder was grasped and elevated from its fossa. The cystic duct and artery were dissected and doubly clipped proximally and distally, dividing them with the scissors. The gallbladder was then shelled from its fossa using electrocautery and brought up and out of the upper midline incision. The abdomen was irrigated with saline until returns were clear. There was no bleeding from the liver bed. Clips were in with no evidence of bleeding. When we were removing the final port, we could see down in the right groin, and she had small, indirect inguinal hernia, which was about 3 mm in size. We removed the remaining trocar port with no evidence of bleeding, closed the supraumbilical and upper midline ports and fascial defects with interrupted 0 Vicryl sutures, and closed the skin at all port sites with subcuticular 4-0 undyed Vicryl. Steri-Strips and sterile bandages were applied.

Pathology Report Later Indicated: Benign tissue

SERVICE CODE(S): _____

ICD-10-CM DX CODE(S): _____

(Answers to every other Case are located in Appendix D . The full answer key is only available in the TEACH Instructor Resources on Evolve.)

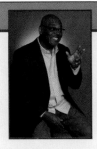

From the Trenches

"The healthcare industry is certification driven. It is highly unlikely that individuals looking for coding positions in healthcare organizations would gain employment as coders without a certification."

ROLANDO RUSSELL

MBA, RHIA, CPC, CPAR

CASE 7-15A   *Outpatient Consultation*

In Case 7-12, you coded a case with extensive inpatient services for Maynard Peters. In this case, you will code these same types of services, except these services are on an outpatient and inpatient basis.

LOCATION: Outpatient, Clinic

PATIENT: Alma Kincaid

PHYSICIAN: Larry Friendly, MD

REASON FOR CONSULTATION: Alma is in the clinic today after being referred to us from Dr. Alanda for a nonhealing gastric ulcer.

HISTORY OF PRESENT ILLNESS: She is a 60-year-old white female who states that she has had an ulcer since March 2000. She has failed medical treatment with both Zantac and Prilosec. She has had several upper endoscopies, which revealed a large ulcer at the greater curvature of the antrum. A biopsy was taken, which was benign. She has also tested negative for *Helicobacter pylori*. There has been no healing of this ulcer since it was discovered. On January 30, she underwent an exploratory laparoscopy. This all turned out to be normal also. She denies any hematemesis. She denies any nausea; however, she is unable to eat secondary to the pain. She states she has been basically living off of Ensure for the past few months and has lost quite a bit of weight. She denies any blood in her stool. She denies any fever or chills.

CURRENT MEDICATIONS:

1. Prilosec, 1 b.i.d. (twice a day)
2. Zantac, 1 b.i.d.

3. Tylenol as needed
4. Tylox as needed for pain

ALLERGIES:

1. Penicillin
2. Toradol

PHYSICAL EXAMINATION: Neck is supple and without lymphadenopathy. There is no supraclavicular or infraclavicular lymphadenopathy. Lungs are distant breath sounds but clear. Heart: S1 (first heart sound) and S2 (second heart sound) heard. No apparent murmurs are noted. Regular rate and rhythm. Abdomen is soft and moderately tender in the epigastric area with palpation. Bowel sounds are positive. Two well-healing port sites from her laparoscopy are noted, with no signs of infection. Extremities: No edema is noted. Dorsalis pedis and posterior tibial pulses are palpable and symmetric.

IMPRESSION: Nonhealing gastric ulcer, failure of medical treatment.

PLAN: At this time, we would like to obtain an upper gastrointestinal series on this patient. This still could be cancer until proven otherwise. Once we have this and re-evaluate, the patient will probably have to undergo a partial gastrectomy. The patient is willing to proceed with this, and she understands the risks and benefits of the procedure. We will discuss this with her after we get the upper gastrointestinal results. We will also have her seen by internal medicine for clearance for surgery.

SERVICE CODE(S): _____

ICD-10-CM DX CODE(S): _____

(Answers to every other Case are located in Appendix D . The full answer key is only available in the TEACH Instructor Resources on Evolve.)

CASE 7-15B *Emergency and Outpatient Record*

LOCATION: Outpatient, Hospital

PATIENT: Alma Kincaid

PRIMARY CARE PHYSICIAN: Leslie Alanda, MD

EMERGENCY DEPARTMENT PHYSICIAN: Paul Sutton, MD

SUBJECTIVE: This 60-year-old white female is currently diagnosed with gastric ulcer and is having workup for potential surgical treatment. She also has gastroesophageal reflux disease.

MEDICATIONS: She is taking Prilosec, Zantac, amitriptyline, and p.r.n. (as needed) GI (gastrointestinal) cocktails.

ALLERGIES: She has allergies to penicillin and Toradol.

She presents acutely in the Emergency Room stating that she is scheduled in the morning for some x-ray procedures for which she has to be NPO (nothing by mouth). She is having significant abdominal discomfort and is wondering whether she can get something for pain until she has the procedures done in the morning. She is scheduled for 8 o'clock; apparently, upper GI. She is also scheduled for a preoperative evaluation by Dr. Green and is going to be seeing Dr. Sanchez. She is a chronic smoker who has chronic obstructive pulmonary disease, being evaluated regarding that prior to surgery.

OBJECTIVE: She is afebrile. Blood pressure is elevated at 159/78. She is obviously uncomfortable. She has tenderness in the abdominal area. There is slight guarding but no rebound tenderness. The ABDOMINAL EXAM is otherwise grossly unremarkable.

ASSESSMENT:

1. Abdominal pain
2. Gastric ulcer

PLAN: We gave her 100 mg (milligram) of Demerol and 100 mg of Vistaril IM (intramuscular), which did afford some improvement. She was discharged with a recommendation to return here if she has increasing problems. Otherwise, plan on following up for evaluation in the morning.

SERVICE CODE(S): _____

ICD-10-CM DX CODE(S): _____

CASE 7-15C *Outpatient Consultation*

Dr. Alanda, Alma Kincaid's primary care physician, requested a consultation from Dr. Green, whose caseload includes many of the critical care patients for the clinic, regarding the pending gastric resection.

LOCATION: Outpatient, Clinic

PATIENT: Alma Kincaid

PRIMARY CARE PHYSICIAN: Leslie Alanda, MD

CONSULTANT: Ronald Green, MD

Dr. Alanda asked me to evaluate the patient for preparation for pending gastric resection. The patient was examined and the chart reviewed.

HISTORY OF PRESENT ILLNESS: She has been having problems with recurrent peptic ulcer disease in spite of therapy with Zantac and Prilosec. She had several endoscopies, which revealed a large ulcer, which was reported to be benign. The patient was also noted to have a slightly elevated CEA (carcinoembryonic antigen) of 11. Two months ago, the patient underwent laparoscopy, which turned out to be normal as well. There were no signs of any lymphadenopathy.

PAST SURGICAL HISTORY:

1. Hysterectomy
2. Tubal ligation

The patient never has problems with surgery or anesthesia.

SOCIAL HISTORY: Positive for smoking. The patient denies alcohol abuse. She smokes about a pack per day, with a total of a 40-pack-a-year history.

FAMILY HISTORY: Negative for colonic carcinoma, premature coronary artery disease, but positive for severe peptic ulcer disease in her sister.

ALLERGIES: Penicillin and Toradol

REVIEW OF SYSTEMS: Negative for melena, hematochezia, and hematemesis

PHYSICAL EXAMINATION: Demonstrates a slender white female in no acute distress. She is uncomfortable, however, because of epigastric discomfort. Her neck is supple. There is no thyromegaly or regional lymphadenopathy. No subclavicular or supraclavicular lymph nodes. ENT is within normal limits. Eyes: Sclerae anicteric. Conjunctivae are pale. Funduscopic exam shows no AV (arteriovenous) nicking, hemorrhages, exudates, or papilledema. Chest is barrel-shaped without dullness to percussion but with rhonchi scattered throughout the lung fields. Prolonged expiratory phase was noted. Cardiac exam: Regular rhythm. Distant heart sounds, 1/6 systolic ejection murmur at the base. Abdomen is soft and tender to palpation. Epigastric area without rebound, tenderness, or guarding. Liver span is 7 cm (centimeter); edge at right costal margin. Aorta diameter is normal. Extremities: No edema, cyanosis, or clubbing. Neurologic exam is nonfocal.

REVIEW OF LABORATORY ANALYSIS revealed hypercalcemia of 10.3, which is probably exaggerated by a low albumin and is likely to be more significant than that. Creatinine is 0.5. AST (aspartate aminotransferase [formerly SGOT]) is 15. Carcinoembryonic antigen is 11.5. *H. pylori* was 4.8 3 months ago.

IMPRESSION/PLAN: Nonhealing peptic ulcer disease. Patient's doctor increased her Prilosec to twice daily and is continuing Zantac at the present dose. In fact, one might increase it to 300 mg (milligram) b.i.d. (twice a day) if necessary. There is certainly need to rule out ZE (Zollinger-Ellison syndrome) and hyperparathyroidism in the source of the patient's nonhealing ulcer. C-terminal PTH (plasma thromboplastin antecedent) will be checked along with ionized calcium. One might plan a parahyperthyroidectomy simultaneous with gastrectomy should patient have high PTH, which I suspect will be the case, although in the case of treatment with H$_2$ blockers and Prilosec, a gastrin level might be elevated. Anyhow, we will check it and make sure that it is not extreme. If the gastrin level is very high, one might consider complete gastrectomy rather than a partial one on the presumption of Zollinger-Ellison syndrome. The patient will be reevaluated after results of the aforementioned tests

Continued

CASE 7-15C—cont'd

are available and scheduled for surgery. Elevated CEA (carcinoembryonic antigen) is bothersome. She has had no colonoscopy for some time; if it is again elevated, one might consider colonoscopy simultaneously during the same admission. I am concerned with her pulmonary status. She is advised to curtail her cigarette consumption as much as possible and to switch to low-tar nicotine cigarettes in the interim. Once she is admitted, therapy with beta-agonists and Atrovent will be immediately initiated, and the patient will be started on incentive spirometry.

Thank you for letting me see this interesting patient. We discussed the aforementioned problem with Dr. Sanchez, who will hold surgery for 1 week until all laboratory analyses are completed. A total of 135 minutes was spent with patient, and going over data; 55 of those minutes were spent consulting the patient.

SERVICE CODE(S): _____

ICD-10-CM DX CODE(S): _____

(Answers to every other Case are located in Appendix D . The full answer key is only available in the TEACH Instructor Resources on Evolve.)

CASE 7-15D *Operative Report, Ulcer and Cholecystitis*

The patient is admitted by Dr. Alanda for an operative procedure for the duodenal ulcer. Dr. Sanchez is the general surgeon who will perform the procedures. You will be reporting a partial gastrectomy with gastrojejunostomy, vagotomy, and cholecystectomy with cholangiogram, with the diagnoses of duodenal ulcer and cholecystitis to support the medical necessity for the three procedures.

LOCATION: Inpatient, Hospital

PATIENT: Alma Kincaid

ATTENDING PHYSICIAN: Leslie Alanda, MD

SURGEON: Gary Sanchez, MD

PREOPERATIVE DIAGNOSIS: Nonhealing duodenal ulcer. Chronic cholecystitis.

POSTOPERATIVE DIAGNOSIS: Nonhealing duodenal ulcer. Chronic cholecystitis.

PROCEDURES PERFORMED:

1. Exploratory laparotomy
2. Partial gastrectomy (antrectomy)
3. Truncal vagotomy
4. Gastrojejunostomy
5. Cholecystectomy with intraoperative cholangiogram

INDICATION: The patient is a 60-year-old female who presented with a nonhealing gastric ulcer. She has had symptoms for about a year. She complains of epigastric pain. She failed medical therapy with Prilosec and therapy for *H. pylori*. Biopsy of the ulcer showed it to be benign. The patient had a negative workup for gastrinoma. Calcium level was also normal. The patient now presents for exploratory laparotomy and partial gastrectomy. The risks and benefits were discussed with the patient in detail. She understood and agreed to proceed.

PROCEDURE: The patient was brought to the operating room. Her abdomen was prepped and draped in a sterile fashion. A midline umbilical incision was made. The peritoneal cavity was entered. Initial inspection of the peritoneal cavity showed normal liver, spleen, colon, and small bowel. There was an ulcer along the first portion of the duodenum just beyond the pylorus with some scarring. There was also an ulcer in the posterior part of the duodenal bulb, which was penetrating to the pancreas. We started dissection along the greater curvature of the stomach. Vessels were ligated with 2-0 silk ties. There was an enlarged lymph node along the

greater curvature of the stomach, which was sent for frozen section. It proved to be a benign lymph node. This was the only enlarged node found during dissection. We then proceeded with truncal vagotomy. The anterior vagus and posterior vagus were identified. They were clipped proximally and distally, and a segment of each nerve was excised and sent for frozen section. A segment of both vagus nerves was excised and confirmed by frozen section. An incision was made around the gastrohepatic ligament. The mesentery along the lesser curvature of the stomach was dissected. The vessels were ligated with 2-0 silk ties along the lesser curvature of the stomach. A Kocher maneuver was performed to aid mobilization. The pancreas was completely normal. No masses were seen in the pancreas. There was penetration of the ulcer in the superior part of the head of the pancreas. Dissection was continued posterior to the stomach. The adhesions posterior to the stomach were taken down. The ulcer was in the posterior segment of the duodenal bulb just beyond the pylorus and it had penetrated the pancreas. All the posterior layer of the ulcer that was left adherent to the pancreas was shaved off. The stomach was divided with the GIA stapler so that the complete antrum would be in the specimen. The duodenum was divided between clamps. The stomach pylorus and first part of the duodenum were sent to pathology for examination. Then the duodenal stump was closed with running suture. Using 3-0 Lembert sutures, the posterior wall of the ulcer was incorporated for duodenal closure. The base of the duodenum was rolled over the ulcer, and it was all-incorporating to the duodenal closure. Our next step was to proceed with cholecystectomy. The gallbladder was separated from the liver, reflected, and taken down, and the gallbladder was divided from the liver with blunt dissection and cautery. The cystic artery was doubly ligated with silk. The cystic duct was identified. The cystic duct and gallbladder junction and gallbladder ducts were identified. Intraoperative cholangiogram was performed showing free flow of bile into the intrahepatic duct and into the duodenum. No leaks were seen. The cystic duct was doubly ligated, and the gallbladder was sent to pathology. The staple line in the proximal stomach was oversewn with 3-0 silk Lembert sutures. A retrocolic isoperistaltic Hofmeister-type gastrojejunostomy was performed on the remaining stomach and loop of jejunum. This was an isoperistaltic end-to-side two-layer anastomosis with 3-0 chromic and 3-0 silk. The stomach was secured to the transverse mesocolon with several interrupted silk sutures to prevent any herniation along the retrocolic space. The anastomosis had a good lumen and good blood supply. There was no twist along the anastomosis. Prior to finishing the anastomosis, a nasogastric tube was placed along the afferent limb

CASE 7-15D—*cont'd*

of the jejunum to decompress the duodenum and prevent blowout of the duodenal stump. Extra holes were made in the NG tube to provide adequate drainage. The anastomosis was marked with two clips on each side, and a Jackson-Pratt drain was placed over the duodenal stump. The peritoneal cavity was irrigated until clear. Hemostasis was adequate. The fascia was then closed with interrupted 0 Ethibond sutures. Skin edges were approximated with staples. Subcutaneous tissues were irrigated before closure. Estimated blood loss throughout the procedure was 200 ml (milliliter), IV (intravenous) fluids: 3400 ml. Urine output: 840 ml.

FINDINGS:

1. Nonhealing benign ulcer in the posterior duodenal bulb penetrating into the head of the pancreas.

2. Partial gastrectomy (antrectomy performed) and excision of the pylorus, first portion of the duodenum along with ulcer.
3. Hofmeister-type retrocolic isoperistaltic gastrojejunostomy.
4. Posterior wall of the ulcer that was penetrating into the pancreas incorporated into closure of the duodenal stump.
5. Truncal vagotomy performed with intraoperative frozen section confirming both vagus nerves.
6. Cholecystectomy performed with normal intraoperative cholangiogram.
7. Jackson-Pratt drain placed over the duodenal stump.

Pathology Report Later Indicated: See Report 7-15F.

SERVICE CODE(S): _____

ICD-10-CM DX CODE(S): _____

(Answers to every other Case are located in Appendix D . The full answer key is only available in the TEACH Instructor Resources on Evolve.)

CASE 7-15E   *Intraoperative Cholangiogram*

LOCATION: Inpatient, Hospital

PATIENT: Alma Kincaid

ATTENDING PHYSICIAN: Leslie Alanda, MD

SURGEON: Gary Sanchez, MD

RADIOLOGIST: Morton Monson, MD

DIAGNOSIS: Chronic cholecystitis

INTRAOPERATIVE CHOLANGIOGRAM: Two views were obtained portably in the Operating Room during the intraoperative cholangiogram. Catheter

is in the cystic duct remnant. No definitive filling defects are seen in the common duct. There is incomplete visualization of the intrahepatic ducts. There is contrast seen within the proximal duodenum without evidence of obstruction.

SERVICE CODE(S): _____

ICD-10-CM DX CODE(S): _____

(Answers to every other Case are located in Appendix D . The full answer key is only available in the TEACH Instructor Resources on Evolve.)

Gastric ulcers (K25/531) are lesions of the stomach that result in the death of the tissue and a defect of the surface as illustrated in **Figures 7-11** and **7-12. Perforated ulcers** are those in which the lesion penetrates the gastric wall, leaving a hole, as illustrated in **Figure 7-11B.** Peptic refers to the gastric juice, pepsin. **Duodenal ulcers** (K26) are lesions of the duodenum. **Peptic ulcers** are lesions of the stomach or the duodenum, which do not necessarily cause necrosis or perforation. The site may be unspecified (K27).

Obstruction must be reported separately with K31.5.

CASE 7-15F   *Pathology Report*

During and following the operative procedure, the surgeon sends specimens of the tissue removed to the pathologist for examination and a written report of documents. The report has been highlighted to assist in coding.

LOCATION: Inpatient, Hospital

PATIENT: Alma Kincaid

ATTENDING PHYSICIAN: Leslie Alanda, MD

SURGEON: Gary Sanchez, MD

PATHOLOGIST: Grey Lonewolf, MD

CLINICAL HISTORY: Nonhealing ulcer gastric ulcer, failure of medical treatment.

A. Gastroepifleur lymph node
B. Anterior vagus nerves
C. Posterior vagus nerves
D. Ulcer bed
E. Gallbladder

TISSUE RECEIVED:

FA. Gastroepifleur lymph node (FS) *(2 cassettes, 1 specimen)*
A. Gastroepifleur lymph node (FS) *(2 cassettes, 1 specimen)*

Continued

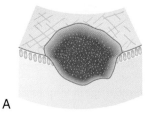

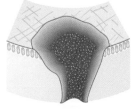

FIGURE 7–11 **A.** Ulcer.
B. Perforated ulcer.

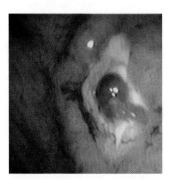

FIGURE 7–12 Ulcer.

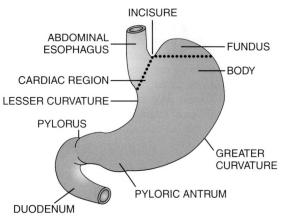

FIGURE 7–13 Parts of the stomach.

CASE 7-15F—cont'd

FB. Anterior vagus (FS)
 B. Anterior vagus (FS)
FC. Posterior vagus (FS)
 C. Posterior vagus (FS)
FD. Ulcer bed (FS)
 D. Ulcer bed (FS)
 E. Gallbladder

GROSS DESCRIPTION:

A. The specimen is labeled with the patient's name and "gastroepifleur lymph node," which consists of a 1.0 × 0.6 × 0.5-cm (centimeter) pink-tan lymph node. The specimen is bisected and processed in toto in two cassettes (1 lymph node).

INTRAOPERATIVE FROZEN SECTION DIAGNOSIS: (1, FS)

Gastriepifleur lymph node: Benign lymph node.

B. The specimen is labeled with the patient's name and "anterior vagus," which consists of two linear pink-tan tissues, up to 6.0 cm in length and 0.1 cm in width. The specimen is processed in toto in two cassettes.

INTRAOPERATIVE FROZEN SECTION DIAGNOSIS: (2, FS)

Peripheral nerve identified.

C. The specimen is labeled with the patient's name and "posterior vagus," which consists of a 0.6-cm pink-tan soft tissue. The specimen is processed in toto in one cassette.

INTRAOPERATIVE FROZEN-SECTION DIAGNOSIS: (3, FS)

Posterior vagus: Peripheral nerve identified.

D. The specimen is labeled with patient's name and "ulcer bed," which consists of a 14 × 8-cm segment of pink-tan stomach with attached fatty tissue along with the lesser and greater curvatures. Multiple lymph nodes are identified on the greater curvature, and these range in size from 0.3 to 1.5 cm in size and are pink-tan. Approximately 2 mm (millimeter) from the distal resection margin, there is a 3 × 2-cm ulcer. Approximately 1.5 cm proximal to this ulcer, there is another

2 × 0.5-cm linear ulcer. The stomach mucosa is pink-tan with no other obvious gross lesions. Representative sections are processed in 19 cassettes.

INTRAOPERATIVE FROZEN-SECTION DIAGNOSIS: (4, FS)

Ulcer bed: Benign ulcer.

E. The specimen is labeled with the patient's name and "gallbladder," which consists of a previously opened collapsed gallbladder 7 × 2.5 × 1 cm. The serosal surface is stained bile green. The wall is 1 to 2 mm (millimeter) thick, and the mucosa is dark green and velvety. No stones accompany the specimen. Representative sections are processed in two cassettes.

MICROSCOPIC DESCRIPTION:

A. Permanent sections confirm the frozen-section diagnosis showing a benign lymph node (micro 1) with mild follicular hyperplasia.
B. Permanent sections confirm the frozen-section diagnosis showing fibrofatty tissue with peripheral nerve segments (micro 2).
C. Permanent sections confirm the frozen-section diagnosis showing fibrofatty tissue with peripheral nerve segments (micro 3).
D. Permanent sections confirm the frozen-section diagnosis showing a benign antral ulcer (stomach ulcer) (micro 4) characterized by fibrinous neutrophilic exudate with underlying granulation tissue and fibrosis with acute inflammatory infiltrates. The region of the ulcer wall is markedly thinned with fibrosis extending in the adjacent perigastric fatty tissue. The adjacent mucosa shows an intact glandular architecture with reactive and regenerative glands. The lamina propria is mildly edematous with mild lymphocytic, plasma cell, and eosinophilic infiltrates. The muscular wall adjacent to the ulcer site shows hypertrophy with scattered lymphoid aggregates and lymphoid follicles. Sections of the linear ulcer show gastric body mucosa with benign ulceration. The adjacent gastric body mucosa shows intact glandular architecture with reactive and regenerative glands showing increased cytoplasmic basophilia with slightly enlarged

CASE 7-15F—cont'd

hyperchromatic nuclei and occasional mitoses. The lamina propria is mildly edematous with mildly increased lymphocytic, plasma cell, and eosinophilic infiltrates. A rare gland shows intraluminal neutrophils. There is submucosal edema with lymphoid aggregates and lymphoid follicles. Random sections of the stomach show intact gastric body-type mucosa. The superficial lamina propria shows mildly increased lymphocytic, plasma cell, and eosinophilic infiltrates. Multiple lymph nodes show mild reactive follicular hyperplasia.

E. Sections of the gallbladder (micro 5) show mild mucosal atrophy and intermuscular fibrosis. There is mild smooth-muscle hypertrophy with an occasional Rokitansky-Aschoff sinus.

DIAGNOSIS:

A. Gastric epifleur lymph node: Mild follicular hyperplasia, benign
B. Peripheral nerve segment, consistent with anterior vagus nerve
C. Peripheral nerve segment, consistent with posterior vagus nerve
D. Partial gastrectomy:
   1. Benign antral ulcer with acute inflammation (DX 1).
   2. Benign gastric body ulcer with acute inflammation (DX 2).
   3. Multiple lymph nodes: mild follicular hyperplasia (DX 3), benign.
E. Gallbladder, excision: chronic cholecystitis (DX 4)

SERVICE CODE(S): _____

ICD-10-CM DX CODE(S): _____

(Answers to every other Case are located in Appendix D . The full answer key is only available in the TEACH Instructor Resources on Evolve.)

CASE 7-15G   *Discharge Summary*

LOCATION: Inpatient, Hospital

PATIENT: Alma Kincaid

ATTENDING PHYSICIAN: Leslie Alanda, MD

REASON FOR ADMISSION: Nonhealing gastric ulcer.

SUMMARY OF HOSPITAL COURSE: The patient is a 60-year-old female with a history of ulcer disease, which failed medical management. She was subsequently referred to Dr. Sanchez for partial gastrectomy. The patient was admitted and taken to the operating room, where she underwent exploratory laparotomy with partial gastrectomy, truncal vagotomy, gastrojejunostomy, and a cholecystectomy with intraoperative cholangiogram. All pathology reports were benign. The patient tolerated the procedure well. She had an epidural in place following this, and she was transferred to the ICU (intensive care unit) for observation postoperatively.

The patient did well in the ICU, and by the following Monday, she was ready for transfer to the floor. By Wednesday, her ileus was resolving, her NG discontinued, and she was started on a diet. By Friday, the patient was tolerating a regular diet. Her Jackson-Pratts were removed.

She was afebrile with stable vital signs and was ready for discharge to home.

DISCHARGE INSTRUCTIONS: Activity as tolerated. Diet as tolerated.

DISCHARGE MEDICATIONS: Tylenol no. 3, 1-2 tablets p.o. (by mouth) q.4h. (every 4 hours) p.r.n. (as needed) pain.

FOLLOW-UP: The patient is to call for an appointment.

CONDITION ON DISCHARGE: Improved

DISCHARGE DIAGNOSES:

1. Nonhealing duodenal ulcer, chronic
2. Chronic cholecystitis

PROCEDURE PERFORMED: Exploratory laparotomy with partial gastrectomy, truncal vagotomy, gastrojejunostomy, and a cholecystectomy with intraoperative cholangiogram.

SERVICE CODE(S): _____

ICD-10-CM DX CODE(S): _____

(Answers to every other Case are located in Appendix D . The full answer key is only available in the TEACH Instructor Resources on Evolve.)

Incisional (Open) Surgical Procedures

Unlike laparoscopic (closed) procedures, which must be viewed through an endoscope during an open procedure, the surgical site is opened to the view of the surgeon. The following are a variety of open surgical procedures for you to code.

CASE 7-16   *Operative Report, Cystectomy*

LOCATION: Inpatient, Hospital

PATIENT: Tiffany Blue

ATTENDING PHYSICIAN: Ronald Green, MD

SURGEON: Gary Sanchez, MD

PREOPERATIVE DIAGNOSIS: Right intra-abdominal cyst on CT (computerized tomography) scan

POSTOPERATIVE DIAGNOSIS: Right descending sigmoid colon area mesenteric cyst

PROCEDURE PERFORMED: Exploratory laparotomy, excision of descending sigmoid colon area mesenteric cyst

ANESTHESIA: General

INDICATIONS FOR PROCEDURE: The patient is a 27-year-old white female who was found to have an abdominal mass in the left lower abdominal

Continued

CASE 7-16—cont'd

area. The patient underwent a CT scan, and Dr. Monson found a cyst in what appeared to be the mesentery of the colon. The patient was taken to the operating room for exploratory laparotomy and excision.

DESCRIPTION OF PROCEDURE: The patient had previously undergone a bowel prep the day before. She was then prepped and draped in the usual manner. She received Mefoxin 2 g intravenously preoperatively. The lower midline abdominal incision was made. The abdomen was entered, and a large cyst was found in the lateral wall along the colon mesentery in the area about the junction of the descending and sigmoid colon. This cyst was then sharply and bluntly dissected free from the surrounding tissues and excised and sent to pathology. Hemostasis was obtained using pressure and Bovie cautery.

Thorough examination of the abdomen was then done. The liver, spleen, stomach, duodenum, and gallbladder all felt within normal limits. The colon and small bowel also appeared within normal limits. The uterus,

both ovaries, and tubes were in place and also appeared within normal limits. There was what may be a small fibroid on the right apex of the uterus. No abnormalities were found. The cyst was sent to pathology.

After thorough examination of the abdomen and no other abnormalities were noted, the appendix also appeared normal and was left in place. The abdominal incision was then closed using a running no. 1 double-stranded suture. The subcutaneous tissues were irrigated and closed with a running 3-0 Vicryl suture. The skin was closed with skin clips. The patient tolerated the operation and returned to recovery in stable condition.

Pathology Report Later Indicated: Benign neoplasm

SERVICE CODE(S): _____

ICD-10-CM DX CODE(S): _____

(Answers to every other Case are located in Appendix D . The full answer key is only available in the TEACH Instructor Resources on Evolve.)

CASE 7-17   *Operative Report, Hemicolectomy*

LOCATION: Inpatient, Hospital

PATIENT: Sally Ortez

ATTENDING PHYSICIAN: Leslie Alanda, MD

SURGEON: Gary Sanchez, MD

PREOPERATIVE DIAGNOSIS: Adenocarcinoma of the ascending colon

POSTOPERATIVE DIAGNOSIS: Perforated adenocarcinoma of the ascending colon with attachment to the lateral abdominal wall.

ANESTHESIA: General

INDICATIONS FOR SURGERY: The patient is a 56-year-old white female who is having difficulties with her bowels. The patient was found to have adenocarcinoma of the ascending colon that was proven by biopsy. The patient is taken to the operating room after a bowel prep yesterday for surgery.

PROCEDURE: The patient was prepped and draped in the usual manner. A midline abdominal incision was made. The patient has had previous surgeries, which included an appendectomy, hysterectomy, cholecystectomy, and radiation therapy to her abdomen for a lymphoma. The patient had adhesions from her multiple previous surgeries and radiation therapy. These adhesions were taken down sharply using the Bovie cautery and Metzenbaum scissors. After this was done, the right colon was elevated using the Bovie cautery to divide the peritoneum on the right lateral gutter. The colon was then brought up into the operative area. The small bowel ileum was adherent down into the pelvis from her previous surgeries. These were taken down using the Metzenbaum scissors; then the small bowel was freed up into the incision area. The dissection was carried out to the transverse colon in about the midpoint of the transverse colon. A Penrose drain was then placed around the transverse colon and also

one around the ileum. During dissection of the cancer from the lateral abdominal wall, the cancer was firmly adherent to the abdominal wall. When this was finally freed up, there was an opening in the colon that appeared to be a perforation of the area of cancer, which had been sealed by the lateral abdominal wall. There was no gross evidence of any tumor on the abdominal wall. The opening in the colon was closed with a 2-0 silk suture. Next the mesentery was scored using the Bovie cautery. The mesentery was clamped and divided using Kelly clamps and tied with interrupted 2-0 silk sutures. After this was completed, the bowel clamp was placed on the proximal ileum and also on the distal colon. Kocher clamps were placed on the specimen side of the ileum and colon. The colon and ileum were then transected, and the specimen was sent to pathology. An end-to-end anastomosis was then done. A two-layer closure was done. Interrupted 3-0 silk sutures were placed on either end of the anastomosis and then the posterior layer was placed. All sutures were placed before they were tied. After this was completed, the inner layer was then run using a running 3-0 Vicryl suture using a locking stitch for the posterior layer and a running stitch on the anterior layer. After this was completed, the bowel clamps were removed. The anterior outer layer was then placed using interrupted 3-0 silk sutures. There was an excellent anastomosis following this procedure. The opening in the mesentery was closed with a running 2-0 Vicryl suture. The operative area was thoroughly irrigated. A few small bleeders were found after the irrigation, and these were controlled by 2-0 silk ties or Bovie cautery. An additional adhesion was taken down from the omentum attached to the pelvis down into the pelvic gutter, and this was freed. After all the adhesions were taken down, the operative area was again thoroughly irrigated. The bowel was returned to the abdomen. The anastomosis was again checked and was excellent. The

CASE 7-17—cont'd

abdominal incision was then closed with a running no. 1 looped PDS suture for the fascia and the peritoneum in a single-layer closure. The subcutaneous tissues were then thoroughly irrigated, and the skin was closed with skin clips. The patient tolerated the operation and returned to recovery in stable condition.

Pathology Report Later Indicated: Adenocarcinoma of both the colon (primary) and abdominal wall neoplasm (secondary)

SERVICE CODE(S): _____

ICD-10-CM DX CODE(S): _____

(Answers to every other Case are located in Appendix D . The full answer key is only available in the TEACH Instructor Resources on Evolve.)

CASE 7-18A *Initial Hospital Service*

The patient, Mary Black, was brought to the hospital emergency room by ambulance from Manytown. Mary recently moved to Manytown to be located closer to her son. Her primary care physician in Manytown is Dr. Gregory Whipple. Dr. Paul Sutton treated the patient in the emergency department and then contacted Dr. Larry Friendly, who admitted the patient to the hospital.

LOCATION: Inpatient, Hospital

PATIENT: Mary Black

ATTENDING PHYSICIAN: Larry Friendly, MD

Please see Dr. Sutton's note. His history was reviewed, the patient was interviewed, and then Dr. Whipple was contacted at Manytown; finally, the patient was examined.

Briefly, I was called about this woman earlier this morning. There was a history of questionable diverticulitis and pneumonia. She was brought in, and the pneumonia seemed to be well treated; however, she developed distention when they tried to feed her. They then did a barium enema, which did not show any diverticulitis. There was diverticulosis but definitely no active diverticulitis. There was question of a lesion at the splenic flexure, and there was no dye going into the small bowel. A CT (computed tomography) scan was done 2 days ago, which showed very distended small bowel and completely collapsed small bowel, and, again, no signs of diverticulitis.

When we went in to do a history and examine the patient, she was very confused. She has a Duragesic patch, which was started, according to Dr. Whipple, because of her abdominal pain. He did not want to stop it during transfer because he wanted the patient to be free of pain during transfer. That was a good decision because the medication worked very well for her pain.

She cannot tell what surgery she has had done. When I talked to Dr. Sutton, he suggested that she had a hysterectomy, some stomach surgery, a right hemicolectomy, and an aortic aneurysm repair; however, the CT that was

done on the outside shows no evidence that aortic surgery ever was done because she has a 4-cm (centimeter) aneurysm that goes down to her iliacs. I am also not clear about the right colon resection because the staples are in the left upper quadrant.

According to the chart, she had *Klebsiella* pneumonia, some hypertension, and underlying renal insufficiency.

PHYSICAL EXAMINATION: She is really quite distended with a silent abdomen. When I push, she does show signs that she is in pain. I reviewed her x-rays with Dr. Monson. There indeed is a questionable lesion at the splenic flexure, but this is where the staples are. It could easily be that what the barium enema is showing is old changes from previous surgery, but obviously there could be another lesion there. I am not even sure whether this was a cancer operation or a benign etiology, and nor was Dr. Sutton. Her CT scan showed massively distended small bowel and completely collapsed small bowel; so she has an obvious complete obstruction. According to the patient, she has not passed any gas for the last 2 days.

ASSESSMENT: She has a severe problem, and the treatment is extremely high risk. If I operate, there is a reasonable chance that she is not going to make it through the perioperative and postoperative periods. I told her this, and she made it very clear that she wanted to go ahead with surgery. It is impossible, however, to get an informed consent from this patient. Apparently, the family is on their way, and I will talk to them when they arrive.

According to Dr. Sutton, the patient and her family had understood that they were coming to town likely for an operation, and they had consented to that, but I do want to hear it from them.

I was worried enough about this patient that I will get Dr. Green involved from critical care preoperatively. He will help us also with her postoperative care.

SERVICE CODE(S): _____

ICD-10-CM DX CODE(S): _____

(Answers to every other Case are located in Appendix D . The full answer key is only available in the TEACH Instructor Resources on Evolve.)

CASE 7-18B   *Operative Report, Laparotomy*

LOCATION: Inpatient, Hospital

PATIENT: Mary Black

ATTENDING PHYSICIAN: Larry Friendly, MD

SURGEON: Gary Sanchez, MD

PREOPERATIVE DIAGNOSIS: Complete small bowel obstruction

POSTOPERATIVE DIAGNOSIS:

1. Ischiorectal hernia with obstruction
2. Enterocolic fistula
3. Intestinal adhesions

PROCEDURE PERFORMED:

1. Exploratory laparotomy and lysis of adhesions
2. Release of small bowel obstruction
3. Takedown of enterocolonic fistula

ANESTHESIA: General anesthesia

IV (INTRAVENOUS) FLUIDS: 3800 ml Crystalloid; 500 ml albumin

URINE OUTPUT: 40 cc (cubic centimeter)

NG TUBE OUTPUT: 1100 cc

COMPLICATIONS: None

INDICATIONS: The patient was referred from her local care facility after having been admitted there for 3 to 4 days with the presence of a nonresolving small bowel obstruction. The patient had multiple intra-abdominal surgeries, including two gastric surgeries for peptic ulcer disease, a right hemicolectomy for benign polyps, and a total abdominal hysterectomy for benign disease. The patient had been having signs of complete bowel obstruction for at least 4 days that did not respond to medical therapy. The patient was transferred to our institution, and after confirming the diagnosis, she was taken to the operating room for exploration.

DESCRIPTION OF PROCEDURE: The patient was informed about indications and alternatives of the procedure. Her family members were informed as well, and she was made a code I. After discussing the situation with the family, we took her to the operating room. An informed written consent was obtained. The patient was placed in the supine position and given general anesthesia. Her abdomen was prepped and draped in the usual sterile fashion. The patient had several surgical scars from previous procedures. A mid-line supra and infraumbilical incision was performed. We gained access to the abdominal cavity from the most superior aspect of the incision. At this area we found heavy adhesions from the small bowel and transverse colon to the anterior abdominal wall. Through a meticulous dissection, we took down the adhesions and were able then to divide the fascia at the midline. In the lower-most aspect, there were many adhesions, and we

were actually able to release the entire small bowel from this area. The patient had a mild amount of straw-colored free fluid inside the abdomen. We subsequently proceeded to perform adhesiolysis, releasing all the small intestine and adhered to the anterior wall to both sides. The transverse colon was also released from the anterior abdominal wall, which gave us exposure of the whole intra-abdominal contents. At this point, we proceeded to perform a formal exploratory laparotomy. The most superior organs of the abdomen were not evaluated because our incision did not extend to this area, and the patient had dense adhesions all over. We did not get to the area of the stomach or the liver. The patient does have evidence of a previous right hemicolectomy with an ileocolonic anastomosis that was localized in the right upper quadrant. We checked the transverse colon, the splenic flexure, and the descending colon including the sigmoid and the rectum, which showed normal characteristics. No evidence of obstruction in the sigmoid area was seen as previously suggested on CT scan. The colon itself looked normal in all its extent.

We proceeded then to inspect the small bowel, starting at the ligament of Treitz. There was dilated small bowel proximally. Approximately at the level of the transition between the jejunum and ileum, there was an area of transition caused by an internal hernia that was created by an enterocolonic fistula from the distal ileum to the colon almost at the area of the anastomosis from the previous right hemicolectomy. To be able to reduce the hernia and decompress the small bowel, we had to take down the fistula itself. Initially we dissected all the inflammatory tissue around this with Metzenbaum scissors. Once we got down to the fistula itself, we fired a GIA 75 across. Both ends of the fistula were completely sealed with no evidence of leak. At this point, we were able to run the small bowel completely. As already mentioned, the fistula was localized in the distal ileum approximately 30 cm (centimeter) away from the ileocecal valve. The area of transition was in the distal jejunum and proximal ileum. The hernia was completely reduced without any difficulty. A 1-cm segment in this area looked somewhat dusky but was definitely viable. This did not prompt us to perform any small bowel resection because once the pressure of the hernia was released, it looked completely viable. The pelvis itself looked normal with an absent uterus. The rest of the exploratory laparotomy was essentially normal. We then irrigated the abdominal cavity copiously until clear returns were obtained. Once this was achieved, we proceeded to close the wound at the level of the fascia with a running stitch of 2-0 nylon, and the skin was closed with staples. The patient tolerated the procedure well without any difficulty.

SERVICE CODE(S): _____

ICD-10-CM DX CODE(S): _____

(Answers to every other Case are located in Appendix D. The full answer key is only available in the TEACH Instructor Resources on Evolve.)

CASE 7-18C   *Discharge Summary*

LOCATION: Inpatient, Hospital

PATIENT: Mary Black

ATTENDING PHYSICIAN: Larry Friendly, MD

DIAGNOSES:

1. Small bowel obstruction diagnosed at the time of transfer. Ischiorectal hernia with obstruction.
2. Enterocolonic fistula.

3. Acute respiratory distress syndrome.
4. Failure to extubate—challenge to extubate, challenge to wean.
5. Atherosclerotic heart disease.

SUMMARY: The patient was admitted for adhesiolysis because of bowel obstruction and underwent surgery. Unfortunately, in the postoperative period, she developed increasing respiratory problems, most likely *Klebsiella pneumoniae* complicated by acute respiratory distress syndrome. She was on prolonged mechanical ventilation but continued to be fairly difficult to

CASE 7-18C—cont'd

wean because of respiratory and muscle fatigue and also problems with a pulmonary toilet. At one time the patient was on pressure support alone, but intermittently she had episodes of heart failure, undoubtedly as a result of high demand of breathing on patients with marginal coronary status and poor left ventricular systolic function. She continues to be a challenge to

wean and is being transferred to Manytown Critical Care Unit for chronic acute care, to be followed by Dr. Green.

SERVICE CODE(S): _____

ICD-10-CM DX CODE(S): _____

(Answers to every other Case are located in Appendix D . The full answer key is only available in the TEACH Instructor Resources on Evolve.)

Crohn's Disease

Crohn's disease is an inflammatory bowel disease (IBD) that is a group of conditions that can affect any portion of the gastrointestinal tract. The disease produces inflammatory lesions, and the type of Crohn's is named for the location of the inflammation, for example, colonic, ileocolonic, small bowel, or upper gastrointestinal Crohn's disease. The inflammation causes pain and diarrhea. The cause of Crohn's disease is unknown, but suspected causes are bacteria, genetics, suppressed immune system, or environmental factors.

The treatment for Crohn's disease is medications, such as the anti-inflammatory drug prednisone, but surgical management

of complications may be necessary for complications such as abscess, fistula, obstruction, or hemorrhage. Surgery is not a cure but is only used to manage complications that arise as a part of the disease process.

Crohn's Disease Diagnosis

Crohn's disease (K50.—), also known as regional enteritis, is a chronic inflammatory disease of the intestines. Classification is based on the location in the small (duodenum, ileum, jejunum) or large (cecum, colon, rectum, anal canal) intestine.

CASE 7-19 *Operative Report, Gastrojejunostomy/Tracheostomy*

Bill Stillman is admitted by Dr. Naraquist, his PCP, for placement of a tracheostomy tube and a feeding tube. Dr. Riddle, Interventional Radiologist, attempted to place a gastrointestinal tube, but the colon was punctured during the procedure. The patient is now scheduled for an open procedure by Dr. Sanchez.

LOCATION: Inpatient, Hospital

PATIENT: Bill Stillman

ATTENDING PHYSICIAN: Leslie Naraquist, MD

SURGEON: Gary Sanchez, MD

PREOPERATIVE DIAGNOSIS: Crohn's disease

POSTOPERATIVE DIAGNOSIS: Crohn's disease

PROCEDURE PERFORMED:

1. Repair of intestinal wound
2. Gastrojejunostomy with no. 18-French Moss tube
3. Tracheostomy with no. 8-Shiley tube

ANESTHESIA: General.

INDICATIONS: The patient is a 61-year-old male with Crohn's disease. He is now on the ventilator, ventilatory dependent, in need of feeding tube placement, and in need of tracheostomy to further assist in weaning the patient from the ventilator. Interventional radiology had attempted to place a feeding tube, but their needle had entered the colon; so he presents today for elective exploration, placement of feeding tube, possible repair of colon, and then tracheostomy. I discussed with the brother the surgery and its risks. He understands and wishes to proceed.

PROCEDURE: The patient was brought to the operating room, placed under general anesthesia, and prepped and draped with Betadine solution. A midline incision with a no. 10 blade and dissection was carried down through subcutaneous tissues using electrocautery. We entered the abdominal cavity sharply and encountered the transverse colon, which was dilated, and we could see a puncture site within the transverse colon. There was a leak of some air from the puncture site but no purulence in the peritoneal cavity. We oversewed the colon with 3-0 silk Lembert sutures. We then evaluated our small bowel anastomoses, and these appeared normal. There was also clear fluid within the peritoneal cavity. We irrigated and removed the clear fluid. We then placed two concentric pursestring sutures on the stomach, made our gastric opening, and then placed a no. 18-French Moss gastrojejunostomy tube through a left upper quadrant stab incision, passed it into the stomach, inflated the balloon, and passed the distal tip around the duodenum to the third portion of the duodenum. We secured our two pursestring sutures and then anchored it to the anterior abdominal wall with 3-0 silk sutures. We then once again closed the midline fascia with a combination of interrupted 0 Vicryl and running 0 PDS. The skin was left open and packed with Kerlix. The patient was then placed in the reverse Trendelenburg position with his neck slightly extended. We made a collar-type incision about two fingerbreadths above the manubrium. We carried our dissection through platysma using electrocautery and then divided the strap muscles along the midline. We encountered the thyroid cartilage and then the first tracheal ring. We placed a tracheal retractor, divided the second and third tracheal rings sharply with a no. 11 blade, withdrew the endotracheal tube above our opening into the trachea, placed a 3-0 Prolene suture on either side of the trachea, and then passed a no. 8-Shiley tracheostomy tube. We

Continued

CASE 7-19—cont'd

insufflated the balloon and had good returns. We then placed trach ties on and sterile dressing. All sponge and needle counts were correct. He tolerated this well and was taken to recovery in stable condition.

SERVICE CODE(S): _____

ICD-10-CM DX CODE(S): _____

(Answers to every other Case are located in Appendix D . The full answer key is only available in the TEACH Instructor Resources on Evolve.)

CASE 7-20A   *Operative Report, Appendectomy*

LOCATION: Inpatient, Hospital

PATIENT: Sally Jacobson

ATTENDING PHYSICIAN: Leslie Alanda, MD

PREOPERATIVE DIAGNOSIS: Acute appendicitis

POSTOPERATIVE DIAGNOSIS: Acute appendicitis

ANESTHESIA: General anesthesia

INDICATION: The patient is a 17-year-old female with insulin-dependent diabetes mellitus who presents with crampy, colicky right lower quadrant abdominal pain and an ultrasound showing a question of appendicitis. Her white count is within normal limits. She continues to have pain in the right lower quadrant. She presents today for elective open appendectomy.

We discussed the risks of bleeding, infection, and possible abscess formation with the patient's mother, and they wish to proceed.

PROCEDURE: The patient was brought to the operating room and prepped and draped sterilely. A right lower quadrant skin incision was made with a no. 10 blade and carried down through subcutaneous tissues using electrocautery. The anterior sheath of the rectus was scored. The rectus retracted medially, and the posterior sheath and peritoneum were grasped with curved clamps and sharply incised, thus allowing entry into the peritoneal cavity. Some serous fluid

was found in the right lower quadrant, and this was aspirated. The cecum was grasped, and the appendix was delivered up and into the wound. The mesoappendix was taken down between the right-angle clamps. The base of the appendix was transected sharply and sent to pathology for examination. The tip was cauterized and inverted into the cecum with a 3-0 silk pursestring suture. Two to three feet of the terminal ileum were explored, with no evidence of Meckel's diverticula. The remainder of the abdominal cavity was within normal limits.

The abdomen was irrigated with saline solution, and then the posterior sheath and peritoneum were closed with running 3-0 Vicryl. The anterior sheath was closed with interrupted 3-0 Vicryl. The skin was closed with subcuticular 4-0 undyed Vicryl. Steri-Strips and sterile bandage were applied.

SPONGE AND NEEDLE COUNT: All sponge and needle counts were correct.

The patient tolerated the procedure well and was taken to recovery in stable condition.

Pathology Report Later Indicated: See Report 7-20B.

SERVICE CODE(S): _____

ICD-10-CM DX CODE(S): _____

(Answers to every other Case are located in Appendix D . The full answer key is only available in the TEACH Instructor Resources on Evolve.)

CASE 7-20B   *Pathology Report*

LOCATION: Inpatient, Hospital

PATIENT: Sally Jacobson

ATTENDING PHYSICIAN: Leslie Alanda, MD

PATHOLOGIST: Grey Lonewolf, MD

CLINICAL HISTORY: Rule out acute appendicitis

TISSUE RECEIVED: Appendix

GROSS DESCRIPTION:

The specimen is labeled with the patient's name and "appendix" and consists of 7.3-cm (centimeter) veriform appendix with attached mesoappendix. The serosal surface is smooth pink-tan. Cut sections

show a white-tan wall with a pinpoint lumen. Representative sections are submitted in two cassettes.

MICROSCOPIC DESCRIPTION:

Cross-sections of appendix show intact mucosal epithelium. No evidence of acute inflammation is seen. There is fibrofatty obliteration of the distal tip.

DIAGNOSIS:

Appendix, excision. Fibrofatty obliteration of the distal tip; no acute inflammation identified.

SERVICE CODE(S): _____

ICD-10-CM DX CODE(S): _____

(Answers to every other Case are located in Appendix D . The full answer key is only available in the TEACH Instructor Resources on Evolve.)

CASE 7-21A   *Hospital Inpatient Service*

In the Impression section of the report, the physician indicates this patient has an abdominal mass with rule out diagnosis. Rule out diagnoses are not reported by outpatient coders, so the abdominal mass would be reported. Also the urinary tract infection requires two codes, one for the "infection" and one for the causative agent "E. coli." Begin your search for both codes under the main term "Infection" in the Index. Always list the "infection" first followed by the infectious agent, which in this case is the E. coli.

LOCATION: Inpatient, Hospital

PATIENT: Dominick Miller

PHYSICIAN: Larry Friendly, MD

The patient is a 69-year-old white male who was admitted to the hospital approximately 5 days ago because of faintness and slight neurologic difficulties. This patient has a history of having multiple strokes in the past. The etiology of the strokes has never been determined. The patient had a CT (computerized tomography) scan at the other facility, which showed evidence of old strokes but nothing new at this time. The patient was initially rehydrated because he was dehydrated, and his condition remained stable. He was also found to have urinary tract infection, greater than 100,000 colonies of *E. coli*. He has been on Unasyn for this problem. The patient improved. On Friday, he stated that he began having abdominal pain and pain in the right lower quadrant area. Because of this continued abdominal pain, the patient was transferred today for further evaluation and treatment of this problem. The patient also has a history of having blood in his stool, and he is also anemic. Because of these findings, the patient needs further evaluation. He is also presently taking Coumadin for his strokes, and this complicates any surgical intervention at this time. The patient is stable. He states that he is hungry and wants to eat and otherwise complains of pain in the right lower quadrant area. The patient has a history of having some type of an endoscopic procedure done about a year and a half ago at the Manytown Hospital. He is not sure whether it was a colonoscopy or a flexible sigmoidoscopy; therefore, we do not know if his right colon was fully evaluated. The patient is again stable at this time.

PAST MEDICAL HISTORY:

OPERATIONS:

1. Bilateral herniorrhaphies
2. TURP (Transurethral Resection of the Prostate)
3. Laparoscopic cholecystectomy

ILLNESSES:

1. Multiple strokes
2. Hypertension
3. Arthritis

MEDICATIONS:

1. Labetolol 200 mg (milligram) t.i.d. (three times a day)
2. Sulindac 200 mg b.i.d. (twice a day)
3. Coumadin 5 mg half a tablet on Mondays, Wednesdays, and Fridays and 1 tablet on the other days
4. Detrol LA 4 mg q.d. (every day) or b.i.d. as needed
5. Colace b.i.d.
6. Multiple vitamins
7. Calcium 600 mg b.i.d.

ALLERGIES: IVP (intravenous pyelogram) dye and sulfa

REVIEW OF SYSTEMS: The patient states that he does not smoke and does not drink. Neuro: The patient denies any history of seizure disorder or headaches. He does have trouble with dizziness and has had multiple strokes in the past. Cardiac: No history of myocardial infarction or congenital heart disease. The patient does have hypertension. Pulmonary: No history of asthma, hay fever, or pneumonia. No hemoptysis. GI (gastrointestinal): The patient denies any nausea, vomiting, diarrhea, or constipation. He has a history of rectal bleeding. The patient has complaints of pain in the right lower quadrant; see present illness. GU (genitourinary): The patient has a urinary tract infection of *E. coli*, which is being treated presently. Hematologic: The patient has received blood transfusions in the past but otherwise presently has not had any recently, even though he is anemic, and he also has rectal bleeding.

EXAMINATION: The patient is a 69-year-old white male. Eyes: Pupils are equal, round, and react to light and accommodation. Ears: TMs (tympanic membranes) are normal. Nose within normal limits. Throat within normal limits. The patient has his own teeth. Neck is supple. No carotid bruits are heard. Lungs: The patient has bilateral basilar rales. Heart: Regular rhythm, grade 2/6 systolic murmur. Abdomen: Normal bowel sounds. The patient has tenderness in the right lower quadrant area and questionable palpable mass in this area.

IMPRESSION:

1. Right lower quadrant mass, rule out ruptured appendicitis, rule out tumor
2. Urinary tract infection of *E. coli*
3. Hypertension

PLAN: The patient will be admitted to the hospital. He will be kept on IV (intravenous) antibiotics. His Coumadin will be stopped. He will undergo a CT scan of his abdomen for evaluation of this mass. The patient is not critical to the point where he requires emergency surgery at this time. We will rehydrate the patient and continue him on IV antibiotics and see whether we can treat this medically and, possibly, if there is an abscess pocket, drain it percutaneously. If this is possible, we will continue on this plan, but if it is not, then the patient may require surgery.

Total time was 40 minutes.

SERVICE CODE(S): _____

ICD-10-CM DX CODE(S): _____

(Answers to every other Case are located in Appendix D. The full answer key is only available in the TEACH Instructor Resources on Evolve.)

CASE 7-21B *Operative Report, Cecectomy*

LOCATION: Inpatient, Hospital

PATIENT: Dominick Miller

PHYSICIAN: Larry Friendly, MD

SURGEON: Gary Sanchez, MD

PREOPERATIVE DIAGNOSIS: Right lower quadrant mass.

POSTOPERATIVE DIAGNOSIS: Inflamed ruptured appendix with mass palpable in the cecum, possibly inflammatory, possibly cancer.

OPERATION PERFORMED: Right cecectomy with anastomosis. Appendectomy.

ANESTHESIA: General

INDICATIONS FOR SURGERY: The patient is a 69-year-old white male who was recently admitted to the hospital with a right lower quadrant mass and tenderness, possible appendicitis. The patient has also been anemic for quite some time, and no etiology could be found for the anemia. The patient was taken to the operating room after bowel prep for surgery.

DESCRIPTION OF PROCEDURE: The patient was prepped and draped in the usual manner. A midline abdominal incision was made. The patient was also receiving Zosyn 4.5 g, and he was given a dose prior to surgery. Examination of the right lower quadrant revealed an inflamed appendix, which appeared to be ruptured, but the cecum was also quite inflamed, and

there is a solid mass in this area. An appendectomy was then performed. It was difficult to ascertain whether or not this mass was inflammatory only or possible cancer. Because of this, a cecectomy was performed. The ascending colon was transected using a GIA stapler followed by the ileum resection. The mesentery was then clamped and divided using Pean clamps and tied with interrupted 2-0 silk sutures. The specimen was sent to pathology, and then a stapled anastomosis was done using the GIA stapler and the TA-60 stapler to close the opening that remained after the stapling procedure. There was excellent anastomosis following this procedure. The staple line was reinforced with several interrupted 3-0 silk sutures. The operative area was thoroughly ir rigated. The opening in the mesentery was closed with a running 3-0 Vicryl suture. The bowel was returned to the abdomen, and the fascia was then closed with running no. 1, double-stranded PDS suture. The subcutaneous tissues were thoroughly irrigated. The skin was left open, and a dressing was applied. The patient tolerated the operation and returned to recovery in stable condition.

Pathology Report Later Indicated: Ruptured appendix; Benign mass, rt lower quadrant

SERVICE CODE(S): _____

ICD-10-CM DX CODE(S): _____

(Answers to every other Case are located in Appendix D . The full answer key is only available in the TEACH Instructor Resources on Evolve.)

CASE 7-21C *Discharge Summary*

You will note that this is a very long discharge summary that details a complex case in which the patient died. Report all of the diagnoses indicated in the Principal Diagnosis and Secondary Diagnosis sections of the report.

LOCATION: Inpatient, Hospital

PATIENT: Dominick Miller

PHYSICIAN: Larry Friendly, MD

SURGEON: Gary Sanchez, MD

INDICATIONS FOR ADMISSION: Abdominal pain with pain mainly in the right lower quadrant.

This 69-year-old gentleman was transferred from another hospital. He was admitted to the other hospital with history of neurological difficulties and feeling faint. Subsequent CT (computerized tomography) showed multiple old strokes but no new infarcts. The patient had a UTI with more than 100,000 colonies of *E. coli* and was subsequently treated with Unasyn at the other hospital. He was also hydrated. At the other hospital, he started having right lower quadrant abdominal pain, for which the patient was transferred to this facility for evaluation and treatment. The patient also had history of having blood in the stool and was taking Coumadin for strokes.

PAST MEDICAL HISTORY on this gentleman is significant for multiple strokes, hypertension, and arthritis.

PAST SURGICAL HISTORY: He underwent laparoscopic cholecystectomy, transrectal resection of prostate, and bilateral inguinal herniorrhaphies in the past.

PHYSICAL EXAMINATION revealed a grade 2.6 systolic murmur and tenderness in the right lower quadrant of the abdomen. Questionable palpable mass was seen in the area. The patient underwent an ultrasound examination of the right lower quadrant, which showed complex structure in the right lower quadrant measuring about 4.3 × 4.1 × 2 cm (centimeter), which does not compress during the ultrasound examination and demonstrates bowel nature. On a few of the views, there is a tubular structure, which may be separate from the more complex-looking area. The complex structure may represent a cecum according to the radiologist's report on the ultrasound examination. These findings could be compatible with a contained perforation. The patient also underwent a CT scan examination of the abdomen and pelvis on 05/03/xx. Findings at this examination include a phlegmonous-type mass density noted in the right lower quadrant adjacent to and cannot be separated from the cecum. This was at least 3 cm in diameter. The differential considerations include inflammation/infection and also a mass arising from the cecum. There is inflammatory change in the inferior aspect of the right lower abdominal musculature. Nonspecific hypodensity is noted in the anterior aspect of the left lobe. Small bilateral pleural effusions with patchy opacity were seen in the lung bases and were compatible with volume loss. The right kidney appears slightly larger than the left, with some stranding noted in the perirenal fat on the right side. The patient also underwent cardiac evaluation prior to surgery. As part of this workup, the patient underwent an echocardiogram, which showed a normal left ventricular size with left ventricular systolic function, mild left ventricular hypertrophy, mild mitral insufficiency without stenosis, and trace tricuspid insufficiency without stenosis. The left ventricular inflow pattern was suggestive of early

CASE 7-21C—cont'd

diastolic dysfunction not borderline. The patient was recommended for acute bacterial endocarditis prophylaxis, which was given prior to surgery.

The patient underwent right cecectomy with primary stapled anastomosis between ileum and ascending colon on Monday. Findings at surgery included an inflamed, ruptured appendix with mass palpable in the cecum, most probably inflammatory, but neoplastic could not be ruled out. Pathologic examination of this resected cecal specimen showed acute inflammation of the appendix, which was severe and extensive, with perforation and excision of inflammation into the mesoappendix and mesocolon with abscess formation. The cecum showed that the acute inflammation was terminal ileum. No evidence of neoplasm in the cecum or in the appendix or ileum was seen. The patient developed spiking temperature immediately after the surgery. The patient was cared for in the major postoperative period in the medical ICU (intensive care unit), where he was given nitroprusside drip and was on arterial monitoring. The patient was transferred back to the floor, where he developed some confusion. His medications were stopped, especially the narcotic analgesics, to help with his confusion. The patient developed chest infection with sputum Gram stain showing gram-positive bacteria and yeast. He was started on IV (intravenous) antibiotics and IV fungal agents on Monday. The patient desatted again on Tuesday. There was evidence of aspiration into the bronchial tree. We found large amounts of gastric contents as part of the suction. The patient had to be intubated and ventilated and was transferred to the surgical care unit on Wednesday as treatment for this aspiration pneumonitis. The patient was started on TPN (total parenteral nutrition) in the meantime. Critical care service was involved in the management of this patient in view of the aspiration pneumonitis and associated problems. The patient continued to be managed on ventilator for his respiratory failure secondary to Pseudomonas pneumonia. The sputum culture showed presumptive Pseudomonas species, which were rare. There was some yeast, but it was not Candida albicans. The patient was started on tube feeds. Subsequently, the patient developed symptoms suggestive of respiratory distress syndrome secondary to the pulmonary insult he had sustained. The patient was managed in the surgical critical care unit all the time and had central venous access for TPN and also resuscitative efforts. The patient had problems with continued pyrexia. The exact source of the pyrexia was not easily ascertained after multiple investigations, and the lines were changed. The patient had a CT scan of the abdomen on Thursday as part of workup for pyrexia.

The CT scan showed at that time that he had pleural effusions that were present even previously. He had scattered fluid throughout the abdomen and pelvis, which was new. There could be some postoperative changes. There was no definite fluid collection noted to suggest an abscess. There were distended bowel loops of both large and small bowel consistent with generalized ileus. There were atelectasis and/or infiltrates at both lung bases, part of which was new.

The patient also underwent a CT scan examination of the paranasal sinuses, which showed some mucosal thickening in most of the ethmoidal sinuses. The bilateral sphenoid sinuses showed considerable mucosal thickening with the possibility of fluid level in either of the sphenoid sinuses. The maxillary sinus showed mucosal thickening, particularly posteriorly. The patient had deteriorating renal function and was started on renal dialysis on Friday. The patient had tunneled hemodialysis catheter placed on the Thursday prior to the start of dialysis. The patient underwent tracheostomy tube placement on Friday without complications. The patient had some altered neurologic status

and subsequently underwent CT scan of the brain on Saturday. This showed questionable low density of the superior margin of the left temporal lobe, which might represent a recent ischemic change. There were no hemorrhages in the brain noted on that study. The patient continued to have hemodialysis performed in the surgical critical care unit. The patient developed failure of the lateral aspect of the left lower extremity for which he underwent a skin biopsy, and the pathology of the lesion showed minimal chronic dermatitis and dermal edema, which was nonspecific and without evidence of cellulitis. The patient continued to spike temperature. The patient continued to have problems with multiple organ systems and was acutely ill and was treated in the surgical critical care unit.

The patient continued to have some intermittent problems with the GI (gastrointestinal) function with KUB (kidney, ureter, bladder) showing persistent small bowel distention consistent with possible obstruction of the persistent ileum. The patient was weaned off the ventilator and was put on trach mask on Tuesday. The patient tolerated this transition. The patient's urine output started to pick up, and the patient was continued on dialysis to augment his renal function. Repeated sputum culture showed Pseudomonas with yeast. The patient underwent CT scan of the abdomen on Wednesday, which showed dilated bowel in the mid-abdomen and pelvis. A portion of this dilated bowel was found to be sigmoid colon. The rectum was also of abnormal appearance, and the wall appears to be thickened. There was stranding about both the kidneys noted. There was abnormal appearance of a loop of bowel in the inferior pelvis, which was most likely sigmoid colon and could be from continued inflammatory or infected change. The patient had a flexible sigmoidoscopy subsequent to this on Friday. The patient had an attempted placement of a GJ catheter by interventional radiology but was not successful due to overlying bowel, and this was tried on Friday. The patient's care transferred to Dr. Alanda on Friday at request of the patient's family. The patient underwent a repeat CT scan of the abdomen, which showed prominently dilated loops of small bowel, the findings of which were worrisome for small bowel obstruction. This obstruction could be traced to the level of the operative site in the right lower quadrant. Free fluid was noted in the pelvis, and infiltrate/volume loss in the lung bases has improved compared with the previous surgery. The patient underwent exploratory laparotomy, adhesiolysis, and closure of enterotomies and multiple serosal tears along the insertion of Moss tube. Findings at surgery included internal hernia with a small bowel loop stuck to the anterior abdominal wall with proximal dilated and distal collapsed small bowel. Multiple small bowel adhesions were noted. Anastomosis was intact. The patient needed increased amount of fluid secondary to the third spacing from the surgery. The patient needed repeat dialysis in view of the significant third spacing. Prior to this surgery, he had a dialysis-free period of about 10 days. The repeat dialysis was initiated after the surgery to clear his fluids secondary to third spacing. The patient was taken off the ventilator. The patient had significant amount of serious fluid draining from this main abdominal wound initially after the surgery, but it reduced over a period of time. The patient was transferred to the floor. The patient was restarted on tube feedings and tolerated them reasonably well. He developed attacks of fast atrial fibrillation and was started on digoxin for it. The patient was restarted on Coumadin for this as part of treatment for atrial fibrillation. The patient's renal function again deteriorated, with urine output falling and patient developing acidosis. The patient became hypotensive with mottling and tachypnea. The

Continued

CASE 7-21C—cont'd

impression was that he might have started developing sepsis and also possible dehydration secondary to dialysis. The patient was given extra fluids; despite these measures, the patient died on Saturday.

PRINCIPAL DIAGNOSIS: Acute appendicitis with perforation and abscess formation

SECONDARY DIAGNOSES:

1. Anemia
2. Hypertension
3. Respiratory failure
4. Renal failure, acute and chronic
5. Postoperative small bowel obstruction due to internal hernia
6. Urinary tract infection secondary to *E. coli*

PROCEDURES PERFORMED:

1. Right colectomy with primary anastomosis
2. Intubation and mechanical ventilation

3. Insertion of central venous catheter
4. Placement of right femoral central line
5. Placement of tunneled triple lumen catheter
6. Placement of hemodialysis catheter
7. Tracheostomy placement
8. Skin biopsy of the cellulitic area over the right hip
9. Flexible sigmoidoscopy
10. Attempt at placement of gastrojejunostomy catheter
11. Exploratory laparotomy and reduction of internal small bowel hernia, lysis of adhesions, repair of multiple enterotomies, and serosal tears with placement of Moss gastrojejunostomy tube
12. Multiple sittings of hemodialysis

SERVICE CODE(S): _____

ICD-10-CM DX CODE(S): _____

(Answers to every other Case are located in Appendix D . The full answer key is only available in the TEACH Instructor Resources on Evolve.)

CASE 7-22   *Operative Report, Placement of Gastrostomy Tube*

This patient, George Powers, returned to the hospital for a procedure to treat a bowel obstruction. The procedure in Case 7-22A is performed during the postoperative period of the previous surgery.

LOCATION: Inpatient, Hospital

PATIENT: George Powers

SURGEON: Gary Sanchez, MD

PREOPERATIVE DIAGNOSIS: Bowel obstruction

POSTOPERATIVE DIAGNOSIS: Bowel obstruction

PROCEDURES PERFORMED:

1. Adhesiolysis and repair of bowel enterotomy
2. Placement of Moss gastrostomy tube

OPERATIVE NOTE: With the patient under general anesthesia, the abdomen was opened, extending the midline incision from below the xiphoid to below the umbilicus. Most of the old incision was open. We were able to get into the abdominal cavity without too much difficulty. There were minimal adhesions to the anterior abdominal wall. There was marked dilatation of the small bowel, and we began by taking down multiple adhesions. There were multiple incidents of serosal tear due to the marked dilatation of the small bowel. Once we got started, we could identify a loop of small bowel that was approximately 6 or 12 inches from the ileocecal valve, which was stuck into the pelvis. The rest of the small bowel was volvulized around this as an internal hernia and was creating the bowel obstruction. There was a clear transition zone from the dilated bowel and to the nondilated bowel. As we worked to take down all these adhesions doing extensive adhesiolysis, we entered the bowel at one point with an enterotomy. Very tough, tenacious, almost stool-like material was within

the small bowel, suggesting that this has been obstructed for quite some time. We attempted to keep all of this out of the abdominal cavity, and we were successful, but we did have some spillage of this tenacious small bowel material. It was so thick that we really could not suction it out of the bowel with the sucker. We had to allow it to run out of the opening in the bowel into a basin as we squeezed; it was too thick to come through a sucker. In any event, we finally got the entire bowel lysed such that we could run through the bowel from the ligament of Treitz to the ileum. We could see that the point of obstruction was not at the anastomotic site, and the anastomosis appeared widely patent. Multiple serosal tears were repaired with interrupted silk sutures. The enterotomy into the bowel was repaired in two layers using an inner layer of Vicryl and an outer layer of interrupted silk. With this accomplished, we copiously irrigated the abdominal cavity and then proceeded to return to the bowel to the abdominal cavity. We then placed a Moss gastrostomy tube into the stomach. This was brought through the anterior abdominal wall through a stab incision, and then a double pursestring was placed into the stomach and the tube introduced. The balloon was inflated, and the distal portion of the tube was threaded through the pylorus into the duodenum. The stomach was tacked up to the anterior abdominal wall. The abdominal cavity was again copiously irrigated with saline, and then the abdomen was closed using running 0 loop nylon. We did tack the sutures around the umbilicus and then left the wound packed with some wet saline gauze. A sterile dressing was applied. The patient tolerated the procedure well and was discharged from the operating room on the ventilator but in stable condition. He went directly to the surgical intensive care unit. At the end of the procedure, all sponges and instruments were accounted for.

SERVICE CODE(S): _____

ICD-10-CM DX CODE(S): _____

(Answers to every other Case are located in Appendix D . The full answer key is only available in the TEACH Instructor Resources on Evolve.)

Hernia

A hernia is a protrusion of tissue or an organ through an abdominal opening. Hernias are named for the type and location of the hernia. Reference a medical dictionary under the main term "hernia" for the various types of hernias, for example, an inguinal hernia (into the inguinal canal) or a sliding hernia (cecum and sigmoid colon that involves the viscera).

Hernias can be strangulated (cut off from the blood supply) or incarcerated (cannot be returned to original location). In a surgical reduction of a hernia, the surgeon returns the hernia to the original location. Sutures and/or mesh may be used to repair the area and provide support. The strangulated hernia may involve an organ, such as the large or small intestine, and

that organ may also require repair. Additional organ repair would be reported in addition to the hernia repair.

Hernia codes are divided based on whether the repair is initial/recurrent, incarcerated/strangulated, patient age, and type (i.e., femoral, inguinal), etc.

Other hernia codes (49591-49596, 49613-49618) are divided based on the type (epigastic, incisional, ventral, umbilical or spigelian), initial or recurrent repair, the size of the defect(s), and the presentation of the hernia (reducible, strangulated or incarcerated). The implantation of mesh or prosthesis is included in the code when performed. The repair is performed open, laparoscopic or robotic.

Diagnosis coding of hernias was discussed prior to Case 7-7.

CASE 7-23A   *Hospital Inpatient Service*

LOCATION: Inpatient, Hospital

PATIENT: Doris Craven

ATTENDING PHYSICIAN: Gary Sanchez, MD

CHIEF COMPLAINT: Right inguinal hernia

HISTORY OF PRESENT ILLNESS: The patient is a 39-year-old female who reports a 1-year history of an intermittent painful lump in the right groin area. She states that it will come out every so often, more frequently toward the end of the day or with exertion. It is painful while it is out; however, she has always been able to reduce it. She did have one episode approximately a week ago when she could not reduce it at first and had to leave work to go home and lie down before it reduced. She saw Dr. Friendly for this problem, and he referred her to us. She has been seen several times in the clinic. She denies any GI (gastrointestinal) symptoms, specifically no nausea, vomiting, or change in bowel habits.

PAST MEDICAL HISTORY: She is essentially healthy. She takes no medications.

ALLERGIES: No known drug allergies.

FAMILY HISTORY: Her father had a cerebral aneurysm; otherwise, family history is unremarkable.

SOCIAL HISTORY: She smokes one pack of cigarettes per day. Rarely uses alcohol.

REVIEW OF SYSTEMS: Negative. Specifically, she denies any syncope, shortness of breath, hemoptysis, chest pain, GI, or GU (genitourinary) symptoms. She denies any muscle or joint pain.

PHYSICAL EXAMINATION: This slender white female is appropriate for stated age. She is afebrile. Stable vital signs. Blood pressure is 112/72. Her weight is 116 pounds. HEENT (head, ears, eyes, nose, throat) is unremarkable. Neck is supple with no masses. Chest: The lungs are clear to auscultation bilaterally. Heart is regular rate and rhythm without murmur. Abdomen has positive bowel sounds, soft without masses. GU: There is no reducible hernia in the right inguinal region. No hernias noted on the left. Extremities: Appropriate pulses, reflexes, and muscle strength. Neurologic: She is grossly intact.

ASSESSMENT: Right inguinal hernia.

PLAN: I discussed the nature of the disease and the treatment options with the patient. The patient understood and wished to proceed with surgical repair in the morning.

TT: 40 minutes

SERVICE CODE(S): _____

ICD-10-CM DX CODE(S): _____

(Answers to every other Case are located in Appendix D . The full answer key is only available in the TEACH Instructor Resources on Evolve.)

CASE 7-23B   *Operative Report, Right Inguinal Hernia Repair*

LOCATION: Inpatient, Hospital

PATIENT: Doris Craven

SURGEON: Gary Sanchez, MD

PREOPERATIVE DIAGNOSIS: Right inguinal hernia

POSTOPERATIVE DIAGNOSIS: Right direct and right indirect inguinal hernias

PROCEDURE PERFORMED: Right inguinal hernia repair

PROCEDURE: The patient was brought to the operating room and placed in the supine position on the operating table. After satisfactory general anesthesia had been induced, the patient's abdomen and groins were prepped and draped in a sterile manner. A short transverse incision was made over the right inguinal area. Subcutaneous tissue was divided sharply. Ties and cautery were used for hemostasis. The external oblique aponeurosis was identified and opened from above downward. The ilioinguinal nerve was identified and protected. The patient had a direct inguinal hernia about 1 cm (centimeter) superior and medial to the internal ring. It was properitoneal fat pushed

through a very small opening about 0.5 cm in size. We reduced this and closed this hole with interrupted Ethibond, which gave a solid closure without tension. We then dissected up the round ligament and ligated it distally. Proximally we then separated the round ligament from a small internal sac. We ligated the round ligament and the sac separately and then closed the internal ring with Ethibond suture in a Bassini repair. This gave us a solid repair with fixed hernias. We then irrigated the wound with Neomycin. Final sponge and needle counts were taken; they were correct. We then closed the external oblique aponeurosis with Vicryl; subcutaneous tissue was closed with chromic and skin with nylon. Blood loss during the procedure was minimal. Sponge and needle counts were correct. The patient tolerated the procedure well and left for the recovery room in stable condition.

Pathology Report Later Indicated: See Report 7-23C.

SERVICE CODE(S): _____

ICD-10-CM DX CODE(S): _____

CASE 7-23C   *Pathology Report*

LOCATION: Inpatient, Hospital

PATIENT: Doris Craven

PHYSICIAN: Gary Sanchez, MD

PATHOLOGIST: Grey Lonewolf, MD

CLINICAL HISTORY: Right inguinal hernia

TISSUE RECEIVED: Round ligament

GROSS DESCRIPTION:

The specimen was labeled with the patient's name and "round ligament" and consists of two membranous pink-tan tissues, 2.0

and 2.5 cm (centimeter) in greatest dimension. Submitted in one cassette.

MICROSCOPIC DIAGNOSIS:

Mesothelial-lined fibrovascular tissue with skeletal muscle, consistent with right inguinal hernia.

SERVICE CODE(S): _____

ICD-10-CM DX CODE(S): _____

(Answers to every other Case are located in Appendix D . The full answer key is only available in the TEACH Instructor Resources on Evolve.)

CASE 7-24A   *Surgical Consultation*

LOCATION: Outpatient, Clinic

PATIENT: Rose Scheibler

PRIMARY CARE PHYSICIAN: Gary Sanchez, MD

CONSULTANT: Ronald Green, MD

CHIEF COMPLAINT: Umbilical hernia

HISTORY OF PRESENT ILLNESS: The patient is an otherwise healthy 35-year-old female who presents with a symptomatic umbilical hernia that has been present for some time. She thinks it may have occurred during work and now is tender when she exercises. It is occasionally tender when she moves patients. She is a nurse. She denies any symptoms of obstruction or incarceration and denies any chronic cough, chronic constipation, or difficulty with urination.

PAST MEDICAL HISTORY:

1. Normal spontaneous vaginal delivery ×3
2. History of hypothyroidism

MEDICATIONS: Synthroid

ALLERGIES: None

REVIEW OF SYSTEMS: Otherwise healthy

PHYSICAL EXAM: Chest is clear. Cardiovascular: Regular rate and rhythm. Abdomen: Soft and nontender. There are no masses. She has an easily reducible umbilical hernia. She has no inguinal hernias. Musculoskeletal: Negative. Extremities: Negative. EENT: Negative. Lymph nodes: Negative.

IMPRESSION: Umbilical hernia

RECOMMENDATIONS/PLAN: I have discussed umbilical hernia repair along with the risks of bleeding, infection, and possible recurrence. She appears to understand and wishes to proceed. Will plan to proceed at her earliest convenience. She states that, due to work, she wishes to have this repaired on Monday. I will make arrangements. Letter to Dr. Sanchez.

SERVICE CODE(S): _____

ICD-10-CM DX CODE(S): _____

(Answers to every other Case are located in Appendix D . The full answer key is only available in the TEACH Instructor Resources on Evolve.)

CASE 7-24B   *Operative Report, Umbilical Herniorrhaphy*

LOCATION: Inpatient, Hospital

PATIENT: Rose Scheibler

SURGEON: Gary Sanchez, MD

PREOPERATIVE DIAGNOSIS: Umbilical hernia

POSTOPERATIVE DIAGNOSIS: Umbilical hernia

PROCEDURE: Umbilical herniorrhaphy

DATE OF OPERATION:

ANESTHESIA: General

INDICATIONS: The patient, a 35-year-old female, noticed increasing periumbilical pain. She has a noticeable bulge that has increased in size over the past several weeks. She denies any symptoms of obstruction or incarceration. She presents today for elective repair. She understands the risks of bleeding, infection, or possible recurrence and wishes to proceed.

PROCEDURE: The patient was brought to the operating room and placed under general anesthesia, prepped, and draped sterilely. An infraumbilical skin incision was made with a no. 15 blade and carried down through the subcutaneous tissues using sharp dissection. We carried the dissection down to the fascia and then dissected the umbilicus free from its fascial attachment. We opened the hernia sac, reduced the hernia contents, and then repaired the fascial defect with interrupted 0 Vicryl sutures. The umbilicus was packed back down to the fascia with a single interrupted 4-0 undyed Vicryl. Steri-Strips and sterile Band-Aids were applied. Sponge and needle counts were correct prior to leaving the operating room. The wound was anesthetized with 30 cc of 0.5% Sensorcaine with epinephrine solution.

Pathology Report Later Indicated: Umbilical hernia

SERVICE CODE(S): _____

ICD-10-CM DX CODE(S): _____

(Answers to every other Case are located in Appendix D . The full answer key is only available in the TEACH Instructor Resources on Evolve.)

Hemic/Lymphatic System

The hemic system is the blood-forming system of the body and includes blood cells and bone marrow. The lymphatic system is the drainage system of the body and is closely related to the blood system. The lymph carries waste from the body to the bloodstream. The system is part of the immune system that protects the body, and as such, the physician assesses the status of the lymphatic system by palpating (feeling) the various lymph nodes that are located throughout the body. Enlarged lymph nodes are a sign of infection.

The lymphatic channels are the vessels throughout which the lymph circulates. The lymph nodes are lymph tissue located along the channel. The lymph nodes can be the site of tumor, such as in Hodgkin disease, which is a malignant tumor of the lymph tissue and spleen. There are several types of non-Hodgkin lymphoma, such as lymphocytic lymphoma and histiocytic lymphoma. Radiation and/or chemotherapy are used to halt the progress of the disease.

The CPT codes for the lymph nodes and lymphatic channels are 38300-38999. Biopsy of nodes is reported based on the method used to obtain the sample (open or percutaneous) and the nodes sampled (cervical, axillary, internal mammary). Biopsy and excision are usually in a separate section, such as Excision and Biopsy, but for these lymph node codes, both an excision and/or a biopsy can be reported with the same code, for example, 38510 Biopsy or excision of lymph node(s); open, deep cervical node(s). Note that the description indicates both biopsy and excision. Also note that the method (open) and node (cervical) are specified in the code.

Laparoscopy can be used to repair retroperitoneal lymph nodes (38570-38572). Resection of the lymph node differs from the excision of a lymph node. Resection is when the nodes as well as the surrounding tissue are removed and excision is only the lymph node(s).

The **spleen** is composed of lymph tissue located in the left upper quadrant (LUQ). The surgical removal of the spleen is a splenectomy, which can be either total or partial. The spleen is sometimes removed due to extensive disease and is reported with 38100-38102. The spleen can be ruptured, as in motor vehicle accidents and then require a splenorrhaphy (38115).

Bone marrow and stem cells (38204-38243) are part of the Hemic and Lymphatic Systems subsection in the CPT, which includes service codes for bone marrow aspirations and transplantation. Most of these codes are for preparation and preservation of marrow and stem cell transplantation.

Diagnosis Coding of Hematopoietic and Lymphatic Neoplasms

Hematopoietic and lymphatic neoplasms do not spread to secondary sites; rather the cells travel through the hemic and lymphatic systems and then occur in multiple sites within the system. All of these sites are considered primary sites. For example, if the diagnosis is lymphosarcoma of the face, axilla, and intra-abdominal lymph nodes, you would report C85.08.

Only assign the C85 codes when the neoplasm originates in the lymphatic or hematopoietic systems. If a neoplasm spreads from another location in the body to the lymph node, C77 code is assigned to indicate the lymph node is a secondary site.

Leukemia is a progressive, malignant disease of the blood-forming organs. Leukemias are reported with codes from C91-C95.

Lymphoid leukemia (C91) is a proliferation of the lymphoblasts (immature lymphocytes) referred to as lymphocytic, lymphoblastic, lymphatic, and lymphogenous leukemia.

Myeloid leukemia (C92) is a proliferation of the myeloblasts (immature myelocytes) referred to as granulocytic, myeloblastic, myelocytic, myelogenous, myelomonocytic, myelosclerotic, and myelosis.

Monocytic leukemia (C93) is a myelogenous leukemia with a blastic phase. The diagnosis of the blastic phase requires greater than 30% myeloblasts in marrow or blood. Patients in blastic phase live an average of 3 to 6 months.

CASE 7-25A   *Operative Report, Axillary Node Dissection*

LOCATION: Inpatient, Hospital

PATIENT: Gloria Polenske

SURGEON: Gary Sanchez, MD

PREOPERATIVE DIAGNOSIS: Left axillary nodes

POSTOPERATIVE DIAGNOSIS: Left axillary nodes, possible malignancy

PROCEDURE PERFORMED: Left axillary node dissection

ANESTHESIA: General

INDICATIONS FOR SURGERY: The patient is a 37-year-old white female who was noted to have left axillary nodes on a physical examination and scan. The patient has a history of having a right breast cancer removed many years ago. The patient is now undergoing left axillary node dissection for diagnosis.

DESCRIPTION OF PROCEDURE: The patient was prepped and draped in the usual manner. She was given a general anesthetic. An incision was made on the lateral border of the pectoralis major muscle. The dissection was carried down into the axilla. Multiple enlarged lymph nodes were identified and excised. All lymph nodes that could be found were removed and sent to pathology. Pathology stated that the lymph nodes were not breast cancer; however, they were highly suspicious for some type of malignancy. Hemostasis was obtained using Bovie cautery and also 3-0 silk ties. The operative area was thoroughly irrigated. The deep layer was closed with a running 3-0 Vicryl suture. The subcutaneous tissue was closed with a running 3-0 Vicryl suture. The skin was closed with 4-0 Vicryl subcuticular stitch. Steri-Strips were applied. The drain was sutured in place using a 3-0 nylon suture. The patient tolerated the operation and returned to recovery in stable condition.

Pathology Report Later Indicated: See Report 7-25B.

SERVICE CODE(S): _____

ICD-10-CM DX CODE(S): _____

(Answers to every other Case are located in Appendix D . The full answer key is only available in the TEACH Instructor Resources on Evolve.)

CASE 7-25B   *Pathology Report*

LOCATION: Inpatient, Hospital

PATIENT: Gloria Polenske

SURGEON: Gary Sanchez, MD

PATHOLOGIST: Morton Monson, MD

CLINICAL HISTORY: History of breast cancer, left axillary nodes

SPECIMEN RECEIVED: A: Left axillary nodes with frozen section. B: Additional axillary nodes, left.

GROSS DESCRIPTION:

A. The specimen is labeled with the patient's name and "left axillary lymph nodes" and consists of a 4 × 2 × 1-cm (centimeter) ovoid fatty lymphoid tissue.

INTRAOPERATIVE FROZEN-SECTION DIAGNOSIS: No evidence of breast carcinoma; rule out lymphoma on permanent sections.

B. The specimen is labeled with the patient's name and "additional axillary nodes, left" and consists of three, up to 2-cm, pieces of tan lymphoid-appearing tissue.

MICROSCOPIC DESCRIPTION:

A. and B. Sections show lymph nodes showing a diffuse proliferation, lymphocytes, which are uniform in size and shape and replace the normal lymphoid architecture. Occasional histiocytic-type cells are scattered throughout the proliferation, and prominent vasculature is noted in the interstitium. Immunohistochemical stain for CD20 shows positive diffusion.

DIAGNOSIS:

A. and B. Small lymphocytic lymphoma, left axillary nodes.

COMMENT: The case was reviewed with Dr. Sanchez.

SERVICE CODE(S): _____

ICD-10-CM DX CODE(S): _____

(Answers to every other Case are located in Appendix D . The full answer key is only available in the TEACH Instructor Resources on Evolve.)

CASE 7-26A *Operative Report, Splenectomy*

LOCATION: Inpatient, Hospital

PATIENT: Morgan Hillard

SURGEON: Gary Sanchez, MD

PREOPERATIVE DIAGNOSIS: Idiopathic thrombocytopenic purpura refractory to medical therapy

POSTOPERATIVE DIAGNOSIS: Same

PROCEDURE PERFORMED: Splenectomy, total *(Figure 7-14)*

HISTORY: This gentleman has ITP refractory to medical therapy. It was elected to do an open splenectomy. It was difficult to consider a laparoscopic splenectomy in a person who has had such severe vascular disease, but more importantly he had perforated diverticulitis with a colon resection and then had an incisional hernia repair with mesh. I felt that the wiser approach would be to do a left-sided Kocher incision and try to stay away from the mesh and away, hopefully, from the adhesions.

PROCEDURE: The patient was given a general anesthetic. He had a Foley catheter inserted. He was prepped and draped while in a supine fashion. We made a left-sided Kocher incision. We looked way into the abdomen. He had a lot of adhesions, but they were below our lower-most incision, so that turned out great. We used the Omni retractor and got everything set up. We then identified a very large spleen. It was about 60% the size of the liver. We lifted up the spleen and brought it through the wound. We identified the major vessels, which we controlled with right angles, and then we divided them. There were short gastric vessels that we dealt with the same way. We then removed the spleen and made sure that there was no tear of the spleen and no chance of splenosis. We then doubly tied all areas and made sure we suture ligated the major vessels in addition to tying them. We then looked along the greater curve. There were two small short gastric vessels that were not bleeding that had been dealt with

during the dissection, but we elected to lift these up and clip them. We had excellent hemostasis at the end. The pancreas looked normal. We looked around and made sure that there were no signs of any accessory spleens. We then irrigated and suctioned out copiously and closed the wound with no. 2 Vicryl stitches in a two-layer fashion. We then irrigated out the wound and put in some staples. We put some 0.25% plain Marcaine into the wound. Telfa, Toppers, and gauze were applied. The patient tolerated this well and went to the recovery room in good condition.

SERVICE CODE(S): _____

ICD-10-CM DX CODE(S): _____

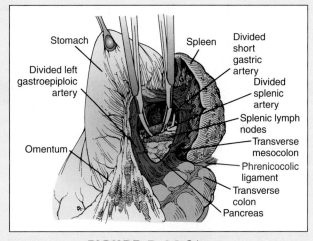

FIGURE 7-14 Splenectomy.

(Answers to every other Case are located in Appendix D . The full answer key is only available in the TEACH Instructor Resources on Evolve.)

CASE 7-26B *Pathology Report*

LOCATION: Inpatient, Hospital

PATIENT: Morgan Hillard

SURGEON: Gary Sanchez, MD

PATHOLOGIST: Morton Monson, MD

CLINICAL HISTORY: Idiopathic thrombocytopenia, purpura

SPECIMEN RECEIVED: Spleen

GROSS DESCRIPTION:

Received in a container labeled "spleen" is a spleen measuring 18 × 9.5 × 6 cm (centimeter) in greatest dimension and weighing 620 g. The surface contains a capsule that is mildly wrinkled and has a gray-purple appearance. The hilum demonstrates small superficial lacerations. The specimen is step-sectioned and demonstrates a uniform red-purple color. A faintly distinct nodular appearance is present. Representative portions are submitted.

The spleen demonstrates a prominent red pulp with congestion of the sinusoids. Scattered follicles showing normal morphology are widely separated by the expanded red pulp. The sinusoids exhibit megakaryocytic and erythroid metaplasia.

DIAGNOSIS:

Spleen, excision: Splenomegaly, marked, with severe congestion. Extramedullary hematopoiesis with megakaryocytic and erythroid hyperplasia.

COMMENT: The above-described findings have been noted in idiopathic thrombocytopenic purpura.

Case reviewed by Dr. Melon from the university.

SERVICE CODE(S): _____

ICD-10-CM DX CODE(S): _____

(Answers to every other Case are located in Appendix D . The full answer key is only available in the TEACH Instructor Resources on Evolve.)

CASE 7-27 *Bone Marrow Biopsy*

In the following report, there were two procedures performed during one operative session. The aspiration procedure is the least intensive procedure.

LOCATION: Inpatient, Hospital

PATIENT: Sammy Schultz

SURGEON: Gary Sanchez, MD

PREOPERATIVE DIAGNOSIS: Anemia, acute renal failure, diffuse skeletal pain

POSTOPERATIVE DIAGNOSIS: Same

PROCEDURE PERFORMED: Bone marrow aspiration and biopsy

DESCRIPTION OF PROCEDURE: The patient was sterilized and anesthetized by standard procedure. One bone marrow core biopsy was obtained from the right posterior iliac crest with moderate to severe discomfort. At the end of the procedure, the patient had no obvious discomfort and no obvious complications. On three different occasions, I attempted to obtain bone marrow aspiration from the right posterior iliac crest and was unsuccessful. It seemed to be a dry tap. I went over to the left posterior iliac crest and was able to obtain some bone marrow aspirate with some minimal to moderate discomfort. Most of the patient's discomfort was from having to lie on his right shoulder because he has been having discomfort there.

At the end of the procedure, the patient had no discomfort, and there was no obvious complication.

SERVICE CODE(S): _____

ICD-10-CM DX CODE(S): _____

(Answers to every other Case are located in Appendix D . The full answer key is only available in the TEACH Instructor Resources on Evolve.)

CASE 7-28 *Bone Marrow Biopsy*

LOCATION: Inpatient, Hospital

PATIENT: George Orwell

SURGEON: Gary Sanchez, MD

PREOPERATIVE DIAGNOSIS: Acute myelogenous leukemia

POSTOPERATIVE DIAGNOSIS: Acute myelogenous leukemia

PROCEDURE PERFORMED: Bone marrow biopsy

PROCEDURE: The patient was sterilized and anesthetized by standard procedure. One bone marrow core biopsy was obtained from the left posterior iliac crest with minimal discomfort. At the end of the procedure, the patient denied discomfort, and there were no obvious complications. I did obtain one bone marrow aspirate from the left posterior iliac crest with minimal to moderate discomfort. At the end of the procedure, the patient denied discomfort, and there were no obvious complications.

Pathology Report Later Indicated: Acute myelogenous leukemia

SERVICE CODE(S): _____

ICD-10-CM DX CODE(S): _____

(Answers to every other Case are located in Appendix D . The full answer key is only available in the TEACH Instructor Resources on Evolve.)

CHAPTER 7   *Auditing Review*

Audit the coding for the following reports.

Audit Report 7.1 Operative Report, Colonoscopy

LOCATION: Inpatient, Hospital

PATIENT: Lori Dubois

SURGEON: Larry Friendly, MD

PREOPERATIVE DIAGNOSES:

1. Left inguinal hernia.
2. Family history of colon cancer.

POSTOPERATIVE DIAGNOSES: Same.

PROCEDURES PERFORMED: Colonoscopy to cecum and left herniorrhaphy.

ANESTHESIA: General.

INDICATIONS FOR SURGERY: This is a 45-year-old Caucasian female who noticed a bulge in her left groin area. It was tender. The patient was found to have a left inguinal hernia, and she was taken to surgery for repair. The patient also had been previously scheduled for a screening colonoscopy, but because she was going to have the anesthetic for the repair, she decided to undergo colonoscopy during surgery. The patient has a long family history of colon cancer.

DESCRIPTION OF THE SURGERY: The patient was given a general anesthetic. She was then placed in the left lateral position. The colonoscope was then passed per rectum. The scope was passed to the cecum. Examinations of the cecum and ascending colon were within normal limits. The transverse and descending colon were within normal limits. The sigmoid, rectosigmoid, and rectum were also within normal limits. The scope was retroflexed. The internal anal area also appeared within normal limits. The scope was then removed. The patient tolerated the procedure.

The patient was then placed in a supine position. She was then prepped and draped in the usual manner. A left skin line hernia incision was made. Dissection was carried down to the round ligament. The round ligament was elevated. The distal end of the round ligament was tied with a 0 Ethibond stick tie suture and then transected. Examination of the round ligament did reveal an indirect hernia sac. There was some fat within the sac. A high ligation of the round ligament and the hernia sac were then done using a 0 Ethibond stick tie suture and a 2-0 silk free tie suture. The sac and the round ligament were transected and sent to Pathology. Next a floor repair was done. The transversalis fascia was sutured to the iliopubic tract using interrupted 0 Ethibond sutures. This completely closed the canal. The sutures were tied. The area was thoroughly irrigated. The incision was then injected with 0.25% Marcaine with Epinephrine; a total of 30 cc was used. The operative area was irrigated. The external oblique fascia was then closed with a running 2-0 Vicryl sutures. The subcutaneous tissue was closed with a running 3-0 Vicryl suture. The skin was closed with a 4-0 Vicryl subcuticular stitch. Steri-Strips were applied. The patient tolerated the operation and returned to recovery in stable condition.

One of the following codes is not reported for this case. Indicate the missing code.

PROFESSIONAL SERVICES:	Inguinal hernia repair, **49505**; Colonoscopy, **45378-51**
ICD-10-CM DX:	Inguinal hernia, **K40.90**; Family history of colon cancer, **Z80.0**
MISSING CODE:	_____

Audit Report 7.2 Operative Report, Small Bowel Resection

LOCATION: Inpatient, Hospital

PATIENT: Edna Holland

SURGEON: Larry Friendly, MD

PREOPERATIVE DIAGNOSIS: Acute abdomen/perforated viscus.

POSTOPERATIVE DIAGNOSIS: Gangrenous segment of small bowel—distal ileum.

PROCEDURE PERFORMED:

1. Exploratory laparotomy.
2. Small bowel resection (approximately 45-50 centimeters) with a stapled side-to-side/functional end-to-end anastomosis.
3. Nasoenteric feeding tube placement (CORFLO).

INDICATION: This is a 65-year-old female who has an acute abdomen. She has been in the hospital for a couple of days with some abdominal pain, as well as an MI. Her CT scan was fairly unremarkable a couple of days ago. Plain film today shows evidence of contrast outside the lumen of the bowel. I was asked this afternoon if I could take her to the operating theater for exploratory laparotomy. After seeing her, evaluating her and reviewing the plain films from today, as well as seeing that on exam she definitely had peritoneal signs, I agreed that she needed to go to the OR and took her to the operating room immediately. I had counseled the patient, as well as the family, to the risks of the procedure. She is a high risk. I am not sure what we are going to find for sure. We discussed multiple possibilities, including bowel resection, colostomy, ileostomy/bowel ostomies, or numerous other potential pathology. We discussed that she was a high risk. She is a very high risk for even intraoperative mortality, very high risk for developing multiple complications including cardiac, pulmonary and systemic problems, and liver problems.

I discussed that these are all potential problems that can occur during this procedure, as well as start afterwards. Chance of recovery from this is quite small; if we do not do anything though, she will succumb to this and die from her current condition. She understood this. Her family history is not characteristic of CMV colitis, biopsied normal terminal ileum. Normal colon otherwise. They understand and wish to proceed with the operation. They also understand that she will remain on a ventilator, at least initially after the procedure.

ANESTHESIA: General.

PROCEDURE: The patient was brought to the operating theater and placed in supine position on the operating table. After receiving general anesthetic, she was prepped and draped in a sterile fashion. A vertical midline incision was made. Dissection was carried down through the subcutaneous tissues, down through the anterior fascia. Peritoneal

Continued

CHAPTER 7—cont'd

cavity was entered. We could see that the omentum was stuck down to the mid and lower abdomen. There was purulent greenish fluid present. Cultures of this were obtained. On peeling back the omentum, we could see that this was stuck over a segment of dead bowel. We ran the small bowel from the ligament of Treitz to the terminal ileum. There was a segment with full-thickness necrosis in it. There was a fibrinous exudate; it varies where the bowel was sticking to this, as well as omentum had been sticking to it. This was in the distal aspect of the ileum. The cecum itself appeared okay. The appendix was normal. Right colon, transverse colon, descending colon and sigmoid colon all appeared normal. No evidence of abnormalities here. While some of the small bowel looked a little bit rough and inflamed from being adjacent to this area, the remainder of this appeared viable. We proceeded with small bowel resection at this time. We marked out our distal aspect on the small bowel. We then made a small window in the mesentery. We then used a TLC-75 stapler and fired this across here. We then scored the mesentery. We did not go too far down on the mesentery because we wished to keep any collaterals open. We took down the mesentery between right angle clamps, transected and ligated with 2-0 Vicryl. We picked another spot on the more proximal bowel that looked viable. We felt that this area was going to be nice and viable and good. We took the mesentery down over to here as already described. The TLC-75 stapler was then used to fire across the small bowel at this segment. It should also be noted that we had checked Doppler flow through the mesentery.

It appeared at these other areas that there was Doppler flow. The total length of the small bowel that was removed was approximately 45-50 cm. At this point, we used staplers. We used the TLC-75 stapler to create our anastomosis. This was done by attaching the anterior mesenteric borders with a couple of 3-0 silk sutures. A couple of enterotomies were made on each side. Succus entericus was aspirated with the sucker. We then inserted the TLC-75 stapler and fired this along the anterior mesenteric border. Hemostasis was present at our anastomotic line. Things looked secure. We used a TA-90 stapler to close off our opening. This was fired. This was then transected off. We placed one more 3-0 silk at the very end of the staple line. Our staple line looked good and secure. We then had Anesthesia inject 1 amp of fluorescein. After a few minutes, we did check with the wood lamp. All segments of small bowel, as well as the colon and stomach, all appeared to be viable with good flow. We had good fluorescein lighting up at our anastomosis. Things looked good here. We then closed our mesenteric defect with 2-0 Vicryl in a running fashion.

One or more codes should not have been reported for this case. Indicate the code(s) incorrectly reported.

PROFESSIONAL SERVICES: Enterectomy of the small intestine with anastomosis, **44120**

ICD-10-CM DX: Perforation of ileum, **K63.1**; Necrosis of intestine, **K55.069**

INCORRECTLY REPORTED CODE(S): _____

Audit Report 7.3 Operative Report, Colonoscopy and Polypectomy

LOCATION: Inpatient, Hospital

PATIENT: Diane Halvorson

SURGEON: Larry Friendly, MD

PRIMARY PHYSICIAN: Frank Gaul, MD

INDICATIONS: A pleasant 52-year-old white female referred by Dr. Gaul for colonoscopy. The patient had a screening flexible sigmoidoscopy and a 3- to 4-mm polyp was at 35 cm and a pedunculated polyp at 20 cm. The patient has no symptoms. Patient believes there is a family history for colon cancer.

FINDINGS: The Pentax video colonoscope was inserted without difficulty to the cecum. The ileocecal valve was identified. The appendiceal orifice was seen. Careful inspection in the cecum, ascending colon, hepatic flexure, transverse colon, splenic flexure, and descending colon revealed no erythema, ulceration, exudate, friability, or other mucosal abnormalities.

The sigmoid colon revealed a 3-mm polyp. This was hot-biopsied and cauterized. No other polyps were seen in the remainder of the descending, sigmoid, or rectum. The patient tolerated the procedure well.

IMPRESSION: A 3-mm pedunculated polyp at about 35 cm, biopsied and cauterized.

PLAN: The patient will return again in one year for surveillance.

PATHOLOGY FINDINGS LATER INDICATED: Benign polyp tissue.

One or more codes should not have been reported for this case. Indicate the code(s) incorrectly reported.

PROFESSIONAL SERVICES: Colonoscopy with biopsy, **45380-59**; Colonoscopy with removal of tumor by hot biopsy forceps, **45384**

ICD-10-CM DX: Sigmoid colon polyp, **D12.5**; Family history of colon cancer, **Z80.0**

INCORRECTLY REPORTED CODE(S): _____

CHAPTER 7—cont'd

Audit Report 7.4 Operative Report, Anal Fissure

LOCATION: Inpatient, Hospital

PATIENT: Annabelle Antman

SURGEON: Larry P. Friendly, MD

PREOPERATIVE DIAGNOSIS: Anal fissure

POSTOPERATIVE DIAGNOSIS: Anal fissure

OPERATIVE PROCEDURE:

1. Sphincterotomy with fissurectomy
2. Pallipectomy with excision of one sentinel tag

ANESTHESIA: Spinal

INDICATIONS: Annabelle is a pleasant 44-year-old female who is post three quadrant hemorrhoidectomy for severe external hemorrhoids. She has an anal fissure as well as a sentinel tag that is quite tender. She presents today for elective sphincterotomy and excision of the sentinel tag. She understands the surgery and the risks of bleeding and infection, possible damage to the sphincter muscles, and wishes to proceed.

DESCRIPTION OF PROCEDURE: The patient was brought to the operating room, given spinal anesthesia, and placed in a jackknife position. We could see the enlarged hemorrhoid/sentinel tag at the 10 o'clock position and the fissure right at the base of this. Anoscope was placed, and we placed a Kelly clamp behind the hypertrophied scarred band of muscle and divided the muscle. We then excised the sentinel tag and fissure then closed the defect with interrupted 3-0 chromic sutures and running locked 3-0 chromic. There were no other internal hemorrhoids, and there were no other fissures. We infiltrated the area with a total of 30 cc of 0.5% Sensorcaine with epinephrine solution and placed four gauze dressings in the area, which we will remove in 30 minutes, and she was taken to recovery in stable condition.

One or more of the following codes are reported incorrectly for this case. Indicate the incorrect code or codes.

SERVICE CODE(S): Sphincterotomy, **46080;** Fissurectomy, **46200;** Excision anal papilla or tag, **46220**

ICD-10-CM DX CODE(S): Anal fissure, **K60.2**

INCORRECT/MISSING CODE(S): _____

Audit Report 7.5 Operative Report, Colon Polypectomy

LOCATION: Outpatient, Hospital

PATIENT: Jeffrey Henrys

SURGEON: Larry Friendly, MD

SCOPE USED: Pentax video colonoscope

MEDICATION GIVEN: Fentanyl 100 mcg IV; Versed 2 mg IV

PREOPERATIVE DIAGNOSIS: Polyp found on flexible sigmoidoscopy

POSTOPERATIVE DIAGNOSIS:

1. Two small 2-mm polyps in the descending sigmoid colon.
2. An 8-mm semipedunculated rectal polyp, snare removed.

PROCEDURE PERFORMED: Colonoscopy with polypectomy

INDICATION: This is a 65-year-old white male referred for colonoscopy. The patient had a screening flexible sigmoidoscopy. He is asymptomatic and was found to have a small colon polyp at 22 cm and a 4-mm polyp in the rectum.

FINDINGS: The Pentax video colonoscope was inserted easily to the cecum. The ileocecal valve was identified. The appendiceal orifice was seen. Careful inspection in the cecum, ascending colon, hepatic flexure, transverse colon, splenic flexure, and descending colon revealed no erythema, ulceration, exudates, friability, or other mucosal abnormalities.

The distal descending sigmoid revealed two small polyps 2-mm or less in size. These were hot biopsied off. The rectum, however, did reveal an 8-mm semipedunculated polyp. This was snared piecemeal. The patient did have one medium- to large-size internal hemorrhoid, now bleeding. The patient tolerated the procedure well.

IMPRESSION:

1. Two diminutive polyps in the descending sigmoid colon, hot biopsied off.
2. An 8-mm semipedunculated polyp in the rectum, snared off.
3. A medium-sized internal hemorrhoid.

PLAN: As the polyps are adenomatous, which is what I suspect they are, the patient can return again in 5 years for surveillance.

PATHOLOGY REPORT LATER INDICATED: Rectal polyp; fragments of villous adenoma, benign

One or more of the following codes are reported incorrectly for this case. Indicate the incorrect code or codes.

SERVICE CODE(S): Sigmoidoscopy, **45330;** Colonoscopy with hot biopsy forceps, **45384;** Colonoscopy with snare technique, **45385**

ICD-10-CM DX CODE(S): Benign neoplasm of rectosigmoid junction, **D12.7;** Benign neoplasm of sigmoid colon, **D12.5**

INCORRECT/MISSING CODE(S): _____

Continued

CHAPTER 7—cont'd

Audit Report 7.6 Operative Report, Laparotomy

LOCATION: Inpatient, Hospital

PATIENT: Stephen Moore

ATTENDING PHYSICIAN: Gary Sanchez, MD

SURGEON: Gary Sanchez, MD

PREOPERATIVE DIAGNOSIS: Massive thoracic and abdominal injuries.

POSTOPERATIVE DIAGNOSIS: Same.

PROCEDURE PERFORMED: Damage control laparotomy (reported as an exploratory laparotomy) with suture of a bleeding liver laceration.

This young man presented with a temperature of 27° C after being involved in a rollover accident. During the transport down, he apparently had an arrest three times. The patient has a 60 systolic blood pressure at this stage. He had not had a collar placed during transport but was controlled on the backboard with his head stabilized. Immediately on arrival in the operating room, a cervical collar was placed. The patient had already been intubated. He had bilateral chest tubes in place.

Once he was on the operating room table, an attempt was made to get chest x-ray, but radiology could not get a plate under the patient. With good function of the chest tubes and the patient's continued severe hypotension, it was elected to proceed with the laparotomy and proceed with further evaluation as the case progressed. As the abdomen was being prepped, anesthesia was giving him fluids and blood and trying to warm him up. All fluids were run in warmers, including the blood that was being infused. Immediately upon having the abdomen prepped and draped, a long midline incision was made; the patient was found to have approximately a liter and one-half of blood present within the abdomen. He was cold. He had an actively bleeding liver tear that was on the dorsum just lateral to the ligament teres. Several 0 chromic sutures were placed through this in figure-of-eight fashion, and this stopped the bleeding. This was done after we had immediately packed both the left and right upper quadrants, as well as the pelvis. After being assured that his bleeding was controlled with the packing, anesthesia was continuously warming him and we used warm irrigation in the abdomen. The chest tubes were draining adequately.

According to anesthesia, the patient still had fixed, dilated pupils. By the end of the procedure, the patient's temperature was up to about 30° C.

As the anesthesia was infusing the blood and fluids and the patient's blood pressure was now coming up, we started looking at each of the quadrants. The patient is found to have a non-expanding hematoma involving the pelvis consistent with a pelvic fracture. This was repacked to make sure there was no active bleeding in this area but there was no active bleeding. The packs were removed from the left upper quadrant slowly. The spleen was then visualized and there was no active bleeding; this was repacked. The right side was then evaluated. Most of the blood was around the liver. The patient had a laceration at the dome of the liver just to the right of the ligamentum teres, and this was oversewn as noted above. At this point, because of the patient's hypothermia and instability, the abdomen was re-packed. A Vac-Pac was quickly placed. The patient's pupils at this stage were still fixed and dilated. There was a question whether the fixed pupils were due to either a primary head injury with an intracranial bleed, or whether this was just a hypoxic-related issue related to the original injury and the 3 arrests during transport. The patient was taken immediately from the operating room to the CAT scanner with neurosurgeon available. CAT scan will be done immediately. If the patient does not have anything intracranial that needs to be fixed immediately, he will be taken to the intensive care unit, where we will continue resuscitation with the warm fluids and blood as necessary. The patient is in critical condition. At the end of the procedure the patient's blood pressure was up in the 80s systolic.

One or more of the following codes are reported incorrectly for this case. Indicate the incorrect code or codes.

SERVICE CODE(S): Exploratory laparotomy, **49000;** Surgical management of liver injury with hemorrhage, **47360**

ICD-10-CM DX CODE(S): Hemorrhage, **R58;** Abdominal distension, **R14.0;** Liver laceration, **S36.113A;** Car accident, **V48.5XXA**

INCORRECT/MISSING CODE(S): _____

(Auditing Review answers with rationales are only available in the TEACH Instructor Resources on Evolve.)

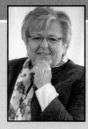

"The career of coding is not only vital but also just plain interesting. Assigning codes to a complex report is not only challenging but also invigorating."

Musculoskeletal System

http://evolve.elsevier.com/Buck/next

(Answers to every other Case are located in Appendix D, with the full answer key only available in the TEACH Instructor Resources on Evolve)
(Auditing Review answers with rationales are only available in the TEACH Instructor Resources on Evolve)

Common musculoskeletal complaints are pain of the neck, knee, shoulder, elbow, wrist, hand, back, hip, ankle, and foot. Conditions commonly related to the musculoskeletal system are sprains, bursitis, tendonitis, dislocations, fractures, nerve entrapments (such as carpal tunnel syndrome), and gout. A physician who specializes in the diagnosis and treatment of musculoskeletal disorders is an **orthopedist.** An **orthopedic surgeon** is one who not only diagnoses and treats musculoskeletal disorders but also performs musculoskeletal surgical procedures, for example, repairs involving the placement of pins, wires, screws, cranial halos, spinal instrumentation, and other fixation devices. Reconstruction surgeries such as hip replacements and other joint replacements are now performed frequently. Endoscopic procedures are often used in the orthopedic specialty. Most major clinics would have orthopedic physician(s)/surgeon(s) on staff, and in other settings the orthopedic services would be provided by an orthopedist in independent practice. Orthopedic physicians frequently receive referrals from other physicians to consult on musculoskeletal conditions.

Arthrocentesis

Arthrocentesis is injection and/or aspiration of a joint and is a commonly used treatment for joint conditions **(Figures 8-1 and 8-2).** A needle is inserted into the joint to anesthetize it. Drugs such as Depo-Medrol (synthetic glucocorticoid) or cortisone can then be injected into the joint, or fluid can be withdrawn. Bundled into the arthrocentesis are the dual services of injection and aspiration. For example, 20610 is reported when a physician withdraws fluid from the knee joint and then injects Depo-Medrol into the knee joint. The drug injected would be reported separately with a HCPCS code. HCPCS J code (drug code) descriptions identify the drug by the generic name, not the brand name. When reporting the drug with a HCPCS code, it is necessary to translate the brand name into the generic name; this is when the cross-reference feature of the Table of Drugs will be useful. For example, if the medical record indicates a Depo-Medrol injection, the Table of Drugs entry for Depo-Medrol (brand name) refers

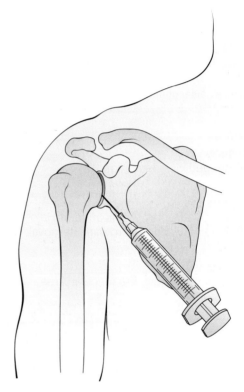

FIGURE 8–1 Arthrocentesis.

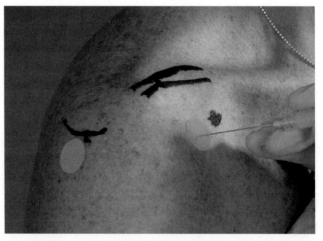

FIGURE 8–2 Arthrocentesis. Orange areas are injection sites.

you to the generic name of the drug, methylprednisolone acetate (J1020-J1040). A current medical drug reference is also often necessary to translate brand names into the generic names to locate the drug in the HCPCS manual.

If fluoroscopic, CT, or MRI guidance is performed, also report 77002, 77012, 77021. Do not report codes 20600-20611 with the ultrasound guidance code 76942. Codes 20604, 20606, 20611 are reported for arthrocentesis, aspiration and/or injection of a joint or bursa procedures performed with ultrasound guidance.

Injections into the tendon sheath or ligament, tendon origin or insertion, or muscle are reported with 20550-20553 and are reported one time per service visit when the same tendon sheath, tendon origin/insertion, or muscle is injected, no matter how many injections were placed in that specific sheath, origin/insertion, or muscle. If, however, a tendon sheath and a tendon insertion were injected, both injections are reported.

■ One sheath, origin/insert, or muscle injected, report one injection code.

■ Multiple sheaths, origins/insertions, or muscle sites injected, report multiple injection codes.

Use modifier -59 (distinct service) when reporting multiple injections during the same service visit to make it clear that documentation indicates that separate services were provided. The drug injected would be reported separately with a CPT or HCPCS code. If image guidance was used during an injection reported with 20550-20553, report the radiographic service separately with 77002, 77021, or 76942.

Fractures

Closed fractures are those in which the bone does not protrude outside the skin and usually include terms such as comminuted, compound, depressed, elevated, fissured greenstick, impacted, linear, simple, or spiral.

Open fractures are those in which the bone does protrude outside the skin and include terms such as compound, infected, missile, puncture, or with foreign body. If the documentation indicates both open and closed fracture terminology, assign an open fracture code. The type of treatment does not necessarily correlate to type of fracture; for example, an open reduction of a closed fracture—meaning that the closed fracture can be repaired by means of an open procedure. The terminology describing the type of fracture and the type of treatment must be carefully abstracted from the documentation to correctly report the fracture type.

Fractures are reported with S codes based on the area of injury, such as fractures of the facial bones, S02, or fracture of lumbar spine and pelvis, S32.

Vertebral column fractures

Vertebral column fractures are reported with S12, S22, S32. Spinal cord injury is reported separately in addition to the fracture code. If the injury was only of the spinal cord, the injury would be reported with one of these codes: S14, S24, and S34. Cervical fractures are reported with S12.1--A for a closed fracture, and S12.1--B for an open fracture. Multiple cervical fractures are reported individually for each vertebral fracture.

Fractures of the rib(s), sternum, larynx, and trachea

Fractures of the upper limbs (S42, S52, S62) are divided by the specific location, as are the fractures of the lower limbs (S72, S82, S92). All fractures codes require a 7th character to indicate the episode of care, such as "A" for the initial encounter, "D" for subsequent encounter, or "S" for sequelae. Not all codes have the same 7th characters available for assignment. Turn to the Tabular to S82 and review all of the 7th characters available for assignment. Also, see instructions in the *Official Guidelines for Coding and Reporting*, Section I.A.4. and 5., for more specific instructions on episode of care. External cause codes are assigned for the length of treatment. A 7th character is assigned to indicate initial encounter, subsequent encounter, or sequela for each encounter as long as the injury or condition is being treated.

External cause codes are only reported at the time of initial episode of care and only if the facility policy indicates that external cause codes will be assigned. If, as per facility policy, external cause codes are assigned, and since fractures usually are a result of an accident of some type, an external cause code would be assigned to indicate the way in which the accident happened (circumstances of the accident).

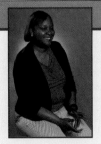

From the Trenches

"In medical coding there has to be a constant commitment to research, data gathering, and asking questions to get to the answer."

LETITIA PATTERSON
MPA, RHIA, CCS-P, CPC, CPMA, CPC-I

CASE 8-1   *Orthopedic Consultation*

Dr. Green sent Janelle Masche to Dr. Almaz, an orthopedic physician/surgeon, for an opinion regarding her right tennis elbow (epicondylitis), which is an overuse syndrome. The lateral epicondyle is the outside bony portion of the elbow where the tendons attach from the muscle to the elbow. Repetitive motion can injure the tendon, causing pain. X-rays are usually normal. Local cortisone may be injected.

LOCATION: Outpatient, Clinic

PATIENT: Janelle Masche

PRIMARY CARE PHYSICIAN: Ronald Green, MD

CONSULTANT: Mohomad Almaz, MD

HISTORY OF PRESENT ILLNESS: The patient is a 52-year-old woman who works in coding at the local hospital. Dr. Green referred her for right tennis elbow.

She explained that her right wrist started hurting about 6 months ago when she was pulling some charts. Then, about 4 months ago, she developed some pain along the lateral aspect of her right elbow. She saw Dr. Green and states that he treated her with an injection. I am unable to find evidence of this injection in the chart, but she explained that it was done probably in 1989. She has also been treated with a tennis elbow strap.

PHYSICAL EXAMINATION: The physical examination today finds that she localizes her pain to the lateral aspect of the right elbow near the lateral humeral epicondyle.

She has pain in the area with dorsiflexion of her wrist against resistance. She has a full range of motion of her right elbow, including supination and pronation. No areas of erythema are noted.

X-rays of her right elbow found the bony architecture to appear essentially within normal limits.

IMPRESSION: Right lateral humeral epicondylitis

RECOMMENDATION: I have elected to inject the tender area over the right lateral humeral epicondyle with 80 mg (milligram) of Depo-Medrol and 1 cc (cubic centimeter) of 1% Xylocaine following Betadine prep. I have asked that she let me know if she has further problems. She understands that a tennis elbow release may be necessary if the pain returns following these injections.

SERVICE CODE(S): _____

HCPCS DRUG CODE: _____

ICD-10-CM DX CODE(S): _____

(Answers to every other Case are located in Appendix D . The full answer key is only available in the TEACH Instructor Resources on Evolve.)

Fixation

Fixation can be internal or external and is used to hold a bone in place. **Internal** fixation is the placement of wires, pins, screws, plates, or rods onto or into the bone to repair bones. **External** fixation is the application of a device that holds the bone in place from the outside. Fasteners are driven into the bone percutaneously, and the external fixation device is attached to the fasteners. **Percutaneous** fixation (skeletal fixation) is a type of external fixation that serves as attachments for traction devices.

Both application and removal of the device are reported with one code. If a physician other than the physician who applied the device removes the device, the removal is reported separately. When reporting a fracture repair with the application of a fixation device, the device is usually reported separately; however, use caution when reporting the repair and application, because some fracture codes include application of devices in the code description (so then you would not report the services separately). Routine adjustment of the device is included in the application code unless the adjustment requires anesthesia.

CASE 8-2   *Operative Report, Application of Halo*

*Dr. Almaz applies a cranial halo to stabilize a C1-C2 fracture, as illustrated in **Figures 8-3** and **8-4**. This is the initial treatment of the injury. Assign an external cause code to indicate how the accident happened.*

LOCATION: Outpatient, Hospital

PATIENT: Ella German

SURGEON: Mohomad Almaz, MD

PREOPERATIVE DIAGNOSIS: Fracture of C1 (first cervical vertebra) and C2 (second cervical vertebra)

POSTOPERATIVE DIAGNOSIS: Fracture of C1 and C2

PROCEDURE PERFORMED: Application of halo

PROCEDURE: The patient's head was prepped and draped. The halo was applied to the head. Lidocaine was used in the area where the pins enter. We then placed the pins and fitted the patient with the rest of the vest. The patient is comfortable. She can get mobilized with the halo. She is 89 years old. You wonder whether she will ever heal after this fall. We will keep her in the halo for 3 to 4 months and see if she heals properly.

SERVICE CODE(S): _____

ICD-10-CM DX CODE(S): _____

(Answers to every other Case are located in Appendix D . The full answer key is only available in the TEACH Instructor Resources on Evolve.)

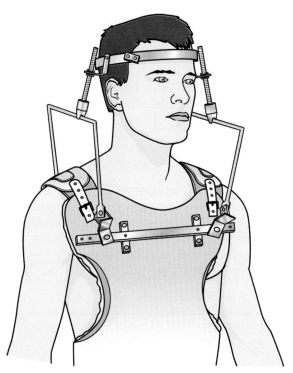

FIGURE 8–3 A cranial halo device.

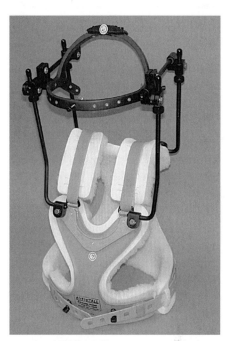

FIGURE 8–4 Halo device.

CASE 8-3 *Operative Report, Hardware Removal*

Removal of hardware is not included in the insertion procedures when the procedure is performed outside the global period, as in this case in which the hardware was placed last year and is being removed now and reported separately. Code the removal service in the following case. (Remember to report the diagnosis with an ICD-10-CM fracture code, indicating aftercare with a 7th character for subsequent care.)

LOCATION: Outpatient, Hospital

PATIENT: Gary Leiser

SURGEON: Mohomad Almaz, MD

PREOPERATIVE DIAGNOSIS: Healed comminuted fracture, right distal radius

POSTOPERATIVE DIAGNOSIS: Healed comminuted fracture, right distal radius

NAME OF OPERATION: Removal of hardware, right distal radius

INDICATIONS FOR SURGERY: This patient had a traumatic distal radius fracture treated last year with a Synthes dorsal distal radius plate.

Because of the risk of atraumatic rupture of the extensor tendons running over the plate, it was elected to remove the plate at this time.

OPERATIVE PROCEDURE: After a suitable general anesthesia was achieved, the patient's right wrist, hand, and forearm were prepped and draped. Before prepping, an arm tourniquet was applied and, after draping, inflated to 250 mmHg (millimeter of mercury). Scar on the dorsal aspect of the wrist was used as the site of the incision. The extensor pollicis longus tendon was incised in line with the tendon. The tendon was then retracted. The extensor retinaculum was elevated off at the plate bone level. The plate was then easily exposed. Screws were removed, and the plate was easily elevated. The wound was then irrigated. Skin edges were infiltrated with 0.5% Marcaine with adrenaline. The retinaculum was closed with 2-0 Tycron, subcutaneous tissue with 3-0 Vicryl, and the skin with interrupted 4-0 nylon horizontal mattress sutures (*this indicates the plate removal was from "deep" layers*). The patient tolerated the procedure well and returned to the recovery room in stable condition.

SERVICE CODE(S): _____

ICD-10-CM DX CODE(S): _____

(Answers to every other Case are located in Appendix D . The full answer key is only available in the TEACH Instructor Resources on Evolve.)

Excision

Throughout the Musculoskeletal System subsection, there are excision codes. These codes are used to report excisions from the deeper levels. Recall that excision codes are also located in the Integumentary System subsection. It is the origin of the excision that differentiates the codes. For example, if a superficial benign lesion was removed from the skin of the leg, the service is reported with a code from 11400-11406 (Integumentary System). If the excision was of a lesion located on the muscle of the leg, the service is reported with 27619 or 27634 (Musculoskeletal System), depending on the size of the tumor (<5 cm, >5 cm). Watch for terms that indicate the origin of the neoplasm, such as melanoma (skin) or sarcoma (connective tissue) to direct you to the correct code selection.

CASE 8-4   *Operative Report, Preauricular Area Excision*

LOCATION: Outpatient, Hospital

PATIENT: Doris Fisher

SURGEON: Mohomad Almaz, MD

PREOPERATIVE DIAGNOSIS: Malignant melanoma, skin of left preauricular area

POSTOPERATIVE DIAGNOSIS: Malignant melanomas with clear margins on the skin of the left preauricular area

PROCEDURE PERFORMED: Wide excision (this indicates radical excision) of malignant melanoma, skin of left preauricular area

ANESTHESIA: General endotracheal with supplementary 1% Xylocaine with 1:800,000 epinephrine

ESTIMATED BLOOD LOSS: Approximately 25 cc (cubic centimeter)

PROCEDURE: The patient's left face and ear were prepped with Betadine scrub and solution and draped in a routine sterile fashion.

The 0.8-cm lesion was excised to include the crus of the left ear in the dissection, because this was the only method to provide at least 2 cm (centimeter) of width around the excision site. We were able to get about 2.5 cm on the anterior excision site and at least 3 cm proximally and distally. We submitted the specimen, tagging the superior aspect with a silk suture, and cauterized the bleeding. A small section of the fascia and muscle was repaired, and then, using separate instrument and gloves, we undermined the skin after the manner of a subcutaneous facelift and brought the skin up, suturing it to the more posterior edge with interrupted 3-0 Prolene. We dressed the wound with Xeroform, Kerlix fluffs, and a Kerlix roll plus Kling. The patient tolerated the procedure well and left the operating table in good condition.

Pathology Report Later Indicated: Malignant melanoma

SERVICE CODE(S): _____

ICD-10-CM DX CODE(S): _____

(Answers to every other Case are located in Appendix D . The full answer key is only available in the TEACH Instructor Resources on Evolve.)

CASE 8-5   *Operative Report, Carbuncle Removal*

*Not all deep tissue excisions are reported with Musculoskeletal System codes. For example, the services in the next case are reported with Integumentary system codes. Note the two diagnoses highlighted in this report. This is another good example of why a coder **must** read the report and not code from the Postoperative Diagnosis section of the report.*

LOCATION: Outpatient, Hospital

PATIENT: Jennifer Carlin

PRIMARY CARE PHYSICIAN: Ronald Green, MD

SURGEON: Gary Sanchez, MD

PREOPERATIVE DIAGNOSIS: Two separate carbuncles, left axilla

POSTOPERATIVE DIAGNOSIS: Two separate carbuncles, left axilla

PROCEDURE PERFORMED: Removal of two separate carbuncles, left axilla. Tissue was submitted for aerobic and anaerobic cultures as well as permanent section.

INDICATION: This patient for the last 6 months has had a couple of carbuncles in her left axilla. They have been observed, and she has been placed on antibiotics. Attempts at drainage have been made, however, without results. Finally, the patient wants to have these tumors removed.

PROCEDURE IN DETAIL: After good MAC, the patient was prepped and draped in the usual sterile fashion. The left arm was adducted to expose the axilla. The two areas were infiltrated separately with 1% lidocaine after the incisions were made over both affected areas, and dissection was carried

down to encompass subdermal and deeper tissue. An inflamed lymph node was also identified, and this was taken with the more superficial tissue. After this, the wounds were irrigated and closed with 4-0 subcuticular stitch. Steri-Strips and sterile dressings were applied. The patient tolerated the procedure well and was returned to the recovery room in good condition.

Pathology Report Later Indicated: Lymph node was negative for neoplastic behavior.

SERVICE CODE(S): _____

ICD-10-CM DX CODE(S): _____

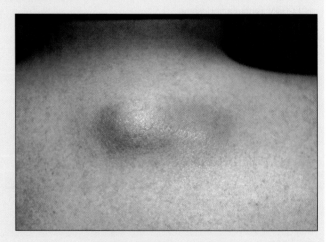

FIGURE 8–5 Carbuncle.

(Answers to every other Case are located in Appendix D . The full answer key is only available in the TEACH Instructor Resources on Evolve.)

CASE 8-6 · *Operative Report, Dissection and Excision*

LOCATION: Outpatient, Hospital

PATIENT: Sara Henre

PRIMARY CARE PHYSICIAN: Ronald Green, MD

SURGEON: Gary Sanchez, MD

PREOPERATIVE DIAGNOSIS: History of palpable right axillary mass

POSTOPERATIVE DIAGNOSIS: History of palpable right axillary mass

OPERATIVE PROCEDURE: Superficial right axillary dissection and excision of lymphatic tissue, 2.9 cm

COMPLICATIONS: None

ESTIMATED BLOOD LOSS: 50 cc (cubic centimeter)

ANESTHESIA: General endotracheal with 30 cc of 0.5% Marcaine augmentation

SPECIMEN: Superficial axillary contents. 1.8-cm mass was identified.

PROCEDURE: After good general endotracheal anesthesia, the patient was prepped and draped in the usual sterile fashion. The arm and axilla were prepped, and the hand and forearm were covered with a stockinette to allow mobilizing. The patient was previously interviewed in the preoperative area, and the palpable mass had been marked with ink. An incision was made over this area, which was in the axillary skin fold just above the axillary hairline, and this was after anesthetizing the skin. Dissection was carried down right under the skin in search of this nodule. We did find a 1.8-cm mass that represented a small lipoma in this area. This was resected. The axillary fascia was identified and incised, and similar fatty tissue was excised upward at the border of the latissimus and then down toward the posterior border of the axilla. An exploring finger was placed up in the axilla up toward the axillary vein, and no palpable adenopathy was noted, nor was there any adenopathy noted when the rest of the axilla was explored with a finger. We did continue to take away small pieces of lymphatic tissue in the entire area where the patient felt the lump and submitted this as axillary fatty and lymphatic contents. The wound was thoroughly irrigated. Bleeding was controlled using electrocautery. The wound was then closed in layers with 3-0 Vicryl and 4-0 Vicryl subcuticular. The patient tolerated the procedure well and was returned to the recovery room in good condition.

Pathology Report Later Indicated: Benign encapsulated lipoma (of subcutaneous breast)

SERVICE CODE(S): _____

ICD-10-CM DX CODE(S): _____

CASE 8-7 · *Operative Report, Nevus Removal*

A congenital nevus is a mole that is present at birth. There is a difference between a small and a giant nevus. Usually a giant congenital nevus is larger than 20 cm, and the small nevus is usually about 1.5 cm. In the CPT manual, the excision codes for nevus are based on the depth of subcutaneous or intramuscular and the size of the tumor.

LOCATION: Outpatient, Hospital

PATIENT: Earl Oukek

PRIMARY CARE PHYSICIAN: Ronald Green, MD

SURGEON: Mohomad Almaz, MD

PREOPERATIVE DIAGNOSIS: Giant congenital nevus, left pectoral region involving the left areola

POSTOPERATIVE DIAGNOSIS: Giant congenital nevus, left pectoral region involving the left areola

PROCEDURE PERFORMED: Excision of giant congenital nevus and portion of areola of the left chest

SURGICAL FINDINGS: A 7 × 4-cm (centimeter) giant congenital nevus (common nevus) involving about 50% of the areola on the left side

ANESTHESIA: General endotracheal plus 4 cc (cubic centimeter) of 0.5% Xylocaine and 1:100,000 epinephrine

COMPLICATIONS: None

SPONGE AND NEEDLE COUNTS: Correct

DESCRIPTION OF THE PROCEDURE: The patient's chest wall was prepped with Betadine scrub and solution and draped in a routine sterile fashion. I injected 4 cc of 0.5% Xylocaine with 1:100,000 epinephrine along the suture line and excised the lesion down to carpus fascia being sure to include the complete dermis and a little subcutaneous fat. We cauterized the bleeders and tagged the superior aspect of the specimen with a silk suture. We closed the wound with subcuticular 3-0 Monocryl and three twists of 6-0 Prolene. One-half-inch Steri-Strips were applied, plus a clavicle strap for immobilization. Estimated blood loss was less than 5 cc. The patient tolerated the procedure well and left the operating room in good condition.

Pathology Report Later Indicated: Benign tissue (chest skin)

SERVICE CODE(S): _____

ICD-10-CM DX CODE(S): _____

(Answers to every other Case are located in Appendix D . The full answer key is only available in the TEACH Instructor Resources on Evolve.)

From the Trenches

"When dealing with health records, it's imperative that you are able to focus on small details when recording and coding patient information. It's vital that you are able to stay focused."

LETITIA PATTERSON
MPA, RHIA, CCS-P, CPC, CPMA, CPC-I

CASE 8-8 *Operative Report, Costovertebral Tumor*

LOCATION: Outpatient, Hospital

PATIENT: Leif Hanson

PRIMARY CARE PHYSICIAN: Leslie Alanda, MD

SURGEON: Mohomad Almaz, MD

PREOPERATIVE DIAGNOSIS: Residual plexiform fibrous histiocytic tumor of left costovertebral angle area

POSTOPERATIVE DIAGNOSIS: Residual plexiform fibrous histiocytic tumor of left costovertebral angle area

PROCEDURE PERFORMED: Excision of plexiform fibrous histiocytic tumor (this is a mast cell tumor) of left costovertebral angle (this is connective tissue of the back) measuring 2.4 cm, and evacuation of hematoma (this is a postoperative hematoma), left costovertebral angle

ANESTHESIA: General endotracheal was with approximately 20 cc (cubic centimeter) of tumescent solution prepared by adding to 1L of Ringer's lactate, 25 cc 2% Xylocaine, 1 cc of 1:100,000 epinephrine, and 3 cc of 8.4% sodium bicarbonate.

ESTIMATED BLOOD LOSS: Negligible

SURGICAL FINDINGS: There was a healing 2.5-cm (centimeter) incision of the left costovertebral angle, and in the subcutaneous space on top of the latissimus dorsi muscle, there was about a 50-cc hematoma that was beginning to organize.

DESCRIPTION OF PROCEDURE: The patient was intubated and turned in the prone position. The area of the left costovertebral angle was prepped with Betadine scrub and solution and draped in a routine sterile fashion. An incision was made 2 cm around in the previous incision site and carried down to the fascia of the muscle, where a hematoma was entered. The skin portion of that lesion (5.1 cm) was removed, and the fascia and a portion of the muscle of the latissimus dorsi were removed secondarily. Bleeding was electrocoagulated, and a no. 7 Jackson-Pratt drain was inserted in the depth of the wound. The wound was closed with interrupted 0 Monocryl for the deep fascia layer and subcuticular 4-0 Monocryl using a few vertical mattress sutures of 3-0 Monocryl. Steri-Strips and Kerlix fluffs plus Elastoplast were applied. The patient tolerated the procedure well and left the operating room in good condition.

Pathology Report Later Indicated: Mast cell tumor

SERVICE CODE(S): _____

ICD-10-CM DX CODE(S): _____

CASE 8-9A *Operative Report, Shoulder Mass Excision*

LOCATION: Outpatient, Hospital

PATIENT: Verner Fox

SURGEON: Mohomad Almaz, MD

PREOPERATIVE DIAGNOSIS: Giant mass of right shoulder

POSTOPERATIVE DIAGNOSIS: Giant mass of right shoulder, probable lipoma

PROCEDURE PERFORMED: Excision of a giant shoulder mass. The mass was excised and measured 14 × 14 cm × 6 cm deep. This was found to be superficial to the trapezius fascia.

DRAIN: One Jackson-Pratt

PROCEDURE IN DETAIL: After good sedation, the area around the giant mass was anesthetized with a total of 60 cc (cubic centimeter) of 0.5% Marcaine with epinephrine. An incision was made along Langer's line over the apex of the mass. Dissection was carried down through the skin down to the mass itself. Very large skin flaps were created in both directions measure 6 inches and 6 inches. The mass was quite adherent, and any fibrous septa were dissected free to mobilize it. Eventually we were able to mobilize the bottom of the mass, and we were able to reflect it back from the fascia. We then dissected it free of its fascial attachments, going medially to laterally. We then removed it from the lateral attachments that were very close to the skin. After the mass was excised, the wound was thoroughly irrigated. Meticulous hemostasis was obtained with electrocautery. A no. 10 flat Jackson-Pratt drain was placed and brought out inferior to the wound. The wound was then closed in two layers with 3-0 Vicryl subdermal and 2-0 nylon mattress sutures. The drain was secured with 0 Prolene and placed to bulb suction. The patient tolerated the procedure well and was returned to the recovery room in good condition.

Pathology Report Later Indicated: See Report 8-9B.

SERVICE CODE(S): _____

ICD-10-CM DX CODE(S): _____

CASE 8-9B *Pathology Report*

LOCATION: Outpatient, Hospital

PATIENT: Verner Fox

SURGEON: Mohomad Almaz, MD

PATHOLOGIST: Morton Monson, MD

CLINICAL HISTORY: Right shoulder mass

SPECIMEN RECEIVED: Right shoulder mass

GROSS DESCRIPTION: The specimen is labeled with the patient's name and "right shoulder mass" and consists of a 635-gm globulated mass of adipose-like tissue. The exterior surgical margins are inked in black. The mass is approximately 14 × 14 × 6 cm (centimeter) in thickness. Cut sections show adipose tissue throughout. Representative sections are submitted in 13 cassettes.

MICROSCOPIC DESCRIPTION: Sections show adipose throughout, intersected by fine strands of fibrous tissue.

DIAGNOSIS: Right shoulder mass: benign lipoma

SERVICE CODE(S): _____

ICD-10-CM DX CODE(S): _____

CASE 8-10   *Operative Report, Tumor Excision*

LOCATION: Outpatient, Hospital

PATIENT: Ervin Gulman

SURGEON: Mohomad Almaz, MD

PREOPERATIVE DIAGNOSIS: Malignant melanoma, left shoulder (6 cm [centimeter])

POSTOPERATIVE DIAGNOSIS: Malignant melanoma, left shoulder (6 cm [centimeter])

PROCEDURE PERFORMED: Radical excision of malignant melanoma, posterior aspect of skin of left shoulder

ANESTHESIA: General endotracheal with supplementary 1% Xylocaine with 1:100,000 epinephrine, approximately 10 cc (cubic centimeter)

ESTIMATED BLOOD LOSS: Negligible

PROCEDURE: The shoulder was prepped with Betadine scrub and solution and draped in the routine sterile fashion. A margin of about 3 cm (centimeter) laterally and medially around the healed incision site was taken, tapering to 4 to 5 cm proximally and distally. The incision was carried down into the muscle fascia, which was included with the specimen. Bleeding was electrocoagulated, and the wound was closed with subcuticular 2-0 Monocryl and some twists and pulley sutures of 2-0 Monocryl in the center of the wound, where the most tension was. Kerlix fluffs and a sling were applied followed by an external Ace bandage. The patient tolerated the procedure well and left the area in good condition.

Pathology Report Later Indicated: Malignant melanoma of shoulder (this is an upper limb)

SERVICE CODE(S): _____

ICD-10-CM DX CODE(S): _____

(Answers to every other Case are located in Appendix D . The full answer key is only available in the TEACH Instructor Resources on Evolve.)

CASE 8-11   *Operative Report, Ganglion Cyst*

LOCATION: Outpatient, Hospital

PATIENT: Lilah Coan

SURGEON: Mohomad Almaz, MD

INDICATIONS FOR PROCEDURE: This patient has had a ganglion cyst of the second web space of the left hand just proximal to the web space but overlying the ulnar side of the A1 pulley (tendon on anterior surface of finger). It has become annoying and occasionally painful.

PREOPERATIVE DIAGNOSIS: Ganglion cyst, left index finger, with protrusion into second web space on the ulnar side

POSTOPERATIVE DIAGNOSIS: Ganglion cyst, left index finger, with protrusion into second web space on the ulnar side

PROCEDURE PERFORMED: Excision of ganglion cyst, left index finger

SURGICAL FINDINGS: A 1-cm (centimeter) diameter more or less dumbbell-shaped ganglion cyst of the left index finger arises from the ulnar side of the A1 pulley and extending into the base of the second web space.

ANESTHESIA: Intravenous block

ESTIMATED BLOOD LOSS: Zero

COMPLICATIONS: None

SPONGE AND NEEDLE COUNTS: Correct

PROCEDURE: Under satisfactory intravenous block anesthesia, the patient's left hand and arm were prepped with Betadine scrub and solution and draped in the routine sterile fashion. Using 2.5-power magnification, two 1-cm-long Z-plasty flaps were marked out beginning at the central limb, which was situated over the site of the mass. After development of the flaps, dissection was carried down to the A1 pulley, which had a ganglion cyst arising from its surface more or less on the ulnar side and extending in an ulnar direction into the area of the base of the second web space. This cyst was dissected free intact. After completion of the ganglion removal and submission for permanent sections, we closed the wound with interrupted 6-0 Prolene sutures with Gillies sutures for the tips of the flaps. After cleaning Betadine off the hand and the arm, dressing consisted of Xeroform, Kerlix, several Kerlix fluffs, Kerlix roll, Kling, Sof-Rol, and an Ace bandage from the fingers to the elbow. The patient tolerated the procedure well and left the operating room in good condition.

Pathology Report Later Indicated: Ganglion cyst, benign

SERVICE CODE(S): _____

ICD-10-CM DX CODE(S): _____

(Answers to every other Case are located in Appendix D . The full answer key is only available in the TEACH Instructor Resources on Evolve.)

Repair, Revision, and Reconstruction

Most of the anatomic subheadings (e.g., Shoulder or Humerus [Upper Arm] Elbow) in the Musculoskeletal System subsection include a Repair, Revision, and Reconstruction category. The procedures are osteoplasty, osteotomies, arthroplasty, tendon transplants or transfers, and various other repairs, revisions, and reconstructive procedures with numerous grafting procedures for bones, tendons, and muscles. Be certain to identify the correct location and extent of the procedure before assigning a code. A good medical dictionary is an important tool as you report muscle repairs, as only by understanding all of the medical terminology in each report can you be certain to report the service accurately.

CASE 8-12   *Operative Report, Rotator Cuff Repair*

This report states that the reconstruction procedure was a repair with acromioplasty. An acromioplasty is the surgical removal of a portion of the acromion (the highest point on the shoulder) to relieve compression of the rotator cuff when the joint moves. The acromioplasty is bundled into the repair procedure and is not reported separately.

LOCATION: Outpatient, Hospital

PATIENT: Casey Chaput

SURGEON: Mohomad Almaz, MD

PREOPERATIVE DIAGNOSIS: Left, nontraumatic, rotator cuff tear

POSTOPERATIVE DIAGNOSIS: Left, nontraumatic, rotator cuff tear

PROCEDURE PERFORMED: Repair of left rotator cuff repair with Neer acromioplasty

ANESTHESIA: General with endotracheal intubation

FINDINGS: The patient was found to have a complete tear of the rotator cuff. This extended from approximately the level of the long head of the biceps around posteriorly about 2 cm (centimeter).

We created an incision over the left acromion in a shoulder-strap fashion and dissected down through the subcutaneous tissue until we identified the acromion. We reflected the deltoid sharply off the anterior and anterolateral aspect of the acromion. We were then able to view the subacromial space, and we immediately noted a large tear in the rotator cuff. We were careful not to split the deltoid more than about 1 cm.

We then thought there was a rather prominent inferior corner to the anterolateral edge of the acromion. We elected to proceed with a Neer acromioplasty. We then removed the inferior corner of the anterolateral aspect of the acromion using an oscillating saw. We smoothed the undersurface of the acromion with a rasp. After thoroughly irrigating the area with saline, we were able to achieve a very nice view of the rotator cuff tear. We found that the rotator cuff had essentially split into two layers, and they were both avulsed from the humeral head from the long head of the biceps around the articular surface about 2 cm. We freshened the edges of the rotator cuff and then created a bony trough along the margin of the articular surface, starting from the long head of the biceps posteriorly about 2 cm. We then used two sutures of no. 1 Nurolon. We passed each suture through the proximal humerus and out through the bony trough. We then entered the rotator cuff and then again through the bony trough such that when we tied the sutures, the rotator cuff was pulled nicely into the bony trough. We thoroughly irrigated this area before we tied the sutures and then abducted the shoulder as the sutures were tied. Again, the rotator cuff was pulled nicely into the trough without undue tension. We then freshened the margins of the acromion and repaired the deltoid back to the acromion with no. 1 Panacryl suture. We closed the subcutaneous tissue using 2-0 Vicryl, and the skin was closed using 4-0 nylon suture. A sterile Xeroform dressing was applied. Then we placed the patient's left arm into a sling with an abduction pillow to keep the arm abducted slightly. She was then taken from the operating room in good condition and breathing spontaneously. The final sponge and needle counts were correct. She was given 1 g of Kefzol intravenously preoperatively and will be continued on 1 g of Kefzol q.8h. for 2 days.

Pathology Report Later Indicated: Benign tissue and bone morsels

SERVICE CODE(S): _____

ICD-10-CM DX CODE(S): _____

(Answers to every other Case are located in Appendix D . The full answer key is only available in the TEACH Instructor Resources on Evolve.)

Sprains and Strains

Sprain and strain do not mean the same thing. A sprain (Figure 8-6) is a ligament injury, and a strain is a muscle/tendon injury.

Coding for sprains and strains is now more specific, as there are separate codes for sprains and strain. The codes for sprains and strains consist of seven characters with the 7th a character of A (initial), D (subsequent), or S (sequelae). For example, coding for a neck sprain vs. strain:

S33.5XXA Sprain lumbar spine, initial encounter

S39.012A Strain of muscle, fascia, and tendon of lower back, initial encounter

S33.5XXD Sprain lumbar spine, subsequent encounter

S39.012D Strain of muscle, fascia, and tendon of lower back, subsequent encounter

S33.5XXS Sprain lumbar spine, sequelae encounter

S39.012S Strain of muscle, fascia, and tendon of lower back, sequelae encounter

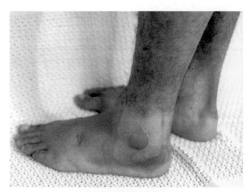

FIGURE 8–6 Ankle sprain.

CASE 8-13A *Consultation, Tendon Rupture*

Since this is the initial episode of treatment of the injury, assign an external cause code to indicate how the injury occurred.

Note that this patient presented to the clinic and a decision was made to admit the patient to the hospital as an inpatient. This fact must be considered when you assign the E&M code.

LOCATION: Outpatient, Clinic

PATIENT: Lyle Conard

ATTENDING PHYSICIAN: Ronald Green, MD

CONSULTANT: Mohomad Almaz, MD

CHIEF COMPLAINT: Right pectoralis major tendon rupture

HISTORY OF PRESENT ILLNESS: This 22-year-old right-hand-dominant student at the University of Manytown presents with an injury of his right pectoralis major that occurred approximately 2 weeks ago. He was doing a bench press at the time and had sudden loss of shape and function of the right pectoralis major. Follow-up examinations confirmed evidence of damage to that tendon.

PAST MEDICAL HISTORY: He had nasal reconstruction done 4 years ago. He has had no other operations. He has had no other ongoing medical concerns.

MEDICATIONS: He takes no medications.

ALLERGIES: He has no allergies.

FAMILY HISTORY: His mother is diabetic, but there have been no other problems within the family for medical concerns.

SOCIAL HISTORY: He is a student living here in Manytown. He is a nonsmoker.

REVIEW OF SYSTEMS: Systems inquiry shows he is otherwise healthy. No weight loss. There is no history of asthma, diabetes, high blood pressure, or cancer. He has no cardiac or pulmonary concerns. There is no hepatic or renal dysfunction. He has no other joint problems related to tendon problems. There are no neurologic, vascular, or skin-related concerns.

PHYSICAL EXAMINATION shows him to have a height of 5 feet 11 inches. Weight of 250 pounds. Blood pressure is 108/80. Head and neck examinations are normal. The chest is symmetrical and clear. The first and second heart sounds are normal; there are no extra heart sounds or murmurs. Abdominal, soft; examination shows no tenderness. Musculoskeletal examination is normal with the exception of the right pectoralis major, which shows obvious evidence of disruption. The neurologic and vascular examinations are normal.

SURGICAL PLAN: The patient will be admitted overnight for repair of the right pectoralis major.

TT: 40 minutes

SERVICE CODE(S): _____

ICD-10-CM DX CODE(S): _____

(Answers to every other Case are located in Appendix D . The full answer key is only available in the TEACH Instructor Resources on Evolve.)

CASE 8-13B *Radiology Report, Shoulder*

This x-ray was done in the clinic prior to admission. Assign an external cause code to indicate how the injury occurred.

LOCATION: Outpatient, Clinic

PATIENT: Lyle Conard

PRIMARY CARE PHYSICIAN: Ronald Green, MD

SURGEON: Mohomad Almaz, MD

RADIOLOGIST: Morton Monson, MD

DIAGNOSIS: Sprain right pectoralis major

RIGHT SHOULDER, ONE VIEW:

FINDINGS: There is no definite evidence for acute fracture or dislocation of the visualized bony structures identified on this examination. The bone mineral density appears to be within normal limits. Please correlate clinically the need for additional more advanced imaging or other evaluation.

SERVICE CODE(S): _____

ICD-10-CM DX CODE(S): _____

(Answers to every other Case are located in Appendix D . The full answer key is only available in the TEACH Instructor Resources on Evolve.)

CASE 8-13C   *Operative Report, Open Tendon Repair*

Assign an external cause code to indicate how the injury occurred. Remember, external cause codes are assigned for the length of treatment for I-10.

LOCATION: Inpatient, Hospital

PATIENT: Lyle Conard

PRIMARY CARE PHYSICIAN: Ronald Green, MD

SURGEON: Mohomad Almaz, MD

PREOPERATIVE DIAGNOSIS: Right shoulder pectoralis major tendon rupture

POSTOPERATIVE DIAGNOSIS: Complete right pectoralis major tendon rupture

PROCEDURE PERFORMED: Open repair, right pectoralis major

CLINICAL HISTORY: This 22-year-old gentleman injured his right pectoralis major while weight lifting approximately 14 days ago. He presented to orthopedics yesterday. It was determined that he had a complete rupture of his right pectoralis major and that surgery was necessary. He was advised that because of the delay there was some further risk if we went any further before having this repaired, and we recommended that surgery be done as soon as possible. After the risks and benefits of anesthesia and surgery were explained to both the patient and his parents, the decision was made to undertake the procedure.

OPERATIVE REPORT: Under general anesthetic, the patient was laid in a beach-chair position on the operating table. He was given 1 g of cefazolin intravenously before the onset of surgery. The right shoulder was prepped and draped in the usual fashion. A deltopectoral incision approximately 10 cm (centimeter) long was made and was deepened through subcutaneous tissue to expose the deltoid fascia. Immediately apparent was that there was complete avulsion of the pectoralis major with retraction of the muscle medially. The tendinous portion of the muscle was quite inflamed and macerated. It was typical of the type of softened tendon we would expect 14 days post injury. The area on the humerus where the tendon had been avulsed was exposed. Just lateral to the biceps tendon, three Mitek super anchors were then placed down into the bone with no. 2 Ethibond sutures coming from them. A series of no. 5 Ethibond sutures were then woven through the tendon medially to act as stay sutures. These allowed us to place traction on the muscle and bring it toward the arm attachment. The no. 2 Ethibond sutures were then placed through tendinous structures from the top to bottom and sewn down into position. The tendon was then further anchored using the no. 5 Ethibond sutures to the surrounding structures laterally. When this was done, there was quite a firm repair. Because of the length of time in contracture, however, the muscle itself was not flexible enough to allow substantial external rotation. The wound was then thoroughly irrigated with normal saline and closed in layers with absorbable suture and Steri-Strips. The wound was then infiltrated with Marcaine and dressed with Vaseline gauze, 4 × 4s, and HypaFix. The arm was then placed in a CryoCuff sling. The patient awakened, was placed on his hospital bed, and was taken to the recovery room in good condition. Estimated blood loss for the procedure was less than 100 cc. The sponge and needle counts were correct.

SERVICE CODE(S): _____

ICD-10-CM DX CODE(S): _____

(Answers to every other Case are located in Appendix D . The full answer key is only available in the TEACH Instructor Resources on Evolve.)

CASE 8-13D   *Discharge Summary*

Assign an external cause code to indicate how the injury occurred. Remember, external cause codes are assigned for the length of treatment for I-10.

LOCATION: Inpatient, Hospital

PATIENT: Lyle Conard

PRIMARY CARE PHYSICIAN: Ronald Green, MD

SURGEON: Mohomad Almaz, MD

FINAL DIAGNOSIS: Right pectoralis major tendon rupture

CLINICAL HISTORY: This 22-year-old gentleman injured his right pectoralis major 2 weeks ago. He was doing a bench press at that time. He had a sudden pain in the right pectoral area.

Surgical examination confirmed that he has complete rupture of the right pectoralis major.

The patient was taken to surgery yesterday for repair of the tendon of the right pectoralis major. No perioperative complications occurred. The patient's pain was controlled with the usual analgesics postoperatively. He was discharged home in the care of his parents today. Arrangements were made for him to be seen by myself in follow-up in 7 to 8 days. He will be sent home with Lorcet for analgesic in the interval.

SERVICE CODE(S): _____

ICD-10-CM DX CODE(S): _____

(Answers to every other Case are located in Appendix D . The full answer key is only available in the TEACH Instructor Resources on Evolve.)

CASE 8-14 *Operative Report, Tendon Repair*

Assign an external cause code to indicate how the injury occurred. In this report, there is no indication of how the injury occurred, so assign an unspecified accident external cause code.

LOCATION: Outpatient, Hospital

PATIENT: Melvin Brodern

ATTENDING PHYSICIAN: Mohomad Almaz, MD

SURGEON: Mohomad Almaz, MD

PREOPERATIVE PROCEDURE: Quadriceps tendon rupture, right knee

POSTOPERATIVE PROCEDURE: Quadriceps tendon rupture, right knee

OPERATIVE PROCEDURE: Repair of quadriceps tendon, right knee

OPERATIVE PROCEDURE: After suitable spinal anesthesia had been achieved, the patient's right knee was prepped and draped in the usual manner. Prior to prepping, a thigh tourniquet was applied. A midline skin incision was made from the inferior pole of the patella to one handbreadth above the superior pole of the patella. The patient had a thickened prepatellar bursa and chronic bursitis. This was partially excised. The quadriceps tendon was exposed. The patient had complete rupture of the quadriceps tendon extending to the medial and lateral retinacula. The interposed clot was removed. Four blocking stitches of no. 5 Ethibond were then placed into the central aspect of the quadriceps tendon. These were passed through drill holes, going from the superior pole of the patella to the inferior pole of the patella. The sutures were then tied over a bone bridge at the inferior pole of the patella securing the main portion of the quadriceps tendon back to the patella. The medial and lateral retinacula tears were then repaired with interrupted no. 1 Panacryl. Before wound closure, a Hemovac drain was inserted into the knee joint. Subcutaneous tissue was then closed with 2-0 Vicryl, and the skin was closed with staples. A fiberglass cylinder cast was then applied. The tourniquet was released before cast application. After tourniquet release, good circulation was noted to return to the foot. The patient tolerated the procedure well and returned to the recovery room in stable condition.

SERVICE CODE(S): _____

ICD-10-CM DX CODE(S): _____

(Answers to every other Case are located in Appendix D . The full answer key is only available in the TEACH Instructor Resources on Evolve.)

CASE 8-15 *Operative Report, Arthroplasty*

LOCATION: Inpatient, Hospital

PATIENT: Jack Baglien

SURGEON: Mohomad Almaz, MD

PREOPERATIVE DIAGNOSIS: Osteoarthritis, right knee

POSTOPERATIVE DIAGNOSIS: Osteoarthritis, right knee

PROCEDURE PERFORMED: Right cemented posterior stabilized total knee arthroplasty

COMPONENTS USED: Duracon size extra-large femur, size large 2 tibia, 9-mm (millimeter) posterior stabilized tibial insert, and 33-mm symmetric patella

OPERATIVE PROCEDURE: After suitable epidural anesthesia had been achieved, the patient's right knee was prepped and draped in the usual manner. Before prepping, the thigh tourniquet was applied, but initially it was not inflated. A long anterior midline skin incision and a long anteromedial arthrotomy were performed. The patient was noted to have marked synovitis in his knee. Once the synovial bleeders, capsular bleeders, and skin bleeders were cauterized, the leg was stripped with an Esmarch, and the tourniquet inflated to 275 mmHg (millimeter of mercury).

A partial fat pad excision was performed. The patella was dislocated laterally. An entry hole was made in the distal femur for the intramedullary alignment rod. Rotation was selected off the interepicondylar axis. Anterior referencing instruments were used. Using the intramedullary alignment, the anterior shim cut and then the distal femoral cuts were performed. The tibia was then subluxed forward. The proximal tibial cut was performed. Nine millimeters of bone were excised, referencing off the intact lateral femur. The extension gap was then measured. The flexion gap was assessed, and a mark was placed on the distal femur to reproduce the identical flexion gap. This indicated the femoral component should be extra-large sized. An extra-large 4-in-1 jig was then applied. Anterior and posterior chamfer cuts were then performed. A trial femur was then placed to fit very well. A trial tibia with a 9-mm insert was placed, and there was excellent alignment and good stability. The patella was then everted and prepared for resurfacing technique using free-hand cuts with a saw. A symmetrical 3-mm trial component was placed and fit quite well. The box was then cut for the posterior stabilized femoral component, and the slot in the tibia was cut for the keel of the tibial component. The wounds were then thoroughly irrigated and dried. Bone graft was placed into the lug holes in the distal femur and the entry hole in the distal femur. The large 2-tibial component was then cemented into place. The extra-large femoral component was cemented into place. A trial tibial insert was in place, and the leg was placed into full extension. The patellar component was then cemented into place. Once the cement was hard, stability was reassessed and found to be very good. A trial component was removed. The knee was carefully examined for any cement debris, which was carefully removed. The actual 9-mm posterior stabilized insert was then placed, and a locking screw was placed. The knee was then thoroughly irrigated. Autotransfusion Hemovac drain was placed. The wound was closed in layers. The capsule was closed with no. 1 Panacryl, the subcutaneous tissue with 2-0 Vicryl, and the skin with staples. A Robert Jones dressing and anterior splint were then applied. Before wound closure, an autotransfusion Hemovac drain was placed. The patient tolerated the procedure well and returned to the recovery room in stable condition.

Pathology Report Later Indicated: Benign bone.

SERVICE CODE(S): _____

ICD-10-CM DX CODE(S): _____

(Answers to every other Case are located in Appendix D . The full answer key is only available in the TEACH Instructor Resources on Evolve.)

Grafts (or Implants)

There are several types of grafts, including bone, tissue (fat, dermis), cartilage, tendon, bone marrow, and fascia lata (the deep fascia of the thigh).

An allograft, also known as an allogeneic graft or a homograft, is body tissue or an organ transplanted from one person to another, including from cadavers. However, an autograft utilizes a person's own bone or tissue that is transplanted from one area of the body to another. The most common site of the body for a bone autograft is the hip.

Late Effects

Sometimes an acute illness or injury leaves a patient with a residual health problem that remains after the illness or injury has resolved. The residual effect or manifestation is coded first, and then the late effects code is assigned to indicate the cause of the residual. An example would be scars (residual) that remain after a severe burn (cause).

In most instances, two codes will be assigned—one code for the **residual** that is being treated (chief complaint) and one code that indicates the **sequelae/late effect** (cause). There is no time limit for the development of a residual. It may be evident at the time of the acute illness, or it may occur months after an injury. It is also possible that a patient may develop more than one residual. For example, a patient who has had a stroke may develop right-sided hemiparesis (paralysis of one side) and aphasia (loss of ability to communicate). However, a person cannot have a current hip fracture (S72.009A) and a late effect of hip fracture (S72.009S) at the same site. The code is either a current injury or a condition caused by a prior injury. (The only exception to this rule is in category I69, Sequelae/Late effects of cerebrovascular disease.)

The late effects code is accessed in the Index under the main term "Sequelae". When reporting codes for late effects of an injury, the initial injury code is reported with the 7th character "S" to indicate sequelae. Report the specific type of sequelae (e.g., scar) followed by the injury code with the 7th character "S."

CASE 8-16   *Operative Report, Fusion with Autograft*

Assign a diagnosis code for the osteoarthritis of the foot and a sequelae/late effects code for the bone fracture of the extremity. Note the "due to old calcaneal fracture," which is the indication for the sequelae/late effects code. Code only the autograft for services provided.

LOCATION: Outpatient, Hospital

PATIENT: Rose Stich

SURGEON: Mohomad Almaz, MD

PREOPERATIVE DIAGNOSIS: Posttraumatic subtalar osteoarthritis, left hindfoot, due to old calcaneal fracture

POSTOPERATIVE DIAGNOSIS: Posttraumatic subtalar osteoarthritis, left hindfoot, due to old calcaneal fracture

PROCEDURE PERFORMED: Left subtalar fusion using moldable autograft obtained from the left iliac crest

OPERATIVE PROCEDURE: After suitable general anesthesia had been achieved, the patient's left iliac crest and left foot and ankle were prepped and draped in the usual manner. Before prepping, a thigh tourniquet was applied but initially not inflated. Bone graft was harvested from the left iliac crest. A 10-cm (centimeter) incision was made and carried down through the subcutaneous fat. The fascia was incised in line with the crest starting about 2 cm back from the anterior-superior iliac spine. Cortical cancellous bone graft was then harvested from the inner table. Defect was packed with

Gelfoam. The wound was closed in layers. The skin was closed with staples.

The leg was then elevated. The tourniquet was inflated. The incision was made from the tip of the fibula to the base of the fourth metatarsal. The distally based flap of the extensor digitorum brevis was elevated off the lateral aspect of the calcaneus. Fat pad and the sinus tarsi were split in line with the skin incision. Anterior process of the calcaneus was excised. The capsule was incised. A lot of thickened synovial tissue was removed. The joint surfaces were noted to be substantially damaged from the old calcaneal fracture. The remaining articular cartilage and scar tissue were removed with a curet and rongeur. The subchondral bone was then carefully burred down to a bleeding surface. Autograft from the iliac crest was then packed in between the bone surfaces. Using an image intensifier, a large-fragment cannulated screw was then placed starting at the talar neck across the posterior face of the subtalar joint into the central aspect of the calcaneal body. Further gap in the fusion at the sinus tarsi area was filled with autograft and allograft. The wound was then closed. Skin was closed with 4-0 nylon. Dressing and a Robert Jones dressing with a posterior fiberglass splint were then applied. The tourniquet was released. Following tourniquet release, good circulation was noted to return to the foot. The patient tolerated the procedure well and returned to the recovery room in stable condition.

SERVICE CODE(S): _____

ICD-10-CM DX CODE(S): _____

(Answers to every other Case are located in Appendix D . The full answer key is only available in the TEACH Instructor Resources on Evolve.)

Fractures

Several methods are employed to repair fractures. Open treatment of a fracture is when a surgeon opens the tissue and the fracture is exposed; the fractured bone can then be visualized by the physician. Closed treatment is when the fracture is repaired without the physician directly visualizing the fracture. Fractures are reported by the specific anatomic site and the reason for the repair. Manipulation is manually returning the bone (pushing or pulling) to proper alignment without an incision. The codes are often divided based on whether or not manipulation was performed in closed treatment of a fracture.

The CPT manual defines the key fracture repair terms as follows:

■ **Closed treatment** describes procedures that treat fractures by one of three methods: (1) without manipulation, (2) with manipulation, or (3) with or without traction.

■ **Manipulation** is a reduction, which is an attempt to maneuver the bone back into proper anatomic alignment.

The physician may bend, rotate, pull, or guide the bone back into position.

■ **Closed treatment without manipulation** is a procedure in which the physician immobilizes the bone with a splint, cast, or other device but without having to manipulate the fracture into alignment first.

■ **Closed treatment with manipulation** is a procedure in which the physician has to reduce (put back in place) the fracture.

■ **Open treatment** is used when the fracture is surgically opened (exposed to the external environment). In this instance, the fracture (bone) is open to view, and internal fixation (pins, screws, etc.) may be used. Open treatment can also mean that a remote site (not directly over the fracture) is opened to place a nail (intramedullary) across the fracture site.

■ **Percutaneous skeletal fixation** describes fracture treatment that is neither open nor closed. In this procedure, the fracture is not open to view, but fixation (e.g., pins) is placed through the skin across the fracture site, usually under x-ray imaging.

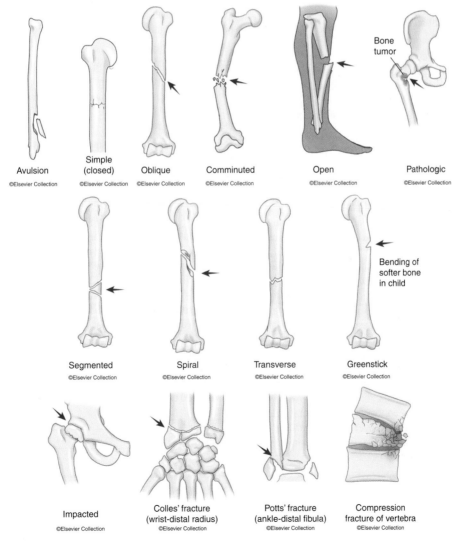

Avulsion	Simple (closed)	Oblique	Comminuted	Open	Pathologic
©Elsevier Collection	©Elsevier Collection	©Elsevier Collection	©Elsevier Collection	©Elsevier Collection	©Elsevier Collection

Bone tumor

Segmented	Spiral	Transverse	Greenstick
©Elsevier Collection	©Elsevier Collection	©Elsevier Collection	©Elsevier Collection

Bending of softer bone in child

Impacted	Colles' fracture (wrist-distal radius)	Potts' fracture (ankle-distal fibula)	Compression fracture of vertebra
©Elsevier Collection	©Elsevier Collection	©Elsevier Collection	©Elsevier Collection

FIGURE 8–7 Types of fractures.

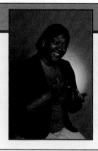

From the Trenches

"You will need to have a basic grasp of medical terminology and human anatomy, in addition to being analytical. Logic and the ability to thoroughly analyze information are also important traits."

LETITIA PATTERSON
MPA, RHIA, CCS-P, CPC, CPMA, CPC-I

CASE 8-17A   *Operative Report, Open Reduction*

Assign an external cause code to indicate how the injury occurred.

LOCATION: Outpatient, Hospital

PATIENT: Doyle Dryhdahl

SURGEON: Mohomad Almaz, MD

PREOPERATIVE DIAGNOSIS: Displaced fracture, right scaphoid

POSTOPERATIVE DIAGNOSIS: Displaced fracture, right scaphoid

OPERATIVE PROCEDURE: Right scaphoid open reduction internal fixation with bone grafting

CLINICAL HISTORY: This gentleman presents with a history of having injured his right scaphoid in 2001 and had an open reduction internal fixation at that time. He had been managing quite well until a week ago, when his arm was hit by a sledgehammer. Follow-up x-rays showed displacement of the scaphoid area. It was unclear whether this was a new fracture or displacement of a nonunion. After the risks and benefits of anesthesia and surgery were explained to the patient, a decision was made to undertake the procedure.

PROCEDURE: Under a general anesthetic, the patient was laid supine on the operating table. The right hand was prepped and draped in the usual fashion. He was given 1 g of cefazolin intravenously before the onset of surgery. A tourniquet was then inflated around the right upper arm to 250 mmHg (millimeter of mercury). We used the same volar incision for access that had been used previously. It was deepened through subcutaneous tissue and down through the scar to expose the volar carpal ligaments, which were then incised longitudinally to allow access to the scaphoid tubercle and the wrist joint. With this done, we were then able to expose the scaphoid fully. We could see that there was some scar tissue present in the area of the fracture. This was all excised to get us down to hard bone. Distally, there was reasonable blood supply. Proximally, it was not clear that there was any evidence of blood supply to the proximal pole. A curet was then used to remove the sclerotic bone along the margins of the area. When this was done, a single K-wire was then introduced across the fracture on the ulnar side to stabilize it. We had to open the bone because there was a tendency toward a humpback deformity. With the gap created, we then removed the Herbert screw that had been placed previously. We then switched

to the AcroMed screw system. A single guide pin was then placed down the central axis of the scaphoid, and we then viewed this with anteroposterior and lateral fluoroscopic imaging. Satisfied that the position of the guide pin was accurate, we then drilled the hole for the AcroMed screw. We measured it and decided that a 20-mm (millimeter) screw would be sufficiently long to stabilize the fracture. A 20-mm AcroMed was then introduced and then held firmly. It gave good support, and the temporary K-wire was then removed and the guide pin removed.

We now had a gap of approximately 1 cm (centimeter) on the volar cortex. We elected to treat this with local graft from the distal radius.

Accordingly, at the proximal end of our incision, the distal radius was exposed through the pronator quadratus. An osteotome was then used to remove a triangular shape bone cortical graft. The cancellous graft was then harvested with a curet.

The cancellous graft was then packed firmly into the cavity of the scaphoid. When this was completed, we had filled the cavity. The cortical graft was then wedged into the defect on the volar cortex of the scaphoid and tamped into place with a bone tamp. When this was completed, we had a very secure solid construct of the volar cortex and the scaphoid was filled with cancellous bone.

The wound was then thoroughly irrigated with normal saline. The volar carpal ligaments were then repaired with 2-0 Vicryl suture. Fascial layers were then closed with absorbable sutures, and the skin was closed with Monocryl. The wound edges were also opposed with Steri-Strips and then infiltrated with Marcaine. The wound was then dressed with Vaseline gauze, 4 × 4s, and sterile Sof-Rol, and a thumb spica splint was then placed on and held in position with Kerlix and an Ace wrap. The patient's arm was then placed in a sling. The tourniquet was deflated after a total of 80 minutes. The patient was then awakened, placed on his hospital bed, and taken to the recovery room in good condition. Estimated blood loss for the procedure was less than 20 cc. The sponge and needle counts were correct.

SERVICE CODE(S): _____

ICD-10-CM DX CODE(S): _____

(Answers to every other Case are located in Appendix D . The full answer key is only available in the TEACH Instructor Resources on Evolve.)

CASE 8-17B *Radiology Report, Wrist*

Assign an external cause code to indicate how the injury occurred.

LOCATION: Outpatient, Hospital

PATIENT: Doyle Dryhdahl

SURGEON: Mohomad Almaz, MD

RADIOLOGIST: Morton Monson, MD

CLINICAL FINDINGS: Displaced fracture, right scaphoid

AP (ANTERIOR POSTERIOR) AND LATERAL VIEWS OF THE RIGHT WRIST PERFORMED INTEROPERATIVELY:

FINDINGS: Screw fixation across a fracture of the right scaphoid

SERVICE CODE(S): _____

ICD-10-CM DX CODE(S): _____

(Answers to every other Case are located in Appendix D . The full answer key is only available in the TEACH Instructor Resources on Evolve.)

CASE 8-18 *Operative Report, Closed Reduction*

Do not report the x-ray service provided; only report the surgeon's service and diagnosis code(s).

LOCATION: Outpatient, Hospital

PATIENT: Scott Laranzo

SURGEON: Mohomad Almaz, MD

DIAGNOSIS: Right hand fourth metacarpal fracture, transverse and displaced. Patient was injured in a fight.

PROCEDURE PERFORMED: Closed reduction, percutaneous pin fixation of right fourth metacarpal fracture

PROCEDURE: Under a satisfactory level of sedation and regional block, the extremity was prepped and draped. At this time, the fracture was

reducible with distraction and manipulation. This was then further augmented with intramedullary retrograde pinning.

This was demonstrated in AP (anterior posterior), lateral, and oblique views to maintain virtually anatomic position. I elected, at this time, to leave the pin proud and dress the pin, and then applied an ulnar gutter spica cast, fiberglass, about the extremity, keeping free and mobile the thumb and the index finger. There were no other complicating events. Fluoroscopy photos were obtained. The patient tolerated the procedure well.

SERVICE CODE(S): _____

ICD-10-CM DX CODE(S): _____

(Answers to every other Case are located in Appendix D . The full answer key is only available in the TEACH Instructor Resources on Evolve.)

CASE 8-19A *Radiology Report, Right Femur*

Becky Bradley fell while walking to her car today and was seen in the emergency department by Dr. Sutton, who called Becky's primary care physician, Dr. Green. Dr. Sutton had ordered an x-ray, and when Dr. Green arrived at the emergency department he reviewed the x-ray. Report Dr. Monson's radiology service. Assume from this point on in this chapter that the health care facility requires external cause codes to be assigned for all initial treatments of injuries. This is a case for good medical terminology because the word "shaft" does not appear in the report. The coder needs to know epiphysis from diaphysis and distal from proximal. Other femur codes mention epiphysis, but none mention diaphysis.

LOCATION: Outpatient, Hospital

PATIENT: Becky Bradley

PRIMARY CARE PHYSICIAN: Ronald Green, MD

EMERGENCY DEPARTMENT PHYSICIAN: Paul Sutton, MD

RADIOLOGIST: Morton Monson, MD

EXAMINATION OF: Right femur

CLINICAL SYMPTOMS: Right leg pain, status post fall while walking to car today

RIGHT FEMUR, TWO VIEWS: No prior studies are available for comparison. There is evidence of an acute fracture involving the proximal diaphysis of the femur. This is severely angulated laterally and anteriorly. It is slightly impacted. Additional acute fractures are not seen, although views of the femur are somewhat limited. The femoral head appears to be seated within the acetabulum. There is some cortical thickening involving the slightly more distal femoral diaphysis. I do not know whether this is from a previous injury or some sort of a benign cortical thickening. I do not see gross destructive change. This should be clinically correlated, however.

CONCLUSION: Acute displaced fracture involving the proximal diaphysis of the right femur. Additional fractures are not seen, although views are somewhat limited. There is also an incidental finding of cortical thickening involving the slightly more distal femoral diaphysis. I believe this is most likely a benign cortical thickening because I do not see obvious destructive change involving the cortex. This could even be sequelae from perhaps a previous injury. This, of course, must be clinically correlated.

SERVICE CODE(S): _____

ICD-10-CM DX CODE(S): _____

(Answers to every other Case are located in Appendix D . The full answer key is only available in the TEACH Instructor Resources on Evolve.)

CASE 8-19B *Orthopedic Consultation, Thigh Pain*

Based on the x-ray and Dr. Sutton's notes (which are not available to you here), Dr. Green decided to admit Becky to the hospital immediately. Dr. Green also contacted Dr. Almaz, an orthopedist, to provide a consultation regarding Becky's care.

LOCATION: Inpatient, Hospital

PATIENT: Becky Bradley

ATTENDING PHYSICIAN: Ronald Green, MD

CONSULTANT: Mohomad Almaz, MD

CHIEF COMPLAINT: Pain, right thigh

HISTORY OF PRESENT ILLNESS: This patient was walking to her car this afternoon and twisted and then developed acute pain in the right thigh. She fell. She had marked deformity of the thigh. X-rays revealed a midshaft fracture of the femur. The patient states that she has had right thigh pain for several months. She has been evaluated by Dr. Sutton. Bone scan was performed last month, and it suggested a stress fracture of both femurs. Right side has been much more symptomatic than the left. She has been prescribed Fosamax and Evista.

PAST MEDICAL HISTORY: History of hypothyroidism. She is taking Synthroid. She has a history of osteoporosis and is taking Fosamax and Evista. Patient denies any history of diabetes, coronary artery disease, or lung problems.

ALLERGIES: Penicillin, which results in a rash.

The patient is using a cane because of her thigh pain.

PHYSICAL EXAMINATION: On examination, she is in moderate distress. Blood pressure was initially 200/104. Pulse is 80 and regular. There is no neck tenderness. She has a contusion on the left frontal area.

There was no loss of consciousness with this fall. She has no chest wall tenderness. Upper extremities are nontender. Left lower extremity is nontender. Right lower extremity has marked shortening and marked deformity of the midthigh. She has good pedal pulses and normal sensation in the foot.

X-rays reveal a transverse fracture of the midshaft of the femur on the right side.

It sounds like she has had some ongoing problems with thigh pain from a stress fracture, and I think she completed the stress fracture this evening. I do not see any evidence on the plane x-ray to suggest anything else going on other than osteoporosis. Certainly she could also have osteomalacia. I see no evidence of any metastatic disease for the femurs.

I recommended to the family that we stabilize this evening with an intramedullary nail. In addition to taking Fosamax and Evista, because of her problems with the left femur, I recommend we add calcitonin, and we should also add a high dose of vitamin D for osteomalacia. If the left side becomes more symptomatic, we may want to consider prophylactic intramedullary nailing.

Operative procedure was discussed with the patient and family. Risks and benefits were discussed and typical postoperative course discussed. I advised that the patient has already lost blood into the femur fracture and may lose further blood with the surgery and may require transfusion. Risks and benefits of transfusion were discussed with the family. All questions were answered.

SERVICE CODE(S): _____

ICD-10-CM DX CODE(S): _____

(Answers to every other Case are located in Appendix D . The full answer key is only available in the TEACH Instructor Resources on Evolve.)

CASE 8-19C *Operative Report, Femur Repair, Intramedullary Nailing*

Becky has been scheduled for repair of her fractured right femur. Report Dr. Almaz's surgical services.

LOCATION: Inpatient, Hospital

PATIENT: Becky Bradley

ATTENDING PHYSICIAN: Ronald Green, MD

SURGEON: Mohomad Almaz, MD

PREOPERATIVE DIAGNOSIS: Transverse midshaft fracture, right femur

POSTOPERATIVE DIAGNOSIS: Transverse midshaft fracture, right femur

PROCEDURE PERFORMED: Intramedullary nailing, right femur

OPERATIVE PROCEDURE: After suitable general anesthesia had been achieved, the patient was positioned on the fracture table for right femoral nailing. The patient's right buttock, thigh, and knee were

prepped and draped. A 7-cm (centimeter) incision was made on the lateral aspect of the buttock. The incision was carried down to fascia. The fascia was split just above the greater trochanter. A guide pin was inserted into the piriformis fossa. A 13-mm (millimeter) reamer was used over the guide pin to establish the entry hole. A guidewire was then easily passed across the fracture site and impacted into the distal femoral metaphysis. Reaming was then done to 14 mm. A 13 × 360-mm Synthes titanium-cannulated nail was then inserted. Proximal and distal locking was performed. The incisions were then irrigated. The wounds were closed in layers, and the skin was closed with staples. Estimated blood loss for the procedure was 100 ml (milliliter). The patient tolerated the procedure well and returned to the recovery room in stable condition.

SERVICE CODE(S): _____

ICD-10-CM DX CODE(S): _____

(Answers to every other Case are located in Appendix D . The full answer key is only available in the TEACH Instructor Resources on Evolve.)

CASE 8-19D *Discharge Summary*

LOCATION: Inpatient, Hospital

PATIENT: Becky Bradley

PRIMARY CARE PHYSICIAN: Ronald Green, MD

PRINCIPAL DIAGNOSIS: Transverse midshaft fracture, right femur, secondary to osteoporosis/osteomalacia.

PRINCIPAL PROCEDURE: Yesterday the patient underwent an intramedullary nailing, right femur.

HISTORY OF PRESENT ILLNESS: The patient had thigh pain for several months. X-rays suggested possible stress fracture, as did bone scan. She was placed on Fosamax and Evista. On the day of admission, she was turning to get into the car and her right femur snapped.

COURSE IN HOSPITAL: She was seen by Dr. Elhart from cardiology for preoperative evaluation regarding her hypertension. He thought her hypertension was up a little bit secondary to pain, but otherwise she was stable for surgery. On the day of admission, she was taken to the operating room and an open intramedullary nailing of the right femur was performed. There were no intraoperative or postoperative complications. She will be seen at the rehabilitation center for continued therapy.

DISCHARGE RECOMMENDATIONS: Remove staples 2 weeks postoperatively. Follow-up is with me in 3 to 4 weeks postoperatively.

SERVICE CODE(S): _____

ICD-10-CM DX CODE(S): _____

(Answers to every other Case are located in Appendix D . The full answer key is only available in the TEACH Instructor Resources on Evolve.)

CASE 8-20A *Orthopedic Consultation, Supracondylar Fracture*

LOCATION: Inpatient, Hospital

PATIENT: Lourene Bohn

PRIMARY CARE PHYSICIAN: Maxamillian Conclave, MD

CONSULTATION: Mohomad Almaz, MD

CHIEF COMPLAINT: Left thigh pain

HISTORY OF PRESENT ILLNESS: The patient is a 54-year-old woman accompanied today by her son. They were referred by Dr. Conclave from Anytown. The patient explained that she was walking in the hallway in her house when she just fell, injuring her left femur. She was brought by ambulance to see Dr. Conclave, who obtained an x-ray that revealed a comminuted displaced supracondylar fracture of her left femur. She was transported here. She is complaining of pain only in her left thigh and denies pain elsewhere. She denies any loss of sensation. She did tell me she had had a stroke, I believe, in 1999, resulting in left-sided weakness. She has regained much of the function of her left arm but still has a weak left leg. She walks with a walker outside but can sometimes get along without the walker at home. She also is a diabetic and recently developed bronchitis. I am told that the ambulance crew had a hard time keeping her sats above 90% on her way here today. This was with the use of oxygen. She lives at home with her husband and one son.

PAST MEDICAL HISTORY reveals that she has no known allergies to medications. She has a history of hypertension along with marked obesity. She had a CVA (stroke/cerebrovascular accident) in 1999. She told me that she has had cellulitis of her legs in the past but not currently.

PHYSICAL EXAMINATION today finds that she is an alert and cooperative, obese woman lying in the supine position. She appears to be fairly comfortable. All extremities are symmetrical. She is able to move her upper extremities and her right leg. She is unable to move her left leg because of pain in her left thigh. She can dorsiflex and plantarflex her toes slightly, although she does not have a full range of motion. She does not have a full range of motion of her ankle. She explains that she has not been able to move her left leg well since she had her stroke in 1999. She does have rather leathery skin involving the distal two thirds of her leg between her knee and her ankle. There are no lacerations or abrasions. I am unable to palpate the dorsalis pedis or the posterior tibialis pulse in her left foot, but the foot is warm and sensation is intact to light touch. She is unable to move her left leg without pain.

X-rays of her left distal femur found that she does have a comminuted supracondylar fracture, which is displaced. It appears that she may have some early osteophytes forming about her left knee. No other fractures are noted.

IMPRESSION:

1. Comminuted displaced supracondylar fracture, left distal femur
2. History of diabetes mellitus
3. History of recent onset bronchitis
4. Obesity
5. History of hypertension
6. Status post cellulitis, lower extremities

RECOMMENDATIONS: I have thoroughly discussed this fracture with her and her son, who accompanied her today. I have recommended that we proceed with an open reduction internal fixation of this supracondylar fracture. I have discussed the procedure along with the risks involved and specifically mentioned the possibility of an infection or the possibility of loss of fixation, malunion, or nonunion. We have also discussed the possibility of a stroke or a heart attack, especially because she has had a previous stroke. Certainly there are very significant risks involved here. They understand this and would like to proceed. We have mentioned other forms of treatment including the possibility of traction; however, due to her size and the length of traction required, I do not think this is a good option. I have asked Dr. Green to see her preoperatively. If he believes that she is an acceptable candidate for surgery, we will plan this for tomorrow. Their questions have been answered.

SERVICE CODE(S): _____

ICD-10-CM DX CODE(S): _____

(Answers to every other Case are located in Appendix D . The full answer key is only available in the TEACH Instructor Resources on Evolve.)

CASE 8-20B   *Operative Report, Supracondylar Fracture*

LOCATION: Inpatient, Hospital

PATIENT: Lourene Bohn

PRIMARY CARE PHYSICIAN: Maxamillian Conclave, MD

ATTENDING: Mohomad Almaz, MD

PREOPERATIVE DIAGNOSIS: Supracondylar fracture, left distal femur

POSTOPERATIVE DIAGNOSIS: Supracondylar fracture, left distal femur

ANESTHESIA: General

FINDINGS: The patient was found to have a markedly comminuted supracondylar fracture. This fracture extended down to the condyles but not between them. We were able to achieve a near anatomic output, but we bone grafted this fracture as well.

PROCEDURE: The patient was brought from the intensive care unit, where she had already been intubated for several days. She was placed under a general anesthetic and then transported carefully to the operating room table. She is a very heavy woman, weighing nearly 300 pounds, and we had to be very careful with her. We padded all bony prominences.

We then prepped the patient's left leg by applying traction to the leg and supporting it during the prep. We prepped with Betadine and then draped it in a sterile fashion.

We then created a longitudinal incision over the anterolateral aspect of her left knee and leg. We carried the dissection down through the subcutaneous tissue and identified the fascia longitudinally. We reflected the vastus lateralis off the lateral intermuscular septum, and we were able to identify the femur and the fracture. We cauterized the perforators as we approached them. We then exposed the lateral femoral condyle, and we could identify the patellofemoral joint. We found that the supracondylar fracture was a markedly comminuted fracture with multiple fragments. We elected first of all to apply a cerclage wire (*an encircling loop*) around the distal fragment to more or less hold this in position as there were some longitudinal cracks, especially over the anterior surface of the distal femur. This seemed to help hold things in position as we manipulated the fracture into a more anatomic position. After having done this, we used the guide for the 95 supracondylar C-arm image intensifier to identify the location of this wire because we certainly could not palpate the distal end of the wire due to her obesity.

We eventually passed a reamer over this guidewire and reamed to a depth of about 65 mm (millimeter). We then placed a 70-mm lag screw across the condyles and eventually attached a 16-hole 95 supracondylar plate. We were able to position this adjacent to the femur quite nicely and hold the fracture in a near anatomic position. We eventually used a second cerclage wire around the femur and removed the first. We used a cable lock to enhance our fixation on the distal fragment. We were able to get two good cancellous screws and this cable lock around the distal fragment. This seemed to provide excellent fixation, together with the lag screw. We placed cortical screws in the remainder of the plate, and this provided again excellent fixation of the proximal fragment as well. These screws were somewhat difficult to insert, and we did end up twisting the heads off two of the screws in midportion of the plate. In the end, however, we obtained excellent fixation of the proximal fragment, and we felt that we had good fixation of the distal fragment as well. There was no motion of the fracture site with range of motion of the knee. The bone at the fracture site, however, appeared to be quite thin, and we will need to be very careful in moving her leg in the future until this fracture heals. We felt that bone grafting this area would be a good idea. We then used cancellous bone chips from the Red Cross and scattered these about the fracture site. There were several of her bone fragments, which we had removed. We were able to place these into the femur as in completing a jigsaw puzzle.

We thoroughly irrigated the area frequently with saline throughout this procedure. We finally tightened the cable lock on the distal fragment at the end of the procedure so that we could be certain that it would be tight after we had inserted all those screws. We crimped the cable and cut off the excess cable.

We then repaired the fascia using 0 Vicryl and the subcutaneous tissue with 2-0 Vicryl. We closed the skin with skin staples. A sterile Xeroform dressing was applied, and we very carefully lifted the leg by lifting behind the distal femur and knee as well as the foot as we applied a knee immobilizer. With the knee immobilizer in place, we were able to transport her back to her hospital bed. She was left intubated and transported to the ICU (intensive care unit). She was given IV (intravenous) antibiotics ahead of time and will be continued on IV antibiotics for several days postoperatively. She tolerated the procedure well.

SERVICE CODE(S): _____

ICD-10-CM DX CODE(S): _____

(Answers to every other Case are located in Appendix D . The full answer key is only available in the TEACH Instructor Resources on Evolve.)

Amputation

An **amputation** is the removal of a limb or an appendage that has been so damaged or diseased that the amputation is the procedure of last resort. Persons with diabetes or vascular disease often have great difficulties with their legs and feet because the blood flow can be so decreased as to cause death to the tissues. In colder climates, frostbite, a condition in which the tissue is frozen and dies, is often a reason for amputation because the necrotic tissue will lead to gangrene and blood poisoning.

CASE 8-21 *Operative Report, Amputation*

LOCATION: Inpatient, Hospital

PATIENT: Edwin Burslie

SURGEON: Loren White, MD

PREOPERATIVE DIAGNOSIS: Gangrene and severe peripheral vascular disease, left leg due to diabetes

POSTOPERATIVE DIAGNOSIS: Gangrene and severe peripheral vascular disease, left leg due to diabetes

PROCEDURE PERFORMED: Left below-knee amputation

ANESTHESIA: Spinal sedation

INDICATIONS: The patient is a 51-year-old male with diabetes and severe peripheral vascular disease who is post left-foot toe amputation by Dr. Sanchez. He has ischemia and gangrene of the foot and had seen Dr. Green, and they talked about a left below-knee amputation. Dr. Sanchez is out of town and asked me to perform the procedure. I discussed this with the patient. Also discussed the possibility of above-knee amputation, postoperative wound infections, and bleeding. He understands all this and wishes to proceed.

DESCRIPTION OF PROCEDURE: The patient was brought to the operating room, given spinal sedation, and then prepped with Betadine solution and draped in sterile fashion. An incision was made approximately 8 cm (centimeter) below the tibial tuberosity on the left leg. With a no. 10 blade, we carried our dissection down through subcutaneous tissues sharply. We raised a posterior flap using popliteal muscles, and our dissection through subcutaneous tissues found multiple enlarged venous bleeders and venous hypertension. We had to tie off nearly all the vessels, and we did this with 3-0 silk and 3-0 Vicryl free-ties. We used a periosteal elevator to elevate the tibial periosteum and divided this with the Gigli saw. We used the bone cutter to divide the fibula and then used sharp dissection to go through the popliteal muscles. We irrigated with saline until returns were clear and then rasped the bone edges so that there was no sharpness, and we assured that the vessels were tied as well as the nerves up above the bone edges themselves. After we had irrigated, we closed the popliteal flap over the top of the tibia and the fibula and did a deep layer of 3-0 Vicryl sutures. The skin was then closed with vertical mattress 3-0 Ethilon. The leg was then packed with fluffs and then wrapped with Ace wrap. All sponge and needle counts were correct. He tolerated this well and was taken to recovery in stable condition.

SERVICE CODE(S): _____

ICD-10-CM DX CODE(S): _____

(Answers to every other Case are located in Appendix D . The full answer key is only available in the TEACH Instructor Resources on Evolve.)

Arthroscopy

Arthroscopy is fast becoming the treatment of choice for many surgical procedures. The incisions are smaller, which decreases the risk of infection and speeds recovery time. Several small incisions are made through which lights, mirrors, and instruments are inserted. The arthroscopy codes are located separately at the end of the Musculoskeletal subsection. If multiple procedures are performed through a scope, they are reported with modifier -51. Bundled into all surgical arthroscopic procedure codes is the diagnostic arthroscopy, so do not unbundle and code a diagnostic arthroscopy and a surgical arthroscopy if both were performed during the same encounter. Do not report separately things performed during a procedure that are considered a part of the procedure, such as shaving, removing, evacuating, casting, splinting, or strapping.

A note preceding the Endoscopy/Arthroscopy codes states, "When arthroscopy is performed in conjunction with arthrotomy, add modifier -51." This note indicates that if a surgeon performs a therapeutic arthroscopy and during the procedure also does an arthrotomy, you can report both services. For example, a physician performs an arthroscopic shaving of the articular cartilage and also does an open capsulotomy (posterior capsular release) of the knee. Both the arthroscopic shaving (29877) and the capsulotomy (27435)

would be reported, and to the least expensive procedure you would add modifier -51 (multiple procedures).

The codes in this subheading are divided according to body area—elbow, shoulder, knee—and then according to the type and extent of procedure performed. An example of type of service is as follows: code 29805 is for an arthroscopy of the shoulder for diagnostic purposes, whereas code 29819 is an arthroscopy of the shoulder for a surgical procedure. Not only are there two different codes for surgical and diagnostic arthroscopy procedures, but also the surgical procedure is significantly more expensive than the diagnostic procedure. Great care must be taken to select the code that correctly describes the services supported in the medical record.

Note the description for code 29805: "Arthroscopy, shoulder, diagnostic, with or without synovial biopsy (separate procedure)." You will find the term "separate procedure" several times in the Endoscopy/Arthroscopy subheading because often an arthroscopic procedure is part of a larger procedure. You cannot report the service of the diagnostic arthroscopy unless it has been performed as an independent, separate procedure. Also note that the parenthetical information following the codes indicates the codes to use if the procedure was performed as an open (incisional) procedure rather than as an endoscopic (closed) procedure.

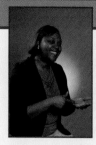

From the Trenches

"Because many hospitals and physicians' offices have made the switch to electronic health records, technology will play an increasingly important role in being successful as a medical coder."

LETITIA PATTERSON
MPA, RHIA, CCS-P, CPC, CPMA, CPC-I

CASE 8-22   *Operative Report, Shoulder*

This is not the first treatment of the injury.

LOCATION: Outpatient, Hospital

PATIENT: Deb Slover

SURGEON: Mohomad Almaz, MD

PREOPERATIVE DIAGNOSIS: Right shoulder pain

POSTOPERATIVE DIAGNOSIS: Normal right shoulder

PROCEDURE PERFORMED: Diagnostic arthroscopy, right shoulder

CLINICAL HISTORY: This 67-year-old woman presents with a history of having fallen on her right side and injuring her right shoulder. She is experiencing severe pain in the shoulder area. X-rays were normal. Preoperative MRI (magnetic resonance imaging) showed no evidence of skeletal or soft-tissue damage. The patient continued to have pain and discomfort. After the risks and benefits of anesthesia and surgery were explained to the patient, the decision was made to undertake the procedure.

OPERATIVE REPORT: Under general anesthetic, the patient was laid in the beach-chair position on the operating table. The right shoulder was examined and found to be stable with full range of motion. The shoulder was then prepped and draped in the usual fashion. A standard posterior arthroscopic portal was created and the camera was introduced into the back of the joint. Inspection of the articular surfaces showed no evidence of damage of the glenoids or the humerus. The anterior ligamentous structures were normal. The biceps attachment and its transit through the joint were normal. Subscapularis was intact with no abnormality. The undersurface of the rotator cuff showed no fraying or inflammation. It was well attached laterally with no evidence of damage. The inferior recess showed no abnormalities.

The camera was then taken out of the glenohumeral joint and placed in the subacromial space. We had excellent visualization of this region. The rotator cuff surface showed absolutely no evidence of fraying or disruption. We had good visualization right out the lateral-most recess. No abnormalities could be identified, and there was no evidence of impingement taking place. The camera was then removed from the subacromial space, and the area was infiltrated with Marcaine. The posterior portal was then closed with absorbable sutures and Steri-Strips, and a Mepore dressing was placed on it. The arm was then placed in a sling; the patient awakened and was placed on her hospital bed and taken to the recovery room in good condition.

SERVICE CODE(S): _____

ICD-10-CM DX CODE(S): _____

(Answers to every other Case are located in Appendix D . The full answer key is only available in the TEACH Instructor Resources on Evolve.)

CASE 8-23   *Operative Report, Debridement*

LOCATION: Outpatient, Hospital

PATIENT: Viola Reynolds

SURGEON: Mohomad Almaz, MD

PREOPERATIVE DIAGNOSIS: Left frozen shoulder

POSTOPERATIVE DIAGNOSIS: Left frozen shoulder adhesive pericapsulitis

PROCEDURE PERFORMED: Arthroscopic debridement, left shoulder. Joint manipulation, left shoulder.

CLINICAL HISTORY: This 73-year-old woman presents with a history of progressive pain and discomfort of her left shoulder. Evaluation confirmed evidence of a left frozen shoulder. After the risks and benefits of anesthesia and surgery were explained to the patient, the decision was made to undertake the procedure.

PROCEDURE: Under general anesthetic, the patient was laid in the beach-chair position on the operating room table. The left shoulder was prepped and draped in the usual fashion. A standard posterior arthroscopic portal was created, and the camera was introduced into the back of the joint. We had excellent visualization. It was immediately apparent that there were substantial inflammation and adhesions throughout the entirety of the joint. Using a switch-stick technique, an anterior portal was created and the 7-mm (millimeter) cannula was then brought in from the front. Using a 4.0 double-biter resector, the synovium was then debrided throughout the entirety of the rotator cuff over the surface of the biceps and the anterior ligamentous structures as well as inferior ligamentous structures. With this completed, the joint was then thoroughly irrigated to remove any blood. The articular surfaces were inspected and were found to be normal. The attachment

CASE 8-23—cont'd

of the biceps was normal, although it had been covered with synovium. Anterior ligamentum structures were free from the subscapularis. The joint was then infiltrated with 80 mg (milligram) of Depo-Medrol and 12 cc of Marcaine. The instruments were removed. The arthroscopic portal was closed with absorbable sutures and Steri-Strips. The joint was then manipulated. Before the manipulation, we had about 90 degrees of elevation passively. After manipulation, evaluation was free up to 180 degrees, and external rotation in an abducted position was possible to 90 degrees, as was internal rotation. Extension was possible to 40 degrees, and adduction was possible to 50 degrees. The wounds were then dressed with Myopore dressing. The patient was then placed in a Cryo/Cuff sling, awakened, placed on her hospital bed, and taken to the recovery room in good condition.

SERVICE CODE(S): _____

ICD-10-CM DX CODE(S): _____

(Answers to every other Case are located in Appendix D . The full answer key is only available in the TEACH Instructor Resources on Evolve.)

CASE 8-24   *Operative Report, Knee Repair*

Before you code this case, let's take a moment to review some of the terms that you will find in this report. The medial meniscus is C-shaped and is wider on the posterior horn (point) than on the anterior horn. The term "medial" means the middle of, and lateral is the farthest point from the middle or midline. A bucket handle tear is a vertical tear in the meniscus, which can be either the medial meniscus or the lateral meniscus. A plica is a fold in the lining of the knee joint, and chondromalacia is softening of the kneecap. Understanding of these terms will be necessary to correctly code this case.

LOCATION: Outpatient, Hospital

PATIENT: Glenn Arch

SURGEON: Mohomad Almaz, MD

PREOPERATIVE DIAGNOSIS: Medial meniscus tear

POSTOPERATIVE DIAGNOSES:

1. Right knee medial meniscus tear (*this is a derangement*)
2. Right knee plica
3. Right knee diffuse chondromalacia, grade 2-3

PROCEDURE PERFORMED: Right knee arthroscopy with partial medial meniscectomy and removal of plica

ANESTHESIA: General

ESTIMATED BLOOD LOSS: Minimal

No drains.

A 36-year-old male suffered with chronic right knee pain. MRI (magnetic resonance imaging) demonstrated a medial meniscus tear.

The patient was taken to surgery today. After an appropriate level of anesthesia was achieved, the right knee was appropriately prepped and draped in an orthopedic manner. We made two portal sites in the knee, one medial and the other lateral to the patellar tendon at the joint line. On examination of the joint, we appreciated that the patient had grade 1-2 chondromalacia involving the patella. On the articulating surface on the femur anteriorly, the patient had grade 2-3, a rather large area about 2 cm (centimeter) in diameter. He had a large plica medially, and this was debrided with a shaver. The medial lateral gutters and patella fascia were cleared of some loose bodies. At the joint space level, I appreciated some cartilage floating around, coming off these various sites of chondromalacia. In the medial compartment, he had a complex posterior horn medial meniscus tear, which was debrided back to the stable tissue. I appreciated that the patient had significant grade 2-3 chondromalacia and a 2-3 × 5-cm area on the weight-bearing surface of the knee, starting with the knee flexed to about 10 degrees. Laterally, the patient had a 1 × 2-cm area of chondromalacia on the weight-bearing surface. The lateral meniscus was probed and considered intact. The anterior cruciate ligament was noted to be intact, as was the remainder of the medial meniscus. We irrigated the knee copiously and injected 20 cc of 0.5% Marcaine to the portal spaces in the joint. We reapproximated the portal sites with interrupted nylon sutures, dressed the knee sterilely, and placed the patient in the knee immobilizer. The patient appeared to tolerate the procedure well and left the operating room in good condition.

SERVICE CODE(S): _____

ICD-10-CM DX CODE(S): _____

(Answers to every other Case are located in Appendix D . The full answer key is only available in the TEACH Instructor Resources on Evolve.)

CASE 8-25A   *Operative Report, Acromioplasty*

In this case, it is not specified if the tear was traumatic or atraumatic. Consider this as a chronic atraumatic tear when you code this case.

LOCATION: Inpatient, Hospital

PATIENT: Else Wavia

SURGEON: Mohomad Almaz, MD

PREOPERATIVE DIAGNOSIS: Right shoulder rotator cuff tear

POSTOPERATIVE DIAGNOSES:

1. Loose body, right shoulder joint
2. A 4-cm (centimeter) rotator cuff tear (*rupture*)
3. Grade 3 osteoarthritis, right shoulder

OPERATIONS PERFORMED:

1. Removal of loose body, right shoulder joint
2. Right shoulder arthroscopic acromioplasty
3. Mini-open right rotator cuff repair

CLINICAL HISTORY: This 81-year-old woman presents with a history of pain and discomfort of her right shoulder. She had undergone an MRI (magnetic resonance imaging) done preoperatively with confirmed evidence of a full-thickness rotator cuff tear. After the risks and benefits of anesthesia and surgery were explained to the patient, the decision was made to undertake this procedure.

PROCEDURE: Under general anesthetic, the patient was laid in a beach-chair position on the operating table. The right shoulder was prepped and draped in the usual fashion. A standard posterior arthroscopic portal was created, and the camera was introduced into the back of the joint. Visualization was good. The undersurface of the rotator cuff was substantially inflamed. The articular surface of the glenoid and humerus showed several areas of substantial degenerative change. There was a full-thickness articular cartilage loss through some smaller segments. There were broader areas of grade 3 articular cartilage change. The biceps tendon was well attached. The anterior labrum was normal.

Using a switching stick technique, an anterior portal was created, and a 7-mm (millimeter) cannula was brought in from the front. Using a 4.0 double-biter resector, the undersurface of the rotator cuff was then debrided. The damaged edges of the glenoid and humeral articular surfaces were then debrided back to a smooth surface. We then found an 8 × 12-mm loose body in the inferior recess. This was then removed without difficulty. (Procedure 1: removed loose body through scope.) The remainder of the inspection of the joint showed no other abnormalities. The camera was then taken out of the glenohumeral joint and placed into the subacromial space. We had good visualization once again. There was fraying on the undersurface of the acromion. A lateral portal was then created, and a 5.5 resector blade was brought in. The undersurface of the acromion was then denuded of soft tissue. A very large anterior bone spur was curving inferiorly. This was then removed, and the undersurface of the acromion was thinned through a depth of approximately 4 mm extending from the acromioclavicular joint over to the lateral margin and from the anterior margin posteriorly for 2.5 cm. When this was completed, the camera was then placed into the lateral portal and the shaver placed posteriorly. Using a "butcher-block technique," the undersurface of the acromion was then smoothed to a flat surface. When this was completed, the camera was then placed so that we could see the rotator cuff more fully. We could see evidence of substantial damage through the central portion of the cuff, although no full-thickness injury could be identified. (Procedure 2: acromioplasty through scope.)

Instruments were removed from the subacromial space. The lateral portal was then extended to a 4-cm incision (Procedure is converted to open), and the deltoid split to expose the rotator cuff. We could now see more fully that there was an area about the size of a silver dollar where the cuff had been substantially thinned and was atrophic. This was then sharply excised. Side-to-side repair was done with a series of no. 2 Panacryl sutures. (Procedure 3: mini-open rotator cuff repair.) When this was completed, the arm was then placed through a range of motion. No further stress appeared on the repair.

The deltoid was then repaired with no. 1 Vicryl suture. The skin was closed in layers with Monocryl suture and Steri-Strips. The wound was then infiltrated with Marcaine and dressed with Mepore dressing. The arm was then placed in a CryoCuff sling. The patient was awakened and placed on her hospital bed and taken to the recovery room in good condition. Estimated blood loss for the procedure was less than 50 cc. The sponge and needle counts were correct.

SERVICE CODE(S): _____

ICD-10-CM DX CODE(S): _____

(Answers to every other Case are located in Appendix D . The full answer key is only available in the TEACH Instructor Resources on Evolve.)

CASE 8-25B   *Operative Report, Debridement and Irrigation*

Else had surgery 2 months ago to repair her torn rotator cuff. The surgeon who performed the cuff repair is now returning her to the operating room for an incision and drainage of the infected wound (previous incision) on her right shoulder within the postoperative period. This wound is a complication of her original surgical procedure and occurs within the postoperative period.

LOCATION: Outpatient, Hospital

PATIENT: Else Wavia

SURGEON: Mohomad Almaz, MD

PREOPERATIVE DIAGNOSIS: Infected wound, right shoulder

POSTOPERATIVE DIAGNOSIS: Infected wound, right shoulder

PROCEDURE PERFORMED: Debridement and irrigation of infected wound, right shoulder

CLINICAL HISTORY: This 81-year-old woman had previously undergone an arthroscopic mini-open repair of a right rotator cuff tear, which I performed. At about the 4-week stage postoperatively, she developed drainage from the wound. This was culture positive for *Staphylococcus aureus*. She was then placed on oral antibiotics and did show some improvement, but there has been persistent drainage for the last 2 weeks without evidence of resolution. Because of the continuation of this problem, the decision was made to undertake the procedure.

ANESTHESIA: General

CASE 8-25B—cont'd

PROCEDURE: Under general anesthesia, the patient was laid in the beach-chair position on the operating table. The right shoulder was prepped and draped in the usual fashion. The anterior 3 cm (centimeter) of the surgical wound was excised. There was fluid drainage from this area. A sinus tract was identified that went down to the anterior acromial area. We followed the tract down. No further purulence could be identified. The rotator cuff was exposed, and the repair was holding well with no evidence of disruption. The edges of the sinus tract area were then fully debrided and then irrigated using a power lavage system and 4 L of normal saline. Once the irrigation

was completed, we repaired the soft tissues around the sinus tract with interrupted no. 1 Vicryl suture and then closed the skin with Monocryl suture. The wound was then dressed with Vaseline gauze, 4 × 4s, and Hypafix. The arm was placed in a sling. The patient was then awakened and placed on her hospital bed and taken to the recovery room in good condition. Estimated blood loss for the procedure was negligible. Sponge and needle counts were correct.

SERVICE CODE(S): _____

ICD-10-CM DX CODE(S): _____

(Answers to every other Case are located in Appendix D . The full answer key is only available in the TEACH Instructor Resources on Evolve.)

CASE 8-26   *Operative Report, Debridement*

This is the initial treatment of this injury. The lesion of the radius is listed first followed by the ligament tear and the external cause code.

LOCATION: Outpatient, Hospital

PATIENT: Anita Aune

SURGEON: Mohomad Almaz, MD

PREOPERATIVE DIAGNOSIS: Right wrist pain

POSTOPERATIVE DIAGNOSES:

1. Partial-thickness chondral lesion, right distal radial articular surface
2. Partial thickness tear, right scapholunate ligament

PROCEDURE PERFORMED: Right wrist arthroscopy and debridement

CLINICAL HISTORY: This 35-year-old woman was involved in a motor vehicle accident. She sustained injuries to both wrists. She has had continuing pain on the right side, and after the risks and benefits of anesthesia and surgery were explained to the patient, the decision was made to undertake this procedure.

PROCEDURE: Under a general anesthetic, the patient was laid supine on the operating table. The right hand was prepped and draped in the usual fashion and placed in the fingertip traction with 10 pounds of weight around the upper arm. A tourniquet was inflated around

the right upper arm after prepping. The joint was infiltrated with saline. Only 3 cc of saline could enter into the joint. The standard 3-4 arthroscopic portal was created, and the camera was introduced into the joint. We had excellent visualization. The undersurface of the carpus showed a small flap tear in the scapholunate junction. The same corresponding region on the distal radial articular surface showed a ridge of heaped-up scar tissue. More ulnarly, the triangular fibrocartilage was inspected and was found to be intact with no evidence of damage through it.

The 6-R portal was created, and a 2.5 full radius resector was then brought in. The surface of the radius was then smoothed to a flat surface, and the flap tear in the scapholunate ligament was debrided. No further abnormalities could be identified. The instruments were then removed, and then the two arthroscopic portals closed with absorbable suture. Wound edges were also closed with Steri-Strips, and then the wound was dressed with Vaseline gauze, 4 × 4s, Kerlix, and an Ace wrap. The tourniquet was deflated, and the patient awoken, placed on her hospital bed, and taken to the recovery room in good condition. Sponge and needle counts were correct.

Pathology Report Later Indicated: Benign lesion of radius.

SERVICE CODE(S): _____

ICD-10-CM DX CODE(S): _____

(Answers to every other Case are located in Appendix D . The full answer key is only available in the TEACH Instructor Resources on Evolve.)

CASE 8-27   *Operative Report, Knee*

This is the initial care for the injury. Darrell was working out in the gymnasium when he attempted to lift a 150-pound weight. Dr. Almaz diagnoses the condition as a dislocation of the patella with fracture of the right knee, and he is performing a repair procedure today. Any dislocation at the same site as a fracture is included in the fracture diagnosis code and not reported separately.

LOCATION: Outpatient, Hospital

PATIENT: Darrell Backer

SURGEON: Mohomad Almaz, MD

PREOPERATIVE DIAGNOSIS: Prepatellar dislocation with osteochondral fracture, inferior pole of patella, right knee

POSTOPERATIVE DIAGNOSIS: Acute patellar dislocation with osteochondral fracture, inferior pole of patella, right knee; an old posterior horn tear, medial meniscus, posterior horn of right knee

PROCEDURE PERFORMED:

1. Right knee arthroscopy and partial arthroscopic lateral meniscectomy
2. Arthrotomy and attempted open reduction and internal fixation of osteochondral fracture, inferior pole of patella, right knee
3. Removal of osteochondral body, right knee

Continued

CASE 8-27—cont'd

OPERATIVE PROCEDURE: After suitable general anesthesia had been achieved, the patient's right knee was prepped and draped in the usual manner. Before prepping, the thigh tourniquet was applied after draping, inflated to 300 mmHg (millimeter of mercury). Inflow cannula was inserted in the suprapatellar pouch on the medial side. Hemarthrosis was evacuated from the knee. Arthroscopic anteromedial and anterolateral portals were established. Thickened inferior plica was noted and excised for visualization of the ACL (anterior cruciate ligament). The ACL was intact and stable to probing. The medial compartment was intact. The articular surfaces were stable with intact medial meniscus. Examination of the lateral compartment revealed a tear on the medial aspect of the posterior horn. Using combination punch and shaver, the torn area was excised. The articular surfaces laterally looked in good shape. Examination of the patellofemoral joint revealed some evidence of tearing of the medial retinacular structures. There was an osteochondral fragment off the inferior pole. This was stuck to the synovium. The shaver was placed. Clot around the fragment was evacuated. The fragment was then mobilized. It looked like there was a reasonable area of osseous tissue on the undersurface of the fragment. The fragment was too large to be manipulated arthroscopically, and it was elected to do an arthrotomy of the knee and possible repair, possible excision.

Arthroscope was removed. Incision was made from the tibial tubercle to about two fingerbreadths above the patella over the midline. A medial arthrotomy was made from the superior pole of the patella to the joint line. The patella was everted. A defect off the inferior aspect of the patella on the inferior tongue of the patella was noted. The osteochondral fragment was retrieved from the knee. The osseous surface covered about 40% of the fragment. Attempts to try to reduce the fragment revealed some plastic deformation of the fragment, but I could not get this to align appropriately. With the deformation of that fragment and the very thin area of osseous component affecting about 40% of the fragment, it was felt that repair would not be something that would have a high likelihood of success. For this reason, the fragment was excised.

Hemovac drain was then inserted. Synovium and the medial patellofemoral ligament were repaired. Medial capsule was repaired and bursa repaired. Skin was closed with 3-0 Vicryl subcuticular sutures and staples. Hemovac drain was inserted through the superolateral portal prior to wound closure. A dressing and a hinged-knee immobilizer with a hinge lock in full extension were then applied. The patient tolerated the procedure well and returned to the recovery room in stable condition.

SERVICE CODE(S): _____

ICD-10-CM DX CODE(S): _____

(Answers to every other Case are located in Appendix D . The full answer key is only available in the TEACH Instructor Resources on Evolve.)

CASE 8-28   *Operative Report, Meniscectomy and Chondroplasty*

LOCATION: Outpatient, Hospital

PATIENT: Doyle Dryhdahl

SURGEON: Mohomad Almaz, MD

PREOPERATIVE DIAGNOSIS: Chondromalacia patella, left knee

POSTOPERATIVE DIAGNOSIS: Chondromalacia patella, left knee; anterior horn tear, lateral meniscus, left knee; focal grade 2 chondromalacia, medial femoral condyle (10 cm [centimeter] in diameter).

PROCEDURE PERFORMED: Left knee arthroscopy, partial arthroscopic lateral meniscectomy, and chondroplasty patella and medial femoral condyle.

PROCEDURE: After suitable general anesthesia had been achieved, the patient's left knee was prepped and draped in the usual manner. Before prepping, a thigh tourniquet was applied; after draping, it was inflated to 300 mmHg (millimeter of mercury). The arthroscope was inserted through an anteromedial portal. Operative anterolateral portal was established. The lateral compartment was examined; it had intact articular surfaces, stable intact meniscus. Examination of the notch revealed some hypertrophic synovium, which was cauterized with the radiofrequency

probe. ACL (anterior cruciate ligament) and PCL (posterior cruciate ligament) were intact. Examination of the medial compartment revealed about a 10-mm (millimeter) diameter area of grade 2 chondromalacia with loose articular cartilage flap and about 20 degrees of flexion. The loose articular cartilage flap was divided with the shaver and further smoothing down with the radiofrequency probe at a very low setting. The patient was noted to have a marked multiple fraying of the anterior horn with multiple tears. Using a combination of punch and shaver, the unstable meniscus was excised and contoured. The meniscus was intact medially. Examination of the patellofemoral joint revealed diffuse grade 3 changes of the lateral facet of the patella but minimal articular cartilage flaps where there was loose collapse at the inferior pole, and these were smoothed with the shaver. The knee joint was then thoroughly irrigated and the arthroscope removed. The tourniquet was released. Following the tourniquet release, good circulation was noted to return to the foot. The patient tolerated the procedure well and returned to recovery room in stable condition.

SERVICE CODE(S): _____

ICD-10-CM DX CODE(S): _____

(Answers to every other Case are located in Appendix D . The full answer key is only available in the TEACH Instructor Resources on Evolve.)

CHAPTER 8 *Auditing Review*

Audit the coding for the following reports.

Audit Report 8.1 Operative Report, Meniscectomy

LOCATION: Outpatient Surgery

PATIENT: Joe Calendar

SURGEON: Mohomad Almaz, MD

DIAGNOSES:

1. Internal derangement, right knee.
2. Impingement syndrome, left shoulder.
3. Arthritic pain complaints, left ankle.

PROCEDURES PERFORMED:

1. Arthroscopic partial medial and lateral meniscectomies.
2. Abrasion chondroplasty of areas of excessive redundant articular cartilage wear, medial femoral condyle, grade II/III. 3. Therapeutic injection, left shoulder subacromial space, 5 cc .25% Marcaine, 20 mg of Kenalog. 4. Arthritic symptoms, left ankle, secondary injection, 5 cc .25% Marcaine and 10 mg of Kenalog.

PROCEDURE: After a satisfactory administration of general anesthesia and with the patient in a supine position, the left shoulder and ankle were addressed under sterile technique undergoing subacromial injection at the shoulder of the above-noted preparation as well as, under sterile technique, anterolateral approach about the ankle, undergoing an injection. This was then followed by prepping and draping of the knee on the right side in a routine manner. Routine arthroscopic portals were established. Upon entering the confines of the knee proper, there was a suprapatellar plical entity that was very broad and stout. This was trimmed back. A medial plical entity secondarily was trimmed back for the sake of visualization of the fat pad. The medial compartment, at this time, had grade II-III arthritic changes about the redundant flap and the articular cartilage of the medial femoral condyle. This was trimmed back to stable margins. There was a degenerative superior surface tear of the meniscus that was loose, redundant, and excursible. At this setting, we trimmed it back to stable margins. The interarticular notch was obscured with fat pad and ligamentum mucosum. These were removed for the sake of visualization. Cruciate structures were, otherwise, unremarkable. The lateral compartment, at this time, showed superficial grade I changes of the lateral tibial plateau and a radial tear of the meniscus. Given its size and localization, after extensive debridement, this was trimmed back to a stable margin. At the completion of this element of the procedure, the knee was injected with 5 cc 0.25% Marcaine and 20 mg of Kenalog. He tolerated the procedures well. Sterile dressings were applied once the portal sites were closed. There were no other complicating events.

One or more of the following codes is reported incorrectly for this case. Indicate the incorrect code(s).

PROFESSIONAL SERVICES: Knee arthroscopy, **29880-RT**; Knee arthroscopy, **20610-59-RT**; Ankle injection, **20605-59-LT**; Plicectomy, **29875-59**

ICD-10-CM DX: Meniscus tear, medial, **S83.241A**; Meniscus tear, lateral, **S83.281A**; Plica syndrome, **M67.51**; Shoulder impingement syndrome, **M75.42**; Shoulder osteoarthritis, **M19.012**; Arthritis, **M19.90**

INCORRECT CODE(S): _____

Audit Report 8.2 Operative Report, Fracture Nailing

Warren Oas was involved in a motorcycle accident when he lost control of the motorcycle he was driving at an excess speed on the highway. He slid into the ditch and received a fracture of the shaft of the right femur.

LOCATION: Inpatient, Hospital

PATIENT: Warren Oas

SURGEON: Mohomad Almaz, MD

ATTENDING PHYSICIAN: Mohomad Almaz, MD

PREOPERATIVE DIAGNOSIS: Winquist type III closed fracture, right femoral shaft.

POSTOPERATIVE DIAGNOSIS: Same.

PROCEDURE: Open locked intramedullary nailing, right femur.

OPERATIVE PROCEDURE: After suitable general anesthesia had been achieved, the patient was transferred from his hospital bed and positioned on the fracture table for right femoral nailing. With the patella pointing towards the ceiling, the femoral neck was assessed for anteversion using the mini C-arm, and there was noted to be about 10-15 degrees of anterior anteversion, suggesting rotational alignment looked pretty good. The patient's right buttock, thigh, and knee were then prepped and draped. A 7.5-cm buttock incision was made. A thigh pin was placed into the pyriformis fossa and advanced into the proximal femoral canal. The DHS reamer was used over the top of the guide pin to establish the entry point. The guidewire was passed through the fracture site. Reaming was then done to 12 mm. A femoral manipulator was then inserted. The fracture was reduced, and the guidewire passed down the femoral canal to the knee. The fracture was then reamed from 9 to 14 mm. A 400 x 13 mm intramedullary nail was then inserted without difficulty. Proximal locking was performed times two and distal locking performed times two. The wound was then thoroughly irrigated. A Hemovac drain was inserted. The wounds were closed in layers. The skin was closed with staples. Dressing was then applied. The patient tolerated the procedure well and returned to the recovery room in stable condition.

One or more of the following codes are reported incorrectly for this case. Indicate the incorrect code or codes.

PROFESSIONAL SERVICES: Femur fracture, **27506-RT**

ICD-10-CM DX: Femur fracture, **S72.301B**; Motorcycle accident, **V28.49**

INCORRECT CODE(S): _____

Continued

CHAPTER 8—cont'd

Audit Report 8.3 Operative Report, Arthroscopy with Synovectomy

LOCATION: Outpatient, Hospital

PATIENT: Joshua Saylor

SURGEON: Mohamad Almaz, MD

PREOPERATIVE DIAGNOSES:

1. Left knee medial femoral condyle fracture.
2. Retained metal, left knee.

POSTOPERATIVE DIAGNOSES: Same.

PROCEDURE PERFORMED: Left knee arthroscopy with synovectomy and metal removal and manipulation under general anesthesia.

ANESTHESIA: General.

ESTIMATED BLOOD LOSS: Minimal.

DRAINS: None.

PROCEDURE: A 42-year-old male is six weeks status post medial femoral condyle fracture on the left. He underwent open reduction internal fixation. After appropriate level of anesthesia was achieved, the left knee was appropriately prepped and draped in orthopedic manner. We made two portals in the knee, one medial and the other lateral to the patellar tendon. Sharp dissection was carried through the skin and blunt dissection was carried into the joint space. On examination of the knee, we appreciated that the patient had extensive scarring in the suprapatellar area and the medial gutter. This was debrided with a shaver. We appreciated some scarring in the femoral notch area, but this was debrided. The patient had a nonfunctioning anterior cruciate ligament tear. The medial and lateral meniscus were probed and felt to be intact. The fracture site was identified. We could appreciate no gross motion with palpation or range of motion across the fracture site. We manipulated the knee, but we could not get more than 45 degrees of flexion. For fear of suffering a fracture or rupture, we did not do any further aggressive manipulation. There was appreciated a metal staple in the femoral notch area. This appeared to be loose. We went ahead and pulled it out through the scope. We repaired the portal sites with interrupted nylon sutures and dressed the wound sterilely. The patient was placed in an Ace wrap. The patient appeared to tolerate the procedure well and left the operating room in good condition.

One or more codes should not have been reported for this case. Indicate the code(s) incorrectly reported.

PROFESSIONAL SERVICES: Arthroscopic debridement of the knee, **29877-LT**; Arthroscopic synovectomy of the knee, **29875-51-LT**; Arthroscopic removal of foreign body from the knee, **29874-51-LT**

ICD-10-CM DX: Disorder of knee joint, **M25.862**; Sequelae of fractured medial femoral condyle, **S72.432S**; Complication of surgery, suture material, **T85.898S**

INCORRECTLY REPORTED CODE(S): _____

Audit Report 8.4 Operative Report, Application of Halo

LOCATION: Outpatient, Hospital

PATIENT: Josh Blake

SURGEON: Mohamad Almaz, MD

PREOPERATIVE DIAGNOSIS: Fracture of C1, C2

POSTOPERATIVE DIAGNOSIS: Fracture of C1, C2

PROCEDURE PERFORMED: Placement of a halo

INDICATION: Fracture occurred when the patient was involved in an unspecified motor vehicle collision. It is known that Mr. Blake was the driver of the vehicle.

PROCEDURE: The patient's head was prepped and draped in the usual manner. The head was shaved. The halo apparatus was applied with screws and four-points. Then the vest was applied. The patient was then discharged to the recovery room to have films taken in the recovery room.

One or more of the following codes are reported incorrectly for this case. Indicate the incorrect code or codes.

SERVICE CODE(S): Application of cranial tongs, caliper or stereotactic frame, **20660**

ICD-10-CM DX CODE(S): Nondisplaced fracture of first cervical vertebra, **S12.001A**; Nondisplaced fracture of second cervical vertebra, **S12.101A**; Occupant injury in car collision, **V49.29XA**

INCORRECT/MISSING CODE(S): _____

Audit Report 8.5 Operative Report, Costovertebral Tumor

LOCATION: Outpatient, Hospital

PATIENT: Casey Wild

PRIMARY CARE PHYSICIAN: Leslie Alanda, MD

SURGEON: Mohamad Almaz, MD

PREOPERATIVE DIAGNOSIS: Lipoma, right lumbar area

POSTOPERATIVE DIAGNOSIS: Lipoma, right lumbar area

PROCEDURE PERFORMED: Excision of lipoma, right lumbar area

ANESTHESIA: General endotracheal with 2 cc of 1% Xylocaine with 1:100,000 epinephrine.

SURGICAL FINDINGS: 3.5-cm diameter subcutaneous lesion sitting on the right latissimus dorsi muscle morphologically resembling a lipoma.

DESCRIPTION OF PROCEDURE: The patient was intubated and turned to a prone position. The lesion was prepped with Betadine scrub and solution and draped in a routine sterile fashion. I injected about 2 cc of 1% Xylocaine with 1:100,000 epinephrine over the site of the lesion and around it. I excised an ellipse of skin that I left attached to the lipoma and carried dissection down to the superficial muscular fascia, from which I separated the lipoma. I cauterized the bleeding and closed the wound with subcutaneous 2-0 Monocryl to close the dead space and subcuticular 3-0 Monocryl. I used Steri-Strips to appose the skin edges and used Kerlix fluffs and Elastoplast for the remainder of the dressing. The patient tolerated the procedure well and left the operating room in good condition.

PATHOLOGY REPORT LATER INDICATED: Lipoma

One or more of the following codes are reported incorrectly for this case. Indicate the incorrect code or codes.

SERVICE CODE(S):   Lesion excision, **11404**

ICD-10-CM DX CODE(S):   Lipoma, **D17.39**

INCORRECT/MISSING CODE(S):   _____

Audit Report 8.6 Operative Report, Tumor Excision

LOCATION: Outpatient, Hospital

PATIENT: Alice Lyon

SURGEON: Mohamad Almaz, MD

PREOPERATIVE DIAGNOSIS: Neuroma (two, each 1.1 cm) right leg

POSTOPERATIVE DIAGNOSIS: Neuroma (two, each 1.1 cm) right leg

PROCEDURE PERFORMED: Excision of two 1.1-cm masses near the right tibial bone

ANESTHESIA: General endotracheal

ESTIMATED BLOOD LOSS: Negligible

SURGICAL FINDING: Two 1.1-cm masses of the right leg overlying the tibia within close proximity to each other.

DESCRIPTION OF PROCEDURE: Under satisfactory general endotracheal anesthesia, the patient's right leg was prepped with Betadine scrub and solution and draped in the routine sterile fashion. A tourniquet was applied. The leg was exsanguinated, and the tourniquet was inflated to 400 mm of pressure. An incision, in continuity, was made to encompass both of the lesions of the medial aspect of the right leg, and these were excised without difficulty. It did appear there was some scarred nerve tissue in the upper region. The wounds were then closed with interrupted 3-0 Prolene, and a dressing of Xeroform, Kerlix fluffs, Kerlix roll, Kling, and an Ace bandage from the toes to the knee was applied. The tourniquet was released, and circulation was intact in the leg following release of the tourniquet. The patient tolerated the procedure and left the area in good condition.

PATHOLOGY REPORT LATER INDICATED: Two 1.1-cm benign neoplasms of the connective tissue of leg.

One or more of the following codes are reported incorrectly for this case. Indicate the incorrect code or codes.

SERVICE CODE(S):   Lesion excision, **11402, 11402-59**

ICD-10-CM DX CODE(S):   Benign neoplasm skin of right lower extremity, **D23.71**

INCORRECT/MISSING CODE(S):   _____

(Auditing Review answers with rationales are only available in the TEACH Instructor Resources on Evolve.)

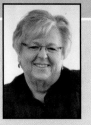

"Take pride in each detail, in each code, in each report because that is what coding is all about. It is a documentation of your best effort."

Respiratory System

http://evolve.elsevier.com/Buck/next

(Answers to every other Case are located in Appendix D, with the full answer key only available in the TEACH Instructor Resources on Evolve)
(Auditing Review answers with rationales are only available in the TEACH Instructor Resources on Evolve)

The respiratory system often reflects diseases in other organ systems of the body. The process of respiration includes not only the lungs but also the diaphragm, the brain (regulates respiration through cerebral regulatory centers), and the cardiovascular system. The physician treating the patient with pulmonary disease must take into consideration a wide variety of pathological considerations. For example, areas of density on a chest x-ray may be caused by pulmonary infection or tumor. Dysfunction of the lungs could represent a systemic disease, such as an embolism or a cardiac disturbance. The physician will begin the diagnostic process with a complete history and physical.

E/M Services

During the history portion of the service, the physician will be seeking information about factors that would have an effect on the patient's lungs, such as exposure to tobacco smoke, pollution, asbestos, coal, and other irritating respiratory factors. A family history of lung disease, such as asthma, allergies, lung cancer, or chronic obstructive lung disease, is significant for making a diagnosis. The personal history includes eliciting information about previous lung infections, such as tuberculosis or pneumonia, and other factors that have an effect on the respiratory system, such as drug abuse or human immunodeficiency virus (HIV). The patient's history of medications is important, as some drugs can affect long-term lung function.

The physical examination will reveal much to the skilled clinician. For example, if there is an absence of breath sounds during inspiration over a certain area of the lung, the absence may indicate **atelectasis** (incomplete expansion of the lung) or a pleural **effusion** (liquid in the pleural space). Tenderness over the sinus area may indicate a sinus infection, or clubbed fingers may indicate lung cancer or cystic fibrosis. Each element in the physical examination is important in the diagnostic process and is noted in the medical documentation.

Common respiratory symptoms are chronic cough, sore throat, and **hemoptysis** (blood in sputum). Conditions of the respiratory system frequently include upper respiratory infection, laryngitis, croup, bronchiolitis, asthma, bronchitis,

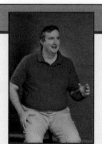

From the Trenches

"A successful coder must stay inquisitive and investigate, but don't overanalyze."

MIKE MCCOLLUM
CPC, COC

chronic obstructive pulmonary disease, pneumonia, atelectasis, and pulmonary embolus. Common procedures include endotracheal intubation, tracheostomy, **thoracentesis,** biopsies, and various endoscopic procedures, such as sinus endoscopy or bronchoscopy. Pulmonary specialty studies include pulmonary function, oxygen saturation, polysomnogram, and sleep studies. X-rays and computerized tomography (CT) scans are often part of the medical documentation for patients with respiratory conditions.

Physicians who specialize in treatment of the nose and throat are otolaryngologists, and physicians who specialize in treatment of the respiratory system are **pulmonologists.**

Enzyme Immunoassay

An EIA (enzyme immunoassay) is screening for strep. *Streptococcus* organisms are classified by means of the Lancefield classification into Groups A through O. The CPT manual divides *Streptococcus* into Groups A and B. Group A is *Streptococcus pyogenes,* which can be a cause of sore throat **(pharyngitis).** A culture allows identification of the cause of the pharyngitis. The patient presents to the laboratory, and laboratory personnel will swab the pharyngeal wall

and tonsillar area. The material on the swab is placed into a medium (culture medium) that allows for the growth of the microorganism over a period of time. Newer methods allow results to be known more quickly; these are termed rapid detection methods and are not cultured (noncultured). Noncultured is also known as primary source, which means that instead of waiting for the overnight incubation, as is required in the cultured method, the swabbed material is incubated with an acid solution or an enzyme that extracts the Group A antigen. EIA that utilizes this fast test method is manufactured in a kit, much like the commercially available pregnancy test kits that are now readily available. A plus sign appears to indicate that *Streptococcus* was detected, and a minus sign appears to indicate that no *Streptococcus* was found in the sample. These results are stated on a laboratory report that is sent to the physician for review.

The diagnosis for the laboratory tests is not stated in the laboratory report; rather, when the service is submitted for reimbursement, the reason for the service is stated as the diagnosis assigned by the physician. Laboratory results are not used for diagnosis unless a physician has interpreted the results.

You can locate the various enzyme immunoassays in the index of the CPT manual under Antigen Detection.

CASE 9-1A   *Evening Clinic, Sore Throat*

LOCATION: Outpatient, Clinic

PATIENT: Cindy Byer

PHYSICIAN: Ronald Green, MD

This established patient presents to the evening clinic on May 9. She relates that she has had a sore throat for 1 day. No fever. No nausea, vomiting, or diarrhea. No significant runny nose or congestion. She has had occasional nonproductive cough, which she attributes to smoking.

EXAMINATION: The patient is an alert, cooperative, 36-year-old white female with a temperature of 99.6° F. AU (both ears) TMs (tympanic membranes) are clear. The nose is inflamed but patent. Sinuses are nontender. The oropharynx is hyperemic. The are no exudates. There is a bit of food debris in the right tonsillar crypt. Neck is supple without significant nodes. Lungs are clear to auscultation. A 4-hour EIA (enzyme immunoassay) strep screen is pending.

ASSESSMENT:

1. Food debris in right tonsil (not significant)
2. Rhinopharyngitis

PLAN: An EIA strep screen is pending. We will call her back with the results but will have her call back if she has not heard from us by 11 o'clock tomorrow morning. Hygiene precautions are discussed, and over-the-counter medication is also discussed. Further treatment pending the results of the strep screen. Total time spent with the patient today was 20 minutes.

SERVICE CODE(S): _____

ICD-10-CM DX CODE(S): _____

(Answers to every other Case are located in Appendix D . The full answer key is only available in the TEACH Instructor Resources on Evolve.)

CASE 9-1B   *Laboratory, Respiratory Cultures*

Dr. Green sends Cindy to the laboratory for an EIA.

LOCATION: Outpatient, Clinic

PATIENT: Cindy Byer

PHYSICIAN: Ronald Green, MD

INDICATION: Rhinopharyngitis

STREP SCREEN EIA (enzyme immunoassay)

SPECIMEN SOURCE: Throat

SPECIAL REQUESTS: None

STREP FA: Negative for group A beta strep by EIA

SERVICE CODE(S): _____

ICD-10-CM DX CODE(S): _____

(Answers to every other Case are located in Appendix D . The full answer key is only available in the TEACH Instructor Resources on Evolve.)

Residents

As a part of the medical resident's education, each resident is required to serve a rotation in a variety of health care settings under the direct supervision of a qualified physician who serves as the resident's supervisor and teacher. When the health care services provided by the resident are not directly reported to all the third-party payers (e.g., Medicare), the HCPCS modifier -GC (performed in part by a resident) or -GE (performed completely by a resident) is sometimes used on the code submitted for the teaching physician to indicate that the resident, under supervision of the teaching physician, performed a portion of the service and that the resident's notes have been considered when reporting the teaching physician's service. For example, in the following case, the teaching physician dictated a history and physical on admitting a patient to the hospital. The resident also dictated a history and physical. The coder uses both the teaching physician's notes and the resident's notes to report the teaching physician's services of a hospital admission.

Most third-party payers will not reimburse a facility for services performed completely by a resident.

CASE 9-2A   *Admission History and Physical (Physician's and Resident's Notes)*

Dr. Dawson admitted Mr. Gulman to the hospital and prepared an admission history and physical. Dr. Grovedahl is a resident being supervised by Dr. Dawson. When completing the audit form for the admission service, place a "✓" on the form to indicate elements Dr. Dawson provided and an "✕" to indicate elements Dr. Grovedahl provided. Dr. Grovedahl performed only part of the service because Dr. Dawson also contributed to the service. Assume that the third-party payer requires the use of the HCPCS modifiers for those services provided in part by a resident.

LOCATION: Inpatient, Hospital

PATIENT: Ervin Gulman

PRIMARY CARE PHYSICIAN: Ronald Green, MD

ATTENDING PHYSICIAN: Gregory Dawson, MD

PHYSICIAN ADMISSION NOTES: The emergency room notified that the patient presented himself there with increasing shortness of breath, and of course he had an abnormal chest x-ray. This is the same patient I tried to talk into coming into the emergency room earlier, and Dr. Green also tried even a week before that, and he has now agreed that perhaps he is sick enough to come in.

He is a patient who is well known to me, so a lot of history is already in the clinic chart. His past medical history, social history, family history, and review of systems are outlined in detail by my resident. Please see the resident's note for complete details of the entrance history and physical.

The patient has significant COPD (chronic obstructive pulmonary disease) with hypoxic, hypercarbic respiratory failure on today's blood gases. He has had diminished appetite for a couple of weeks and dry mouth, and he is too short of breath really to eat well. He is on home O_2 (report dependence on supplemental oxygen with a V code), and he has been on Avalax since the 10th. Before that he had a week's worth of antibiotics as well, but I do not know what they were. No fevers, sweats, or chills were present. He had increasing malaise, and he had some fever, with a temperature of 101° F to 102° F before admission.

The time I saw the patient revealed a very ill-appearing white male. HEENT (head, ears, eyes, nose, throat) is benign. No blood in the nose or posterior pharynx. The neck is supple without adenopathy. No JVD (jugular vein distention). Thyroid is not palpably enlarged. Lungs have diminished air movement everywhere, with rales in the right. No wheezes, rhonchi, or rubs. Heart shows a heart rate of about 110. I thought it was regular, without an S3 (third heart sound) or S4 (fourth heart sound). No diastolic sounds, clicks, or rubs; maybe a grade 1 murmur over the fourth intercostal, but his heart is so fast I am not sure what exactly I am hearing at this point. Abdomen is benign without hepatosplenomegaly. Normal bowel sounds are present. No bruits are heard in either flank. No masses are palpable, nontender, somewhat distended and tympanitis but within the range of normal. Neurologically he is awake and alert. Extremities show no edema, rashes, clubbing, cyanosis, or tremor except some ecchymosis in his upper arms, probably from steroid use. Neurologic: Cranial nerves II-XII are intact, and there is symmetrical strength in all four extremities. A detailed exam is not done because of his respiratory distress. Lymphatics: There are no nodes in the neck, clavicular, or axillary area.

IMPRESSION:

1. Acute pneumonia, organism unknown with secondary acute bronchospasm superimposed in a patient with significant COPD and respiratory failure. He will be admitted for antibiotic use and bronchodilator therapy, and we will have to look more into this hypercarbia. If the problem gets too great, we might have difficulty because this patient did not tolerate the BiPAP mask because of claustrophobia.

2. Chronic anxiety: In fact, that is why he is on BuSpar. We will try to get into him as soon as we can, but I do not really want to do it right today because of the elevated pCO_2 (partial pressure of carbon dioxide) (not reported).

LOCATION: Inpatient, Hospital

PATIENT: Ervin Gulman

PRIMARY CARE PHYSICIAN: Ronald Green, MD

ATTENDING PHYSICIAN: Gregory Dawson, MD

RESIDENT: Mandy Grovedahl, MD

CHIEF COMPLAINT: Increasing shortness of breath and malaise

HISTORY OF PRESENT ILLNESS: This 73-year-old male was seen in Dr. Green's office 1 week ago to follow up on pneumonia. The patient had been taking quinolone for a week for a pneumonia that had been diagnosed approximately 2 weeks previously when he had presented with cough, fever, chills, and shortness of breath. Since then, those symptoms have resolved. The patient complained of a decreased appetite at home and complaining of a dry mouth. He is on home O_2 and has been on Avelox since the 10th when he went to the office to see Dr. Green. Over the past 2 days he has complained of increasing shortness of breath, increasing malaise, temperature 101° F to 102° F yesterday. He denies any nausea, vomiting, or diarrhea.

PAST MEDICAL HISTORY:

1. Severe chronic obstructive pulmonary disease
2. Congestive heart failure
3. Elevated PSA (prostate specific antigen) in the past

Continued

CASE 9-2A—cont'd

MEDICATIONS:

1. BuSpar 10 mg (milligram) b.i.d. (twice a day).
2. Lasix 40 mg q.d. (every day).
3. Ibuprofen 1 tab p.r.n. (as needed).
4. Albuterol 0.5% nebulizer q.6h. (every 6 hours).
5. AeroBid inhalers 4 puffs b.i.d.
6. Albuterol sulfate 0.5 mg with each nebulizer treatment.
7. Serevent 2 puffs q.12h.
8. Atrovent 2 puffs q.i.d. (four times a day).

ALLERGIES: Aspirin

PAST SURGICAL HISTORY: Right jaw repair following a broken jaw. No other surgeries.

FAMILY HISTORY: Father passed away at age 86 of congestive heart failure. Mother passed away at age 78 of colon cancer. The patient has three brothers and one sister alive. Two brothers have pacemakers. One sister has COPD.

SOCIAL HISTORY: Patient one pack daily × 45-year smoker. He quit approximately 15 years ago. He does have a history of heavy drinking in the past but denies any current use. He currently lives in Manytown with his wife.

REVIEW OF SYSTEMS: Constitutional: The patient indicates that there was an 18-pound weight loss approximately 2 months ago secondary to some fluid overload. He denies any headaches. He has had a decreased appetite in the past week or so, and he sleeps well with no problems. Eyes: Denies any history of glaucoma and has no eye pain or blurry or double vision. Ears, nose, mouth, and throat: No hearing problems reported. No bleeding from the nose or mouth. Cardiovascular: Denies palpitations. Denies any pressure or racing heartbeat. He does complain of some substernal chest pain off and on with exertion, last experienced approximately 1 week ago. Respiratory: Chronic cough, which is productive of white sputum. Dyspnea on exertion. GI (gastrointestinal): No history of ulcers. No digestive problems. He has had some positive stools recently. GU (genitourinary): History of prostate problems. Positive burning with urination recently. Skin: Complaint of dryness around the nares. No rashes. No nonhealing lesions. Musculoskeletal: No arthritis. No complaints of joint pain. No loss of

muscle strength. Psych: Patient does have a history of anxiety secondary to shortness of breath. Neuro: No epilepsy or history of seizures. Hematology: Patient states he bruises easily. He does not have a bleeding problem. Endocrine: No kidney problems. No thyroid problems.

PHYSICAL EXAMINATION: Vitals: Pulse 105. Blood pressure 132/157. O_2 saturation on 3L nasal cannula is 82% to 89%. Respirations are mid 20s to 30s. Temperature 36.8° C. HEENT: Normocephalic and atraumatic. Extraocular movements are intact. Neck is soft. No cervical adenopathy. Pharynx is without erythema. There are no oral lesions. Cardiovascular: Tachycardia. No murmurs, rubs, or gallops heard. Respiratory: Diminished air movement in bilateral bases. Minimal respiratory wheeze heard. No rhonchi or rales appreciated. Abdomen: Soft, positive bowel sounds, nondistended. The patient complains of positive tenderness to palpation over the right upper quadrant. Musculoskeletal: Strength is 5/5 and equal bilaterally upper and lower extremities. Extremities: No clubbing, cyanosis, or edema. Full range of motion times four. Neuro: Cranial nerves II-XII grossly intact. Sensation is intact.

LABORATORY: Sodium 142, potassium 4.4, chloride 96, CO_2 greater than or equal to 41.8, BUN (blood urea nitrogen) 17, creatinine 0.7, and glucose 129. Calcium 8.9. White blood cells 9.7, hemoglobin 15.6, and platelets 202. ABGs (arterial blood gases) from this morning: pH (potential of hydrogen) 7.439, pCO_2 (partial pressure of carbon dioxide) 52.9, pO_2 (oxygen pressure) 55.2, bicarbonate 35.1, O_2 saturation 94% on 3L nasal cannula from 9:30 this morning, when he came in through the emergency department. Chest x-ray from 2 weeks ago revealed extensive opacities on the right side, awaiting results of x-ray from the emergency room this morning. I will review those this afternoon with Dr. Dawson.

ASSESSMENT/PLAN: Pneumonia right-sided in someone with COPD. Patient is oxygen dependent due to chronic respiratory failure. He has been placed on Claforan, Zithromax, and Solu-Medrol as well as a variety of breathing treatments. We will monitor labs, ABGs, and x-ray. See orders for remainder.

SERVICE CODE(S): _____

ICD-10-CM DX CODE(S): _____

(Answers to every other Case are located in Appendix D . The full answer key is only available in the TEACH Instructor Resources on Evolve.)

CASE 9-2B   *Radiology Report, Chest*

This radiology report indicates that there were two parts to the chest film (upper and lower); however, this is a single view (anteroposterior, front to back). It is the number of views that is reported.

LOCATION: Inpatient, Hospital

PATIENT: Ervin Gulman

PRIMARY CARE PHYSICIAN: Ronald Green, MD

ATTENDING PHYSICIAN: Gregory Dawson, MD

RADIOLOGIST: Morton Monson, MD

EXAMINATION OF: Chest

CLINICAL SYMPTOMS: Pneumonia, COPD (chronic obstructive pulmonary disease), and chronic respiratory failure

PORTABLE CHEST: SINGLE VIEW: FINDINGS: Study is compared today with the study dated 2 weeks ago. Cardiac monitor leads overlie the

patient. This chest film is obtained in two parts—one contains the upper portion of the chest, the second the lower portion of the chest. Cardiac silhouette is prominent but stable. Pulmonary vasculature also mildly prominent but stable. The left lung appears relatively clear. There is some linear opacity, left infrahilar area, consistent with segmental volume loss. Opacity is seen in the right lung with some mild sparing of the right apex. This is a mixed interstitial and alveolar pattern with a more focal area of opacity in the right mid-lung extending to the lateral chest wall. Pleural density is seen along the right lateral chest wall, and there is an unusual lucency over the right heart border. Osseous structures are stable.

IMPRESSION:

1. Increasing consolidation in the right mid-lung and infiltrate in the right lung base. Clinical correlation is suggested.
2. Pleural density is new since previous exam on the right, likely related to a pleural effusion. Again, clinical correlation is suggested. These findings may represent an acute infiltrate likely secondary to

CASE 9-2B—cont'd

infectious process, but it can also be seen with other etiologies, such as pulmonary embolism.

3. There is an unusual lucency over the right lung base adjacent to the heart border. This may represent aerated lung against consolidation, but other etiologies, including pneumatocele,

could have this appearance, and clinical correlation suggests the need for further imaging.

SERVICE CODE(S): _____

ICD-10-CM DX CODE(S): _____

CASE 9-2C   *Radiology Report, Chest*

Dr. Monson suggested further imaging, and based on that recommendation, Dr. Dawson ordered a posteroanterior (PA) and lateral chest x-ray.

LOCATION: Inpatient, Hospital

PATIENT: Ervin Gulman

PRIMARY CARE PHYSICIAN: Ronald Green, MD

ATTENDING PHYSICIAN: Gregory Dawson, MD

EXAMINATION OF: Chest

CLINICAL SYMPTOMS: Pneumonia, COPD (chronic obstructive pulmonary disease), and chronic respiratory failure

PA (POSTERIOR/ANTERIOR) AND LATERAL CHEST X-RAY, 9:15 AM: Previous portable upright only yesterday

CLINICAL INFORMATION: There is cardiomegaly, as there has been on previous x-rays for this patient. The vascular markings on the left are within normal limits. On the left, there is what appears to be interstitial fibrosis, mid-lung and base. No left effusion suggested. On the right, there is abnormal density throughout the right lung that is interstitial in nature and could be unilateral failure pattern. That is less confluent than it was in the right upper lobe compared with the previous report. The remainder of the right lung (mid-lung and base) shows no change

from previous report. There is blunting of the right costophrenic angle and the right posterior sulcus suggesting a small effusion that is stable. There is some pleural density along the right lateral chest wall and over the apex that is assumed to be scarring. There is degenerative change of the thoracic spine, mild. No destructive lesion or fracture is seen.

IMPRESSION:

1. Cardiomegaly stable
2. No vascular congestion on the left. The left lung shows scar but no active parenchymal disease and no left effusion.
3. On the right, there is a pleural scar along the right lateral chest wall and over the apex.
4. There is abnormal interstitial finding throughout the entire right lung except for the apex. That is abnormal and is new compared with the previous film, indicating that it is an acute finding. It could be a unilateral failure pattern. It could be interstitial pneumonia. There is slightly improved aeration in the periphery of the right upper lobe compared with the film taken 2 days ago. The remainder of the chest is stable.
5. Suggestion of small effusion on the right.

SERVICE CODE(S): _____

ICD-10-CM DX CODE(S): _____

(Answers to every other Case are located in Appendix D . The full answer key is only available in the TEACH Instructor Resources on Evolve.)

CASE 9-2D   *Thoracic Medicine/Critical Care Progress Report*

Note that the physician changed the diagnosis from "pneumonia" to "pneumonia, interstitial-type," which is in the inner spaces of the lung linings. Since the outpatient coder reports only those diagnosis(es) stated on that current report being coded, the diagnoses for this patient will need to reflect this more current diagnosis.

LOCATION: Inpatient, Hospital

PATIENT: Ervin Gulman

PRIMARY CARE PHYSICIAN: Ronald Green, MD

ATTENDING PHYSICIAN: Gregory Dawson, MD

The patient has a right-lung pneumonia, interstitial-type; COPD (chronic obstructive pulmonary disease) and chronic respiratory failure. Yesterday's x-ray showed maybe some clearing. The sputum culture so far is not very helpful. The Gram stain does show evidence of gram-positive disease with moderate gram-positive cocci and moderate gram-positive cocci in clusters. He is taking Claforan and Zithromax, which should cover that. He seems to be responding and is a little more energetic.

OBJECTIVE: He has been afebrile since he has been here. HEENT (head, ears, eyes, nose, throat): Benign. Neck: Supple without JVD (jugular vein distention). Chest: Symmetrical. Rales on the right. Very distant breath sounds. Left sounds pretty good. I do not hear any rales, anyway, but again, distant breath sounds. Heart: S1 (first heart sound) and S2 (second heart sound) are regular with a grade 1/6 murmur at the fourth interspace near the sternum that really does not radiate much. Abdomen: soft. Benign without hepatosplenomegaly. Extremities: No clubbing. No edema.

The patient is a significant CO_2 (carbon dioxide) retainer but does not really tolerate BiPAP much at all, and he tried that in the past. He seems to be quite claustrophobic and just cannot do it. I will put him back on his BuSpar, put him back on his Lasix today 40 mg (milligram) a day, and we will continue the rest of the drugs. We will start physical therapy with him a little bit to see if we cannot get him moving. His Solu-Medrol is every 6; go down to every 8 today. I would like to discharge him after a good 5 days of antibiotics, as I am sure the x-ray is better.

SERVICE CODE(S): _____

ICD-10-CM DX CODE(S): _____

(Answers to every other Case are located in Appendix D . The full answer key is only available in the TEACH Instructor Resources on Evolve.)

CASE 9-2E *Thoracic Medicine/Critical Care Progress Report*

LOCATION: Inpatient, Hospital

PATIENT: Ervin Gulman

PRIMARY CARE PHYSICIAN: Ronald Green, MD

ATTENDING PHYSICIAN: Gregory Dawson, MD

The patient has significant COPD (chronic obstructive pulmonary disease), is oxygen dependent, and has chronic respiratory failure. He had an extensive right-lung pneumonia, interstitial type, basically sparing the apex. Gram stain showing gram-positive *cocci* in the chains and clusters. No pathogen was grown. He is actually doing better. He was able to walk in the hallway a little bit.

EXAMINATION: He has fewer rales. He still has a little bit of wheeze. His weight, however, has gone up. He has some edema in his legs. We will have to give him some Lasix today. I am sure this is fluid retention from steroids. He weighs about 3 pounds more now than he did on the 27th (186 pounds).

The plan is to finish out this week with steroids. I will taper him off so he will be done on the 2nd. With any luck, he can be discharged on the 3rd. Recheck a chest x-ray tomorrow. Recheck his oxygen level. He gets a little dizzy when he stands up, and that may be from hypercarbia, which he is prone to have. Hopefully things are improving enough that we can get him home on Friday.

SERVICE CODE(S): _____

ICD-10-CM DX CODE(S): _____

(Answers to every other Case are located in Appendix D . The full answer key is only available in the TEACH Instructor Resources on Evolve.)

CASE 9-2F *Thoracic Medicine/Critical Care Progress Note*

On this report the physician indicates that the interstitial is now clear, so the diagnosis for the pneumonia is no longer the interstitial type.

LOCATION: Inpatient, Hospital

PATIENT: Ervin Gulman

PRIMARY CARE PHYSICIAN: Ronald Green, MD

ATTENDING PHYSICIAN: Gregory Dawson, MD

The patient is here for pneumonia that is clearing on x-ray. Interstitially clear. On exam, it is clearing. He is symptomatically better and is afebrile. On exam, he still has a few rales at the base. Very distant breath sounds, but he has extremely severe COPD (chronic obstructive pulmonary disease). His O_2 (oxygen) requirement is back down to his usual 2 L (liter). His pO_2 (oxygen pressure) 60, pCO_2 (partial pressure of carbon dioxide) 77, pH (potential of hydrogen) 7.38, and that is his usual set of blood gases. He still has a little edema on exam. Heart shows a regular flow as well as a regular rhythm.

DISPOSITION: We will switch from IV (intravenous) antibiotics to oral antibiotics. If he is doing this well tomorrow, I can discharge him at that time, and with any luck we can get him discharged tomorrow and home.

SERVICE CODE(S): _____

ICD-10-CM DX CODE(S): _____

(Answers to every other Case are located in Appendix D . The full answer key is only available in the TEACH Instructor Resources on Evolve.)

CASE 9-2G *Discharge Summary*

LOCATION: Inpatient, Hospital

PATIENT: Ervin Gulman

PRIMARY CARE PHYSICIAN: Ronald Green, MD

ATTENDING PHYSICIAN: Gregory Dawson, MD

The patient was admitted with pneumonia, increasing shortness of breath, and failure to thrive. He had been treated as an outpatient for similar things but has gradually declined and become quite fatigued and increasingly short of breath. He had acute pneumonia, unknown organism, at the time of admission. I do not think our cultures helped much in identifying a causative organism. His case was gradual slow improvement. He was able to take care of himself a little bit, and he was able to be discharged.

The Gram stain suggested a streptococcal or even a streptococcal organism with moderate gram-positive *cocci* in pairs and gram-negative *cocci* in clusters, but no cultures actually revealed pathogenic diagnosis.

We finally were able to discharge him today to his home under the care of his family.

MEDICATIONS: he was discharged with were:

1. Albuterol nebulizer four times a day and then q.3h. (every 3 hours) p.r.n. (as needed)
2. BuSpar 10 mg (milligram) q.d. (every day)
3. Vantin 200 mg b.i.d. (twice a day)
4. Atrovent four times a day with the albuterol
5. Theo-Dur 200 mg q.d.
6. Oxygen

The Vantin will be discontinued on the 5th after his dose on that day. Follow-up will be in a week in the office to repeat his chest x-ray. His O_2 (oxygen) was set at 4 L (liter) with 2 L continuously.

DISCHARGE DIAGNOSES:

1. Pneumonia
2. Chronic respiratory failure
3. Chronic obstructive pulmonary disease, O_2 dependent

SERVICE CODE(S): _____

ICD-10-CM DX CODE(S): _____

(Answers to every other Case are located in Appendix D . The full answer key is only available in the TEACH Instructor Resources on Evolve.)

CASE 9-3A   *Thoracic Medicine/Critical Care Consultation*

Dr. Dawson was called to the emergency department for a consultation regarding Kurt Troy, who presented with pulmonary edema and respiratory failure. During the consultation, Dr. Dawson decided to admit Mr. Troy to the hospital. The consultation then becomes a hospital admission and is reported as an admission, not as a consultation, even though you will note that the report is titled a consultation. Dr. Dawson admitted the patient and is the attending physician. The ventilation services are bundled into the E/M codes and are not to be reported separately. This patient has a myriad of problems; when reporting the diagnoses, report the chief reason(s) the patient reported for this service. In Case 9-3, you will find the diagnoses highlighted for you to illustrate how the diagnosis changes slightly from report to report.

LOCATION: Inpatient, Hospital

PATIENT: Kurt Troy

ATTENDING PHYSICIAN: Gregory Dawson, MD

CHIEF COMPLAINT: Pulmonary edema **(Figure 9-1)** with respiratory failure

HISTORY OF PRESENT ILLNESS: This is a 57-year-old male admitted through the emergency department at 6:04 AM in respiratory distress

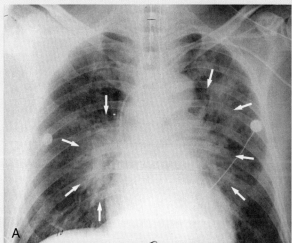

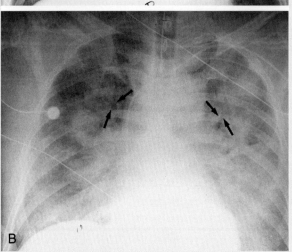

FIGURE 9–1 Pulmonary edema.

leading to intubation. The patient did vomit in the emergency department and was suctioned with possible aspiration. The patient has no significant cardiac arrhythmia since intubation, and no CPR (cardiopulmonary resuscitation) was performed in the emergency room. The patient is currently on a vent with settings of tidal volume 650, rate 21, PEEP (positive end expiratory pressure) 7, FIO_2 (forced inspiration oxygen) 50%, SIMV (synchronized intermittent mandatory ventilation) mode PSV (pressure supported ventilation) of 15. Family reports that the patient had complained of chest pain and pressure and severe back pain in the previous 2 days since falling a week ago. He was seen in the emergency room on that date. CT (computerized tomography) and x-ray were done and indicated that there were some lumbar spine transverse process fractures. The patient also hit his head in the fall, but there was no loss of consciousness.

PAST MEDICAL HISTORY:

1. COPD (chronic obstructive pulmonary disease)
2. Atherosclerotic heart disease with CABG (coronary artery bypass graft) performed 10 years ago
3. History of silent MI 10 years ago
4. Chronic congestive cardiomyopathy
5. Congestive heart failure
6. Questionable hypertension
7. Increased cholesterol
8. Diabetes diagnosed in February of last year

CURRENT MEDICATIONS IN HOSPITAL:

1. Cozaar 10 mg (milligram) b.i.d. (twice a day)
2. Nitroglycerin IV (intravenous) titration
3. Midazolam IV titration
4. Bumex 1 mg q.6h.
5. Morphine IV 2-4 mg p.r.n.

ALLERGIES: No known drug allergies

PAST SURGICAL HISTORY:

1. Coronary artery bypass graft 10 years ago
2. Hemorrhoid surgery sometime in the past

SOCIAL HISTORY: The patient lives at home with wife and daughter. He smoked one pack per day × 41 years, quit 1 year ago. No alcohol.

FAMILY HISTORY: Father with history of multiple MIs after the age of 55, congestive heart failure, and pacemaker. Mother passed away when patient was 15.

REVIEW OF SYSTEMS: Not obtainable at this time other than above from family, as patient is sedated.

EXAMINATION: VITAL SIGNS: Afebrile (98), pulse 72, blood pressure 127/69, O_2 (oxygen) saturation 98% on 50% FIO_2, and rate 21. GENERAL: The patient is a 57-year-old white male who appears his stated age; he is well nourished and well hydrated. CARDIOVASCULAR: S1 (first heart sound) and S2 (second heart sound); no murmur appreciated. ECG (electrocardiogram) indicates a rate of 85 and left bundle-branch block. Cardiac enzymes × 1 indicate CK (creatine kinase) of 378, MB of 4, and troponin I of 0.3. Cardiac enzymes will be repeated in triplicate. PULMONARY: Diminished breath sounds at bilateral bases. ABGs (arterial blood gases) were drawn at 10:30 AM indicating a pH (potential of hydrogen) of 7.409, pCO_2 (partial pressure of carbon dioxide) of 35.0, O_2 saturation 99.6%, pO_2 (oxygen pressure) is 213.3, and bicarb is 21.7.

Continued

CASE 9-3A—cont'd

FIO$_2$ was set at 50% with PEEP of 7, pressure support of 15, and rate of 21 during this draw. (The preceding are the ventilator settings.) Chest x-ray done in the emergency department indicated congestive heart failure and infiltrate. Antibiotics have been started secondary to the likely aspiration. GI (gastrointestinal) and GU (genitourinary): Soft, positive bowel sounds, nontender, and nondistended. Foley catheter and nasogastric tube in place. ELECTROLYTES: Sodium 133, potassium 5.1, chloride 94, creatinine 1.1, BUN (blood urea nitrogen) 30, magnesium 2.2. ENDOCRINE: Blood glucose 233 this AM; insulin sliding scale has been implemented, and Accu-Chek will be done every 4 hours. INFECTIOUS DISEASE: We have ordered cultures for blood, urine, and sputum. Antibiotics have been started. NEUROLOGICAL: The patient is sedated at this time.

DISPOSITION: Likely aspiration, questionable angina of 5 days' duration, leading to flash pulmonary edema. Cardiology has been consulted. Echo for left ventricular function. Added a third set of cardiac enzymes to be drawn. Aspirin now 325 mg. Blood, urine, sputum, cultures, and sensitivities ordered. Morphine drip at 1 mg continuous with 0.5-mg bolus q. 10 minutes p.r.n. (as needed). Begin Unasyn. Change vent settings to PEEP of 5, drop tidal volume to 600; recheck ABGs (arterial blood gases) in 30 minutes.

SERVICE CODE(S): _____

ICD-10-CM DX CODE(S): _____

(Answers to every other Case are located in Appendix D . The full answer key is only available in the TEACH Instructor Resources on Evolve.)

CASE 9-3B   *Thoracic Medicine/Critical Care Progress Note*

LOCATION: Inpatient, Hospital

PATIENT: Kurt Troy

ATTENDING PHYSICIAN: Gregory Dawson, MD

The patient is on ventilator with aspiration and acute pulmonary edema and respiratory failure. His chest x-ray is now clearing up. He still has some clutter, but it is much better than it was. He still has residual changes of pulmonary edema pattern, right greater than left, but much better and his oxygenation is better.

REVIEW OF SYSTEMS/PHYSICAL EXAM:

CARDIOLOGY REVIEW OF SYSTEMS: Fairly stable. Blood pressures are holding their own, with systolic in the 110 range and diastolic in the 50 range with sinus rhythm of about 80. Troponins have not really risen very much. I think the highest we had was 0.8 and is now down to 0.6, so I do not think we had an acute MI, just a troponin leak. No S3 (third heart sound) or S4 (fourth heart sound). I do not appreciate any murmurs. Echocardiogram, however, shows a really depressed left ventricular function down to 10% to 15%. Right ventricular pressure is 45, which is mild pulmonary hypertension. He shows marked hypokinesis of the septum. He has some calcification of the aortic leaflets and mitral leaflets, and apical and periapical segments are also severely hypokinetic and probably akinetic. We have a really bad pump.

PULMONARY SYSTEM REVIEW was just excellent. The pH (potential of hydrogen) is 7.53, pCO$_2$ (partial pressure of carbon dioxide) 29, pO$_2$ (oxygen pressure) 152. On exam, he has a few scattered rales, much improved over his initial exam.

GASTROINTESTINAL SYSTEM REVIEW: He has really low residuals. Abdomen is soft and nontender. No ascites.

GENITOURINARY SYSTEM REVIEW: He had 1.7 L (liter) more out than in with a creatinine clearance exceeding 100. He has no edema on exam.

ENDOCRINOLOGY: Blood sugars are holding their own at 152.

ELECTROLYTES: Potassium is a little low; we will have to replace that. Sodium 135, potassium 3.2, chloride 102, CO$_2$ (carbon dioxide) 21.8, calcium 7.2, magnesium 1.6, phosphorus 2.4; we will have to replace that as well.

HEMATOLOGIC: White count is coming down, but it is still high at 15,530. Hemoglobin is 15.8 with normal platelets of 178,000.

INFECTIOUS DISEASE: White count is coming down. Cultures so far have not grown much. There is a gram-negative *Diplococcus*, but it is rarely seen on Gram stain and may be causative organism, and he is on Unasyn anyway, and he has been afebrile.

NEUROLOGIC: He is too sedated right now.

DISPOSITION: We will not start any tube feedings because I think we will be extubating him this afternoon. Will try to wean him off the ventilator. Will replace his potassium. Dr. Elhart will be by later to see him and adjust his medications. At this point, I think the reason for the flash pulmonary edema was really poor cardiac function.

We spent a total of 45 minutes discussing the case with Dr. Elhart and discussing with the family, examining the patient, reviewing his labs, especially digging up the microbiology, reviewing his x-rays, writing the orders, and dictating the note. This is a pivotal day for this patient. He seems to be getting better but has such precarious cardiac function that it still makes him a critical care patient, and it is somewhat tedious to make decisions. Mostly, we will spend all day today watching how he responds to the ventilator changes, because his cardiac function is so precarious that just the extra work of breathing might be enough to cause more trouble with pulmonary edema. So we may have to go slower than I expect.

SERVICE CODE(S): _____

ICD-10-CM DX CODE(S): _____

(Answers to every other Case are located in Appendix D . The full answer key is only available in the TEACH Instructor Resources on Evolve.)

CASE 9-3C *Radiology Report, Chest*

LOCATION: Inpatient, Hospital

PATIENT: Kurt Troy

ATTENDING PHYSICIAN: Gregory Dawson, MD

EXAMINATION OF: Chest

CLINICAL SYMPTOMS: Follow-up congestive heart failure

REFERRING DR: None stated

PORTABLE CHEST: ONE VIEW: 5:00 AM. Comparisons are made with the previous study taken on admission at 5:00 AM. The heart is enlarged. Central vascularity is mildly prominent. Endotracheal tube lies at the level of the aortic arch. Nasogastric tube transverses the esophagus and lies beyond our field of view within the region of the stomach. Effusions are not seen.

CONCLUSION:

1. There is persistent cardiomegaly, perhaps slightly worsened compared with the previous study. Central vessels are also mildly prominent.
2. Multiple support apparatuses as discussed above.

SERVICE CODE(S): _____

ICD-10-CM DX CODE(S): _____

CASE 9-3D *Thoracic Medicine/Critical Care Progress Note*

LOCATION: Inpatient, Hospital

PATIENT: Kurt Troy

ATTENDING PHYSICIAN: Gregory Dawson, MD

The patient was seen and examined at 8:30 AM. He remains unresponsive secondary to sedation. The acute pulmonary edema is improved on x-ray following diuresis.

Vitals: Pulse 95. Blood pressure 111/53. O_2 (oxygen) saturation 97% on 35% FIO_2 (forced inspiration oxygen); rate is 15. Patient is afebrile (98.6° F). Cardiovascular: Regular rate and rhythm. No edema is noted. Ejection fraction is 15% per echo done by cardiology in April. Cardiac enzymes are negative ×3. Pulmonary: Decreased breath sounds, scattered rales. Improved chest x-ray this morning with decreased infiltrate. ABG (arterial blood gases) at 8 AM shows a pH (potential of hydrogen) of 7.465, pCO_2 (partial pressure of carbon dioxide) of 35.6, pO_2 (oxygen pressure) of 125.1, bicarbonate of 25.1, FIO_2 40%, rate of 17 with PEEP (positive end-expiratory pressure) of 5, and PFV (peak flow volume) of 15. Gastrointestinal: Soft with positive bowel sounds; nondistended. Nasogastric tube residuals of 10 cc (cubic centimeter) and 10 cc, respectively. GU (genitourinary): Foley in place. Good urine output: 1396/3100. Endocrine: Serum glucose 152. Accu-Cheks of 137/145 today.

No insulin necessary. Electrolytes: Sodium 135, potassium 3.2, chloride 102, CO_2 (carbon dioxide) 21.8, BUN (blood urea nitrogen) 27, creatinine 1.1, and calcium 7.2. The patient had 40 mEq of potassium chloride in the NG tube ×2 doses this morning. Potassium will be redrawn at noon. Hematologic: White blood cells 15.5, down from a high of 17.3. Hemoglobin 15.8, hematocrit 45.6, and platelet count 178. PT (prothrombin time) is 12.8. INR (International Normalized Ratio) 1.1 and PTT (partial thromboplastin time) 24.9. Infectious Disease: Continue antibiotics until sensitivity is back on the sputum culture. Blood culture and urine culture show no growth. The patient is afebrile. White blood cell count is dropping. Neurologic: The patient is sedated, but minimally responsive. Integumentary: Normal.

DISPOSITION: Change the vent settings to rate of 10 and draw ABG in 30 minutes. Begin weaning the patient from the vent. Anticipate extubation this afternoon. Will see the patient after extubation. Await identification and sensitivity on sputum culture. Cardiology is following the cardiomyopathy. Discontinue Versed drip.

SERVICE CODE(S): _____

ICD-10-CM DX CODE(S): _____

CASE 9-3E *Thoracic Medicine/Critical Care Progress Note*

LOCATION: Inpatient, Hospital

PATIENT: Kurt Troy

ATTENDING PHYSICIAN: Gregory Dawson, MD

The patient is doing well. He had no major events during the night. He was extubated yesterday and transferred out to the floor. He has been walking and eating. His main complaint was back pain, which seems to have been helped by Tylenol.

He denies nausea or vomiting. He is having bowel movements.

PHYSICAL EXAMINATION: He is afebrile. Blood pressure 150/46, heart rate 87 per minute. Respirations 18 per minute. Saturations 100% on 3 L (liter). LUNGS: Clear bilaterally. Regular rate and rhythm; no murmur. Soft and nontender abdomen. No sacral or lower extremity edema, no clubbing. The patient is awake, alert, and oriented times three. No focal neurologic deficit.

IMPRESSION:

1. Congestive heart failure and respiratory failure, improved, status post extubation
2. Pulmonary edema
3. Back pain from questionable vertebral fractures without neurologic deficits

PLAN:

1. Taper oxygen
2. Discontinue Triamterene
3. Tylenol 650 mg (milligram) p.o. (by mouth) q.6h. (every 6 hours)
4. Possible discharge tomorrow. Will discuss with Dr. Elhart in the morning

Patient and his family who accompany him today agree with this plan.

SERVICE CODE(S): _____

ICD-10-CM DX CODE(S): _____

(Answers to every other Case are located in Appendix D. The full answer key is only available in the TEACH Instructor Resources on Evolve.)

CASE 9-3F   *Radiology Report, Chest*

LOCATION: Inpatient, Hospital

PATIENT: Kurt Troy

ATTENDING PHYSICIAN: Gregory Dawson, MD

EXAMINATION OF: Chest

CLINICAL SYMPTOMS: Follow-up congestive heart failure, pulmonary edema, respiratory failure

REFERRING DR: None stated

ONE-VIEW CHEST: 7:50 PM. Single AP (anterior posterior) view was obtained of the chest yesterday at 7:50 PM. Comparison study is the previous day. Endotracheal tube and nasogastric tube have been removed. There is again cardiac enlargement. Pulmonary vascularity is mildly prominent. Along the perihilar and infrahilar regions, there are some hazy density and increased markings. Suspect these findings relate to congestive changes. These findings are generally similar compared with the previous day. Suggest continued progress studies.

SERVICE CODE(S): _____

ICD-10-CM DX CODE(S): _____

CASE 9-3G   *Discharge Summary*

LOCATION: Inpatient, Hospital

PATIENT: Kurt Troy

ATTENDING PHYSICIAN: Gregory Dawson, MD

The patient was admitted with acute respiratory distress secondary to pulmonary edema. His course included intubation and being on the ventilator. He was extubated after the pulmonary edema came under control. He has severe cardiac disease, and ejection fraction was quite diminished. He was able to be discharged.

DISCHARGE DIAGNOSES:

1. Acute respiratory failure secondary to acute pulmonary edema
2. Congestive cardiomyopathy
3. Congestive heart failure

DISCHARGE MEDICATIONS:

1. Tylenol 650 mg (milligram) q.6h. p.r.n. (as needed)
2. Furosemide 40 mg q.d. (every day)
3. Cozaar 100 mg b.i.d. (twice a day)
4. Protonix 40 mg q.d.

He was to resume his Imdur, Lanoxin, Glucovance, Atrovent, Maxair, Serevent, and Lipitor as he was taking at home prior to admission.

Follow-up was arranged with his primary care physician, Dr. Green, Thursday after discharge to get a basic metabolic panel before that visit. He is to see Dr. Elhart in a month after discharge for medication review. Dr. Elhart will probably elect to use Coreg later when he is stable and use a graduated increasing dose as is customary for severe congestive heart failure. I also advised him not to use ibuprofen because it has some salt retention properties and can aggravate the underlying congestive heart failure by the salt and water retention properties and is also nephrotoxic, especially in low cardiac output states, and he should probably stay off of all NSAIDS (nonsteroidal antiinflammatory drugs). I will be glad to see him as necessary, but my duty was mainly for ICU (intensive care unit) critical care while he was in the hospital.

SERVICE CODE(S): _____

ICD-10-CM DX CODE(S): _____

(Answers to every other Case are located in Appendix D . The full answer key is only available in the TEACH Instructor Resources on Evolve.)

CASE 9-4   *ENT Consultation*

Dr. Dawson requested an ENT consultation to assess the viability of tracheostomy for a ventilator-dependent patient.

LOCATION: Inpatient, Hospital

PATIENT: Bea Fore

ATTENDING PHYSICIAN: Gregory Dawson, MD

CONSULTANT: Jeff King, MD

Thank you for asking me to see the patient in consultation.

CHIEF COMPLAINT: Respiratory failure

HISTORY: The patient is a 60-year-old who suffered a left hip fracture 2 weeks ago. She underwent an open reduction internal fixation and required intubation. Postoperatively, she developed pneumonia and some ARDS (acute or adult respiratory distress syndrome). She has been ventilated since that time. Any attempts to wean her have been unsuccessful, and it is recommended that she have a tracheostomy to facilitate weaning and tracheal pulmonary toileting.

PAST MEDICAL HISTORY:

1. Hypertension
2. CVA (stroke/cardiovascular accident)
3. Diabetes
4. Bronchitis
5. Cellulitis of the lower extremity
6. Coronary artery disease
7. Coronary catheter
8. Renal artery stenosis
9. Right carotid stenosis
10. Obesity
11. Chronic obstructive pulmonary disease

MEDICATIONS:

1. Albuterol
2. Colace
3. Insulin

CASE 9-4—cont'd

4. Multi-vites
5. Vasotec
6. Procrit
7. Morphine PCA (patient-controlled analgesia)
8. Protonix

HABITS: She smokes one pack per day and has an approximately 30-pack-year history. She does not drink alcohol. She has been off work on disability.

ALLERGIES: No known drug allergies

SOCIAL HISTORY: She is married. I was able to speak to her husband today. I understand she has six children.

PHYSICAL EXAMINATION: She is intubated and ventilated. She is not responding to me today. She has an NG tube in place for feeding. Blood pressure is 140/50. Pulse is 99. Respiratory rate is 15 on the vent. She is saturating at 92%. She is afebrile. Examination of her neck reveals a very thick short neck with a lot of adipose tissue. Landmarks are very difficult to palpate.

LABORATORY: She had some increased LFTs (liver function tests). Her hemoglobin was 8.8, red blood cell count 292, hematocrit 28.2, and platelets 264.

IMPRESSION: Chronic respiratory failure

PLAN: We will arrange to perform a tracheostomy procedure for her tomorrow or Wednesday. We will need to arrange for her to be n.p.o. (nothing by mouth) and to have her insulin adjusted appropriately. Thank you again for allowing me to participate in her care.

SERVICE CODE(S): _____

ICD-10-CM DX CODE(S): _____

CASE 9-5   *Consultation/Transfer of Care*

Dr. Elhart requested a consultation from Dr. Dawson due to bouts of V. tach, wheezing, chest pain, and possible pulmonary edema.

LOCATION: Inpatient, Hospital

PATIENT: Arlo Dockray

ATTENDING PHYSICIAN: Marvin Elhart, MD

CONSULTANT: Gregory Dawson, MD

The patient is a 71-year-old Caucasian male who was admitted 6 days ago for severe shortness of breath, which was thought to be related to pneumonia. During his hospitalization, the patient has been complaining of chest pain across his chest, radiating to his jaw and right neck. He had a cardiac perfusion scan that was normal, with an ejection fraction of 70%. He had a neck CT (computed tomography) scan, which was negative for any abscesses.

The patient was doing well. Today he was walking in his room, and suddenly everybody was rushing into the room because he was in V. tach (ventral tachycardia) for 30 seconds; however, the patient did not lose his pulse and was totally asymptomatic. His heart rate stayed at around 110 to 130 per minute.

The patient complained of chest pain across his chest later, which was radiating to the shoulders and to the jaw. He received two doses of sublingual nitroglycerin with resolution of the pain. He continues to wheeze, however.

He has been progressively short of breath over the last 2 or 3 weeks. He cannot walk across the room without feeling short-winded. He also has orthopnea and PND (paroxysmal nocturnal dyspnea).

Apparently the patient had coronary artery disease and had an angiogram in the past, probably 2 years ago or so, by Dr. Elhart. According to the patient, there was some coronary artery disease, but he was not amenable to any intervention.

PAST MEDICAL HISTORY:

1. COPD (chronic obstructive pulmonary disease)
2. Type 2 diabetes since 1957
3. Coronary artery disease as mentioned
4. Pancreatic insufficiency, on pancreatic enzymes
5. Benign prostatic hyperplasia
6. Depression
7. History of pulmonary hypertension
8. Gastroesophageal reflux disease
9. Fibromyalgia and osteoarthritis
10. Status post pacemaker placement
11. Partial resection of the colon, appendectomy, and cholecystectomy
12. History of CVA (stroke/cardiovascular accident)
13. Hyperlipidemia
14. History of mitral and tricuspid regurgitation on echocardiogram
15. History of tuberculosis in the past
16. Left upper lobectomy for tuberculosis
17. Rotator cuff repair
18. Two back surgeries
19. Hypertension

ALLERGIES: No known drug allergies.

SOCIAL HISTORY: The patient never smoked. He lives with his wife in Manytown. He does not use alcohol or drugs.

FAMILY HISTORY: Brother had a heart attack at age 36. Mother had enlarged heart. Father died of natural causes.

REVIEW OF SYSTEMS: General: No fever, chills, or night sweats. Respiratory: Dry cough with wheezing. Cardiovascular: Orthopnea, PND (paroxysmal nocturnal dyspnea), exertional dyspnea, and generalized edema. GI (gastrointestinal): No heartburn, abdominal pain, constipation, diarrhea, hematemesis, or hematochezia, but he has been feeling bloated. ENT: Tinnitus bilaterally, which is chronic. Eyes: Negative. Skin: Negative. Neuro: Headache, but that is nonfocal. No neurologic deficits. No motor weakness, numbness, or tingling. Musculoskeletal: Arthralgias. No arthritis. GU (genitourinary): No frequency, urgency, hesitancy, hematuria, or dysuria.

CURRENT MEDICATIONS include the following:

1. Albuterol ipratropium treatments
2. Serevent
3. Amlodipine 5 mg (milligram) q.d. (every day)
4. Pancreatic enzymes

Continued

CASE 9-5—cont'd

5. Aspirin 325 mg q.d.
6. Sinemet q.h.s. (each bedtime)
7. Lasix 40 mg b.i.d. (twice a day)
8. Isosorbide 50 mg q.d.
9. Metoprolol XL 50 mg q.d.
10. Protonix 40 mg q.d.
11. Paxil 20 mg q.d.
12. Actos 45 mg q.d.
13. Prednisone 30 mg q.d.
14. Vitamin E
15. Lovenox 40 mg daily
16. Regular insulin and Lantus insulin
17. Bumex 0.5 mg was given stat at 6:00 PM
18. Zithromax 500 mg q.d.
19. Claforan 1g q.8h.

EXAMINATION: He is wheezing. His wheezing is audible. His blood pressure is in the 120s to 130s systolic and 60s diastolic. Heart rate is 137, atrial fibrillation with PVCs (premature ventricular contraction). He has engorged neck vein distention. I cannot see his JVP because of the engorgement in his neck veins. He is pleasant and talkative and responds nicely. Respiratory rate is probably 25 to 27 per minute. Lungs: Bilateral wheezes, decreased air entry in the left side but no obvious crackles. He has generalized edema, 2 in the lower extremities, no clubbing. He had some sacral and abdominal wall edema. No organomegaly. Positive bowel sounds are noted. The patient is awake and oriented × 3. No focal neurological deficits. Motor power 5/5 bilaterally. He has trace pulses in the extremities.

ECG (electrocardiogram) shows PVC and atrial fibrillation. No Q waves. No ST (sinus tachycardia) elevations or T-wave inversions.

Potassium from this morning was 4.5, with bicarb of 34.

IMPRESSION:

1. Wheezing, probably chronic obstructive pulmonary disease and questionable pneumonia

2. Questionable pulmonary edema
3. Engorged neck veins, probably secondary to pulmonary hypertension and right ventricular hypertrophy
4. Diastolic dysfunction on previous echocardiogram with mitral regurgitation
5. Normal cardiac perfusion
6. Multiple PVCs and nonsustained V. tach, which all precipitated after Bumex therapy; this could be related to hypomagnesemia or hypokalemia.
7. Status post pacemaker
8. Generalized edema, which could be related to the diastolic dysfunction. I suspect that the prednisone and Actos have exacerbated that.

PLAN:

1. The patient was transferred to the intensive care unit.
2. Stat x-ray has been ordered.
3. Stat labs including troponin, CPK (creatine phosphokinase), magnesium, potassium, and phosphorus were ordered.
4. We will plan to control his heart rate with Cardizem.
5. Will get albuterol nebulizers.
6. We will repeat troponins in the morning.
7. We will consult cardiology in the morning.
8. Per discussion with the patient, he is code level I. In case of cardiopulmonary compromise, he will be fully resuscitated. If he stays on the ventilator more than 4 to 5 days and if we decide that the chances of his survival are minimal, the patient will be withdrawn from life support.

The patient seems to understand and agrees with the above plan.

SERVICE CODE(S): _____

ICD-10-CM DX CODE(S): _____

Discussion

There are a number of questionable and probable diagnoses listed under the Impression section of the report, such as probable chronic obstructive pulmonary disease and questionable pneumonia. Outpatient coders do not report probable, suspected, questionable, rule out, or working diagnoses. Only code symptoms or confirmed diagnoses: wheezing (R06.2) and edema (R60.9—this is the generalized edema indicated in point 8 of the Impression section of the report, not the questionable pulmonary edema indicated in point 2). Also in point 4 of the Impression section, the physician indicates the patient has mitral regurgitation. When referencing the Index, under the term "Regurgitation, mitral valve," a cross-reference directs the coder to "Insufficiency, mitral, I34.0," so the regurgitation is not reported separately, as it is included in I34.0.

(Answers to every other Case are located in Appendix D . The full answer key is only available in the TEACH Instructor Resources on Evolve.)

Medicine Services

The pulmonary specialty uses laboratory procedures to diagnose and treat patients with respiratory problems. Codes in the range 94010-94621 and 94680-94781 are for diagnostic procedures, and codes 94625-94668 are for therapeutic or diagnostic treatments. It is helpful to the coder to note treatment or procedure next to the code in the margin of the CPT manual to help distinguish easily between the diagnostic and therapeutic codes. Usually these procedures are conducted by a technician who is trained in administration of the test or the treatment. The technician provides these services under the supervision of a physician, usually a pulmonologist.

Many of the codes in the Pulmonary subsection (94010-94799) are **component codes,** which means that both the professional and technical components are included in the code unless the code description specifies otherwise. If the code description is for the entire procedure and only the technical component of the procedure is provided, use the -TC modifier with the code; if only the professional component is provided, you would use -26 modifier with the code.

Pulmonary function tests are performed to evaluate the mechanical ability of the respiratory system and the effectiveness with which the system can exchange carbon dioxide and oxygen. The components of the pulmonary function tests are spirometry, lung volume determinations, and diffusion capacity.

Spirometry

A common procedure that has many variations is a **spirometry**, which measures breathing capacity. Spirometry is one of the best tests available for early detection of many lung disorders. The spirometer takes readings (spirogram) of the patient's breathing and then compares the readings to normal values. The tests are usually administered by a technician under the supervision of a physician. A printout of the results (strip) is then produced for interpretation by the physician. The physician analyzes the results and prepares a written report.

Spirometry can be performed in the laboratory (94010/94060) or be patient-initiated. For procedures performed in the pulmonary laboratory, the technician measures the patient's breathing capacities. **Patient-initiated spirometry** (94014-94016) results in the same measurements but involves the submission of the data via telephone transmission from the patient's location to the pulmonary laboratory. The data is then reviewed for any sign of problems. The patient-initiated procedure represented in 94014 includes the technician instructing the patient on the use of the machine, graphic recordings, analysis of the data, periodic recalibration of the machine, and physician review and interpretation of results for a 30-day period. 94015 represents only the recording component for the patient-initiated procedure, and 94016 is for only the review and interpretation of the results. Patient-initiated spirometry is used to measure the strength of the lung function.

The spirometry report uses many assessments, such as the following:

- Forced vital capacity (FVC)—The maximum volume a patient can exhale after a maximum inspiration (volume the patient breathes out)
- Forced expiratory volume (FEV1)—Volume that can be expired at the first second after a maximum inhalation
- Forced expiration ratio (FEV1/FVC)—Forced expiratory volume divided by forced vital capacity. Normal would be that the patient could exhale about 75% to 80% of the air the patient inhaled.
- Peak expiratory flow rate (PEFR)—The fastest speed at which the patient can expel air from the lungs at a maximum effort
- Total lung capacity (TLC)—Lung volume following a maximum inspiration

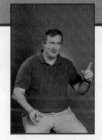

From the Trenches

"Communication and a willingness to adapt and grow are keys to a successful career as a medical coder."

MIKE MCCOLLUM
CPC, COC

Bronchospasm is the constriction of airways of the lung by a spastic contraction of the muscles of the bronchial area. These contractions obstruct airflow and are an indicator of lung disorders, such as asthma and allergy. There are many bronchospasm agents, such as histamine, methacholine, antigen, or gas. A spirometry is administered before and after a bronchodilator to measure the patient's lung capacities before the bronchodilator and after the bronchodilator and is reported with 94070. The bronchodilators are reported separately with 99070.

A complete spirometry (94070) includes:

1. Flow volume loop
2. Prebronchodilator flow rates
3. Postbronchodilator values
4. Maximal (ventilation) values [MVV] as in 94200

The bronchospasm is not to be confused with an inhalation bronchial challenge test. An **inhalation bronchial challenge test** (95070) is the inhalation of various substances to which the patient is thought to be allergic. The patient's bronchial response is then measured. The test does not include the pulmonary function tests necessary to assess the patient's response, only the inhalation of the substance. The function test that would subsequently be administered would be reported separately.

Although each physician establishes what is to be included in his or her complete pulmonary function test, it would include spirometry, lung volume determination, and diffusing capacity. A complete pulmonary function test would often include the following:

94010 Spirometry

This is the basic spirometry. For example, a patient presents with a history of cigarette smoking of 25 years duration. The patient complains of shortness of breath. The physician orders a spirometry to determine if there is decreased lung function.

94060 Spirometry with Bronchodilator

The basic spirometry is performed, and then bronchodilators are administered before and after the test to determine if the values increase after bronchodilator administration.

94070 Spirometry with Agents

This is the basic spirometry but with multiple determinations (measures/values) and the administration of irritating agents, such as cold air or methacholine.

Prebronchodilator and postbronchodilator values are assessments of lung function before a bronchodilator (such as albuterol or Ventolin—the facility reports these separately with 99070) and after a bronchodilator administration to determine if the lung function is significantly improved after administration of medication to expand the lumina of the air passages of the lungs.

94727 FRC (Functional Residual Capacity), Also Known as a Nitrogen Washout (Lung Volume Determination)

Functional residual capacity is also known as a nitrogen washout and measures the lung volume at the end of normal exhalation. The residual volume (RV) cannot be measured by spirometry because that is the air that remains in the lungs after exhalation. The determination of the residual (remaining) air is calculated by subtracting the expiratory reserve volume (ERV) from the functional residual capacity. Not being able to adequately exhale the air in the lungs is a sign of pulmonary disorder, such as emphysema. The physician interpretation of the results and preparation of the report are included in the services.

94726 TGV (Thoracic Gas Volume), Also Known as Plethysmography Lung Volume or Lung Volumes, Includes (Spirometry)

Thoracic gas volume (TGV) is a pulmonary function test that is known as plethysmography lung volume or lung volumes. The test uses various methods to assess the lung function and includes the residual volume or the amount of air that remains in the patient's lungs after exhaling. The assessment includes the volume of a single breath, air trapping (air caught in a collapsed bronchial branch), and airway collapse (closure of a branch or branches of the bronchial tree). The collapse or trapping is caused by bronchial walls that have been weakened by disease.

A nitrogen washout measures residual capacity or residual volume, air remaining in the lungs after exhalation. If a nitrogen washout is performed, do not report 94726 (thoracic gas volume); rather, report 94727 (functional residual capacity).

94729 DLCO (Diffusion Capacity of Carbon Monoxide), Also Known as Transfer Factor (Diffusing Capacity)

A DLCO is a diffusion spirometry. The DLCO is also referred to as transfer factor. A spirometry measures the mechanical properties of the lungs, but the DLCO measures the ability of the lungs to perform gas exchange. The patient inhales a gas that usually consists of helium and carbon monoxide with air. The mixture is held in the lungs for a few seconds. During that time, the lungs diffuse the mixture into the pulmonary blood. The patient then exhales and a sample is taken, and the resulting measurement indicates the diffusing capacity of the lungs. This assessment is especially useful in diagnosing interstitial lung disease, which occurs in the interspaces of the lung. 94729 is an add-on code and reported in conjunction with codes 94010, 94060, 94070, 94375, and 94729-94728.

94726/94728 Airway Resistance (Lung Volume Determination)

Airflow in the respiratory tract encounters resistance when the air molecules are slowed because of collisions with the sides of the ducts. Bronchial constriction or obstruction results in a decrease in the size of the bronchial airway and increases airway resistance. A determination of the resistance to airflow is measured by the air exhaled from the lungs in a single breath.

CASE 9-6   *Pulmonary Function Study*

You will be reporting only the physician portion of the service. In this case, the diagnoses that you are to report have been highlighted. The five reportable services of this study are indicated for you by the name of the study having been placed after each element in the Interpretation section of the report. Note that the components of the spirometry are not indicated in consecutive order in this report and often are not in order; rather, items 1, 2, 7, 8, and 9 are all parts of the spirometry. You will be coding another pulmonary function study in Case 9-9A without any indicators, so study this report carefully to ensure that you can identify the various elements of the study without the indicators.

LOCATION: Outpatient, Clinic
PATIENT: Hag Ulrich

CASE 9-6—cont'd

PHYSICIAN: Gregory Dawson, MD

ENTRANCE DIAGNOSIS: Dyspnea in a patient who has a 67.5-packs-per-year history of smoking and has a nonproductive cough. Gave good consistent effort.

INTERPRETATION:

1. Flow volume loop has mild concavity toward the volume axis, well-preserved inspiratory limb, reduced flow rates. (spirometry)
2. No significant change after bronchodilator. (spirometry)
3. Lung volumes are normal without evidence of hyperinflation. (also known as functional residual capacity)
4. Single-breath lung volumes are also normal without hyperinflation. (functional residual capacity)
5. There is significant dynamic airway collapse. (gas volume)
6. Transfer factor is reduced to 52% of predicted, suggesting reduced alveolar capillary membrane surface area and/or V/Q mismatching. (carbon monoxide, diffusion capacity)
7. Prebronchodilator flow rates have a pattern consistent with mild chronic obstructive pulmonary disease. (spirometry)

8. Postbronchodilator values show no significant change, and the same conclusion can be reached. (spirometry)
9. The MVV (maximum voluntary ventilation) is abnormal prebronchodilator and postbronchodilator. Between that and a normal FEV1 (forced expiratory volume in one second), I expect a reasonably normal exercise tolerance. (spirometry)
10. Airway resistance is normal. (resistance to airflow)

OVERALL IMPRESSION: COPD (chronic obstructive pulmonary disease) of mild degree; no significant reversibility. It does not explain this patient's complaint of being short of breath after any exertion, and it would probably be reasonable to get a methacholine challenge after the patient quits smoking to see whether he has bronchospastic disorder. One can assume that kind of complaint with his smoking history and that he probably already does have a bronchospastic component.

SERVICE CODE(S): _____

ICD-10-CM DX CODE(S): _____

(Answers to every other Case are located in Appendix D . The full answer key is only available in the TEACH Instructor Resources on Evolve.)

Sleep Studies

Sleep studies are performed to assist the physician in diagnosing sleep disorders. These tests are conducted for 4 or more hours, and the physician reviews, interprets the results, and prepares a written report. Polysomnography (many sleep recordings) differs from sleep studies in that it includes an electroencephalogram, electrooculogram, and an electromyogram. Other sleep study components (parameters) may be electrocardiography, airflow, ventilation and respiration effort, gas exchanges, extremity muscle activity, snoring, and other parameters as outlined in the Sleep Testing notes (95800-95811, 95782-95783) in the CPT manual.

Somnolence is an unnatural sleepiness or drowsiness that is often an entrance diagnosis for patients who undergo sleep studies.

Symptoms, Signs, and Ill-Defined Conditions

Subjective observations are those that are reported by the patient to the physician, such as drowsiness. The physician has not, at the point when the patient presents with the complaint, diagnosed the reason for the drowsiness. The physician may order a sleep study to assist in the diagnosis process. Reporting the diagnoses for these types of subjective observations directs the coder to either the chapter specific to the body area or to Chapter 18 of the ICD-10-CM, Symptoms, Signs and Abnormal Clinical and Laboratory Findings not Elsewhere Classified (R00-R99). If the reason for the symptom has been identified by the physician, the Chapter 18 codes cannot be assigned as the primary diagnosis because these codes report symptoms, signs, and ill-defined conditions; but if the reason for the symptoms has not been identified by the physician, the Chapter 18 codes would be assigned as the primary diagnosis. If the physician indicates contrasting or comparative conditions may be responsible for the condition, the symptom is reported as the primary diagnosis, because at that point no more definitive diagnosis has been stated. Once the cause or related condition is identified, the symptom cannot be reported as the primary diagnosis, since a more definitive diagnosis is then known.

Symptoms as Diagnoses

General symptoms are listed in categories R42-R69.

Symptoms involving the nervous and musculoskeletal systems are reported with R25-R29. For example, abnormal involuntary movements (R25.9) or lack of coordination (R27.9).

Symptoms involving the skin and other integumentary tissue are reported with R20-R23. For example, localized swelling upper limb (R22.3-) or cyanosis (R23.0).

Symptoms concerning nutrition, metabolism, and development are reported with R63.8. For example, anorexia (R63.0) or polyphagia (excessive eating) (R63.2).

Symptoms involving the head and neck are reported with R22/R51. For example, headache (R51.9) or swelling, mass or lump in neck (R22.1).

Symptoms involving the cardiovascular system are reported with R00-R03. For example, unspecified tachycardia (R00.0).

Symptoms involving the respiratory system and other chest symptoms are reported with R04-R09. For example, tachypnea (R06.82) or chest pain (R07.9).

Symptoms involving the digestive system are reported with R10-R19. For example, nausea and vomiting (R11.0) or dysphagia [difficulty swallowing] (R13.19).

Symptoms involving the urinary system are reported with R30-. For example, dysuria (R30.0) or incontinence (R32).

Other symptoms involving the abdomen and pelvis are reported abdomen pain (R10.9) and abdominal tenderness (R10.829).

Nonspecific Abnormal Findings

Categories R70-R97 are used to report abnormal findings that are nonspecific. For example, R73.09 is assigned to nonspecific findings on examination of the blood, such as abnormal glucose level. Sometimes the physician will indicate that the red blood cell count is abnormal but will not indicate what the abnormality is due to, or may document a differential diagnosis (such as, "either iron deficiency anemia [D50.9] or pernicious anemia [D51.0]"). Review the categories within the R70-R97 range now so you are familiar with the types of codes contained there.

CASE 9-7A   *Overnight Oxygen Desaturation Study*

Report the physician services for the following oxygen saturation levels during a 7-hour sleep study that was attended by a technologist.

LOCATION: Outpatient, Hospital

PATIENT: Sheldon Boucher

PHYSICIAN: Gregory Dawson, MD

ENTRANCE DIAGNOSIS: Somnolence.

The patient began the study at 2114 hours on 1 L with a baseline O_2 (oxygen) saturation of 91%. Between 2300 and 2330 hours, the patient had a significant period of time when the O_2 saturation was as low as 80%. The continuous printout is not really very helpful. At that time, oxygen was then turned up to 1 L and remained there through the rest of the night; the rest of the night his O_2 saturation was above 90%.

It appears that this patient needs 1 L via nasal prongs to control oxygenation. There was only one episode through the night, but it was for quite some time.

SERVICE CODE(S): _____

ICD-10-CM DX CODE(S): _____

(Answers to every other Case are located in Appendix D . The full answer key is only available in the TEACH Instructor Resources on Evolve.)

CASE 9-7B   *Nocturnal Polysomnogram*

At a later date, the patient also has a nocturnal polysomnogram but one without CPAP (continuous positive airway pressure).

LOCATION: Outpatient, Hospital

PATIENT: Sheldon Boucher

PHYSICIAN: Gregory Dawson, MD

ENTRANCE DIAGNOSIS: Somnolence

PROCEDURE PERFORMED: Nocturnal polysomnogram without CPAP titration.

The study began at approximately 2200 hours, continued through to about 0615 hours the next morning for a total of 480.5 minutes in bed, 411 minutes asleep, sleep latency of 26.5 minutes, and 92 arousals. Heart rate of 60 while awake and 50 while asleep. Had only four respiratory

CASE 9-7B—cont'd

events throughout the night. This gives him a respiratory disturbance index of less than five events per hour; anything over 5 is considered moderate to severe. After a total of four episodes, they were all hypopnea; the longest duration was 18 seconds. The lowest saturation was 89%. Heart rate was 45. We did measure some sinus bradycardia. He had no myoclonic leg jerks noted. He had grade 3 snoring that was intermittent, most prominent on his back and the first third of the night.

Because he did not have a significant enough problem, no CPAP was titrated. He had a UPPP (uvuloplatopharyngoplasty) in 2000 and that seems to have been effective.

SERVICE CODE(S): _____

ICD-10-CM DX CODE(S): _____

CASE 9-7C   *Multiple Sleep Latency Study*

Sheldon presents to the clinic 3 days later for a multiple sleep latency study.

LOCATION: Outpatient, Hospital

PATIENT: Sheldon Boucher

PHYSICIAN: Gregory Dawson, MD

ENTRANCE DIAGNOSIS: Somnolence

This was performed this morning. He had four separate naps, each of 20 minutes' duration. The first two naps he had a sleep latency

of 5 minutes for the first one, 9 minutes for the second time, and did not go to sleep at all the third and fourth time. He had no REM stages with any of these naps.

This is a negative study for narcolepsy. It does show the patient is sleep deprived, however (sleep deprivation is reported with a Z code).

SERVICE CODE(S): _____

ICD-10-CM DX CODE(S): _____

CASE 9-8   *Sleep Study*

Charlie Grove presents to the clinic for a sleep study.

LOCATION: Outpatient, Hospital

PATIENT: Charlie Grove

PHYSICIAN: Gregory Dawson, MD

STUDY PERFORMED: Nocturnal polysomnogram with CPAP (continuous positive airway pressure) titration.

ENTRANCE DIAGNOSIS: Daytime somnolence and obstructive sleep apnea.

The study began at about 2230 hours and continued to about 0530 hours the next morning, for a total of 444 minutes in bed, 271 minutes of sleep, with a sleep latency of 26.5 minutes. He had 275 arousals. He had a heart rate of 80 while awake, 78 while asleep, and it took 2 hours to document the severity of the disease. During that first 2 plus hours, he had a total of 46 respiratory events, for a respiratory disturbance index of 31.7; anything over 5 is considered significant. He had a heart rate of 90 while awake and 78 while asleep. The longest duration of any of these events was 39 seconds. The lowest O_2 saturation was 83%, and

the lowest heart rate was 70, showing hypoxic and some cardiac effect of these events. He also had 109 myoclonic leg jerks, 97 associated with arousal. He had grade 3 to 4 snoring in all sleep positions, but on his back the snoring was much more significant.

Once it was decided that the patient had severe significant sleep apnea, CPAP was titrated with a nasal mask and was not tolerated; full-face mask not tolerated for more than 5 minutes; BiPAP was also not tolerated. The patient experienced nasal obstruction with a claustrophobic feeling and just could not tolerate the masks.

The patient was also up to the bathroom about five times, which may be a direct effect of the significant obstructive sleep apnea.

During the rest of the night, he had many more events. The patient has obvious severe significant obstructive apnea.

The patient is intolerant of BiPAP and CPAP, so I would recommend referral to ENT for their consideration of a surgical procedure.

SERVICE CODE(S): _____

ICD-10-CM DX CODE(S): _____

CASE 9-9A   *Pulmonary Function Study*

In the following case, you will be reporting services that include pulmonary function study, consultation, operation, pathology, radiology, and several types of evaluation and management services.

Ellen Zutz is a patient who presents to the pulmonary function laboratory for an assessment for her dyspnea. Dr. Dawson will supervise and interpret the results of this testing.

LOCATION: Outpatient, Clinic

PATIENT: Ellen Zutz

PHYSICIAN: Gregory Dawson, MD

ENTRANCE DIAGNOSIS: Dyspnea in a patient who smokes 600 packs a year and has a nonproductive cough. Gave good consistent effort.

INTERPRETATION:

1. Flow volume loop has mild concavity toward the volume axis, well-preserved inspiratory limb, and reduced flow rates.
2. No significant change after bronchodilator.
3. Lung volumes are normal without evidence of hyperinflation.
4. Single-breath lung volumes are also normal without hyperinflation.
5. There is no significant dynamic airway collapse (air trapping).
6. Transfer factor is quite reduced to 50% of predicted, suggesting reduced alveolar capillary membrane surface area and/or V/Q mismatching.
7. Prebronchodilator flow rates have a pattern consistent with mild chronic obstructive pulmonary disease/emphysema.
8. Postbronchodilator values show no significant change, and the same conclusion can be reached.
9. The MVV (maximum voluntary ventilation) is abnormal prebronchodilator, normal postbronchodilator. Between that and a normal FEV1 (forced expiratory volume in one second), I expect a reasonably normal exercise tolerance.
10. Airway resistance is normal.

OVERALL IMPRESSION: Chronic obstructive pulmonary disease/emphysema of mild degree, no significant reversibility. It does not explain this patient's complaint of being short of breath after any exertion, and it would probably be reasonable to get a methacholine challenge after the patient quits smoking to see whether she has bronchospastic disorder. One can assume with that kind of complaint and with her smoking history that she probably already does have a bronchospastic component.

SERVICE CODE(S): _____

ICD-10-CM DX CODE(S): _____

(Answers to every other Case are located in Appendix D . The full answer key is only available in the TEACH Instructor Resources on Evolve.)

CASE 9-9B   *Cardiothoracic Consultation*

LOCATION: Outpatient, Clinic

PATIENT: Ellen Zutz

PRIMARY CARE PHYSICIAN: Gregory Dawson, MD

CONSULTANT: Gary Sanchez, MD

REASON FOR CONSULTATION: Right lung lesion

HISTORY OF PRESENT ILLNESS: This 62-year-old long-term smoker was seen by Dr. Elhart last October for angina. At that time, a chest x-ray showed an ill-defined density in the right mid-lung, which prompted a CT (computerized tomography) scan, which confirmed the lesion. There also appeared to be some hilar and subcarinal adenopathy. The patient has had progressive shortness of breath over the last 6 months with a dry cough. She has not had any hemoptysis at this juncture; however, she did have hemoptysis during episodes of pulmonary embolism several years ago. The patient uses four pillows for her gastroesophageal reflux disease and has some ankle edema. Skin testing 4 years ago for tuberculosis was negative. She has not had any other exposures of which she is aware. The patient has a 54-year history of smoking up to two to three packs a day and is currently smoking one-half pack of cigarettes per day. She does have some night sweats.

PAST MEDICAL HISTORY:

1. Numerous pulmonary emboli resulting in vena caval ligation.
2. Previous coronary angioplasties, the last angiogram being done last October, which showed total occlusion of the right coronary artery with good left ventricular function but with inferior dyskinesis.
3. Hypercholesterolemia.

PREVIOUS OPERATIONS: Two lumbar laminectomies with vena caval ligation, appendectomy, and hysterectomy.

ALLERGIES: Morphine, which causes swelling, and to penicillin, which causes a rash.

CURRENT MEDICATIONS:

1. Aspirin 325 mg (milligram) q.d. (every day).
2. Combivent 2 puffs b.i.d. (twice a day) to t.i.d. (three times a day)
3. Lipitor 10 mg q.d.
4. Covera HS 240 mg q.d.
5. Nitroglycerin as needed. She states that she takes the nitroglycerin one or two times per month.

SOCIAL HISTORY: The patient is married and lives in Manytown, where she is a postal clerk. She does not drink.

CASE 9-9B—cont'd

FAMILY HISTORY: Positive for emphysema and coronary artery disease.

REVIEW OF SYSTEMS: Cardiovascular: See above. Respiratory: See above. GI (gastrointestinal): See above. Musculoskeletal: Normal. Other than noted above is noncontributory.

PHYSICAL EXAMINATION: The patient is a 186-pound, 5 feet 5 inch female in no apparent distress. Blood pressure is 130/72. Heart rate is 90. The jugular venous pressure is normal. Carotids are 2, equal, and quiet. CHEST is clear and equal. The patient does have an occasional dry cough during conversation. HEART has a regular rhythm with a rate of 90 without murmur, rub, or gallop. ABDOMEN is obese without organomegaly, masses, or tenderness. EXTREMITIES show no clubbing, cyanosis, or edema. There are no varicosities. Pulses are intact peripherally. The patient is grossly neurologically intact.

Chest x-ray shows normal cardiothoracic ratio. There is an ill-defined mass in the right mid-lung field that extends nearly to the parietal pleura. This is confirmed by CT scan, which also shows some borderline adenopathy in the subcarinal area and right hilar area. Pulmonary function tests show a mid-expiratory flow rate of 109% of predicted with a mid-expiratory flow rate of 65% of predicted, and a maximal ventilatory volume of 78% of predicted. Her DLCO (diffuse capacity of lungs) is 52%. Echocardiogram done in October showed an ejection fraction of 55% with moderate LV (left ventricle) hypertrophy somewhat asymmetric in the septal area along with inferior dyskinesis.

LABORATORY done today showed a pO_2 of 72.6 with a pCO_2 of 41.9. Metabolic panel was essentially normal. PT (prothrombin time) was 10.8 and PTT (partial thromboplastin time) was 31.5. Hematocrit was 42.2 with 214,000 platelets.

IMPRESSION: Ill-defined mass in the right mid-lung field not amenable to bronchoscopy or CT-guided needle biopsy diagnosis.

DISPOSITION: The patient will be admitted in 2 days for elective right thoracoscopy and possible right thoracotomy and biopsy. Operation complications including blood transfusion, risks, and alternatives were discussed with the patient and her family.

SERVICE CODE(S): _____

ICD-10-CM DX CODE(S): _____

(Answers to every other Case are located in Appendix D . The full answer key is only available in the TEACH Instructor Resources on Evolve.)

CASE 9-9C   *Operative Report, Lung Mass*

Up until this report, the patient's diagnosis was that of a chest mass, but the pathology report that accompanies 9-9C indicates neoplasm of the middle and upper lobes of the lung. Rather than reporting one diagnosis code for the middle lobe neoplasm and another code for the upper lobe neoplasm, use the code for the lung neoplasm of contiguous sites, because the upper and middle lobe are connected or contiguous.

LOCATION: Inpatient, Hospital

PATIENT: Ellen Zutz

ATTENDING PHYSICIAN: Gregory Dawson, MD

SURGEON: Gary Sanchez, MD

PREOPERATIVE DIAGNOSIS: Right lung mass

POSTOPERATIVE DIAGNOSIS: Right lung mass

PROCEDURE PERFORMED: Right upper and right middle lobectomy with biopsy of four hilar lymph nodes

INDICATIONS: This 62-year-old female with a recent cough and shortness of breath was noted on chest x-ray to have a vague right mid-lung field lesion, which was confirmed by CT (computerized tomography) scan. There was some hilar adenopathy as well.

FINDINGS AT SURGERY: Lymph nodes from the hilum were biopsied times four, all of which were negative on frozen section. The inferior pulmonary ligament area, the azygous area, and the paratracheal area were all devoid of lymph nodes. The lesion was deep within the confines of the right upper lobe and appeared to cross the minor fissure into the right middle lobe.

DESCRIPTION OF PROCEDURE: The patient was brought to the operating room and placed in the supine position under general intubation anesthesia with a double-lumen tube. The patient was rolled in her left lateral decubitus position with the right side up. The chest was entered through the sixth intercostal space anterior axillary line with a thoracoscope. Gentle exploration of the right hemithorax showed no evidence of gross tumor implants on the parietal pleura. Retraction of the right lower lobe, however, did show evidence of what appeared to be tumor under the visceral pleura in the right upper lobe. A portion of the right middle lobe had been incorporated into this tumor mass. General exploration of all the lymph node–bearing areas really disclosed only mildly enlarged lymph nodes in the hilum. These were biopsied and sent for frozen section; all were benign. A standard right upper and right middle lobectomy utilizing the arterial first technique was carried out. The arteries were encircled with 0 silk, ligated, and clipped. The pulmonary vein was ligated distally and stapled proximally. The fissures between the upper and lower lobe were divided by several applications of the GIA automatic stapling machine. The bronchus was then skeletonized and clamped. Forced insufflation of the endotracheal tube produced good expansion of the right lower lobe. Following this, the staples were fired, and the right upper and right middle lobes were removed in one piece. These were submitted for frozen-section diagnosis, which showed adenocarcinoma. The chest was then checked for hemostasis and irrigated thoroughly with antibiotic solution and closed over two 36-French atrium chest tubes in the usual fashion. Sterile compression dressings were applied, and the patient returned to the postanesthesia care unit recovery room in satisfactory condition after application of an epidural anesthetic by Dr. Larson. Sponge count and needle count correct × 2.

Dr. Dawson will be assuming all postoperative care for this patient.

Pathology Report Later Indicated: See Report 9-9D

SERVICE CODE(S): _____

ICD-10-CM DX CODE(S): _____

(Answers to every other Case are located in Appendix D . The full answer key is only available in the TEACH Instructor Resources on Evolve.)

CASE 9-9D *Pathology Report*

PATIENT: Ellen Zutz

ATTENDING PHYSICIAN: Gregory Dawson, MD

SURGEON: Gary Sanchez, MD

PATHOLOGIST: Grey Lonewolf, MD

CLINICAL HISTORY: Lung mass, right side

SPECIMEN RECEIVED:

A. Hilar lymph nodes, right with FS (frozen section)
B. Hilar lymph node, right no. 2 with FS
C. Right upper and middle lobe with FS

GROSS DESCRIPTION:

A. The specimen is labeled with the patient's name and "right hilar lymph nodes" and consists of three red-brown lymph nodes, 1.0 cm, 1.0 cm (centimeter), and 1.4 cm in greatest dimension. These were submitted in one cassette.

INTRAOPERATIVE FROZEN SECTION DIAGNOSIS: Right hilar lymph nodes, (3): Benign lymph nodes as per Dr. Lonewolf.

B. The specimen is labeled with the patient's name and "right hilar lymph nodes" and consists of 0.5 cm, 0.8 cm, and 1.0 cm in greatest dimension red-brown lymph nodes. Submitted in one cassette.

INTRAOPERATIVE FROZEN SECTION DIAGNOSIS: Right hilar lymph nodes, (3): Benign lymph nodes as per Dr. Lonewolf.

C. The specimen is labeled with the patient's name and "right upper and middle lobe" and consists of a 360 g upper and middle lobe segment. Suture marks the location of tumor, and this area is inked black. Cut sections show a scirrhous gray-tan mass, 2.5 × 2.0 × 2.0 cm. Remaining lung tissue is red-brown. Surgical margins are grossly uninvolved by tumor. Possible lymph nodes are submitted in cassettes C2-C3 (second cervical vertebra-third cervical vertebra). Tumor is submitted in cassettes C4-C8 (fourth cervical vertebra-fifth cervical vertebra). Random section of red-brown lung is submitted in

C9, and pleural surface is submitted in C10. Representative sections are submitted in 10 cassettes.

INTRAOPERATIVE FROZEN SECTION DIAGNOSIS: Right upper and middle lobe tumor: Adenocarcinoma as per Dr. Lonewolf.

MICROSCOPIC DESCRIPTION:

A. Permanent sections confirm the frozen-section diagnosis of three perihilar lymph nodes negative for metastatic tumor.
B. Permanent sections confirm the frozen-section diagnosis of adenocarcinoma. Sections show infiltrating sheets of neoplastic cells with rudimentary gland formation. The neoplastic cells contain enlarged pleomorphic vesicular nuclei with prominent nucleoli and mitoses scattered throughout. There is surrounding fibrosis with chronic inflammation and anthracotic pigment and hemosiderin deposition. Tumor cells also follow the outline of the alveolar walls in areas. Tumor extends to the pleural surface, which is inked black. Additional perihilar lymph nodes are examined and are all negative for metastatic tumor. Tumor does not involve the surgical margin. Adjacent lung shows dilated alveoli containing extravasated red cells and hemosiderin-laden macrophages. There is anthracotic pigment deposition in some areas.

DIAGNOSIS:

A. Right hilar lymph nodes, (3): Benign lymph nodes, negative for metastatic tumor.
B. Right upper and middle lobe, lung:
   Infiltrating adenocarcinoma, moderately differentiated, forming a mass approximately 2.5 × 2.0 × 2.5 cm, extending to the pleural surface. Tumor does not involve the surgical margin.
   Twelve perihilar lymph nodes are negative for metastatic tumor.

SERVICE CODE(S): _____

ICD-10-CM DX CODE(S): _____

(Answers to every other Case are located in Appendix D. The full answer key is only available in the TEACH Instructor Resources on Evolve.)

CASE 9-9E *Thoracic Medicine/Critical Care Note*

LOCATION: Inpatient, Hospital

PATIENT: Ellen Zutz

CONSULTANT: Ronald Green, MD

ATTENDING PHYSICIAN: Gregory Dawson, MD

I have been asked to give an opinion on this patient regarding the care of her emphysema and to assist in weaning the patient off the ventilator. I have seen the patient as an outpatient, the first time in February at the request of Dr. Dawson because of abnormal chest x-ray. That was worked up and thought to be a cancer of the lung. Eventually we sent the patient to Dr. Sanchez, and he operated on her, taking her right upper lobe and her right middle lobe.

The patient is alert and oriented postoperatively and doing well.

For details of all the past medical history, social history, family history, and review of systems, please refer to my physician's assistant note where they are outlined in detail. The patient has also had a pulmonary function study, which showed obstructive disease of a mild degree. She is doing fine at this point just with a bilobectomy.

PHYSICAL EXAMINATION/REVIEW OF SYSTEMS:

CARDIAC SYSTEM REVIEW: Blood pressures are good at 120s-110s/60s. Pulse rate of 90.

PULMONARY SYSTEM REVIEW: Chest is clear. Chest x-ray looks pretty good. The pO$_2$ (oxygen pressure) is 80.8 on 40%, pH (potential of hydrogen) 7.34, and pCO$_2$ (partial pressure of carbon dioxide) 48.

GI SYSTEM REVIEW: Abdomen is soft and benign. I heard one bowel sound, so they are really quite hypoactive. Nontender. No hepatosplenomegaly.

GU SYSTEM REVIEW: She weighs 200 pounds. Baseline weight was 184 pounds taken from our scale in the clinic. No edema. BUN (blood urea nitrogen) 10, creatinine 0.7, and her fluid input yesterday was 4348 in and 510 out.

ELECTROLYTES: Sodium 140, potassium 4.9, and chloride 104.

HEMATOLOGY: White count 11,560, hemoglobin 12.6, and platelets 246,000.

ENDOCRINOLOGY: Glucose 141.

CASE 9-9E—cont'd

INFECTIOUS DISEASE: She is afebrile. Sputum is nonexistent. I do not think we have any evidence of active infection at this point.

DISPOSITION: I will try to wean her off the ventilator, and with any luck we can get her extubated later this afternoon. We will have to watch her electrolytes. I would be glad to monitor along if so requested. This looks like it might be relatively easy to get the patient off the ventilator.

SERVICE CODE(S): _____

ICD-10-CM DX CODE(S): _____

(Answers to every other Case are located in Appendix D . The full answer key is only available in the TEACH Instructor Resources on Evolve.)

CASE 9-9F   *Radiology Report, Chest*

Atelectasis is incomplete expansion of the lung.

LOCATION: Inpatient, Hospital

PATIENT: Ellen Zutz

ATTENDING PHYSICIAN: Gregory Dawson, MD

RADIOLOGIST: Morton Monson, MD

EXAMINATION OF: Chest x-ray

CLINICAL SYMPTOMS: Follow-up atelectasis

PORTABLE AP (ANTERIOR POSTERIOR) CHEST, SINGLE VIEW, 5:00 AM: FINDINGS: Comparison is made with yesterday morning's portable AP chest. Right ileojejunal catheter with tip in the right atrium. The patient has been extubated (ventilator status discontinued). Two right chest tubes are again seen. Small amount of subcutaneous emphysema has resolved. No appreciable change was seen in the heart size and pulmonary vascularity given the difference in technique. Area of atelectasis in the left lower lobe is somewhat more prominent. There may be a left mid-lung infiltrate, which is more prominent. This could be due to patient rotation. The left costophrenic angle is not included on the film. Strand of fibrosis or linear atelectasis, right perihilar region, is unchanged. Postoperative change is right thoracotomy.

SERVICE CODE(S): _____

ICD-10-CM DX CODE(S): _____

(Answers to every other Case are located in Appendix D . The full answer key is only available in the TEACH Instructor Resources on Evolve.)

CASE 9-9G   *Thoracic Medicine/Critical Care Progress Report*

Dr. Dawson was called out of town and has asked Dr. Green to assume the postoperative care for this patient. The official transfer was documented in the medical record. When reporting the postoperative care services for Dr. Green, you would report the CPT code for the surgical procedure (lung lobectomy) along with modifier -55, Postoperative Management Only.

LOCATION: Inpatient, Hospital

PATIENT: Ellen Zutz

ATTENDING PHYSICIAN: Ronald Green, MD

The patient was extubated yesterday from her surgery. She had a bilobe lobectomy for cancer of the middle lobe and lower lobe and underlying emphysema. This morning, on a simple mask, her pO_2 (oxygen pressure) was 58, pCO_2 (partial pressure of carbon dioxide) was up to 66.5, pH (potential of hydrogen) 7.26. Just from using BiPAP (bilevel positive airway pressure) 40%, her pO_2 was 54, pCO_2 was down to 58, and the pH (potential of hydrogen) was better at 7.31.

PHYSICAL EXAMINATION/REVIEW OF SYSTEMS: The patient was a bit sleepy but sitting on the edge of the bed, cooperating well with the mask; so we do not have to worry about intubation, at least at this time. Pulse, 90.

CARDIAC SYSTEM REVIEW: Blood pressures are excellent, I have 120s to 140s over diastolic of 60s. No S3 (third heart sound) or S4 (fourth heart sound). I do not appreciate any murmurs.

PULMONARY SYSTEM REVIEW: Please see above. On exam, she has a few rales scattered about. Chest, symmetrical. Chest x-ray shows increased vascular markings, more on the left than the right.

GI SYSTEM REVIEW: She does have some bowel sounds. She has been started on a clear liquid diet. Abdomen is nontender.

GU SYSTEM REVIEW: BUN (blood urea nitrogen) 8, creatinine 0.6. She had 2992 in yesterday and 1720 out. She weighs 194.3 pounds today. Her baseline weight is 186 pounds.

ENDOCRINOLOGY: Glucose 142.

ELECTROLYTES: Sodium 134, potassium 4.2, chloride 97, CO_2 32.2, calcium 8.1, magnesium 1.8, and phosphorus 3.2.

HEMATOLOGY: White count is 16,280, hemoglobin 12, and platelets 137.

INFECTIOUS DISEASE: She is afebrile. So far the cultures are negative, and she remains on cefazolin at this point. Chest tube output is 140 over the last 8 hours.

DISPOSITION: Use the BiPAP mask. Adjust it for eating, and if she is more awake she can just have the prongs on. Otherwise, if she is asleep, we will have to use the BiPAP mask. Check her labs in the morning. She is just a little bit volume overloaded, so I will try just a little bit of Bumex today and cut down her IV (intravenous) fluids.

SERVICE CODE(S): _____

ICD-10-CM DX CODE(S): _____

(Answers to every other Case are located in Appendix D . The full answer key is only available in the TEACH Instructor Resources on Evolve.)

CASE 9-9H *Radiology Report, Chest*

This is a single-view x-ray.

LOCATION: Inpatient, Hospital

PATIENT: Ellen Zutz

ATTENDING PHYSICIAN: Ronald Green, MD

RADIOLOGIST: Morton Monson, MD

EXAMINATION OF: Chest

CLINICAL SYMPTOMS: Follow-up left lower lobe pneumonia

PORTABLE UPRIGHT SITTING CHEST, 5:00 AM: Previous is from yesterday 5 AM. There is cardiomegaly as there has been. The vascular markings on the right are normal. On the left, there are some accentuated perihilar markings and some peripheral lung markings that are decreasing compared with yesterday and likely represent resolving failure pattern. They do not have the appearance of pneumonia. No atelectatic change is seen on left and no pleural effusion on left. In the interval since yesterday, the two chest tubes have been removed from the right hemithorax. There is small apical pneumothorax on the right. There is elevation of right hemidiaphragm. There is no atelectatic change or effusion. There is some prominence of the right paratracheal tissue, stable.

IMPRESSION:

1. Interval removal of right chest tubes. Small apical pneumothorax seen currently.
2. Right paratracheal soft tissue remains.
3. Cardiomegaly.
4. Accentuated parahilar markings on the left and some in the left lung periphery indicating this is respiratory failure rather than a pneumonia or pneumonitis. Overall there is improvement, left aeration, since previous examination of yesterday.

SERVICE CODE(S): _____

ICD-10-CM DX CODE(S): _____

(Answers to every other Case are located in Appendix D . The full answer key is only available in the TEACH Instructor Resources on Evolve.)

Pulmonary Stress Test

There are three types of tests performed to check pulmonary function. The exercise test is performed to check for bronchospasm and reported with 94617. The pulmonary stress test is also known as the 6-minute walk test and is reported with 94618 and the cardiopulmonary exercise testing is reported with 94621. The pulmonary stress test measures the workload and heart rate while also measuring the oxygen desaturation level. This type of test is conducted to measure the degree of hypoxemia that occurs with exertion. The cardiopulmonary exercise testing measures the oxygen uptake and production. This type of test is used to distinguish between cardiac and pulmonary causes of shortness of breath **(dyspnea),** to determine the level of ambulatory oxygen a patient requires, and to develop a safe exercise program for a patient with cardiac or pulmonary conditions as well as other conditions in which this more complex measurement is required.

Pulmonary stress tests are usually conducted with electrocardiographic monitoring. Because they are performed both at the outpatient clinic setting and the outpatient hospital setting, the use of modifier -26 is a consideration. When the clinic physician performs the study at the clinic, the global procedure is reported; but when the physician performs the study in an outpatient department at the hospital, the physician's services are reported with -26.

CASE 9-9I *Pulmonary Function Study*

LOCATION: Inpatient, Hospital

PATIENT: Ellen Zutz

ATTENDING PHYSICIAN: Ronald Green, MD

PROCEDURE PERFORMED: Walking O_2 (oxygen) saturation study because of dyspnea

Study began with an O_2 saturation of 90%, 89% on room air. With just a small exercise of up to 0.5 minutes, she had an O_2 saturation of 87, 86, 84, and 85%. In fact, it took 4 L per minute by nasal prongs to move the O_2 saturation above 89%. The highest I got was 92. Borg scale was rated as 1. Highest heart rate was 91. She was able to walk 500 feet. The patient walked at a good pace.

The patient does have reasonable exercise tolerance for so soon after a lobectomy, but she has significant oxygen desaturation and requires 4 L/min by nasal prongs with minimal exertion.

SERVICE CODE(S): _____

ICD-10-CM DX CODE(S): _____

(Answers to every other Case are located in Appendix D . The full answer key is only available in the TEACH Instructor Resources on Evolve.)

CASE 9-9J *Discharge Summary*

LOCATION: Inpatient, Hospital

PATIENT: Ellen Zutz

ATTENDING PHYSICIAN: Ronald Green, MD

HOSPITAL COURSE: This 62-year-old white female was noted on chest x-ray to have a lesion in her right lung. It was followed up for a short time and appeared to be somewhat denser. She was therefore submitted for a thoracic surgical consultation. After extensive preoperative evaluation by Dr. Sanchez, she was considered to be a suitable candidate for a thoracotomy. She underwent a right upper and right middle lobectomy for a stage I adenocarcinoma that appeared to be in the right upper lobe with extension across the fissure to the right middle lobe. The patient was maintained overnight in the ICU (intensive care unit), after which she was extubated and transferred to the ambulatory ward. The epidural was removed on the second postoperative day, and the chest tubes were removed on the fourth postoperative day. From that point on, with an episode of atrial fibrillation occurring the fifth day postoperatively, she was treated with digoxin and diltiazem with resolution. She did have short bursts of atrial fibrillation, however, the day prior to discharge; therefore, she was begun on oral anticoagulation, anticipating that she

may continue to have episodes of atrial fibrillation after discharge. On the seventh postoperative day, the patient was discharged home and given a return appointment to see me in 2 weeks for a chest x-ray, rhythm strip, and prothrombin time.

MEDICATIONS at the time of discharge:

1. Digoxin 0.25 mg (milligram) p.o. (by mouth) q.d. (every day)
2. Diltiazem 120 mg p.o. q.6h.
3. Ipratropium bromide inhalers.
4. Coumadin 5 mg p.o. q.d.
5. Percodan as needed for pain

FINAL DIAGNOSIS:

1. Stage I adenocarcinoma, right upper and middle lobe
2. Atrial fibrillation
3. Emphysema

SERVICE CODE(S): _____

ICD-10-CM DX CODE(S): _____

(Answers to every other Case are located in Appendix D . The full answer key is only available in the TEACH Instructor Resources on Evolve.)

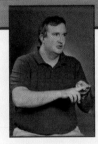

From the Trenches

"For a medical coder it doesn't matter where you start, but you must always be working toward a long term goal."

MIKE MCCOLLUM
CPC, COC

Septoplasty and Turbinates

The nasal septum divides one side of the nose from the other and is often deviated (crooked). **Septoplasty** is the surgical treatment for a deviated septum to relieve obstruction. The surgeon incises the mucous membrane inside the nose that covers the septum. The cartilage and bone are then elevated and portions of the septum are removed, straightened, or repaired. The mucous membrane is then returned to the normal position, and the nose is splinted and/or packed.

A septoplasty may be combined with a turbinate reduction or resection. Turbinates are the bones located inside of the nose; they are divided into three sections—inferior, middle, and superior, as illustrated in **Figure 9-2**. A resection is removal of an inferior turbinate bone and is reported with 30140. Turbinate reduction is performed to return the normal nasal airway by removal of turbinate tissue and is reported with 30140. Turbinate tissue will again develop after reduction, and as such the reduction may need to be repeated.

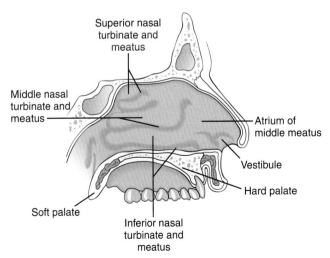

FIGURE 9-2 Superior, inferior, and middle nasal turbinates.

CASE 9-10   *Operative Report, Septoplasty, Turbinate Reduction, and Tonsillectomy*

This report is an excellent example of the need to correlate the CPT procedure code with a diagnosis code that supports the reason for the service. In the following case, the surgeon performed a septoplasty, turbinate reduction, and tonsillectomy. There must be a diagnosis code to support the reason each was performed; for example, the septoplasty (CPT code) was performed due to a deviated septum (diagnosis code); the turbinates were reduced (CPT code, this was bilateral) due to hypertrophy of the turbinates (diagnosis code), and the tonsillectomy (CPT code) was performed due to tonsil hypertrophy (diagnosis code). Each service has a supporting diagnosis and therefore substantiates why the procedure was performed (medical necessity). You may also code the sleep apnea as it indicates respiratory difficulties.

LOCATION: Inpatient, Hospital

PATIENT: Art Schear

PHYSICIAN: Gregory Dawson, MD

PREOPERATIVE DIAGNOSES:

1. Obstructive sleep apnea
2. Nasal obstruction
3. Septal deviation
4. Bilateral inferior turbinate hypertrophy
5. Hypertrophic tonsils

POSTOPERATIVE DIAGNOSES:

1. Obstructive sleep apnea
2. Nasal obstruction
3. Septal deviation
4. Bilateral inferior turbinate hypertrophy
5. Hypertrophic tonsils

PROCEDURES PERFORMED:

1. Septoplasty
2. Bilateral inferior turbinate mucosal reduction with radiofrequency
3. Tonsillectomy

ANESTHESIA: General endotracheal anesthesia

INDICATION: The patient is a 16-year-old male with documented obstructive sleep apnea. He also has a prior history of severe nasal obstruction due to a traumatic injury to his nose. Examination reveals a significant septal deviation with inferior turbinate hypertrophy. He also has very hypertrophic tonsils. At this point, we will correct his nasal airway and also increase his oral airway by removing his tonsils and see if that will help his sleep apnea. If there is any residual sleep apnea, he may be treated with nasal CPAP (continuous positive airway pressure) or, if he is unable to tolerate that, further airway expansion surgery.

DESCRIPTION OF PROCEDURE: After parental consent was obtained, the patient was taken to the operating room and placed on the operating table in the supine position. After an adequate level of general endotracheal anesthesia was obtained, the patient was turned and draped in the appropriate manner for nasal surgery. The patient's nose was packed with cotton pledgets and soaked with 4% cocaine. After several minutes, 1% Xylocaine with 1:100,000 units epinephrine was infiltrated into the septum bilaterally. It was also infiltrated into the inferior turbinates bilaterally. The nasal hairs were trimmed. Then, utilizing a right hemitransfixion incision, the mucoperichondrium and mucoperiosteal flaps were elevated. The deviated portion of the cartilaginous bony septum was then removed. Spurs off the maxillary crest were also removed. Hemostasis was achieved with suction cautery along the maxillary crest and then with FloSeal. Attention was then focused on the inferior turbinate. The anterior mucosa was treated with a radiofrequency needle to 500J on each side. The hemitransfixion incision was then closed with interrupted 4-0 chromic suture. A quilting suture of 4-0 plain gut was then performed. Silastic splints were then placed on both sides of the nasal septum and secured with nylon suture. The nose was then packed bilaterally with nasal packs, which consisted of Merocel sponge covered with a gloved finger coated with Bacitracin ointment. This was inflated with local solution. The patient was then repositioned for tonsillectomy. The McIvor mouth gag was placed, allowing visualization of the tonsil. Attention was first focused on the left tonsil. The Dean retractor was placed in the superior pole, and tonsil was retracted toward the midline. Then, utilizing a harmonic scalpel at power level III, the tonsil was removed in its entirety from a superior-to-inferior direction. Hemostasis was achieved from spot suction cautery. The similar procedure was then performed on the right tonsil. The tonsillar fossa was then irrigated with saline. There was no bleeding. Tension of the mouth gag was then released. Reinspection showed no active bleeding. The anterior and posterior pillars of the superior aspect of the tonsillar fossa were then reapproximated with interrupted 3-0 chromic suture and figure-of-eight closure. Subsequent reinspection showed no active bleeding. Mouth gag was then removed. Prior to removal of mouth gag, 1% Xylocaine with 1:100,000 units epinephrine was infiltrated into the retromolar and soft palate areas bilaterally. The patient tolerated the procedure well. There was no break in technique. The patient was extubated and taken to the postanesthesia care unit in good condition.

FLUIDS ADMINISTERED: 1800 cc of RL

ESTIMATED BLOOD LOSS: Less than 50 cc

PREOPERATIVE MEDICATION: 1 g Ancef and 12 mg (milligram) Decadron IV (intravenous)

SERVICE CODE(S): _____

ICD-10-CM DX CODE(S): _____

(Answers to every other Case are located in Appendix D . The full answer key is only available in the TEACH Instructor Resources on Evolve.)

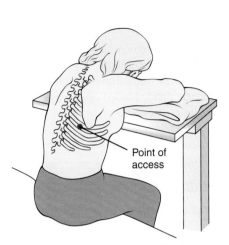

FIGURE 9-3 Patient in position for a thoracentesis.

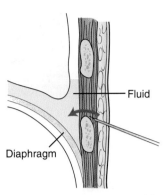

FIGURE 9-4 After administration of local anesthesia, a needle is inserted between the ribs, and fluid is withdrawn (thoracentesis).

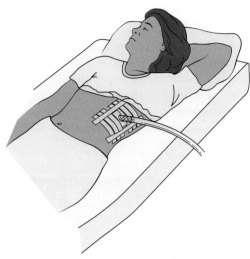

FIGURE 9-5 A chest tube may be inserted after thoracentesis to allow further drainage of fluid.

Thoracentesis

Thoracentesis is accomplished by having the patient sit with arms supported, as illustrated in **Figure 9-3**; local anesthesia is administered, a needle is inserted (**Figure 9-4**) between the ribs, and fluid is withdrawn. Thoracentesis is performed to withdraw fluid from the pleural space that has accumulated as a result of a variety of conditions, such as congestive heart failure, pneumonia, tuberculosis, or carcinoma.

Thoracentesis may also be performed to insert a chest tube as an indwelling method of draining the accumulated fluid in the pleural space (pleural effusion), as illustrated in

Figure 9-5. Local anesthesia is administered, and a small incision is made through the skin, fat, and muscle. The hole is then enlarged by using an instrument, and the tube is inserted into the pleural space. A suture is placed through the skin and tied to the tube. The tube is then secured with tape. The fluid is withdrawn by means of a suction device called a multichamber water-seal suction tube. This therapeutic procedure may be performed when the patient's pleural space contains air or gas (pneumothorax), blood (hemothorax), or a large amount of fluid (pleural effusion). These conditions can be caused by trauma, can be secondary to another disease process, or can occur spontaneously.

CASE 9-11   *Operative Report, Thoracentesis*

The physician in this report performed not only the thoracentesis but also the professional portion of the ultrasound guidance.

LOCATION: Inpatient, Hospital

PATIENT: Rod Foster

ATTENDING PHYSICIAN: Ronald Green, MD

SURGEON: Gregory Dawson, MD

EXAMINATION OF: Thoracentesis

CLINICAL SYMPTOMS: Possible infected pleural effusion

THORACENTESIS: The patient is a 57-year-old male with extensive medical history including persistent fevers of unknown etiology. The patient also has pneumococcal pneumonia, right middle lobe, and COPD (chronic obstructive pulmonary disease). Thoracentesis was requested by Dr. Green.

Prior to start of the study, the procedure was explained to the patient's brother, including the risks, complications, and alternatives. The patient's brother understood and consented to the exam.

The patient was prepped and draped in the usual sterile fashion. Using sterile technique under ultrasound guidance following administration of local anesthesia (1% lidocaine), a 19-gauge Yueh sheath needle was advanced into the inferior aspect of the right pleural space. Approximately 750 cc of clear yellow fluid was removed, and a specimen was sent to the lab for analysis. There is no evidence of pneumothorax.

IMPRESSION: Pleural effusion. Removed was 750 cc of clear fluid from the right pleural space as described above.

SERVICE CODE(S): _____

ICD-10-CM DX CODE(S): _____

(Answers to every other Case are located in Appendix D . The full answer key is only available in the TEACH Instructor Resources on Evolve.)

Tracheostomy

A tracheostomy is a procedure that can be performed as an emergency procedure, or it may be planned. A planned tracheostomy is performed to provide the patient with ventilation support. There are two approaches to a tracheostomy—transtracheal or cricothyroid, based on the location of the incision. The incision for the transtracheal tracheostomy goes across the trachea, and the incision for the cricothyroid tracheostomy goes vertically over the cricothyroid.

Tracheostomies are reported based on whether the procedure was a planned or an emergency procedure. The emergency procedure codes are further divided based on the approach. The planned procedure codes are divided based on the age of the patient as younger than 2 years or 2 and over.

From the Trenches

"Medical coders must demonstrate competency and the ability to adapt to changing technology."

MIKE MCCOLLUM
CPC, COC

CASE 9-12   *Operative Report, Tracheostomy*

This patient is 58 years old.

LOCATION: Inpatient, Hospital
PATIENT: Sally Gross
PHYSICIAN: Gregory Dawson, MD
PREOPERATIVE DIAGNOSIS: Failure to extubate, prolonged intubation
POSTOPERATIVE DIAGNOSIS: Chronic respiratory failure
PROCEDURE PERFORMED: Tracheostomy, planned
ANESTHESIA: General endotracheal

PROCEDURE IN DETAIL: Following informed consent from the patient's daughter, Charlene, the patient was taken to the operating room and placed supine on the operating room table. The appropriate monitoring devices were placed on the patient, and general anesthesia was induced. She was already orally intubated with a size 8 endotracheal tube. The neck was prepped and draped in the usual sterile fashion. The patient had a shoulder roll placed beneath her shoulders, and her neck was extended. Great care was taken so that there was not too much tension on the neck, and there was not.

The neck was marked. It was then injected with approximately 3 cc of 1% Xylocaine with 1:100,000 epinephrine. A scalpel was used to incise in a horizontal fashion through the skin. Cautery dissection was used to cauterize between the strap muscles down to the level of the thyroid isthmus. The patient had a very thin neck but surprisingly wide and thick thyroid isthmus, approximately 1 inch wide. Blunt dissection was used to dissect between the thyroid isthmus, and it was divided and tied off. Bleeders were all well controlled before proceeding further.

The cricoid cartilage was identified. A cricoid hook was placed into it. The inner space between the second and third thyroid cartilage was then incised with a no. 15 blade scalpel. Metzenbaum scissors were then used to enlarge this incision. A size no. 8 cuffed Shiley trach tube was then placed into the trachea following partial removal of the endotracheal tube. The cuff was then inflated. A good CO_2 (carbon dioxide) return was then appreciated on the monitor. The Shiley trach tube was then sutured in position. A piece of Xeroform gauze was then placed beneath the flange of the Shiley. The patient tolerated the procedure well. She was transferred to recovery in good condition. Estimated blood loss was less than 5 cc.

SERVICE CODE(S): _____
ICD-10-CM DX CODE(S): _____

(Answers to every other Case are located in Appendix D. The full answer key is only available in the TEACH Instructor Resources on Evolve.)

Endoscopic Procedures

Endoscopic procedures utilize a scope that is placed through an existing body opening, or a small incision is made into the body through which the scope is passed. Endoscopic procedures are often used in the diagnosis and treatment of respiratory conditions. When coding endoscopic procedures, be certain you code to the full extent of the procedure and the correct approach. The full extent is the farthest point to which the scope is passed.

When multiple procedures are performed, the surgeon may do one procedure with a scope and another procedure without a scope.

When multiple endoscopic procedures are performed through the scope during the same operative session, place the most resource-intensive procedure first and the subsequent procedure(s) to follow with modifier -51. There are, however, many bundled procedures in the respiratory codes, so be certain not to unbundle services that can be reported with one code.

CASE 9-13   *Operative Report, Septoplasty, Turbinoplasty, and Ethmoidectomy*

This report has several procedures performed during one operative session, which is not uncommon. Code each of the services while watching for bundled surgical services. Just because there are six items under the Procedure Performed section of the report does not mean there were six separate procedures performed. Only by reading the report can you correctly code the operative procedures. The ethmoidectomy is the most resource-intensive procedure performed during this operative session.

LOCATION: Outpatient, Hospital

SURGEON: Gregory Dawson, MD

PATIENT: Lucy Chang

PREOPERATIVE DIAGNOSES:

1. Septal deviation
2. Hypertrophic inferior turbinates
3. Enlarged (hypertrophic) ethmoid air cells

POSTOPERATIVE DIAGNOSES:

1. Septal deviation
2. Hypertrophic inferior turbinates
3. Enlarged ethmoid air cells

PROCEDURE PERFORMED:

1. Septoplasty
2. Turbinoplasty
3. Left intranasal anterior ethmoidectomy
4. Left intranasal posterior ethmoidectomy
5. Left intranasal removal of middle turbinate
6. Bilateral inferior turbinoplasty

OPERATIVE NOTE: The patient is a 39-year-old woman who was seen in the office and diagnosed with the above condition. She had a significant septal deviation to the right. The ethmoid air cells had overgrown on the opposite side, which meant that they had to be removed to allow the septum to assume a more midline position. She was admitted through the same-day surgery department and taken to the operating room, where she was administered general anesthetic by intravenous injection. She was then intubated endotracheally. The patient was draped in the usual fashion. Pledgets were placed in the nose with 4 cc (cubic centimeter) of 4% cocaine solution. After a short interval, the pledgets were removed and the 4-mm (millimeter) scope (indicates endoscopic procedure) was inserted in the left side. The roots of middle turbinate and uncinate were injected with 1% lidocaine with epinephrine. The middle turbinate was medialized. The large anterior ethmoid bulla was taken down, and we went posteriorly into the ethmoid cells and removed a medial portion of the anterior and posterior ethmoid cells (indicates ethmoidectomy). The root of the middle turbinate was identified, and the turbinate scissors were used to resect (left turbinoplasty) this, creating space for the septum to move over. We then packed this with some Afrin-soaked strip gauze. The left side of the septum was injected with 1% lidocaine with epinephrine. A left hemitransfixion incision was created, and a mucoperichondrial flap was elevated on this side. This extended posteriorly over the perpendicular place of ethmoid and vomer. We then separated the cartilaginous bony septum with the Freer elevator. We removed the deviated portion of the bony septum posteriorly, and then the cartilaginous portion was removed, leaving the dorsal strip and caudal portion of 1 cm (centimeter) inside for tip support (indicates septoplasty). Flap was laid back into position and sewed up with interrupted 4-0 chromic suture, and plain gut sutures were then used to quilt the septum in multiple places. Silastic stents were then placed on either side of the septum and secured with a single 3-0 nylon suture. The inferior turbinates were then medialized; these were large and redundant (left turbinate). Approximately two-thirds of the turbinate was left in place. The mucosa overlying this turbinate was then treated with electrocautery in several locations, and effective blanching was achieved. The Afrin gauze was then removed, from the ethmoid area, and this side of the nose was packed with Bacitracin-soaked strip gauze. The inferior turbinate on the right side was then medialized, and again the inferior portion was resected (right turboplasty). The mucosal portion of the remaining turbinate was then treated with electrocautery, and effective blanching was achieved. This side of the nose was then packed with the same Bacitracin-soaked strip gauze. The patient was then allowed to recover from the general anesthetic and taken to the postanesthesia care unit in stable condition. There were no complications from this procedure.

SERVICE CODE(S): _____

ICD-10-CM DX CODE(S): _____

(Answers to every other Case are located in Appendix D . The full answer key is only available in the TEACH Instructor Resources on Evolve.)

CASE 9-14 *Operative Report, Ethmoidectomy and Antrostomy*

In this surgical session, the surgeon performed three procedures, each of which is highlighted in the Procedure Performed section of the report.

LOCATION: Outpatient, Hospital

PATIENT: Inez Epley

PHYSICIAN: Gregory Dawson, MD

PREOPERATIVE DIAGNOSIS: Recurrent acute left-sided sinusitis and left conchal bullosa, left nasal obstruction

POSTOPERATIVE DIAGNOSIS: Recurrent acute left-sided sinusitis and left conchal bullosa, left nasal obstruction

PROCEDURE PERFORMED: Left functional endoscopic sinus surgery and removal of left conchal bullosa (this is a concha bullosa resection). The patient also had left anterior ethmoidectomy and left maxillary antrostomy.

ANESTHESIA: General endotracheal anesthesia

PROCEDURE IN DETAIL: Following informed consent from the patient, she was taken to the operating room and placed supine on the operating room table. The appropriate monitoring devices were placed on the patient, and general anesthesia was induced. She was orally intubated without difficulty. The left nasal cavity was packed with Afrin-soaked gauze. This was removed after 5 minutes. The patient was draped in the usual sterile fashion. The lateral nasal wall on the left-hand side was injected with approximately 2 cc of 1% Xylocaine with 1:100,000 units epinephrine. The widened left middle turbinate was also injected with 1 cc of the same. Following adequate time for the injection to take effect, a sickle knife was used to incise through the central portion of the left middle turbinate. The lateral half of the conchal bullosa was removed using Wilde forceps. A nice left maxillary sinus antrostomy was then created. The shaver was used to trim the mucosal edges. The anterior ethmoid air cells were opened using the Wilde forceps. The shaver was used to trim some of the mucosa within the left anterior ethmoid air cells. The area was then packed with Afrin-soaked gauze. After 5 minutes it was removed. There was no further bleeding. A stent was then placed into the left ostial meatal complex. The nasopharynx was then suctioned of blood.

The patient was then allowed to recover from general anesthetic and was transferred to the recovery room in good condition. She tolerated the procedure well.

ESTIMATED BLOOD LOSS: Less than 50 cc

SERVICE CODE(S): _____

ICD-10-CM DX CODE(S): _____

(Answers to every other Case are located in Appendix D . The full answer key is only available in the TEACH Instructor Resources on Evolve.)

CASE 9-15A *Thoracic Medicine and Critical Care Consultation*

This case contains many reports for a patient who was admitted to the hospital and received a wide variety of services to diagnose and treat his condition.

LOCATION: Inpatient, Hospital

PATIENT: Virgil Zejdlek

ATTENDING PHYSICIAN: Ronald Green, MD

CONSULTANT: Gregory Dawson, MD

This is a patient who is well known to me from the past. I was asked to see the patient again today to comment on his abnormal chest x-ray; actually the patient has already had a biopsy taken. I went to pathology, and we saw on preliminary results poorly differentiated carcinoma. They are having a lot of trouble determining whether it is a non–small cell or small cell. I think we have to wait for the special stains and the core biopsy to come out for a better diagnostic label. The patient does describe dysphagia and shortness of breath. He may need drainage of the pleural fluid again, but we will see how that goes in the future. Right now I think we will let Dr. Green know what is going on with the abnormal CT (computerized tomography) scan and take a look at the esophagus. He may actually have a lung cancer that has spread through the esophagus. I will let oncology know that they should see whether he could be started on a chemotherapy program of radiation, depending on the final diagnosis.

For a detailed review of the past medical history, social history, family history, and review of systems, please refer to my notes from last time just a little less than a month ago and Dr. Green's note where they are outlined in detail.

PHYSICAL EXAMINATION: On examination, the patient is alert and able to give his own history. Neck is supple. Lungs have diminished breath sounds, in fact more so on the left than the right. Heart shows a regular rhythm without an S3 (third heart sound). Abdomen is benign. Extremities show some trace edema. Chest, symmetrical. Back, straight.

IMPRESSION: Poorly differentiated carcinoma of the lung with pleural effusion that may have to be drained again because of the shortness of breath, although he says it is better today than it has been. He is lying flat on his side at this time. I did talk to Dr. Green, who is his primary care physician at this point. We will get in touch with oncology and Dr. White to see what we can offer this patient. He may have some real problems here. I would be happy to follow along if so requested.

CYTOLOGY REPORT of the aspirate confirmed the pleural effusion was not malignant.

SERVICE CODE(S): _____

ICD-10-CM DX CODE(S): _____

(Answers to every other Case are located in Appendix D . The full answer key is only available in the TEACH Instructor Resources on Evolve.)

CASE 9-15B   *Thoracic Medicine and Critical Care Progress Report*

Dr. Green transferred care of Virgil Zejdlek to Dr. Dawson, who now is the attending physician. Dr. Dawson continues to update Dr. Green regarding the patient's care by indicating that Dr. Green is the primary care physician, and as such Dr. Green will receive copies of Dr. Dawson's documentation regarding Mr. Zejdlek. Note that for the diagnosis for this report, Dr. Dawson has indicated that the carcinoma is of either the lung or esophagus. As such, as an outpatient coder you cannot report the diagnosis code for the specific site of the carcinoma; rather, you will report the unspecified site.

LOCATION: Inpatient, Hospital

PATIENT: Virgil Zejdlek

PRIMARY CARE PHYSICIAN: Ronald Green, MD

ATTENDING PHYSICIAN: Gregory Dawson, MD

The patient is here with a poorly differentiated carcinoma of either the lung or esophagus. The patient has been experiencing shortness of breath for some time now. Dr. Friendly is going to be scoping the patient today to see what the distal esophagus looks like, and we have some CT (computerized tomography) scan evidence that there may be some involvement of that. We still do not have a final pathology of the poorly differentiated carcinoma; that will be coming hopefully today or tomorrow. He still has shortness of breath. I think the fluid has reaccumulated. I will check on that today with PA (posterior/anterior) and lateral and left lateral decubitus, and if he has more fluid coming back down, perhaps CT surgery can place a chest tube at this time. We will see if we cannot get it drained more. Chest is barrel-shaped. The chest today sounds like there may be more fluid in there, at least the level of diminished breath sounds seems to be higher, so we will get that ordered today. I am basically waiting for laboratory results to come back. .

SERVICE CODE(S): _____

ICD-10-CM DX CODE(S): _____

(Answers to every other Case are located in Appendix D . The full answer key is only available in the TEACH Instructor Resources on Evolve.)

CASE 9-15C   *Thoracic Medicine and Critical Care Progress Report*

LOCATION: Inpatient, Hospital

PATIENT: Virgil Zejdlek

PRIMARY CARE PHYSICIAN: Ronald Green, MD

ATTENDING PHYSICIAN: Gregory Dawson, MD

The patient has cancer of the lung. We were not sure originally whether it was cancer of lung to esophagus or esophagus to lung, but this is lung to esophagus and has a pleural effusion with it. The patient is still experiencing shortness of breath. Yesterday I received chest x-rays looking for extensive left pleural effusion. I think it is a small amount of fluid that is freely flowing, as you can tell by the lateral decubitus. Most of what we see of tumor mass and atelectatic lung surrounding the tumor mass extends into the mediastinum. I do not think a thoracentesis would be of much help at this point. There was some controversy whether or not the patient had free air in the abdomen, but after consulting with our radiologist, I do not believe that is the problem. I do not think it exists. I think we are just being fooled by the air bubble in either the colon or the stomach. The patient is too out of shape for that. The patient does have some chest pain, but I think it is the same chest discomfort he had when he came in that was pleuritic associated with the mass. ECG (electrocardiogram) done this morning shows sinus rhythm, LVH (left ventricular hypertrophy), and no acute changes anyway. Cardiac enzymes are pending. I did contact Dr. Eagle. He says the patient needs radiation therapy and chemotherapy. I will let the radiation therapists and Dr. Eagle work out who does what to whom first. At this point, unless a pleural effusion becomes larger, I do not think a repeat thoracentesis would be of much help at this point. If it does become larger, I think at that time perhaps a chest tube might be of some help, because I think there is going to be a recurrent problem. I talked to the patient about this. I stated that I would be out of town and I would have to sign off the case until I get back. I would be glad to see him again in the future if so requested.

SERVICE CODE(S): _____

ICD-10-CM DX CODE(S): _____

(Answers to every other Case are located in Appendix D . The full answer key is only available in the TEACH Instructor Resources on Evolve.)

CASE 9-15D   *Radiology Report, Chest*

Note in this report that the reason for the service is primarily the pleural effusion, not the carcinoma of the lung. This means that you should report the pleural effusion code first and the neoplasm code second.

LOCATION: Inpatient, Hospital

PATIENT: Virgil Zejdlek

PRIMARY CARE PHYSICIAN: Ronald Green, MD

ATTENDING PHYSICIAN: Gregory Dawson, MD

EXAMINATION OF: Chest

CLINICAL SYMPTOMS: Follow-up of pleural effusion. Primary carcinoma lung

PA (POSTERIOR/ANTERIOR) AND LATERAL CHEST WITH A LEFT LATERAL DECUBITUS VIEW OF THE CHEST: FINDINGS, TOTAL 3 VIEWS: This examination is compared to a prior chest radiograph. The heart size appears prominent but unchanged compared with the prior examination. The pulmonary vascular markings appear within normal limits. Left-sided pleural effusion is present at this examination. On the decubitus views, at least a portion of this is believed to layer out.

There is focal opacity present within the left mid and left lower lung zones, which is similar in appearance to the prior examination. There is radiographic evidence of COPD (chronic obstructive pulmonary disease). Mild patchy right infrahilar opacity is also noted. There is an unusual lucency seen to overlie the central portion of the epigastric region of the upper abdomen. This may be within bowel; however, the possibility of free intraperitoneal air cannot be excluded, and further evaluation with decubitus, supine, and upright views of the abdomen is recommended.

IMPRESSION:

1. Left-sided pleural effusion as described above. At least a portion of this is felt to layer out.
2. Focal opacity is seen within the left mid and left lower lung zone, which is similar to the prior examination. This may relate to atelectasis or infiltrate with underlying lesions not excluded.
3. Unusual lucency seen in the epigastric region. Additional evaluation with dedicated abdominal films is recommended.

SERVICE CODE(S): _____

ICD-10-CM DX CODE(S): _____

(Answers to every other Case are located in Appendix D . The full answer key is only available in the TEACH Instructor Resources on Evolve.)

CASE 9-15E   *Operative Report, Esophagogastroduodenoscopy*

In this report, the surgeon passes a flexible endoscope through the patient's mouth and obtains a duodenal biopsy. However, note that in addition to this procedure, the surgeon also dilates the esophagus. This is a manual dilation using a Maloney (rubber tube filled with tungsten or mercury) dilator. There are two types of mechanical bougies used for esophageal dilation: Savary dilator (stiff, yet somewhat flexible plastic) and the Maloney. Both types are graded in millimeters (mm) and French (1F = mm). The goal of the dilation is to disrupt any strictures by stretching them. Modifier -59 is added to indicate that the dilation was performed manually rather than via the endoscope as a distinct procedure, because an endoscopic dilation would be bundled into the endoscopy code and is not usually reported separately.

LOCATION: Inpatient, Hospital

PATIENT: Virgil Zejdlek

PRIMARY CARE PHYSICIAN: Ronald Green, MD

ATTENDING PHYSICIAN: Gregory Dawson, MD

SURGEON: Larry Friendly, MD

PREOPERATIVE DIAGNOSIS: Dysphagia

POSTOPERATIVE DIAGNOSIS: An ulcerated stricture area in the upper esophagus consistent with either squamous cell carcinoma of the esophagus or consistent with extrinsic metastases or local invasion.

PROCEDURE PERFORMED: Esophagogastroduodenoscopy with biopsy and esophageal dilation with Maloney dilator.

INDICATIONS: This 77-year-old white male was referred by Dr. Dawson for endoscopy. The patient has poorly differentiated carcinoma of the lung just diagnosed. He has had dysphagia, anorexia, and 30-pound weight loss.

PREOPERATIVE MEDICATION: Demerol 50 mg (milligram) IV (intravenous); Versed 2 mg IV

FINDINGS: The flexible Pentax video pediatric endoscope was passed without difficulty into the oropharynx. Immediately seen at 30 cm (centimeter) was what looked like the gastroesophageal junction. At about 31 cm there was an ulcerated strictured area to 34 cm. The area did allow passage of the pediatric endoscope. The patient had discomfort as we passed through the area. The gastroesophageal junction was actually seen at 42 cm. Inspection of the esophagus at this level did not reveal erythema, ulceration, exudate, friability, or other mucosal abnormalities. The stomach proper was entered, and the endoscope advanced into the stomach. There was a large amount of food present, but the patient was fasting post midnight. We were able to advance through the pylorus; however, we did not see any obstruction, and I did not pass beyond the duodenum. The retroflexion revealed a large amount of food. Inspection of the antrum and body from what we could see did not show any abnormalities except the large amount of food. We then, on withdrawal, reviewed the area again in the upper esophagus and performed multiple biopsies. We then removed the endoscope and passed a no. 46 French-Maloney dilator with only minimal resistance noted. The patient tolerated the procedure well.

IMPRESSION: Ulceration in the upper third of esophagus [this "upper third" is necessary to correctly assign the diagnosis code], distance at about 3 cm with some stricturing dilated with a Maloney dilator no. 46-French. This lesion could be the primary source, or it could be secondary with metastases or extrinsic involvement of the esophagus. We will await biopsies.

Pathology Report Later Indicated: Secondary squamous cell carcinoma

SERVICE CODE(S): _____

ICD-10-CM DX CODE(S): _____

(Answers to every other Case are located in Appendix D . The full answer key is only available in the TEACH Instructor Resources on Evolve.)

CASE 9-15F *CT-Guided Lung Biopsy*

LOCATION: Inpatient, Hospital

PATIENT: Virgil Zejdlek

PRIMARY CARE PHYSICIAN: Ronald Green, MD

ATTENDING PHYSICIAN: Gregory Dawson, MD

INTERVENTIONAL RADIOLOGIST: Edward Riddle, MD

EXAMINATION OF: CT (computerized tomography)-guided lung biopsy

CLINICAL SYMPTOMS: Lung mass

CT-GUIDED LUNG BIOPSY: The patient is a 77-year-old male with mediastinal and left lung mass. CT-guided lung biopsy was requested by Dr. Dawson.

The patient was prepped and draped in the usual sterile fashion. The mass in the left lobe was again localized. Using sterile technique from a left posterolateral standpoint, three separate core biopsies were obtained utilizing an 18-gauge ASAP Medi-Tech biopsy device. Suspicious cells were noted, and a definite diagnosis is pending.

The patient tolerated the procedure well. The patient denied shortness of breath or chest pain. There is no evidence of pneumothorax on the immediate post-biopsy CT study or on the 3-hour and 5-hour post-biopsy chest x-rays.

IMPRESSION: Three separate core biopsies of the left lung mass utilizing an 18-gauge ASAP Medi-Tech biopsy device as described above.

Pathology Report Later Indicated: See Report 9-15G

SERVICE CODE(S): _____

ICD-10-CM DX CODE(S): _____

(Answers to every other Case are located in Appendix D . The full answer key is only available in the TEACH Instructor Resources on Evolve.)

CASE 9-15G *Pathology Report*

Cytology is the study of cells that have been obtained by brushing or washing. Find direction to the correct code for this service by referencing the index of the CPT manual under the heading Cytopathology, Fluid.

LOCATION: Inpatient, Hospital

PATIENT: Virgil Zejdlek

PRIMARY CARE PHYSICIAN: Ronald Green, MD

ATTENDING PHYSICIAN: Gregory Dawson, MD

PATHOLOGIST: Grey Lonewolf, MD

CLINICAL HISTORY: Large mass left lung mediastinal area, concurrent

GROSS DESCRIPTION: Pleural effusion, two diff quiks, six prepared smears

SPECIMEN RECEIVED: Lung touch prep, left, mass

SPECIMEN ADEQUACY: Specimen satisfactory for cytologic evaluation

DIAGNOSIS: Malignant cells suggestive of undifferentiated neoplasm

COMMENTS: The malignant cells show some subjective features reminiscent of small cell carcinoma, but nuclear size is more compatible with non–small cell carcinoma. Cytology correlates with accompanying histology specimen.

SERVICE CODE(S): _____

ICD-10-CM DX CODE(S): _____

(Answers to every other Case are located in Appendix D . The full answer key is only available in the TEACH Instructor Resources on Evolve.)

CASE 9-15H *Ultrasound Marking for Thoracentesis*

LOCATION: Inpatient, Hospital

PATIENT: Virgil Zejdlek

PRIMARY CARE PHYSICIAN: Ronald Green, MD

ATTENDING PHYSICIAN: Gregory Dawson, MD

RADIOLOGIST: Morton Monson, MD

EXAMINATION OF: Ultrasound marking for thoracentesis

CLINICAL SYMPTOMS: Pleural fluid

ULTRASOUND MARKINGS FOR THORACENTESIS: Left hemithorax was marked in the visualized area of the largest amount of pleural fluid on the left. Distance from the skin surface to the central portion of the fluid equals 6 cm (centimeter).

SERVICE CODE(S): _____

ICD-10-CM DX CODE(S): _____

(Answers to every other Case are located in Appendix D . The full answer key is only available in the TEACH Instructor Resources on Evolve.)

CASE 9-15I   *Operative Report, Thoracentesis*

LOCATION: Inpatient, Hospital

PATIENT: Virgil Zejdlek

PRIMARY CARE PHYSICIAN: Ronald Green, MD

ATTENDING PHYSICIAN: Gregory Dawson, MD

PREOPERATIVE DIAGNOSIS: Right pleural effusion with unknown cause

POSTOPERATIVE DIAGNOSIS: Right pleural effusion with unknown cause

PROCEDURES PERFORMED:

1. Diagnostic thoracentesis
2. Four quadrant pleural biopsy (This indicates the number of biopsies you will be reporting.)
3. Pleural drainage with a small-caliber temporary chest tube

PROCEDURE: With the usual Betadine scrub to the area previously marked by ultrasound, the area was anesthetized with approximately 15 cc (cubic centimeter) of 1% lidocaine, and then a 21-gauge needle was inserted into the space. Fluid was removed for appropriate bacteriologic, hematologic, and chemical analysis.

Once this was accomplished, a larger tube using a Cope pleural biopsy needle was inserted into the space, and four quadrants were biopsied and sent for appropriate pathological specimens. Once that was accomplished, using a small-caliber temporary chest tube from the Cook as well as the pneumothorax set, the space was entered and 1.5 L of bloody fluid was removed. A small bandage was attached afterward. There was no pain involved, and the chest x-ray will be taken afterward to assure ourselves we had a reasonable effect without any ill consequences.

Pathology Report Indicated: See Report 9-15J

SERVICE CODE(S): _____

ICD-10-CM DX CODE(S): _____

(Answers to every other Case are located in Appendix D . The full answer key is only available in the TEACH Instructor Resources on Evolve.)

CASE 9-15J   *Pathology Report*

Report the cytopathology services provided by Dr. Lonewolf.

LOCATION: Inpatient, Hospital

PATIENT: Virgil Zejdlek

PRIMARY CARE PHYSICIAN: Ronald Green, MD

ATTENDING PHYSICIAN: Gregory Dawson, MD

PATHOLOGIST: Grey Lonewolf, MD

CLINICAL HISTORY: Large mass, left lung and mediastinum, pleural effusion, concurrent cytology

SPECIMEN RECEIVED: Left-lung fine needle biopsy (This is a fine needle core biopsy [FNB], which involves tissue. This is not an FNA [fine needle aspiration], which would involve fluid obtained via needle.)

GROSS DESCRIPTION: Submitted in formalin, labeled with patient's name and "left lung FNB" are core needle fragments of white to brown tissue measuring less than 0.25 cc in aggregate. Submitted in toto.

MICROSCOPIC DESCRIPTION: Sections show tiny core needle fragments of fibrous tissue featuring nests of infiltrating poorly differentiated neoplastic cells. There is a surrounding desmoplastic response. The tumor cells show high nuclear/cytoplasmic (N/C) ratios and moderate nuclear enlargement. Focal nests demonstrate cells with a small to moderate amount of pink cytoplasm and vesicular nuclei.

DIAGNOSIS: Lung, left, fine needle biopsy: Invasive poorly differentiated non–small cell carcinoma, fragments of.

SERVICE CODE(S): _____

ICD-10-CM DX CODE(S): _____

(Answers to every other Case are located in Appendix D . The full answer key is only available in the TEACH Instructor Resources on Evolve.)

CASE 9-15K   *Oxygen Desaturation Study*

This is an oxygen sleep study being performed to diagnose somnolence.

LOCATION: Inpatient, Hospital

PATIENT: Virgil Zejdlek

PRIMARY CARE PHYSICIAN: Ronald Green, MD

ATTENDING PHYSICIAN: Gregory Dawson, MD

ENTRANCE DIAGNOSIS: Somnolence

The patient started the study at 2100 and was continued until 0515 the next morning. He was on room air at the beginning, but his O_2 (oxygen) saturation dropped to 87%, and he was started on 1 L. I cannot tell from the tracing how long he was at 87% before starting 1 L (liter) per minute.

This was continued through the rest of the night, and his O_2 saturation stayed about 90%. He was intermittently observed. (This indicates attendance by technology.) No apneas were seen. No snoring was noted on intermittent observations. Lowest O_2 saturation recorded looks like 83%, and it appears that 3% of his time was spent with O_2 saturations in the 80s, and 97% of his time was spent with O_2 saturations 90% or better. That is because most of the night was done with 1 L per minute by nasal prongs.

It appears that the patient does desaturate significantly with sleep, and it appears that it is 87%. The lowest was 83%.

SERVICE CODE(S): _____

ICD-10-CM DX CODE(S): _____

(Answers to every other Case are located in Appendix D . The full answer key is only available in the TEACH Instructor Resources on Evolve.)

CASE 9-15L *Radiology Report, Chest*

LOCATION: Inpatient, Hospital

PATIENT: Virgil Zejdlek

PRIMARY CARE PHYSICIAN: Ronald Green, MD

ATTENDING PHYSICIAN: Gregory Dawson, MD

EXAMINATION OF: Chest

CLINICAL SYMPTOMS: Pneumothorax, pleural effusion

ONE-VIEW CHEST, 4:00 PM: AP (anterior posterior) portable view obtained of the chest at 4:00 PM. Comparison study is from 5 days prior. Pleural effusion on the left appears decreased. There now appears to be left pneumothorax seen superiorly and laterally. This is as marked on the film. There is left basilar/retrocardiac opacity. There appears to be some patient rotation. There are superimposed cardiac leads. Cardiac silhouette is not appreciably changed. There is volume loss on the left.

IMPRESSION:

1. Left pleural effusion appears decreased since prior study. There appears to be residual pleural fluid and there is left basilar opacity. There now appears to be pneumothorax on the left. There is volume loss of the left.
2. Cardiac silhouette appears stable.
3. Not mentioned above, there is some oral contrast noted in the upper abdomen.

SERVICE CODE(S): _____

ICD-10-CM DX CODE(S): _____

(Answers to every other Case are located in Appendix D . The full answer key is only available in the TEACH Instructor Resources on Evolve.)

CASE 9-15M *Operative Report, Thoracostomy*

LOCATION: Inpatient, Hospital

PATIENT: Virgil Zejdlek

PRIMARY CARE PHYSICIAN: Ronald Green, MD

ATTENDING PHYSICIAN: Gregory Dawson, MD

SURGEON: Gary Sanchez, MD

PREOPERATIVE DIAGNOSIS: Left pleural effusion

POSTOPERATIVE DIAGNOSIS: Left pleural effusion

NAME OF OPERATION: Left tube thoracostomy

HISTORY OF PRESENT ILLNESS: The patient is a 77-year-old man who was recently admitted with right-sided chest pain and shortness of breath. Chest x-ray revealed a moderate- to large-sized left pleural effusion. A CT (computerized tomography) scan revealed the presence of a large left pulmonary mass as well as significant subcarinal adenopathy or mass effect. Thoracentesis was performed and the left pleural effusion was drained; however, it recurred after only 24 hours. Cardiothoracic surgery was consulted to discuss the option of tube thoracostomy. The above findings were explained to the patient. The prognosis as well as the risks and benefits of continued observation versus repeat thoracentesis versus tube thoracotomy were discussed at length. His questions concerning his options for therapy were answered.

He appeared to understand the above findings, and after our discussion expressed a desire to proceed with tube thoracotomy and gave written consent to proceed.

OPERATIVE FINDINGS: Approximately 700 cc (cubic centimeter) of clear, yellow-red fluid was removed from the left pleural cavity.

DESCRIPTION OF PROCEDURE: The patient was brought to the procedure room and placed on a cart in the decubitus position. The left side was up. The left side of the chest was then prepped and draped in the usual sterile fashion. Local anesthesia was accomplished using 15 cc of 1% Xylocaine. A 2-cm (centimeter) incision was made in the mid-axillary line in approximately the seventh intercostal space. Using a Kelly clamp, subcutaneous tunnel was created. Additional lidocaine was injected and the intercostal muscles separated, and the left pleural cavity was entered. A 32-French chest tube was then inserted into the left pleural cavity and secured in place with a 2-0 silk stitch. The chest tube was placed on 20 cm of water suction, and a sterile dressing was applied. The patient tolerated the procedure quite well. A postprocedure chest x-ray was ordered.

SERVICE CODE(S): _____

ICD-10-CM DX CODE(S): _____

Discussion

This was an excellent case from which to learn how choosing the diagnoses changes from one report to another based on the service being provided to the patient. Inpatient coders would consider all of the diagnoses stated by all of the physicians when reporting the inpatient hospital services for this patient upon discharge. The outpatient coder reports the diagnosis(es) that was/were the primary reason(s) for the encounter.

(Answers to every other Case are located in Appendix D . The full answer key is only available in the TEACH Instructor Resources on Evolve.)

CASE 9-16A *Emergency Department Report*

Dr. Sutton provides not only the E/M service but also places this patient on a ventilator. The intubation (placing the tube into the trachea) is included in the initial ventilator services and not reported separately. You can locate the directions to the ventilator codes in the index of the CPT manual under "Ventilation Assist."

LOCATION: Inpatient, Hospital

PATIENT: Reen Hesse

PHYSICIAN: Paul Sutton, MD

SUBJECTIVE: The patient is an 80-year-old male in acute respiratory distress. He is from the New York City area and was just about to take a train to go there today. He had sudden onset of shortness of breath and presents now because of it. He denies any chest pain or tightness. He has had no recent cough. He is bringing up frothy sputum as he arrives here.

PAST MEDICAL HISTORY:

Surgical:

1. Bypass surgery
2. Angioplasty and stent
3. Pacemaker

Illnesses: The patient has a previous history of congestive heart failure and has been intubated in the past, most recently 4 months ago with this same problem.

FAMILY HISTORY, SOCIAL HISTORY, and REVIEW OF SYSTEMS were not obtainable for this patient.

OBJECTIVE: This alert 80-year-old male appears to be in acute respiratory distress. Oxygen saturation is 72%. Blood pressure is 210/107. Respirations are 36. Pulse is 120. Telemetry shows a paced wide complexed rhythm. HEENT (head, ears, eyes, nose, throat): Frothy pink sputum coming out of his mouth. NECK is supple without lymphadenopathy. His jugular veins are full. Respirations are labored. LUNGS: Rales throughout. HEART: Rapid rate and rhythm. ABDOMEN: Soft and nontender with normal bowel sounds. EXTREMITIES: No peripheral edema is noted. No clubbing.

ASSESSMENT: Acute pulmonary edema

PLAN: He was immediately given Lasix 80 mg (milligram) IV (intravenous), given Nitro spray, and started on a Nitro drip. We gave him a few minutes to try to turn around. He was on 100% oxygen. He did not turn around and, in fact, he looked worse. We then talked about intubation with him and his wife and proceeded with it. He was bagged. He was given Versed IV, and he then was given succinylcholine 100 mg IV. He was then intubated without difficulty with an 8.0 ET tube to 24 cm (centimeter). Breath sounds were heard bilaterally. CO_2 (carbon dioxide) monitoring device confirmed placement. The patient was placed on the ventilator and transported to ICU (intensive care unit) in reasonably stable condition.

SERVICE CODE(S): _____

ICD-10-CM DX CODE(S): _____

(Answers to every other Case are located in Appendix D . The full answer key is only available in the TEACH Instructor Resources on Evolve.)

CASE 9-16B *Thoracic Medicine/Critical Care Consultation*

Reen was admitted to the hospital onto Dr. Elhart's service. Dr. Elhart immediately requested a consultation from Dr. Dawson regarding the patient's respiratory condition.

LOCATION: Inpatient, Hospital

PATIENT: Reen Hesse

ATTENDING PHYSICIAN: Marvin Elhart, MD

CONSULTANT: Gregory Dawson, MD

I have been asked by Dr. Elhart to see the patient for ICU (intensive care unit) care. The patient was admitted with pulmonary edema, respiratory failure; he has chronic renal disease and is on Dr. Elhart's service, I would assume for the chronic renal disease as well as respiratory failure, but that was secondary. The patient looks like he had a myocardial infarction with elevated troponins, CK-MBs (creatine kinase-methylene blue), CPKs (creatine phosphokinase), and CKs (creatine kinase). His pulmonary edema has started to clear. He was adjusted on the ventilator this morning. The CPAP (continuous positive airway pressure) went from 6 o'clock to 8 o'clock, and then he got too short of breath and went back on the ventilator. Since then he has diuresed more, and I have him on CPAP at present. He is doing quite well, with a respiratory rate of 19 with good oxygenation. I think we have a fair chance of getting him extubated today.

The patient was visiting with relatives here in Manytown. He was trying to move some luggage, started to get diaphoretic, and did not

feel well, and it started to become difficult to breathe. The wife felt he was gurgling, and he was sent to the emergency room, where he was found to be in pulmonary edema, intubated, and placed on a ventilator.

The patient is intubated and on a ventilator, so I do not have a good family history, social history, past medical history, past surgical history, or review of systems. I got some things from the chart and some things from his wife. The patient's wife is fairly sure that he had stenting of the LAD (left anterior descending coronary artery) done last year. We will send for those records. He had a coronary artery bypass graft done before that. It sounds fairly extensive. It seems to have been in 1989. He had at least three grafts, and the cardiologist has this outlined pretty well and what was done at that point. He also had a pacemaker. He has a history of renal artery disease status post renal artery stenosis, history of hypertension, dyslipidemia, bradycardia, and chronic renal disease. He apparently has had some trouble with dye toxicity from angiogram done a year ago and did not quite get over it. I guess there was partial clearing. It is difficult to tell without the records what went on.

PHYSICAL EXAMINATION at the time I saw the patient reveals a patient who is alert, on a ventilator, and able to answer questions, yes and no anyway. He certainly cannot verbalize it. HEENT (head, ears, eyes, nose, throat): Benign. No blood was found in the posterior pharynx or the nose. NECK is supple. No JVD (jugular vein distention). LUNGS actually show rales bilaterally but in the bases, not in the rest of the areas. HEART shows S1 (first heart sound) and

CASE 9-16B—cont'd

S2 (second heart sound) are regular without an S3 (third heart sound) or S4 (fourth heart sound). There is a systolic murmur at the fourth interspace midclavicular line that is somewhat difficult to hear. It is somewhat vague and soft, but I think it is present. ABDOMEN is soft and benign without hepatosplenomegaly. Normal bowel sounds are present. No bruits heard in either flank; no masses palpable; nontender. EXTREMITIES show no edema, rashes, clubbing, cyanosis, or tremor. LYMPHATIC SYSTEM: No nodes in the neck, clavicular, or axillary area.

IMPRESSION:

1. Acute myocardial infarction with acute pulmonary edema and acute respiratory failure.
2. Chronic renal failure. You can see that on today's material his BUN (blood urea nitrogen) and creatinine levels are climbing. I am not sure

what the plan is at this point. I am waiting for cardiology to come by, but I think I can get him extubated later this afternoon. I will check his sputum. He does have a fair amount to suction and it is somewhat thick, so I will make sure he does not have an infection. He is already on Unasyn for any sort of aspiration that might have occurred, although it is not well documented. We will check a 24-hour urine for creatinine clearance, get the records from the Manytown hospital to see what actually was done there, and then check on his lab in the morning. I will wait for Dr. Elhart to come by before we have any other plans, but hopefully the patient will be extubated here shortly.

SERVICE CODE(S): _____

ICD-10-CM DX CODE(S): _____

CASE 9-16C   *Radiology Report, Chest*

This x-ray was taken the day after admission.

LOCATION: Inpatient, Hospital

PATIENT: Reen Hesse

ATTENDING PHYSICIAN: Marvin Elhart, MD

RESPIRATORY CARE: Gregory Dawson, MD

RADIOLOGIST: Morton Monson, MD

EXAMINATION OF: Chest

CLINICAL SYMPTOMS: Follow-up acute pulmonary edema

PORTABLE AP (ANTERIOR POSTERIOR) CHEST, 5:00 AM: FINDINGS: Comparison is made with yesterday morning's portable AP chest. Sternotomy with mediastinal clips. No appreciable change in the heart size or pulmonary vascularity given the difference in technique. Lungs are clear.

SERVICE CODE(S): _____

ICD-10-CM DX CODE(S): _____

(Answers to every other Case are located in Appendix D . The full answer key is only available in the TEACH Instructor Resources on Evolve.)

CASE 9-16D   *Radiology Report, Chest*

LOCATION: Inpatient, Hospital

PATIENT: Reen Hesse

ATTENDING PHYSICIAN: Marvin Elhart, MD

RESPIRATORY CARE: Gregory Dawson, MD

RADIOLOGIST: Morton Monson, MD

EXAMINATION OF: Chest

CLINICAL SYMPTOMS: Acute MI (myocardial infarction), pulmonary edema, acute respiratory failure, and renal disease

PORTABLE AP (ANTERIOR POSTERIOR) CHEST X-RAY: FINDINGS: The cardiac silhouette is upper normal to mildly prominent but stable. Mild interstitial prominence remains in the infrahilar areas, but no other significant interval change is noted.

SERVICE CODE(S): _____

ICD-10-CM DX CODE(S): _____

(Answers to every other Case are located in Appendix D . The full answer key is only available in the TEACH Instructor Resources on Evolve.)

CASE 9-16E   *Thoracic Medicine/Critical Care Progress Report*

LOCATION: Inpatient, Hospital

PATIENT: Reen Hesse

ATTENDING PHYSICIAN: Marvin Elhart, MD

RESPIRATORY CARE: Gregory Dawson, MD

This is a follow-up for this patient with acute respiratory failure. He was extubated yesterday. He apparently had a cardiac catheterization in the

past, and his kidneys were bad enough that they thought he might need dialysis, but then he recovered; but he certainly recovered incompletely because BUN (blood urea nitrogen) today is 72, creatinine 2.6, and creatinine clearance is pending. Interestingly enough, potassium is low at 2.8, so we will replace that with oral potassium. We will check his basic metabolic panel in the morning and transfer him to the floor on telemetry. He does not want anything done here. He wants to go

Continued

CASE 9-16E—cont'd

home by train, which is probably not the best idea because there is no guarantee that what happened to him this time will not happen again.

PHYSICAL EXAMINATION: CHEST: Clear. Chest x-ray looks pretty good too. HEART: Regular rhythm. ABDOMEN: Benign. EXTREMITIES: No edema. No clubbing.

LABORATORY DATA: All in good shape. Sputum showed greater than 25 white cells, less 10 squamous. No bugs were seen, so it may be just inflammation rather than true infection.

MEDICATIONS: He is on Unasyn at this point. We stopped the Unasyn today and put him on Augmentin. There is some question about whether he aspirated on it, but I certainly do not see anything on x-ray right now.

He is going to be talking to Dr. Elhart later today to decide what to do about whether to discharge or have the study done here. The patient is really 4+ positive that he wants to go back home in case things go wrong with his kidneys. At least he is at home and can undergo the dialysis closer to home. He is most comfortable with the situation there as well as with his surroundings there, so we will leave that up to Dr. Elhart and the patient. But I still think it is a somewhat risky idea, so I imparted that to the patient of those particular ideas. Otherwise, he can be discharged at cardiology's leisure.

SERVICE CODE(S): _____

ICD-10-CM DX CODE(S): _____

(Answers to every other Case are located in Appendix D . The full answer key is only available in the TEACH Instructor Resources on Evolve.)

CASE 9-16F *Discharge Summary*

Dr. Elhart discharges the patient.

LOCATION: Inpatient, Hospital

PATIENT: Reen Hesse

ATTENDING PHYSICIAN: Marvin Elhart, MD

RESPIRATORY CARE: Gregory Dawson, MD

The patient was admitted with acute pulmonary edema, respiratory failure, and chronic renal disease. The patient looked like he has had myocardial infarction with elevated troponins. The patient was extubated after the pulmonary edema. Discussions with the patient and his family indicated that he did not want anything further done. He wanted further cardiac care done at home. We arranged for him to be discharged, and he was discharged Tuesday. It was advised that he have a cardiac

catheterization to determine the extent of his myocardial infarction and whether anything could be fixed, but this is on top of somebody with chronic renal disease who most likely would suffer from the toxic effects of the dye and would probably have some difficulty with renal failure post cardiac catheterization if everything went wrong. Please see my drug note that outlined the drugs the patient was on when he was sent home.

DISCHARGE DIAGNOSES:

1. Subendocardial infarction
2. Congestive heart failure
3. Acute pulmonary edema with acute respiratory failure

SERVICE CODE(S): _____

ICD-10-CM DX CODE(S): _____

(Answers to every other Case are located in Appendix D . The full answer key is only available in the TEACH Instructor Resources on Evolve.)

CASE 9-17 *Operative Report, Bronchoscopy*

There are only two services for this report—a bronchial brushing and a lavage. The washing is designated as a "(separate procedure)" and is only reported if it is the only procedure performed. Note that the diagnosis is going to be an abnormal radiological examination of the lung.

LOCATION: Inpatient, Hospital

PATIENT: Mary Ellen Gavisconi

ATTENDING PHYSICIAN: Marvin Elhart, MD

RESPIRATORY CARE: Gregory Dawson, MD

PREOPERATIVE DIAGNOSIS: Abnormal chest/lung x-ray

POSTOPERATIVE DIAGNOSIS: Inflammatory secretions

PROCEDURE PERFORMED: Fiberoptic bronchoscopy, cell washings, cell brushings, and bronchoalveolar lavage.

PROCEDURE: For details of the drugs used and the amounts of drugs used, please refer to the bronchoscopy report sheet. The patient was already intubated and on the ventilator. She was sedated as per ICU (intensive care unit) protocol. She was also given some drugs prior to that. Please refer, again, to the bronchoscopy report sheet.

The patient was monitored throughout the procedure with electrocardiography, O_2 (oxygen) saturations, and ventilator monitoring. These were all within parameters, and no real adverse effects were noted with those various monitoring services.

Once the patient had been sedated, the bronchoscope was introduced into the endotracheal tube. The distal portion of the trachea, the carina, and all the airways were examined both right and left. All the airways were patent and entered. The trachea and the carina were basically normal. The trachea is about 2 cm (centimeter) above the carina. The right and left lungs were also examined. All segments were patent and entered, and no

CASE 9-17—cont'd

masses were seen. The right lower lobe had some crowding and swelling and some inflammatory changes, but they were relatively mild. I did not see any obvious purulent material. There were excess secretions, but they did not appear thick and discolored. This area was brushed and washed and was also subjected to bronchoalveolar lavage in the right lower lobe. (This procedure now has become a surgical procedure and is no longer an exploratory procedure.) These specimens were sent for appropriate pathological, cytologic, and bacterial studies. Hopefully the results will be back tomorrow. The patient suffered no ill effects from this procedure. She was left in the ICU for monitoring.

SERVICE CODE(S): _____

ICD-10-CM DX CODE(S): _____

(Answers to every other Case are located in Appendix D . The full answer key is only available in the TEACH Instructor Resources on Evolve.)

CASE 9-18A   *Operative Report, Bronchoscopy*

LOCATION: Outpatient, Hospital

PATIENT: Greg Encore

PHYSICIAN: Gregory Dawson, MD

PREOPERATIVE DIAGNOSIS: Abnormal chest x-ray. We are considering, by history, coccidioidomycosis pneumonia. So far, we are not getting much back for confirmation of this, and this procedure is being done to confirm that diagnosis.

POSTOPERATIVE DIAGNOSIS: Abnormal superior segment, left lower lobe, consistent with either inflammation or tumor or both.

PROCEDURE PERFORMED: Fiberoptic bronchoscopy, transbronchial biopsies, bronchial biopsies, cell washings, cell brushings, and bronchoalveolar lavage superior segment of left lower lobe.

For details of drugs used and the amounts of drugs used, please refer to the bronchoscopy report sheet. The patient was intubated already on a Vaughn cycle ventilator (*ventilator dependent*), sedated, and paralyzed per ICU (intensive care unit) protocol for the respiratory failure. An additional drug was given with atropine 0.5. The patient was monitored throughout the procedure with electrocardiograph, O_2 (oxygen) saturations, blood pressure, and the usual ICU monitoring with no real adverse problems. The ventilator was monitored by one of the respiratory therapists to ensure that we had adequate volume and adequate oxygenation.

Once the patient was firmly sedated with the usual ICU medications for his respiratory failure, the bronchoscope was introduced through the endotracheal tube. The part of the trachea we saw in the carina appeared to be within normal limits. In the right lung, all segments were patent and entered, and no masses were seen. The left upper lobe was also patent, and all segments were entered and no masses were seen. In the left lower lobe, the superior segment was deformed, closed, had blood in it, and was friable consistent with inflammation, tumor, or both.

Multiple biopsies, brushings, and washings were done in the area as well as sheath brushings looking specifically for coccidioidomycosis and not only that, a BAL was performed on this segment with a "mini-BAL" apparatus. Biopsies were then done in this same area: the superior segment of the left lower lobe, both transbronchially and bronchially.

The patient tolerated the procedure well. No adverse effects were noted. We will check a chest x-ray shortly to assure ourselves that there are no problems there. Follow-up will be a little later, when we get the results back.

Pathological Findings: See Report 9-18B.

SERVICE CODE(S): _____

ICD-10-CM DX CODE(S): _____

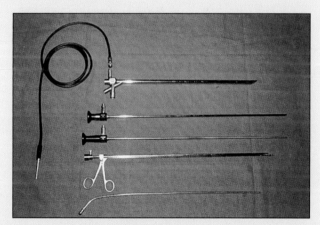

FIGURE 9-6 Bronchoscopy equipment.

(Answers to every other Case are located in Appendix D . The full answer key is only available in the TEACH Instructor Resources on Evolve.)

CASE 9-18B   *Pathology Report, Cytology*

LOCATION: Outpatient, Hospital

PATIENT: Greg Encore

PHYSICIAN: Gregory Dawson, MD

PATHOLOGIST: Morton Monson, MD

CLINICAL HISTORY: Possible coccidia

SPECIMEN RECEIVED:

A. Bronch brush tip, left lower lobe
B. Bronchial biopsy, left lower lobe

GROSS DESCRIPTION:

A. Received in a container labeled "brush tip" is a brush tip with a scant amount of tan-red material. The specimen is totally submitted as A.
B. Received in a container labeled "biopsy" are four fragments of tan-gray tissue measuring 0.2 to 0.3 cm (centimeter) in greatest dimension. The specimen is totally submitted as B.

MICROSCOPIC DESCRIPTION:

A. The bronchial brushings contain rare scattered large atypical cells with hyperchromatic angulated nuclei. Some contain prominent nucleoli. Very small scattered areas show glands lined by similar cells.
B. The bronchial biopsies of the left lower lobe contain irregularly outlined and complex glands lined by enlarged pleomorphic cells. The cells contain hyperchromatic irregularly outlined and angulated nuclei. There is a dense supporting fibrous stroma that shows multiple foci of coagulation necrosis.

DIAGNOSIS:

A. Bronchial brushings, left lower lobe: Malignant cells are present, consistent with adenocarcinoma.
B. Bronchial and transbronchial biopsies, left lower lobe: Adenocarcinoma, well to moderately differentiated.

SERVICE CODE(S): _____

ICD-10-CM DX CODE(S): _____

(Answers to every other Case are located in Appendix D . The full answer key is only available in the TEACH Instructor Resources on Evolve.)

CHAPTER 9 *Auditing Review*

Audit the coding for the following reports.

Audit Report 9.1 Overnight Oxygen Desaturation Study

LOCATION: Outpatient, Hospital

PATIENT: Robert Longworth

PHYSICIAN: Gregory Dawson, MD

INDICATIONS: COPD

The study was an overnight oxygen desaturation study to fine-tune this patient's oxygen prescription.

The study began at 2236 hours and continued to about 6 o'clock the next morning.

This study was intermittently observed. He had no apneic spells on intermittent observation. His O_2 saturation remains above 90% on 2 liters.

However, for one-half hour between 4:45 and 5:15 in the morning, the O_2 saturation dropped down to as low as 82%.

I suspect it requires 3 liters/minute nasal prongs to keep this patient's O_2 saturation above 90%. He was admitted at this time with congestive heart failure, and I think we have to be a bit more precise in his oxygen therapy, so I would recommend 3 liters/minute while this patient sleeps.

One of the following codes is reported incorrectly for this case. Indicate the incorrect code.

PROFESSIONAL SERVICES: O_2 oximetry, **94760-26**

ICD-10-CM DX: Chronic obstructive pulmonary disease, **J44.9**; Congestive heart failure, **I50.9**

INCORRECT CODE: _____

Audit Report 9.2 Walking O_2 Desaturation Study

LOCATION: Office

PATIENT: Robert Longworth

PHYSICIAN: Gregory Dawson, MD

INDICATIONS: COPD

This is a walking O_2 desaturation done because the patient is hypoxemic and has dyspnea, and we are trying to fine-tune the patient's oxygen prescription.

The study was done for 6 minutes with EKG monitoring. The patient was able to walk without stopping for the 6 minutes. He went 450 feet. Oxygen saturation started out at 1 liter with his O_2 saturation at 90%. It immediately dropped to 89%, to 87%, required 1 and then 2 liters, and then dropped down to 86% and required 3 liters/minute by nasal prongs

from that point on. This was verified later also by a physical therapist who walked the patient on 2 liters and found that he required 3 liters to keep O_2 saturation above 90%.

OVERALL IMPRESSION: This patient has hypoxemia with relatively mild exercise although he went to a Borg scale of 2, which is mild for him, and requires 3 liters/minute nasal prongs to maintain O2 saturation above 90%.

One of the following codes is reported incorrectly for this case. Indicate the incorrect code.

PROFESSIONAL SERVICES: Pulmonary stress test, **94621**; Electrocardiography, **93000-26**

ICD-10-CM DX: Chronic obstructive pulmonary disease, **J44.9**

INCORRECT CODE: _____

Audit Report 9.3 Pulmonary Function Study

LOCATION: Outpatient, Hospital

PATIENT: Jan Wagner

PHYSICIAN: Gregory Dawson, MD

ENTRANCE DIAGNOSIS: Dyspnea. Patient has a 33-pack-a-year history of smoking and has a cough due to smoking. She gave good consistent effort.

INTERPRETATION:

1. The flow volume loop has a reasonably normal configuration of both inspiration and expiratory limb.
2. No significant change after bronchodilator.
3. Plethysmographic lung volumes are normal without evidence of hyperinflation.
4. Single breath lung volumes are also normal without evidence of hyperinflation.
5. There is no significant dynamic airway collapse (air trapping).
6. Transfer factor is at the low end of normal but still normal.
7. Pre-bronchodilator flow rates have a pattern consistent with mild COPD/ emphysema, but it is really trivial. It is actually very close to the normal and probably falls within the normal range, and calling it COPD might be overreading it.
8. Post-bronchodilator values show no significant change, and the same conclusion can be reached.
9. The MVV is normal both pre- and post-bronchodilator. Between that and the normal FEV1, I would expect normal exercise tolerance.
10. Airway resistance is normal.

OVERALL IMPRESSION: This is basically a normal study with the trivial exception as noted above.

Continued

CHAPTER 9—*cont'd*

One or more of the following codes are reported incorrectly for this case. Indicate the incorrect code or codes.

PROFESSIONAL SERVICES: Pulmonic spirometry, **94060-26**; Diagnostic pulmonology, **94727-26**; Diagnostic pulmonology, **94726-26**; Diagnostic pulmonology, **94729-26**; Diagnostic pulmonology, **94728-26**

ICD-10-CM DX: Shortness of breath, **R06.02**; Smokers' cough, **J41.0**; Tobacco dependence, **Z87.891**

INCORRECT CODE(S): _____

Audit Report 9.4 Sleep Study

LOCATION: Outpatient, Hospital

PATIENT: Liz Charles

PHYSICIAN: Gregory Dawson, MD

STUDY PERFORMED: Nocturnal polysomnogram without CPAP titration

ENTRANCE DIAGNOSIS: Somnolence

This is a fully attended, multichannel nocturnal polysomnogram, giving the patient 386.6 minutes in bed, 317 minutes asleep with 61 arousals through the night, which is above the normal. It looks like she had some difficulty with sleep maintenance. She had sleep onset at 18.5 minutes, REM latency 171.5 minutes, again a little bit prolonged. She had 27 respiratory events through the night, a mixture of obstructive apneas and obstructive hypopneas with a respiratory disturbance index of 5.1. Anything over 5 is considered moderate to severe. The longest duration of any one event was 34 seconds. O_2 sat was between 76 and 95%, with 29% of the time spent with O_2 sats less than 88%. Heart rate varied between 55 and 113, somewhat varying with the obstructive events. The patient had grade 1-2 snoring noted, and respiratory disturbance events were most evident in REM while supine. All five stages of sleep were represented. Basically the only thing abnormal was a reduced amount of REM.

OVERALL IMPRESSION: This 42-year-old patient has significant obstructive sleep apnea based on the respiratory disturbance index of 5.1, whereas anything over 5 is considered moderate to severe, plus the amount of time that the patient spent hypoxic, at less than 88%. 29% of the time was spent that way. So I suspect that the patient does have significant obstructive sleep apnea. We will need a second sitting to do the CPAP titration.

The overall impression is obstructive sleep apnea.

One or more of the following codes is/are reported incorrectly or missing in this case. Indicate the incorrect or missing code or codes.

SERVICE CODE(S): Polysomnography, **95811**

ICD-10-CM DX CODE(S): Somnolence, **R40.0**

INCORRECT/MISSING CODE(S): _____

Audit Report 9.5 Operative Report, Septoplasty, Turbinate Reduction, and Tonsillectomy

LOCATION: Inpatient, Hospital

PATIENT: Brad Nelson

PHYSICIAN: Gregory Dawson, MD

PREOPERATIVE DIAGNOSIS:

1. Septal deviation.
2. Bilateral inferior turbinate hypertrophy.
3. Nasal obstruction.
4. Chronic tonsillitis.

POSTOPERATIVE DIAGNOSIS: Same

PROCEDURES PERFORMED:

1. Septoplasty
2. Bilateral inferior turbinate outfracture
3. Tonsillectomy

ANESTHESIA: General endotracheal anesthesia

DESCRIPTION OF PROCEDURE: Following informed consent from the patient, he is taken to the operating room and placed supine on the operating room table. The appropriate monitoring devices were placed on the patient, and general anesthesia was induced. He was orally intubated without difficulty. He was draped in the usual sterile fashion.

The right and left nasal cavities were packed with Afrin-soaked gauze. It was removed after 5 minutes. The right and left nasal septum was injected with approximately 3 cc of Xylocaine with epinephrine on each side. Evaluation of the nasal cavity did indicate significant bilateral inferior turbinate hypertrophy. There was quite a significant left septal deviation and spur, mostly posteriorly on the left-hand side.

A #15 blade scalpel was used to make an incision on the anterior end of the left nasal septum. A mucoperiosteal and mucoperichondrial flap was then elevated. It was elevated over the septal spur and deviation on the left-hand side. The Freer elevator was then used to incise the cartilage and remove a 1 × 2-cm strip of cartilage from the posterior, inferior aspect of the nasal septum. Care was taken to maintain at least 1 and $^1/_2$ cm of anterior and dorsal nasal cartilage to provide tip support. This amount of cartilage was easily maintained. Once the strip of cartilage was removed, some of the bony vomer had to be removed using the small Wilde forceps. Following this, the left nasal septum was significantly straighter.

The butter knife was then used to outfracture both left and right inferior turbinates. Following this, the nasal airway was significantly improved. 4-0 Chromic catgut suture was used to close the anterior left nasal septum incision. Doyle splints were then placed into the right and left nasal cavities and sutured to the right nasal septum anteriorly.

The patient was repositioned for tonsillectomy. The McIvor mouth gag was placed. The left tonsil was removed by incising its mucous membranes superior and anterior, dissecting it down to its base, removing it with a tonsillar snare. A pack was placed. The right tonsil was removed by incising its mucous membranes superior and anterior,

CHAPTER 9—cont'd

dissecting this tonsil down to its base, and removing it with a tonsillar snare. Bismuth pack was placed. Packs were removed. The peritonsillar area was injected with 1% Xylocaine with epinephrine. Following this, electrocautery was used to obtain good hemostasis on both sides. The nasopharynx was examined, and no evidence of significant adenoids was noted. The oral cavity was washed well with saline. When good hemostasis was noted to be present in the tonsillar fossae, they were painted with viscous Xylocaine. The patient was then awakened from his anesthetic and returned to the recovery room in stable condition. Prognosis immediate and remote is good.

ESTIMATED BLOOD LOSS: 25 cc

PREOPERATIVE MEDICATION: Keflex 500 mg p.o. q.i.d. for 10 days. We will remove the stent in 2 weeks' time. I also provided a prescription for Percocet.

One or more of the following codes are reported incorrectly for this case. Indicate the incorrect code or codes.

SERVICE CODE(S): Therapeutic nasal fracture, **30930**; Septoplasty, **30520**; Tonsillectomy, **42825**
_____

ICD-10-CM DX CODE(S): Chronic tonsillitis, **J35.01**; Hypertrophy nasal turbinates, **J34.3**; Deviated septum, **J34.2**
_____

INCORRECT/MISSING CODE(S): _____

Audit Report 9.6 Operative Report, Tracheostomy

LOCATION: Inpatient, Hospital

PATIENT: Andrew McGregor

PHYSICIAN: Gregory Dawson, MD

PREOPERATIVE DIAGNOSIS:

1. Aspiration pneumonia
2. Ventilator dependent
3. Prolonged intubation with inability to extubate
4. Quadriplegia

POSTOPERATIVE DIAGNOSIS:

1. Aspiration pneumonia
2. Ventilator dependent
3. Prolonged intubation with inability to extubate
4. Quadriplegia

PROCEDURES PERFORMED: Tracheostomy, planned

ANESTHESIA: General endotracheal anesthesia

INDICATION: This is a 58-year-old male who has been ventilator dependent and has had prolonged intubation. Attempts at weaning off the ventilator have been unsuccessful. The patient is also being treated for aspiration pneumonia. He has quadriplegia.

DESCRIPTION OF PROCEDURE: After consent was obtained, the patient was taken to the operating room and placed on the operating room table in the supine position. After an adequate level of general endotracheal anesthesia was obtained, the patient was positioned for tracheostomy. The patient's neck was prepped with betadine prep and then draped

in a sterile manner. A curvilinear incision was marked approximately a fingerbreadth above the sternal notch in an area just below the cricoid cartilage. This area was then infiltrated with 1% Xylocaine with 1:100,000 units epinephrine. After several minutes, sharp dissection was carried down through the skin and subcutaneous tissue. The subcutaneous fat was removed down to the strap muscles. Strap muscles were divided in the midline and retracted laterally. The cricoid cartilage was then identified. The thyroid gland was divided in the midline with the Bovie and then the two lobes retracted laterally. This exposed the anterior wall of the trachea. The space between the second and third tracheal ring was then identified. This was infiltrated with local solution. A cut was then made through the anterior wall. The endotracheal tube was then advanced superiorly. An inferior cut into the third tracheal ring was then made to make a flap. This was secured to the skin with 4-0 Vicryl suture. A #6 Shiley cuffed tracheotomy tube was placed. This was secured to the skin with ties as well as the tracheostomy strap. The patient was then turned over to anesthesia.

The patient tolerated the procedure well, there was no break in technique, patient was extubated and taken to the Medical Critical Care Unit in stable condition. Fluids administered 500 cc of RL. Estimated blood loss less than 5 cc.

One or more of the following codes are reported incorrectly for this case. Indicate the incorrect code or codes.

SERVICE CODE(S): Tracheostomy, **31603**
_____

ICD-10-CM DX CODE(S): Pneumonia, **J18.9**; Ventilator status, **Z99.11**

INCORRECT/MISSING CODE(S): _____

(Auditing Review answers with rationales are only available in the TEACH Instructor Resources on Evolve.)

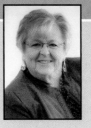

"When in doubt, ask questions. Never leave a code if there is any question. Ask the provider or another coder."

Urinary, Male Genital, and Endocrine Systems

http://evolve.elsevier.com/Buck/next

(Answers to every other Case are located in Appendix D, with the full answer key only available in the TEACH Instructor Resources on Evolve)
(Auditing Review answers with rationales are only available in the TEACH Instructor Resources on Evolve)

Urinary System

Common urinary symptoms are nocturia, polyuria, hematuria, proteinuria, dysuria, oliguria, urinary **incontinence,** and enuresis. Often treated urinary conditions include hypercalciuria (urinary stones caused by the body's inability to process calcium properly), renal failure, pyelonephritis, and infections as well as kidney and bladder cancer. A physician who specializes in the diagnosis and treatment of conditions of the urinary system is a **urologist.** A urologist also specializes in male genitourinary conditions and often treats patients with prostatitis, benign prostatic hyperplasia, and prostate cancer. Urology is classified as a surgical subspecialty. A **nephrologist** specializes in the treatment of conditions of the kidney and has special education and training in kidney disease and dialysis therapy as well as transplantation. Nephrology is a subspecialty of internal medicine.

Chronic Renal Failure

Chronic renal failure is a progressive loss of kidney function that causes the kidneys to overcompensate by excessive straining (hyperfiltration) within the remaining **nephrons** (filtering units). In time, this leads to further loss of function. When 70% or more of the kidney function is lost, the patient begins to experience renal failure. One of the diagnostic methods used to determine the cause of the failure or the extent of damage is a biopsy in which a fine needle is percutaneously inserted into the kidney and a sample of tissue is withdrawn for analysis.

Diagnosis Coding

For a refresher on diagnosis coding for renal failure, refer back to the information that appears before Case 1-8 in Chapter 1.

CASE 10-1 *Operative Report, Kidney Biopsy*

The patient in this case was in chronic renal failure with blood (hematuria) and excess protein (proteinuria) in her urine. Dr. Avila performs a percutaneous kidney biopsy. Report only Dr. Avila's service.

LOCATION: Outpatient, Hospital
PATIENT: Maria Ace
SURGEON: Ira Avila, MD
RADIOLOGIST: Morton Monson, MD
PROCEDURE PERFORMED: Kidney biopsy
INDICATIONS: Chronic renal failure, hematuria, and proteinuria
DESCRIPTION OF PROCEDURE: The patient was placed in the prone position. The right kidney was visualized using ultrasound provided by

Dr. Monson. The skin was prepped in the usual fashion. One-percent lidocaine was used for local anesthesia. Multiple core biopsies were obtained under real ultrasound guidance using an 18-gauge biopsy gun without difficulty. Multiple core biopsies were obtained and were sent for light electromicroscopy and immune fluorescence.

The patient tolerated the procedure well and without immediate complications. She will be sent back to the procedure area to be monitored in 6 hours with repeat hemoglobin on her.

Pathology Report Later Indicated: Renal cell adenocarcinoma, primary

SERVICE CODE(S): _____
ICD-10-CM DX CODE(S): _____

Discussion

Note how in this case the hematuria and proteinuria were not reported because a more definitive diagnosis was stated as primary, malignant neoplasm of the kidney. Also remember that the kidney is a paired organ, and as such, needs the -RT modifier to indicate the kidney on the right side.

(Answers to every other Case are located in Appendix D . The full answer key is only available in the TEACH Instructor Resources on Evolve.)

Nephrostomy Tube

A nephrostomy tube is a small, flexible tube that is placed into one or both kidneys to drain urine when the kidney is not filtering properly. The tube can be placed temporarily, such as when a patient is being prepared for removal of a large kidney stone, or permanently, such as when the kidney is unable to excrete urine on its own. The **ureter** may also be blocked by a stone, tumor, infection, or scarring. In some settings, the interventional radiologist would conduct these placements or replacements of nephrostomy tubes using ultrasound or x-ray to locate the kidney.

CASE 10-2A   *Radiology Report, Nephrostogram*

At times, the kidney of a patient with a nephrostomy tube will require examination by means of contrast being injected into the kidney using the existing nephrostomy tube. Dr. Avila referred Richard Arco to Dr. Monson for an x-ray due to a bloody discharge from Richard's nephrostomy tube. Dr. Monson provided the injection procedure and supervision or interpretation. The diagnoses codes for this case will be for a complication of a urinary catheter and ureter obstruction.

LOCATION: Outpatient, Hospital

PATIENT: Richard Arco

SURGEON: Ira Avila, MD

RADIOLOGIST: Morton Monson, MD

EXAMINATION OF: Nephrostogram

CLINICAL SYMPTOMS: Bloody drainage from nephrostomy tube

NEPHROSTOGRAM: HISTORY: A 69-year-old man presents with a longstanding right nephrostomy tube. Recently he has had blood drainage from the nephrostomy tube. The patient's creatinine is 2.5, PT (prothrombin time) 23.1, INR (International Normalized Ratio) 4.0, and PTT (partial thromboplastin time) 52.9. Hemoglobin is stable at 10.7 (last Monday it was 10.6).

FINDINGS: Nephrostogram was performed and compared with the prior study of last month. The patient had been doing well until several days ago, when he started to experience bloody discharge. The patient describes a situation where the tube may have been retracted while he was sleeping.

INR is 4.0. Nephrostogram was performed and is basically unremarkable. There continues to be distal right ureter obstruction (this is the indication of the ureter obstruction), and the lower pole calyces are not well identified, and they were not present previously as well. There may be a single calyx (not a reported diagnosis as it is not confirmed), which is not seen today. The locking pigtail mechanism is at the edge of the renal pelvis and was advanced several centimeters into a more secure position in the mid to distal renal pelvis. There is no evidence of extravasation or clot within the collecting system. With the patient's coagulation times as abnormal (this is a diagnosis of abnormal blood chemistry, but it is not reported because it is not the reason the service is being provided; rather, it is an incidental finding) as they currently are, I felt it was not worth any risk of losing access, and we would just leave the current tube in position. We agree that discontinuing Coumadin at least for a time is worthwhile in hopes of normalizing his coagulation times so that we could discontinue the current problem. The bloody discharge is a serosanguineous fluid. It is mixed with both urine and blood. There were really only a few minimal clots that came with gravity drainage from this. Once the patient's coagulation times are normalized, we will follow this closely, and perhaps at that time we will plan to do other interventions. Again, the patient's hemoglobin is stable. It is 10.7 today and was 10.6 on last Monday.

IMPRESSION: Nephrostogram is basically unremarkable. See above comments.

SERVICE CODE(S): _____

ICD-10-CM DX CODE(S): _____

(Answers to every other Case are located in Appendix D . The full answer key is only available in the TEACH Instructor Resources on Evolve.)

CASE 10-2B   *Operative Report, Nephrostomy Tube Exchange*

The patient in this case requires replacement of a previously placed nephrostomy tube. The diagnosis is the reason for the service, which in this case will be a Z code for attention to an artificial opening. No guidance is mentioned in this report; however, there was a radiologic exam performed.

LOCATION: Outpatient, Hospital

PATIENT: Richard Arco

SURGEON: Ira Avila, MD

EXAMINATION OF: Right nephrostomy tube exchange

CLINICAL SYMPTOMS: Routine exchange of nephrostomy tube

RIGHT NEPHROSTOMY TUBE EXCHANGE: HISTORY: A 69-year-old man presents for routine exchange of nephrostomy tube.

FINDINGS: The patient was prepped and draped in the standard fashion. Through the existing no. 8-French nephrostomy tube, contrast was

infused (injection procedure done by radiologist) and demonstrated sharp calyces and a well-formed renal pelvis with normal flow of control into the distal right ureter to the level of the uterovesical junction, which is the known site of obstruction. There is no evidence of contrast extending into the bladder. No filling defects or calculi were evident. Then, with standard wire and catheter exchange techniques, the no. 8-French nephrostomy tube was exchanged for a new no. 8-French nephrostomy tube. The locking mechanism pigtail was in the right renal pelvis. There were no complications. The patient tolerated the procedure well. The patient did not receive conscious sedation.

IMPRESSION: Successful exchange of no. 8-French right nephrostomy tube. The patient requires routine 3-month exchanges of right nephrostomy tube.

SERVICE CODE(S): _____

ICD-10-CM DX CODE(S): _____

(Answers to every other Case are located in Appendix D . The full answer key is only available in the TEACH Instructor Resources on Evolve.)

Nephrectomy

A **nephrectomy** is the partial or total removal of the kidney that may be performed due to disease or in those instances when the patient is donating a kidney (a total removal). The procedure can be performed as an open approach (50220-50240) or as a laparoscopic procedure (50543, 50545, or 50548, which includes a donor nephrectomy).

Urinary System Subcategories

Open the CPT manual to the Urinary System subsection. There are the following categories:
Kidney
Ureter (kidney to bladder)
Bladder
Urethra (bladder to external body)

It is very important to know the anatomy of the urinary system when coding from the subsection. It is all too easy to report the wrong code, as all of the categories have many of the same types of subcategories. For example, it is easy to report the wrong code when reporting a procedure of the ureter(s) or the urethra. Make certain you are in the correct category before assigning a code. Also, write in your CPT manual next to Ureter (50600-50980) "kidney(s) to bladder" and next to Urethra (53000-53899) "bladder to external body." These types of notes will personalize your coding manuals and make them more helpful to use.

Urinary System Cysts

Code Q61.0- is assigned to **congenital cysts** of the kidney. M28.1 is assigned to **acquired cysts** of the kidney (peripelvic [lymphatic] cyst), and a **ureteral polyp** and **ureterocele** is reported with N28.89. If there is no diagnostic statement as to whether the cyst is congenital or acquired, assign an acquired diagnosis.

Reference "Cyst, kidney, acquired" in the index of the ICD-10-CM to be referred to N28.1 and to locate the other codes under that term, such as "Cyst, kidney, congenital Q61.00."

If the condition is an acquired calculus of the kidney or ureter, code N20.- is assigned. If the calculus is a congenital condition, assign Q63.8. If there is no diagnostic statement as to whether the calculus is congenital or acquired, assign an **acquired** diagnosis code. This is because in the Index of the ICD-10-CM, under the main term "Calculus, kidney," there is a subterm for "congenital," so unless the stone was specifically stated as congenital, it would be coded as acquired, even though there is no acquired terminology in the Index under the term "calculus."

Further congenital abnormalities of the urinary system include:

Q60.-	Renal agenesis (absence of an organ) or dysgenesis
Q61.-	Cystic kidney disease (cysts of kidney)
Q62.--	Obstructive defects of the renal pelvis and ureter
Q63.3-	Other specified anomalies of the kidney or ureter (includes calculus) and kidney abnormalities (horseshoe kidney)
Q64.1-	Exstrophy (turning inside out) of the urinary bladder
Q64.3-	Atresia (absence of external opening) and stenosis of urethra and bladder neck
Q64.4	Anomalies of urachus (connects urinary bladder with umbilicus in fetus)
Q64.5-Q64.79	Other anomalies of the bladder and urethra (such as hernia of bladder and prolapse of bladder)

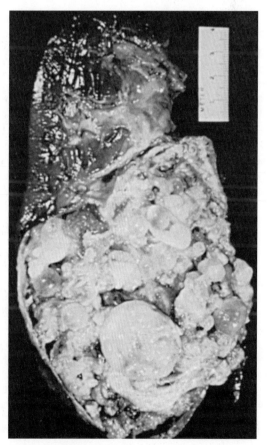

FIGURE 10–1 Urinary cysts.

Renal Calculus

Renal calculus is a kidney stone and often causes excruciating pain. Stones form due to structural disorders, metabolic abnormalities, or recurrent urinary tract infections. Structural abnormalities such as cysts of the kidney (polycystic kidney disease), obstructions, and malformed kidneys predispose stone formation. Metabolic conditions (e.g., hypercalciuria and hyperuricemia) that increase the body's production of calcium increase the chances of kidney stone. Most stones are composed of calcium and magnesium, although stones of other constituents are not uncommon.

Stones are very small, with a usual diameter of 1.5 cm or smaller. X-ray (KUB), CT scan, or ultrasound may be useful to visualize the stone. Stones usually pass spontaneously but on occasion may require intervention. Methods of removal include pharmaceuticals that dissolve calcium-based stones, percutaneous removal, transurethral ureteroscopy, extracorporeal shock wave lithotripsy (ESWL), or even open surgical removal. ESWL is the use of ultrasound to shatter the stone so the fragments will then usually pass spontaneously.

Urodynamics

Urodynamics is used to study how the bladder stores and releases urine, such as the bladder capacity and ability of the bladder to empty completely. Circular muscles **(sphincters)** close tightly around the urethra to prevent the leakage of

---

CASE 10-3   *Operative Report, Nephrectomy*

LOCATION: Inpatient, Hospital

PATIENT: Rosa Alvarado

SURGEON: Ira Avila, MD

PREOPERATIVE DIAGNOSIS: Multicystic, dysplastic left kidney

POSTOPERATIVE DIAGNOSIS: Multicystic, dysplastic left kidney

PROCEDURE PERFORMED: Left laparoscopic radical nephrectomy

CLINICAL NOTE: The patient was found to have a multicystic, dysplastic kidney on investigation for abdominal pain. There are multiple complex cysts of this kidney. It is grossly enlarged. There is no way to determine whether there are malignant changes. It is decided to proceed with attempt at laparoscopic nephrectomy for removal of this. Renogram showed the primary dominant kidney to be the right kidney.

OPERATIVE NOTE: The patient was given a general endotracheal anesthetic, prepped, and draped in the left flank position. Foley catheter was placed, and an orogastric tube was placed. Hassan trocar was placed two fingerbreadths above and lateral to the umbilicus at the lateral margin of the rectus fascia. Two further 12-mm (millimeter) ports were placed in the right lower quadrant under visual guidance, and a 5-mm port was placed in the subcostal position in the anterior axillary line.

The colon was mobilized off the kidney. The kidney was grossly enlarged. Cysts could be seen bulging through perirenal fat.

The kidney was mobilized, and the renal hilum was identified. The ureter was identified just below the lower pole of the renal kidney, where it was doubly clipped and divided and used for retraction. A single renal vein and renal artery were identified. The renal artery was in a posterior superior position. This was triply clipped on the patient's side and doubly on the specimen side and divided. The linear GIA was then utilized to clip the renal vein. It was decided to try to spare the adrenal gland, and therefore Gerota's fascia superior to the kidney was taken, but the adrenal gland was left in situ. A harmonic scalpel was used for mobilization. Multiple collateral vessels were around the kidney and desmoplastic reaction. At one point during mobilization, the cyst was entered and the contents spilled. These were evacuated during suction. Then the wound was irrigated at this point and then subsequently. The specimen was ultimately mobilized and freed. It was placed in a large lap sac, and the lap sac was brought through the Hassan trocar site. The wound was draped with clean towels, and the kidney was morselized using the sponge forceps. All cyst fluid was suctioned from the bag and sent for cytologic evaluation. A total of 600 cc (cubic centimeter) of fluid was obtained. The specimen was also sent for pathology. A small pale nodule was identified during the morselization, and this was sent separately as the renal mass.

Gown and gloves were changed; green towels were removed and Hassan trocar reintroduced. The wound was thoroughly irrigated using 1 L of Kefzol/heparin in normal saline. Hemostasis was ensured. The 12-mm trocar sites were closed using a GraNee needle and 2-0 Vicryl. Peritoneum and external oblique fascia were closed in the Hassan trocar site using 2-0 Vicryl. Skin was closed with subcuticular Dexon. Sponge and needle counts were reported correct. The patient tolerated the procedure well and was transferred to the recovery room in good condition.

ESTIMATED BLOOD LOSS: 100 cc

Pathology Report Later Indicated: Multiple, benign renal cysts

SERVICE CODE(S): _____

ICD-10-CM DX CODE(S): _____

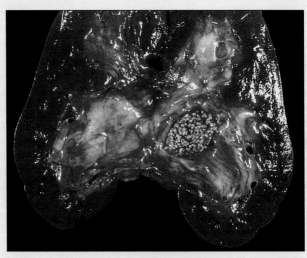

FIGURE 10–2 Kidney stone.

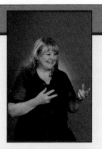

From the Trenches

"A successful medical coder must be able to think outside of the box."

MELANIE MARTIN

CPC

CASE 10-4   *Operative Report, ESWL*

LOCATION: Outpatient, Hospital

PATIENT: Juan Santos

SURGEON: Ira Avila, MD

PREOPERATIVE DIAGNOSIS: Left renal calculus

POSTOPERATIVE DIAGNOSIS: Left renal calculus

PROCEDURE PERFORMED: Left ESWL (extracorporeal shock wave lithotripsy)

CLINICAL NOTE: This gentleman came in with renal colic, and a stent was placed. He had his anticoagulation reversed and presents now for ESWL.

The patient was given a general laryngeal mask anesthetic, prepped, and draped in the supine position. Stone was targeted and shock head engaged. A total of 2400 shocks at maximum KV and stone partial fragmentation and dissolution could be seen. The patient tolerated the procedure well and transferred to the recovery room in good condition. He will be seen in follow-up in 2 weeks' time for KUB (kidney, ureter, bladder).

SERVICE CODE(S): _____

ICD-10-CM DX CODE(S): _____

(Answers to every other Case are located in Appendix D . The full answer key is only available in the TEACH Instructor Resources on Evolve.)

---

urine (incontinence). If the urinary problem is related to nerve damage, electrodes (electromyographic [EMG] electrodes) may be placed into the urethra and rectum to assess the response of these muscles. When EMG electrodes are used as a part of the urodynamic study, they are reported separately. Another component of the urodynamic assessment may be a cystometrogram (CMG), in which a small catheter is placed into the bladder and warm water is placed into the bladder to measure the capacity of the bladder. Leak point pressure can also be assessed by means of the CMG when the patient coughs with a full bladder. The CMG can also measure the pressure required to urinate with a voiding pressure study (VCUG) that is reported separately. X-ray or ultrasound (video urodynamics) may also be used to image the filling and emptying of the bladder. Contrast material is added to the liquid that is used to fill the bladder to enhance the image.

The notes preceding the Urodynamic codes 51725-51798 indicate that if the physician only interprets the results or operates the equipment, modifier -26 is to be added to identify that only the professional component of the service was provided. When codes in this category are reported without -26, that use indicates that the professional and technical components of the service were provided. If, however, the urodynamic assessment was provided by a clinic physician in the outpatient department of the hospital, the hospital would report the technical component and the physician would report the professional component with the -26 modifier.

CASE 10-5 *Urodynamic Assessment*

The following report indicates the components that are to be coded with bold typeface. You are reporting the professional component of the service, so remember to use the correct modifier (-26) to indicate only the professional component of the service. Because there are multiple procedures, you will need to indicate that with a modifier. Remember to place the modifiers on the code in descending order with the highest-numbered modifier first followed by the lower-numbered modifier.

LOCATION: Outpatient, Hospital

PATIENT: Elva Sexton

SURGEON: Ira Avila, MD

DIAGNOSIS: Chronic renal failure

This lady is referred for urodynamic assessment prior to renal transplantation. Previous attempts were unsuccessful in that she was having what appeared to be a significant hypoglycemic episode and was referred to the emergency room. I have not heard of any follow-up from our emergency department in this regard. The patient presents now.

Uroflow: (This is the uroflowmetry service.)

Maximum flow: 17 ml/sec (milliliter/second)
Average flow: 5.4 ml/sec
Voided volume: 64 cc (cubic centimeter)
Voiding pattern is normal.

Cystometrogram: (This is the cystometrogram service.)

Urethral and rectal catheters were placed. **EMG** electrodes applied. The patient was placed in a semisitting position.

The first sensation of bladder filling after 161 cc
Normal desire to void 289 cc
Strong desire to void 369 cc
Maximum cystometrogram capacity 520 cc

No evidence of uninhibited bladder contractions was seen. **Leak point pressure** (This is the voiding pressure study of the bladder.) was not established with Valsalva in excess of 80 cm (centimeter) of water. The patient could not void with the Foley catheter in situ. She did void by Valsalva. Pressure flow showed no evidence of obstruction. EMG activity was normal.

Once the catheter was removed, the patient was able to void easily without evidence of Valsalva and voided to completeness.

ASSESSMENT: No evidence of uninhibited bladder contractions. Normal bladder capacity. The patient was unable to void with catheter in situ, but normal uroflow study and post EMG voiding suggest normal detrusor function.

SERVICE CODE(S): _____

ICD-10-CM DX CODE(S): _____

(Answers to every other Case are located in Appendix D . The full answer key is only available in the TEACH Instructor Resources on Evolve.)

Stress Incontinence

Stress incontinence is involuntary loss of urine that is usually associated with activities that increase the bladder pressure, such as coughing, sneezing, or exercising. This is a condition that most often occurs in women due to physical changes resulting from pregnancy, childbirth, and menopause. The pelvic floor muscles that support the bladder become weakened and the bladder moves downward (prolapses), preventing the muscles (sphincters) that would force the urethra shut from contracting properly, resulting in leakage. After more conservative treatments have failed, surgery may be used to alleviate the incontinence, such as a wing sling that holds the bladder up and returns it to normal position.

CASE 10-6 *Operative Report, Urethropexy*

LOCATION: Outpatient, Hospital

PATIENT: Jan Barens

SURGEON: Ira Avila, MD

PREOPERATIVE DIAGNOSIS: Stress incontinence

POSTOPERATIVE DIAGNOSIS: Stress incontinence

PROCEDURE PERFORMED: Anterior urethropexy

CLINICAL NOTE: The patient is a 59-year-old woman who has stress incontinence. She is undergoing oophorectomy and colposuspension for enterocele. She also has a hypermobile urethra.

PROCEDURE: The patient was already open and had undergone bilateral oophorectomy by Dr. Sanchez. Prior to apical suspension, I was asked to perform her anterior urethropexy.

The Foley catheter was in situ. With a finger in the vagina, the urethra was identified and sutures were placed bilaterally at the mid-portion of the urethra 1 cm (centimeter) lateral and at the bladder neck 2 cm lateral. These sutures were then suspended to Cooper's ligament bilaterally. The sutures were tied down to elevate the urethra to the horizontal position. One finger could be passed between the urethra and the symphysis anteriorly. Hemostasis was ensured.

SERVICE CODE(S): _____

ICD-10-CM DX CODE(S): _____

(Answers to every other Case are located in Appendix D . The full answer key is only available in the TEACH Instructor Resources on Evolve.)

Bladder Rupture

The bladder is ruptured when pressure is placed on a distended bladder. This type of injury is often associated with seatbelt injury in which extreme force results in a compression rupture and most often results in a laceration of the dome of the bladder. The bladder is repaired by means of suture repair (cystorrhaphy) of the resulting lacerations either by percutaneous or open abdominal surgical approach.

CASE 10-7 *Operative Report, Intraperitoneal Bladder Rupture*

This is an internal injury to the bladder as a result of a fall from a ladder that required a complicated repair. The injury is the primary diagnosis followed by an external cause code to indicate how the injury happened.

LOCATION: Inpatient, Hospital

PATIENT: Racio Ruiz

SURGEON: Ira Avila, MD

PREOPERATIVE DIAGNOSIS: Intraperitoneal bladder rupture

POSTOPERATIVE DIAGNOSIS: Intraperitoneal bladder rupture

PROCEDURE PERFORMED: Repair of retroperitoneal bladder rupture

INDICATIONS: This is a 22-year-old man who sustained an intraperitoneal bladder rupture secondary to a fall from a ladder.

ANESTHESIA: General

PROCEDURE: The patient was brought to the operative theater and placed in the supine position on the operating table. After receiving a general anesthetic, he was prepped and draped in a sterile fashion. A vertical midline incision was made from a little above the umbilicus down to the pubis. Dissection was carried down through the subcutaneous tissues and through the anterior fascia. The peritoneal cavity was entered sharply. Some blood clots down in the pelvis were seen overlying the bladder. This area was packed off. We then examined the rest of the abdomen. There were no blood or fluid collections elsewhere. We did not extend the incision all the way up to the top, so it was difficult to get good visualization of the liver and the spleen; however, there was no blood in this area, and palpation of them revealed no abnormalities. The stomach felt normal. Orogastric tube showed good placement. The small bowel was run from the ligament of Treitz to the terminal ileum. This was fine. The appendix was present and normal. The colon was grossly normal throughout its length. Some stool was present. No gross abnormalities were seen down to the pelvis. We had to remove the packing. There were some blood clots setting in the bladder itself. He had a fairly long laceration (indicates complexity) that was for the most part vertical and went fairly close to the superior anterior aspect and continued about two thirds of the way down, pretty much right over the dome (indicates complexity). We inspected the inside of the bladder. No other lesions or lacerations could be identified. We then closed this in two layers (indicates complexity). The inner layer was a 3-0 Vicryl in a running fashion. We then imbricated all of this with interrupted sutures of 3-0 Vicryl through the serosa/peritoneum. There was another bit of lateral laceration that was not full thickness but involving just the serosa. This was also repaired with interrupted sutures of 3-0 Vicryl in a Lembert fashion. This was to the left side, and there was also another short one to the right side. We made sure that each of the corners/apexes had a three-corner stitch placed. We then gently filled the bladder with 250 cc of methylene blue/normal saline solution. No leaks were identified. We then allowed everything to flush back out and irrigated out the pelvis and the abdomen. Clear returns were present. We again looked down the pelvis to be sure there were no other injuries. He currently has a no. 18-French three-way catheter in place. Instead of placing a suprapubic tube, I think it would be easier to manage him with this Foley catheter, and we will plan to take this out in 2 to 3 weeks' time. He will be allowed to go home with a leg bag. We then pulled down the omentum over the small bowel. We closed the fascia with no. 1 looped PDS in a running fashion. The wound was irrigated out. The skin was then closed with staples. Sterile dressings were applied. The patient tolerated the procedure well and went to the recovery room in stable condition.

SERVICE CODE(S): _____

ICD-10-CM DX CODE(S): _____

(Answers to every other Case are located in Appendix D . The full answer key is only available in the TEACH Instructor Resources on Evolve.)

Hydronephrosis

Hydronephrosis is an increase in the size of the renal pelvis and calyces and may have a variety of causes, such as obstruction by tumor or stricture in the urinary system. This is a serious condition that, if unattended, can lead to infection and subsequent sepsis. A cystoscopic examination of the urinary system may be performed to ensure that the collection system is free of obstruction. Fluoroscopic examination may also be performed during the procedure and is reported separately on an hourly basis.

CASE 10-8   *Operative Report, Cystoscopy*

*In the following case Dr. Avila provided **both** the cystoscopic and fluoroscopic examination of the kidney. The physician also reports the bilateral retrograde pyelogram.*

LOCATION: Outpatient, Hospital

PATIENT: Beth Childs

SURGEON: Ira Avila, MD

PREOPERATIVE DIAGNOSIS:

1. Right hydronephrosis
2. Hematuria

POSTOPERATIVE DIAGNOSIS:

1. Mild hydronephrosis
2. No evidence of obstruction
3. Possible old vesicoureteral reflux

PROCEDURE PERFORMED: Cystoscopy, bilateral retrograde pyelogram under fluoroscopic control

CLINICAL NOTE: The patient is a 79-year-old woman who presented with microhematuria (blood seen with microscope). Ultrasound showed mild right hydronephrosis.

OPERATIVE NOTE: The patient was prepped and draped in the lithotomy position, given IV (intravenous) sedation, and the urethra was anesthetized with 2% Xylocaine generally. The patient was cystoscoped. The urethra was normal. There was no evidence of bladder neoplasia. Ureteric orifices and ureters were fairly lateral but appeared normal in shape and size. Bilateral retrograde pyelogram was performed, which showed normal collecting system on the left-hand side. The right system was indeed hydronephrotic, but no evidence of filling defect or calculi was identified. The system drained well on fluoroscopic images. I wonder if she may have had mild reflux at a younger age because of this appearance. At any rate, there was no evidence of inflammation or neoplasia or other significant abnormality. The patient tolerated the procedure well. She will be followed up in the clinic in 3 months' time.

SERVICE CODE(S): _____

ICD-10-CM DX CODE(S): _____

(Answers to every other Case are located in Appendix D . The full answer key is only available in the TEACH Instructor Resources on Evolve.)

Bladder Stones

There are several types of bladder stones: secondary, migrant, and endemic. **Secondary** stones are those that are formed due to a bladder condition, such as obstruction or infections.

Migrant stones originate in the kidney and pass out through the bladder, sometimes becoming lodged in the bladder or ureter. **Endemic** stones are caused by nutritional deficiencies and are uncommon in the United States. Symptoms of a bladder stone are pain and hematuria.

CASE 10-9   *Operative Report, Ureteroscopic Stone Extraction*

*The following case involves the removal of a ureteral calculus by means of ureteroscope and insertion of a stent using fluoroscopic imaging. Dr. Avila provided **both** the scoping procedure and the fluoroscopic imaging supervision and interpretation. Read the notes in the CPT manual following 52351 for reporting of radiological supervision and interpretation.*

LOCATION: Outpatient, Hospital

PATIENT: Oscar Adkins

SURGEON: Ira Avila, MD

PREOPERATIVE DIAGNOSIS: Left ureteral calculus

POSTOPERATIVE DIAGNOSIS: Left ureteral calculus

PROCEDURE PERFORMED: Left ureteroscopic stone extraction and stent insertion under fluoroscopic control

CLINICAL NOTE: The patient is a 37-year-old man with a 3¹/₂-week history of intermittent left renal colic. He now has significant urinary frequency.

PROCEDURE: The patient was prepped and draped in the lithotomy position after being given a general endotracheal anesthetic. A 21-French cystoscope was passed per urethra under direct vision. The

urethra was normal. The prostate showed mild lateral lobe enlargement and mild outlet obstruction with mild bladder trabeculation. The bladder mucosa was normal without evidence of inflammation or neoplasia. The left ureteral orifice appeared quite narrow. A Terumo guidewire was advanced up the left ureter under fluoroscopic control and beyond the stone in the distal left ureter. Again, attempts to pass the rigid ureteroscope without prior ureteral dilation were unsuccessful because of significant ureteral stenosis. A 6-French balloon dilation catheter was then placed, and the distal ureter was dilated under fluoroscopic control. This was withdrawn, and then the patient was ureteroscoped using 6- and 7-French rigid ureteroscopes. The stone was visualized, grasped with a helical basket, and withdrawn intact. Because of significant ureteral edema from stone impaction, it was decided to stent the patient. A 6-French 28-cm (centimeter) Bard inlay stent was then placed under fluoroscopic control in the usual fashion. The guidewire was withdrawn and the bladder drained. A B and O suppository was placed rectally. The patient tolerated the procedure well and was transferred to the recovery room in good condition.

Pathology Report Later Indicated: Ureteral calculus

SERVICE CODE(S): _____

ICD-10-CM DX CODE(S): _____

(Answers to every other Case are located in Appendix D . The full answer key is only available in the TEACH Instructor Resources on Evolve.)

CASE 10-10   *Operative Report, Stent Insertion and TURP*

*Radi Riley has metastatic prostate cancer with liver metastases. There is concern that the cancer is blocking his ureters and has resulted in hydronephrosis. Dr. Avila is going to open the ureter by means of a cystoscope and place a stent to improve his kidney function. Dr. Avila places the cystoscope into the meatus, through the urethra, and into the bladder with guidance and attempts to correct the obstruction of the left and right ureters. Dr. Avila provided **both** the guidance and procedure portions of this service.*

LOCATION: Inpatient, Hospital

PATIENT: Radi Riley

SURGEON: Ira Avila, MD

PREOPERATIVE DIAGNOSIS: Left ureteral obstruction

POSTOPERATIVE DIAGNOSIS: Recurrent prostate cancer with bilateral ureteral obstruction. (Ureter obstruction is the third listed diagnosis.) Liver metastasis.

PROCEDURE PERFORMED: Cystoscopy. (Cystourethroscopy with resection of the prostate is the primary procedure.) Attempted left ureteral stent insertion. Right ureteral stent insertion (Cystourethroscopic insertion of ureteral stent is the second procedure.) under fluoroscopic control. (The professional component of the fluoroscopic guidance is the third procedure.) Transurethral (electrosurgical) resection of recurrent prostate cancer.

CLINICAL NOTE: The patient has known extensive prostate cancer (primary neoplasm) with multiple liver metastases (secondary neoplasm). He has responded well to initial antiandrogens but now is on Decadron for androgen-resistant prostate cancer. He is noted to have left hydronephrosis, and it was decided to try to stent the left ureter after discussion with the daughter and patient. Obviously, his disease is progressing and his long-term outcome is dismal, but over the short term, we had hoped to preserve some renal function.

OPERATIVE NOTE: The patient was given IV (intravenous) sedation and prepped and draped in the lithotomy position. The flexible cystoscope was passed per urethra. The urethra was normal. Prostate fossa was open. There was increased size in the lesions over the left ureteric orifices from just a couple weeks ago when he was last cystoscoped. I could not identify the orifice; several attempts were unsuccessful. The rigid cystoscope was then employed, and again I was unable to identify the orifice. A guidewire was advanced up the right ureteric orifice under fluoroscopic control. The cancer seemed to be encroaching quite quickly on the right orifice, and therefore it was thought best to stent it.

The patient was stented using a 6-French 26-cm (centimeter) stent under fluoroscopic control in the usual fashion. The rectoscope was then introduced into the bladder under direct vision. The area of recurrent tumor overlying the left ureteral orifice was resected. Careful inspection was carried out down to the point where I could just begin to see paravesical fat. A ureteric orifice and ureter could not be identified, and therefore the procedure was terminated at this time. The area was cauterized and chips were evacuated from the bladder. Hemostasis was achieved. A 22 three-way catheter was inserted into the bladder and placed for continuous bladder irrigation.

I will have to have a straightforward discussion with the patient and his daughter with regard to any further intervention. We could proceed with left nephrostomy tube insertion and subsequent antegrade stenting or just leave him with this solitary ureteral stent and change this on a regular basis.

SERVICE CODE(S): _____

ICD-10-CM DX CODE(S): _____

(Answers to every other Case are located in Appendix D . The full answer key is only available in the TEACH Instructor Resources on Evolve.)

Urethral and Ureteral Strictures

Strictures (narrowing) result in frequent, slow urination and can lead to infection. The treatment of a stricture is based on the type and duration of the stricture. The narrowing can be alleviated by means of excision using a cystoscopic knife or dilation (stretching). For example, during a cystourethroscopy with ureteral meatotomy, the surgeon inserts a scope through the urethra and bladder and makes an **incision** of the ureter into the bladder (52290). Compare this procedure to 52281, which is also a cystourethroscopy but one that widens the urethra by dilating a urethral stricture/stenosis by means of a **balloon** catheter. Note 52281 specifies "male or female."

CASE 10-11   *Operative Report, Meatotomy*

Keith Hanshaw is a 5-year-old boy who has been diagnosed with urethral stenosis (narrowing) and requires a meatotomy to open the urethral area to allow normal urine flow.

LOCATION: Outpatient, Hospital

PATIENT: Keith Hanshaw

SURGEON: Ira Avila, MD

PREOPERATIVE DIAGNOSIS: Urethral meatal stenosis

POSTOPERATIVE DIAGNOSIS: Urethral meatal stenosis

PROCEDURE PERFORMED: Urethral meatotomy and cystoscopy

ANESTHESIA: General mask

PROCEDURE: The patient was given a general mask anesthetic as well as a caudal block for postoperative pain control. He was prepped and

draped in the lithotomy position. The meatus was calibrated and found to be tight at the 8-French level. A meatotomy was then performed in a ventral position in the standard fashion. Then 4-0 chromic sutures were placed to reapproximate urethral and penile skin. The patient was then cystoscoped using a 9-French instrument. Urethra was normal. Sphincter was intact. The prostate was not obstructed. There were no posterior urethral valves. The ureteric orifices were normal. The trigone was normal. The bladder mucosa was normal. The bladder was drained and the cystoscope withdrawn. The patient tolerated the procedure well and was transferred to the recovery room in good condition.

SERVICE CODE(S): _____

ICD-10-CM DX CODE(S): _____

(Answers to every other Case are located in Appendix D . The full answer key is only available in the TEACH Instructor Resources on Evolve.)

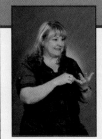

From the Trenches

"A successful medical coder must continuously network, pay attention, and keep an open mind."

MELANIE MARTIN
CPC

Male Genital System

A urologist is also a specialist in the diagnosis and treatment of male genital system conditions. Common conditions are benign prostatic hyperplasia, neoplasm of the prostate, and testicular **hydrocele.** Services include procedures of the penis, testis, epididymis, tunica vaginalis, scrotum, vas deferens, spermatic cord, seminal vesicles, and prostate.

Hemangioma

A **hemangioma** is a benign tumor that commonly occurs in infants and children, although it may occur in patients of any age. See **Figure 10-3.** The tumor is formed of blood vessels and can be difficult to remove because of the vascularity of the mass. The mass may be removed by means of electrodesiccation, application of chemicals, application of liquid nitrogen, cryothermal instrument, laser beam, or blunt excision. Codes for destruction of lesions of the penis, such as condyloma, papilloma, and herpetic vesicle, are included in the Destruction category of codes (54050-54065). These codes can be located in the Index of the CPT manual under the heading of "Penis" or "Destruction, Penis."

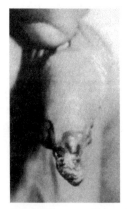

FIGURE 10-3 Hemangioma.

Diagnosis Coding of Hemangioma

Hemangiomas are reported with D18.-- based on the site (such as skin, intracranial, retina, intra-abdominal, other, or unspecified). You can locate codes for hemangioma in the Index under the main term "Hemangioma" and subtermed by location.

CASE 10-12 *Operative Report, Resection*

Report Dr. Avila's surgical services.

LOCATION: Outpatient, Hospital

PATIENT: Harold Arin

SURGEON: Ira Avila, MD

PREOPERATIVE DIAGNOSIS: Penile mass

POSTOPERATIVE DIAGNOSIS: Probable large hemangioma with vascular malformation and superficial dorsal venous complex, penis

PROCEDURE PERFORMED: Resection of large penile vascular mass

CLINICAL NOTE: This 23-year-old gentleman presents with a 1-month history of increased tender dorsal penile mass. Ultrasound, CT (computerized tomography), and MRI (magnetic resonance imaging) have all shown this to be a solid lesion. No flow has been documented within it, and it is suggested that it might be a sarcoma. It is fluctuant and soft, and I wonder whether it might be vascular, but this has not been confirmed on previous imaging.

OPERATIVE NOTE: The patient was given a general endotracheal anesthetic, prepped, and draped in a supine position. An incision was made overlying this large dorsal penile mass at the base of the penis. Just beneath the skin, a large vein was encountered that bled and was dealt with by isolating it and ligating it with 3-0 chromic ligatures. The mass was large, approximately 10 cm (centimeter) in greatest diameter. There was extensive neovascularity, and on further dissection, it was noted that this appeared to be a large hemangioma rising from superficial veins outside Buck's fascia. Extensive care and mobilization were undertaken. This, again, was a very vascular lesion, and I took care to identify all perforating vessels and individually ligated them with chromic ligature. Intraoperative photographs were obtained of the mass showing its extensive vascularity and its location. Frozen section of the mass was obtained that showed no malignant cells. Once the mass was resected, there was a very large cavity. Subcutaneous tissues were closed with 4-0 chromic and skin ultimately with subcuticular Dexon. Compression dressing was applied. The patient tolerated the procedure well and was transferred to the recovery room in good condition.

Pathology Report Later Indicated: Benign hemangioma

SERVICE CODE(S): _____

ICD-10-CM DX CODE(S): _____

(Answers to every other Case are located in Appendix D . The full answer key is only available in the TEACH Instructor Resources on Evolve.)

Balanitis and Circumcision

Balanitis is an inflammation of the glans penis, and **phimosis** is a constriction of the preputial orifice that does not allow for the foreskin to fold back over the glans. See **Figure 10-4**. **Circumcision** is incision of the foreskin and removal of a portion of the foreskin. The CPT codes for circumcision (54150-54161) are divided based on the method of circumcision (clamp or surgical excision) and whether the patient is a neonate or other than a neonate.

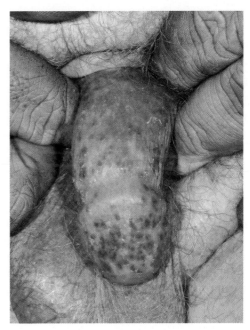

FIGURE 10–4 Balanitis.

CASE 10-13   *Operative Report, Circumcision*

LOCATION: Outpatient, Hospital

PATIENT: Harlen Mata

SURGEON: Ira Avila, MD

PREOPERATIVE DIAGNOSIS: Recurrent candidiasis, balanitis, and phimosis

POSTOPERATIVE DIAGNOSIS: Recurrent candidiasis, balanitis, and phimosis

PROCEDURE PERFORMED: Circumcision

PROCEDURE: This 2-year-old male child was given general mask anesthetic as well as caudal block for postoperative pain control. He was prepped and draped in the supine position, foreskin retracted, and preputial adhesions broken down. Circumcision was performed using a dorsal slit technique. Hemostasis was achieved with judicious use of electrocautery and chromic ties. Prepuce was re-anastomosed to the penile skin using 5-0 chromic catgut. Vaseline gauze dressing was applied. The patient tolerated the procedure well and was transferred to the recovery room in good condition.

Pathology Report Later Indicated: Benign penile tissue

SERVICE CODE(S): _____

ICD-10-CM DX CODE(S): _____

(Answers to every other Case are located in Appendix D . The full answer key is only available in the TEACH Instructor Resources on Evolve.)

CASE 10-14   *Operative Report, Biopsy*

Azoospermia, sometimes documented as male infertility, is the absence of sperm and can be caused by many conditions, including neoplasm of the testes. Biopsies of the testis can be accomplished by means of percutaneous biopsy or open incision biopsy. Code the following services provided to John Ibarra.

LOCATION: Outpatient, Hospital

PATIENT: John Ibarra

SURGEON: Ira Avila, MD

PREOPERATIVE DIAGNOSIS: Azoospermia

POSTOPERATIVE DIAGNOSIS: Azoospermia

PROCEDURE PERFORMED: Bilateral testicular biopsies

PROCEDURE: The patient was given a general mask anesthetic and prepped and draped in the supine position. Bilateral testicular cord blocks were performed with a 50% mixture of 0.5% Marcaine and 2% Xylocaine with epinephrine. Beginning on the right side, a scrotal incision was made. The tunica vaginalis was identified and opened, and a stay stitch was placed in the testis. A small incision was made, and tubules delivered, resected, and sent for permanent resection. The testis was closed with 3-0 Vicryl, the tunica vaginalis with 3-0 chromic, and skin with 3-0 chromic.

The procedure was repeated in identical fashion on the contralateral side. The patient tolerated the procedure well. Dressings were applied. Scrotal support was applied. He will be contacted when the results are available. A discharge prescription for Tylenol no. 3 was given.

Pathology Report Later Indicated: Benign testicular tissue

SERVICE CODE(S): _____

ICD-10-CM DX CODE(S): _____

(Answers to every other Case are located in Appendix D . The full answer key is only available in the TEACH Instructor Resources on Evolve.)

Vasectomy

A **vasectomy** is a method of permanent birth control for men that is nearly 100% effective. Sperm are produced in the testicles and mix with seminal fluid to form semen. A vasectomy intersects (cuts) the vas deferens and blocks the sperm from mixing with the seminal fluid. During ejaculation the sperm-free seminal fluid is ejected. If a vasectomy is an incidental procedure conducted at the time of a more major procedure of the area, the vasectomy is not reported separately but is bundled into the more major procedure.

If the only reason the patient presents is for sterilization, a Z code is assigned to indicate an encounter for the purpose of sterilization.

CASE 10-15   *Operative Report, Vasectomy*

LOCATION: Outpatient, Hospital

PATIENT: Jessy Arley

SURGEON: Ira Avila, MD

PROCEDURE NOTE: The patient is in for a vasectomy having undergone counseling earlier today. He was placed in a supine position, and the scrotal area was shaved. Under sterile technique, the scrotal area was prepped with Betadine, and the sterile drapes were applied. The right vas was localized and under sterile technique was infiltrated with 1% Xylocaine. The vas was externalized, and 1.5-cm (centimeter) portion of the tube was removed. Proximal and distal stumps were doubly ligated with 4-0 silk. A small blood vessel in the skin was oozing and was clamped. Attention was directed to the left side, where a similar procedure was performed. With hemostasis intact, the proximal and distal stumps on the left were retracted into the scrotum, and attention was directed to the right side, where there was slight oozing from the skin edge. With pressure, this did resolve, and the proximal and distal stumps were retracted into the scrotum.

CASE 10-15—*cont'd*

ASSESSMENT: Vasectomy

PLAN: The patient had been given the postvasectomy instruction sheet, and Bacitracin and gauze dressing were applied. He is to apply antibiotics a couple of times a day with gauze. He was given an instruction sheet to have sperm counts done in 2 months' time and to take contraceptive precautions in the meantime.

Pathology Report Later Indicated: Benign vas deferens tissue

SERVICE CODE(S): _____

ICD-10-CM DX CODE(S): _____

(Answers to every other Case are located in Appendix D . The full answer key is only available in the TEACH Instructor Resources on Evolve.)

Hydrocele

Hydrocele (Figure 10-5) is an accumulation of fluid caused by trauma, infection, or tumor; treatment can include surgical excision of the hydrocele. **Epididymitis** is inflammation of the epididymis; treatment can include surgical excision of the epididymis.

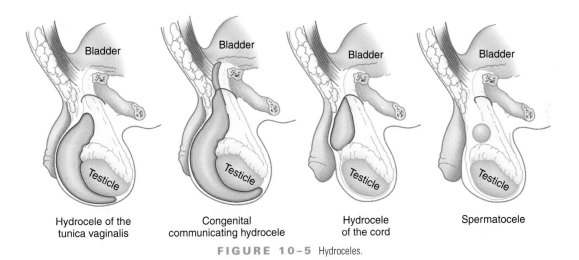

Hydrocele of the tunica vaginalis   Congenital communicating hydrocele   Hydrocele of the cord   Spermatocele

FIGURE 10–5 Hydroceles.

CASE 10-16   *Operative Report, Resection Hydrocele and Epididymectomy*

This service includes a unilateral excision of epididymis and a unilateral excision of hydrocele. Remember to use the correct HCPCS modifier to indicate on which side the surgery was performed. The diagnoses codes must support the reason for each of these two services. See Figure 10-6 for illustration.

LOCATION: Outpatient, Hospital

PATIENT: Dwain Frost

SURGEON: Ira Avila, MD

PREOPERATIVE DIAGNOSIS: Recurrent left hydrocele, chronic epididymitis

POSTOPERATIVE DIAGNOSIS: Recurrent left hydrocele, chronic epididymitis

PROCEDURE PERFORMED: Resection of left hydrocele and left epididymectomy

CLINICAL NOTE: This gentleman has a recurrent left hydrocele and chronic epididymal pain. On examination, he is very tender in his epididymis. I have discussed options with him. He has requested a left epididymectomy and repair of the hydrocele.

He is aware of the potential risks associated with this procedure, including infection, chronic pain, and testicular atrophy.

PROCEDURE: The patient was given general endotracheal anesthetic and prepped and draped in the supine position. A left ilioinguinal nerve block was performed with a 50% mixture of 2% Xylocaine and 0.5% Marcaine with epinephrine. A scrotal incision was made and the testis delivered. There were dense adhesions of the pseudohydrocele sac around the scrotum; these were liberated using electrocautery. The sac was then opened and resected. The epididymis was buried beneath scar tissue. With electrocautery and sharp and blunt technique, the epididymis was identified and resected, and hemostasis was ensured. I could not identify the testicular artery, but I do not believe it was involved. Hemostasis was ensured, and the testis returned to the scrotum. A ¼-inch Penrose drain was left through a separate stab wound and sutured to the skin with 3-0 Prolene. The scrotum was closed in two layers with 3-0 chromic. A supportive dressing was applied. The patient tolerated the procedure well and was discharged in good condition. He will be seen next week in the clinic for drain removal.

Pathology Report Later Indicated: Benign epididymis tissue

SERVICE CODE(S): _____

ICD-10-CM DX CODE(S): _____

(Answers to every other Case are located in Appendix D . The full answer key is only available in the TEACH Instructor Resources on Evolve.)

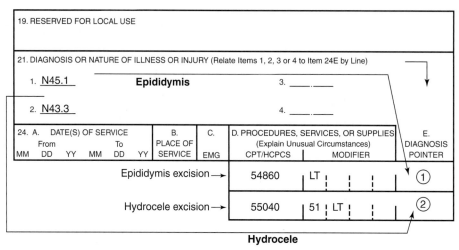

FIGURE 10–6 Diagnosis supports medical necessity for each service.

Prostate-Specific Antigen

Prostate-specific antigen (PSA) is secreted by the epithelial cells of the prostate gland (including cancerous cells), and an elevation in the levels of PSA in the blood indicates an abnormality of the prostate gland. The screening test is used to detect potential problems in the prostate gland and to follow the progress of prostate cancer. A reading greater than 4 mg/ml is abnormal and generally indicates that a prostate biopsy would be performed. A biopsy may be obtained transrectally and often includes the use of ultrasound to ensure correct placement of the biopsy forceps. The ultrasound is reported in addition to the biopsy code. The biopsy may also be obtained by an incisional approach.

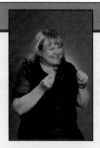

From the Trenches

"As medical coders are unique, working in the medical coding field gives you the sense of belonging."

MELANIE MARTIN
CPC

CASE 10-17 | *Transrectal Ultrasound for Prostate Volume Determination and Biopsy*

The surgeon provides both the biopsy of the prostate and the professional component of the ultrasonic determination of the prostate size. The diagnosis for this service is an elevated PSA. You can find direction to the code in the Index under the main term "Elevated" and subterm "prostate specific antigen."

LOCATION: Outpatient, Hospital
PATIENT: Ray Engert
SURGEON: Ira Avila, MD

PREOPERATIVE DIAGNOSIS: Elevated PSA (prostate-specific antigen)

POSTOPERATIVE DIAGNOSIS: Elevated PSA

CLINICAL NOTE: The patient has a PSA of 6.5 and a benign-feeling prostate.

PROCEDURE NOTE: The patient was placed in the left lateral position, and the ultrasound probe was introduced. Prostate volume was determined at 50.7 g (gram). Some calcifications are found in the right lobe, with no obvious hypoechogenic abnormality. The base of the prostate was infiltrated with 1% Xylocaine, and random biopsies were performed in the

CASE 10-17—cont'd

usual fashion. The patient tolerated the procedure well. He was discharged in good condition and will be contacted when results are available.

Pathology Report Later Indicated: Benign prostate tissue

SERVICE CODE(S): _____

ICD-10-CM DX CODE(S): _____

(Answers to every other Case are located in Appendix D . The full answer key is only available in the TEACH Instructor Resources on Evolve.)

Prostate Cancer

Prostate cancer is the second most common malignancy in men (skin cancer is first), and it is also the second leading cause of death (lung cancer is first). PSA screening and transrectal ultrasound with biopsy are two important diagnostic tools in early diagnosis of prostate cancer. Staging for cancer is a process of assigning a stage (level of invasion) to a cancer. Two staging methods are the Whitmore-Jewett method and the TNM (tumor, nodes, metastases) method, as illustrated in **Figures 10-7** and **10-8**. A prostatectomy is the surgical removal of a portion of or the entire prostate, and reporting of the procedure is based on the extent of the procedure and the approach used. A **retropubic** approach (55831-55845) is one in which the incision is made in the lower abdomen behind the pubic arch. With a **perineal** approach (55801-55815), the incision is made in the skin between the scrotum and the anus. A **suprapubic** approach (55821) is above the pubic arch.

In the index of the CPT manual, locate the main term "Prostate" and subterm "Excision." Note that there are subterms for partial, perineal, radical, retropubic, suprapubic, and transurethral. Partial and radical are the **extent of the procedure.** Perineal, retropubic, and suprapubic are **surgical**

WHITMORE-JEWETT STAGES:

Stage A is clinically undetectable tumor confined to the gland and is an incidental finding at prostate surgery.
   A1: well-differentiated with focal involvement
   A2: moderately or poorly differentiated or involves multiple foci in the gland

Stage B is tumor confined to the prostate gland.
   B0: nonpalpable, PSA-detected
   B1: single nodule in one lobe of the prostate
   B2: more extensive involvement of one lobe or involvement of both lobes

Stage C is a tumor clinically localized to the periprostatic area but extending through the prostatic capsule; seminal vesicles may be involved.
   C1: clinical extracapsular extension
   C2: extracapsular tumor producing bladder outlet or ureteral obstruction

Stage D is metastatic disease.
   D0: clinically localized disease (prostate only) but persistently elevated enzymatic serum acid phosphatase
   D1: regional lymph nodes only
   D2: distant lymph nodes, metastases to bone or visceral organs
   D3: D2 prostate cancer patients who relapse after adequate endocrine therapy

FIGURE 10-7 Whitmore-Jewett stages.

TNM STAGES:

Primary Tumor (T)
TX: Primary tumor cannot be assessed
T0: No evidence of primary tumor
T1: Clinically inapparent tumor not palpable or visible by imaging
   T1a: Tumor incidental histologic finding in 5% or less of tissue resected
   T1b: Tumor incidental histologic finding in more than 5% of tissue resected
   T1c: Tumor identified by needle biopsy (e.g., because of elevated PSA)
T2: Tumor confined within the prostate
   T2a: Tumor involves half a lobe or less
   T2b: Tumor involves more than half of a lobe, but not both lobes
   T2c: Tumor involves both lobes; extends through the prostatic capsule
T3a: Unilateral extracapsular extension
T3b: Bilateral extracapsular extension
T3c: Tumor invades the seminal vesicle(s)
T4: Tumor is fixed or invades adjacent structures other than the seminal vesicle(s)
   T4a: Tumor invades any of bladder neck, external sphincter, or rectum
   T4b: Tumor invades levator muscles and/or is fixed to the pelvic wall

Regional lymph nodes (N)
NX: Regional lymph nodes cannot be assessed
N0: No regional lymph node metastasis
N1: Metastasis in a single lymph node, 2 cm or less in greatest dimension
N2: Metastasis in a single lymph node, more than 2 cm but not more than 5 cm in greatest dimension; or multiple lymph node metastases, none more than 5 cm in greatest dimension
N3: Metastasis in a single lymph node more than 5 cm in greatest dimension

Distant metastases (M)
MX: Presence of distant metastasis cannot be assessed
M0: No distant metastasis
M1: Distant metastasis
   M1a: Nonregional lymph node(s)
   M1b: Bone(s)
   M1c: Other site(s)

FIGURE 10-8 TNM stages.

---

approaches that can be either laparoscopic or by means of an open surgical site. Transurethral is a surgical **technique** by means of an endoscope. This means the coder has to identify the correct approach or technique as well as the extent of the procedure. For example, 55840-55845 are for radical (extent) retropubic (approach) prostatectomies. If a laparoscopic retropubic (surgical approach) radical (extent) prostatectomy was performed, the service is reported with 55866.

CASE 10-18   *Operative Report, Prostatectomy*

Donald Berry's prostate biopsy indicated carcinoma of the prostate. Dr. Avila has scheduled a bilateral pelvic lymphadenectomy and prostatectomy.

LOCATION: Inpatient, Hospital

PATIENT: Donald Berry

SURGEON: Ira Avila, MD

PREOPERATIVE DIAGNOSIS: Carcinoma of the prostate

POSTOPERATIVE DIAGNOSIS: Carcinoma of the prostate

OPERATIVE PROCEDURE: Bilateral pelvic lymph node dissection and radical retropubic prostatectomy

CLINICAL NOTE: This 65-year-old man presented with a PSA (prostate-specific antigen) of 8.1. He has a 100 g prostate, and 1 of 10 cores was positive for a Gleason's 6/10 carcinoma and T4A on the TNM.

PROCEDURE NOTE: The patient was given a spinal anesthetic with epidural assist. He was prepped and draped in the supine position. A no. 20-French Foley catheter was then inserted into the bladder and placed to straight drainage. A lower abdominal midline incision was made. The retropubic space was entered. The Omni retractor was used for exposure. Bilateral pelvic lymphadenectomy was performed in the usual fashion. Obturator nerves were identified and spared. The lymph nodes were small and benign in palpation and therefore were sent for permanent resection. The endopelvic fascia was opened bilaterally. The prostate was extremely large, and the parapelvis very narrow, which made it difficult for mobilization. There was not much of a superficial venous complex. Dorsal venous complex was surrounded with a McDougal clamp, doubly ligated distally with no. 1 silk, and oversewn proximally with 0 chromic. Puboprostatic ligaments were divided sharply. The dorsal venous complex was then divided with electrocautery. The

urethra was identified and divided anteriorly with a scalpel. The catheter was withdrawn, clamped, and divided, and the urethra was divided posteriorly. The prostate was densely adherent to the Denonvilliers fascia. A small tear in the prostate was created at the apex. This was recognized and repaired. The prostate was then mobilized using blunt dissection technique. Bilateral nerve-sparing technique was employed. Neurovascular bundles were dissected off the prostate using sharp dissection techniques and 2-0 chromic suture ligatures for hemostasis. Denonvilliers fascia was opened posteriorly to identify the seminal vesicles and ampulla. These were dissected near the base of the seminal vesicles in which they were individually clipped and divided. Lateral pedicles were taken with 0 chromic suture ligatures. The bladder neck was opened anteriorly. The bladder, ureteric orifices, and then trigone were identified, and the bladder neck was divided posteriorly and the specimen removed. Hemostasis was ensured with 2-0 chromic suture ligatures. The bladder neck was closed in a tennis racquet fashion using 2-0 chromic. Mucosa was inverted using 4-0 chromic and urethra to re-anastomose the bladder neck over a 20-French Foley catheter using 2-0 Monocryl sutures. A 10-mm (millimeter) Jackson-Pratt drain was left through a right lower quadrant stab wound and sutured to the skin using 2-0 Prolene. The fascia was closed with clips with no. 1 Vicryl, subcutaneous tissues with 2-0 chromic, and the skin with 4-0 subcuticular Dexon. Dressings were applied. The patient tolerated the procedure well. Estimated blood loss was 450 cc. Sponge and needle counts were reported as correct. The patient was transferred to the recovery room in good condition.

Pathology Report Later Indicated: Adenocarcinoma prostate, primary

SERVICE CODE(S): _____

ICD-10-CM DX CODE(S): _____

(Answers to every other Case are located in Appendix D . The full answer key is only available in the TEACH Instructor Resources on Evolve.)

Staging

Staging is assigning a level of invasion to cancer patients based on the information available. Staging is used in the development of a treatment plan. There are two staging methods: Whitmore-Jewett staging, developed in 1956, and the TNM, developed in 1992. The TNM is more detailed than the Whitmore-Jewett (see **Figures 10-7** and **10-8**).

CASE 10-19   *Operative Report, Lymphadenectomy, Prostatectomy, and Plastic Repair*

This prostatectomy includes an additional element of plastic repair of the bladder neck (cystourethroplasty), which is included in the prostatectomy.

LOCATION: Inpatient, Hospital

PATIENT: Rex Kaat

SURGEON: Ira Avila, MD

PREOPERATIVE DIAGNOSIS: Carcinoma of the prostate

POSTOPERATIVE DIAGNOSIS: Carcinoma of the prostate

PROCEDURE: Bilateral pelvic lymphadenectomy with frozen section, radical retropubic prostatectomy, and plastic repair of bladder neck.

CLINICAL NOTE: This man was found to have poorly differentiated diffuse adenocarcinoma of the prostate after presenting with a PSA (prostate-specific antigen) of 7.8 and an abnormal digital rectal examination.

PROCEDURAL NOTE: The patient was given a spinal anesthetic and prepped and draped in the supine position. A 20-French Foley catheter was inserted into the bladder and placed to straight drainage. A lower abdominal midline incision was made. The Omni retractor was used for exposure.

CASE 10-19—cont'd

The retropubic space was entered. Bilateral pelvic lymphadenectomy was performed, and obturator nerves were identified and spared. There were palpable abnormalities in the right pelvic lymph nodes; therefore, both sets of nodes were sent for frozen section, and results were benign.

Endopelvic fascia was then opened bilaterally. Puboprostatic ligaments were divided. Dorsal venous complex surrounded with no. 1 silk distally and oversewn proximally with 0 chromic. This was then divided using electrocautery. Urethra was identified and divided anteriorly; catheter was withdrawn, clamped, and divided; and then the urethra was divided posteriorly. There was significant fibrotic reaction at the prostatic apex with adhesions to Denonvilliers fascia. A non–nerve-sparing technique was used, and neurovascular bundles were taken widely, particularly on the left. During dissection of the apex, a small piece of the prostate was torn, and this was sent separately, labeled as prostatic apex.

Neurovascular bundles were controlled with 0 chromic suture ligatures. Lateral pedicles were taken of 0 chromic suture ligatures. Seminal vesicles were dissected to the base, where they were clipped and divided along with the ampulla of the vas. Bladder neck was opened anteriorly, ureteric orifice identified, and the bladder neck divided posteriorly. The specimen was sent for permanent resection. Hemostasis was achieved with 2-0 chromic. The bladder neck was closed in a tennis racquet fashion using 2-0 chromic and mucosa inverted using 4-0 chromic. Urethra was re-anastomosed to the bladder neck using five 2-0 Monocryl sutures in the usual fashion. Fresh 20-French Foley catheter was placed prior to closure of the bladder neck. A 10-mm (millimeter) Jackson-Pratt drain was left through a right lower quadrant stab wound and sutured to the skin with 2-0 Prolene. Fascia was closed with no. 1 Vicryl in a running fashion, subcutaneous tissues with 2-0 chromic, and skin with 4-0 subcuticular Dexon. Steri-Strips were applied. Estimated blood loss was 500 cc (cubic centimeter). Sponge and needle counts were reported as correct.

Pathology Report Later Indicated: N3 metastasis and T4a primary adenocarcinoma of the bladder neck. (Refer to Figure 10-8, entries "T4a" and "N3" to determine the results of the pathologic examination.)

SERVICE CODE(S): _____

ICD-10-CM DX CODE(S): _____

(Answers to every other Case are located in Appendix D . The full answer key is only available in the TEACH Instructor Resources on Evolve.)

Cryoablation

Cryoablation (use of super-cold liquid) is used to freeze the prostate, destroying all living tissue of the gland. Ultrasound guidance is included in the procedure and is not reported separately for the placement of the cryoprobes into the prostate. Several probes are inserted using guidance, and then a substance such as nitrogen is inserted through the probes. The area may be allowed to thaw and then is refrozen (termed *cycles*) one or more times to ensure that no viable prostatic tissue remains. The probes are removed and the puncture sites closed with stitches.

CASE 10-20   *Operative Report, Cryoablation of Prostate*

This case demonstrates the use of cryoablation. In the index of CPT manual, locate direction to the codes under the main term "Ablation" or "Destruction."

LOCATION: Outpatient, Hospital

PATIENT: Dean Jailor

SURGEON: Ira Avila, MD

PREOPERATIVE DIAGNOSIS: Recurrent primary prostate cancer

POSTOPERATIVE DIAGNOSIS: Recurrent primary prostate cancer

PROCEDURE PERFORMED: Cryoablation of prostate, insertion of suprapubic catheter, and cystoscopy

CLINICAL NOTE: This gentleman had radiation therapy for adenocarcinoma of the prostate. Unfortunately, he has developed a recurrence and has a biopsy-proven adenocarcinoma. Biopsies from the right mid-region of the prostate were positive. Options were discussed. The patient was cleared preoperatively for surgery. He decided to proceed with cryoablation. He is aware of the risks of incontinence and rectal injury.

ANESTHESIA: General

PROCEDURE: The patient was given a general endotracheal anesthetic and was prepped and draped in the lithotomy position. An 18-French Foley catheter was placed in the bladder to straight drainage. A transrectal probe was introduced. Prostate volume was returned at 28.5 g (gram). A six-probe freeze was selected. Using the quick stick method, sheaths were placed under ultrasound guidance. Following placement of the sheaths, temperature probes were then placed in the left and right neurovascular bundles, apex, external sphincter, and Denonvilliers fascia. The patient then underwent cystoscopy after removal of the Foley catheter with the flexible instrument. The urethra was normal. The external sphincter probe appeared to be in good position. The bladder was inspected, and no evidence of violation of the bladder was seen. A 12-French Cook suprapubic catheter was then placed in trocar fashion under endoscopic guidance and secured to the skin.

A guidewire was left in the bladder, and over this guidewire the urethra-warming catheter was placed. Continuous bladder irrigation was achieved by running warm saline through the suprapubic and out through the urethra-warming catheter.

Continued

CASE 10-20—cont'd

A two-cycle probe freeze was undertaken. The first cycle had a very rapid freeze, and the second cycle was more prolonged. (Please see operative note for detailed records of freeze times and temperature.) The external sphincter temperature never reached less than 0° C (Celsius). The freeze was monitored both digitally as well as radiographically with ultrasound.

The probes were withdrawn after full thaw. Two active thaw cycles were undertaken. The perineal incisions were then closed with 3-0 plain catgut subcuticular sutures. The suprapubic catheter was left in situ. Urethral catheter was not placed at the end of the case. The patient

tolerated the procedure well and was transferred to the recovery room in good condition.

SERVICE CODE(S): _____

ICD-10-CM DX CODE(S): _____

(Answers to every other Case are located in Appendix D . The full answer key is only available in the TEACH Instructor Resources on Evolve.)

Endocrine System

An **endocrinologist** is a physician who specializes in the diagnosis and treatment of conditions of the endocrine system. Conditions include goiter, diabetes mellitus, ketoacidosis, hypothyroidism, thyroiditis, adrenal insufficiencies, calcemia, kalemia, natremia, and various fluid imbalances. Endocrine conditions that require surgery may be diagnosed by an endocrinologist, but usually a general surgeon performs the surgical procedure, which is often excision of a lesion.

The CPT codes for the thyroid gland include only one code for an incision (60000). The remaining codes are for excisions (60100-60281) based on the extent of the procedure, except for 60300 (aspiration or injection of thyroid cyst) and 60100 (thyroid biopsy by core needle). If the aspiration biopsy of the thyroid is performed by fine needle, report with code range 10004-10021 depending on the type of imaging guidance, if performed.. The codes in the range 60500-60699 are primarily for excision of the parathyroid, thymus, adrenal, pancreas, and carotid body, with two codes for laparoscopic procedures (60650-60659). Often the diagnosis will be a neoplasm or mass of the gland, pancreas, or carotid body, which explains the predominance of the excision codes.

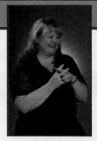

From the Trenches

"Certification is important especially if you want to work in a hospital. Having a certification solidifies that you have an excellent understanding of medical coding."

MELANIE MARTIN
CPC

CASE 10-21 *Operative Report, Left Thyroid Mass*

Yolanda Saldivar had an enlarged thyroid gland that biopsy indicated was benign. She continues to have edema, and Dr. Avila referred her to Dr. Sanchez for a possible thyroidectomy.

LOCATION: Inpatient, Hospital

PATIENT: Yolanda Saldivar

PRIMARY CARE PHYSICIAN: Ira Avila, MD

SURGEON: Gary Sanchez, MD

PREOPERATIVE DIAGNOSIS: Left thyroid mass

POSTOPERATIVE DIAGNOSIS: Left thyroid mass, right thyroid nodules

PROCEDURE PERFORMED: Total thyroidectomy **(Figure 10-9)**

OPERATIVE NOTE: The patient is a 29-year-old woman who was seen in the office and diagnosed with the above-named condition. The decision was made in consultation with the patient to undergo the above-named procedure. The risks and benefits of surgery were discussed prior to the operation. Informed consent was obtained. The patient had a history of previous lymphoma. She has undergone mantle radiation. She was concerned that the masses could represent cancer.

She was admitted through the inpatient surgery program and taken to the operating room, where she was administered a general anesthetic

CASE 10-21—cont'd

by intravenous injection. She was then intubated endotracheally. She was prepped and draped in the usual sterile fashion. The anterior neck was injected with 1% lidocaine with epinephrine. An 8-cm (centimeter) transverse skin incision was created with a no. 15 blade through the skin and subcutaneous tissue. We dissected down to the platysma, which was also incised sharply with the no. 15 blade. Subplatysmal flaps were elevated superiorly to the thyroid notch and inferiorly to the sternal notch. Gelpi retractor was then placed in the wound and expanded. The midline straps were grasped on either side of the midline using electrocautery. The straps were divided from the thyroid notch down to the sternal notch area. We then retracted the straps on the left side and dissected over the gland and identified a large mass **(Figure 10-10)**. The trachea was identified midline above and below the isthmus. We then identified the superior pole, the vessels were clamped and ligated, and 2-0 and silk sutures were used to tie off the pole vessels. The gland was then rotated medially, and the inferior pole was identified. These vessels were then ligated and tied with the same 2-0 silk suture. We dissected in a subscapular fashion and identified the superior and inferior parathyroid glands. These were reflected down. The recurrent laryngeal nerve was then identified and traced medially to its insertion. The gland was then elevated off this area. The isthmus was divided midline with Kelly clamps and tied with the same 2-0 silk suture. Once the gland was pedicled on the thyroid, the remaining Berry's ligament was removed, and the gland was sent to the pathologist for tissue identification. The quick section identification suggested an adenomatous lesion. We then elevated the straps off the right side of the thyroid, and there were at least two prominent nodules on this side. These nodules were quite firm, and both were about 1 cm large. The decision was made at this point, given the aforementioned history and the patient's previous expressed desire to have these lesions removed, to go ahead with removal of the right thyroid gland. We dissected in a subcapsular fashion on this side. Superior vessels were again identified, clamped, and ligated. Silk ties (2-0) were used to tie off the superior pole vessels. Again, the inferior vessels were identified and tied off. We rotated the gland medially and dissected in a subcapsular fashion to identify the superior parathyroid gland. The recurrent laryngeal nerve was somewhat difficult to find. We dissected carefully along its usual course and identified it, tucked underneath the trachea. We were able to dissect this clearly, and it was preserved right to its entranceway into the larynx. We then removed the remaining thyroid off this area and incised the remaining Berry's ligament. The gland was then sent to the pathologist for identification. The wound was thoroughly irrigated. Careful hemostasis was achieved. Two pieces of Surgicel were placed on either side in the gutter areas. We then placed two medium Hemovac drains through separate stab incisions. These were secured with 2-0 silk suture. The straps were then re-approximated with interrupted 4-0 Vicryl suture. The skin was then closed in two layers; the first layer was an interrupted 4-0 Vicryl suture, and the second layer was a running subcuticular 5-0 Prolene suture. The wound was then reinforced with Steri-Strips. The patient was then allowed to recover from the general anesthetic and taken to the post-anesthesia care unit in a stable condition. No complications occurred during this procedure.

Pathology Report Later Indicated: Benign colloid nodule

SERVICE CODE(S): _____

ICD-10-CM DX CODE(S): _____

(Answers to every other Case are located in Appendix D . The full answer key is only available in the TEACH Instructor Resources on Evolve.)

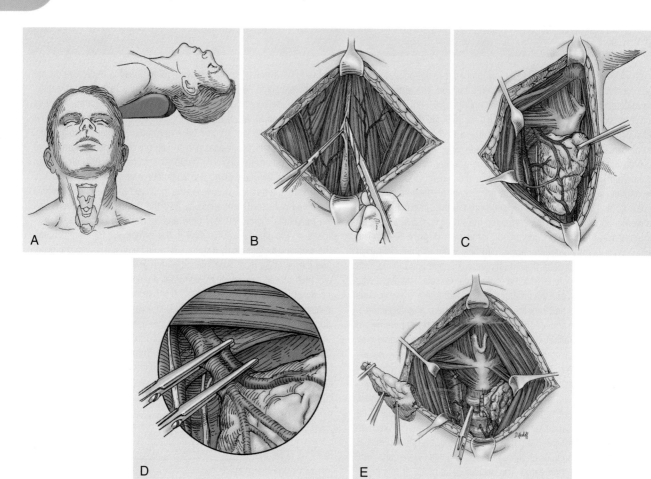

FIGURE 10-9 Thyroidectomy.

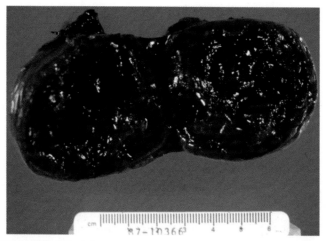

FIGURE 10-10 Mass removed from thyroid lobe during a total thyroidectomy.

CASE 10-22A   *Operative Report, Excision of Right Carotid Body Tumor*

The excision is of a tumor of the carotid body.
Electroencephalography (EEG) is used during this procedure and is reported separately.

LOCATION: Inpatient, Hospital

PATIENT: Delores Janus

SURGEON: Gary Sanchez, MD

PREOPERATIVE DIAGNOSIS: Right carotid body tumor

POSTOPERATIVE DIAGNOSIS: Frozen section confirmed a right carotid body tumor with tortuous internal and external carotids that have been displaced by tumor mass with multiple blood vessels feeding this tumor mass, rising from the external carotid, all ligated individually. The tumor was highly vascularized.

OPERATIVE PROCDURE: Excision of right carotid body tumor

ANESTHESIA: General endotracheal with EEG (electroencephalogram) monitoring.

The patient tolerated the procedure well.

COMPLICATIONS: None

NEEDLE AND SPONGE COUNTS: Needle and sponge counts appear correct. No adverse EEG changes were noted during the procedure.

ESTIMATED BLOOD LOSS: 125 cc. No drains were placed. Incision was closed.

INDICATION FOR PROCEDURE: The patient, on a workup for another problem, was dubiously noted to have what looked like a carotid body tumor on CT (computerized tomography) scan. Subsequently an angiogram was done to examine this further. This confirmed our suspicions and also showed that the blood supply was derived mostly from the external carotid. Consent was obtained for operative intervention. The procedure, indication, risks, benefits, and alternatives were discussed at length with the patient. She understood and wished to proceed.

OPERATIVE TECHNIQUE: The patient was brought to the operating room and placed supine on the operating room table. General endotracheal anesthesia was administered under EEG monitoring. We then proceeded to prep the neck, lower face, and upper chest with Betadine and draped them off in a sterile fashion. We proceeded with proper placement of her neck, somewhat extended to provide adequate exposure. We proceeded with her incision anterior to the sternocleidomastoid. We extended this through skin and subcutaneous tissues and the platysma muscle down to the sternocleidomastoid and then subsequently retracted the sternocleidomastoid laterally and exposed the jugular vein, which was quite large and had many tributaries. These tributaries were doubly ligated on the large ones and also retracted laterally. The common carotid was identified, dissected down onto the common carotid, and a vessel loop placed around the common carotid dissection, subsequently carried distally. We identified the internal and external carotids and also placed vessel loops around this. On the external carotid, we identified the superior thyroid, placed a vessel loop around this, and followed this further. Another branch of the external carotid was noted to be feeding the tumor mass between external and internal carotid; multiple small feeding vessels were also identified and were individually ligated. We used bipolar cautery to dissect some of the tissue because this was very hypervascular. The tumor was well circumscribed, although it caused a lot of hypervascularity around it. We were able to dissect this off, identified and preserved the hypoglossal nerve, and identified and preserved the vagus nerve posteriorly. Also, after taking the mass out and sending it for frozen section, we had confirmation that this was a carotid body tumor. We will await permanent sections. Hemostasis was good. We then irrigated. Once we were satisfied with this procedure, we closed the platysma muscles with running 3-0 Vicryl sutures and closed the skin with 4-0 Vicryl subcuticular running sutures. We applied Steri-Strips and sterile dressings. The patient tolerated the procedure well without complications. On awakening in the operating room, she was able to move all extremities. She will be transferred to the surgical critical care unit for further observation and recovery.

Pathology Report Later Indicated: See Report 10-22B.

SERVICE CODE(S): _____

ICD-10-CM DX CODE(S): _____

(Answers to every other Case are located in Appendix D . The full answer key is only available in the TEACH Instructor Resources on Evolve.)

CASE 10-22B   *Pathology Report*

LOCATION: Outpatient, Hospital

PATIENT: Delores Janus

SURGEON: Gary Sanchez, MD

PATHOLOGIST: Grey Lonewolf, MD

CLINICAL HISTORY: Patient has right carotid body mass. She has a history of thyroid cancer.

SPECIMEN RECEIVED: Carotid body tumor with FS (frozen section)

GROSS DESCRIPTION: The specimen is labeled with the patient's name and "right carotid body mass" and consists of a 3.5 × 2.8 × 1.4-cm (centimeter) red-brown tissue weighing 8.5 g (gram). The tumor is inked black. Cut sections show a solid red-brown center. The specimen is submitted in five cassettes.

INTRAOPERATIVE FROZEN-SECTION DIAGNOSIS: Right carotid body tumor. Paraganglioma (carotid body tumor)

MICROSCOPIC DESCRIPTION: Permanent sections confirm the frozen-section diagnosis of carotid body tumor. The lesion appears relatively well circumscribed, partially surrounded by a hyalinized fibrous capsule. The tumor is composed of nests (Zellballen) of polygonal cells with areas of trabeculae of fibrous tissue. The tumor cells have abundant granular eosinophilic cytoplasm and predominantly round to ovoid nuclei showing some focal

Continued

CASE 10-22B—cont'd

pleomorphism and hyperchromatism. Mitoses are scant. Vascular invasion is not seen.

DIAGNOSIS: Right carotid body mass: carotid body paraganglioma

COMMENT: It is almost impossible histologically to judge the clinical course of a carotid body tumor by its histology, even though these tumors are seldom malignant. Mitoses, nuclear pleomorphism, and even vascular invasion are unreliable markers of malignancy. Close clinical follow-up needed because these tumors may recur.

SERVICE CODE(S): _____

ICD-10-CM DX CODE(S): _____

(Answers to every other Case are located in Appendix D . The full answer key is only available in the TEACH Instructor Resources on Evolve.)

CHAPTER 10   *Auditing Review*

Audit the coding for the following reports.

Audit Report 10.1 Operative Report, Lymphadenectomy with Prostatectomy

Martin Glass is admitted to the hospital by Dr. Avila for a retropubic radical prostatectomy.

LOCATION: Inpatient, Hospital

PATIENT: Martin Glass

SURGEON: Ira Avila, MD

ATTENDING PHYSICIAN: Ira Avila, MD

PREOPERATIVE DIAGNOSIS: History of adenocarcinoma of the prostate

POSTOPERATIVE DIAGNOSIS: History of adenocarcinoma of the prostate

PROCEDURE PERFORMED: Bilateral pelvic lymphadenectomy with radical retropubic prostatectomy

PROCEDURE: Please see the preoperative note for indications of the procedure as well as full informed consent. The patient underwent a general anesthetic and was put in a modified frog-leg position. Anesthesia preparation included a central venous line, arterial line, and an epidural catheter. After this was achieved, a midline was deepened down through skin and generous subcutaneous tissue to the midline. This was opened along the lines of the incision midline. The retropubic space was entered and developed. The pelvic lymphadenectomy was then performed. This was carried along the usual lines. The lateral extension was the external iliac vein. Tissues surrounding that vein were brought down and around the muscle wall to include the obturator group, preventing injury to the obturator artery, vein, and nerve. Proximally we went to the circumflex iliac branches, including the node of Cloquet, and then used clips across the trunks of the lymphatics. Distally or proximally on the patient, we proceeded to the bifurcation of the iliac vein, ending the dissection at that point. Again, the lymphatic trunks were clipped. Each package was delivered and sent to pathology for frozen section analysis. With the result of negative nodes, we proceeded with surgical removal of the prostate. This was performed in standard fashion. The Thompson retractor was used with modifications under padded retractors throughout the procedure. This allowed adequate exposure. The margin between the lateral and endopelvic fascia was opened in anteromedial fashion to the puboprostatic ligaments, which were opened. The patient's size was fairly good; he had a large prostate so the

visualization in the apical area of the prostate was not great. We finger dissected along the superficial venous complex, reaching the apex of the prostate on each side. The McDougall clamp was placed through the fascia under the superficial venous complex but anterior to the urethra. Space was created there. A TIA-46 stapler was used to staple across the superficial venous complex. The urethra was exposed and opened anteriorly. Sutures at 10 and 2 o'clock were placed, 2-0 chromic, outside to in. The rest of the urethra was mobilized after the catheter was brought up and out of the wound and used for traction device after it was cut. The urethra was incised, and sutures were placed at the 4 and 8 o'clock positions likewise. Apex of the prostate was mobilized using sharp and blunt dissection, carrying it down to the lateral pelvic fascial leavers. These were separated using sharp and blunt dissection off the lateral aspect of the prostate. Clips were used for the small bleeding vessels encountered. The lateral pedicle was then mobilized between clamps and ligated with 0 chromics, each side. Care was again taken to avoid the neurovascular bundle apparatus. The prostate was mobilized anteriorly and the Denonvilliers' fascia was opened over the seminal vesicles. Those were dissected posteriorly. The bladder neck was then incised down just behind the prostate. Because of the large medial lobe on the prostate, we had to open the bladder neck somewhat more than normal. We exposed the trigone but did not approach it. The prostate was dissected posteriorly off the bladder neck using sharp and blunt dissection. The seminal vesicles were then approached anteriorly as was the ampulla of the vas. Each was cross-clamped and ligated. Final hemostasis was achieved at this point with the prostate removed. We everted the urothelium and closed the bladder neck slightly. We then brought sutures concomitantly from inside to out, at 2, 10, 4, and 8 o'clock. An 18-silcone catheter was placed in the bladder, and the sutures were tied down. Hemovac drains were placed, and the wound was closed with double-stranded running nylon. Skin clips were placed, and the drains were secured. He tolerated the procedure well overall.

One or more of the following codes are reported incorrectly for this case. Indicate the incorrect code or codes.

PROFESSIONAL SERVICES:	Prostatectomy, **55840**; Pelvic lymphadenectomy, **38870-50**
ICD-10-CM DX:	Prostate neoplasm, **C61**
INCORRECT CODE(S):	_____

Audit Report 10.2 Operative Report, Varicocele Ligation

LOCATION: Outpatient, Hospital

PATIENT: Joseph Schaff

SURGEON: Ira Avila, MD

PREOPERATIVE DIAGNOSES:

1. Bilateral varicoceles.
2. Infertility.

POSTOPERATIVE DIAGNOSES: Same.

PROCEDURE PROPOSED: Laparoscopic bilateral varicocelectomy.

PROCEDURE PERFORMED: Attempted laparoscopy and bilateral inguinal exploration and varicocele ligation.

CLINICAL NOTE: This gentleman has infertility with seminal abnormalities consistent with varicocele. He has bilateral varicoceles on ultrasound and on physical examination. Options were discussed. I offered him a laparoscopic, possible open varicocele ligation. He is obese, and I thought it may be somewhat of a challenge to perform the laparoscopy.

PROCEDURE NOTE: The patient was given a general endotracheal anesthetic, the bladder drained with a 16-French Foley. Using the Bladeless Trocar System, an incision was made at the subumbilical space and

Continued

CHAPTER 10—cont'd

the 12-French trocar passed with the 0-degree camera under direct vision. I was unable to safely enter the peritoneum space although I did pass through the fascia without difficulty. I found myself in the properitoneal space with no ability to enter the peritoneum safely. I therefore abandoned the procedure. Fascial defect was closed with 2-0 Vicryl.

Bilateral inguinal incisions were made, cords identified at the level of the external ring where they were isolated and elevated on a Penrose drain, external fascia of the cord opened, vas identified and isolated. The artery was also identified. Veins were isolated, resected, and ligated with 3-0 silk. Cords were returned to the canals. The procedure was repeated in an identical fashion on both sides. Subcutaneous tissue was closed with 3-0 chromic, skin with subcuticular 4-0 Dexon; 0.25% Marcaine

with epinephrine was instilled into all the wounds for postop analgesic. The subcutaneous tissues were all closed with 4-0 Vicryl. Steri-Strips were applied. The patient tolerated the procedure well and was transferred to the recovery room in good condition.

*One or more codes should **not** have been reported for this case. Indicate the code(s) incorrectly reported.*

PROFESSIONAL SERVICES: Laparoscopic ligation, **55550-52**; Bilateral inguinal varicocele ligation, **55530-50**

ICD-10-CM DX: Varicocele, **I86.1**; Laparoscopic procedure converted to open, **Z53.31**

INCORRECTLY REPORTED CODE(S): _____

Audit Report 10.3 Operative Report, Lithotripsy

LOCATION: Inpatient, Hospital

PATIENT: Harvey Samuelson

SURGEON: Ira Avila, MD

PREOPERATIVE DIAGNOSIS: Right ureteral and renal calculi.

POSTOPERATIVE DIAGNOSIS: Same.

PROCEDURES PERFORMED: Right rigid and flexible ureteroscopy, laser lithotripsy, stone extraction, stent insertion under fluoroscopic control with retrograde pyelography.

CLINICAL NOTE: This 55-year-old gentleman had a staghorn calculus of his right kidney. He has had multiple treatments. He continues to have stones adjacent to a stent in the lower ureter, as well as a few small fragments remaining in the kidney.

PROCEDURE NOTE: The patient was given a general laryngeal mask anesthetic, prepped and draped in the lithotomy position. A #21 French cystoscope was passed into the bladder under direct vision. The stent was visualized, grasped and removed to the urethral meatus. A guidewire was advanced up the stent and the stent completely removed. The #7 French rigid ureteroscope was then utilized. The stones in the distal ureter were targeted and engaged with the holmium

laser and a 20-micrometer fiber with a maximum energy of 5 watts. The stones were fragmented and then using a basket were withdrawn. A second guidewire was passed up the ureter under fluoroscopic control and a flexible ureteroscope then advanced up into the kidney. Using the holmium laser the stones in the lower and middle calix were targeted and fragmented. Large fragments were trapped in the basket and withdrawn to the distal ureter where they were further fragmented using the holmium laser and the fragments extracted. The fragments remaining in the kidney were no bigger than 1 to 2 mm.

A 6 French 26 cm stent was then placed under fluoroscopic control in the usual fashion. The bladder was drained, stones retrieved. A B&O suppository was placed rectally. The patient tolerated the procedure well and was transferred to the recovery room in good condition.

One or more codes should not have been reported for this case. Indicate the code(s) incorrectly reported.

PROFESSIONAL SERVICES: Cystourethroscopy lithotripsy, **52353-RT**; Cystourethroscopy with insertion of indwelling ureteral stent, **52332-51-RT**; Urinary tract x-ray, **74400-26**

ICD-10-CM DX: Calculus of the kidney and ureter, **N20.2**

INCORRECTLY REPORTED CODE: _____

Audit Report 10.4 Operative Report, ESWL

LOCATION: Outpatient, Hospital

PATIENT: Allen Athens

SURGEON: Ira Avila, MD

PREOPERATIVE DIAGNOSIS: Right renal calculus with stent

POSTOPERATIVE DIAGNOSIS: Right renal calculus with stent

PROCEDURE PERFORMED: Right ESWL, cystoscopy, stent removal

CLINICAL NOTE: This gentleman has had a large stone burden bilaterally; he is now here for his third and hopefully, final ESWL treatment to these stones. He has no further stones left in the left kidney. He has one residual stone in the right with the stent in situ.

PROCEDURE NOTE: The patient was placed on the lithotripsy table and administered a general anesthetic. The stone was targeted, shock head engaged. Total of 2400 shocks at maximum kV of 24 were administered to the stone. Good fragmentation was noted. The patient was then

CHAPTER 10—cont'd

prepped and draped in the supine position. The urethra was anesthetized with 2% Xylocaine jelly. The patient was cystoscoped with the flexible instrument; stent was visualized, grasped, and removed intact. He tolerated the procedure well and was transferred to the recovery room in good condition. He will be seen in six weeks' time for follow-up KUB and to make arrangements for metabolic workup.

One or more of the following codes are reported incorrectly for this case. Indicate the incorrect code or codes.

SERVICE CODE(S):   Cystourethroscopy with lithotripsy, **52353**

ICD-10-CM DX CODE(S):   Kidney stone, **N20.0**

INCORRECT/MISSING CODE(S):   _____

Audit Report 10.5 Operative Report, Urethropexy

LOCATION: Outpatient, Hospital

PATIENT: Irene Ash

SURGEON: Ira Avila, MD

PREOPERATIVE DIAGNOSIS: Incontinence

POSTOPERATIVE DIAGNOSIS: Incontinence

PROCEDURE PERFORMED: Urethropexy

CLINICAL NOTE: The patient is a 60-year-old woman who has been suffering from stress incontinence for quite some time now. She has made the decision to proceed with surgery to correct this situation.

PROCEDURE: The patient was brought to the operating room and placed on the operating table in the supine position and prepped and draped. A small horizontal incision is made in the abdomen just above the symphysis pubis. The bladder was then suspended by placing sutures bilaterally at the mid-portion of the urethra 1 cm lateral and at the bladder neck 2 cm lateral. The sutures were then suspended to the Cooper's ligament bilaterally. The urethra was then elevated to the horizontal position. One finger could be passed between the urethra and the symphysis anteriorly. Hemostasis was achieved, and the incision was then closed in layers. The patient was turned over to the recovery area in stable condition.

One or more of the following codes are reported incorrectly for this case. Indicate the incorrect code or codes.

SERVICE CODE(S):   Anterior urethropexy or vesicourethropexy, **51841**

ICD-10-CM DX CODE(S):   Urinary incontinence, **R32**

INCORRECT/MISSING CODE(S):   _____

Audit Report 10.6 Operative Report, Cystoscopy

LOCATION: Outpatient, Hospital

PATIENT: Eileen Lab

SURGEON: Ira Avila, MD

PREOPERATIVE DIAGNOSIS: Left ureteral calculus

POSTOPERATIVE DIAGNOSIS: Left ureteral calculus

PROCEDURE PERFORMED: Cystoscopy, bilateral retrograde pyelograms, left ureteroscopy, stone extraction.

PROCEDURE: The patient was given a general laryngeal mask anesthetic, prepped, and draped in the lithotomy position. The patient was cystoscoped using a 21-French instrument. There was no evidence of urethral or bladder abnormality. Bilateral retrograde pyelograms were performed that showed normal collecting system of the right-hand side. There was only a minimal suggestion of a filling defect in the distal ureter on the left. There was minimal dilation of the left collecting system, and clear urine could be seen effluxing from both orifices. Because her symptoms were so classic for a stone, I decided to ureteroscope the patient anyway. A stiff Terumo guidewire was advanced up the ureter under fluoroscopic control and then followed this with a 7-French rigid short ureteroscope without prior ureteral dilation. Just at the level of Waldeyer's fascia, a stone was visualized. This was entrapped in a helical basket and withdrawn under visual guidance. Repeat ureteral inspection showed no evidence of abrasion or edema; therefore, it was decided not to stent the patient. The bladder was drained and cystoscope withdrawn. B&O suppository was placed rectally. She tolerated the procedure well and was transferred to the recovery room in good condition. She will be discharged later today. Follow-up will be arranged for ultrasound in 3 months' time.

One or more of the following codes are reported incorrectly for this case. Indicate the incorrect code or codes.

SERVICE CODE(S):   Cystourethroscopy with FB removal, **52310**; Cysto-urethroscopy, **52000-51**

ICD-10-CM DX CODE(S):   Kidney stone, **N20.0**

INCORRECT/MISSING CODE(S):   _____

(Auditing Review answers with rationales are only available in the TEACH Instructor Resources on Evolve.)

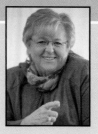

Female Genital System and Maternity Care/Delivery

http://evolve.elsevier.com/Buck/next

(Answers to every other Case are located in Appendix D, with the full answer key only available in the TEACH Instructor Resources on Evolve)
(Auditing Review answers with rationales are only available in the TEACH Instructor Resources on Evolve)

Female Genital System

Female genital disorders are treated by all types of physicians, such as family medicine, internal medicine, and other types of primary care physicians. A **gynecologist** specializes in female genital diagnoses and treatment. Often, the gynecologist is an obstetric and gynecology specialist (OB/GYN), and patients are referred to the specialist for more complex diagnosis, treatment, and/or delivery. For example, an established patient presents to her primary care physician with complaints of spotting between menstrual cycles. The physician examines the patient, obtains a Pap smear, and based on abnormal test results refers the patient to a gynecologist with a request for a cervical biopsy.

Common reproductive presenting complaints are dysmenorrhea (painful menstruation), abnormal vaginal bleeding, abnormal Pap smears, nipple discharge, vaginal discharge, and pelvic pain. Conditions often treated are fibrocystic breast disease, female genital system cancer, vaginitis, cervicitis, sexually transmitted diseases, endometriosis, menopause, premenstrual syndrome, infertility, and pregnancy. Frequently performed office procedures include Pap smear, **colposcopy,** and cervical biopsy, as well as implantation of contraceptives such as an intrauterine device, Norplant, and diaphragms.

Evaluation and Management

OB/GYN physicians provide the same types of E/M services as other physicians, such as office visits, hospital services, and consultations, and these services are reported with E/M codes.

Pains and Other Female Genital Organ Symptoms Pains and other symptoms associated with the female genital organs **(N94)** include dyspareunia (difficult or painful sexual intercourse, N94.1-), vaginismus (painful vaginal spasms due to involuntary contractions, N94.2), mittelschmerz (painful ovulation, N94.0), dysmenorrhea (painful menstruation, N94.4), premenstrual tension syndrome (premenstrual syndrome [PMS], N94.3), pelvic congestion syndrome (chronic pelvic pain, N94.89), stress incontinence (urine leakage on stress, such as coughing or sneezing, N39.3), other specified symptoms associated with the female genital organs (N94.89) (symptoms such as perineal swelling, palpable uterus, etc.), and unspecified symptoms (N94.9) (such as generalized pain).

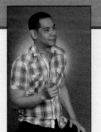

From the Trenches

"Now is the best time to begin a career in medical coding because of all the dynamic changes that are happening within the industry. If you join now, you will have a good chance at participating in the development of health information management for years to come."

PETER EDU
MD, CPC, CCS, CHDA, CDEO, CPC-I
AHIMA - APPROVED ICD-10 CM/PCS TRAINER
AHIMA - ICD-10 AMBASSADOR

CASE 11-1   *Emergency Department Services*

Dr. Sutton provided an emergency department service for Rachel Grey.

LOCATION: Outpatient, Hospital

PATIENT: Rachel Grey

PHYSICIAN: Paul Sutton, MD

SUBJECTIVE: The patient is a 26-year-old female with complaint of low abdominal pain. In reality, she points to the right adnexal region. She states that she had excruciating pain earlier today that caused her to bend over in discomfort. She states that the pain was bad; it was like spasm. She was unable to straighten up. At the time, she felt like there was a bump at the site, and the pain at this time went away after she took ibuprofen. She denies any pain at this time. With further questioning she denies any vaginal discharge or itching. No dysuria. She does state that in August she quit taking contraceptive pills because she would not quit smoking; so this was discontinued. She had her period September 15. With further questioning she does admit to having a similar pain almost 4 weeks ago at the same site. She denies any fever or chills.

OBJECTIVE: On examination, this is a pleasant female in no acute distress. She is afebrile (98.5). Vital signs are stable. HEENT (head, ears, eyes, nose, throat) is unremarkable. Lungs are clear. Cardiovascular is regular. Abdomen is soft. Normotensive bowel sounds. No organomegaly. On palpation over the right adnexal region, there is mild tenderness. No palpable masses. No suprapubic tenderness. No costovertebral angle.

Pregnancy test declined. Urinalysis unremarkable.

ASSESSMENT: Right adnexal pain, rule out mittelschmerz.

PLAN: Reassurance is given. After talking to the patient regarding ovulatory pain, she does feel that this possibly may be the etiology. She feels comfortable right now without any pain whatsoever. Instructions for her to take ibuprofen 600 to 800 mg (milligram) every 8 hours as needed should the pain return. If it is ovulatory pain, this may dissipate when her menstrual cycle kicks in off the contraceptive pill. If she continues to have problems, she is to follow-up with her primary care physician. Patient is agreeable to this.

SERVICE CODE(S): _____

ICD-10-CM DX CODE(S): _____

(Answers to every other Case are located in Appendix D . The full answer key is only available in the TEACH Instructor Resources on Evolve.)

Surgical Procedures

The gynecologist may prefer to perform the required surgical procedures himself or herself, whereas other gynecologists diagnose and treat patients but prefer to have a general surgeon perform surgical procedures, such as a hysterectomy. Because the reproductive system is so closely related to the urinary system, urologists also work closely with gynecologists. For example, an older female patient with prolapsing uterus may have a bladder displacement. A gynecologist would repair the prolapsing uterus, and the urologist would return the bladder to the original position.

A **hysterectomy** is the surgical removal of the uterus. The CPT hysterectomy codes are divided based on the approach (abdominal or vaginal) and the secondary procedures that are performed at the same time, such as surgical removal of the ovaries or fallopian tubes. For the **abdominal approach** hysterectomy, the abdomen is incised and opened to the view of the surgeon. For a **vaginal approach** hysterectomy, the surgeon makes an incision in the vagina around the cervix and removes the uterus and/or ovaries/fallopian tubes (salpingo-oophorectomy) through the incision. The cuff of the vagina is then closed with sutures. **Laparoscopic approach** is the insertion of a scope through the abdomen, and the surgical procedure is completed by means of surgical instrumentation manipulated through ports. A **hysteroscope** can also be used in conjunction with a laparoscope, as illustrated in **Figure 11-1**.

Menopausal and Postmenopausal Disorders

Menopausal and postmenopausal disorders (N95) include premenopausal menorrhagia (excessive bleeding associated

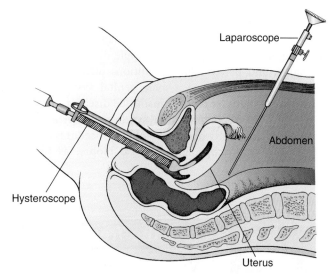

FIGURE 11–1 Hysteroscopy/laparoscopy.

with onset of menopause, N92.4), postmenopausal bleeding (menstrual bleeding after menopause, N95.0), symptomatic or female climacteric state (irregular ovarian and estrogen level fluctuation, N95.10), postmenopausal atrophic vaginitis (decreased levels of estrogen resulting in inflammation of the vagina, N95.2), symptoms associated with artificial menopause (result of drug-induced or surgical menopause, N95.8), other specified menopausal or postmenopausal disorders (N95.8), and unspecified menopausal or postmenopausal disorders (N95.9).

CASE 11-2A   *Consultation, Postmenopausal Bleeding*

Dr. Green's patient, Gladys Hardy, is seen in consultation by Dr. Martinez for postmenopausal bleeding.

LOCATION: Outpatient, Clinic

PATIENT: Gladys Hardy

ATTENDING PHYSICIAN: Ronald Green, MD

CONSULTANT: Andy Martinez, MD

This is a 62-year-old white female gravida 2, para (to bring forth) 2, 0, 0, 2, who is postmenopausal and is referred by Dr. Green to render an opinion regarding postmenopausal bleeding. Papanicolaou smear last year in July. Mammograms unknown.

REASON FOR THE VISIT: The patient has a chief complaint of postmenopausal bleeding.

Evaluation by Dr. Green, including pelvic ultrasound, demonstrates the uterus to be enlarged for age with multiple calcifications suggesting residuals of prior fibroid and thickened endometrium with what appears to be a 3.2 × 3.3 × 2.3-cm (centimeter) solid mass endometrium with some surrounding fluid.

Differential diagnoses are endometrial polyp, localized hyperplasia, and even malignancy. Endometrial sampling for further evaluation is highly recommended.

The right ovary is normal in size and texture. The left ovary is not well visualized, probably due to atrophy.

MEDICATIONS: Multivitamins and calcium

MEDICAL PROBLEMS:

Illnesses: None

Injuries: None

Surgeries: None

ALLERGIES: No known drug allergies

TOBACCO: None. ALCOHOL: None.

SOCIAL HISTORY: The patient is a retired bookkeeper.

The above was discussed with the patient.

FAMILY HISTORY: Positive for colon cancer, breast cancer, and heart disease. Negative for hypertension, cholesterol, diabetes, osteoporosis, and ovarian cancer.

REVIEW OF SYSTEMS: The patient is positive for eyeglasses, arthritis of the left shoulder, the above genitourinary symptoms, pelvic relaxation, stress urinary incontinence, and postmenopausal bleeding.

GYNECOLOGY EXAMINATION: Blood pressure is 110/68. Height $63^1/_2$ inches. Weight is 138 pounds. Neck: Supple.

Nonpalpable thyroid. Breasts: Negative for masses, discharge, or tenderness. Breasts are symmetrical. Pelvic: Adult female genitalia, marital vagina, cervix multiparous, and uterus 6 weeks. Midline adnexa negative. Rectal: Deferred. Musculoskeletal, within normal limits.

IMPRESSION: Postmenopausal bleeding with abnormal pelvic ultrasound and symptomatic pelvic relaxation.

PLAN: Hysteroscopy with fractional D&C (dilation and curettage). Subsequent to the D&C, the patient will probably require a total abdominal hysterectomy with bilateral salpingo-oophorectomy and Burch urethrovesical neck suspension in conjunction with Dr. Sanchez (surgery) with possible staging for malignancy. The risks, benefits, indications, and alternatives to surgery have been discussed with the patient and her daughter. The patient gives informed consent and elects to proceed with surgery. The patient is scheduled for surgery 3 days from now. Dr. Green's preoperative history and physical are reviewed, and he feels she is "okay" for anesthesia and procedure as planned. The patient does have advanced directives.

Written report was sent to Dr. Green by Dr. Martinez stating that, in his opinion, the patient will need hysteroscopy with a fractional D&C and possibly a total abdominal hysterectomy.

SERVICE CODE(S): _____

ICD-10-CM DX CODE(S): _____

(Answers to every other Case are located in Appendix D . The full answer key is only available in the TEACH Instructor Resources on Evolve.)

Colposcopy

A **colposcope** is illustrated in **Figure 11-2** and is used to examine the vagina and cervix as illustrated in **Figure 11-3**. A colposcopy is an examination and/or biopsy of the vaginal and cervical areas and is most often an office procedure.

A **hysteroscope** is a scope that is inserted through the vagina and cervix and into the uterus. A hysteroscopy is a procedure performed in an operating room because of the danger for possible uterine perforation and/or hemorrhage.

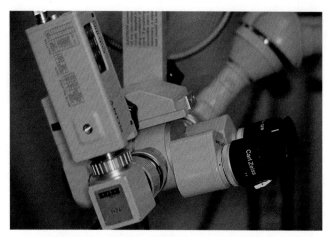

FIGURE 11–2 Office colposcope with beam splitter.

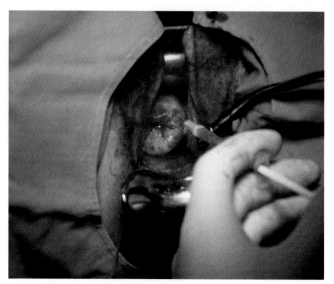

FIGURE 11–3 Colposcopy.

CASE 11-2B   *Operative Report, Hysteroscopy*

Dr. Martinez schedules a hysteroscopy for Gladys, which becomes a hysterectomy. During the hysterectomy procedure, it is found that Gladys has extensive gallbladder calcification. Dr. Sanchez is called into the operating room to assess the gallbladder, and he recommends that the gallbladder be removed during this operative session (Operative Report 11-2C). Before surgery, the patient had signed a consent form to proceed with the cholecystectomy if it were warranted. Report the services of Dr. Martinez for the following:

LOCATION: Inpatient, Hospital

PATIENT: Gladys Hardy

ATTENDING PHYSICIAN: Ronald Green, MD

SURGEON: Andy Martinez, MD

PREOPERATIVE DIAGNOSIS: Postmenopausal bleeding with abnormal pelvic ultrasound

POSTOPERATIVE DIAGNOSIS: Grade 1, stage I endometrial cancer and porcelain gallbladder

PROCEDURE PERFORMED: Hysteroscopy with fractional dilation and curettage by Dr. Martinez. Exploratory laparotomy with lysis by Dr. Sanchez. Total hysterectomy and bilateral salpingo-oophorectomy by Dr. Martinez. Cholecystectomy by Dr. Sanchez.

ANESTHESIA: General laryngeal mask

ESTIMATED BLOOD LOSS: 350 cc

URINE OUTPUT: 220 cc

FLUIDS: 2700 cc

COMPLICATIONS: Perforation of uterus at time of hysteroscopy and D&C (dilation and curettage)

PROCEDURE: The patient was prepped and draped in a lithotomy position under general laryngeal mask anesthesia. The weighted speculum was placed in the vagina. The anterior lip of the cervix was grasped with a single-tooth tenaculum. The Kevorkian curet was then used to obtain endocervical curettings. There was thick brown mucous material present. The uterus then sounded to a depth of 8 cm (centimeter). The cervical os (opening) was then serially dilated to allow passage of a hysteroscope. The hysteroscope was then passed into the uterine cavity. With poor visualization of the uterine contents, it became apparent that there was a perforation (report accidental puncture during surgery based on this comment) in the posterior uterine cavity. The instruments were removed from the vagina. The patient was then placed in a supine position, and a Foley catheter was placed. The abdomen was prepped and draped. A vertical incision was made in the lower abdomen (this is where the procedure converted to a TAH [total abdominal hysterectomy]). The fascia was divided in the midline. The peritoneum was entered and the incision was extended vertically. Palpation of the abdominal cavity revealed an abnormally hard, fixed lesion in the right upper quadrant by the liver that was suspicious for metastatic malignancy. The incision was extended. The bowel was packed out of the operative field using a self-retaining retractor and laparotomy sponges. An adhesiolysis was required to mobilize the sigmoid off the posterior uterine wall. The uterus was grasped and elevated. The round ligaments were cross-clamped, divided, and ligated with 0 Vicryl suture ligature. The bladder flap was created using sharp and blunt dissection and reflected inferiorly. The ureters were attempted to be visualized bilaterally. The right ovary was adherent to the pelvic sidewall, and then the utero-ovarian ligament was clamped, divided, and ligated with 0 Vicryl suture ligature. The left infundibulopelvic ligament was doubly clamped, divided, and ligated with 0 Vicryl free tie and 0 Vicryl suture ligatures. The uterine vessels were skeletonized. The bladder was advanced from the operative field. The broad ligaments were stepwise fashioned down to the uterosacral-cardinal ligament complex using 0 Vicryl suture. The vaginal cuff was reapproximated using 0 Vicryl figure-of-eight sutures times three. The operative was inspected and was hemostatic. The right adnexa was then grasped, and

CASE 11-2B—cont'd

adhesiolysis was performed to allow mobilization of the left adnexa. The infundibulopelvic ligament was then doubly clamped, divided, and ligated and then surgically excised from the pelvic sidewall. Operative sites were inspected and were hemostatic. The pelvis and abdomen were liberally irrigated. See Dr. Sanchez's dictation for cholecystectomy. At completion of this procedure, hemostasis was observed in the operative site. The omentum was brought down anteriorly. The fascia and peritoneum were closed with 0 Vicryl internal interrupted retention sutures and 0 PDS continuous suture. The incision was irrigated. The skin was closed with staples. All sponges and needles were accounted for at completion of the

procedure. The patient left the operating room in apparent good condition having tolerated the procedure well. The Foley catheter was patent and draining clear yellow urine at completion of the procedure.

Pathology Report Later Indicated: Grade I, endometrial cancer with minimal myometrial invasion. Focal areas of FIGO (International Federated Gynecological Oncology) grades 2 and 3 with focal invasion limited to the inner third of the myometrium.

SERVICE CODE(S): _____

ICD-10-CM DX CODE(S): _____

(Answers to every other Case are located in Appendix D . The full answer key is only available in the TEACH Instructor Resources on Evolve.)

CASE 11-2C *Operative Report, Cholecystectomy*

Dr. Sanchez removes the diseased gallbladder of this patient during the same operative session as the hysterectomy performed by Dr. Martinez. Report the services of Dr. Sanchez in the following:

LOCATION: Inpatient, Hospital

PATIENT: Gladys Hardy

ATTENDING PHYSICIAN: Ronald Green, MD

SURGEON: Gary Sanchez, MD

PREOPERATIVE DIAGNOSIS: Porcelain gallbladder

POSTOPERATIVE DIAGNOSIS: Porcelain gallbladder

PROCEDURE PERFORMED: Open cholecystectomy

INDICATION: This is a 62-year-old female on whom Dr. Martinez had performed a hysterectomy. This was done in regard to endometrial cancer. Please see his operative note for specific details. Briefly, it had been a D&C (dilation and curettage) and hysteroscopy, but a perforation of the uterus had occurred. He then converted to an open procedure for the hysterectomy. During this time, on exploration of the abdomen, it was noted that she had a contracted, rock-hard porcelain gallbladder present. I was called in for evaluation of this. Please see my intraoperative consult dictation regarding this. I recommended removal of her porcelain gallbladder because of the potential malignancy being present.

PROCEDURE: The abdomen had already been opened through a vertical midline incision. This went from a little way above the umbilicus down to the pubic symphysis. To get adequate exposure of the gallbladder and liver, we had to extend the incision superiorly some. Then, with the use of a Balfour retractor and the upper arm, we were able to get good exposure. Laps were packed on top of the liver to bring it down. We were able to dissect out the neck of the gallbladder, the cystic duct, and the cystic artery. The cystic artery was ligated with 4-0 silks. It was then transected. We then dissected all the way around the cystic duct. We then took down the gallbladder out of the gallbladder fossa using cautery. We clamped the cystic duct just above the common duct. We identified the junction. It was transected and handed off the table as specimen. We doubly ligated the cystic duct stump then with 3-0 Vicryl. Hemostasis was achieved. Dr. Martinez then came back in to finish the closure of the wound. Again, this is an abbreviated dictation.

I met with the patient's family member postoperatively and did discuss the removal of her gallbladder and the reason for the decision regarding this. Her questions were answered. She understood and was glad that the gallbladder was removed at this time.

Pathology Report Later Indicated: Extensive calcification of gallbladder, benign

SERVICE CODE(S): _____

ICD-10-CM DX CODE(S): _____

(Answers to every other Case are located in Appendix D . The full answer key is only available in the TEACH Instructor Resources on Evolve.)

CASE 11-2D *Oncology Consultation*

Dr. Green requests that Dr. White, oncologist, provide his opinion about the patient's uterine cancer.

LOCATION: Inpatient, Hospital

PATIENT: Gladys Hardy

ATTENDING PHYSICIAN: Ronald Green, MD

CONSULTANT: Rapheal White, MD, Oncology

REASON FOR CONSULTATION: Endometrial uterine carcinoma

HISTORY OF PRESENT ILLNESS: The patient is a 62-year-old white woman who had been seen at the beginning of May by Dr. Martinez for vaginal

bleeding. Evaluation included D&C (dilation and curettage). She has had perforation of the uterus. Surgery of total abdominal hysterectomy had been performed for tumor of the uterus. Porcelain gallbladder had been found and this had been also removed. Postoperatively, she has recovered relatively promptly, started feeding, and has had bowel movements. She required fluid support and because of this she probably has developed tachycardia in the range of 175 with blood pressure dropped from 160 systolic to 120. She had been treated with digoxin and diltiazem and had been transferred to the surgical ICU (intensive care unit) and started on esmolol. Electrolytes also had been replaced. At this point, she gives no specific complaints. She feels somewhat depressed and scared by the whole situation.

Continued

CASE 11-2D—cont'd

PAST MEDICAL HISTORY: Past medical history has been insignificant. She has had no illnesses, injuries, or surgeries.

Her only medications have been multivitamins and calcium.

SOCIAL HISTORY: She is a retired bookkeeper. Lives together with her husband in Manytown. There is no history of tobacco abuse or alcohol abuse.

She has no known allergies.

FAMILY HISTORY: Notable above for colon cancer and breast cancer. There is also heart disease in the family. No significant history of dyslipidemia, diabetes, osteoporosis, or history of ovarian cancer.

REVIEW OF SYSTEMS: Except for the events in the hospital associated with tachyarrhythmia, she has had no chest pain, cough, shortness of breath, nausea, or vomiting. Constitutional: There is no history of any significant weight loss. Appetite has been good. There is no history of fevers. HEENT (head, ears, eyes, nose, throat): She uses glasses. No significant change in vision. No blurred or double vision. No change in hearing or swallowing problems. No new headaches. No new neck stiffness. She has arthritis of the left shoulder that has been present for a long time. Respiratory: She has had no history of exposure to tuberculosis. No pneumonia. No chronic history of any shortness of breath, cough, or expectoration. No hemoptysis. Cardiovascular: No significant prior history. No palpitations or chest pain. Gastrointestinal: No history of abdominal pain. No history of gastroesophageal reflux, regurgitation, peptic ulcer disease, or recent change significant of bowel habits. No melena or hematochezia. No mucus in the stool. Genitourinary: She has had complaints of stress urinary incontinence. Gynecologic: There is postmenopausal bleeding for which she had surgery. She is para (to bring forth) 2. She has had uncomplicated deliveries. She has a son and daughter who are living close by and essentially healthy. She has not been on hormonal replacement treatment. Musculoskeletal: She has complaints consistent with osteoarthritis, pain mainly in the left shoulder that had been present for a long time. Neurologic: No history of stroke, seizures, loss of consciousness, paresis, tingling, or numbness. Hematologic: No history of easy bruising or bleeding prior to the postmenopausal bleeding. No history of blood transfusions. Lymphatic: No history of lymph node enlargement. Endocrine: No history of polydipsia. No cold or heat intolerance. Immunologic: No history of hives or recurrent frequent infections. Psychiatric: No history of major depression or psychosis.

PHYSICAL EXAMINATION: She is alert and oriented times three; was in apparent distress while in the ICU. Blood pressure at present in the range of 122-150/70-80. Pulse is in the range of 79; it reaches 120-130 at times. Respiratory rate is 16. She is afebrile. Normocephalic and atraumatic. Eyes: PERRLA (pupils equal, round, reactive to light and accommodation). No jaundice. No extraocular muscle movement. No sinus tenderness. Clear oral and nasal mucosa. Tongue and uvula midline. No pharyngeal exudates, erythema, or thrush. The ear canals are clear. The neck is supple. No JVD (jugular vein distention). Trachea midline. Nonpalpable thyroid. No palpable cervical, supraclavicular, axillary, or inguinal lymph nodes. Lungs are clear to auscultation and percussion bilaterally. Heart: S1 (first heart sound) and S2 (second heart sound). No gallop or rub. No significant murmur. Breast exam: No palpable mass or nipple discharge. The abdomen is soft and nondistended. Bowel sounds are present, hypoactive. Difficult to examine, she has had recent surgery but no palpable masses or organomegaly. Extremities: There is no cyanosis, clubbing, or edema. Pulses are present. Neurologic: There are no focal motor, sensory, or cranial nerves II-XII deficits. Muscle tone and reflexes are grossly within normal range. She shows appropriate insight and judgment. Mood is somewhat depressed. Affect is grossly normal.

Her ECG (electrocardiogram) and monitor slips have shown episodes of V-tach (ventricular tachycardia), episodes of atrial fibrillation, and some slowed PR (pulse rate) intervals. Dr. Martinez has considered WPW (Wolff-Parkinson-White syndrome).

LABORATORY DATA: White blood cell 15.27, hemoglobin 12.4, hematocrit 35.2, platelets 186, and normal red cell indices. Differential: Increased neutrophils 88.6%, decreased lymphocytes 5.7%, monocytes 5%, eosinophils 0.6, and basophils 0.1%. Basic metabolic panel: potassium 3.5, glucose 123, and calcium 7.4. The rest is within normal range. PT/INR (prothrombin time/International Normalized Ratio) today has been 13 and 1.2. Magnesium was normal at 1.7, and phosphorus decreased to 0.3. Urine culture has been done but is not available yet. LDH (lactate dehydrogenase) was 143. Troponin had been 0.08. The pathology result from the surgery has concluded with endocervical curettings and benign endocervical mucosa; the uterus has shown endometrial adenocarcinoma endometrioid-type, predominantly grade 1 with focal areas of FIGO (International Federated Gynecological Oncology) grades 2 and 3 with focal invasion limited to the inner third of the myometrium. Left ovary, fallopian tube, no pathologic diagnosis. Multiple intramural and subserosal leiomyomata showing the myometrium, benign, right ovary and fallopian tube portion of benign ovary and fallopian tube. The gallbladder has shown extensive calcification.

ASSESSMENT: A 62-year-old patient has had recent surgery at this point and is in critical condition, namely because of cardiac arrhythmias probably related to fluid overload related also to medications. She has been started in the hospital on Peri-Colace, Zoloft, azithromycin, cefotaxime, and Zofran, and Tylenol has been given. In terms of the uterine cancer, the cancer seems to be early stage. As per the available data, the tumor is T1B, N0, M0, the stage is IB endometrioid carcinoma, low grade in most of the tumor. No evidence of any intravascular, perineural spread. These are also associated, most likely, with stress leukocytosis as well as electrolyte abnormalities. The patient at this point is still in critical condition in terms of her cardiac function. She has been monitored. Anticoagulation has been planned considering relatively prolonged hospital stay, and at this point she is bedridden in the ICU. Dr. Green has started replacement of electrolytes and anticoagulation. She has been kept n.p.o. (nothing by mouth) with consideration of possible ileus. Aside from this, her immediate problems, which will be managed by Dr. Green in terms of the uterine cancer, the only disturbing factor is the fact that there was perforation of the uterus during D&C, which may have caused some spilling of tumor cells in the pelvic area. Still this is not a justifiable consideration for any additional adjuvant treatment. The recommendation in her case would be after stabilization of her condition in several weeks to perform CT (computerized tomography) scans to evaluate for any pelvic, periaortic, possible adenopathy, which at her stage of cancer is not very likely. As there was tumor spilling, the risk for recurrence of such an early stage uterine cancer is minimal, and studies would be indicated in less than 10% over 5 years. Considering these facts, no additional treatment would be recommended; yet a cautious approach with obtaining of imaging studies, CT scan of pelvis and abdomen could be considered once she is stable, and if those are negative, further follow-up could be done on a clinical basis. The patient herself is not willing to proceed with any aggressive treatment, which again in her case is not recommended and most likely will not be needed in the future either. She will need regular gynecological follow-up as well as mammograms as per guidelines. I would be glad to follow up with her in 1 to 2 months when she would be able to have the CT scans done. I appreciate the opportunity to see this pleasant lady, who in terms of her uterine cancer would have very likely good prognosis.

SERVICE CODE(S): _____

ICD-10-CM DX CODE(S): _____

CASE 11-2E *Discharge Summary*

LOCATION: Inpatient, Hospital

PATIENT: Gladys Hardy

PRIMARY CARE PHYSICIAN: Ronald Green, MD

ATTENDING PHYSICIAN: Ronald Green, MD

PRINCIPAL DIAGNOSES:

1. Endometrial uterine adenocarcinoma
2. Porcelain gallbladder

POSTOPERATIVE DIAGNOSIS: Wolff-Parkinson-White syndrome

OPERATIVE PROCEDURE: Hysteroscopy with fractional dilatation and curettage converted to a total abdominal hysterectomy with bilateral salpingo-oophorectomy, open cholecystectomy, lysis of adhesions, open biopsy frozen section of ovary and fallopian tube, arterial line insertion, and postoperative fluid overload.

CONSULTANTS: Drs. Martinez, Sanchez, White, and Orbitz.

IDENTIFICATION HISTORY OF PRESENT ILLNESS: The patient had preoperative history and physical by Dr. Green.

PREOPERATIVE GYN NOTE: The patient is a 62-year-old white female, gravida 2, para (to bring forth) 2, who is postmenopausal with postmenopausal bleeding. Pap smear 11/03. Mammogram unknown.

REASON FOR THE VISIT: The patient had a chief complaint of postmenopausal bleeding. Evaluation by Dr. Monson (radiology), including pelvic ultrasound, demonstrates the uterus to be enlarged for age with multiple calcifications suggesting residuals of prior fibroid and thickened endometrium with what appears to be a 3.2 × 3.3 × 2.3-cm (centimeter) solid mass in the endometrium with some surrounding fluid. Differential diagnoses are endometrial polyp, localized hyperplasia, and even malignancy. Endometrial sample for further evaluation is highly recommended. The right ovary is normal size and texture. The left ovary is not well visualized, probably due to atrophy.

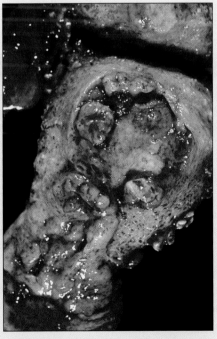

FIGURE 11-4 Endometrial adenocarcinoma.

MEDICATIONS: Multivitamins and calcium

MEDICAL PROBLEMS: None

ILLNESSES: None

INJURIES: None

SURGERY: None

ALLERGIES: No known drug allergies

TOBACCO: None. ALCOHOL: None.

SOCIAL HISTORY: The patient is a retired bookkeeper.

FAMILY HISTORY: Positive for colon cancer, breast cancer, and heart disease.

REVIEW OF SYSTEMS: The patient is positive for eyeglasses, arthritis of left shoulder, the above genitourinary findings, pelvic relaxation, stress urinary incontinence, and postmenopausal bleeding.

EXAMINATION: Blood pressure is 110/68. Height: 63½ inches. Weight: 138 pounds. Neck is supple. Nonpalpable thyroid. Breasts negative for masses, discharge, or tenderness. Breasts are symmetrical. Pelvic: Adult female genitalia, marital clean vagina. Cervix multiparous. Adnexa negative. Rectal: Deferred. BUS (Bartholin's, urethra, and Skene's glands) within NORMAL LIMITS. Some pelvic relaxation is noted.

IMPRESSION: Postmenopausal bleeding with abnormal pelvic ultrasound and symptomatic pelvic relaxation.

HOSPITAL COURSE: During the hysteroscopy and D&C (dilation and curettage), it was noted that there was perforation of the uterus, at which time the procedure was converted to a total abdominal hysterectomy and bilateral salpingo-oophorectomy. During that time there was noted to be a gelatinous mass posterior to the uterus, which was sent to pathology. At the time of frozen-section pathologic evaluation, it was determined that the endocervical curettings were benign endocervical mucosa. Uterus, left fallopian tube, and ovary resection with endometrial adenocarcinoma endometrioid-type: Predominantly grade 1 with focal areas of FIGO (International Federated Gynecological Oncology) grades 2 and 3 with focal invasion limited to the inner third of the myometrium. Left ovary and fallopian tube resection: No pathologic diagnosis. Multiple intramural and subserosal leiomyomata showing extensive hyalinization with focal calcification. Focal adenomyosis: Myometrium, benign. Right ovary and fallopian tube: Portion of benign ovary and fallopian tube. Gallbladder excision: Extensive calcification of the gallbladder. The cytologic washings returned atypical cells; cannot rule out malignancy.

The hospital course continued with the patient developing problems with fluid overload, at which time Dr. Orbitz (nephrology) was consulted, and he determined that the patient had Wolff-Parkinson-White syndrome, which was aggravated by the stress of surgery. The patient also had frequent episodes of atrial fibrillation and was anticoagulated, and he thought she should remain anticoagulated until she was further evaluated in 4 to 6 weeks. She was discharged on Toprol XL 100 daily, and he thought she should stay on the beta-blocker indefinitely. She should also have a Holter monitor done in 4 to 6 weeks. Then if she is in sustained sinus rhythm at that time, it would be reasonable to remove the anticoagulation. The patient was discharged postoperative day 8 with instructions to return to the clinic in 1 week for incision check and in 4 weeks for postoperative evaluation. A consultation was arranged with oncology, who felt that she would not require additional treatment; yet they recommend a cautious

Continued

CASE 11-2E—cont'd

approach with obtaining imaging studies, CT (computerized tomography) scan of the pelvis and abdomen every 3 months times 1 year. The patient was not willing to proceed with any aggressive treatment at the time of discharge.

DISCHARGE MEDICATIONS:

1. Metoprolol 50 mg (milligram) q.12h.
2. Coumadin 1 tablet q.d. (every day) at 1 PM
3. Tylenol p.r.n. (as needed)

This narrative discharge summary is being sent to Dr. White to render an opinion regarding recommendations about further treatment for this cancer relative to perforation of the uterus at time of D&C hysteroscopy (tumor cells spilled into abdomen). We will also send copies of the cytology and slides for that evaluation. I spent a total of 45 minutes providing this discharge service for this patient.

SERVICE CODE(S): _____

ICD-10-CM DX CODE(S): _____

(Answers to every other Case are located in Appendix D . The full answer key is only available in the TEACH Instructor Resources on Evolve.)

From the Trenches

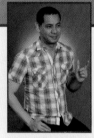

"Openness and adaptability to change and a willingness to learn new skills are keys to success as a coder."

PETER EDU
MD, CPC, CCS, CHDA, CDEO, CPC-I
AHIMA - APPROVED ICD-10 CM/PCS TRAINER
AHIMA - ICD-10 AMBASSADOR

Pelvic Pain

Pelvic pain is a common gynecologic complaint and can have many origins, for example, pregnancy-related pelvic pain, pelvic inflammatory disease (PID), dysmenorrhea (painful menstruation), endometriosis, and pelvic adhesions. The pelvic pain can also indicate a nongynecologic etiology, and so the OB/GYN physician is alert to differential diagnoses from other organ systems. Gastrointestinal-related pelvic pain could indicate appendicitis, irritable bowel syndrome, or inflammatory bowel disease. Urology-related pelvic pain could indicate urinary tract infection or renal stones. Musculoskeletal-related pelvic pain could indicate strain, contusion, fracture, or radiating pain from a herniated disc or arthritic condition of the spine.

CASE 11-3A   *History and Physical Examination*

The patient in this case, Gloria Rhodes, has been experiencing pelvic pain and dysmenorrhea. She is admitted by Dr. Martinez for a hysterectomy.

LOCATION: Inpatient, Hospital

PATIENT: Gloria Rhodes

ATTENDING PHYSICIAN: Andy Martinez, MD

CHIEF COMPLAINT: Pelvic pain and pain with periods

HISTORY: This lady is a 39-year-old married white female, gravida 2, para (to bring forth) 2. Her LMP (last menstrual period) was May 14, and she received an injection of Depo-Provera at 200 mg (milligram) IM (intramuscular) on May 17. The patient has a longstanding history of endometriosis dating back 10 years ago when she had bilateral ovarian cystectomies for endometriosis. She was then treated with danazol for 6 months. She had a laparoscopy with lysis of adhesions 8 years ago, at which time the right ovary was mildly adherent to the pelvic side wall but was broken up somewhat with dissection, and she had some small bowel adherent to the left ovary. She was then treated on multiple cycles of

Klonopin citrate because of luteal-phase deficiency but failed to conceive. She has undergone repeat laparoscopy with exploratory laparotomy and pelvic adhesiolysis having had bowel and pelvic adhesions, and she had resection of several areas of endometriosis. At that point, the patient continued to try to get pregnant but was having more problems with pain, and therefore it was treated with oral contraceptives and nonsteroidal anti-inflammatory drugs. The patient did spontaneously conceive and delivered her second child. She was not having much success in alleviating her symptoms of dysmenorrhea and dyspareunia; therefore, she was begun on continuous oral contraceptives in the form of Demulen 1/50. This did result in the expected amenorrhea, and her symptoms were initially controlled fairly well. She then started having more in the way of cramping and pain; however, dyspareunia had improved. At this point, she is being brought in for definitive surgery because of persistent pelvic pain and cramping.

CURRENT MEDICATIONS: Calcium 1000 mg q.d. (every day)

ALLERGIES: None

REVIEW OF SYSTEMS: She has occasional lower abdominal cramping, but this is improved somewhat since her injection of Depo-Provera on May 17.

CASE 11-3A—cont'd

She has no URI (upper respiratory infection) symptoms or cough. No GI (gastrointestinal) or GU (genitourinary) symptoms. No vaginal discharge. Cardiovascular, negative.

FAMILY HISTORY: Her dad has maturity-onset diabetes, coronary artery disease, and hypertension, but he is living. Paternal grandfather and grandmother had heart problems. Her mom is in good health. She had two maternal aunts with breast cancer, and there are other types of cancer in her mother's siblings, the specifics of which are unknown.

SOCIAL HISTORY: Habits: Occasional alcohol. Very rarely does she smoke a cigarette.

PAST SURGICAL HISTORY:

1. Eight years prior, laparoscopy, exploratory laparotomy with adhesiolysis
2. Ovarian cystectomy and appendectomy
3. Diagnostic laparoscopy

PHYSICAL EXAMINATION: Weight is 148 pounds. Blood pressure is 100/60. HEENT (head, ears, eyes, nose, throat) unremarkable. Neck has no masses. Lungs are clear to auscultation. Heart has a regular rhythm without audible murmurs or gallops. Breasts are negative. Abdomen shows a laparoscopy scar and Pfannenstiel scar. Vulva and vagina are normal. Cervix is parous. Uterus is anterior and normal size. Adnexa reveal tenderness on the left but not on the right. On rectovaginal examination, there is some extreme nodularity on the left side of the cul-de-sac. Extremities show no phlebitis.

LABORATORY STUDIES: Preop laboratory work taken on the date of examination shows the urinalysis to be normal. White count is 5440. Hemoglobin is 13.6 g (gram).

PREOPERATIVE DIAGNOSIS: Endometriosis with chronic dysmenorrhea and pelvic pain.

OPERATIVE PLAN: She is scheduled for a total abdominal hysterectomy and bilateral salpingo-oophorectomy in the morning. The patient will receive a mechanical and antibiotic bowel prep, and she will also have ureteral catheters placed preoperatively by Dr. Avila. The patient understands the potential complications, including infections, bleeding, bowel, bladder, and ureteral injury. Potential complications of blood clot formation and pulmonary emboli are also discussed with the patient. She understands the necessity of the operation, its intended outcome, and risks and agrees to proceed as planned.

A total time of 55 minutes with spent on this patient today.

SERVICE CODE(S): _____

ICD-10-CM DX CODE(S): _____

(Answers to every other Case are located in Appendix D . The full answer key is only available in the TEACH Instructor Resources on Evolve.)

Endometriosis

Endometriosis is a condition for which no clear cause has been identified. Endometrial tissue is expelled from the uterus into the body and can implant onto a variety of organs. Classification is based on the site of implant of the endometrial tissue. Category N80 is used to classify the condition based on the specific site of implantation. For example, N80.10- is endometriosis of the ovary, and N80.50 is endometriosis of the intestine. Often the endometriosis is of several locations, and these multiple locations, if documented, are reported.

CASE 11-3B   *Operative Report, Ureteral Stents*

Report Dr. Avila's services.

LOCATION: Inpatient, Hospital

PATIENT: Gloria Rhodes

ATTENDING PHYSICIAN: Andy Martinez, MD

SURGEON: Ira Avila, MD

PREOPERATIVE DIAGNOSES:

1. Expressed desire of the operating gynecologist to insert indwelling ureteral stents for ease of dissection of the anticipated enlarged adherent uterus
2. Gynecologic diagnosis of uterine endometriosis

POSTOPERATIVE DIAGNOSIS: Same

PROCEDURE PERFORMED: Cystourethroscopy, insertion of bilateral ureteral catheters

TECHNIQUE OF THE PROCEDURE: After general anesthesia, and after the abdomen and genitalia had been prepped and draped in the usual fashion, the patient was placed in the dorsolithotomy position. The genitalia were examined and proved to be essentially unremarkable. The urethra was instrumented with a no. 24-French Panendoscope sheath, and, using the Foroblique and right-angle lenses, inspection of the entire cavity showed no indication of any pathologic lesion. There is slight indention on some of the bladder incident to the uterine impression. The two ureteral orifices appear to be essentially unremarkable. The left ureteral orifice was catheterized with a no. 6-French Whistle Tip catheter with ease. The catheter was advanced to approximately 25 cm (centimeter) on the left side. Attention was then directed to the right side, and the right ureteral orifice was catheterized with a no. 6-French Whistle Tip catheter. The catheter was placed at approximately 24 cm. The bladder was then entered, and the Panendoscope sheath was withdrawn. A no. 18-French 5-ml (milliliter) balloon Foley catheter was then inserted into the bladder and left indwelling to the Foley catheter. The two ureteral catheters were anchored with no. 1 black silk. The two ureteral catheters and the Foley catheters were then connected to straight drainage, and the patient was removed from the dorsolithotomy position. Dr. Martinez, the patient's gynecologist, then proceeded with a total abdominal hysterectomy and bilateral salpingo-oophorectomy.

SERVICE CODE(S): _____

ICD-10-CM DX CODE(S): _____

(Answers to every other Case are located in Appendix D . The full answer key is only available in the TEACH Instructor Resources on Evolve.)

CASE 11-3C *Operative Report, Hysterectomy*

Report the services of Dr. Martinez.

LOCATION: Inpatient, Hospital

PATIENT: Gloria Rhodes

ATTENDING PHYSICIAN: Andy Martinez, MD

SURGEON: Andy Martinez, MD

PREOPERATIVE DIAGNOSIS: Endometriosis with resultant chronic pelvic pain

POSTOPERATIVE DIAGNOSIS: Same with mild pelvic adhesions

PROCEDURES PERFORMED:

1. Total abdominal hysterectomy with bilateral salpingo-oophorectomy
2. Cystoscopy with placement of ureteral catheters (Dr. Avila)

ANESTHESIA: General endotracheal

SURGICAL INDICATIONS: This patient is a 39-year-old, gravida 2, para (to bring forth) 2, who has had multiple operations in the past for endometriosis. She had recently been tried on hormonal suppression for her symptoms of pain, and this initially worked; however, she has had breakthrough bleeding and quite bothersome discomfort. At this point in time, she had elected definitive surgery.

OPERATIVE FINDINGS: The uterus was normal size. There were a lot of anterior cul-de-sac adhesions over the bladder and anterior surface of the uterus. There were some adhesions between the left tube and ovary and the posterior aspect of the left broad ligament. The right adnexa was free of any significant adhesions. Both ovaries were small, but she had been on hormonal suppression for the past several months.

PROCEDURE: After Dr. Avila did a cystoscopy and placed ureteral catheters, the patient was placed in the supine position and the abdominal area was prepped and draped. The abdomen was opened through a Pfannenstiel incision. A Balfour retractor was placed. The adhesions in the anterior cul-de-sac and left adnexa were separated with Metzenbaum scissors. The bowel was packed off out of the pelvis with wet lap sponges. The uterus was elevated with Pean clamps. The left round ligament was clamped, divided, and suture ligated. All sutures heretofore are 1-0 Vicryl unless otherwise indicated. The round ligament was suture ligated and tagged. The peritoneum lateral to the left infundibulopelvic ligament was opened with Metzenbaum scissors, isolating the left ovarian vasculature. This pedicle was then clamped, divided, and doubly tied, first with a free tie and then a stick tie medial to the free tie. The anterior leaf of the left broad ligament was opened with Metzenbaum scissors. These structures were treated identically on the right side. The bladder was dissected free from the lower uterine segment and cervix with blunt and sharp dissection. The uterine artery pedicles were skeletonized on both sides with Metzenbaum scissors. The uterine artery pedicles were clamped with curved Rogers clamps, cut, and suture ligated with fixation sutures of a Heaney type. The cardinal ligaments were taken with straight Heaney-Ballantine clamps, cut, and suture ligated. The vaginal angles were clamped with curved Rogers clamps and incised, and then the apex of the vagina was incised across with right-angle scissors, removing the uterus, which was then handed off. Kocher clamps were placed in the vaginal apex and mucosa for identification. Angle sutures at both right and left angles were placed and then the middle of the vagina closed with several figure-of-eight sutures of 1-0 Vicryl. There was a small bit of oozing on the underside of the bladder, and this was isolated and oversewn with 3-0 Vicryl on a GI (gastrointestinal) needle. A small piece of Hemopad was then placed over the vaginal cuff. The bladder flap was loosely approximated over the vaginal cuff with a mattress suture of 3-0 Vicryl. The pelvis was irrigated with saline. There was no bleeding noted at this time. The sponges were removed and, with sponge and needle counts correct, attention was directed toward closure. The peritoneum was closed with a running 2-0 Vicryl. A medium Hemovac drain was placed subfascially to exit below the right side of the incision. The fascia was then closed with running locked 1-0 Vicryl using two strands, one from either side to the middle. The skin was closed with staples and the drain sutured to the skin with Prolene. Blood loss estimated by anesthesia was 175 ml (milliliter). Specimen to pathology was the uterus with attached tubes and ovaries. Final sponge and needle counts were correct.

Pathology Report Later Indicated: See Report 11-3D.

SERVICE CODE(S): _____

ICD-10-CM DX CODE(S): _____

(Answers to every other Case are located in Appendix D . The full answer key is only available in the TEACH Instructor Resources on Evolve.)

CASE 11-3D *Pathology Report*

LOCATION: Inpatient, Hospital

PATIENT: Gloria Rhodes

ATTENDING PHYSICIAN: Andy Martinez, MD

SURGEONS: Ira Avila, MD, and Andy Martinez, MD

PATHOLOGIST: Grey Lonewolf, MD

CLINICAL HISTORY: Endometriosis

TISSUE RECEIVED: UTO

GROSS DESCRIPTION:

The specimen is labeled with the patient's name and "uterus, tubes, and ovaries" and consists of a 143-g (gram) chordate uterus with attached fallopian tubes and ovaries. The serosal surface is smooth pink-tan. The cervix is white-tan, patent, and transverse. The endometrium is 0.2 cm (centimeter) thick and light tan. The myometrium is 1.8 cm deep and trabeculated pink-tan.

The right ovary is 4.0 × 2.7 × 2.2 cm. Attached is a 6.0-cm segment of fallopian tube, which includes the distal fimbriated end. Cut sections show multiple fluid-filled cysts ranging from 0.3 to 1.0 cm in greatest dimension. An occasional cyst is filled with blood. The ovarian parenchyma is pink-tan. Cut sections of fallopian tube show cylindrical white-tan tissue. Representative sections of right ovary and fallopian tube are submitted in cassettes 8-10.

The left ovary is 3.5 × 3.1 × 1.3 cm. Attached is a 5.2-cm segment of fallopian tube, which includes the distal fimbriated end. Cut sections of ovary show pink-tan parenchyma and two fluid-filled cysts, 0.3 and 1.0 cm in greatest dimension. Representative sections of left ovary and fallopian tube are submitted in cassettes 11-13.

CASE 11-3D—cont'd

Representative sections of the entire specimen are submitted in 13 cassettes.

MICROSCOPIC DESCRIPTION:

Sections of cervix show benign squamous metaplasia overlying cervical glands, some of which are cystically dilated. The cervical stroma contains foci of lymphocyte and plasma cell infiltrates. There is a small focus of microglandular hyperplasia. The endometrium appears relatively thin and inactive and contains small tubular glands lined by a single layer of cuboidal epithelium. Occasional glands are cystically dilated. The surrounding endometrial stroma appears focally edematous but is otherwise unremarkable. The superficial myometrium contains a rare focus of endometrial glands and stroma. The remaining myometrium is histologically unremarkable.

Sections of the right ovary and left ovary contain multiple follicular cysts, some of which are focally hemorrhagic. Other cysts are also present and are lined by a flattened epithelium. The right ovary contains a large hemorrhagic cyst lined by one to three layers of cuboidal epithelium. The wall contains numerous decidualized cells. The remaining ovarian parenchyma contains a spindled stroma with corpora albicantia scattered throughout. Foci of hemosiderin-laden macrophages are present. The serosal surface of the right ovary shows attached fibrous adhesions. The serosal surface of the left and right ovary also contains occasional foci of small endometrial glands and stroma. Some show hemorrhage with hemosiderin-laden macrophages. Cross-sections of left and right fallopian tube are unremarkable.

DIAGNOSIS:

Uterus, bilateral fallopian tubes, and ovaries, excision:

1. Mild chronic cervicitis with squamous metaplasia
2. Benign nonsecretory endometrium
3. Adenomyosis
4. Left and right fallopian tubes: No diagnostic abnormality
5. Left and right ovaries: Endometriosis

SERVICE CODE(S): _____

ICD-10-CM DX CODE(S): _____

(Answers to every other Case are located in Appendix D . The full answer key is only available in the TEACH Instructor Resources on Evolve.)

CASE 11-3E   *Discharge Summary*

LOCATION: Inpatient, Hospital

PATIENT: Gloria Rhodes

ATTENDING PHYSICIAN: Andy Martinez, MD

DISCHARGING SERVICE: Gynecology

HISTORY: This female is a 39-year-old gravida 2, para (to bring forth) 2, who has had multiple surgical treatments as well as medical treatment for endometriosis. Despite treatment with oral contraceptives and nonsteroidal anti-inflammatories, she continued to have pelvic pain and dyspareunia. At this time, she is brought in for definitive surgery because of persistent pelvic pain and cramping.

PAST SURGICAL HISTORY revealed laparoscopy 6 years ago with an exploratory laparotomy and adhesional lysis. Ten years ago, she had an ovarian cystectomy and an appendectomy. Five years ago, she had a diagnostic laparoscopy. Preoperative hemoglobin was 13.6 g (gram).

PERTINENT FINDINGS ON ADMISSION were limited to the pelvis. The vulva and vagina were normal. The cervix was parous. The uterus was anterior and normal in size. Adnexa revealed tenderness on the left side, but not on the right. On rectovaginal exam, there was some extreme nodularity on the left side of the cul-de-sac. This area was quite tender.

HOSPITAL COURSE: On the day of admission, the patient underwent a total abdominal hysterectomy with bilateral salpingo-oophorectomy after placement of ureteral catheters by Dr. Avila. At the time of surgery, she had a lot of adhesions in the anterior cul-de-sac over the bladder and adhesions between the left tube and ovary and the posterior aspect of the left broad ligament. The right adnexum was free of any significant adhesions. Pathology revealed adenomyosis in the uterus and endometriosis on both left and right ovaries. Postoperatively, she had no significant problems. She had a singular temperature elevation at 38.2 on the evening of surgery but after that remained essentially afebrile (*no fever*). Hemoglobin postoperatively on the first day was 12.2 g. She was discharged on the third postoperative day to return to the clinic in 2 weeks for follow-up.

DISCHARGE DIAGNOSES:

1. Endometriosis of uterus and ovaries
2. Chronic pelvic pain secondary to endometriosis
3. Pelvic adhesions secondary to endometriosis
4. Adenomyosis
5. Cervicitis

PRINCIPAL PROCEDURE: Abdominal hysterectomy with bilateral salpingo-oophorectomy

ADDITIONAL PROCEDURE: Cystoscopy with placement of ureteral catheters

SERVICE CODE(S): _____

ICD-10-CM DX CODE(S): _____

(Answers to every other Case are located in Appendix D . The full answer key is only available in the TEACH Instructor Resources on Evolve.)

Dysfunctional Uterine Bleeding

Dysfunctional uterine bleeding (DUB) is irregular bleeding not caused by an organic condition. In the normal cycle, the endometrial lining builds up during the proliferation phase due primarily to estrogen until ovulation. The secretory phase of the cycle follows with sloughing of the endometrial lining. With a dysfunctional cycle, the estrogen can continue to stimulate the buildup of the endometrial lining, causing an abnormal thickening that can lead to intermittent sloughing of the endometrial lining or DUB. Polycystic ovarian disease (PCOD or Stein-Leventhal syndrome) is a condition that can lead to DUB. This dysfunctional bleeding can also be caused by low levels of estrogen in relationship to the progesterone, for example, with low-estrogen oral contraceptive pills (OCP). The dysfunction can be irregular and/or unpredictable and/or heavy bleeding.

The constant stimulation of the endometrium with estrogen can lead to hypertrophy of the endometrium and then to endometrial cancer. A hysterectomy is the treatment of last resort for chronic DUB. The dysfunctional bleeding may also be caused by polyps, ovulation, fibroids, cancer, cervicitis, PID (pelvic inflammatory disease), or certain bleeding conditions.

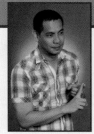

From the Trenches

"The most rewarding part about being a medical coder is knowing that you have indirectly touched a patient's life without them even knowing it."

PETER EDU

MD, CPC, CCS, CHDA, CDEO, CPC-I

AHIMA - APPROVED ICD-10 CM/PCS TRAINER

AHIMA - ICD-10 AMBASSADOR

CASE 11-4A   *Operative Report, Hysterectomy*

LOCATION: Inpatient, Hospital

PATIENT: Charlotte Sweet

ATTENDING PHYSICIAN: Andy Martinez, MD

SURGEON: Andy Martinez, MD

PREOPERATIVE DIAGNOSIS: Dysfunctional uterine bleeding

POSTOPERATIVE DIAGNOSIS: Dysfunctional uterine bleeding

PROCEDURE PERFORMED: Subtotal abdominal hysterectomy

PREAMBLE: The patient is a 32-year-old gravida 4, para (to bring forth) 3, SA 1 who presented with a history of irregular menstrual bleeding. The patient had tried oral contraceptive pills to see if this would cause any improvement in her menses, but no improvement was noted. Trial of Provera also failed to cause any improvement in the cycles. The patient stated that she was done with her childbearing, and she requested definitive therapy in the form of abdominal hysterectomy. The ovaries were to be conserved given the patient's age. The patient did have prior surgeries, including repair of a bicornuate uterus, as well as two cesarean sections in the past.

PROCEDURE NOTE: The patient was taken to the operating room, and spinal anesthetic was administered. The patient was then prepped and draped in the usual manner in supine position. A Foley catheter was inserted.

A Pfannenstiel incision was made through the pre-existing scar. There was lots of scarring of the fascia, and this was taken down sharply. The peritoneal cavity was then entered without incident. Upon inspection of the pelvis, the bladder was noted to be quite firmly adherent to the uterus anteriorly. Bicornuate shape of the uterus was noted. Both fallopian tubes and ovaries appeared normal to inspection.

The uterus was grasped, and round ligaments were identified bilaterally. These were then suture ligated using 0 Vicryl. The anterior release of the broad ligament was then sharply entered to create the bladder flap. This was quite adherent mostly on the left-hand side. Bladder was then taken down away from the front of the cervix using sharp dissection. Again, the bladder was found to be quite densely adherent to the cervix, particularly on the left-hand side. Bleeding was encountered while trying to take the bladder down. At this point then, attention was directed toward the adnexa. Blunt finger dissection was used to create a hole in the broad ligaments to allow for placement of Heaney clamps bilaterally across the fallopian tubes and utero-ovarian ligaments. These pedicles were then cut and suture ligated with 0 Vicryl. Free tie was placed around each pedicle first so that these pedicles would be doubly ligated. At this point then, the uterine arteries were skeletonized bilaterally. Heaney clamps were then used to clamp the uterine arteries bilaterally, and pedicles were cut and suture ligated with 0 Vicryl. At this point, the cervix was palpated, and it was quite long and deep into the pelvis. Since the bladder was so adherent anteriorly given the patient's previous surgeries, the decision was made just to complete a subtotal hysterectomy and leave the cervix in place to minimize patient morbidity. The fundus of the uterus was therefore sharply excised. The remaining cervical stump was then grasped using Kochers. Any remaining endometrium was cauterized at the level of the cervix. The cervical stump was then oversewn using

CASE 11-4A—cont'd

0 Vicryl. Good hemostasis was ensured. At this point, the pelvis was washed with sterile water. Bleeding site was identified on the right utero-ovarian pedicle, and this was suture ligated with 0 Vicryl. Good hemostasis was then ensured aside from a small amount of oozing, which persisted from the bladder. A small piece of Surgicel was therefore placed at the level of the bladder flap for this. The packs and retractors were then removed. The fascia was closed using running 0 Vicryl. The skin was then reapproximated using staples.

The patient tolerated the procedure well and went to the recovery room in good condition. There were no complications. The estimated blood loss was 250 cc.

Pathology Report Later Indicated: See Report 11-4B.

SERVICE CODE(S): _____

ICD-10-CM DX CODE(S): _____

(Answers to every other Case are located in Appendix D . The full answer key is only available in the TEACH Instructor Resources on Evolve.)

CASE 11-4B *Pathology Report*

LOCATION: Inpatient, Hospital

PATIENT: Charlotte Sweet

ATTENDING PHYSICIAN: Andy Martinez, MD

SURGEON: Andy Martinez, MD

PATHOLOGIST: Grey Lonewolf, MD

CLINICAL HISTORY: Dysfunctional uterine bleeding. Concurrent case exists.

TISSUE RECEIVED: Uterus

GROSS DESCRIPTION:

The specimen is labeled with the patient's name and "uterus" and consists of a 70-g (gram), heart-shaped uterus, 7.5 × 5.0 × 3.2 cm (centimeter). The cervix is not attached. The serosa surface is a smooth pink-tan. The endometrium appears hemorrhagic and is 0.4 cm thick.

The myometrium is pink-tan and 2.4 cm in thickness. Representative sections are submitted in four cassettes.

MICROSCOPIC DESCRIPTION:

The endometrial lining consists of tubular glands lined by stratified columnar epithelium. Foci of endometrial glands and stroma are present within the myometrium.

DIAGNOSIS:

Bicornuate uterus, subtotal hysterectomy:

1. Proliferative phase endometrium (endometriosis of uterus)
2. Adenomyosis

SERVICE CODE(S): _____

ICD-10-CM DX CODE(S): _____

(Answers to every other Case are located in Appendix D . The full answer key is only available in the TEACH Instructor Resources on Evolve.)

CASE 11-5 *Operative Report, Dilatation and Curettage*

LOCATION: Inpatient, Hospital

PATIENT: Mary Moore

ATTENDING PHYSICIAN: Andy Martinez, MD

SURGEON: Andy Martinez, MD

PREOPERATIVE DIAGNOSIS: Irregular uterine bleeding

POSTOPERATIVE DIAGNOSIS: Irregular uterine bleeding

OPERATIVE PROCEDURE: Hysteroscopy and dilatation and curettage of the uterus

ANESTHESIA: General

SURGICAL INDICATIONS: This patient is a 41-year-old multiparous female who had been having irregular, abnormal, and prolonged bleeding since June of this year. Ultrasound suggested a small myoma on the right side of her uterus.

OPERATIVE FINDINGS: The uterus was 7.5 cm (centimeter) deep. The cavity was symmetrical without evidence of polyps or submucous myomas.

DESCRIPTION OF PROCEDURE: After introduction of general anesthesia, the patient was placed in the dorsolithotomy position, after which the perineum and vagina were prepped and bladder straight catheterized. The patient was then draped. The cervix was grasped with a single-tooth tenaculum, and sharp endocervical curettage was done. The endocervical canal was then dilated to 7 cm with Hegar dilators. A 5.5-mm (millimeter) Olympus hysteroscope was introduced and the cavity inspected. The hysteroscope was withdrawn, and then a sharp endometrial curettage was done. Blood loss was 5-10 cc. Specimen to pathology: Endocervical and endometrial curettings. The patient tolerated the procedure well and returned to the recovery room in stable condition.

Pathology Report Later Indicated: Primary endometrial cancer

SERVICE CODE(S): _____

ICD-10-CM DX CODE(S): _____

(Answers to every other Case are located in Appendix D . The full answer key is only available in the TEACH Instructor Resources on Evolve.)

Maternity Care/Delivery

The gestation of a fetus takes approximately 266 days or 40 weeks; but when the **estimated date of delivery (EDD)** is calculated, 280 days are often used, counting the time from the **last menstrual period (LMP).** The gestation is divided into three time periods, called trimesters. The trimesters are as follows:

- 1st   less than 14 weeks 0 days
- 2nd   14 weeks 0 days to less than 28 weeks 0 days
- 3rd   28 weeks 0 days until delivery

When a maternity case is uncomplicated, the service codes normally include the **antepartum** care, delivery, and **postpartum** care in the global package. **Antepartum care** is considered to include both the initial and subsequent history and physical examinations; blood pressures; patient's weight; routine urinalysis; fetal heart tones; and monthly visits to 28 weeks of gestation, biweekly visits from gestation weeks 29 through 36, and weekly visits from week 37 to delivery when these services are provided by the same physician/physician group. If the patient is seen by the same physician/physician group for a service other than those identified as part of antepartum care (59425-59426), you would report that service separately using evaluation and management codes.

Delivery includes admission to the hospital, which includes the admitting history and examination, management of an uncomplicated labor, and delivery that is either vaginal or by cesarean section (including any episiotomy and use of forceps). If the labor or delivery is complicated by medical problems, those services may be separately reported with an E&M code.

Included in postpartum care are the hospital visits and/or office visits for 6 weeks after a delivery. If the postpartum care is complicated or if services are provided to the patient during the postpartum period but the services are not generally part of the postpartum care, you would report those services separately.

Routine Obstetric Care

There are four codes that describe the global routine obstetric care, which includes the antepartum care, delivery, and postpartum care based on the delivery:

59400	Vaginal delivery
59510	Cesarean delivery
59610	Vaginal delivery after a previous cesarean delivery
59618	Cesarean delivery following an attempted vaginal delivery after previous cesarean delivery

If the physician provided only a portion of the global routine obstetric care, the service is reported with codes that describe that portion of the service as delivery only or postpartum care only based on the delivery method. For example, if the physician provided only the delivery portion of the service, you would report the service with the following:

59409	Vaginal delivery only
59514	Cesarean delivery only
59612	Vaginal delivery only, after previous cesarean delivery
59620	Cesarean delivery only, following an attempted vaginal delivery after previous cesarean delivery

If the global obstetric care is provided and twins are delivered vaginally, codes 59409 or 59612 are used in addition to the global code, with modifier -51 (Multiple Procedures) added. Some third-party payers prefer billing the global code with modifier -22 (Increased Procedural Services) added. If a global obstetric care is provided and both twins are delivered by cesarean, most payers will allow only one code (59510) with modifier -22 added to report both deliveries. If the global obstetric care is provided when one twin is delivered vaginally and then the second twin is delivered cesarean, you would report the cesarean delivery with the global code (59510 or 59618) for the first twin and the second twin with a code for vaginal delivery only (59409 or 59612) with modifier -59 added.

At the time of delivery, the patient may request permanent sterilization, such as a tubal ligation. These procedures may be conducted at the time of delivery (such as when a cesarean is performed) or shortly after the delivery during the same hospitalization. These procedures may be performed by the OB/GYN or by another physician, such as a general surgeon.

Third-party payers would usually include a tubal ligation at the time of delivery in the surgical bundle for the delivery.

Admission for Normal Delivery Admission for normal delivery is reported with O80/650 but is only assigned when a single liveborn is the outcome of a completely normal (Z37.0), spontaneous vaginal delivery after the completion of 38 to 42 weeks of gestation. The newborn presents head first (cephalic presentation) with only minimal or with no assistance. No instrumentation (forceps) or fetal manipulation (such as rotation to cephalic presentation) would be required during a normal delivery. An episiotomy (surgical incision into the perineum and vagina to prevent tearing during delivery) may be performed, and the delivery can still be assigned to O80/650. A completely normal, spontaneous vaginal delivery with no complications before, during, or after delivery (O80) with the outcome of a single liveborn (Z37.0) must be reported together.

CASE 11-6A *Operative Report, Sterilization*

Susan requests a tubal ligation shortly after delivering her child. Report Dr. Sanchez's services. A code is assigned to report the sterilization.

LOCATION: Inpatient, Hospital

PATIENT: Susan Hillard

ATTENDING PHYSICIAN: Andy Martinez, MD

SURGEON: Gary Sanchez, MD

PREOPERATIVE DIAGNOSIS: Desire for sterilization

POSTOPERATIVE DIAGNOSIS: Desire for sterilization

PROCEDURE PERFORMED: Postpartum bilateral tubal ligation

ANESTHESIA: General

SURGICAL INDICATIONS: This patient is a 43-year-old female who delivered her fourth child yesterday by vaginal delivery and desired permanent sterilization by tubal interruption.

PROCEDURE: After induction of general anesthesia, the patient was in the supine position, and the abdomen was prepped and draped. A transverse subumbilical incision was made, and then dissection was carried down bluntly to the fascia, which was picked up with small Kocher clamps, nicked in the midline with a scalpel, and then incised vertically with Mayo scissors. Army-Navy retractors were placed inside the fascial edges, and the peritoneum was identified and entered without incident. A vein retractor was used to elevate the right fallopian tube, which was then grasped with Babcock clamps and marched to its fimbriated end. The mesosalpinx underneath the ampullary portion was opened with Bovie cautery, and then the tube was cross-clamped across the ampullary portion. Then the mesosalpinx underneath this was cross-clamped. The lateral portion of the tube, including the fimbriated end, was excised. Pedicles were doubly tied with 2-0 Vicryl. An identical procedure was carried out on the left tube. The fascia was closed with a running locked 2-0 Vicryl and the skin with subcuticular 4-0 Vicryl. Blood loss was less than 5 cc. Specimens to pathology—segments of right and left fallopian tubes. The patient tolerated the procedure well and returned to the recovery room in stable condition.

Pathology Report Later Indicated: Benign right and left fallopian tubes

SERVICE CODE(S): _____

ICD-10-CM DX CODE(S): _____

(Answers to every other Case are located in Appendix D . The full answer key is only available in the TEACH Instructor Resources on Evolve.)

CASE 11-6B *Discharge Summary*

Susan was subsequently discharged 3 days after admission by her attending physician, Dr. Martinez.

LOCATION: Inpatient, Hospital

PATIENT: Susan Hillard

ATTENDING PHYSICIAN: Andy Martinez, MD

SUMMARY OF HOSPITALIZATION: The patient was admitted with a history of 37 weeks' pregnancy. She was having some leaking membranes and some contractions. The patient was stable on admission. She had a spontaneous vaginal delivery 3 days ago. Both baby and mother were healthy. On postnatal day 1, the patient had a tubal ligation done by Dr. Sanchez. The postoperative and postpartum period was uneventful. The patient was stable. Vital signs: Temperature 36° C, pulse 72, respirations 20, blood pressure 105/72. The patient was discharged today.

DISCHARGE INSTRUCTIONS: Activity level: Pelvic rest for 6 weeks; no heavy weight lifting for 6 weeks. Diet: Regular.

MEDICATIONS: Pain control medication p.r.n. (as needed)

FOLLOW-UP in 6 weeks.

CONDITION ON DISCHARGE: Patient's condition was improved. Bleeding and pain were minimal. Vital signs were stable.

DISCHARGE DIAGNOSIS: Postpartum day 2 with postoperative tubal ligation day 1.

SERVICE CODE(S): _____

ICD-10-CM DX CODE(S): _____

(Answers to every other Case are located in Appendix D . The full answer key is only available in the TEACH Instructor Resources on Evolve.)

Echography

Ultrasound and sonography both describe echography, which is often used in the care of pregnancies. **Figure 11-5** illustrates an ultrasound of a single fetus. Radiology codes 76801-76828 describe transabdominal ultrasound of the obstetrical pelvis with the exception of 76817, which describes a transvaginal ultrasound. Codes 76801 and 76802 describe ultrasound using real-time imaging documentation that is performed during the first trimester. 76802 is an add-on code that is used to report each additional gestation, which means that if the ultrasound detected twins, both 76801 and 76802 would be reported. These codes indicate a survey of the fetus, placenta, amniotic fluid, gestational sac, maternal uterus, and adnexa. Pay special attention to reporting these trimester-specific codes. Codes 76805 and 76810 are similar to 76801 and 76802 but are assigned for echography after the first trimester (described as 14 weeks 0 days). Included in 76805 and 76810 is an assessment of the number of fetuses, measurement of the amniotic sac, fetal anatomy, umbilical cord insertion, placenta, and amniotic fluid, which is a more detailed assessment than the 14-weeks-or-less codes. Note that 76810 is an add-on code used only with 76805.

An examination focused on taking an ultrasound to assess one or more elements is described in 76815. For example, if the fetal heart beat is being assessed, 76815 would be reported. Note that the code is reported only once even though multiple elements noted in the code description are provided. So, if the fetal heartbeat and the fetal position were assessed, 76815 would be reported only once for both of the assessments.

Be certain to read the notes for the Pelvis, Obstetrical codes (76801-76828) before coding echographic services provided to the obstetrical patient.

Cesarean Section

Cesarean delivery is referred to as C-section, cesarean, or CD and is the surgical removal of the fetus through an abdominal

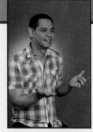

From the Trenches

"As a medical coder, you are at the intersection of the healthcare business and clinical medicine. This allows you to see the difficulties of each side and contribute to the resolution of issues between the two sides."

PETER EDU
MD, CPC, CCS, CHDA, CDEO, CPC-I
AHIMA - APPROVED ICD-10 CM/PCS TRAINER
AHIMA - ICD-10 AMBASSADOR

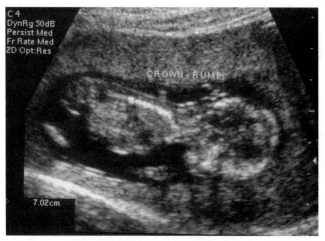

FIGURE 11–5 Ultrasound of fetus.

incision. Cesarean is used when a vaginal delivery would endanger either the mother or the child. A vaginal birth may be possible on subsequent deliveries and is referred to as VBAC, vaginal birth (or delivery) after a previous cesarean delivery. Cesarean delivery codes are divided in the CPT manual based on whether the procedure is a cesarean (59510-59515) or a vaginal delivery after a previous cesarean (59610-59614) or a cesarean delivery after an attempted vaginal delivery when the mother previously delivered a baby by means of cesarean (59618-59622). The codes are subdivided based on the type of services provided, such as postpartum care or delivery only, etc.

CASE 11-7A   *Real-Time Ultrasound*

This case will give you an opportunity to better understand how the ultrasound is used in obstetrical care as this patient has a variety of ultrasound services.

Beth is sent to Dr. Martinez for maternity/delivery care based on abnormal echography by her hometown physician. Dr. Martinez has assumed the patient's care for the duration of her pregnancy and has seen Beth in the clinic where he scheduled her for an ultrasound at the radiology department at the hospital.

LOCATION: Outpatient, Hospital

PATIENT: Beth Lariat

PRIMARY CARE PHYSICIAN: Andy Martinez, MD

RADIOLOGIST: Morton Monson, MD

OBSTETRICAL ULTRASOUND: I have a report from an outside ultrasound from Denver Clinic dated 8 weeks ago. I do not have those films, however. That report states "a 2-cm (centimeter) isoechoic 'mass' with a hypoechoic rim seen along the external aspect of the placenta." A single living intrauterine pregnancy is identified in breech presentation. Average sonographic gestational age is 22 weeks 6 days. Since the previous examination, there has been 8 weeks 1 day, with interval growth of 8 weeks. Fetal cardiac activity identified at 140 beats per minute. Fetal motion is identified. Examination is technically difficult and fetal screen is limited. This is due to fetal lie and patient body habitus. No images were submitted of the fetal heart since this cannot be adequately visualized. There is limited visualization of the posterior fossa/cisterna magna region. The placenta is noted to be anterior. There is an approximately 6-cm hyperechoic area seen at the junction of the uterus and placenta anteriorly and measures up to 6 cm in greatest length.

CASE 11-7A—cont'd

This is worrisome for an area of hemorrhage/abruption. I do not have any color flow of this area, however. No placenta previa is identified.

IMPRESSION:

1. A single living intrauterine pregnancy is identified with average sonographic gestational age 22 weeks 6 days. Suggest the patient return to complete fetal anatomic survey (i.e., fetal four-chamber heart and posterior fossa/cisterna magna).
2. Hyperechoic area seen, a malformation of the placenta (this is the diagnosis) along the junction along the anterior aspect of the

placenta and uterus measuring up to 6 cm in greatest dimension. This is worrisome for an area of hemorrhage/abruption. Other etiologies are not completely excluded. Suggest the patient return for reassessment of this area over a short interval. Per outside report, there was a 2-cm isoechoic lesion reported previously. Dr. Martinez was not immediately available, and a preliminary report was given to his nurse.

SERVICE CODE(S): _____

ICD-10-CM DX CODE(S): _____

(Answers to every other Case are located in Appendix D . The full answer key is only available in the TEACH Instructor Resources on Evolve.)

CASE 11-7B   *Sonogram*

Approximately 7 weeks after the ultrasound in 11-7A, Dr. Martinez orders a sonogram to assess fetal development.

LOCATION: Outpatient, Hospital

PATIENT: Beth Lariat

PRIMARY CARE PHYSICIAN: Andy Martinez, MD

RADIOLOGIST: Morton Monson, MD

FOLLOW-UP OB (OBSTETRICS) SONOGRAM:

HISTORY: Interval growth, placental mass. Last menstrual period is uncertain; estimated menstrual age is 29 weeks 5 days. There is a comparison, which is not the latest, but is used for calculating interval growth. The latest comparison to the ultrasound of 7 weeks prior to follow up the "placental mass."

FINDINGS: Anterior to the placenta is a thin, more linear, hyperechoic focus anterior to the placenta at the placental uterine interface, which is not measured on today's examination, although grossly appears less prominent. Etiology as previously mentioned is uncertain. This could be due to a focus of resolving hemorrhage. The current biparietal diameter, head circumference, abdominal circumference, and femur length measurements correspond to an average estimated gestational age of 33 weeks 4 days. Estimated fetal weight 2002 g (gram). Fetal motion and cardiac activity are demonstrated with a heart rate of 141 beats per minute. Adequate interval growth.

SERVICE CODE(S): _____

ICD-10-CM DX CODE(S): _____

(Answers to every other Case are located in Appendix D . The full answer key is only available in the TEACH Instructor Resources on Evolve.)

CASE 11-7C   *Operative Report, Cesarean Section*

Dr. Martinez admits Beth to the hospital and schedules a cesarean section. He'll follow the patient postpartumly as well.

LOCATION: Inpatient, Hospital

PATIENT: Beth Lariat

ATTENDING PHYSICIAN: Andy Martinez, MD

SURGEON: Andy Martinez, MD

PREOPERATIVE DIAGNOSIS: Previous cesarean section

POSTOPERATIVE DIAGNOSES:

1. Previous cesarean section
2. Macrosomia
3. Breech presentation

PROCEDURE PERFORMED: Repeat low transverse cesarean section

FINDINGS: Viable infant male with Apgars of 8 and 9. The infant's weight is 4206 g (gram). Maternal anatomy normal, including uterus, ovaries, and tubes. She did have significant scarring and adhesions in the subcutaneous tissue as well as subfascially.

ESTIMATED BLOOD LOSS: Approximately 800 cc

COMPLICATIONS: None

ANESTHESIA: Spinal anesthetic with Duramorph

TECHNIQUE: The patient was prepped and draped in the usual fashion. A Pfannenstiel incision was made. I did remove a nevus that looked somewhat inflamed and was oozing. It was right on the incision. The nevus was removed at that time. (This nevus is also reported as a diagnosis.) This was to be sent to pathology. I sharply dissected down to the rectus fascia. The fascia was then incised in the midline. I used sharp and cautery for dissection of this subcutaneous tissue laterally and anteriorly in a U-shape. The fascia was also incised with Mayo scissors laterally and anteriorly in a U-shape. Kocher clamps were placed on the superior and inferior aspect of the fascia, removing it from the underlying rectus muscles in the midline. The fascia was removed both sharply and with cautery. I entered the peritoneum sharply by tenting the peritoneum. The peritoneal incision was extended superiorly and inferiorly by blunt lateral traction. At this point, the lower uterine segment was identified. The anterior serosa of the lower uterine segment was incised. The incision was extended laterally and anteriorly in a U-shape with Metzenbaum scissors. Bladder flap was developed at this time.

CASE 11-7C—cont'd

The lower uterine segment was incised. The incision was extended laterally and anteriorly in a U-shape with bandage scissors. The infant was found to be in a breech presentation with double footling presentation. (This will have an effect on the diagnosis code.) The infant was delivered through the uterine incision without problems or complications. The cord was clamped and cut. The infant was handed to the nursery team standing by. The placenta was manually removed intact with three vessels. On inspection, the placenta had appeared normal. The uterus was exteriorized and wiped clean with a moist lap. The fascial incision was then repaired in a running locking layer. There was good hemostasis. The posterior cul-de-sac was irrigated. The uterus was placed back into the abdomen. Both right and left gutters were irrigated. On inspection of the uterine incision, there was good hemostasis. The fascia was then closed in a running fashion with 0 Vicryl. The subcutaneous tissue was irrigated, and the skin was closed with staples. All needle, sponge, and instrument counts were correct. The patient was stable in the recovery room. She will be transferred to floor status when she meets criteria.

Pathology Report Later Indicated: Benign nevus

SERVICE CODE(S): _____

ICD-10-CM DX CODE(S): _____

Discussion

In report 11-7C, the Preoperative Diagnosis and the Postoperative Diagnosis sections of the report indicate a previous cesarean section delivery. The outcome of delivery, single liveborn, is reported with Z37.0.

ICD-10-CM: Code O34.21- reports previously delivered by cesarean section.

The presentation was breech **(Figure 11-6),** which is a malposition or wrong position. Any position other than cephalic (head first) is a malposition or malpresentation.

Malpositions are reported with O64.8. Category O64 requires 7 characters with the 7th character "0" assigned for single gestations and multiple gestations where the fetus is unspecified. The 7th characters "1" through "9" identify the number of gestations.

Macrosomia is excessive birth weight.

There are two codes in ICD-10-CM to report excessive birth weight: P08.0, Exceptionally large newborn with a birth weight over 4500 grams (9 pounds 15 ounces) and P08.1, Heavy for gestational age, 4000–4499 grams (8 lb 13 oz to 9 lb 14 oz). These codes are only assigned for the infant. Cesarean delivery due to oversize fetus is reported with O36.6. The 7th character "0" is assigned for single gestations and multiple gestations where the fetus is unspecified. The 7th characters "1 through 9" identify the number of gestations.

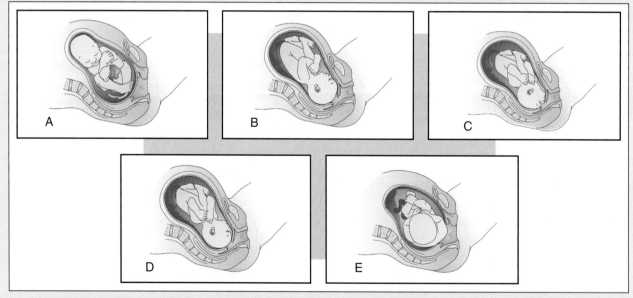

FIGURE 11–6 Five types of malposition and malpresentation of the fetus: **A,** Breech. **B,** Vertex. **C,** Face. **D,** Brow. **E,** Shoulder.

(Answers to every other Case are located in Appendix D . The full answer key is only available in the TEACH Instructor Resources on Evolve.)

CASE 11-7D   *Discharge Summary*

LOCATION: Inpatient, Hospital

PATIENT: Beth Lariat

ATTENDING PHYSICIAN: Andy Martinez, MD

REASON FOR ADMISSION: Low transverse C-section

The patient had a low transverse C-section secondary to breech and macrosomia. Patient had a previous C-section a few years ago. The patient's hospital course was unremarkable. On postoperative day 3, the patient was tolerating diet, having good urine output, but with mild pain that was well controlled. The patient had flatus and bowel movements. Vital signs remained stable.

Physical examination remained unremarkable.

The patient was discharged on postoperative day 3. Hemoglobin 10.6.

INSTRUCTIONS TO PATIENT ON DISCHARGE: The patient is to follow up with me in 6 weeks' time.

DISCHARGE MEDICATIONS:

1. Peri-Colace 100 mg (milligram) 2 p.o. (by mouth) q.d. (every day), #20 given
2. Ibuprofen 200 mg q.6h. p.r.n. (as needed)
3. Percocet 1 tablet q.4h. (every 4 hours)

Prior to discharge, patient's staples were removed.

FINAL DIAGNOSIS: Status post low transverse cesarean section secondary to macrosomia and breech presentation.

DISPOSITION ON DISCHARGE: Stable

SERVICE CODE(S): _____

ICD-10-CM DX CODE(S): _____

(Answers to every other Case are located in Appendix D . The full answer key is only available in the TEACH Instructor Resources on Evolve.)

CASE 11-8A   *Admission History and Physical*

Dr. Martinez admits a patient who will undergo a cesarean section. The diagnoses for this patient will include the gestation code to indicate twins, a code for the premature rupture of the membrane, a code for the malpresentation in multiple gestation, and a Z code to indicate multiple gestation placenta status.

LOCATION: Inpatient, Hospital

PATIENT: Joan Corcoran

ATTENDING PHYSICIAN: Andy Martinez, MD

CHIEF COMPLAINT: Spontaneous rupture of membranes

HPI: This is a 24-year-old female with twin gestation, who now presents to labor and delivery with spontaneous rupture of membranes. The patient has had essentially an uneventful twin gestation and is currently at 34-3/7 weeks. Yesterday evening, she started having contractions. At 4 o'clock this morning, she had spontaneous rupture of membranes. Rupture produced clear fluids. There was no meconium or blood noted. After rupture, the patient's contractions intensified and frequency increased. She presented to labor and delivery in active labor. Cervical exam revealed dilation of 3 cm (centimeter) with 100% effacement and breech presentation of the first twin. The patient was immediately notified of the risks, benefits, consequences, and alternatives to delivery by cesarean section. The patient is a consenting adult and elected to go forth with the procedure immediately. Dr. Sanchez was notified and will be performing the procedure.

OB (OBSTETRICS) HISTORY:

1. 07/89 male, 8 pounds 2 ounces, 41 weeks, 17 hours labor, SVD (spontaneous vaginal delivery)
2. 07/94 male, 8 pounds 1 ounce, 40 weeks, 24 hours labor, SVD
3. 10/98 SAB (spontaneous abortion) at 10 weeks
4. 02/01 SAB at 11 weeks

PAST MEDICAL HISTORY:

1. D&C (dilation and curettage)

ALLERGIES: SULFA, develops a rash.

FAMILY HISTORY: Father had an MI at age 65. He also had bladder cancer. Mother was noted to have ovarian cancer. No known birth defects in the family. She has three brothers and two sisters, all healthy.

SOCIAL HISTORY: Unremarkable. Nonsmoker. Nondrinker.

MEDICATIONS: Prenatal vitamins

REVIEW OF SYSTEMS: As above

PHYSICAL EXAM: Afebrile at 98° F. Vital signs are stable. BP is 120/80. General: Mild distress with contractions. Skin: Warm, dry, and pink. HEENT (head, ears, eyes, nose, throat): Unremarkable. No nystagmus. Acuity is normal. Peripheral vision normal. Lungs are clear. CVS: S1 (first heart sound) and S2 (second heart sound), regular rate and rhythm without murmur, rub, or gallop. Abdomen: Soft and nontender. Gravida. Palpable contractions. Cervix: 3 cm/100%/-1/breech. Extremities: No edema. No rash. No calf tenderness. Neurologic: Nonfocal.

LABORATORY AND TESTS: A positive, antibody negative, rubella immune, hepatitis B surface antigen negative, HIV (human immunodeficiency virus) negative, Pap smear negative, hemoglobin 12.2, and group B negative.

ASSESSMENT:

1. A 34-3/7 weeks' twin gestation in active labor.
2. Breech presentation.
3. Prior history of spontaneous abortions.

PLAN: The patient will be admitted to labor and delivery. Dr. Sanchez has been notified, and a cesarean section will be performed. The patient has been notified of the risks, benefits, consequences, and alternatives to the treatment. She is a consenting adult and elects to go forth with the procedure.

She will have a permit signed and does wish to have a tubal ligation as well. This was also discussed in great depth.

SERVICE CODE(S): _____

ICD-10-CM DX CODE(S): _____

(Answers to every other Case are located in Appendix D . The full answer key is only available in the TEACH Instructor Resources on Evolve.)

CASE 11-8B   *Operative Report, Cesarean Section*

In this report, you will report the diagnoses of the twin pregnancy, breech delivery due to the malposition of the first infant, premature labor with delivery, multiple gestation placenta status (Z code), twins as the outcome of delivery (Z code), and sterilization (Z code).

LOCATION: Inpatient, Hospital

PATIENT: Joan Corcoran

ATTENDING PHYSICIAN: Andy Martinez, MD

SURGEON: Gary Sanchez, MD

PREOPERATIVE DIAGNOSIS: Uterine pregnancy at 34 weeks 4 days with twin gestation, spontaneous rupture of membranes, in active labor with breech presentation of the first twin. Multiparity, desires permanent sterilization.

POSTOPERATIVE DIAGNOSIS: Uterine pregnancy at 34 weeks 4 days with twin gestation, spontaneous rupture of membranes, in active labor with breech presentation of the first twin. Multiparity, desires permanent sterilization.

PROCEDURE PERFORMED: Primary low transverse cervical segment cesarean section with postpartum tubal ligation.

ANESTHESIA: Spinal

ESTIMATED BLOOD LOSS: 800 cc

URINE OUTPUT: 125

FLUIDS: 2000

COMPLICATIONS: None

FINDINGS: Two viable female infants with breech presentation of Infant B. Infant A weighed 5 pounds 6.2 ounces with Apgar of 9 at 1 minute and 9 at 5 minutes. Infant B had Apgar of 9 at 1 minute and 9 at 5 minutes weighing 4 pounds 12 ounces.

PROCEDURE: The patient was prepped and draped in the supine position with left lateral displacement of the uterine fundus under spinal anesthesia with Foley catheter indwelling. A transverse incision was made in the lower abdomen. The fascia was divided laterally. The rectus muscles were divided in the midline. The peritoneum was entered in a sharp manner. The incision was extended vertically. The bladder flap was created using sharp and blunt dissection and reflected inferiorly. The uterus was entered in a sharp manner in the lower uterine segment. The incision was extended laterally with blunt traction. The membranes were ruptured, and the buttocks of the first infant was grasped and delivered. The infant was delivered to the chest, the arms were swept forward, and the head was delivered spontaneously. The infant was bulb suctioned while the cord was doubly clamped and divided. The infant was given to the intensive nursery staff in apparent good condition. Palpation of the second infant revealed that it was breech. The hips were grasped; membranes were ruptured. The infant was delivered to the chest, the arms were swept forward, and the head was delivered spontaneously. The infant was bulb suctioned while the cord was being doubly clamped and divided. The infant was given to the intensive nursery staff in apparent good condition. The placenta was manually expressed. The uterus was delivered from the abdominal cavity and placed on a wet lap sponge. A dry lap sponge was used to ensure that the remaining products of conception were removed. The cervical os (opening) was ensured to be patent with ring forceps. The uterine incision was closed with 0 Vicryl interlocking suture in two layers with the second layer imbricating the first. Figure-of-eight sutures were also placed as required for hemostasis. The operative site was irrigated and hemostatic. The bladder flap was reapproximated using 2-0 Vicryl continuous sutures. The left tube was then identified in its entirety, including fimbriated end. It was grasped in its midportion and elevated. The mesosalpinx was transected using the Bovie. Approximately 3 cm (centimeter) of tube was isolated and excised. The proximal end of the distal portion and the distal end of the proximal portion were ligated with 0 chromic suture. Operative sites were inspected and were hemostatic. The uterus was placed back within the abdominal cavity. Pelvic gutters were irrigated. Operative sites were inspected and were hemostatic. The anterior peritoneum was reapproximated using 2-0 Vicryl continuous suture. The incision was irrigated. The skin was closed with staples. All sponges and needles were accounted for at the completion of the procedure. The patient left the operating room in apparent good condition having tolerated the procedure well. The Foley catheter was patent and draining clear yellow urine at completion of the procedure.

SERVICE CODE(S): _____

ICD-10-CM DX CODE(S): _____

CASE 11-8C   *Discharge Summary*

In this discharge report, you will report the diagnoses of the twin pregnancy, breech delivery due to the malposition of the first infant, multiple gestation placenta status (Z code), twins as the outcome of delivery (Z code), and sterilization (Z code).

LOCATION: Inpatient, Hospital

PATIENT: Joan Corcoran

ATTENDING PHYSICIAN: Andy Martinez, MD

HOSPITAL COURSE: The patient had a low transverse C-section secondary to a twin gestation as well as bilateral tube ligation. The patient's hospital course was unremarkable. The patient tolerated a diet well, had flatus. Lochia was minimal. Pain was well controlled.

Vital signs remained stable. Physical examination was unremarkable and unchanged. The patient was sent home on postoperative day 3. Prior to discharge staples were removed.

Hemoglobin 12.4.

DISCHARGE INSTRUCTIONS: The patient is to follow up in 2 weeks' and 6 weeks' time with Dr. Sanchez.

DISCHARGE MEDICATIONS: Percocet and ibuprofen

FINAL DIAGNOSES:

1. Status post low transverse cesarean section secondary to twin gestation.
2. Bilateral tubal ligation.

CONDITION ON DISCHARGE: The patient is discharged in stable condition.

SERVICE CODE(S): _____

ICD-10-CM DX CODE(S): _____

According to the *Official Guidelines for Coding and Reporting*, codes in the range O00-O9A are assigned to report complications of pregnancy, childbirth, and the puerperium. It is the physician's responsibility to document if the condition being treated is not complicating pregnancy, and if no such documentation is present to indicate the condition is **not** complicating the pregnancy, the condition is considered to be complicating the pregnancy. Sequencing of pregnancy complication codes take priority over codes from other chapters. The complication codes O00-O9A are only used on the **mother's** record, not on the newborn's record.

Additional codes from other chapters may be assigned in conjunction with the pregnancy complication codes to further specify the condition. For example, if the pregnant patient has diabetes, assign a O24.- (pregnancy complicated by diabetes); but this code alone does not indicate the type of diabetes, and as such assign E13.9 to give further specificity to the type of diabetes. Another example would be if the pregnant patient presented with nausea with vomiting, a complication code for pregnancy complicated by vomiting (O21.8) would be reported.

Some of the pregnancy complication categories (O20-O24 and O30-O92) require the use of additional characters/digits to indicate whether the encounter is antepartum or postpartum and whether a delivery has occurred during that encounter.

In an episode of care in which no delivery occurred, the first-listed diagnosis should correspond to the principal complication of the pregnancy that was the reason for the encounter. If there is more than one complication, and all were treated or monitored, all complications are listed before codes from other chapters and any one may be sequenced first.

If the pregnancy was incidental to the encounter, Z33.1, incidental pregnancy state, is reported.

CASE 11-9A   *OB/GYN Consultation*

This complex case will be quite detailed and provide you an opportunity to code many services that are provided to this patient. The patient is pregnant and presents for care because of nausea with vomiting and diarrhea, which is a complication of pregnancy. The patient also has diabetes with nephropathy that will be reported. The diabetes is another complication of this pregnancy as is the chronic hypertension.

LOCATION: Inpatient, Hospital

PATIENT: Patricia Garrison

ATTENDING PHYSICIAN: George Orbitz, MD

CONSULTANT: Andy Martinez, MD

CHIEF COMPLAINT: Nausea, vomiting (complication of pregnancy), and diarrhea

HISTORY OF PRESENT ILLNESS: This patient is pregnant and has been followed by Dr. Orbitz. I got a message to see the patient by orders from the ward secretary. However, I was not sure exactly the reason for the consultation since there had been no direct contact from the admitting physician as to what I was expected to do at this time. She had an insulin reaction 2 days ago, came to the emergency room, and then was discharged. She then had some nausea, vomiting, and diarrhea. She has had no vaginal bleeding or cramping. She is 30 weeks' gestation.

PHYSICAL EXAMINATION: On examination, the fundus is palpable, slightly above the symphysis pubis. I cannot hear tones with the Doppler; however, there is a lot of static electricity interference. An ultrasound was obtained, which showed the baby to be viable gestational size.

The patient's pregnancy is complicated by type 1 insulin-dependent diabetes (complication of pregnancy) with diabetic nephropathy and chronic hypertension (complication of pregnancy).

DIAGNOSES:

1. Intrauterine pregnancy
2. Probable gastroenteritis
3. Type 1 diabetes mellitus with diabetic nephropathy

PLAN: I have been asked by Dr. Orbitz to assume attending for this patient, to which I have agreed.

SERVICE CODE(S): _____

ICD-10-CM DX CODE(S): _____

(Answers to every other Case are located in Appendix D . The full answer key is only available in the TEACH Instructor Resources on Evolve.)

CASE 11-9B *Duplex Venous Examination*

Because you are reporting outpatient services, you do not consider the diagnoses from the previous report. This report, 11-9B, is assigned diagnoses based on the documentation within this one report. The first-listed diagnosis is, therefore, the complication of pregnancy (other specified complication) followed by the code for the leg swelling, which gives specifics to the type of complication. The thrombophlebitis cannot be reported as it is a "rule out" diagnosis that was not confirmed.

LOCATION: Inpatient, Hospital

PATIENT: Patricia Garrison

ATTENDING PHYSICIAN: Andy Martinez, MD

INTERVENTIONAL RADIOLOGIST: Edward Riddle, MD

EXAMINATION OF: Duplex venous examination

CLINICAL SYMPTOMS: Rule out deep venous thrombosis

DUPLEX VENOUS EXAMINATION: Patient is a 28-year-old with leg swelling (complication of pregnancy) and possible DVT (deep vein thrombosis). She is an OB (obstetrics) patient.

Both legs were examined with the duplex scanner in CW (clockwise) and imaging modes. We checked the veins at the common femoral, superficial femoral, popliteal, saphenous, and posterior tibial levels. We checked for spontaneous flow, phasicity, augmentation, and compressibility. The above were all normal.

CONCLUSION: No evidence of thrombophlebitis

SERVICE CODE(S): _____

ICD-10-CM DX CODE(S): _____

(Answers to every other Case are located in Appendix D . The full answer key is only available in the TEACH Instructor Resources on Evolve.)

CASE 11-9C *Ultrasound*

The reason for this service is an antenatal screening reported with a Z code.

LOCATION: Inpatient, Hospital

PATIENT: Patricia Garrison

ATTENDING PHYSICIAN: Andy Martinez, MD

RADIOLOGIST: Morton Monson, MD

EXAMINATION OF: Limited obstetrical ultrasound (*this is a fetal testing ultrasound*)

CLINICAL SYMPTOMS: Amniotic fluid volume

LIMITED OBSTETRICAL ULTRASOUND: Comparison is made with the previous study outlined in 11-9B. Estimated gestational age by last menstrual period is 29 weeks 2 days.

A single intrauterine pregnancy is seen in cephalic presentation with longitudinal lie. Amniotic fluid index is at the upper norm. The amniotic

fluid index is 22.6. The placenta is posterior and grade 1 with no indication of previa. Detailed measurements were not obtained. Detailed anatomical survey was not performed. Fetal heart rate is 129 beats per minute and fetal motion is noted.

CONCLUSION:

1. Limited obstetrical sonogram for amniotic fluid index only. A single intrauterine pregnancy is seen in cephalic presentation with longitudinal lie.
2. Amniotic fluid volume is at the upper norm. The amniotic fluid index is also at the upper norm at 22.6.
3. Fetal heart rate is 129 beats per minute and fetal motion is noted.

SERVICE CODE(S): _____

ICD-10-CM DX CODE(S): _____

(Answers to every other Case are located in Appendix D . The full answer key is only available in the TEACH Instructor Resources on Evolve.)

CASE 11-9D *Biophysical Profile*

The documentation indicates the reason for this service is the diabetes that is complicating the pregnancy (see Clinical Symptoms section). A code is also required to indicate the type of diabetes.

LOCATION: Inpatient, Hospital

PATIENT: Patricia Garrison

ATTENDING PHYSICIAN: Andy Martinez, MD

INTERVENTIONAL RADIOLOGIST: Edward Riddle, MD

CLINICAL SYMPTOMS: Fetal biophysical profile, based on mother's diabetes, type 1.

BIOPHYSICAL PROFILE: FINDINGS: Single active intrauterine gestation is identified in longitudinal lie and cephalic presentation. Placenta is

predominantly posterior in location and, as visualized, appears within normal limits. Cervical os (opening) area is difficult to visualize due to fetal head position. Please see previous dictations. The non-stress testing revealed fetal heart rate recorded at 126 beats per minute. Fetus receives scores of 2 for fetal breathing movements, fetal movements, fetal tone, and amniotic fluid volume. AFI (amniotic fluid index) on today's exam is 21.8, which places this between the 50th and 95th percentile but closer to 95th percentile; 95th percentile would be 23.8 cm (centimeter). The amniotic fluid index has been mildly prominent for the last several readings. Please see previous dictations.

IMPRESSION: Biophysical profile score is 8 out of 9. Please see additional above comments.

SERVICE CODE(S): _____

ICD-10-CM DX CODE(S): _____

CASE 11-9E   *Doppler Umbilical Arterial*

There are two complications of pregnancy codes needed for this case, as well as codes to describe the diabetes in more detail.

LOCATION: Inpatient, Hospital

PATIENT: Patricia Garrison

ATTENDING PHYSICIAN: Andy Martinez, MD

RADIOLOGIST: Morton Monson, MD

EXAMINATION OF: Umbilical arterial Doppler

CLINICAL SYMPTOMS: History of renal nephropathy due to diabetes type 1 and chronic hypertension, complicating pregnancy. The initial report talks about chronic hypertension, so I believe she had hypertension before she was pregnant.

UMBILICAL ARTERIAL DOPPLER: FINDINGS: Limited evaluation was performed. A single active intrauterine gestation is identified in longitudinal lie in cephalic presentation with fetal heart rate recorded at 121 beats per minute. Relatively normal-appearing umbilical arterial waveform is present. Three umbilical artery Doppler tracings were done with systolic-to-diastolic ratio would be less than 4.2. Previous umbilical arterial ratios were 3.2, 3.7, 2.5, and 4 days prior. The AFI (amniotic fluid index) on today's exam is measured at 50th percentile.

SERVICE CODE(S): _____

ICD-10-CM DX CODE(S): _____

(Answers to every other Case are located in Appendix D . The full answer key is only available in the TEACH Instructor Resources on Evolve.)

CASE 11-9F   *OB Ultrasound*

LOCATION: Inpatient, Hospital

PATIENT: Patricia Garrison

ATTENDING PHYSICIAN: Andy Martinez, MD

RADIOLOGIST: Morton Monson, MD

EXAMINATION OF: Limited OB (obstetrics) ultrasound

CLINICAL SYMPTOMS: Estimated fetal weight; preterm labor

LIMITED OB ULTRASOUND: FINDINGS: A single active intrauterine gestation in longitudinal lie and cephalic presentation is identified. Average gestational age is 32 weeks 4 days. This represents interval

growth of 23 weeks 1 day and chronological growth of 22 weeks 3 days. Fetal heart rate is recorded at 128 beats per minute. Systolic/diastolic ratios of the umbilical artery on today's exam were measured at 4, 3.4, and 3.4, which is within normal limits. Normal for 33 weeks would be 4.2 or less.

IMPRESSION: Normal interval growth and normal umbilical arterial ratio.

SERVICE CODE(S): _____

ICD-10-CM DX CODE(S): _____

(Answers to every other Case are located in Appendix D . The full answer key is only available in the TEACH Instructor Resources on Evolve.)

CASE 11-9G   *OB Ultrasound*

This report is the interpretation of the ultrasonic guidance procedure for the amniocentesis. See case 11-9H for the amniocentesis procedure.

LOCATION: Inpatient, Hospital

PATIENT: Patricia Garrison

ATTENDING PHYSICIAN: Andy Martinez, MD

RADIOLOGIST: Morton Monson, MD

EXAMINATION OF: OB (obstetrics) ultrasound for amniocentesis

CLINICAL SYMPTOMS: Check lung maturity; follow-up

OB ULTRASOUND FOR AMNIOCENTESIS: Numerous comparisons are available, including umbilical arterial Doppler from 2 days ago and biophysical profiles from 5 days ago. Fetal motion is noted by the technologist. Fetal heart rate prior to the procedure is 129 beats per minute. After the procedure, it was 143 beats per minute. It is noted by the technologist that Dr. Martinez retrieved approximately 20 cc of clear amniotic fluid. No immediate complications were encountered. Incidental note of a nuchal cord. Umbilical arterial ratios are 2.9, 2.8, and 2.6. Normal for a 34-week fetus is less than 4.1.

SERVICE CODE(S): _____

ICD-10-CM DX CODE(S): _____

(Answers to every other Case are located in Appendix D . The full answer key is only available in the TEACH Instructor Resources on Evolve.)

CASE 11-9H *Operative Report, Amniocentesis*

Note how in this report the patient's chronic hypertension is not documented. In the outpatient setting, you report only those diagnoses that are stated in the documentation and only those that are being treated or monitored.

LOCATION: Inpatient, Hospital

PATIENT: Patricia Garrison

SURGEON: Andy Martinez, MD

PREOPERATIVE DIAGNOSES:

1. Intrauterine pregnancy at 32 plus weeks
2. Insulin-dependent diabetes, type 1
3. Diabetic nephropathy

POSTPROCEDURE DIAGNOSES:

1. Intrauterine pregnancy at 32 plus weeks
2. Insulin-dependent diabetes, type 1
3. Diabetic nephropathy

DATE OF PROCEDURE:

PROCEDURE PERFORMED: Amniocentesis

ANESTHESIA: None

INDICATIONS: The patient is a 28-year-old with a complicated pregnancy who has been on bed rest because of diabetic nephropathy. Due to the fact that the fetus might be in a hostile environment, we felt that accelerated pulmonary maturity might be a possibility. Therefore, at this time we elected to go with amniocentesis to help us manage her pregnancy. She had been fully informed of the risks and benefits of the procedure prior to proceeding.

DESCRIPTION OF PROCEDURE: Ultrasound scanning was done by the technologist, and placenta was posterior. We prepped the abdomen and draped it. We used a sterile covered ultrasound transducer with guide and located a pocket of fluid. The 20-gauge needle was inserted. As we got into the uterus, the baby moved into the area; therefore the needle was immediately withdrawn. The fetus was palpated a little bit, and we stimulated the baby and it moved out of the area. We then repositioned the transducer and we were able to drop into the pocket of amniotic fluid and withdrew 20 cc of clear yellow amniotic fluid. The fluid was sent for maturity studies. The patient tolerated the procedure without difficulty.

SERVICE CODE(S): _____

ICD-10-CM DX CODE(S): _____

(Answers to every other Case are located in Appendix D . The full answer key is only available in the TEACH Instructor Resources on Evolve.)

CASE 11-9I *OB Ultrasound*

LOCATION: Inpatient, Hospital

PATIENT: Patricia Garrison

ATTENDING PHYSICIAN: Andy Martinez, MD

RADIOLOGIST: Morton Monson, MD

EXAMINATION OF: Obstetric ultrasound follow-up

CLINICAL SYMPTOMS: Fetal weight, umbilical artery Doppler, estimated menstrual age 34 weeks 2 days

OBSTETRICAL ULTRASOUND FINDINGS: Single active intrauterine gestation, cephalic presentation, longitudinal lie. Average sonographic gestational age is 34 weeks 4 days. Estimated fetal weight is 2345 g (gram).

Fetal cardiac activity at 158 beats per minute. Fetal motion was present during this study. Since the previous study, where the estimated sonographic gestational age was 9 weeks 3 days, there has been interval growth of 25 weeks 1 day in a 23-week 2-day interval. Umbilical arterial Doppler shows normal waveform with systolic/diastolic ratios of 2.1, 3.5, and 3.5. Normal-appearing amount of amniotic fluid. Amniotic fluid index measures 12.3 cm (centimeter), which is within normal limits. Placenta is in a posterior location with no evidence of placenta previa seen.

SERVICE CODE(S): _____

ICD-10-CM DX CODE(S): _____

(Answers to every other Case are located in Appendix D . The full answer key is only available in the TEACH Instructor Resources on Evolve.)

CASE 11-9J *Operative Report, Cesarean Section*

When this patient was admitted, Dr. Orbitz was the attending physician. Dr. Martinez was brought in as a consultant and then care was transferred from Dr. Orbitz to Dr. Martinez, who then became the attending. Dr. Martinez is performing the cesarean section and the necessary postpartum care. For the diagnoses, the record indicates there were complications of pregnancy, diabetic nephropathy, a cesarean delivery in addition to Z codes for the outcome of delivery and sterilization.

LOCATION: Inpatient, Hospital

PATIENT: Patricia Garrison

SURGEON: Andy Martinez, MD

PREOPERATIVE DIAGNOSES:

1. Intrauterine pregnancy, 33 weeks
2. Insulin-dependent diabetes with diabetic nephropathy
3. Desire for sterilization
4. Previous cesarean section

POSTOPERATIVE DIAGNOSES:

1. Intrauterine pregnancy, 33 weeks
2. Insulin-dependent diabetes with diabetic nephropathy
3. Desire for sterilization
4. Previous cesarean section

PROCEDURE PERFORMED:

1. Repeat low transverse cervical cesarean section
2. Bilateral tubal ligation

CASE 11-9J—cont'd

ANESTHESIA: Subarachnoid block

SURGICAL INDICATIONS: The patient is a 28-year-old gravida 2, para (to bring forth) 1 with an EDC (estimated date of conception) of 08/01, who had been hospitalized for the past several weeks with hypertension and diabetes. Her condition appeared to be worsening, her diabetes was suddenly poorly controlled, and she was having epigastric pain. Her platelet count and AST (aspartate aminotransferase [formerly SGOT]) was normal preoperatively. She had a previous C-section. She also desired permanent sterilization by tubal interruption.

OPERATIVE DESCRIPTION: After induction of subarachnoid block anesthesia, a Foley catheter was placed and the Venodynes were placed as well. The abdomen was prepped and draped. The abdomen was opened through a Pfannenstiel incision. When we separated the rectus muscles, it became apparent that there was very little room as there was so much scarring of the fascia; therefore, a Maylard incision was done by separating the bellies of the rectus muscles transversely. Retractors were placed over the bladder. There was a poor bladder flap, but we dissected some of the bladder downward. An incision was made in the low transverse part of the uterus and entering the uterus was accomplished by blunting with a Kelly clamp. A finger was introduced into the uterus to guide a bandage scissors for a low transverse incision. The infant's head was delivered through the incision, and the muscles were so tight that we were having a little difficulty extracting the head; therefore, I removed my hand and put a Murless retractor behind the head and then the baby was easily delivered. The cord was clamped and cut, and then a segment of cord was sent off for gases. The placenta was then delivered manually. The uterus was closed in two layers, first with a running locked 0 Vicryl, followed by a running horizontal Lembert 0 Vicryl. The pelvis was then irrigated with saline. A few small bleeders were bovie coagulated. The right fallopian tube was elevated and the fimbriated end identified. The mesosalpinx underneath the ampullary portion was opened with bovie, and then the lateral mesosalpinx was cross-clamped on the lateral tube. The lateral portion of the tube, including the fimbriated end, was then excised and pedicles were doubly tied with 2-0 Vicryl. An identical procedure was carried out on the left tube. With sponge and needle counts correct, attention was directed toward closure. The rectus muscles were closed with a series of mattress sutures of 0 Vicryl. A medium Hemovac drain was placed subfascially. The fascia was closed with running locked 0 Vicryl using two strands, one from either side to the middle and tied independently. The skin was then closed with staples, and the drain was sutured to the skin with silk.

BLOOD LOSS ESTIMATION: 400-500 cc (cubic centimeter)

SPECIMEN TO PATHOLOGY: Placenta

FINAL SPONGE AND NEEDLE COUNTS: Correct

The patient tolerated the procedure well and returned to the recovery room in stable condition. After the child was extracted, we did start some magnesium sulfate.

Pathology Report Later Indicated: See Report 11-9K.

SERVICE CODE(S): _____

ICD-10-CM DX CODE(S): _____

(Answers to every other Case are located in Appendix D . The full answer key is only available in the TEACH Instructor Resources on Evolve.)

CASE 11-9K *Pathology Report*

LOCATION: Inpatient, Hospital

PATIENT: Patricia Garrison

ATTENDING PHYSICIAN: Andy Martinez, MD

PATHOLOGIST: Grey Lonewolf, MD

CLINICAL HISTORY: Type 1 diabetic nephropathy, 33 weeks, unstable; hypertension, unstable; repeat C-section; desires sterilization

SPECIMEN RECEIVED: A: Placenta, third trimester. B: Left fallopian tube. C: Right fallopian tube.

GROSS DESCRIPTION: The specimens were received in three containers:

A. In the container labeled "placenta" is a discoid-shaped placenta measuring 17 × 17 × 3 cm (centimeter) in greatest dimension and weighing 410 g (gram). An umbilical cord measuring 7 cm in length inserts 4 cm from the closest margin. The membranes are smooth, shiny, tan-gray, and translucent. The chorionic surface is unremarkable. On the maternal surface, lacerations extend from short distance into the parenchyma. The parenchyma is uniformly spongy and pink-red on sectioning. On sectioning, the umbilical cord demonstrates three vessels. Multiple representative sections of placenta, umbilical cord, and membranes are submitted.

B. In the container labeled "left tube" is a cylindrical tan tissue segment measuring 2.8 cm in length and 0.6 cm in diameter. The specimen is step-sectioned and totally submitted as "B."

C. In the container labeled "right tube" is a cylindrical tan tissue segment measuring 2.8 cm in length and 0.8 cm in diameter. The specimen is step-sectioned and totally submitted as "C."

MICROSCOPIC DESCRIPTION:

A. The umbilical cord demonstrates three vessels within a normal supporting Wharton's jelly. The placenta demonstrates well-vascularized third-trimester villi. The membranes show normal morphology.
B. The left fallopian tube demonstrates normal morphology. (1 specimen)
C. The right fallopian tube demonstrates normal morphology. (1 specimen)

DIAGNOSIS:

A. Placenta, umbilical cord, and membranes: No pathologic diagnosis.
B. Left fallopian tube segment: No pathologic diagnosis.
C. Right fallopian tube segment: No pathologic diagnosis.

SERVICE CODE(S): _____

ICD-10-CM DX CODE(S): _____

(Answers to every other Case are located in Appendix D . The full answer key is only available in the TEACH Instructor Resources on Evolve.)

CHAPTER 11 *Auditing Review*

Audit the coding for the following reports.

Audit Report 11.1 Operative Report, Hysterectomy

LOCATION: Inpatient, Hospital

PATIENT: Angela Swenson

SURGEON: Andy Martinez, MD

PREOPERATIVE DIAGNOSIS: Endometrial carcinoma.

POSTOPERATIVE DIAGNOSIS: Same.

PROCEDURE PERFORMED: Total laparoscopic hysterectomy with laparoscopic staging, including para-aortic lymphadenectomy, bilateral pelvic and obturator lymphadenectomy, and washings.

ANESTHESIA: General, endotracheal tube.

HISTORY: The patient was recently found to have a grade II endometrial cancer. She was counseled to undergo laparoscopic staging. During the laparoscopy, the uterus was noted to be upper limits of normal size, with normal-appearing right fallopian tubes and ovaries. No ascites was present. On assessment of the upper abdomen, the stomach, diaphragm, liver, gallbladder, spleen, omentum, and peritoneal surfaces of the bowel were all unremarkable in appearance.

DESCRIPTION OF PROCEDURE: The patient was brought into the operating room with an intravenous line in place, and anesthetic was administered. She was placed in a low anterior lithotomy position using Allen stirrups. The vaginal portion of the procedure included placement of a ZUMI uterine manipulator with a Koh colpotomy ring and a vaginal occluder balloon. The laparoscopic port sites were anesthetized with intradermal injection of 0.25% Marcaine. There were five ports placed, including a 3-mm left subcostal port, a 10-mm umbilical port, a 10-mm suprapubic port, and 5-mm right and left lower quadrant ports. The Veress needle was placed through a small incision at the base of the umbilicus, and a pneumoperitoneum was insufflated without difficulty. The 3-mm port was then placed in the left subcostal position without difficulty, and a 3-mm scope was placed. There were no adhesions underlying the previous vertical midline scar. The 10-mm port was placed in the umbilicus, and the laparoscope was inserted. Remaining ports were placed under direct laparoscopic guidance. Washings were obtained from the pelvis, and the abdomen was explored with the laparoscope, with findings as noted.

Attention was then turned to lymphadenectomy. An incision in the retroperitoneum was made over the right common iliac artery, extending up the aorta to the retroperitoneal duodenum. The lymph node bundle was elevated from the aorta and the anterior vena cava until the retroperitoneal duodenum had been reached. Pedicles were sealed and divided with bipolar cutting forceps. Excellent hemostasis was noted. Boundaries of dissection included the ureters laterally, common iliac arteries at uterine crossover inferiorly, and the retroperitoneal duodenum superiorly with careful preservation of the inferior mesenteric artery. Right and left pelvic retroperitoneal spaces were then opened by incising lateral and parallel to the infundibulopelvic ligament with the bipolar cutting forceps. The retroperitoneal space was then opened and the lymph nodes were dissected, with boundaries of dissection being the bifurcation of the common iliac artery superiorly, psoas muscle laterally, inguinal ligament inferiorly, and the anterior division of the hypogastric artery medially. The posterior boundary was the obturator nerve, which was carefully identified and preserved bilaterally. The left common iliac lymph node was elevated and removed using the same technique.

Attention was then turned to the laparoscopic hysterectomy. The right infundibulopelvic ligament was divided using the bipolar cutting forceps. The mesovarium was skeletonized. A bladder flap was mobilized by dividing the round ligaments using the bipolar cutting forceps, and the peritoneum on the vesicouterine fold was incised to mobilize the bladder. Once the Koh colpotomy ring was skeletonized and in position, the uterine arteries were sealed using the bipolar forceps at the level of the colpotomy ring. The vagina was transected using a monopolar hook (or bipolar spatula), resulting in separation of the uterus and attached tubes and ovaries. The uterus, tubes, and ovaries were then delivered through the vagina, and the pneumo-occluder balloon was reinserted to maintain pneumoperitoneum. The vaginal vault was closed with interrupted figure-of-eight stitches of 0-Vicryl using the Endo-Stitch device. The abdomen was irrigated, and excellent hemostasis was noted. The insufflation pressure was reduced, and no evidence of bleeding was seen. The suprapubic port was then removed, and the fascia was closed with a Carter-Thomason device and 0-Vicryl suture. The remaining ports were removed under direct laparoscopic guidance, and the pneumoperitoneum was released. The umbilical port was removed using laparoscopic guidance. The umbilical fascia was closed with an interrupted figure-of-eight stitch using 2-0 Vicryl. The skin was closed with interrupted subcuticular stitches using 4-0 Monocryl suture. The final sponge, needle, and instrument counts were correct at the completion of the procedure. The patient was awakened and taken to the postanesthesia care unit in stable condition.

One or more of the following codes are reported incorrectly for this case. Indicate the incorrect code or codes.

PROFESSIONAL SERVICES: Laparoscopic radical hysterectomy with bilateral total pelvic lymphadenectomy and para-aortic lymph node sampling, with removal of tubes and ovaries, **58548**

ICD-10-CM DX: Cancer of the endometrium, **C53.1**

INCORRECT CODE(S): _____

Audit Report 11.2 Operative Report, Hysteroscopy with Polypectomy

LOCATION: Inpatient, Hospital

PATIENT: Elizabeth Coe

SURGEON: Andy Martinez, MD

PREOPERATIVE DIAGNOSIS: Postmenopausal bleeding with probable polyp seen on saline sonohistogram.

POSTOPERATIVE DIAGNOSIS: Postmenopausal bleeding with endometrial polyp seen at hysteroscopy.

PROCEDURE PERFORMED: Hysteroscopy with polypectomy and dilation and curettage.

PREAMBLE: The patient is a 59-year-old postmenopausal woman seen with persistent postmenopausal bleeding. She had an endometrial biopsy carried out two years ago which showed benign nonsecretory endometrium. She had a saline sonohistogram carried out which showed evidence of uterine fibroids, but also 1 cm endometrial lesion suspicious for polyp. Decision was, therefore, made to proceed with hysteroscopy for polypectomy and dilation and curettage.

OPERATIVE FINDINGS: Endometrial polyp seen arising from the left cornual region. Otherwise, benign uterine cavity.

PROCEDURE: The patient was taken to the operating room, and a general anesthetic was administered. The patient was then prepped and draped in the usual manner in lithotomy position, and the bladder was emptied with a straight catheter.

A weighted speculum was placed to allow for visualization of the cervix, which was grasped anteriorly using single toothed tenaculum. The uterus was then sounded to 9 cm in depth. The cervix was dilated to allow for insertion of the diagnostic hysteroscope. The uterine cavity was then inspected. Immediately apparent was a polyp arising from the left cornual region. Remainder of uterine cavity was inspected and appeared to be benign. Minimal endometrial tissue was otherwise present.

At this point then, the hysteroscope was removed, and polyp forceps was placed within the uterus. Attempt was made to grasp the polyp, but this could not be grabbed with the polyp forceps. Therefore, a sharp curet

was used, and the polyp was thereby obtained and removed. A small amount of endometrial tissue was also obtained by curettage. Once this had been completed, the hysteroscope was reinserted and the cavity was reinspected. It was confirmed that the polyp was removed. Otherwise, the endometrial canal then appeared normal. At this point, the procedure was terminated. Tenaculum was removed and good hemostasis was ensured at the cervix. The patient tolerated this procedure well. There were no complications. Fluid in was 325 cc and was equal to fluid out at the end of the procedure. Estimated blood loss was minimal.

One or more codes should not have been reported for this case. Indicate the code(s) incorrectly reported.

PROFESSIONAL SERVICES: Hysteroscopy with polypectomy and D&C, **58558**; Hysterosalpingography, **74740-26**

ICD-10-CM DX: Postmenopausal bleeding, **N95.0**; Endometrial polyp, **N84.0**

INCORRECTLY REPORTED CODE(S): _____

Audit Report 11.3 Operative Report, Cesarean Section

Report Dr. Sanchez's delivery service.

LOCATION: Inpatient, Hospital

PATIENT: Patricia Garrison

ATTENDING PHYSICIAN: Andy Martinez, MD

SURGEON: Andy Martinez, MD

PREOPERATIVE DIAGNOSES:

1. Term intrauterine pregnancy.
2. Fetal pelvic disproportion.

POSTOPERATIVE DIAGNOSES: Same.

PROCEDURE PERFORMED: Primary low transverse cervical cesarean section

ANESTHESIA: Lumbar epidural

SURGICAL INDICATIONS: The patient is a 27-year-old primigravida who had been admitted for labor induction by myself. She had very slow progress in the desultory, latent, and early active phase and arrested at 4-5 cm and, at most, -2 station. This was despite good contractions with internal uterine pressure catheter.

OPERATIVE FINDINGS: The infant was a male weighing 3180 g (7 pounds 0.2 ounces) with Apgar scores of 9 at one minute and 9 at five minutes. The amniotic fluid was clear. The tubes and ovaries were normal. The infant had barely gotten into the pelvis and was occiput posterior. There was a degree of deflection of the fetal head as well.

OPERATIVE DESCRIPTION: The patient had a lumbar epidural during labor, and this was topped off. Foley catheter was placed as well as Venodynes. The patient was prepped and draped. The abdomen was opened through a Pfannenstiel incision. The bladder flap was opened, and the bladder dissected downward with the hand. A small incision

was made in the myometrium of the lower uterine segment, and then entry into the uterus was accomplished with blunt dissection using a Kelly clamp. A finger was introduced into the uterus to guide a bandage scissors for a low transverse incision. The infant was then delivered, and the mouth and nose were suctioned with a bulb syringe, cord was clamped and cut, and the infant handed to the ICN staff. The placenta was delivered manually. The uterus was closed in two layers, first with a running locked 0 Vicryl and then a running horizontal Lembert 0 Vicryl, the first layer using two strands, one from either side to the middle and tied independently. There was a little extra bleeding from the left side of the uterine incision that was secured with a figure-of-eight 0 Vicryl. The pelvis was then irrigated with saline. The uterine incision was reinspected and was dry. With sponge and needle counts correct, attention was directed toward closure. The peritoneum was loosely approximated in the midline with three mattress sutures of 2-0 Vicryl. A medium Hemovac drain was placed subfascially. The fascia was closed with running 0 Vicryl using two strands, one from either side to the middle and tied independently. The skin was closed with staples and the drain sutured to the skin with silk. A sterile dressing was applied. Blood loss estimation was 800 to 1000 cc. Specimen to pathology: None. Final sponge and needle counts correct. The patient tolerated the procedure well and returned to the recovery room in stable condition.

One of the codes is not reported for this case. Indicate the missing code.

PROFESSIONAL SERVICES: Cesarean delivery, **59515**

ICD-10-CM DX: Cesarean section for inertia of uterus during active phase, **062.1**; Obstructed labor due to occipitoposterior position, **O64.0XX0**

MISSING CODE: _____

Continued

CHAPTER 11—cont'd

Audit Report 11.4 Operative Report, Hysteroscopy

LOCATION: Inpatient, Hospital

PATIENT: Margaret Hill

ATTENDING PHYSICIAN: Ronald Green, MD

SURGEON: Andy Martinez, MD

PREOPERATIVE DIAGNOSIS: Postmenopausal bleeding

POSTOPERATIVE DIAGNOSIS: Postmenopausal bleeding

PROCEDURE PERFORMED: Hysteroscopy with fractional dilatation and curettage

ANESTHESIA: General endotracheal

ESTIMATED BLOOD LOSS: Less than 25 cc

IRRIGATION: 400 cc used, 400 cc recovered

FLUIDS: 1,000 cc

FINDINGS: Uterus sounded to 4 inches and the cervix descends to the opening. The patient has a second-degree cystocele and a first-degree rectocele with gaping introitus.

PROCEDURE: The patient was prepped and draped in the lithotomy position under general endotracheal anesthesia, and the bladder was straight catheterized. A weighted speculum was placed in the vagina and the anterior lip of the cervix was grasped with a single-toothed tenaculum. The Kevorkian curet was then used to obtain endocervical curettings. The uterus was then sounded to a depth of 4 inches. The cervical os was then dilated to allow passage of the hysteroscope. The hysteroscope was then used to document intrauterine morphology. There was an endometrial polyp present. The cervical os was then serially dilated further to allow passage of a sharp curet. Stone polyp forceps were used to remove the endometrial polyp. The sharp curet was then used to sample the endometrial cavity, with scant return of tissue. The tenaculum was removed from the cervix. The tenaculum site was oversewn with 3-0 chromic figure-of-eight suture. The weighted speculum was removed from the vagina. All sponges and needles were accounted for at the completion of the procedure. The patient tolerated the procedure well, and when she left my care, she was doing well. The patient was then turned over to Dr. Sanchez for the gallbladder surgery.

PATHOLOGY REPORT LATER INDICATED: Benign endometrial polyp

One or more of the following codes are reported incorrectly for this case. Indicate the incorrect code or codes.

SERVICE CODE(S): Hysteroscopy, **58555;** Dilation and curettage, **58120-51**

ICD-10-CM DX CODE(S): Postmenopausal bleeding, **N95.0**

INCORRECT/MISSING CODE(S): _____

Audit Report 11.5 Operative Report, Hysterectomy

LOCATION: Inpatient, Hospital

PATIENT: Brenda Black

ATTENDING PHYSICIAN: Andy Martinez, MD

SURGEON: Andy Martinez, MD

PREOPERATIVE DIAGNOSIS: Marked atypical endometrium hyperplasia

POSTOPERATIVE DIAGNOSIS: Marked atypical endometrium hyperplasia

PROCEDURE PERFORMED: Total abdominal hysterectomy with lysis.

FINDINGS: Small bowel adherent to anterior abdominal wall, ovaries and tubes absent bilaterally.

PROCEDURE: The patient was prepped and draped in the supine position under general endotracheal anesthesia with Foley catheter indwelling. A vertical incision was made in the lower abdomen. The fascia was divided in the midline, and the peritoneum was entered in a sharp manner and the incision extended vertically. Pelvic washings were obtained for cytology. The patient had the small bowel that was adherent to the right lateral side wall, which may have been impacted by an abdominal retractor. The small bowel was then lifted and a window was noticed between the small bowel and the peritoneum, and this was incised with Metzenbaum scissors without difficulty. The bowel was then packed out of the operative field using a self-retaining retractor and laparotomy sponges. The uterus was then grasped and elevated. There were no tubes and ovaries noted bilaterally. The round ligaments were cross-clamped, divided, and ligated with 0 Vicryl suture ligature. The bladder flap was created using sharp and blunt dissection and reflected inferiorly. The uterine vessels were then skeletonized, doubly clamped, divided and ligated with 0 Vicryl suture ligature times two. The bladder flap was advanced from the operative field. The broad ligaments were cross-clamped, divided, and ligated with 0 Vicryl suture ligature in a stepwise fashion down to uterosacral cardinal ligament complex. The vagina was entered from the right side. The vagina was incised immediately adjacent to the cervix, and the surgical specimen was removed intact and sent out for frozen pathologic evaluation. The vaginal angles were sutured to the uterosacral cardinal ligament complex for support using 0 Vicryl modified Richardson suture. The vaginal cuff was whip stitched using Vicryl interlocking suture. The vaginal cuff was reapproximated using 0 Vicryl interrupted figure-of-eight sutures. The operative site was inspected, irrigated, and was hemostatic. The right ureter could be easily traced throughout its course. The left ureter was more obscure but did not appear to be involved in the surgical site. After irrigation, the sponge and instruments were removed from the abdominal cavity. The omentum was brought down anteriorly. The fascia and peritoneum were reapproximated using 0 Vicryl interrupted internal retention sutures. The fascia was then reapproximated using 0 PDS continuous suture. At the completion of suturing with the PDS, the 0 Vicryl internal retentions were then secured. The operative site was irrigated. The Bovie was used for hemostasis. The skin was reapproximated with staples. A pressure dressing was applied. All sponge and needles were accounted for at the completion of the procedure. The patient left the operating room in apparent good condition, having tolerated the procedure well. The Foley catheter was patent and draining clear yellow urine at the completion of the procedure.

PATHOLOGY REPORT LATER INDICATED:

1. Hyperplasia of uterus endometrium
2. Intramural leiomyoma of uterus (this is a benign tumor)
3. Endometrial polyp
4. Nabothian cyst of cervix
5. Adenomyosis of uterus

One or more of the following codes are reported incorrectly for this case. Indicate the incorrect code or codes.

SERVICE CODE(S): Myomectomy, **58140**

ICD-10-CM DX CODE(S): Endometrial hyperplasia, **N85.00**

INCORRECT/MISSING CODE(S): _____

CHAPTER 11—cont'd

Audit Report 11.6 Operative Report, Sterilization

LOCATION: Inpatient, Hospital

PATIENT: Tara Loud

ATTENDING PHYSICIAN: Andy Martinez, MD

SURGEON: Gary Sanchez, MD

PREOPERATIVE DIAGNOSIS: Desire for sterilization

POSTOPERATIVE DIAGNOSIS: Desire for sterilization

PROCEDURE PERFORMED: Bilateral tubal ligation, modified Pomeroy technique

ANESTHESIA: General

INDICATION: The patient is a 32-year-old gravida 3, para 3, who underwent spontaneous vaginal delivery yesterday and affirmed her request for permanent sterilization. Risks and benefits of surgery were discussed with the patient and she elected to proceed with the surgery.

TECHNIQUE: The patient was taken to the operating room where epidural anesthesia was found to be inadequate, and she was therefore given general anesthesia, prepped and draped in the normal sterile fashion. An approximately 15-mm transverse infra-umbilical incision was made with the scalpel, and blunt dissection to the fascia was made with Kelly clamp. The fascia was grasped between two Kocher clamps, tented up, and entered sharply. The incision was extended bilaterally for about 10 mm. Then the peritoneum was identified, grasped with two hemostats, tented up, and entered sharply to expose the uterus. Then the right fallopian tube was identified, grasped with a Babcock clamp, walked out to its fimbriated end, re-grasped approximately 3 cm from the corneal region, and the avascular portion of the mesosalpinx was identified and perforated under the fallopian tube with a Mosquito. A length of 0 plain gut was drawn back through the proximal followed by distal ends, and an approximately 3-cm segment of tube was tied and the intervening segment of fallopian tube was excised. The luminal ends were identified and found to be hemostatic. Then a similar procedure was carried out on the left. Following this, the fascia was closed in a running fashion with 0 Vicryl, and the skin was reapproximated with 4-0 Vicryl in subcuticular stitch. The patient tolerated the procedure well. Sponge, lap, and needle counts were correct. The patient was taken to recovery in stable condition.

One or more of the following codes are reported incorrectly for this case. Indicate the incorrect code or codes.

SERVICE CODE(S): Fallopian tube ligation, **58600-50**

ICD-10-CM DX CODE(S): Triplet pregnancy, **O30.109**

INCORRECT/MISSING CODE(S): _____

(Auditing Review answers with rationales are only available in the TEACH Instructor Resources on Evolve.)

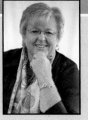

"There is always room in coding for development! If you have an outpatient coding certification, prepare for another type of certification. Keep expanding your skills by learning about other areas of coding."

Nervous System

http://evolve.elsevier.com/Buck/next

(Answers to every other Case are located in Appendix D, with the full answer key only available in the TEACH Instructor Resources on Evolve)
(Auditing Review answers with rationales are only available in the TEACH Instructor Resources on Evolve)

The nervous system is divided into the sympathetic nervous system and the parasympathetic nervous system, as illustrated in **Figures 12-1** and **12-2**. A **neurologist** is a physician who treats and diagnoses conditions of the nervous system, including the spinal cord, brain, nerves, and muscles. Common neurologic disorders are dizziness, tremor, paresthesia (abnormal touch sensation), stroke, altered mental states, headache, seizure, sleep disorders, and neuralgia. The neurologist uses a variety of diagnostic tools, including magnetic resonance imaging (MRI), computed axial tomography (CAT or CT), electroencephalography (EEG), and EMG/NCV (electromyography/nerve conduction velocity). A **neurosurgeon** is a surgeon who specializes in surgical procedures or treatment of conditions of the nervous system, such as lumbar puncture, brain tumor, head injury, hematoma, and disc herniation.

Twist Drill or Burr Holes

Twist drill or burr holes are the opening of the skull to relieve pressure, to insert monitoring devices, or to place tubing or inject contrast material. The placement of these holes leaves the skull intact except for the hole, which is repaired at a later time. This procedure is also termed "trephine." The CPT codes for these procedures (61105-61253) are based on the reason for the hole (such as implantation of catheter or pressure device, biopsy, aspiration of hematoma, etc.) and, in some instances, the location of the hole (such as supratentorial or infratentorial). The tentorium is a tented sheet of dura mater that covers the cerebellum. **Supratentorial** is above the tentorium of the cerebellum and **infratentorial** is beneath the tentorium of the cerebellum. For the purposes of coding, supratentorial is the part of the brain above the cerebellum, and infratentorial is the part of the brain beneath the cerebellum.

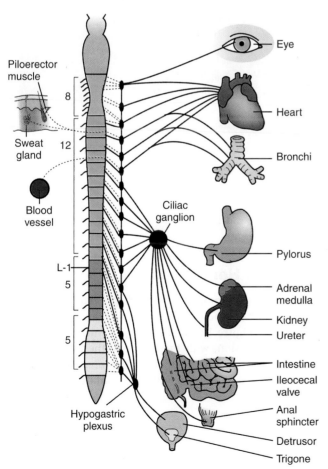

FIGURE 12–1 Sympathetic nervous system.

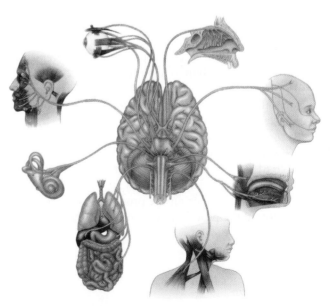

FIGURE 12–2 Parasympathetic nervous system.

CASE 12-1   *Operative Report, Ventriculostomy*

Dick is a patient in the intensive care unit of the hospital. He has an obstructive hydrocephalus as a result of an intracerebral hemorrhage. Report the services of Dr. Pleasant.

LOCATION: Inpatient, Hospital

PATIENT: Dick Dawn

ATTENDING PHYSICIAN: Timothy Pleasant, MD

SURGEON: Timothy Pleasant, MD

PREPROCEDURE DIAGNOSIS: Obstructive hydrocephalus, secondary to intracerebral hemorrhage

POSTPROCEDURE DIAGNOSIS: Obstructive hydrocephalus, secondary to intracerebral hemorrhage

PROCEDURE PERFORMED: Ventriculostomy

OPERATIVE NOTE: While in the intensive care unit, the patient was noted to be deteriorating neurologically and suffering from obstructive hydrocephalus. The right side of the scalp was shaved, prepped, and draped in the usual sterile manner. A small incision was made in the midpupillary line approximately 10 cm (centimeter) behind the supraorbital rim. The standard hole was then fashioned. The dura was then punctured, and a catheter was inserted uneventfully into the right lateral ventricle. Bloody CSF (cerebrospinal fluid) was immediately obtained and was noted to be under high pressure. It was then externalized through the subcutaneous tissue and through another wound. The original wound was then sutured, and a sterile dressing was applied. There were no operative complications.

SERVICE CODE(S): _____

ICD-10-CM DX CODE(S): _____

(Answers to every other Case are located in Appendix D . The full answer key is only available in the TEACH Instructor Resources on Evolve.)

Craniotomy

A **craniotomy** is the surgical removal of a section of bone and is referred to as a **bone flap (Figure 12-3).** Removal of the bone is done in preparation for an operative procedure of the brain. The removed bone is returned to the original site at the end of the procedure. If tissue or bone is removed and not returned to the original site, the procedure is a craniectomy. For example, when a blood clot is removed and the bone flap is replaced, that is a craniotomy. If, however, a portion of the brain was removed due to a disease or condition, the procedure is a craniectomy. The craniotomy or craniectomy is performed for conditions such as trauma, infection, tumor, and aneurysm.

Codes 61510-61530 report the removal or treatment of brain tumor(s), abscess, or cyst in which a portion of the skull bone is removed, procedure performed, bone replaced, and the bone then stabilized in place **(Figure 12-5).**

- 61510-61516 are used to report these types of procedures when they are performed supratentorially (above the tentorium of the cerebellum).
- 61518-61524 are used when performed infratentorially (below the tentorium of the cerebellum).
- 61526-61530 are used when performed transtemporally (across the temporal lobe).

If stealth is used during the procedure, it is reported in addition to the procedure with 61781 if the procedure is intradural and 61782 if the procedure is extradural. A full description of stealth is presented before Case 12-3.

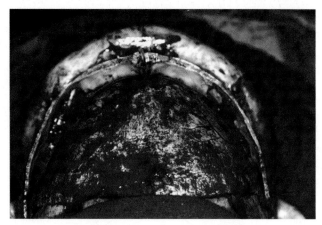

FIGURE 12-3 Craniotomy.

Subdural Hematoma

A subdural **hematoma** is a hemorrhage characterized by a collection of blood between the dura mater and the arachnoid membrane **(Figure 12-4).** A subdural hematoma is often a result of contusion, with the source of the bleeding being an artery or vein. If the hematoma ruptures the arachnoid membrane, the condition is termed **subdural hygroma.**

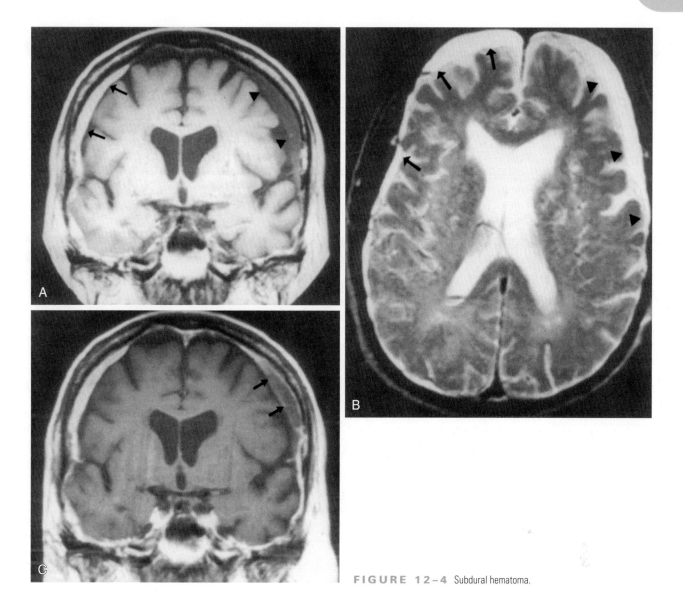

FIGURE 12–4 Subdural hematoma.

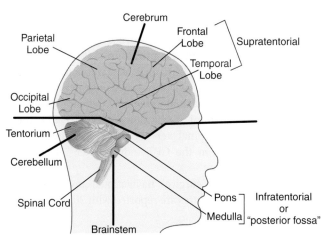

FIGURE 12–5 Cerebral hemisphere and tentorium.

Subdural hematomas caused by trauma (such as head injuries) are categorized according to the presentation after injury: hyperacute (less than 24 hours), acute (1-3 days), early subacute (3-7 days), late subacute (more than 7 days), or chronic (more than 3 weeks). Other causes of subdural hematoma are artery or vein abnormalities (arteriovenous malformation) as a result of shunting procedures or a lumbar puncture, neoplasm, hypertension, hemodialysis, intracranial operations, infections, or as a result of bleeding disorder (such as hemophilia).

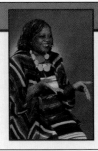

From the Trenches

"Passing the exam is the first step. Getting into a particular specialty, perfecting it, and becoming experienced will enable you to obtain a higher salary in the future. EXPERIENCE is key!"

HARVEY L. JOHNSON
CPC, CPMA, CBCS, CEHRS

CASE 12-2 | *Operative Report, Osteoplastic Craniotomy*

The following craniotomy is for the purpose of removal of a subdural hematoma.

LOCATION: Inpatient, Hospital

PATIENT: Larry Colter

ATTENDING PHYSICIAN: Timothy Pleasant, MD

SURGEON: Timothy Pleasant, MD

PREOPERATIVE DIAGNOSIS: Acute subdural hematoma, left side

POSTOPERATIVE DIAGNOSIS: Acute subdural hematoma, left side

PROCEDURE PERFORMED: Osteoplastic craniotomy

ANESTHESIA: General anesthesia

PROCEDURE: Under general anesthesia, the left head was prepped and draped in the usual manner after having been placed in Mayfield pins. Hemoclips and Dandy clips were utilized on the scalp edges.

Part of the temporalis muscle was taken down. Two burr holes and a circumferential flap were made. The bone was elevated. The dura was incised in an inverted U-shaped fashion. We saw acute clot; probably 45-50 cc of clot was irrigated from the frontal, temporal, and posterior parietal areas (indicates supratentorial; *see* Figure 12-2). Having cleaned it out, there was no free bleeder that I saw. I placed a piece of Gelfoam on the brain and then began closure of the dura with 3-0 Vicryl; this was done. A little patch was necessary; we used temporalis fascia. We tacked up the dura, replaced the bone flap, and utilized Wurzburg plates and burr hole cover. Having secured this, we then closed the scalp with 2-0 Vicryl on the galea with surgical staples on the skin, with a Hemovac drain having been applied prior to closure.

SERVICE CODE(S): _____

ICD-10-CM DX CODE(S): _____

(Answers to every other Case are located in Appendix D . The full answer key is only available in the TEACH Instructor Resources on Evolve.)

Stealth Surgery

Stealth surgery is computer-assisted surgery that produces three-dimensional images and uses infrared intraoperative guidance, which enables location of tumors of the brain and spinal cord with great accuracy. The technology is the same as that of the B22 Stealth Bomber. A CT of the patient's brain is input into the stealth computer to use as a road map during surgery. The computer tracks the surgical instruments being used by the surgeon during the operation by means of an infrared sensor that is located over the operating table. The computer then translates these instrument movements into a three-dimensional image for the surgeon to view. There is a red *x* located on the screen indicating the location of the tumor or area of damage. The technology is accurate to within 1 mm and greatly decreases damage to the brain during these invasive procedures. When stealth technology is utilized during a procedure (and the technology is used with a wide variety of procedures, not just brain surgery), you report the use of the technology in addition to the primary procedure. This technology is referred to in the CPT manual as stereotaxis, which is the method used to precisely locate areas of the brain. There are two codes to report cranial stereotaxis, depending on if the procedure was intradural or extradural (61781/61782). There is one code to report spinal stereotaxis (61783). The code for sterotaxis is located in the CPT index under "Stereotaxis, Computer Assisted."

Computer-assisted surgical navigational procedures for musculoskeletal procedures are reported with 20985.

CASE 12-3A   *Operative Report, Craniectomy*

The label of a procedure (such as, craniectomy or craniotomy) does not mean that the title is the exact procedure. The following procedure is the removal of a tumor and an intracranial clot by means of a craniectomy. Sometimes, the report title might state craniotomy when a craniectomy was performed. Only careful reading of the entire report will reveal the exact procedure and ensure accurate coding. See Figure 12-6 for location of ventricle.

LOCATION: Inpatient, Hospital

PATIENT: Erika Witt

ATTENDING PHYSICIAN: Timothy Pleasant, MD

SURGEON: Timothy Pleasant, MD

PREOPERATIVE DIAGNOSIS: Recurrent tumor, intracranial clot

POSTOPERATIVE DIAGNOSIS: Recurrent tumor, intracranial clot

PROCEDURE PERFORMED: Craniotomy, removal of tumor, and removal of intracranial clot

ANESTHESIA: General

PREOPERATIVE NOTE: This patient has been forewarned about her condition and that we are operating on a marginally reserve patient, that we do not know what the results will be but will certainly try to remove the tumor and the clot to improve the situation.

This case was done under Stealth protocol (reported separately). We utilized a localizer, and we were able to show that the tumor cavity was totally entered and the tumor and clot were removed.

PROCEDURE: Under general anesthesia, the patient was placed in Mayfield pins. The head was prepped and draped in the usual manner. An inverted U-shaped incision was made. The previous craniotomy was opened up, and the dura was incised. We got into the ventricle. We removed what looked like yellow tumor, which was necrotic tissue. We removed a large intracranial clot as well and cleaned out the ventricular area. There was tumor or clot in the temporal lobe as well as in the lateral ventricle. I could see the foramen of Monro. I could clean out the entire cavity. This wound was irrigated; on the raw surface a piece of Gelfoam was placed after coagulation was achieved. The dura was then closed with Duragen. The bone flap was replaced with 22 wires, and the scalp wound was then closed in layers with 3-0 Vicryl on the galea and surgical staples on the skin. A dressing was applied. The patient was discharged to the recovery area.

Pathology Report Later Indicated: See 12-3B.

SERVICE CODE(S): _____

ICD-10-CM DX CODE(S): _____

(Answers to every other Case are located in Appendix D . The full answer key is only available in the TEACH Instructor Resources on Evolve.)

CASE 12-3B   *Pathology Report*

LOCATION: Inpatient, Hospital

PATIENT: Erika Witt

ATTENDING PHYSICIAN: Timothy Pleasant, MD

SURGEON: Timothy Pleasant, MD

PATHOLOGIST: Grey Lonewolf, MD

CLINICAL HISTORY: Recurrent meningioma with intracerebral hemorrhage

SPECIMEN RECEIVED: Meningioma

GROSS DESCRIPTION:

The specimen is labeled with the patient's name and "meningioma" and consists predominantly of blood clot with a few fragments of gray-tan lobulated tissue, 1 and 5 cm (centimeter) in greatest dimension. Representative sections are submitted in 6 cassettes.

MICROSCOPIC DESCRIPTION:

Sections of brain show areas of reactive gliosis with associated focal fibrosis, hemosiderin-laden macrophages, and foamy macrophages. Areas of recent hemorrhage with blood clot and focal areas of necrosis are also seen. A neoplastic infiltrate is not identified.

DIAGNOSIS:

Brain, frontal cortex, excision: Benign brain tumor showing reactive gliosis with areas of fibrosis, foamy macrophages, and foci of necrosis and accompanying blood clot.

SERVICE CODE(S): _____

ICD-10-CM DX CODE(S): _____

(Answers to every other Case are located in Appendix D . The full answer key is only available in the TEACH Instructor Resources on Evolve.)

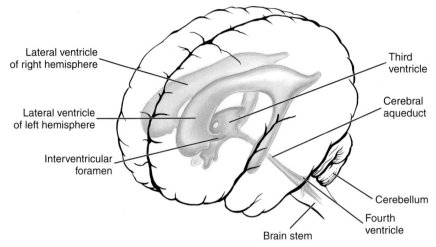

FIGURE 12-6 Ventricles of the brain.

CASE 12-4 | *Operative Report, Craniotomy*

The removal of this tumor is conducted through a bone flap.

LOCATION: Inpatient, Hospital

PATIENT: Arlene Samuels

ATTENDING PHYSICIAN: Timothy Pleasant, MD

SURGEON: Timothy Pleasant, MD

PREOPERATIVE DIAGNOSIS: Right temporal parietal frontal brain tumor

POSTOPERATIVE DIAGNOSIS: Glioblastoma multiforme

PROCEDURE PERFORMED: Osteoplastic craniotomy with removal of tumor in temporal lobe, frontal lobe, and middle cerebral artery complex (contiguous [adjoining] sites).

ANESTHESIA: General

PROCEDURE: Under general anesthesia, the patient's head was prepped and draped in the usual manner. A question mark incision was made in the front of the ear up to the frontal area. The skin flap was turned down. The temporalis muscle was incised. We then did an osteoplastic craniotomy with burr holes and craniotome. The flap was turned. The dura was incised. We then made an incision into the superior temporal lobe. The plan was to resect the temporal lobe to get into the tumor and stay away from the middle cerebral complex and also to decompress her on the frontal lobe as well since the tumor was going into the frontal lobe. I got into the tumor and sent specimen for biopsy and then began the gradual dissection. I encountered some bleeding, probably from middle cerebral artery branches. I had to take a few with silver clips, perhaps two to three. Otherwise, we left the sylvian vein intact and decompressed the area (decompression is bundled into tumor removal). We got into the tumor cavity and took as much visual tumor as we could. The bed was then dried. I irrigated the wound well. I placed a piece of Gelfoam over the raw surface of the brain and began closure of the dura with 3-0 Vicryl. The bone flap was replaced with two straight four-holed Wurzburg plates. Hemovac was placed, and the scalp was closed in layers utilizing 3-0 Vicryl on the galea with surgical staples on the skin. Dressing was applied. The patient was discharged to PAR (postanesthesia recovery).

Pathology Report Later Indicated: Glioblastoma multiforme

SERVICE CODE(S): _____

ICD-10-CM DX CODE(S): _____

(Answers to every other Case are located in Appendix D . The full answer key is only available in the TEACH Instructor Resources on Evolve.)

CASE 12-5 *Operative Report, Pterygocraniotomy and Cranioplasty*

An operating microscope is used in this procedure and is reported separately. Simple aneurysms are any that are 15 millimeters or less.

LOCATION: Inpatient, Hospital

PATIENT: Brett Richards

ATTENDING PHYSICIAN: Timothy Pleasant, MD

SURGEON: Timothy Pleasant, MD

PREOPERATIVE DIAGNOSIS: Subarachnoid hemorrhage secondary to right posterior communicating artery aneurysm

POSTOPERATIVE DIAGNOSIS: Subarachnoid hemorrhage secondary to right posterior communicating artery aneurysm, 12 mm (millimeter)

PROCEDURE PERFORMED: Right pterygocraniotomy with microsurgical clipping of right posterior communicating artery aneurysm and cranioplasty

DESCRIPTION OF PROCEDURE: The patient was taken to the operating room and placed under general endotracheal anesthesia. The right scalp (This indicates an intracranial approach as versus a cervical approach.) was then shaved, prepped, and draped in the usual sterile manner. A modified Souttar bicoronal incision was then outlined in the skin and subcutaneous tissue and was infiltrated with lidocaine with epinephrine. The skin was incised, and sharp dissection was carried through subcutaneous tissue. LeRoy-Raney clips were then applied to the skin edges and the galeacutaneous flap was elevated and reflected anteriorly. Temporalis muscle was then incised and reflected anteriorly, and a free bone flap was fashioned using a Midas burr. A generous craniectomy was carried out on the squamous portion of the temporal bone and the lateral sphenoid wing. Twenty-five grams of mannitol had been given prior to skin incision, and dura was noted to be moderately tense. A horseshoe-shaped dural flap was then fashion based inferiorly. Great care was taken to preserve the Sylvian vein. Only a small amount of cerebral edema was noted at this point. The anterior inferior aspect of the Sylvian fissure was then split, and the CSF (cerebrospinal fluid) was released. This portion of the procedure was somewhat tedious and allowed for brain retraction. The right olfactory nerve was then visualized and protected. The optic nerve was then identified as well as the proximal portion of the intracranial carotid artery. Fixed retractors were then placed, and the remainder of the procedure was carried out using microsurgical technique. The carotid cistern was opened using an arachnoid knife. The proximal portion of the intracranial carotid was then dissected free with thickened hemorrhagic arachnoid. Great care was exercised to minimize retraction on the temporal lobe. An aneurysm was noted in the proximal third of the intracranial and carotid artery immediately proximal to the bifurcation. (This indicates the intracranial aneurysm was in the carotid circulation.) Carefully dissecting the neck of the aneurysm revealed the origin of the anterior choroidal artery immediately distal to the neck. The dome of the aneurysm appeared to be immersed in scar and was largely immobile. After adequately dissecting the neck (This "neck" is the neck of the aneurysm, not the patient's neck.) and allowing for passage of microdissectors along the tract of the clip, the straight clip was selected. Clipping of the aneurysm then proceeded uneventfully. Post clipping, the internal carotid artery was noted to be widely patent, and the anterior choroidal artery was also visualized and noted to be unaffected by the aneurysm clip. Hemostasis was then ensured. The exposed brain was lined with a single layer of Surgicel. The area was generously irrigated with a body-temperature saline. The dura was closed using a running silk suture. The dural tacking sutures were also applied. The bone cap was secured and a cranioplasty was carried out for the squamous portion of the temporal bone and the lateral sphenoid wing. Muscle flap of the temporalis muscle was then repaired using interrupted Vicryl sutures. The galea was closed using interrupted Vicryl sutures, and sutures were utilized for the skin. Steri-Strips and sterile dressing were applied to the wound. The patient tolerated the procedure well. The patient was noted to be moving all extremities in the operating room and was transferred to the recovery room in satisfactory condition.

SERVICE CODE(S): _____

ICD-10-CM DX CODE(S): _____

(Answers to every other Case are located in Appendix D . The full answer key is only available in the TEACH Instructor Resources on Evolve.)

CASE 12-6 *Operative Report, Craniectomy*

LOCATION: Inpatient, Hospital

PATIENT: Suzanne Tracy

ATTENDING PHYSICIAN: Timothy Pleasant, MD

SURGEON: Timothy Pleasant, MD

PREOPERATIVE DIAGNOSIS: Brain tumor

POSTOPERATIVE DIAGNOSIS: Brain tumor

PROCEDURE PERFORMED: Craniectomy and removal of temporal lobe tumor

ANESTHESIA: General

Stealth protocol was utilized in doing this tumor. It was utilized in localizing the tumor.

PROCEDURE: Under general anesthesia, the patient was placed in the supine position. The head was turned to the right. The head was prepped and draped. The phaser was utilized to localize the tumor and to place it into the Stealth machine. Having done this, we then prepped and draped the patient. We made a linear incision extending from the temporal pole, having localized the tumor on the surface of the skin with the pointer. I then incised the skin and incised the temporalis fascia and muscle. I divided it. I then proceeded to perform a burr hole and a small

Continued

CASE 12-6—*cont'd*

craniectomy over the right temporal lobe tip. This having been done, we then incised the dura. This tumor was attached to the dura, and I removed the tumor; it was the size of a walnut. This was undermined from the surrounding brain with patties. There was no bleeding. This came out very easily. We then utilized Duraplast to repair the dura. We were utilizing 4-0 Nurolon. The bone edges were packed with some beeswax, and the dural edges were cauterized. The Duraplast having been placed, I then put a piece of Gelfoam on this, and I approximated the temporalis muscle and temporalis fascia with 0 Vicryl. I utilized 2-0 Vicryl on the galea. Surgical staples on the skin. Tight dressing was applied, and the patient was discharged to recovery.

Pathology Report Later Indicated: Benign neoplasm, meninges

SERVICE CODE(S): _____

ICD-10-CM DX CODE(S): _____

(Answers to every other Case are located in Appendix D . The full answer key is only available in the TEACH Instructor Resources on Evolve.)

Cranioplasty

Cranioplasty is the repair of a cranial defect. The surgeon uses autograft (from the patient) bone that is shaped and grafted into the defect area. If the defect is larger or more complicated than the surgeon can repair by bone grafting, a prosthetic plate may be used. Sometimes the plate is used as the foundation on which the surgeon places surgical cement to fill in an area of defect. The CPT codes in the cranial repair category (62000-62148) are divided based on the type of repair and in some codes, the extent of the repair (see 62140 for defects up to 5 cm in diameter).

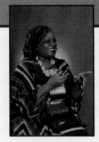

From the Trenches

"Medical coding will continue to be the back bone of a successful billing process."

HARVEY L. JOHNSON
CPC, CPMA, CBCS, CEHRS

CASE 12-7   *Operative Report, Cranioplasty*

LOCATION: Inpatient, Hospital

PATIENT: Sylvia Reagan

ATTENDING PHYSICIAN: Timothy Pleasant, MD

SURGEON: Timothy Pleasant, MD

PREOPERATIVE DIAGNOSIS: Cranial deformity

POSTOPERATIVE DIAGNOSIS: Cranial deformity

PROCEDURE PERFORMED: Cranioplasty

PREOPERATIVE NOTE: This is a patient who has had a cranial defect because she had a bone removed. She was in cerebral swelling post aneurysm clipping and she survived. Now she is set up to have repair of the 10-cm (centimeter) cranial defect. An expander had been placed in this defect before.

PROCEDURE: The patient's head was prepped and draped in the usual manner. An incision was made in the skin. The expander was removed. There was a plate in there. We were able to use this as a base to pour the methylmethacrylate cement. This was fashioned over the steel mesh. Afterward, this was formed to fill the defect out. We utilized the burr to shape it to the defect. We then closed the wound in one layer utilizing 2-0 Prolene on the scalp. A dressing was applied, and the patient was discharged to the PAR (postanesthesia recovery).

SERVICE CODE(S): _____

ICD-10-CM DX CODE(S): _____

(Answers to every other Case are located in Appendix D . The full answer key is only available in the TEACH Instructor Resources on Evolve.)

Shunts

A shunt is a passage from one area to another that diverts fluid from one area to another. There are many different types of shunts. A ventricular shunt is a catheter that is placed into the ventricle of the brain to drain cerebrospinal fluid (CSF) into the peritoneal cavity. **Figure 12-7** illustrates a ventriculoperitoneal shunt. If the catheter becomes damaged or otherwise obstructed, the shunt is replaced. The diagnosis is a complication of a catheter device.

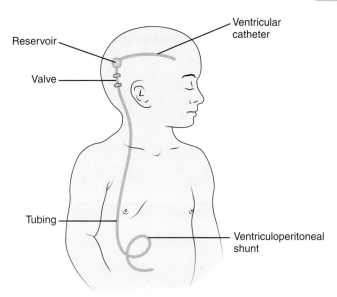

FIGURE 12–7 Ventriculoperitoneal shunt.

CASE 12-8   *Operative Report, Shunt Repair*

This is a report of a shunt obstruction, which represents a diagnosis of a mechanical complication of a shunt, specifically a ventricular catheter device (T85.-).

LOCATION: Inpatient, Hospital

PATIENT: Dean Rob

ATTENDING PHYSICIAN: Timothy Pleasant, MD

SURGEON: Timothy Pleasant, MD

PREOPERATIVE DIAGNOSIS: Shunt obstruction

POSTOPERATIVE DIAGNOSIS: Fracture of shunt

PROCEDURE PERFORMED: Repair of shunt. Replacement of ventricular catheter and valve.

ANESTHESIA: General

Under general anesthesia, the patient's right head was prepped and draped in the usual manner. The entire abdomen and neck were draped.

We were planning to possibly replace the entire shunt. After incising over the head and the shunt in the right posterior parietal area, it was obvious what the problem was. I incised the skin, turned down the flap, and the ventricular end of shunt had fractured from the shunt valve. I removed the valve. I removed the ventricular end and replaced it with a Delta One valve and 6 cm (centimeter) of ventricular shunt tubing and connected it up to the peritoneal catheter. It flowed easily. We did not inspect the peritoneal end, hoping that this would do and solve the problem. The fluid flowed freely into the peritoneal cavity. What I think happened here was the child probably hit his head and fractured the tube.

PROCEDURE: After reconnecting the shunt, we then closed the galea with 2-0 Vicryl interrupted and 4-0 nylon sutures on the skin. A dressing was applied. The patient was discharged to the PAR (postanesthesia recovery).

SERVICE CODE(S): _____

ICD-10-CM DX CODE(S): _____

(Answers to every other Case are located in Appendix D . The full answer key is only available in the TEACH Instructor Resources on Evolve.)

Lumbar Puncture

A lumbar puncture is also termed a spinal tap. This procedure obtains cerebrospinal fluid by means of a needle inserted into the subarachnoid space in the lumbar region, as illustrated in **Figure 12-8**. The patient is positioned so the space between the vertebrae is as wide as possible. Any interspace can be used for the procedure, but L5-S1 is the largest and is most often used as the site of withdrawal. The CSF fluid is used for diagnoses of various conditions. Commonly assessed are the appearance, protein, sugar, serology, cell count, and at times bacterial and fungal cultures of fluid.

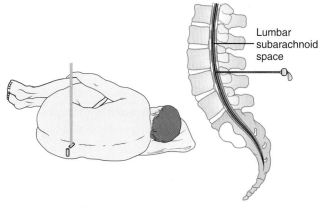

FIGURE 12–8 Lumbar puncture.

CASE 12-9 | *Operative Report, Lumbar Puncture*

LOCATION: Inpatient, Hospital

PATIENT: Larry Swope

ATTENDING PHYSICIAN: Timothy Pleasant, MD

SURGEON: Timothy Pleasant, MD

INDICATION: Vascular headache

PROCEDURE PERFORMED: Diagnostic lumbar puncture

PROCEDURE: Following Betadine prep, local anesthetic was instilled in the L3-4 (third lumbar vertebra-fourth) interspace. A #20-gauge needle was then inserted in this interspace and advanced until it entered the subarachnoid space on the second pass. Opening pressure was 110 mm (millimeter) of water. Five centimeters of crystal-clear fluid was obtained and sent to the laboratory for routine diagnostic studies, including viral culture. The patient tolerated the procedure well. He was given instructions as to how to avoid post–lumbar tap headache.

SERVICE CODE(S): _____

ICD-10-CM DX CODE(S): _____

(Answers to every other Case are located in Appendix D . The full answer key is only available in the TEACH Instructor Resources on Evolve.)

Pump Implantation

Pumps are implanted into the body to dispense various drugs. For example, in Case 12-10A, a baclofen pump is being implanted. Baclofen is a drug that decreases the frequency and severity of muscle spasms and can be administered orally or intrathecally. Intrathecal baclofen therapy (ITB therapy) is a long-term delivery of baclofen via a titanium disc that is 3 inches in diameter and delivers the baclofen directly into the spinal fluid (intrathecal). The pump is programmable with a telemetry wand that is used on the outside of the body, as illustrated in **Figure 12-9**, to adjust the dosage. There are two procedures performed when implanting a pump—the implantation of the pump (62360-62370) and the catheter that leads from the pump to the spinal column or brain (62350-62355). The pump is refillable, and the refilling and maintenance are reported separately with 95990 or 95991. A **laminectomy** (excision of a posterior arch of a vertebra) may be performed when implanting the pump system and requires the selection of a code to indicate the dual procedures of implantation and excision (62351).

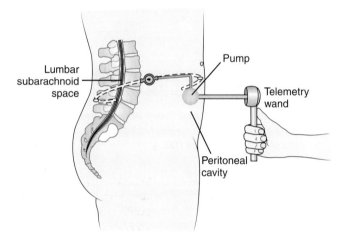

FIGURE 12–9 Lumbo-peritoneal shunt.

CASE 12-10 | *Operative Report, Pump Implantation*

The pump used in this case is programmable.

LOCATION: Inpatient, Hospital

PATIENT: Ross Lowell

ATTENDING PHYSICIAN: Timothy Pleasant, MD

SURGEON: Timothy Pleasant, MD

PREOPERATIVE DIAGNOSIS: Spasticity secondary to multiple sclerosis

POSTOPERATIVE DIAGNOSIS: Spasticity secondary to multiple sclerosis

PROCEDURE PERFORMED: Implantation of Medtronic baclofen pump

ANESTHESIA: General

PROCEDURE: Under general anesthesia, the patient's spine, side, and right abdomen were prepped and draped in the usual manner. The procedure started as follows: Having draped the patient, we then incised the skin over the spinous processes of L2 (second lumbar vertebra), L3 (third lumbar vertebra), and L4 (fourth lumbar vertebra) paramedian and got down to the fascia; here I was able, with a spinal needle, to insert the needle into the subarachnoid space, got good backflow, and placed the catheter into the subarachnoid space, obtaining good CSF (cerebrospinal fluid) flow. I put a clamp on it, and then began the anchoring of the tubing in the paramedian area by securing the tubing to the plastic insert, which holds the tubing to the fascia. We secured this with 2-0 silk. I then went to the anterior right quadrant and made an incision there for acceptance of the pump. This pump was placed into the pocket after using blunt dissection. I then passed the tubing from the posterior to the anterior incision using the trocar. I then had good CSF flow. I connected this

CASE 12-10—cont'd

to the baclofen pump utilizing the prescribed technique for doing same, that is, anchoring it with sutures. I anchored the pump with two sutures to the fascia and then began closure of the wounds. Both wounds were closed watertight with 2-0 Vicryl in the subcutaneous tissue, 2-0 plain in the subcuticular tissue, and surgical staples on the skin. A dressing was applied. The patient was discharged to PAR (postanesthesia recovery).

SERVICE CODE(S): _____

ICD-10-CM DX CODE(S): _____

(Answers to every other Case are located in Appendix D . The full answer key is only available in the TEACH Instructor Resources on Evolve.)

CASE 12-11A   *Preoperative Consultation*

The patient in this case is scheduled to have a baclofen infusion pump implanted, and Dr. Pleasant has requested a consultation prior to surgery by Dr. Green to ensure that there are no contraindications to the procedure. The reason for this service is the cerebral palsy.

LOCATION: Inpatient, Hospital

PATIENT: Foy Crow

ATTENDING PHYSICIAN: Timothy Pleasant, MD

CONSULTATION: Ronald Green, MD

PROCEDURE: Intrathecal catheter placement for baclofen infusion

MEDICATIONS: None

ALLERGIES: None

PAST MEDICAL HISTORY: Cerebral palsy. No previous surgeries. No medical problems.

FAMILY HISTORY: Heart disease in grandparents. There is no diabetes or cancer.

SOCIAL HISTORY: He just recently moved back to Manytown. He is living in his own townhouse. He does have disabilities related to his cerebral palsy. He has been having more problems with speech.

REVIEW OF SYSTEMS: The patient is denying any fevers, chills, cough, sore throat, or allergy problems. He sleeps well except the pain that he gets from the left arm. He is not having any constipation or diarrhea. He denies any dysuria or change in urinary frequency. He is not bothered by a rash. He has no history of blood clots or bleeding disorder.

PHYSICAL EXAMINATION: The patient appears in no acute distress. His speech is very difficult to understand. There is some drooling when trying to talk. His blood pressure is 140/94. HEENT (head, ears, eyes, nose, throat): The oropharynx membranes are moist. There is no exudate. The ears have normal landmarks. Nares are pink. Neck is supple. No tenderness. No adenopathy. No carotid bruits. Heart is regular; S1 and S2. Lungs: He has good aeration. No wheezes. No crackles. Abdomen is soft and nontender. The left arm is prompted forward and has minimal motion. Extremities do not reveal any pedal edema. There is no cyanosis. Chest x-ray does not reveal any infiltrate. Urinalysis is pending. CBC (complete blood count) is pending.

ASSESSMENT: Cerebral palsy

PLAN: The patient has no contraindications to the planned surgery. He has average surgical risks. We are awaiting the laboratory results. Total time spent with patient for this consult today was 35 minutes.

SERVICE CODE(S): _____

ICD-10-CM DX CODE(S): _____

(Answers to every other Case are located in Appendix D . The full answer key is only available in the TEACH Instructor Resources on Evolve.)

CASE 12-11B   *Operative Report, Intrathecal Catheter Placement*

Even though you know from previous reports that this patient has cerebral palsy, this specific report does not indicate that. You therefore report the reason for the service as the dystonia as documented in the report. In this operative report, the surgeon is implanting a temporary, non-programmable Bard pump. It is not uncommon for a temporary pump that cannot be programmed to be implanted and then, if the patient responds well to the temporary pump, the pump is removed and replaced with a permanent, programmable pump. A programmable pump can be adjusted to deliver a set amount of medication.

LOCATION: Inpatient, Hospital

PATIENT: Foy Crow

ATTENDING PHYSICIAN: Timothy Pleasant, MD

SURGEON: Timothy Pleasant, MD

PREOPERATIVE DIAGNOSIS: Symptomatic torsion dystonia

POSTOPERATIVE DIAGNOSIS: Symptomatic torsion dystonia

PROCEDURE PERFORMED: Placement of a Bard port with intrathecal placement of catheter

ANESTHESIA: General anesthesia

PROCEDURE: Under general anesthesia, the patient's back was prepped and draped. The C-arm was introduced. We then placed a needle into the subarachnoid space. This was with a Tuohy needle. We then threaded the catheter in up to T1-T2 (thoracic vertebra 1-2), got good back flow, removed the needle, and then undercut by the plastic tubing so that we could place a trocar, which would come around the right flank. This was done. The path of least resistance was made, and the incision was made over the right quadrant. The plastic catheter was then connected to the Bard port and secured. The wound was then closed. The patient was to have a trial at infusion of medications in the Bard pump, to be brought back at a later date for removal and placement of a Synchro pump. The wound was closed in layers utilizing 4-0 nylon sutures on the skin, and a dressing was applied.

SERVICE CODE(S): _____

ICD-10-CM DX CODE(S): _____

(Answers to every other Case are located in Appendix D . The full answer key is only available in the TEACH Instructor Resources on Evolve.)

CASE 12-11C *Operative Report, Removal of Bard Port*

The temporary Bard port was replaced with a programmable Medtronic pump. This was a staged procedure, which alerts you to the need for a modifier. Dr. Sanchez is a partner of Dr. Pleasant.

LOCATION: Inpatient, Hospital

PATIENT: Foy Crow

ATTENDING PHYSICIAN: Timothy Pleasant, MD

SURGEON: Gary Sanchez, MD

PREOPERATIVE DIAGNOSIS: Symptomatic torsion dystonia

POSTOPERATIVE DIAGNOSIS: Symptomatic torsion dystonia

PROCEDURE PERFORMED: Removal of Bard; placement of Sofamor-Danek Medtronic pump delivery system for intrathecal medication.

PROCEDURE: The skin over the abdomen was prepped and draped. The previous incision was incised. The Bard pump was removed. A pocket was made in the right quadrant of the abdomen by undermining the subcutaneous fat. The pump was then anchored and connected to the catheter securely with 4-0 nylon sutures. Having done this, we then closed the wound in layers utilizing 3-0 Vicryl on the subcutaneous tissue with 2-0 plain in the subcuticular tissue and 4-0 nylon sutures, interrupted mattress, on the skin. A dressing was applied.

SERVICE CODE(S): _____

ICD-10-CM DX CODE(S): _____

(Answers to every other Case are located in Appendix D . The full answer key is only available in the TEACH Instructor Resources on Evolve.)

CASE 12-11D *Discharge Summary*

In this discharge report, the documentation indicates both the cerebral palsy and the dystonia, and both are therefore reported as the diagnoses.

LOCATION: Inpatient, Hospital

PATIENT: Foy Crow

ATTENDING PHYSICIAN: Timothy Pleasant, MD

PRINCIPAL DIAGNOSES:

1. Cerebral palsy secondary to encephalopathy
2. Severe symptomatic torsion dystonia and spasticity
3. Now status post intrathecal catheter placement with intrathecal baclofen pump

NEUROSURGEON: Timothy Pleasant, MD

PREOPERATIVE CONSULTATION: Ronald Green, MD

ALLERGIES: None

PRINCIPAL PROCEDURE: Placement of Bard with intrathecal placement of catheter by Dr. Sanchez under general anesthesia.

Removal of Bard, placement of Medtronic pump delivery system for intrathecal medication, model #87, serial #L550, and #063, implanted catheter length 30 inches, implanted catheter volume 0.168, internal implanted tubing in baclofen pump 0.26.

HOSPITAL COURSE: The patient has done well during his hospitalization. An intrathecal catheter and a Bard were placed intraoperatively. Catheter tip T1 (thoracic vertebra 1) to T2. The catheter was attached to the Bard. The patient was started on his intrathecal baclofen test dose with an initial dose of 100 mcg per 24 hours. He tolerated this well without complications. He noted improvement in dystonia. On day 2 of his hospital stay, his total daily dose of baclofen was increased to 175 mcg (microgram) per 24 hours at 9:40 AM. He had no difficulties with this. At 5:28 PM, on day 2, the dose was increased to 225 mcg per 24 hours with continued positive benefits. On day 3, the total daily dose was increased to 300 mcg per 24 hours with continued positive results and no side effects. On day 4, the Bard was surgically removed and a definitive intrathecal baclofen pump was placed. The patient was given a priming bolus and started on 360 mcg per day. He had no difficulties with this, and on day 5, the total dose was increased to 375 mcg per day. Overall, he has noted a marked decrease in dystonia. He is now able to feel his left fingertips and has decreased pain in his left elbow and resolution of pain in his left shoulder. He does have some mild discomfort across the anterior aspect of the right elbow that may be secondary to position during surgery.

He has had difficulty with urinary retention post both operations and required straight catheter. Volumes have been significant at greater than 700-900 cc. Once he is able to stand, this does improve. He had some initial difficulties with abdominal distention secondary to gas. This has resolved. He does use a Dulcolax suppository p.r.n. (as needed). Initial pain management was with Demerol. When given 75 mg (milligram) IV (intravenous), he was slightly sedated and required a small amount of O_2 (oxygen). When given only 25 mg this did not control his pain but for 45 minutes, when given 35-50, this was sufficient. He also took additional Toradol p.r.n. for pain, and pain management has been good.

He did have initial headache post the initial surgery felt to be spinal leak of CSF (cerebrospinal fluid) in origin as occurred when he sat up, resolved when he laid down. A blood patch was done on day 5, and this is much better. Today he did have some mild light-headedness after straight catheter for urinary residual, and this is resolving with supine position.

The patient has participated in dystonia monitoring by physical therapy and occupational therapy, and they noted an improvement.

The patient will be transferred to the Manytown Rehabilitation Hospital today for continued rehab services status post intrathecal baclofen pump placement and to monitor and increase dosage. Will continue

CASE 12-11D—cont'd

with occupational therapy, physical therapy, and speech evaluation. Will increase dose as necessary.

DISCHARGE DIET: Regular

DISCHARGE MEDICATIONS:

1. Intrathecal baclofen, currently 375 mcg per day
2. IV has been discontinued
3. Tylenol 650 mg q.4-6h. p.o. (by mouth) p.r.n.
4. Bisacodyl suppository 10 mg p.r.n.
5. Ibuprofen 600 mg p.o. p.r.n.
6. Physostigmine to take at bedside 0.7 to 2 mg if needed for inadvertent overdose of baclofen.

PHYSICAL EXAMINATION: Lungs are clear to auscultation. Regular rate and rhythm. Abdomen is soft and nontender. Abdominal incision site is good. No redness or warmth is noted. Neurologically, marked decrease in dystonia.

SERVICE CODE(S): _____

ICD-10-CM DX CODE(S): _____

(Answers to every other Case are located in Appendix D . The full answer key is only available in the TEACH Instructor Resources on Evolve.)

Laminotomy and Foraminotomies

Laminotomies and laminectomies are two of the most frequently performed surgeries used in treatment of herniated discs, spinal trauma, aneurysm correction, and removal of spinal cord tumors. The procedures involve an incision over the operative area and removal of a portion of the bone of the vertebrae (lamina). The bulging or damaged portion of the disc is then removed. Foraminotomy is removal of a portion of the vertebra to relieve pressure on the foramina (that area of the channel in which the nerves are located). If a laminotomy and foraminotomy are performed at the same session, only the laminotomy is reported because the code descriptions for the laminectomies include foraminotomy. If the procedures are performed on both sides of the vertebra, modifier -50 is used to indicate a bilateral procedure was performed.

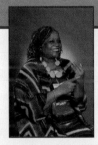

From the Trenches

"Pay close attention to ALL documentation within the patient's chart, relative to that particular day of service."

HARVEY L. JOHNSON
CPC, CPMA, CBCS, CEHRS

CASE 12-12A   *Radiology Report, Lumbar Spine*

Prior to surgery for laminectomies and foraminotomies, Dr. Pleasant orders an x-ray. The reason for this service is the herniation (displacement) of an intervertebral disc.

LOCATION: Inpatient, Hospital

PATIENT: Todd Osmond

ATTENDING PHYSICIAN: Timothy Pleasant, MD

RADIOLOGIST: Grey Lonewolf, MD

EXAMINATION OF: Lumbar spine

CLINICAL SYMPTOMS: Lumbar laminectomy, herniated disc L3-4 (third lumbar vertebra-fourth), L5-S1

LATERAL TWO VIEW OF LUMBAR SPINE: COMPARISON: Comparison is made to a previous lateral view of the lumbar spine dated 2 months ago. For the purposes of this examination, it will be assumed that there are five lumbar-type vertebral bodies. There is evidence of previous fusion of the L4 and L5. Surgical instruments are seen posterior to the L4 vertebral segment. A surgical probe is seen to extend anteriorly from the surgical instruments. The distal tip lies posterior to the superior endplate of L4.

SERVICE CODE(S): _____

ICD-10-CM DX CODE(S): _____

(Answers to every other Case are located in Appendix D . The full answer key is only available in the TEACH Instructor Resources on Evolve.)

CASE 12-12B *Operative Report, Laminotomies and Foraminotomies*

LOCATION: Inpatient, Hospital

PATIENT: Todd Osmond

ATTENDING PHYSICIAN: Timothy Pleasant, MD

SURGEON: Timothy Pleasant, MD

PREOPERATIVE DIAGNOSIS: Herniated disc L3-4 (third lumbar vertebra-fourth) on the right and the left

POSTOPERATIVE DIAGNOSIS: Herniated disc L3-4 on the right and the left

PROCEDURE PERFORMED: Bilateral laminotomies and foraminotomies at L3-4 with removal of the disc from the right and left side. Application of an allograft, 2.5 cc (cubic centimeter) on each side.

ANESTHESIA: General

PROCEDURE: The patient was placed in a prone position. The back was prepped and draped in the usual manner. The previous incision was incised. The erector spinae muscles were dissected from the lamina. About three or four retractors were placed in the wound. We isolated the L3-4 interspace via x-ray. Laminotomies were performed with foraminotomies on the left and the right side. The ligamentum flavum was very hypertrophic. The facets were hypertrophic. We took these down. Retracted on the nerve root and got the disc space. Here is what happened on the left side: There was a disc material on the body of L4. I took this down, went into the disc space, and removed much degenerating material. On the right side, I did the same thing. The disc here was on the body of L3. We took it down, took the midline fragments down. I was satisfied that I had cleaned out the disc space. There was no compression on the nerve roots. Passed a hockey stick up and medially and down and medially into the foramen. The dura was well compressed. Irrigated the wound well. After this, we then put Gleotec about 2.5 cc on the right and on the left side. No drains were utilized. The lumbodorsal fascia was approximated with double knotted 0 chromic, 0 Vicryl as well, 2-0 plain in the subcutaneous tissue, and surgical staples on the skin. A dressing was applied. The patient was discharged to the PAR (postanesthesia recovery).

SERVICE CODE(S): _____

ICD-10-CM DX CODE(S): _____

(Answers to every other Case are located in Appendix D . The full answer key is only available in the TEACH Instructor Resources on Evolve.)

CASE 12-12C *Discharge Summary*

LOCATION: Inpatient, Hospital

PATIENT: Todd Osmond

ATTENDING PHYSICIAN: Timothy Pleasant, MD

SURGEON: Timothy Pleasant, MD

The patient presented with unbearable left leg pain. He apparently had stopped smoking and drinking and had a herniated L3-4 (third lumbar vertebra-fourth) disc. He wanted to go ahead with surgery. He was preoperatively prepped by Dr. Green. Cardiovascular system had a heart murmur.

HOSPITAL COURSE: The patient underwent a bilateral laminectomy, foraminotomy, and removal of disc at L3-4. His postoperative course is uneventful. He has a little drainage from the wound, but I think that will seal; it is clear. His leg pain is gone. I will see him on Thursday for a wound check. He is discharged with Percocet for pain.

FINAL DIAGNOSIS: Herniated disc at L3-4

PROCEDURE PERFORMED: Bilateral laminotomy, foraminotomy, and removal of disc.

SERVICE CODE(S): _____

ICD-10-CM DX CODE(S): _____

(Answers to every other Case are located in Appendix D . The full answer key is only available in the TEACH Instructor Resources on Evolve.)

CASE 12-13 *Operative Report, Hemilaminectomy and Foraminotomy*

One type of nerve pain is radiculopathy, which is pain emanating from the root of the nerve, that is, the part of the nerve that exits the spinal cord and enters the body. In this case, the surgeon performs a hemilaminectomy, which is the removal of only one side of the vertebral lamina due to radiculopathy (nerve disease).

LOCATION: Inpatient, Hospital

PATIENT: Tana Thrall

ATTENDING PHYSICIAN: Timothy Pleasant, MD

SURGEON: Timothy Pleasant, MD

PREOPERATIVE DIAGNOSIS: Intractable left S1 (first heart sound) radiculopathy

CASE 12-13—cont'd

POSTOPERATIVE DIAGNOSIS: Intractable left S1 radiculopathy

PROCEDURE PERFORMED: Left L4-5 (fourth lumbar vertebra-fifth) and L5-S1 redo hemilaminectomy and foraminotomy

PROCEDURE: The patient was taken to the operating room and placed under general endotracheal anesthesia. She was then rotated into the prone position on chest rolls with the arms extended over the head. The lumbar region was shaved, prepped, and draped in the usual sterile manner. The proposed vertical midline incision was then infiltrated with lidocaine with epinephrine. The skin was incised, and sharp dissection was carried through the subcutaneous tissue. The fascia was then incised and subperiosteal dissection was undertaken on the left. X-ray localization confirmed the proper position. There was a generous amount of scar noted at L4-5 that was gradually removed, dissecting along the bone. Dissection proceeded until the left L-4 nerve root could be safely identified, tracking through the neural foramen. The L4 nerve root was well decompressed. The next level was then approached. A generous amount of fusion mass was noted at L5-S1.

This was removed with a drill and then with #45-Kerrison punch. The L5-S1 nerve roots were then identified. The L5-S1 foramen was noted to be moderately stenotic, and a generous decompression was undertaken. In addition, the left S1 nerve root appeared to be slightly compromised by bone, displacing it slightly medially. This nerve was then fully decompressed. On completion, the L4, L5, and S1 nerve roots had all been visualized and were noted to be well decompressed. Hemostasis was then ensured. The epidural space was lined with a single layer of Surgicel and fat graft. The wound was closed with interrupted layers of 4-0 Vicryl subcuticular stitch for skin. Steri-Strips and sterile dressing were applied to the wound. The patient tolerated the procedure well and was transferred to the recovery room in good condition.

SERVICE CODE(S): _____

ICD-10-CM DX CODE(S): _____

(Answers to every other Case are located in Appendix D . The full answer key is only available in the TEACH Instructor Resources on Evolve.)

CASE 12-14A   *Radiology Report, Disc Repair*

LOCATION: Inpatient, Hospital

PATIENT: Sara Vasek

ATTENDING PHYSICIAN: Timothy Pleasant, MD

RADIOLOGIST: Grey Lonewolf, MD

EXAMINATION OF: Four lumbar films for lumbar laminectomy

CLINICAL SYMPTOMS: Disc herniation

FOUR LUMBAR FILMS FOR LUMBAR LAMINECTOMY: FINDINGS: No comparisons. On the image labeled #1, there is a metallic marker seen posteriorly at the L2 (second lumbar vertebra) level superior endplate, assuming there are five lumbar-type vertebral bodies. On the image

labeled #2, there is a metallic density seen posteriorly with the thin metallic rod pointing at the L1 level and the other metallic hardware at the L1-2 level. On the film labeled #3, a posterior metallic hardware is again noted. The most cephalad metallic density is at the L2-3 level, and the thinner caudal metallic density is at the L3-4 level. Film labeled #4 demonstrates metallic densities, and they are located at the L1-2 and L4-5 levels.

SERVICE CODE(S): _____

ICD-10-CM DX CODE(S): _____

(Answers to every other Case are located in Appendix D . The full answer key is only available in the TEACH Instructor Resources on Evolve.)

CASE 12-14B   *Operative Report, Discectomies and Foraminotomies*

LOCATION: Inpatient, Hospital

PATIENT: Sara Vasek

ATTENDING PHYSICIAN: Timothy Pleasant, MD

SURGEON: Timothy Pleasant, MD

PREOPERATIVE DIAGNOSIS: Herniated nucleus pulposus, L1-2 (first lumbar vertebra-second) and herniated nucleus pulposus, L4-5 with back pain, left-sided leg pain, and corresponding radiculopathies.

POSTOPERATIVE DIAGNOSIS: Herniated nucleus pulposus, L1-2 and herniated nucleus pulposus, L4-5 with back pain, left-sided leg pain, and corresponding radiculopathies and left L2-3 disc herniation.

PROCEDURE PERFORMED: Left L1-2, L2-3, and L4-5 discectomies with foraminotomies, and a left L3-4 foraminotomy.

ANESTHESIA: General endotracheal

COMPLICATIONS: Nil

A Hemovac drain was placed.

HISTORY: This is a 32-year-old white female who underwent previous left-sided laminotomies and foraminotomies by me. This was for left-sided neurogenic claudication and spinal stenosis. She did extremely well with this operation; however, she developed a sudden onset of back pain and left-sided leg pain. An MRI (magnetic resonance imaging) scan

Continued

CASE 12-14B—cont'd

was obtained, and it revealed a large disc herniation eccentric to the left at L1-2. It also showed some disc degeneration and foraminal stenosis eccentric to the left, interestingly at all levels of the lumbar spine, L2-3, L3-4, and L4-5. She also had a disc herniation with facet hypertrophy and circumferential stenosis at L4-5. Her symptoms were only on the left.

Indications, alternatives, risks, and benefits of surgery were discussed in detail. The patient was consented for a left-sided L1-2 and a left L4-5 discectomy with lumbar exploration.

The patient was brought to the operating theater and identified. General endotracheal anesthesia was induced. Intravenous antibiotics were given. The region in the low back was prepped and draped in a sterile fashion. A localizing x-ray was obtained after placement of a spinal needle. The old incision was utilized and marked using a skin marker. The region of the incision was infiltrated with 1.5% Xylocaine with epinephrine. A vertical midline incision was made through the old incision using a #10 blade scalpel. Hemostasis was achieved using Bovie electrocautery. Subcutaneous and subcuticular tissues were divided using Bovie electrocautery. The self-retaining retractors were placed. The dorsal lumbar fascia was incised using Bovie electrocautery. The paraspinal musculature and multifidi were reflected off of the spinous process and laminae of L1-2, L2-3, L3-4, and L4-5 using Bovie electrocautery, Cobb elevators, and sponges.

Our attention was directed at entry into the L1-2 space on the left. Using the straight and curved curettes, ligamentum flavum and scar tissue was resected from the superior edge of the inferior lamina of L1 and the inferior edge of the superior lamina of L2. There was a lot of dense scar adherent to the bone. I then redirected and went to the L2-3 space and did a general foraminotomy.

Ligamentum flavum and scar tissue were resected and removed and curetted from the superior edge of the inferior lamina of L3 and the inferior edge of the superior lamina of L2. A general foraminotomy was then fashioned using 3- and 5-mm (millimeter) Kerrison punches. The disc seemed to be humped up, and there was an extruded fragment compressing the nerve from below. This disc fragment was removed,

and disc material was removed in a piecemeal fashion and handed off as specimen. Copious amounts of saline irrigation were utilized until the supernatant was clear. We had entry into the L2-3 space. A large laminotomy was fashioned. The scar adhesions were resected. I then readdressed the L1-2 interspace. A foraminotomy was fashioned using 3- and 5-mm Kerrison punches. The ball-ended probe could pass without let or hindrance. Copious amounts of saline irrigation were utilized. The exiting nerve root and thecal sac were retracted medially. The disc was incised. A large disc fragment presented itself once the annulus was incised. This was handed off as specimen. We alternated between curettes and pituitary punches and handed disc material off as specimen. Copious amounts of saline irrigation were utilized until the supernatant was clear.

Our attention was directed at the L4-5 interspace on the left. A foraminotomy was fashioned. The superior edge of the inferior lamina of L5 (fifth lumbar vertebra) and the inferior edge of the superior lamina of L4 were curetted and scar tissue was resected. We entered into the space created with resection of the soft tissue and performed a generous foraminotomy and laminotomy. The thecal sac and exiting nerve root were retracted off as specimen. I directed my attention to L3-4 and proceeded to perform a small foraminotomy. The ball-ended probe could pass without let or hindrance. This lady tolerated surgery well. There were no intraoperative complications. A Hemovac drain was placed.

Hemostasis was achieved using Bovie electrocautery and bipolar electrocautery. Dorsal lumbar fascia and the paraspinal musculature were reapproximated using double-knotted chromic suture. Subcutaneous tissues were reapproximated using 2-0 Vicryl. Hemovac drain was placed and carried out through a separate stab incision. The skin was reapproximated using staples. All counts were correct and verified.

Pathology Report Later Indicated: See Report 12-14C.

SERVICE CODE(S): _____

ICD-10-CM DX CODE(S): _____

(Answers to every other Case are located in Appendix D . The full answer key is only available in the TEACH Instructor Resources on Evolve.)

CASE 12-14C   *Pathology Report*

LOCATION: Inpatient, Hospital

PATIENT: Sara Vasek

ATTENDING PHYSICIAN: Timothy Pleasant, MD

SURGEON: Timothy Pleasant, MD

PATHOLOGIST: Grey Lonewolf, MD

CLINICAL HISTORY: Disc herniation

SPECIMEN RECEIVED: Lumbar disc

GROSS DESCRIPTION: The specimen is labeled with the patient's name and "disc" and consists of approximately 5 g (gram) of fibrous fragments.

MICROSCOPIC DESCRIPTION: Sections show disc tissue.

DIAGNOSIS: Disc tissue, benign

SERVICE CODE(S): _____

ICD-10-CM DX CODE(S): _____

(Answers to every other Case are located in Appendix D . The full answer key is only available in the TEACH Instructor Resources on Evolve.)

CASE 12-14D   *Radiology Report, Lumbar Spine MRI*

LOCATION: Inpatient, Hospital

PATIENT: Sara Vasek

ATTENDING PHYSICIAN: Timothy Pleasant, MD

SURGEON: Timothy Pleasant, MD

RADIOLOGIST: Grey Lonewolf, MD

EXAMINATION OF: Lumbar spine MRI (magnetic resonance imaging)

CLINICAL SYMPTOMS: Herniated disc

LUMBAR SPINE MRI WITH and WITHOUT CONTRAST: TECHNIQUE: T1 (thoracic vertebra 1), T2, and fat-saturated postcontrast T1 sagittal images were acquired. T1, T2, and postcontrast T1 axial images were acquired from L1 (first lumbar vertebra) to S1 (first sacral vertebra). No prior studies are provided for comparison.

FINDINGS: The conus is normal.

The T11-12 disc space is desiccated with an inferior endplate Schmorl's node and mild anterior spurring.

The T12-L1 disc space is unremarkable.

At L1-2, there is a peripherally enhancing left anterolateral epidural soft-tissue process. A left laminotomy with a peripherally enhancing fluid collection is noted. The disc space is desiccated with bulging. There is no enhancement abnormality within the disc space.

At L2-3, there is a left laminotomy, facetectomy, and foraminotomy with a peripherally enhancing fluid collection in the surgical bed. Enhancing epidural and perineural tissues are noted. Sagittal images show some bright enhancing T2 signal in the left hemisphere of the disc space, without associated endplate changes. Within the left lateral recess of L3 is a peripherally enhancing collection having long T1/long T2 signal. For example, compare postcontrast axial image #16 with T2-weighted axial image #16 and precontrast image #16.

At L3-4, there is a left laminectomy and inferior facetectomy with enhancing granulation tissue in the surgical bed. The disc space is desiccated with bulge and mild spurring.

At L4-5, there is a left laminectomy and partial facetectomy with enhancing epidural granulation tissue. Right ligamentum flavum is redundant. Right lateral recess is moderately to markedly stenotic. Moderate to marked degenerative disease is present in the right facet joint. Right neural foramen is moderately to markedly stenotic. The left neural foramen is amply patent.

At L5-S1, there is advanced bilateral degenerative facet disease with disc desiccation with bulge.

IMPRESSION:

1. Left laminectomies and/or facet postoperative changes including L1-2 through L4-5.
2. Peripherally enhancing mass in the left L3 lateral recess has indeterminate etiology. Given findings of recent surgery, packing material or postoperative fluid collection is considered. A free fragment of peripherally enhancing disc material could have a similar appearance.
3. Enhancing in the left hemisphere of the L2-3 disc space in conjunction with bright T2 signal intensity may represent postoperative change.
4. Multilevel degenerative disc disease.
5. Moderate to marked right L4-5 foraminal stenosis.
6. Peripherally enhancing soft tissue at the dorsal aspect of the L1-2 disc space has uncertain significance. This finding likely represents acute postoperative change; however, clinical correlation is suggested. Acute postoperative change has been described in the literature as mimicking residual or recurrent disc herniation.

SERVICE CODE(S): _____

ICD-10-CM DX CODE(S): _____

(Answers to every other Case are located in Appendix D . The full answer key is only available in the TEACH Instructor Resources on Evolve.)

CASE 12-14E   *Radiology Report, Lumbar Spine MRI*

LOCATION: Inpatient, Hospital

PATIENT: Sara Vasek

ATTENDING PHYSICIAN: Timothy Pleasant, MD

SURGEON: Timothy Pleasant, MD

RADIOLOGIST: Grey Lonewolf, MD

EXAMINATION OF: Lumbar MRI (magnetic resonance imaging)

CLINICAL SYMPTOMS: Herniated disc, recent surgery

MAGNETIC RESONANCE EXAMINATION OF THE LUMBAR SPINE was performed utilizing a combination of T1 (thoracic vertebra 1), gradient echo, and fast spin-echo (fat suppressed) T2-weighted sequences. Appropriate sequences were also performed following intravenous infusion of contrast material.

The patient has had multiple surgical procedures with surgery at almost every level in the lumbar region from L1-2 (first lumbar vertebra-second) to L4-5.

Unfortunately, the patient was moving during the acquisition of some sequences.

At L1-2, there does appear to be abnormal soft-tissue mass to the left of midline, with compression on the dural sac. It certainly has the appearance of disc herniation. However, one also needs to realize that large disc herniation can appear very similarly following surgery as it did prior to surgery, even with removal of the disc.

At L2-3 and L3-4, I believe there has been entry to the spinal canal on the left. There is bulging of the intervertebral disc, and there are underlying bone bars at both levels, and there is indentation of the dural sac, but I doubt that there is evidence of overt disc herniation at this time. I do not feel there is significant stenosis, although the dural sac is small at both levels. I believe there has been previous satisfactory decompression.

At L4-5, I believe there is significant spinal stenosis circumferentially. There might also be a small disc herniation at L4-5 to the left of midline.

I do not believe there is significant abnormality directly at L5-S1.

IMPRESSION: The patient has had multiple surgical procedures. She had recent very extensive surgery. Essentially, there does appear to be residual disc herniation at L1-2 to the left of midline. As noted above,

Continued

CASE 12-14E—cont'd

it needs to be remembered that an appearance of large disc herniation might not change in the immediate postoperative period, even though the disc has been removed. This would not explain the right lower extremity pain.

Continued spinal stenosis at L4-5 with possible small disc herniation to the left of midline.

Previous decompression at L2-3 and L3-4. I believe decompression is satisfactory. I do not believe there is evidence of disc herniation at these levels.

I do not believe there is significant abnormality at L5-S1.

SERVICE CODE(S): _____

ICD-10-CM DX CODE(S): _____

(Answers to every other Case are located in Appendix D . The full answer key is only available in the TEACH Instructor Resources on Evolve.)

Spinal Fusion

Spinal fusion is the fixation of two or more vertebrae together that is performed to provide stabilization to the spinal column. The fusion may be done for degenerative conditions such as spondylolisthesis in which one disc slips over the one below (slipped disc) or for congenital abnormalities. Fusions are reported with codes from the Musculoskeletal System, Spine (Vertebral Column), Arthrodesis (22548-22632) based on the approach used.

The approach is the access location, such as anterior (front), posterior (back), anterolateral (to one side of the front), or posterolateral (to one side of the back). Often a spinal evoked potential monitoring, which is an electroencephalogram (EEG) and monitors the electrical activity of the brain, will be conducted intraoperatively and is reported separately.

If a biomechanical device, such as bone dowel or cage, is applied at the time of surgery, the application of the device is reported separately with add-on codes 22853-22859.

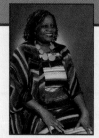

From the Trenches

"Keeping abreast of ongoing changes and attending pertinent seminars and conferences are the keys to success as a medical coder."

HARVEY L. JOHNSON
CPC, CPMA, CBCS, CEHRS

CASE 12-15   *Operative Report, Cage Fusion*

This patient has a degeneration of an intervertebral disc.

This case involves the use of a bone graft from a cadaveric donor and is known as an allograft.

LOCATION: Inpatient, Hospital

PATIENT: Carmen Schultz

ATTENDING PHYSICIAN: Timothy Pleasant, MD

SURGEON: Timothy Pleasant, MD

PREOPERATIVE DIAGNOSIS: Severe degenerative disc disease at L5-S1 (fifth lumbar vertebra-first sacral vertebra)

POSTOPERATIVE DIAGNOSIS: Severe degenerative disc disease at L5-S1

PROCEDURE PERFORMED: L5-S1 anterior intervertebral cage fusion with spinal evoked potential monitoring (evoked potential somatosensory study is reported separately)

ANESTHESIA: General endotracheal anesthesia

OPERATIVE NOTE: The patient was taken to the operating room and placed under general endotracheal anesthesia. The abdomen was then prepped and draped in the usual sterile manner. Anterior exposure was obtained. After exposure had been obtained and x-ray localization was provided, anterior intervertebral cage fusion was performed using standard technique. A 13 × 20 BAK (Bagly and Kuslich) cage was placed uneventfully between the L5 and S1 vertebral bodies under x-ray guidance. Cancellous bone was packed into the BAK cages in the standard fashion. Hemostasis was ensured, and the wound was closed in standard fashion.

SERVICE CODE(S): _____

ICD-10-CM DX CODE(S): _____

(Answers to every other Case are located in Appendix D . The full answer key is only available in the TEACH Instructor Resources on Evolve.)

CASE 12-16 *Operative Report, Halo Vest Placement and Repair*

Now here is a case to challenge your coding abilities. Reference the "Procedure Performed" section of the report to identify the number of procedures to be coded, noting that there are two segments to report for the fixation and fusion. Then read the report and ensure that the procedures are those identified in the "Procedure Performed" section. Assume this is the initial care of this fracture. There will be a CPT for the fracture treatment, arthrodesis, autograft, skeletal fixation, cranial halo, and the evoked potentials. Assign a diagnosis code for the fracture and an external cause for the fracture circumstances.

LOCATION: Inpatient, Hospital

PATIENT: Tim Brent

ATTENDING PHYSICIAN: Timothy Pleasant, MD

SURGEON: Timothy Pleasant, MD

PREOPERATIVE DIAGNOSIS: Unstable C5 (fifth cervical vertebra) fracture with spinal deformity and upper extremity weakness

POSTOPERATIVE DIAGNOSIS: Unstable C5 fracture with spinal deformity and upper extremity weakness

PROCEDURE PERFORMED:

1. Halo vest placement
2. Posterior segmental fixation C4 through C6 with Halifax clamps
3. Open correction of cervical fracture
4. Posterior cervical fusion C4 through C6 using bone autograft and right iliac crest graft
5. Evoked potential monitoring of upper extremity

ANESTHESIA: General endotracheal anesthesia

OPERATIVE NOTE: The patient was taken to the operating room and placed under general endotracheal anesthesia. This was done fiberoptically. On completion of the successful intubation, the patient was then placed in a four-pin halo vest. This was done maintaining an in-line cervical traction using standard technique after neutral position on chest rolls. The posterior cervical region as well as the area surrounding the left iliac crest were then shaved, prepped, and draped in the usual sterile manner. The left iliac crest graft was harvested first. This was done through a standard incision. The split-thickness graft with a generous amount of cancellous bone was harvested. The wound was then closed in interrupted layers after hemostasis had been ensured. The posterior cervical region was then incised. Sharp dissection was carried out through the subcutaneous tissue. The fascia was incised and a subperiosteal dissection was undertaken from C4 through C6. Great care was utilized to avoid stripping the muscle from C3 and C7 in an attempt to minimize any chance of incorporating growing fusion at these levels. The superior aspect of the hemilamina of C4 and the inferior aspect of the hemilamina of C6 were then carefully exposed using curettes. Halifax clamps were then fashioned and secured from C4 through C6. The area of C5 was noted to be fractured in multiple places, including the facet joints bilaterally and the lamina. The Halifax clamp construct was then assembled uneventfully and was noted to be secure. The lamina was then decorticated with a cutting burr, and the cancellous and cortical bones were utilized to complete the posterior cervical fusion. Halifax clamping ensured proper correction of the slight cervical deformity, and throughout the procedure, the evoked potential monitoring (electrodes placed on the scalp electrically stimulate nerves and results are recorded and reported separately) was noted to be normal. Hemostasis was then ensured. The wound was closed in interrupted layers with staples for the skin.

SERVICE CODE(S): _____

ICD-10-CM DX CODE(S): _____

(Answers to every other Case are located in Appendix D . The full answer key is only available in the TEACH Instructor Resources on Evolve.)

CASE 12-17 *Operative Report, Discectomy*

This case is another challenge for you to take on. Read the report carefully to ensure that you are reporting all the various components of the service. There will be a code for each of the discectomies, corpectomy, allograft, spinal fusion, arthrodesis, skeletal fixation, and evoked potentials.

LOCATION: Inpatient, Hospital

PATIENT: Liz Neil

ATTENDING PHYSICIAN: Timothy Pleasant, MD

SURGEON: Timothy Pleasant, MD

PREOPERATIVE DIAGNOSIS: Cervical disc displacement, C4-5 (fourth cervical vertebra-fifth cervical vertebra) and C5-6

POSTOPERATIVE DIAGNOSIS: Spinal stenosis, cervical disc displacement, C4-5 and C5-6

PROCEDURES PERFORMED:

1. Cervical discectomy, C4-5 and C5-6
2. Corpectomy, C5
3. Placement of allograft from C4 to C6
4. Placement of arthrodesis 34-mm (millimeter) plate from C4 to C6

ANESTHESIA: General

This case was done under sensory evoked potential monitoring.

PROCEDURE: Under general anesthesia, the patient was placed in the supine position. The head was turned to the left. The neck was prepped and draped in the usual manner.

An incision was made in a linear fashion along the medial border of the sternocleidomastoid, and then dissecting the platysma, we got by the omohyoid and onto the prevertebral fascia. We then localized the C4-5 and C5-6 interspace and took an x-ray (reported by radiologist).

Continued

CASE 12-17—cont'd

I then sectioned the anterior longitudinal ligament and prepared myself for the discectomy, in which I incised the C4-5 disc space and the C5-6 disc space and removed as much disc material as I could. Then, with an air drill, I did a corpectomy, made a trough in this middle of C5 about 3 mm above the anterior longitudinal ligament. Having done this, I worked with curets and various Kerrison rongeurs to remove all the disc and to take the ridges off C4 and C5 as well as complete the corpectomy. This having been done, I was satisfied that I could see the dura and took out the disc fragments. There was no penetration to see the posterior longitudinal ligament, but we cleaned out this area well so that we could provide acceptance of the graft. I then fashioned a graft from the bone bank. (Literally, a bank of donated bone that is used to reduce the trauma to the patient that is receiving the bone. This is an allograft. Bone is the second most transplanted tissue [blood is first]). With gentle

extraction on the neck, I was able to place the bone graft so that the surfaces of C4 and C6 having been curetted and that cancellous bone was applied to the cancellous bone. Having done this, at this point, we then did the Synthes plate. We placed a 34-mm plate onto the body of C4 and C6 utilizing screws. We put screws into the body of C6 as well as C4 and into the graft. We took an x-ray (reported by radiologist) and felt it was secure and adequate. We irrigated the wound, placed a Hemovac drain in the wound, and closed the wound in layers utilizing a 2-0 chromic on the platysma, 2-0 plain on the subcutaneous tissue, and 3-0 interrupted mattress sutures on the skin. A dressing was applied. The patient was discharged to the PAR (postanesthesia recovery).

SERVICE CODE(S): _____

ICD-10-CM DX CODE(S): _____

(Answers to every other Case are located in Appendix D . The full answer key is only available in the TEACH Instructor Resources on Evolve.)

Neurology and Neuromuscular Procedures

Electroencephalography (EEG) is an important and frequent diagnostic tool used in neurology, as is EMG/NCV (electromyography/nerve conduction velocity). You have coded the EEG in several of the cases in the chapter, but the following reports will give you an additional opportunity to code these reports. The nerve conduction velocity study is one in which electrical impulses are applied to one end of the nerve and the time it takes to travel to the other end of the nerve is measured. Damaged peripheral nerves can be identified by means of this study. When these studies are done at the hospital, remember to use the professional component only modifier.

CASE 12-18 *Electroencephalogram Report*

LOCATION: Outpatient, Hospital

PATIENT: Reed Tolbert

REQUESTING PHYSICIAN: Ronald Green, MD

INDICATION: Convulsions

PHYSICIAN: Timothy Pleasant, MD

The patient was drowsy and asleep during much of this bedside EEG (electroencephalogram). The recording was requested for follow-up of a seizure, which occurred 2 months ago.

MEDICATIONS:

1. Albuterol
2. Atrovent
3. Epoetin
4. Bacitracin
5. Flagyl
6. Nystatin
7. Diflucan
8. Fosphenytoin
9. Gentamicin
10. Piperacillin
11. Protonix

While the patient was awake, the background activity was somewhat poorly organized and consisted of varying mixtures of 15-16 Hz beta and some 8-10 Hz alpha, with amplitudes of 25-35 uV.

Stages I and II of sleep were observed; vertex waves and sleep spindles appear normal.

Hyperventilation and photic stimulation were not performed.

IMPRESSION: This is a minimally abnormal EEG because of somewhat poor organization of the background while the patient was awake. No epileptogenic activity was seen.

SERVICE CODE(S): _____

ICD-10-CM DX CODE(S): _____

(Answers to every other Case are located in Appendix D . The full answer key is only available in the TEACH Instructor Resources on Evolve.)

CASE 12-19 *Electroencephalogram Report*

LOCATION: Outpatient, Hospital

PATIENT: Brian Wheaton

REQUESTING PHYSICIAN: Ronald Green, MD

PHYSICIAN: Timothy Pleasant, MD

TECHNICAL STATEMENT: This is a 21-channel digital recording using the International 10-20 electrode placement system. Three channels were devoted to monitoring the eye movements and EEG (electroencephalogram). The patient was unresponsive (reported diagnosis).

ELECTROGRAPHIC DATA: Background is low amplitude 4 to 5 Hz theta activity. A more prominent high amplitude, polymorphic delta rhythm of 2 to 3 Hz persists throughout the record. This delta activity is more prominent throughout the frontal regions.

During activation with tactile and sound stimuli, delta activity is accentuated and the background frequency increases minimally to 7 Hz. Theta activity is slightly more developed over the right hemisphere. In the absence of activation, background amplitude declines considerably.

The heart rate was 114 beats per minute.

CLINICAL INFORMATION: Severe head trauma 19 days prior. Episodes of seizure-like activity (convulsions are a reported diagnosis) in the last few days; treated with Dilantin.

CLINICAL INTERPRETATION: This is an abnormal record (reported diagnosis) due to markedly slow background with continuous delta activity. The symmetry of stimulus-induced frequency is not significant. No epileptiform activity is detected.

OPINION: Although epileptiform activity is not present in this record, the episodes of tremulousness are highly suggestive of autonomic overflow phenomenon. I recommend continued anti-seizure medications on a prophylactic basis.

The findings seem to be consistent with severe encephalopathy.

SERVICE CODE(S): _____

ICD-10-CM DX CODE(S): _____

(Answers to every other Case are located in Appendix D . The full answer key is only available in the TEACH Instructor Resources on Evolve.)

CASE 12-20 *Electrodiagnostic Evaluation Summary Report*

This is a nerve conduction study in which each study (motor nerve and sensory nerve for each nerve tested) is reported separately.

LOCATION: Outpatient, Hospital

PATIENT: Lynn Jie

REQUESTING PHYSICIAN: Ronald Green, MD

PHYSICIAN: Timothy Pleasant, MD

CLINICAL SYMPTOM: Left arm pain

MOTOR NERVE STUDY
Left Median Nerve

Rec Site: APB STIM SITE	Lat (ms)	Norm Lat	Amp (mV)	Dist (mm)	C.V. (m/s)	Norm C.V.
Wrist	3.7	4.2	3.8	60		
Elbow	7.7		0.167	220	55.0	49

Left Ulnar Nerve

Rec Site: ADM STIM SITE	Lat (ms)	Norm Lat	Amp (mV)	Dist (mm)	C.V. (m/s)	Norm C.V.
Wrist	2.7	3.6	12.0	60		
B. Elbow	6.5		4.7	230	60.0	48
A. Elbow	8.3		0.667	120	68.5	

Continued

CASE 12-20—cont'd

SENSORY NERVE STUDY
Left Median Nerve

Rec Site: Index	Lat (ms)	Norm Lat	Amp (uV)	Dist (mm)	C.V. (m/s)	Norm C.V.
STIM SITE						
Wrist	3.1	3.6	25.3	130	42.6	48

Left Ulnar Nerve

Rec Site: 5th digit						
STIM SITE						
Wrist	3.0	3.1	4.3	110	37.0	48

Left Median-MP Nerve

Rec Site: Wrist						
STIM SITE						
Midpalm	1.6	1.9	40.0	60	37.8	

SUMMARY/INTERPRETATION:

FINDINGS:

1. Normal left median nerve sensory conduction studies including both antidromic and orthodromic techniques
2. Normal left median nerve motor conduction study
3. Normal left ulnar nerve sensory conduction study
4. Normal left ulnar nerve motor conduction study

IMPRESSION: Normal left upper extremity nerve conduction study per standard interpretation criteria

Thanks for the opportunity to have provided you this information. The findings have been briefly reviewed with the patient in the clinic today. Please let me know if you have further questions or if I might be able to provide further information.

SERVICE CODE(S): _____

ICD-10-CM DX CODE(S): _____

(Answers to every other Case are located in Appendix D . The full answer key is only available in the TEACH Instructor Resources on Evolve.)

CHAPTER 12 *Auditing Review*

Audit the coding for the following reports.

Audit Report 12.1 Operative Report, Debridement

This service took place during the postoperative period of a previous surgery performed by Dr. Pleasant.

LOCATION: Inpatient, Hospital

PATIENT: Brady Grady

ATTENDING PHYSICIAN: Timothy Pleasant, MD

SURGEON: Timothy Pleasant, MD

PREOPERATIVE DIAGNOSIS: Infected scalp and infected craniotomy wound

POSTOPERATIVE DIAGNOSIS: Rejection of hardware, rejection of bone plate, and cerebrospinal fluid leak; suture rejection

PROCEDURE PERFORMED: Debridement of craniotomy wound, removal of hardware, removal of bone, removal of sutures, irrigation of wound, and placement of drain

ANESTHESIA: General

PROCEDURE: Under general anesthesia, the patient was placed in the prone position. The head was prepped and draped in the usual manner. The previous craniotomy wound was incised. We turned the flap down. What I did here was I removed the hardware, which was present, plus the screws, bony plate, and any sutures. I then placed a piece of Gelfoam on top of the wound and closed the wound in layers after irrigating the wound, placing a Hemovac drain in the wound, and achieving hemostasis with Bovie and roughing up the tissues with a curet. The scalp was then closed in one layer with 2-0 Prolene sutures, mattress-type fashion. A dressing was applied. After this, a subarachnoid drain was placed. The patient was transferred to the ICU for care.

One of the following codes is reported incorrectly for this case. Indicate the incorrect code.

PROFESSIONAL SERVICES: Plate removal, **62143-78**

ICD-10-CM DX: Orthopedic complication, **T84.7XXA**

INCORRECT CODE: _____

Audit Report 12.2 Operative Report, Plate Removal

LOCATION: Inpatient, Hospital

PATIENT: Robin Taylor

ATTENDING PHYSICIAN: Timothy Pleasant, MD

SURGEON: Timothy Pleasant, MD

DIAGNOSIS: Need for removal of failed Zephyr plate, cervical

PROCEDURE PERFORMED: Removal of failed Zephyr plate

PROCEDURE NOTE: Under general anesthesia, the patient's right neck was prepped and draped in the usual fashion. The previous incision was incised. With lateral dissection, I got on to the common carotid artery and the vein, retracting it laterally. With finger dissection, I was able to get on to the plate (this is anterior instrumentation), made a little hole in the adhesive tissue, and then took off the tissues that were adherent to the plate. There was no pus visible. We exposed the upper and lower parts of the plate, placed retractors in the wound, unscrewed the plate,

and removed it. We cultured the base of the wound. We looked at the fusion site. There was no collection of pus here. It was hard to tell if she had effusion or not, but certainly there was fibrous tissue here. Having removed the plate, we then cleaned the wound, irrigated the wound, put a Hemovac drain in the wound, and then closed the wound in layers utilizing 2-0 chromic in the platysma with 2-0 plain in the subcutaneous tissue and surgical staples on the skin. A dressing was applied. The patient was discharged to the recovery room and back to the Intensive Care Unit.

One of the following codes is reported incorrectly for this case. Indicate the incorrect code.

PROFESSIONAL SERVICES: Spinal instrumentation removal, **22852**

ICD-10-CM DX: Orthopedic complication, **T84.498D**

INCORRECT CODE: _____

Audit Report 12.3 Operative Report, Ventriculostomy

LOCATION: Inpatient, Hospital

PATIENT: Andy Haugen

SURGEON: Frank Gaul, MD

PREOPERATIVE DIAGNOSIS: Infected shunt.

POSTOPERATIVE DIAGNOSIS: Infected shunt.

PROCEDURES PERFORMED:

1. Removal of ventricular catheter from the right occipital region.
2. Right frontal ventriculostomy.

INDICATIONS: This is a 20-month-old male who presented with

hydrocephalus. A ventriculoperitoneal shunt was placed. The peritoneal catheter eroded through the diaphragm into the chest, and the patient developed pneumonia and shunt infection. The shunt needs to be removed and a ventricular drain placed to successfully treat the infection.

DESCRIPTION OF PROCEDURE: The patient was taken to the operating room and underwent induction of general endotracheal anesthesia in the supine position. The head was rotated 60 degrees to the left side and was appropriately padded. The right frontal and posterior scalp was shaved, and the right sides of the head, neck, and chest were sterilely prepped and draped. An approximately 0.5 cm incision was made approximately 1 cm anterior to the right coronal suture approximately 2 cm off the midline to the right. A retractor was placed using the TPS drill. A small burr hole was made in the bone. Bleeding bone edges were waxed. The

Continued

CHAPTER 12—cont'd

dura was coagulated and incised with an #11 blade. The pia arachnoid was coagulated. The ventricular catheter was passed into the right frontal horn a total distance of 5 cm. It was tunneled subcutaneously and exited in the right temporal area. It was then connected to an external drainage bag. There was copious CSF flow prior to connecting it to the bag. At this point, the previous right occipital incision was opened, and the valve and ventricular catheter were removed in one piece. A small incision was made in the neck and chest and the peritoneal catheter was removed.

A piece of Gelfoam was then placed. All of the wounds were closed with interrupted 3-0 Vicryl in the deep layer. The right frontal incision was closed on the skin with a 3-0 nylon and the right occipital incision was closed with a running 3-0 chromic. The patient tolerated the procedure well without apparent complication. Sponge, instrument, and needle counts were correct.

*One of the codes is **not** reported for this case and/or missing a modifier. Indicate the missing code and/or modifier.*

PROFESSIONAL SERVICES: Removal of ventriculoperitoneal shunt, **62256-RT**; Burr hole for right frontal ventriculostomy, **61210-RT**

ICD-10-CM DX: Infected ventriculoperitoneal shunt, **T85.79XA**; Displacement of ventricular intracranial shunt, **T85.02XA**; Hydrocephalus, **G91.9**

MISSING CODE AND/OR MODIFIER: _____

Audit Report 12.4 Operative Report, Craniotomy

LOCATION: Inpatient, Hospital

PATIENT: Shawn Moore

ATTENDING PHYSICIAN: Timothy Pleasant, MD

SURGEON: Timothy Pleasant, MD

PREOPERATIVE DIAGNOSIS: Parietal left brain tumor

POSTOPERATIVE DIAGNOSIS: Parietal left brain tumor

PROCEDURE PERFORMED: Craniotomy with removal of tumor

The Stealth was utilized for localization of the tumor. Coordinated in real-time with the MRI, which had been done the previous day.

PROCEDURE: The head was placed into the Mayfield pins. Fiducials having been placed on the head, the Stealth was then utilized to mark topographically the area of the tumor. The scalp was then marked for our skin incision. This having been done, the fiducials were removed, and the head was prepped and draped in the usual manner. An inverted U-shaped incision was made over the site of the tumor, and the burr hole was done. The bone flap was then elevated. The dura was incised so that the flap came down on the sinus. Having exposed the brain and having utilized the navigator to localize the tumor, we now incised over the tumor, got into the tumor. This was grayish tissue, hard, gritty. This was sent for frozen section. This came back as gemistocytic astrocytoma, so this was, in my opinion, a glioblastoma multiforme. I then removed the tumor with the coagulator and the Bovie. This came out very nicely. We utilized the Stealth probe to make sure that we had gone deep enough and around the cavity of the tumor. Remembering that this was on the left side, we did not want to produce a deficit but stayed within the context of the tumor, achieved adequate hemostasis after the tumor cavity had been cleaned out of its tumor. I then placed a piece of Gelfoam over the raw surface of the brain, and we then closed the dura with 4-0 Nurolon. We then re-applied the bone flap with screws and a small burr hole cover. A Hemovac drain was placed above the bone, and the scalp was approximated with 2-0 Vicryl on the galea and surgical staples on the skin. A dressing was applied. The patient was discharged to the recovery room.

PATHOLOGY REPORT LATER INDICATED: Malignant neoplasm of brain

One or more of the following codes are reported incorrectly for this case. Indicate the incorrect code or codes.

SERVICE CODE(S): Burr hole brain biopsy, **61140**

ICD-10-CM DX CODE(S): Neoplasm of unspecified behavior of brain, **D49.6**

INCORRECT/MISSING CODE(S): _____

Audit Report 12.5 Operative Report, Re-Do Craniectomy

LOCATION: Inpatient, Hospital

PATIENT: Jake Ark

ATTENDING PHYSICIAN: Timothy Pleasant, MD

SURGEON: Timothy Pleasant, MD

PREOPERATIVE DIAGNOSIS: Recurrent atraumatic epidural hematoma

POSTOPERATIVE DIAGNOSIS: Recurrent atraumatic epidural hematoma

PROCEDURE PERFORMED: Re-do craniectomy, enlargement of previous craniectomy and removal of clot and tacking of dura.

ANESTHESIA: General

PREOP NOTE: This patient had his epidural hematoma removed a couple of days ago and had a repeat CT scan. There is re-accumulation here. I have decided to take him back to surgery and enlarge the craniectomy and possibly get at a bleeder that may have been missed or maybe re-accumulation from the scalp, which was quite oozy.

CHAPTER 12—*cont'd*

PROCEDURE: Under general anesthesia, the patient was placed in the outrigger with the left side up. The staples were removed. The previous incision was incised, and there was obvious clot. I removed the clot. I enlarged the craniectomy with the craniotome. There were some surface bleeders on the dura. I utilized Gelfoam in the corners underneath the bone. I then tacked up the dura with 4-0 Nurolon, utilizing about 6-8 tacking sutures, and was satisfied the clot had been removed and there was no active bleeding. I then placed a Hemovac drain in the wound, closed the wound in layers utilizing 0 Vicryl on the galea with surgical staples on the skin. Dressing was applied. The patient was discharged to the SCCU.

One or more of the following codes are reported incorrectly for this case. Indicate the incorrect code or codes.

SERVICE CODE(S): Evacuation of hematoma by craniotomy or craniectomy, **61312**

ICD-10-CM DX CODE(S): Postprocedural infarct, **I97.821;** Extradural hemorrhage, **I62.1;** Stenosis of right middle cerebral artery, **I66.01**

INCORRECT/MISSING CODE(S): _____

Audit Report 12.6 Operative Report, Shunt Placement

LOCATION: Inpatient, Hospital

PATIENT: Cory Rhode

ATTENDING PHYSICIAN: Timothy Pleasant, MD

SURGEON: Timothy Pleasant, MD

PREOPERATIVE DIAGNOSIS: Hydrocephalus and myelomeningocele

POSTOPERATIVE DIAGNOSIS: Hydrocephalus and myelomeningocele

PROCEDURE PERFORMED: Placement of left ventriculoperitoneal shunt

INDICATION: This is a 4-month-old child who presented with a bacterial shunt infection. The shunt was externalized, and after the spinal fluid was sterilized with antibiotics, it was electively decided to place a new shunt on the opposite side.

PROCEDURE: The patient was taken to the operating room and underwent induction of general endotracheal anesthesia in the supine position. At that point, the left side of the head was shaved, and the left head, neck, and abdomen were prepped and draped. A 3-cm midline skin incision was made just above the umbilicus after infiltrating the skin with ¼% Xylocaine without Epinephrine. The skin and subcutaneous tissues were sharply divided using blunt dissection with the Senn retractors. The midline fascia was identified. This was cut with a #15 blade. The properitoneal fat was dissected bluntly out of the way, and the peritoneum was grasped with a hemostat. It was cut with the scissors, and hemostats were applied around the peritoneum. A red rubber catheter was placed into the peritoneal cavity. I next made a horseshoe-shaped incision in the left occipital region and reflected the scalp flap. I then burred a 0.50-cm diameter hole in the left occipital region. The dura was coagulated and incised with a #11 blade, as was the pia/arachnoid. I then made a subcutaneous tunnel from the scalp down to the abdomen and passed the peritoneal catheter. Prior to doing this, I flushed it with normal saline. I used a low-profile Delta I level valve and connected this to the distal catheter. I flushed the valve with normal saline prior to connecting it. I secured this with a silk ligature. I then took a ventricular catheter with a stylet in place and passed it into the occipital horn. I felt an ependymal pop and then withdrew the stylet and advanced the catheter a total length of 8 cm. Copious CSF spontaneously flowed. I then connected this to the valve, and I pulled the distal tubing so that the valve would lie nicely in the subcutaneous pocket in the left occipital region. The connections were all secured with 3-0 silk. The catheter was tacked down at its exit point of the skull with 3-0 silk. I then placed the distal tubing into the peritoneal cavity after verifying that there was good flow while pumping the shunt. I then closed the pursestring suture in the abdomen. I closed the abdomen in layers with interrupted 3-0 and 2-0 Vicryl. The skin was closed with a running 4-0 Prolene stitch. Benzoin and ¼-inch Steri-Strips were placed. The galea was closed with interrupted 3-0 Vicryl on the scalp, and the skin on the scalp was closed with 4-0 chromic. Bacitracin and a dressing were applied. The patient tolerated the procedure well without apparent complications. Sponge, instrument, and needle counts were correct times two. He was taken to the recovery room in stable condition. I would note that after the shunt was placed, I snipped the suture and removed the ventriculostomy from the right occipital region. There were no complications.

One or more of the following codes are reported incorrectly for this case. Indicate the incorrect code or codes.

SERVICE CODE(S): Removal with replacement of CSF shunt, **62258**

ICD-10-CM DX CODE(S): Varices, **I85.09XA;** Spina bifida, **Q05.4**

INCORRECT/MISSING CODE(S): _____

(Auditing Review answers with rationales are only available in the TEACH Instructor Resources on Evolve.)

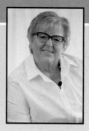

"Believe in yourself and strive to be the best version of yourself. Make this life matter."

Eye and Auditory Systems

http://evolve.elsevier.com/Buck/next

(Answers to every other Case are located in Appendix D, with the full answer key only available in the TEACH Instructor Resources on Evolve)
(Auditing Review answers with rationales are only available in the TEACH Instructor Resources on Evolve)

Eye

An **ophthalmologist** is a physician who specializes in medical and surgical care of the eye and visual system. The ophthalmologist provides a full spectrum of care, including the diagnosis and medical treatment of eye disorders and diseases, prescription of eyeglasses, routine eye exams, a variety of eye and visual system surgery, and management of eye problems that are caused by systemic illnesses, such as diabetic retinopathy. Ophthalmologists can be doctors of osteopathy (DO) or medical doctors (MD). Optometrists and opticians perform eye examinations, but they are not physicians and cannot perform surgery.

Common conditions diagnosed and treated by an ophthalmologist are conjunctivitis, corneal ulceration, corneal foreign body removal, optic neuritis, retinopathy, refractive error correction, macular degeneration, glaucoma, **cataracts,** and blepharitis.

Eye Examinations

During an eye examination, the physician assesses the visual acuity of the patient. This is accomplished by using a hanging wall chart that the patient reads from a distance of 20 feet. The patient covers one eye and reads the smallest character on the chart. Each eye is tested independently (i.e., one is covered while the other is used to read). The charts are marked with a number at the end of each line (e.g., 100, 200) that provides a comparison of that patient's vision with that of persons with normal vision. The larger the number, the worse the acuity. For example, 20/100 means that the patient can see at 20 feet what a normal patient could see at 100 feet. A visual acuity chart displaying the classification and descriptions of visual acuity is illustrated in **Figure 13-1.**

The definitions of a new patient and an established patient are the same as for all patients (less than 3 years since being treated by that physician or another physician of the same specialty who belongs to the same practice group, established; more than 3 years, new). There are two new patient codes and two established patient codes for eye examinations (92002-92014). There are extensive notes before the codes that must be read before coding eye examinations. These notes describe the intermediate, comprehensive, and special ophthalmologic services and should be read prior to coding ophthalmologic services.

Classification		Levels of Visual Impairment					Additional Descriptors Which May Be Encountered
"Legal"	WHO*	Visual Acuity and/or Visual Field Limitation (Whichever Is Worse)					
	(Near-) normal vision	Range of Normal Vision					
		20/10 2.0	20/13 1.6	20/16 1.25	20/20 1.0	20/25 0.8	
		Near-Normal Vision					
			20/30 0.7	20/40 0.6	20/50 0.5	20/60 0.4 0.3	
	Low vision	Moderate Visual Impairment					Moderate low vision
		20/70	20/80 0.25	20/100 0.20	20/125 0.16	20/160 0.12	
		Severe Visual Impairment					Severe low vision, "Legal" blindness
		20/200 0.10	20/250 0.03	20/320 0.06	20/400 0.05		
		Visual field: 20 degrees or less					
Legal Blindness (U.S.A.) both eyes	Blindness (WHO) one or both eyes	Profound Visual Impairment					Profound low vision, Moderate blindness
		20/500 0.04	20/630 0.03	20/800 0.025	20/1000 0.02		
		Count fingers at: less than 3 m (10 ft)					
		Visual field: 10 degrees or less					
		Near-Total Visual Impairment					Severe blindness, Near-total blindness
		Visual acuity: less than 0.02 (20/1000)					
		Count fingers: 1 m (3 ft) or less					
		Hand movements: 5 m (15 ft) or less					
		Light projection, light perception					
		Visual field: 5 degrees or less					
		Total Visual Impairment					Total blindness
		No light perception (NLP)					

*WHO = World Health Organization
Visual acuity refers to best achievable acuity with correction.
Non-listed Snellen fractions may be classified by converting to the nearest decimal equivalent, e.g., 10/200 = 0.05, 6/30 = 0.20.
CF (count fingers) without designation of distance, may be classified to profound impairment.
HM (hand motion) without designation of distance, may be classified to near-total impairment.
Visual field measurements refer to the largest field diameter for a 1/100 white test object.

FIGURE 13-1 Visual acuity chart.

CASE 13-1   *Clinic Progress Note, Eye Examination*

The cataract is determined to be a "juvenile" cataract (as opposed to "senile"), based on the age of the patient at the time of onset.

LOCATION: Outpatient, Clinic

PATIENT: Jay Bender

PHYSICIAN: Rita Wimer, MD

Today I saw Jay, who is now 21 years old. I last saw him 6 years ago when he had a corneal ulcer in his right eye. This is now cleared, and he has noticed that he cannot see well. He can read well, but he cannot see down the road. The last time I saw him, he was 20/30 in the right and 20/25 in the left. Now he is 20/80 in the right and 20/50 in the left, and

this cannot be improved with refraction. His near-vision correction is still 20/25 OU (both eyes). The pressures are 12 OU.

The patient has a normal corneal anterior chamber and iris but with very slow dilating pupils. There is no pseudoexfoliation, but there are dense juvenile nuclear cataracts in both eyes, the right greater than the left. From what I can see in the retina, the macula, optic nerve, and peripheral retina, they are normal. I counseled him for cataract surgery of his right eye first and then the left eye, the need for postoperative correction, a 4- to 6-week recovery time, and the type of procedure; we will see him in surgery on the last Monday of the month.

SERVICE CODE(S): _____

ICD-10-CM DX CODE(S): _____

(Answers to every other Case are located in Appendix D . The full answer key is only available in the TEACH Instructor Resources on Evolve.)

CASE 13-2   *Clinic Progress Note, Eye Examination*

Dr. Wimer uses a B-scan ultrasound to assess the status of Rex's retina while doing an eye examination. The ultrasound is reported in addition to the examination. There is an external cause code that will be assigned to this case. Report the medications given to the patient intramuscularly and intravenously with HCPCS codes. Do not report the drops that were placed in the patient's eye, ointment, or patch.

LOCATION: Outpatient, Clinic

PATIENT: Rex Dagg

PHYSICIAN: Rita Wimer, MD

Today, I saw Rex, a 68-year-old, a new patient to me, who was wrapping a couch with a bungee cord in preparation for moving the couch, when the cord snapped and the metal fitting hit him in his left eye squarely. He has pain and loss of vision and was seen in the ED (emergency

department); there was no light perception, and there was blood in the anterior chamber and a nonmoving pupil.

He was sent to me, and I saw that he was 20/20 in the right and had bare light perception in the left. The pressure was 33, and there was 25% hyperemia and a vitreous hemorrhage. B-scan showed no detachment or separation of the optic nerve. I gave him 60 of Toradol IM (intramuscular) for pain and started him on Cosopt 2 drops and Iopidine 1% two drops and gave him 500 of Diamox IV (intravenous) push. Within a few minutes his pressure had reduced to 22, and the vision improved to finger counting and facial features. I placed atropine ointment, TobraDex patch, and Telfa over his eye and had him on strict bed rest without work. We will see him again in 24 hours.

SERVICE CODE(S): _____

ICD-10-CM DX CODE(S): _____

(Answers to every other Case are located in Appendix D . The full answer key is only available in the TEACH Instructor Resources on Evolve.)

Cataracts

There are various types of cataracts, such as senile cataracts linked to the aging process, and many location areas for formation of a cataract, such as anterior or posterior polar cataracts. See **Figure 13-2**. Reference the term "cataract" in a medical dictionary to see the various types of cataracts. Cataract removal and lens replacement (66830-66990) use three different approaches:

- Extracapsular cataract extraction (ECCE): Removing the hard nucleus in one piece, then removal of the soft cortex in multiple pieces. Extracapsular is on the outside of the eyeball chamber.
- Intracapsular cataract extraction (ICCE): Total removal, which removes the cataract in one piece. Intracapsular is inside the eyeball chamber.
- Phacoemulsification: Dissolves the hard nucleus by means of ultrasound and then the soft cortex is removed in one piece.

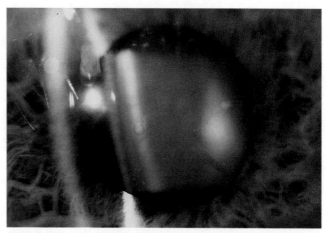

FIGURE 13-2 Cataract.

CASE 13-3   *Clinic Progress Note, Senile Cataracts*

As you code the services for this report, the choice of code for the cataract will be based on the age of the patient.

LOCATION: Outpatient, Clinic

PATIENT: Margo Himon

PHYSICIAN: Rita Wimer, MD

DIAGNOSIS: Senile cataracts.

FINDINGS: This 69-year-old established patient is in for an exam. Vision is 20/50 and 20/70. Failed driver's license eye examination.

See visual findings as noted. Glass prescription as encircled. Slight improvement in right eye can be obtained by increasing prescription by 0.50 to 0.75 sphere. Applanation reading is 16 bilateral. Medications are listed. Drives daytime only.

TREATMENT: Six to eight months' fundus. Copy of glass prescription for right lens change. Driver's license form filled out.

SERVICE CODE(S): _____

ICD-10-CM DX CODE(S): _____

(Answers to every other Case are located in Appendix D . The full answer key is only available in the TEACH Instructor Resources on Evolve.)

CASE 13-4   *Operative Report, Senile Cataracts*

Phacoemulsification is used in the following cataract surgery.

LOCATION: Outpatient, Hospital

PATIENT: Ingrid Cady

ATTENDING PHYSICIAN: Rita Wimer, MD

SURGEON: Rita Wimer, MD

PREOPERATIVE DIAGNOSIS: Senile nuclear cataract, right eye

POSTOPERATIVE DIAGNOSIS: Senile nuclear cataract, right eye

PROCEDURE PERFORMED: Extracapsular cataract extraction by phacoemulsification **(Figure 13-3)**, right eye (model SI40RB, +14.5 diopters, serial no. 38982) and implantation of intraocular lens.

ANESTHESIA: Topical

ESTIMATED BLOOD LOSS: Minimal

COMPLICATIONS: None

PROCEDURE: In the operating room, a drop of lidocaine 4%-MPF was applied to the eye. The patient was prepped and draped in the usual sterile fashion for an intraocular procedure of the right eye. A lid speculum was placed. A Weck-cel soaked with lidocaine 4%-MPF was placed at the limbus, both in the area of the planned phaco incision and planned side port incision. A keratome was used to enter the chamber at the arcade. A small amount of preservative-free lidocaine 1% was injected in the anterior chamber. The aqueous was exchanged with viscoelastic material, and a side port incision was made with a 15-degree angle blade. A continuous tear capsulotomy was made with a bent needle and the Utrata forceps. The nucleus was hydrodissected and removed with phacoemulsification using an ultrasound time of 2.4 minutes and a phaco percentage of 15%. The remaining cortical material was removed with irrigation and aspiration. The

capsule was polished and vacuumed as indicated. A small additional amount of lidocaine 1% was again injected into the anterior chamber. Viscoelastic was used to deepen the chamber, and the posterior chamber intraocular lens was unfolded into the capsular bag and dialed into position. Irrigation and aspiration were used to remove the remaining viscoelastic. The globe was pressurized and the cornea hydrated to ensure a good seal. The wound was tested and found to be watertight. TobraDex drops were placed on the surface of the eye. The patient left the operating room in stable condition without complications, having tolerated the procedure well.

SERVICE CODE(S): _____

ICD-10-CM DX CODE(S): _____

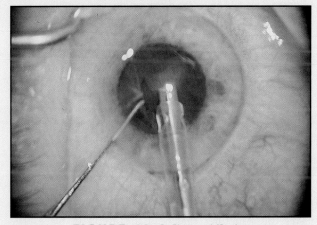

FIGURE 13-3 Phacoemulsification.

(Answers to every other Case are located in Appendix D . The full answer key is only available in the TEACH Instructor Resources on Evolve.)

Photocoagulation

Photocoagulation is the use of laser to seal leaky blood vessels, destroy abnormal blood vessels, destroy abnormal tissue at the back of the eye, and seal retinal tears. The procedure is an office procedure that does not usually require anesthesia other than eyedrops.

Diabetic retinopathy is a condition that manifests by leakage from blood vessels in the retina, causing swelling, which results in decreased vision. Photocoagulation is the treatment of choice for sealing off the leaking vessels.

The Index and Tabular indicate E11.319 for diabetes type 2 with retinopathy.

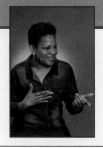

From the Trenches

"A successful medical coder is someone who is able to multi-task and work independently."

YAKIMA FLEMING
MSNM, RHIA, CPC

CASE 13-5A   *Clinic Progress Note, Eye Examination*

LOCATION: Outpatient, Clinic

PATIENT: Carl Kerrie

PHYSICIAN: Rita Wimer, MD

Today I saw this new patient, who is nearly completely blind and deaf. The patient is accompanied by his son, who translated. The patient had glasses at one time but ceased to wear them because they did not help. He noticed that his vision has come down some but noticed no flurries. He has had type 1 diabetes for about 10 years.

Today, when I saw him, he was 20/40 OU (both eyes) with a pressure of 9 on the right and 11 on the left. There was normal pupillary time and a question of rubeosis on the left. The lens and vitreous were clear on both eyes. The patient had extensive preproliferative and frank

neovascularization elsewhere but not on the disc of the left eye only. There are numerous exudates and abortive efforts at neovascularization nasal and superior to the disc. The peripheral retinas are flat, and the macula shows some wrinkle on the left but is free on the right. The optic nerve is normal on the right, and there is no proliferative neuropathy in the right eye. This patient is insulin dependent.

We are dealing with a preproliferative diabetic retinopathy that needs panretinal photocoagulation as soon as possible. We have set up the treatment soon, and this will be started and commenced within the next few days.

SERVICE CODE(S): _____

ICD-10-CM DX CODE(S): _____

(Answers to every other Case are located in Appendix D . The full answer key is only available in the TEACH Instructor Resources on Evolve.)

CASE 13-5B   *Clinic Progress Note, Photocoagulation*

Refer to Report 13-5A for the diagnosis information on this patient.

LOCATION: Outpatient, Clinic

PATIENT: Carl Kerrie

PHYSICIAN: Rita Wimer, MD

PROCEDURE: Photocoagulation, left eye

DIAGNOSIS: Type 1 diabetic retinopathy, insulin-dependent. The patient presents today for a photocoagulation treatment: VA (visual acuity) 20/60-2, SC (without refraction correction) 20/30-1, OP 608, 0.1 sec, 200, 400. Follow-up is in 2 weeks in the office.

SERVICE CODE(S): _____

ICD-10-CM DX CODE(S): _____

Ectropion and Entropion

Ectropion is a condition in which the lower eyelid **droops** due to age, excessive exposure to the sun, or gravity that relaxes the structures that hold the eyelid in place. The punctum is the drain hole on each lid, near the nose, that drains the tears. However, when the eyelid droops, the tears do not drain naturally into the nose. This leads to deterioration of the protective covering of the eye and results in burning, itching, irritation, and discomfort. Repair of ectropion is reported with codes from the 67914-67917 range. The ectropion repair codes include repair of one eye; if two eyes are done, report the service with modifier -50 to indicate bilateral.

Entropion is a condition in which the lower eyelid turns **inward**. See **Figure 13-4**. The eyelashes and skin of the eyelid then rub against the cornea and conjunctiva, which leads

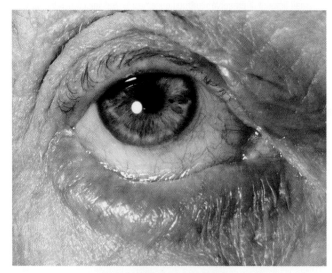

FIGURE 13–4 Entropion.

to excessive tearing, crusting eyelid, discharge, impaired vision, and irritation of the cornea. Repair of entropion is reported with codes from the 67921-67924 range. The entropion repair codes include repair of one eye; if two eyes are done, report the service with modifier -50 to indicate bilateral.

Some third-party payers require the use of the HCPCS modifiers on the service codes:

E1   upper-left eyelid
E2   lower-left eyelid
E3   upper-right eyelid
E4   lower-right eyelid

CASE 13-6   *Operative Report, Entropion and Ectropion Repair*

Use HCPCS modifiers when reporting the services for this patient.

LOCATION: Outpatient, Hospital

PATIENT: Robert Vobr

ATTENDING PHYSICIAN: Rita Wimer, MD

PREOPERATIVE DIAGNOSIS:

1. Upper lid entropion, both eyes; lower lid ectropion, both eyes
2. Graves' disease
3. Status post chemical decompression for Graves' disease
4. Chronic exposure, keratitis secondary to diagnoses 1, 2, and 3
5. Chronic conjunctivitis secondary to diagnoses 1, 2, 3, and 4

POSTOPERATIVE DIAGNOSIS:

1. Upper lid entropion, both eyes; lower lid ectropion, both eyes
2. Graves' disease
3. Status post chemical decompression for Graves' disease
4. Chronic exposure, keratitis secondary to diagnoses 1, 2, and 3
5. Chronic conjunctivitis secondary to diagnoses 1, 2, 3, and 4

OPERATIONS PERFORMED:

1. Upper lid entropion repair, both eyes
2. Lower lid ectropion repair, both eyes

ANESTHESIA: MAC

INDICATION: The patient has had progressive increase of upper lid entropion and lower lid ectropion, ptosis, and a number of other problems secondary to eye disease related to thyroid disease. The excess tissue is now interfering with his vision.

DESCRIPTION OF PROCEDURE: After the patient was placed on the operating room table, the skin to be resected on the upper lid was marked out with a blue sterile marking pen, as was the lower lid. There was a fishtail superiorly and lateral oblique inferiorly. This was infiltrated with Xylocaine 2%, 0.75% Marcaine, and bicarbonate. It was on a 25-gauge needle, and a total of 40 cc was used throughout the procedure. The 15 Bard-Parker blade then dissected the skin to be resected superiorly on the upper lids. This was freehand dissected, and a 2-mm (millimeter) strip of orbicularis was removed. The lateral, central, and medial fat pads were isolated, clamped, cut, and cauterized on the upper lids. The wound was reapproximated without supratarsal fixation using 6-0 nylon black suture to create a 2-mm ectropion of the upper lids. The lower lids were cut out with a 15 Bard-Parker blade through the marked incision. The fat pads centrally, medially, and laterally were identified, clamped, cut, cauterized, and allowed to retract. The amount of skin to be resected inferiorly was determined by the up-eye/open-mouth position, and this was mainly a lateral resection. The wounds were then closed with 6-0 nylon sutures. Maxitrol ointment and Telfa strips were laid on all four lids and half patches so the eyes remained open. There were no complications.

SERVICE CODE(S): _____

ICD-10-CM DX CODE(S): _____

(Answers to every other Case are located in Appendix D . The full answer key is only available in the TEACH Instructor Resources on Evolve.)

Epiphora

Epiphora is a condition in which there is excessive production of tears. Acute epiphora is caused by allergies, foreign bodies, obstruction, or another associated condition. This type of epiphora resolves with treatment. Chronic epiphora is the excessive tearing that does not resolve with treatment. The chronic condition is most commonly caused by a malaligned eyelid, an obstructed lacrimal duct, or an ocular surface disorder. Surgical intervention sometimes is required to open the lacrimal duct by means of a nasal probe.

CASE 13-7   *Operative Report, Nasolacrimal Duct Probing*

Use HCPCS or CPT modifiers when reporting the service for this patient. Epiphora is excessive tearing that is mainly due to obstruction of the lacrimal passage.

LOCATION: Outpatient, Hospital

PATIENT: Peggy Crase

ATTENDING PHYSICIAN: Rita Wimer, MD

PREOPERATIVE DIAGNOSIS:

1. Epiphora, both eyes
2. Nasolacrimal duct obstruction, both eyes

POSTOPERATIVE DIAGNOSIS:

1. Epiphora, both eyes
2. Nasolacrimal duct obstruction, both eyes

PROCEDURE PERFORMED: Nasolacrimal duct probing, both eyes

ANESTHESIA: General anesthesia

INDICATIONS: This 32-month-old white female was referred by Dr. Peterson after an allergy workup to investigate her chronic otitis media, PE (pressure equalization) tubes times two, and the chronic epiphora that she has had in both eyes since birth. The mother was counseled as to the success of probing at this age and the possible reoperations that may be needed.

PROCEDURE: After the patient was placed under suitable anesthesia via the mask, a small punctum dilator was used to dilate the punctum inferiorly and superiorly. These were found to be very tight and occluded. A 2-0 Bowman probe could be passed only through the inferior system with difficulty on both sides. The C-loop could not be irrigated. Probing could not be attempted because of a large bony obstruction that resisted all efforts to pass the tube. There was no fluorescein removed in the nose. TobraDex drops were placed in the eyes. The procedure was complete, and the patient was sent to the recovery room. The patient will be referred for further ENT (ears, nose, throat) consultation and to Dr. Lorabi for the possibility of a white cell deficiency that is causing these chronic infections or other immune problems. There were no complications.

SERVICE CODE(S): _____

ICD-10-CM DX CODE(S): _____

(Answers to every other Case are located in Appendix D . The full answer key is only available in the TEACH Instructor Resources on Evolve.)

Ear

Office Services

Otolaryngologists are physicians trained in the medical and surgical management and treatment of patients with diseases and disorders of the ear, nose, and throat (ENT) and are often referred to as ENT physicians. There are many subspecialty areas in otolaryngology, such as pediatric otolaryngology, otology or neurotology (ears, balance, and tinnitus), allergy, facial plastic and reconstructive surgery, head and neck, laryngology, and rhinology. Some otolaryngologists limit their practices to one area, and others practice across all areas.

Because an otolaryngologist specializes in the ears, nose, and throat, there is a wide range of conditions that are treated, such as cerumen removal (69209-69210), ear infections, sinusitis, septal deviation, laryngitis, and pharyngitis.

CASE 13-8A   *Clinic Progress Note, Sore Throat*

Report both the E/M and lab service. A hint for looking up the strep screen in the CPT index is that it is a bacterial culture.

LOCATION: Outpatient, Clinic

PATIENT: Leah Charles

PHYSICIAN: Rita Wimer, MD

SUBJECTIVE: The patient is a 3½-year-old girl who was seen by me 4 months ago, and today presents with her parents to the clinic. Her mother states that both her brother and sister have been on medication for the second time because of being positive for strep. The patient started complaining of a sore throat 2 days ago. She is also complaining of some ear pain. She does have an ALLERGY to SULFA. Mother noticed a rash on the side of her lips just the other day.

OBJECTIVE: On general appearance, the patient is alert. She does not appear to be in acute distress. Temperature is 99.9° F. Weight is 13.6 kg (kilogram). HEENT (head, ears, eyes, nose, throat): Both TMs (tympanic membranes) are clear. Her PE (pressure equalization) tube is out in the canal on the left. Oropharynx is erythematous. Also, along her lip she does have some erythematous lesions with golden crust and consistent with impetigo. Neck has shotty (like a pellet) cervical nodes bilaterally but is supple. Heart reveals a regular rate and rhythm without murmur. Lungs are clear to auscultation bilaterally. Her abdomen is soft.

IMPRESSION:

1. Pharyngitis, rule out strep
2. Impetigo

CASE 13-8A—cont'd

PLAN:

1. Keflex 250 mg (milligram)/5 cc (cubic centimeter) ³/₄ teaspoon orally, three times daily × 10 days.
2. We will also do a strep screen as well, today.

SERVICE CODE(S): _____

ICD-10-CM DX CODE(S): _____

(Answers to every other Case are located in Appendix D . The full answer key is only available in the TEACH Instructor Resources on Evolve.)

CASE 13-8B   *Clinic Progress Note, Well Child Care*

Three months later, Leah again is brought to the clinic by her mother. The first-listed diagnosis is the otitis media, but you will also need to report a Z code to indicate that the purpose of this visit was a medical examination for admission to preschool.

LOCATION: Outpatient, Clinic

PATIENT: Leah Charles

PHYSICIAN: Rita Wimer, MD

SUBJECTIVE: The patient is an almost 4-year-old girl who presents to the clinic with her parents for well child care and Head Start physical. Mother states that she was seen 1 month ago when they noted fluid in one of her ears. Mother does not notice any problems with the patient's hearing or speech development. She has not had a runny nose, cough, or fever. She eats well from the four food groups and has no problems with constipation or diarrhea.

OBJECTIVE: On general appearance, the patient is alert and does not appear to be in any acute distress. Temperature is 97.7° F. Weight is 15.8 kg (kilogram), which places her right at the 50th percentile. Height is 97.8 cm (centimeter), which places her right beneath the 25th percentile. Blood pressure is 90/60. HEENT (head, ears, eyes, nose, throat): PERRLA (pupils equal, round, reactive to light and accommodation). EOMI (extraocular movement intact). Discs are sharp. Right TM does have some fluid present behind it. The left TM is nice and clear. Oropharynx is unremarkable. Neck is supple. Heart reveals a regular rate and rhythm. Lungs are clear to auscultation bilaterally, and her abdomen is soft. GU (genitourinary): Normal female genitalia. Extremities have full range of motion. Back reveals a straight spine. Hearing was checked and is normal bilaterally. Vision is 20/25 bilaterally.

IMPRESSION: Female almost 4 years old with right serous otitis media.

PLAN: I recommended following up with the patient in 2 months to ensure that the fluid has gone. Prescribed amoxicillin, 20 mg (milligram), q.8h. (every 8 hours). If it has not at that point, we may need to look into further ways of management. Mother was in agreement with this.

SERVICE CODE(S): _____

ICD-10-CM DX CODE(S): _____

(Answers to every other Case are located in Appendix D . The full answer key is only available in the TEACH Instructor Resources on Evolve.)

From the Trenches

"To advance in the medical coding field, a medical coder must stay abreast of the coding guidelines, rules and regulations and stay productive."

YAKIMA FLEMING
MSNM, RHIA, CPC

Myringotomy and Tympanostomy

The eustachian tube connects the middle ear to the back of the throat and allows for drainage of any fluid that may collect there. When a eustachian tube dysfunctions, fluid collects in the middle ear. The tube can become inflamed from allergies or infection. Eustachian tube dysfunction is a fairly common condition in children because the eustachian tube has not always matured to the level of normal function and therefore does not work as well as it does in an adult. The condition prevents air from entering the middle ear, so pressure builds up in the middle ear. Surgical intervention is a **myringotomy**

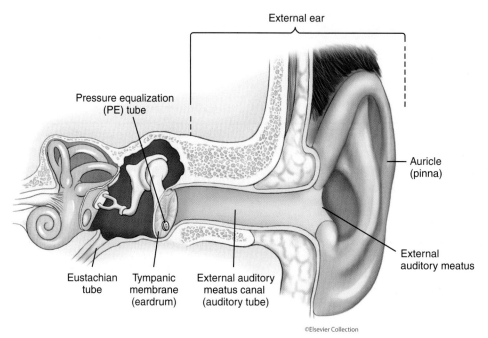

External ear

Pressure equalization
(PE) tube

Auricle
(pinna)

External
auditory meatus

Eustachian
tube

Tympanic
membrane
(eardrum)

External auditory
meatus canal
(auditory tube)

©Elsevier Collection

FIGURE 13–5 Placement of pressure equalization (PE) tube.

(incision into the tympanic membrane) and reinflation of the eustachian tube or insertion of a small plastic or metal tube (PE [pressure equalization] tube) that allows the fluid to drain **(tympanostomy).** See **Figure 13-5** for an illustration of the placement of a PE tube. The tubes may later be removed or fall out naturally, or sometimes they are just left in place.

A myringotomy is the incision and draining of fluid from the middle ear. A tympanostomy is the incision and placement of tubes to drain fluid from the middle ear. If the ventilation tubes are removed due to a complication, the diagnosis is reported based on the reason for the complication, such as an infection.

CASE 13-9   *Operative Report, Pressure Equalization Tube Removal*

LOCATION: Outpatient, Hospital

PATIENT: Ann Sjol

ATTENDING PHYSICIAN: Jeff King, MD

PREOPERATIVE DIAGNOSIS:

1. Retained PE (pressure equalization) tubes
2. Obstructed PE tubes

POSTOPERATIVE DIAGNOSIS:

1. Retained PE tubes
2. Obstructed PE tubes

PROCEDURE PERFORMED: Removal of bilateral PE tubes

OPERATIVE NOTE: The patient is a 7-year-old female who has had PE tubes in for a prolonged period. Recently, she has had problems with recurrent infections and persistent fluid. She has granulation on both tubes. A decision

was made to remove these in the operating room. She was admitted through the same-day surgery program and taken to the operating room, where a general anesthetic was administered via inhalation. A 4-mm (millimeter) speculum was inserted in the right ear. Wax was removed from the canal. The tube was visualized. Using cup forceps, this tube was removed. There was granulation tissue around the opening. Two drops of Cortisporin were applied. The speculum was removed and inserted on the opposite side. Again, wax was removed from the canal. The PE tube was removed with cup forceps. Again, granulation tissue seemed to close the perforation nicely. Two drops of Cortisporin were applied here. The speculum was removed. The patient was allowed to recover from the general anesthetic and taken to the postanesthesia care unit in stable condition. There were no complications during this procedure.

SERVICE CODE(S): _____

ICD-10-CM DX CODE(S): _____

(Answers to every other Case are located in Appendix D . The full answer key is only available in the TEACH Instructor Resources on Evolve.)

CASE 13-10   *Operative Report, Tonsillectomy, Adenoidectomy, and Myringotomy*

In the following case, a myringotomy and a tonsillectomy/adenoidectomy (the most resource-intense) are performed.

LOCATION: Outpatient, Hospital

PATIENT: Dustin Boyle

ATTENDING PHYSICIAN: Jeff King, MD

PREOPERATIVE DIAGNOSES:

1. Chronic adenotonsillitis
2. Adenotonsillar hypertrophy
3. Chronic serous otitis media

POSTOPERATIVE DIAGNOSES:

1. Chronic adenotonsillitis
2. Adenotonsillar hypertrophy
3. Chronic serous otitis media

PROCEDURE PERFORMED:

1. Myringotomy bilaterally
2. Tonsillectomy and adenoidectomy

OPERATIVE NOTE: The patient is a 15-year-old boy seen in the office and diagnosed with the above condition. The decision was made in consultation with his family to take him to the operating room to undergo the above-named procedures.

PROCEDURE: The patient was admitted through the same-day surgery program and taken to the operating room, where he was administered general anesthetic by intravenous injection. He was then intubated endotracheally. A 4-mm (millimeter) speculum was inserted into the right ear, and wax was removed from the canal. An anterior/inferior incision was created, and a small amount of fluid was removed. The speculum was removed and inserted in the opposite ear. Again, wax was removed from the canal. An anterior/inferior incision was created. This middle ear cavity was dry. The speculum was removed.

The patient was turned 90 degrees. The Jennings gag was placed into the mouth and expanded. This was secured to a Mayo stand. Two red rubber catheters were placed through the nose, brought out through the mouth, and secured with snaps. A laryngeal mirror was placed into the nasopharynx, and the adenoid tissue was identified. This was removed with a suction cautery in a systematic fashion. Once this was completed, the red rubbers were released and brought out through the mouth. The right tonsil was grasped with an Allis forceps and retracted medially. Using the harmonic scalpel, the capsule was identified laterally. The tonsil was removed from its fossa in an inferior-to-superior fashion. Once this was completed, the bed was inspected. One small area was cauterized. The left tonsil was grasped with an Allis forceps and retracted medially. Again, the capsule was identified laterally with the harmonic scalpel. The tonsil was removed from its fossa in a superior-to-inferior fashion. Once this was completed, the bed was inspected. No bleeding was noted. Three tonsil sponges were then soaked with 1% Marcaine and epinephrine; one was placed in the nasopharynx and one in each tonsil bed. These were left in position for 5 minutes. At the end of the interval, they were removed. The beds were inspected, and no further bleeding was noted. The gag was released and removed from the mouth. The TMJ (temporomandibular joint) was checked. The patient was allowed to recover from the general anesthetic and taken to the postanesthesia care unit in stable condition. There were no complications during this procedure.

Pathology Report Later Indicated: Benign tonsil and adenoid tissue.

SERVICE CODE(S): _____

ICD-10-CM DX CODE(S): _____

(Answers to every other Case are located in Appendix D . The full answer key is only available in the TEACH Instructor Resources on Evolve.)

CASE 13-11   *Operative Report, Tube Removal*

In this case, both a removal of impacted PE tube and tympanostomy are performed.

LOCATION: Outpatient, Hospital

PATIENT: Will Boyle

ATTENDING PHYSICIAN: Jeff King, MD

PREOPERATIVE DIAGNOSIS: Impacted left PE (pressure equalization) tube

POSTOPERATIVE DIAGNOSIS: Impacted left PE tube

PROCEDURE PERFORMED:

1. Removal of impacted PE tube, left ear
2. Placement of new PE tube, left ear

OPERATIVE NOTE: Will is a patient who was seen in the office with a diagnosis of the above-named condition. A decision was made in consultation with the family for the above-named procedure.

The patient was admitted through same-day surgery department and taken to the operating room, where he was administered a general anesthetic by inhalation. A 3.5-mm (millimeter) speculum was inserted into the right ear. A small amount of wax was removed. The speculum was removed and inserted into the left ear. The impacted PE tube was then removed. There was some granulation tissue around this site. We created a new site posteriorly within some tympanosclerotic plaque. A new PE tube was inserted. The patient was then allowed to recover from the general anesthetic and taken to the postanesthesia care unit in stable condition. There were no complications during this procedure.

SERVICE CODE(S): _____

ICD-10-CM DX CODE(S): _____

(Answers to every other Case are located in Appendix D . The full answer key is only available in the TEACH Instructor Resources on Evolve.)

CASE 13-12   *Operative Report, Myringotomy and Tympanostomy*

The patient's bilateral nasolacrimal duct obstruction is congenital.

LOCATION: Outpatient, Hospital

PATIENT: Karen Vince

SURGEON: Jeff King, MD

PREOPERATIVE DIAGNOSIS:

1. Bilateral nasolacrimal duct obstruction
2. Bilateral cerumen impaction
3. Right otitis media with effusion with nonfunctional pressure equalization tube

POSTOPERATIVE DIAGNOSIS:

1. Bilateral nasolacrimal duct obstruction
2. Bilateral cerumen impaction
3. Acute right otitis media with effusion with nonfunctional pressure equalization tube

PROCEDURE PERFORMED:

1. Bilateral nasolacrimal duct dilation
2. Left endoscopic nasal examination with inferior turbinate fracture
3. Bilateral microscopic ear examination with cleaning of the left and right ear
4. Right myringotomy with tympanostomy tube placement

ANESTHESIA: General endotracheal anesthesia

INDICATION: A 10-year-old female with bilateral nasolacrimal duct obstruction (congenital). The patient is now here for treatment. She has very narrow nasal anatomy. She also has bilateral cerumen impactions that do not allow for ease of access for examination of her ears for the status of her PE (pressure equalization) tubes.

DESCRIPTION OF PROCEDURE: After consent was obtained, the patient was taken to the operating room and placed on the operating table in a supine position. After an adequate level of general endotracheal anesthesia was obtained, the patient was draped in an appropriate manner and the nasolacrimal duct dilation performed, bilaterally. The nose was packed with cotton pledgets soaked with 0.25% Neo-Synephrine. Attention was first focused on the left eye. The left nasal cavity was examined endoscopically. The turbinate was infractured to allow access to the inferior meatus. The turbinate was then repositioned to its normal position and the nose packed with the pledgets soaked with the Neo-Synephrine solution. Attention was then focused on the right. A similar procedure was performed; however, endoscopic examination and turbinate outfracture were not necessary on that side. The right side was then packed with the pledgets soaked with the Neo-Synephrine solution. Attention was then focused on the ears. Using the ear speculum and microscope, the left ear canal was cleared of cerumen. It was functional, and there were no abnormalities on that side. Attention was then focused on the right side, where the ear canal was again cleared of cerumen impaction. Subsequent examination showed an extruded PE tube lying on the tympanic membrane with surrounding cerumen and squamous debris. This was removed. Subsequently, a myringotomy incision was placed in the anterior-inferior quadrant. A large amount of mucoid effusion was suctioned. A bobbin tympanostomy tube was then placed without difficulty. Corticosporin Otic suspension and a cotton ball were then placed in the right ear. The nasal packs were then removed. There was no bleeding. The patient tolerated the procedure well. There was no break in technique. The patient was extubated and taken to the postanesthesia care unit in good condition.

FLUIDS ADMINISTERED: 50 cc (cubic centimeter) of RL

ESTIMATED BLOOD LOSS: Less than 20 cc

PREOPERATIVE MEDICATION: 4 mg (milligram) of Decadron IV (intravenous)

SERVICE CODE(S): _____

ICD-10-CM DX CODE(S): _____

(Answers to every other Case are located in Appendix D . The full answer key is only available in the TEACH Instructor Resources on Evolve.)

CASE 13-13   *Operative Report, Tympanoplasty*

The patient in this case has a history of chronic otitis media and cholesteatoma and presents for reconstruction of the tympanic membrane with ossicular chain. Use an HCPCS National Level II modifier to denote which ear the procedure is being performed on.

LOCATION: Inpatient, Hospital

PATIENT: Neil Fraser

ATTENDING PHYSICIAN: Jeff King, MD

PREOPERATIVE DIAGNOSES:

1. Right moderate conductive hearing loss
2. History of right ear cholesteatoma, status post tympanoplasty and mastoidectomy

POSTOPERATIVE DIAGNOSES:

1. Right moderate conductive hearing loss (Discontinuity of ear ossicles)
2. History of right ear cholesteatoma, status post tympanoplasty and mastoidectomy

PROCEDURE PERFORMED: Right tympanoplasty with ossicular reconstruction using a Kurt titanium partial ossicular replacement prosthesis

ANESTHESIA: General endotracheal anesthesia

INDICATION: A 12-year-old male with history of right chronic otitis media and cholesteatoma. He has undergone tympanoplasty and mastoidectomy. This resulted in a moderate conductive hearing loss. The patient has not shown any evidence of recurrent disease, and the patient is in now for re-exploration and reconstruction if no cholesteatoma is found.

CASE 13-13—cont'd

DESCRIPTION OF PROCEDURE: After parental consent was obtained, the patient was taken to the operating room and placed on the operating table in a supine position. After an adequate level of general endotracheal anesthesia was obtained, the patient was positioned for surgery on the right ear. The patient's right ear was prepped with Betadine prep and draped in a sterile manner. One-percent Xylocaine with 1:100,000 U of epinephrine was infiltrated into the preauricular, tragus, postauricular area, and then in the ear canal. The speculum was secured with a speculum holder. The mastoid cavity was clean. A tympanomeatal flap was then elevated. The chorda tympani nerve was identified and preserved. There was no evidence of recurrent cholesteatoma. The posterior aspect of the tympanic membrane was thin. This was elevated off the head of the stapes. No incus was present. The long process of the malleus was present, but there was no head of the malleus. The stapes was mobile, and there was a round window reflex. Attention was then focused on the tragus, where a cartilage and perichondrium graft was harvested in standard fashion. That incision was closed with interrupted 6-0 rapid absorbing gut suture. The Kurz titanium partial replacement prosthesis was selected. Sizers were placed to determine the appropriate length. This was determined to be 2.5 mm (millimeter). Dry Gelfoam was placed in the middle ear. The prosthesis was then placed on top of the stapes superstructure. Cartilage and perichondrium were then placed on top of this to act as an interface between the titanium and the thin drum remnant and also to reinforce the drum remnant. The tympanomeatal flap was then brought back over this and brought onto the canal wall and facial ridge. Gelfoam soaked with Physiosol was then placed on this. The proximal ear canal was then filled with Bacitracin ointment. A cotton ball coated with Bacitracin ointment was placed in the conchal bowl area, and then a Band-Aid dressing was applied. The patient tolerated the procedure well, and there was no break in technique. The patient was extubated and taken to the postanesthesia care unit in good condition.

FLUIDS ADMINISTERED: 1600 cc of RL

ESTIMATED BLOOD LOSS: Less than 10 cc

SERVICE CODE(S): _____

ICD-10-CM DX CODE(S): _____

(Answers to every other Case are located in Appendix D . The full answer key is only available in the TEACH Instructor Resources on Evolve.)

CHAPTER 13   *Auditing Review*

Audit the coding for the following reports.

Audit Report 13.1 Operative Report, Tympanostomy

LOCATION: Outpatient, Hospital

PATIENT: MacAlister Knutson

SURGEON: Dr. Marsh.

PREOPERATIVE DIAGNOSIS:

1. Chronic otitis media with effusion.
2. Adenoiditis.

POSTOPERATIVE DIAGNOSIS: Same.

PROCEDURES PERFORMED:

1. Bilateral tympanostomy with placement of Ventilation tubes.
2. Adenoidectomy.

PROCEDURE: After this 10-year-old patient was placed under an anesthetic with a mask inhalant, the nasopharyngeal area was examined, and a moderate plus amount of adenoids were noted to be present. The patient was then intubated and following this, the right external auditory canal was cleared of wax and prepped with Betadine, and a radial incision was made in the anterior-inferior quadrant. The serous fluid was suctioned from behind the drum, and a 0.39 mm ventilation tube was placed. The left canal was then cleared of wax and prepped with Betadine. A radial incision was made in the anterior-inferior quadrant, and serous fluid was suctioned from behind this drum. A 0.39 mm ventilation tube was placed. The McIvor mouth gag was inserted, and following this, adenotome was used to remove her adenoids along with a curet. The nasopharynx was then visualized, examined, and palpated to be sure that the adenoids had been removed. Once this was completed, a Bismuth pack was placed. The pack was then removed and electrocautery was used to obtain good hemostasis in the nasopharynx. The nasal cavities were then irrigated and cleaned well with normal saline along with the oral cavity, and once the nasopharynx was rechecked and adequate hemostasis was present, the patient was awakened from anesthetic and returned to the Recovery Room in a stable condition. Prognosis immediate remote is good. Estimated blood loss 20 cc.

One or more of the following codes are reported incorrectly for this case. Indicate the incorrect code or codes.

PROFESSIONAL SERVICES: Adenoidectomy **42830**; tympanostomy with tubes **69436-50-51**

ICD-10-CM DX: Hypertrophic adenoids, **J35.2**; Chronic otitis media with effusion, **H65.493**

INCORRECT CODE(S): _____

Audit Report 13.2 Operative Report, Blepharoplasty

LOCATION: Inpatient, Hospital

PATIENT: Sharon Mann

SURGEON: Rita Wimer, MD

PREOPERATIVE DIAGNOSIS: Bilateral upper eyelid dermatochalasis.

POSTOPERATIVE DIAGNOSIS: Bilateral upper eyelid dermatochalasis.

PROCEDURE: Bilateral upper lid blepharoplasty.

ANESTHESIA: Lidocaine with l:100,000 epinephrine.

This 65-year-old female demonstrates conditions described above of excess and redundant eyelid skin with puffiness and has requested surgical correction. The procedure, alternatives, risks, and limitations in this individual case have been very carefully discussed with the patient. All questions have been thoroughly answered, and the patient understands the surgery indicated. She has requested this corrective repair be undertaken, and the consent was signed. The patient was brought into the operating room and placed in the supine position on the operating table. An intravenous line was started, and sedation anesthesia were administered IV after preoperative P.O. sedation. The patient was monitored for cardiac rate, blood pressure, and oxygen saturation continuously.

The excess and redundant skin of the upper lids producing redundancy and impairment of lateral vision was carefully measured, and the incisions were marked for fusiform excision with a marking pen. The surgical calipers were used to measure the supratarsal incisions so that the incision was symmetrical from the ciliary margin bilaterally.

The upper eyelid areas were bilaterally injected with 1% Lidocaine with 1:100,000 epinephrine for anesthesia and vasoconstriction. The plane of injection was superficial and external to the orbital septum of the upper and lower eyelids bilaterally.

The face was prepped and draped in the usual sterile manner. After waiting a period of approximately ten minutes for adequate vasoconstriction, the previously outlined excessive skin of the right upper eyelid was excised with blunt dissection. Hemostasis was obtained with a bipolar cautery. A thin strip of orbicularis oculi muscle was excised in order to expose the orbital septum on the right. The defect in the orbital septum was identified, and herniated orbital fat was exposed. The abnormally protruding positions in the medial pocket were carefully excised and the stalk meticulously cauterized with the bipolar cautery unit. A similar procedure was performed exposing herniated portion of the nasal pocket. Great care was taken to obtain perfect hemostasis with this maneuver. A similar procedure of removing skin and taking care of the herniated fat was performed on the left upper eyelid in the same fashion. Careful hemostasis had been obtained on the upper lid areas. The lateral aspects of the upper eyelid incisions were closed with a couple of interrupted 7-0 blue Prolene sutures.

At the end of the operation the patient's vision and extraocular muscle movements were checked and found to be intact. There was no diplopia, no ptosis, and no ectropion. Wounds were reexamined for hemostasis, and no hematomas were noted. Cooled saline compresses were placed over the upper and lower eyelid regions bilaterally.

The procedures were completed without complication and tolerated well. The patient left the operating room in satisfactory condition. A follow-up appointment was scheduled, routine post-op medications prescribed, and post-op instructions given to the responsible party.

The patient was released to return home in satisfactory condition.

One or more of the following codes are reported incorrectly for this case. Indicate the incorrect code or codes.

PROFESSIONAL SERVICES: Blepharoplasty **15823-50**

ICD-10-CM DX: Cosmetic surgery, **Z41.1**; Dermatochalasia, **H02.834** (left upper), **H02.831** (right upper)

INCORRECT CODE(S): _____

Audit Report 13.3 Operative Report, Conjunctivoplasty

LOCATION: Inpatient, Hospital
PATIENT: Judy Bachmeier
SURGEON: Rita Wimer, MD
PREOPERATIVE DIAGNOSIS: Blind painful eye, right eye, with conjunctival scarring.

POSTOPERATIVE DIAGNOSES:

1. Blind painful eye, right eye, with conjunctival scarring.
2. Microcornea, right eye.

OPERATIONS PERFORMED:

1. Evisceration with temporary implant, right eye.
2. Conjunctivoplasty, right eye.
3. Frost suture for temporary tarsorrhaphy.

ANESTHESIA: General.
ESTIMATED BLOOD LOSS: Minimal.
COMPLICATIONS: None.
DESCRIPTION OF OPERATION: With the patient in the supine position, in the operating room, after satisfactory anesthesia had been achieved, the patient was prepped and draped for surgery in the usual sterile manner. One gram first-generation cephalosporin was given during the surgery intravenously. A lid speculum was placed, and peritomy was performed as best as possible given severe perilimbal scarring. We then initiated the conjunctivoplasty, carefully unrolling and dissecting the conjunctiva back around the muscle insertion to carefully release scar bands and to maximize the length of the conjunctiva, to maximize the sizes of the fornices.

After this meticulous procedure had been performed and hemostasis assured, we then entered the posterior limbus with a Supersharp knife

and excised the corneoscleral button. We then carefully eviscerated the intraocular contents and scraped the scleral bag. Meticulous hemostasis was assured with electrocautery. Q-tips were used to remove residual retinal and uveal fragments. A 61-mm sphere was seen to fit in the bag without undue tension.

Once hemostasis was assured, we then closed the sclera with interrupted #4-0 Vicryl horizontal mattress sutures, overlapping sclera about 3 mm and burying the knots. We then removed small dog ears medially and laterally, as a relaxing incision of the sclera. Further relaxing incisions were made in the posterior sclera. Subsequently, we then reclosed Tenon and conjunctiva in a single layer with a running #6-0 chromic suture.

At the end of the procedure, after hemostasis was assured, sterile Polysporin Ophthalmic ointment was applied along with medium-sized conformer, which was seen to fit nicely. This was followed by Frost suture consisting of #6-0 silk going to the tarsal plates of the upper and lower eyelids to achieve temporary eyelid closure. This was followed by a pressure patch. The patient was then returned to the recovery room in good condition.

One or more codes should not have been reported for this case. Indicate the code(s) incorrectly reported.

PROFESSIONAL SERVICES: Evisceration of ocular contents, **65093-RT**; Conjunctivoplasty without graft, **68330-51-RT**; Frost suture, **67875-51-RT**

ICD-10-CM DX: Eye pain, **H57.11**; Conjunctival scarring, **H11.241** Microcornea, **Q13.4**

INCORRECTLY REPORTED CODE(S): _____

Audit Report 13.4 Operative Report, Cataract Extraction

LOCATION: Outpatient, Hospital
PATIENT: Guy Parker
ATTENDING PHYSICIAN: Rita Wimer, MD
SURGEON: Rita Wimer, MD
PREOPERATIVE DIAGNOSIS: Senile nuclear cataract, right eye
POSTOPERATIVE DIAGNOSIS: Senile nuclear cataract, right eye
PROCEDURE PERFORMED: Cataract extraction by phacoemulsification, right eye (Model AR40E, +21.5 diopters, serial #90402)
ANESTHESIA: Topical
ESTIMATED BLOOD LOSS: Minimal
COMPLICATIONS: None
PROCEDURE: In the OR, a drop of lidocaine 4%-MPF was applied to the eye. The patient was prepped and draped in the usual sterile fashion

for an intraocular procedure of the right eye. A lid speculum was placed. A Weck-cel soaked with lidocaine 4%-MPF was placed at the limbus both in the area of the planned phaco incision and planned side-port incision. A keratome was used to enter the chamber at the arcade. A small amount of preservative-free lidocaine 1% was injected into the anterior chamber. The aqueous was exchanged with viscoelastic material, and a side-port incision was made with a 15-degree angle blade. A continuous tear capsulotomy was made with a 15-degree angle blade. A continuous tear capsulotomy was made with a bent needle and the Utrata forceps. The nucleus was hydrodissected. Phacoemulsification was used to remove the nucleus using an ultrasound time of 2 minutes, 22 seconds, and effective phaco time of 5.93 seconds. Irrigation and aspiration were used to remove the remaining cortical material. The capsule was polished and vacuumed as indicated. A small additional amount of non-preserved lidocaine 1% was again injected into the anterior chamber. The chamber was

Continued

deepened with viscoelastic, and the posterior chamber intraocular lens was injected into the capsule bag and dialed into position. The remaining viscoelastic material was removed with irrigation and aspiration. The globe was pressurized, and the cornea was hydrated to ensure a good seal. The wound was tested and found to be watertight. Zymar and Pred Forte 1% drops were placed on the surface of the eye. The patient left the operating room in stable condition without complications, having tolerated the procedure well.

One or more of the following codes are reported incorrectly for this case. Indicate the incorrect code or codes.

SERVICE CODE(S):   Cataract removal, **66982**

ICD-10-CM DX CODE(S):   Cataract, right eye, **H25.011**

INCORRECT/MISSING CODE(S): _____

Audit Report 13.5 Operative Report, Entropion with Mini-Blepharoplasty

LOCATION: Outpatient, Hospital

PATIENT: Peter Win

ATTENDING PHYSICIAN: Rita Wimer, MD

SURGEON: Rita Wimer, MD

PREOPERATIVE DIAGNOSIS:

1. Entropion, right lower lid.
2. Chronic eye pain.
3. Chronic conjunctivitis.
4. Chronic exposure keratitis.
5. #2, #3, and #4 secondary to #1

POSTOPERATIVE DIAGNOSIS:

1. Entropion, right lower lid.
2. Chronic eye pain.
3. Chronic conjunctivitis.
4. Chronic exposure keratitis.

PROCEDURE PERFORMED: Tarsal wedge resection right lower lid

ANESTHESIA: MAC

INDICATIONS: This 75-year-old white male has had multiple suffering episodes of red, sore, painful, infected, and irritated eye secondary to entropion of his right lower lid. He was counseled for repair to relieve his symptoms.

PROCEDURE: After the patient was prepped and draped in the usual sterile fashion for ophthalmic surgery, the area we marked was infiltrated with Xylocaine 2% with 0.75% Marcaine and bicarbonate. A 6-mm equilateral triangle base-down was made on the tarsal surface of the right lower lid, the middle one-third, and a 12-mm equilateral triangle base-up was made in the right lateral canthus inferior to the lesion. The tarsal plate triangle was taken first from the inside with a chalazion clamp exposed to control bleeding. A 6-mm triangle was removed, saving the superior point only. This was closed with interrupted 5-0 chromic gut sutures tied anteriorly and one tied posteriorly. The skin surface, anterior side, was closed with two 5-0 chromic sutures. The 12-mm equilateral triangle at the right lower lateral canthus was then cut with a #15 Bard Parker blade down to the fascia. The skin and muscle were cut away. Cautery was used, and this was closed with interrupted 4-0 silk. Maxitrol ointment, Telfa pad, and patch were applied. The patient was sent to the recovery room. There were no complications.

One or more of the following codes are reported incorrectly for this case. Indicate the incorrect code or codes.

SERVICE CODE(S):   Blepharoplasty, **15820**

ICD-10-CM DX CODE(S):   Entropion, **H02.002**

INCORRECT/MISSING CODE(S): _____

Audit Report 13.6 Operative Report, Tube Removal

LOCATION: Outpatient, Hospital

PATIENT: Chad Allen

ATTENDING PHYSICIAN: Jeff King, MD

PREOPERATIVE DIAGNOSIS: Obstructed PE tubes

POSTOPERATIVE DIAGNOSIS: Same

PROCEDURE PERFORMED: Removal of PE tubes

ANESTHESIA: General

OPERATIVE NOTE: The patient is a 9-year-old male who has had PE tubes in for a prolonged period. Recently, he has had problems with recurrent infections and fluid. He has granulation on both tubes. A decision was made to remove these in the operating room.

PROCEDURE: He was admitted through the same-day surgery program and taken to the operating room, where general anesthetic was administered via inhalation. A 4-mm speculum was inserted in the right ear. Wax was removed from the canal. The tube was visualized. Using cup forceps, this tube was removed. There was granulation tissue around the opening. Two drops of Cortisporin were applied. The speculum was removed and inserted in the left ear. Again, wax was removed from the canal. The PE tube was removed with cup forceps. Again, granulation tissue seemed to close the perforation nicely. Two drops of Cortisporin were applied. The speculum was removed. The patient was allowed to recover from the general anesthetic and taken to the postanesthesia care unit in stable condition. There were no complications noted during the procedure.

One or more of the following codes are reported incorrectly for this case. Indicate the incorrect code or codes.

SERVICE CODE(S):   Removal of FB from ear canal, **69205**

ICD-10-CM DX CODE(S):   Otitis externa, **H60.399**

INCORRECT/MISSING CODE(S): _____

(Auditing Review answers with rationales are only available in the TEACH Instructor Resources on Evolve.)

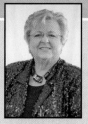

"You are at the end of this step of your advanced studies! Congratulations! You have expanded your toolkit of skills, just what all great coders seek to do."

Anesthesia

http://evolve.elsevier.com/Buck/next

(Answers to every other Case are located in Appendix D, with the full answer key only available in the TEACH Instructor Resources on Evolve)
(Auditing Review answers with rationales are only available in the TEACH Instructor Resources on Evolve)

Introduction

This chapter will provide an overview of the types of anesthesia services and some important factors to consider when reporting anesthesia services. You will learn about the role of the anesthesia professional in providing anesthesia care, pain management, and critical care to patients. Moderate (conscious) sedation and patient-controlled analgesia will be reported. You will also note that preceding some cases, there are notes of explanation regarding the type of anesthesia used in the case and some specific coding considerations when reporting that specific type of anesthesia.

Anesthesia

Anesthesia is the administration of drugs to induce the loss of the ability to sense pain. Often, the term "anesthesia" is used to refer to general anesthesia, but the term also includes regional, local with intravenous sedation, and local anesthesia. An anesthetist is a specialist in perioperative medicine who provides care to a patient prior to, during, and immediately after surgery. This care includes the evaluation and preparation of a patient for anesthesia service. The anesthetist plans the type of anesthesia and then cares for the patient during the surgical procedure by monitoring blood pressure, heart rate and rhythm, breathing, temperature, kidney function, and level of consciousness and analgesia. The anesthetist can also administer drugs for analgesia (pain relief) before, during, and after the procedure.

Additionally, the anesthetist is responsible for any adjustments to the anesthesia plan, medications, fluids (blood volume and electrolytes), and other parameters to ensure a pain-free and safe surgical experience for the patient. The anesthetist provides postoperative care during the patient's time in the recovery room. The anesthetist may be a physician (anesthesiologist, also referred to as MDA [Medical Doctor of Anesthesia]) or a nonphysician practitioner trained to administer anesthesia, such as a CRNA (Certified Registered Nurse Anesthetist).

Types of Anesthesia

Anesthesia commonly refers to general, regional, local with IV sedation, and local. These types of anesthesia, as well as Monitored Anesthesia Care (MAC), are summarized in the following pages. **General** anesthesia is a state of total unconsciousness resulting from the administration of a variety of drugs that can produce different effects to ensure unconsciousness, amnesia, analgesia, and muscle relaxation. Many general anesthetics are gases or vapors administered by mask or endotracheal tube (ET, a tube inserted through the nose or mouth into the trachea) along with intravenous medications. **Regional** or **conduction** anesthesia includes central and peripheral techniques that block nerves to large areas or body parts:

Central Technique

- Epidural anesthesia: The injection of drugs into the epidural space (between the dura and the vertebrae and their supporting ligaments). The drug(s) block the nerves from and near the spinal cord. Epidurals can be a single dose of anesthetic drugs or continuous dose administered through a catheter into the epidural space.
- Spinal anesthesia: The injection of drugs into the subarachnoid space (into the cerebrospinal fluid). This type of anesthesia is fast acting because the drugs directly bathe the nerves originating from the spinal cord. As with the epidurals, a spinal can be a single dose of anesthetic drugs or continuous dose administered through a catheter into the subarachnoid space.
- Neuraxial anesthesia: This type is usually a continuous epidural used for labor/delivery.

Peripheral Technique

- Plexus blocks, such as a brachial plexus block, block the nerves of the shoulder and arm.
- Single nerve blocks, such as an axillary nerve block, are often used for hand surgery. Nerve blocks can be by a single dose of anesthetic drugs or continuous through a catheter, such as a femoral nerve block (64447) or a continuous femoral nerve block (64448).

Intravenous Regional Technique (Bier Block)

- A tourniquet is placed on the arm or leg, and the tourniquet is inflated. Local anesthesia is then injected into a vein. The drug diffuses into the tissues and blocks the peripheral nerves and nerve endings in the extremity. The tourniquet keeps the drugs in the extremity and prevents systemic distribution. This technique is often used for hand surgery. Usually, intravenous sedation is administered in conjunction with a Bier block.
- Field block is a subcutaneous injection of anesthetic into an area bordering the field to be anesthetized. The drug blocks the peripheral nerves to a small area or body part.

Local anesthesia is the application of an anesthetic agent directly to the area. Local anesthesia techniques include:

■ Surface anesthesia is the application of local anesthesia spray or solution to skin or mucous membranes.

■ Infiltration is an injection of anesthetic, such as Xylocaine, into the tissues to be anesthetized.

MAC does not specifically describe minimal, moderate, or deep sedation. Rather, it is a service in which an anesthesiologist cares for a patient during a diagnostic or therapeutic procedure. It includes a pre-op, intra-op, and post-op service. MAC providers must be qualified and credentialed to perform anesthesia services and be prepared to convert to general anesthesia if necessary. MAC includes assessment and management of potential problems that might occur during the procedure, including rescuing the patient's airway should it be compromised by drugs that may have been administered. MAC includes support of the patient's vital functions and may include administration of necessary sedatives, anesthetics, or analgesics. MAC includes postprocedural services as well, such as returning the patient to full consciousness and management of pain side effects that may have resulted from medications administered during the procedure.

Anesthesia Care and Bundled Services/Procedures

The various types of anesthesia care have been reviewed, and now it is time to review the various component services/procedures that are considered integral to the anesthesia care. Procedures that are not bundled into the anesthesia codes and may be reported separately are discussed in the subsection below in Anesthesia Care and Separately Reported Services.

Anesthesia care includes the following services:

■ Preoperative evaluation

■ Preparation of patient for anesthesia, including placement of monitoring devices and IV lines

■ Placement of airway, nasogastric tube

■ Administration of anesthetic, fluids, blood, and other medications

■ Intraoperative care including
  ■ Monitoring of physiological parameters (blood pressure, heart rate, respirations, temperature, EEG, ECG [EKG], vascular Doppler flow, oximetry, etc.)
  ■ Ventilation management
  ■ Cardiopulmonary resuscitation
  ■ Blood sampling and interpretation of lab data (arterial blood gases, hematology, chemistries, etc.)
  ■ Nerve stimulation to determine localization of nerve or paralysis
  ■ Postoperative anesthesia recovery care

These services are included in the anesthesia code and are not reported separately.

Anesthesia services are reported with CPT codes 00100-01999 with modifiers that describe the patient's physical status, concurrency, and other factors that affect anesthesia care and reimbursement. The Anesthesia section of the CPT manual is used by the anesthesiologist/anesthetist to report the provision of anesthesia services. In addition to the

00100-01999 codes, Qualifying Circumstances that affect the anesthesia care are reported with CPT codes 99100-99140. The Qualifying Circumstances codes are located in the Medicine Section, as well as the Anesthesia Section, of the CPT manual and will be addressed a little later in this chapter.

When anesthesia is administered by the physician/surgeon who also performs the procedure/surgery, the anesthesia CPT codes are not used. Rather, the physician reports the anesthesia service by appending modifier -47 to the CPT code that describes the diagnostic or surgical procedure performed.

Anesthesia codes are divided first by anatomic site and then by the specific type of procedure. The last four subsections in Anesthesia—Radiological Procedures, Burn Excisions or Debridement, Obstetric, and Other Procedures—are not by anatomic division. The Radiological Procedures codes are used to report anesthesia services when radiologic services are provided to the patient for diagnostic or therapeutic reasons.

To select the correct anesthesia CPT code, the operative report is essential. Based on the operative report, the coder determines the procedure(s) performed. The correct CPT is selected by referencing the index of the CPT manual and then the code in the Anesthesia section. The coder may also have access to the American Society of Anesthesiologists (ASA) Crosswalk or an encoder with the crosswalk embedded. A crosswalk is a document that indicates which CPT anesthesia codes are reported with the various CPT procedure codes. The coder enters the CPT procedure code and the crosswalk will display the anesthesia code that corresponds to that particular CPT procedure code.

When multiple procedures are performed, with the aid of the ASA *Relative Value Guide*, the coder determines which code carries the highest base unit value and assigns that code. Only one anesthesia code can be reported when multiple procedures are performed.

Anesthesia Care and Separately Reported Services

Additional services/procedures may be performed during anesthesia care and may be reported separately. These include, but are not limited to:

■ Arterial line

■ Swan Ganz catheter

■ Central venous line

■ Nerve block for postoperative pain relief

■ Epidural catheter insertion for postoperative pain control

The time spent performing these separately reportable (billable) services must not be included in the time reported for the anesthesia. For example, the time to establish a Swan Ganz catheter is reported separately, and therefore the time it took to establish the catheter placement is not included in the total anesthesia time.

When an epidural is used specifically for postoperative pain control, it is separately reported with 62324-62327. There must be an order from the surgeon requesting post-op pain management by the anesthesiologist to report the service. The documentation in the medical record must indicate the medical necessity and the intent for postoperative pain management. The time spent providing the epidural procedure is reported separately and therefore not included in the anesthesia total time. If, however, a nerve block is used as the means to provide regional anesthesia for the performance of the surgical procedure, then the nerve block is not reported separately but is considered included in the anesthesia care (00100-01999).

If an epidural catheter is used to provide regional anesthesia during a procedure and is left in place for postoperative pain control, it is not reported separately. The daily management of the epidural (01996) on a subsequent day after surgery can be reported separately.

Codes from the Evaluation and Management and the Surgery sections of the CPT manual are used to report pain management and critical care services/procedures. The assignment of these codes will be discussed later in this chapter.

Base Units

Base units are assigned to the anesthesia care codes (00100-01999) and are referred to as BUV (base unit value). BUVs vary by CPT code and increase in value as the procedures become more complex. The American Society of Anesthesiologists (ASA) assigns the BUVs and publishes the values in the ASA *Relative Value Guide*. The ASA *Relative Value Guide* is commonly accepted among payers. The CMS also assigns and publishes a list of BUVs. Most of the BUVs published by CMS coincide with the ASA BUVs, but in some cases the base units vary.

For the cases you will be coding in this chapter, refer to **Figure 14-1** for an example of the BUVs that are assigned to the anesthesia codes.

Physical Status Modifiers

The second type of modifying unit used in the Anesthesia section is the Physical Status Modifiers. These modifiers are used to indicate the patient's condition at the time anesthesia was administered. The Physical Status Modifier not only indicates the patient's condition at the time of anesthesia but also identifies the level of complexity of services provided. For instance, anesthesia service to a gravely ill patient is much more complex than the same type of service to a normal, healthy patient. The Physical Status Modifier is not assigned by the coder; rather, it is determined by the anesthesiologist and documented in the anesthesia record. The Physical Status Modifier begins with the letter "P" followed by a number from 1 to 6. The relative value for -P1, -P2, and -P6 is zero because these conditions are considered not to affect the service provided.

P1	Normal healthy patient (0 base units)
P2	Patient with mild systemic disease (0 base units)
P3	Patient with severe systemic disease (1 base unit)
P4	Patient with severe systemic disease that is a constant threat to life (2 base units)
P5	Moribund patient who is not expected to survive (3 base units)
P6	Declared brain-dead patient whose organs are being removed for donor purposes (0 base units)

Every anesthesia code reported must have an accompanying Physical Status Modifier, whereas Qualifying Circumstances codes may or may not be reported (see following section).

Concurrent Care Modifiers

Some third-party payers require additional modifiers to indicate how many cases an anesthesiologist is directing or supervising at one time. A certified registered nurse anesthetist (CRNA) may administer anesthesia to patients under the direction of a licensed physician, or they may work independently depending on the state law. When an anesthesiologist is directing the provision of anesthesia in more than one case at a time, modifiers are used to indicate the context and number of cases that are being reported concurrently (at the same time). **Medical direction** is when an anesthesiologist is directing CRNAs or AAs (anesthesia assistants) while 2-4 cases are performed concurrently. **Medical supervision** is when CRNAs or AAs are administering anesthesia in more than four concurrent cases and the anesthesiologist is not present on induction or present to perform oversight/direction for the cases. Also, if there are four concurrent cases being performed and the anesthesiologist is providing medical direction but is called away (such as for an emergency intubation), the medical direction by the anesthesiologist ends, and the medical supervision begins because the anesthesiologist is no longer available to direct the cases.

The MDA's medical direction is reported with -QY or -QK modifier, and medical supervision is reported with modifier -AD. The CRNA service, whether directed or supervised, would be reported with modifier -QX. The CRNA service would be reported as medical direction regardless of the number of concurrent procedures directed or supervised by the anesthesiologist. The CRNA is always reimbursed at the medically directed rate as long as the anesthesiologist is involved with the CRNA in providing the anesthesia service.

Sometimes the services of two anesthetists (both MDA and CRNA) are medically necessary. Examples of situations requiring two anesthetists would be when managing an emergency patient during surgery, a patient has severe multiple injuries, a patient with a ruptured AAA (abdominal aorta aneurysm), etc. In these cases, the MDA's services are considered to be personally performed (-AA required), and the CRNA's services are considered to be independently performed (-QZ required).

The following modifiers are among the most commonly used:

-AA	Anesthesia services performed personally by anesthesiologist
-AD	Medical supervision by a physician: More than four concurrent anesthesia procedures
-QK	Medical direction of two, three, or four concurrent anesthesia procedures involving a qualified individual
-QX	Certified registered nurse anesthetist (CRNA) service, with medical direction by a physician
-QY	Anesthesiologist medically directs one CRNA
-QZ	CRNA service, without medical direction by a physician

Concurrency Scenarios	Who Reports	Modifier Appended
Personally performed by an MDA	MDA	-AA
MDA and CRNA services are each medically necessary in anesthesia care	MDA	-AA
	CRNA	-QZ
MDA medically directing 1 CRNA	MDA	-QY
	CRNA	-QX
MDA medically directing CRNAs during 2-4 concurrent cases	MDA	-QK
	CRNA	-QX
MDA medically supervising a CRNA (either >4 concurrent cases or the MDA is performing procedure that does not allow for involvement required at the medically directed rate)	MDA	-AD
	CRNA	-QX
CRNA without medical direction	CRNA	-QZ

Positioning

Another aspect that may impact the anesthesia charge and reimbursement is unusual positioning. When the patient is placed in a position other than supine or lithotomy or when procedures require field avoidance (change in the way anesthesia is administered so as to avoid contaminating or obstructing the surgical field, such as that used around the head, neck, or shoulder girdle), the anesthesia BUV is 5 regardless of a lesser BUV assigned to the anesthesia code. For example, anesthesia code 00164 has a BUV of 4 (refer to Fig. 14-1). If field avoidance or unusual positioning is required, the BUV would be 5 rather than 4. You would not add the BUV 4 for the procedure and 5 for the field avoidance together.

Qualifying Circumstances

At times, anesthesia is provided in situations that make the administration of the anesthesia more difficult. These types of cases include those that are performed in emergency situations and those dealing with patients of extreme age and include services performed during the use of controlled hypotension (low blood pressure) or the use of hypothermia (low body temperature). The Qualifying Circumstances codes are five digits that begin with 99 and are add-on codes that cannot be used alone but must be used in addition to another code. The Qualifying Circumstances codes are used only to provide additional information and are reported in addition to the anesthesia procedure code.

The Qualifying Circumstances codes are located in two places in the CPT manual—the Medicine section and the guidelines of the Anesthesia section. In both locations, the plus symbol is located before the codes (99100-99140) to indicate their status as add-on codes.

In some cases, more than one Qualifying Circumstances code may apply and can be reported. For example, a surgical procedure performed on a patient of extreme age (99100) in which the anesthesia is complicated by an emergency condition (99140). The Qualifying Circumstances codes

are not subject to the concurrency and physical status modifiers.

There are differing payer guidelines for qualifying circumstances. For example, some payers may limit the reporting of qualifying circumstances to only the directing anesthesiologist. **Throughout this chapter, apply this limitation when reporting Qualifying Circumstances.**

The Qualifying Circumstances codes are as follows:

CPT	Definition
99100	Anesthesia for patient of extreme age, younger than 1 year, or older than 70
99116	Anesthesia complicated by utilization of total body hypothermia
99135	Anesthesia complicated by utilization of controlled hypotension
99140	Anesthesia complicated by emergency conditions

Anesthesia Time

Anesthesia time is important to anesthesia coding and reimbursement because the charge and reimbursement increases based on the time reported. Anesthesia time is defined as the period of time in which the anesthesia provider is with the patient furnishing continuous anesthesia care. It begins when the anesthesia provider begins to prepare the patient and ends when the anesthesia provider is no longer furnishing services and the patient is safely placed under postoperative care. There may be interruptions in the care, and when that is the case, you can add the blocks of time together.

Time spent performing procedures that are separately billable is NOT to be included in the anesthesia time reported with the anesthesia CPT code.

Calculation of Charge/Payment

This is payer-specific information that is not contained in the CPT manual but is included in this text for the benefit of exposing you to the formula commonly used to calculate charges and payment for anesthesia services. Generally, such calculation is accomplished by means of a computer program and is not manually calculated by coding or billing personnel. The formula commonly recognized by providers and payers is:

$$(\text{base units} + \text{time units} + \text{modifying factors}) \times \text{conversion factor} = \text{charge}$$

One unit of time is equal to 15 minutes, but again this varies by payer. Time units are determined by dividing the total anesthesia time in minutes by 15. As such, the formula would be:

$$(\text{base units} + [\text{time/15min}]) + \text{modifying factors}$$
$$(\text{PS} + \text{QC}) \times \text{conversion factor} = \text{charge}$$

Summary

The following steps are necessary in assigning codes for anesthesia care:

1. Determine the surgical procedures performed and the corresponding anesthesia CPT codes
2. Select the most comprehensive anesthesia code by determining which procedure has the highest BUV
3. Determine if unusual positioning or field avoidance was used because if there were fewer than 5 BUVs, you can add additional BUVs
4. Assign physical status modifier
5. Assign concurrency modifier
6. Determine the anesthesia time as indicated in the medical record
7. Calculate the charge based on the payer's definition of a unit
8. Determine if additional procedures were performed that are separately billable
   a. Arterial line
   b. Swan Ganz catheter
   c. CVP
   d. Procedure performed for PO pain management
9. Add any appropriate Qualifying Circumstances add-on codes

Pain Management

Generally, acute postoperative pain is managed by the surgeon, but when necessary, the surgeon may refer postoperative pain management (i.e., continuous epidural catheter infusion or nerve block) to an anesthesia provider. The surgeon must document the referral and the reason for the referral in the medical record. The anesthesia provider's medical record documentation must demonstrate the medical necessity and intent of the epidural/nerve block as specifically for postoperative pain control. For example, the insertion of a continuous lumbar epidural catheter (62326) to infuse pain medication following a surgery known to be very painful postoperatively, such as a hemicolectomy or a joint replacement. As described in the "Anesthesia Care and Separately Reported Services" subsection on the next page, there are situations where the insertion of the epidural is not separately reported but rather is considered to be included in the anesthesia care code (00100-01999).

The daily management of the epidural that is subsequent to the day of surgery is to be reported with 01996. This code is used to report daily management; therefore, it can only be reported once per day. This code is not necessarily time based.

Outside the anesthesia care setting, the anesthesiologist may be requested by the surgeon or attending physician to consult on the pain management of a patient. These settings can include but are not limited to hospital inpatient acute care units, including labor/delivery, outpatient departments, clinics, and skilled nursing facilities. When a consult occurs and all required elements are performed and documented (such as documentation of request, consultant's opinion and services rendered, and a report sent to the requesting physician), the anesthesia professional would use the inpatient or outpatient consultation E/M codes to report the service. Additionally, if a procedure is performed (such as nerve block or epidural injection), a surgical CPT code would be used.

An anesthesiologist may also be a specialist in the control of chronic pain and may work in pain clinics to treat patients with terminal illnesses (such as cancer), chronic pain, or injury.

Obstetrics

The codes for reporting anesthesia care in obstetric services are 01958-01969. Let's take a closer look at the various components of these services.

Labor

When neuraxial anesthesia (spinal or epidural anesthesia) is provided for labor, it is reported with 01967.

There are many different methods for determining the appropriate charge for labor epidurals. Some examples include:

- (Base unit + patient face-to-face time units) × conversion factor = $. The face-to-face time would include catheter insertion, adjustment of dose, management of adverse events, repositioning or replacement of the catheter, delivery, and removal of catheter.
- Single flat fee with no variation. This is usually determined by the provider and should be representative of the time and effort involved.
- Variable fee (other than using the [BU+TU] × CF formula) based on the amount of time (such as 0 to < 2 hours, 2 to 6 hours, > 6 hours).

Delivery

When anesthesia is provided for delivery only (no labor anesthesia provided), the codes are either 01960 (vaginal) or 01961 (cesarean).

When anesthesia is provided for cesarean delivery after a trial of labor under neuraxial labor anesthesia, the cesarean anesthesia is reported as 01967 for the neuraxial labor anesthesia and +01968 for the cesarean delivery anesthesia.

Hysterectomy

Anesthesia for hysterectomy following delivery is reported with 01962, 01963, or +01969.

Urgent hysterectomy following delivery: 01962.

Cesarean hysterectomy without labor analgesia/ anesthesia: 01963.

Cesarean hysterectomy following neuraxial labor anesthesia: 01967 for the labor anesthesia and +01969 for the hysterectomy.

Critical Care

Critical care anesthesia professionals have expertise necessary for stabilizing and, if necessary, preparing critically injured or ill patients for emergency surgery by managing the airway, performing cardiac/pulmonary resuscitation, advanced life support, and pain control. When critical care is provided intraoperatively or in the postoperative recovery area, the care is not separately reported because it is considered to be part of the anesthesia care service (00100-01999), with some exceptions as noted previously. When an anesthesiologist provides critical care (such as intubation, central venous [CVP] line/catheter insertion, or resuscitation) that is not associated with anesthesia care, the critical care may be reported separately.

Moderate (Conscious) Sedation

Types of sedation include minimal (anxiolysis), moderate, and deep. Moderate or conscious sedation (CS) is different than minimal sedation (anxiolysis). Deep sedation and monitored anesthesia care are reported with anesthesia section CPT codes 00100-01999 (only when provided by anesthesia personnel).

Moderate sedation provides a decreased level of consciousness that does not put the patient completely to sleep. This level of consciousness allows the patient to breathe without assistance and to respond to stimulation and verbal commands. It can be provided by either the physician performing the procedure or by another physician. The Anesthesia section CPT codes are not used to report moderate sedation. The codes used to report this type of conscious sedation (moderate) are located in the Medicine section (99151-99157).

The moderate sedation codes include:

- Assessment of the patient
- IV access and administration of fluids to keep the IV access open
- Administration of the sedative agent
- Maintenance of sedation
- Monitoring of oxygen saturation, heart rate, and blood pressure
- Recovery

If the moderate sedation is provided by the same physician who is also performing the procedure, a trained observer is required to be present during the use of the conscious sedation to assist the physician in monitoring the patient. The service is reported with codes 99151-99153.

In the facility setting (i.e., hospital, ambulatory surgery center, skilled nursing facility), when moderate sedation is provided by a physician other than the physician performing the procedure, codes 99155-99157 are reported.

When anesthesia services (general, epidural, spinal, deep sedation, etc.) are required and provided by another physician or anesthesia professional, the use of an anesthesia CPT code is appropriate.

The conscious sedation codes are divided based on the age of the patient (under 5 or 5 and over), time (first 15 minutes and each additional 15 minutes), and whether the service is provided by the same physician performing the diagnostic or therapeutic service or by another physician.

Moderate sedation methods are much less debilitating than is the complete loss of consciousness. For example, for a colonoscopy, a physician could administer an intravenous sedation, such as meperidine (Demerol), morphine, or diazepam (Valium). The patient would be monitored closely as the medication is administered so that the appropriate level of sedation is reached. The patient would have this procedure in an outpatient setting and, without complications, would be able to go home after the procedure.

Patient-Controlled Analgesia

Patient-controlled analgesia (PCA) is a system that allows the patient to self-administer an analgesic drug intravenously by depressing a button on a pump that holds the drug. In this way the patient controls the amount of drug and the frequency of administration.

Anesthesia Services in the Hospital Setting

If a hospital bills for anesthesiologist's and/or CRNA's services, it would bill the professional service component on a separate form (CMS1500 or 837-P). The codes assigned for the professional component of the anesthesia services would be the same whether the anesthesia staff were employed by the facility or were independent. The CMS-1450 (UB-04) or 837-I would include all the charges for the OR, laboratory, supplies, drugs, recovery room, room and board, etc. The hospital bill may or may not include a line item billing for anesthesia. The charges that

From the Trenches

"The possibilities of medical coding are endless as long as you are flexible and willing to learn."

JOHNNA FLOYD
CPMA, CPCO, CRC, CPC, CPC-P

CPT Code	BUV	CPT Code	BUV	CPT Code	BUV	CPT Code	BUV
00100	5	00580	20	00934	6	01652	10
00102	6	00600	10	00936	8	01654	8
00103	5	00604	13	00938	4	01656	10
00104	4	00620	10	00940	3	01670	4
00120	5	00625	13	00942	4	01680	3
00124	4	00626	15	00944	6	01710	3
00126	4	00630	8	00948	4	01712	5
00140	5	00632	7	00950	5	01714	5
00142	4	00635	4	00952	4	01716	5
00144	6	00640	3	01112	5	01730	3
00145	6	00670	13	01120	6	01732	3
00147	6	00700	4	01130	3	01740	4
00148	4	00702	4	01140	15	01742	5
00160	5	00730	5	01150	10	01744	5
00162	7	00731	5	01160	4	01756	6
00164	4	00732	6	01170	8	01758	5
00170	5	00750	4	01173	12	01760	7
00172	6	00752	6	01200	4	01770	6
00174	6	00754	7	01202	4	01772	6
00176	7	00756	7	01210	6	01780	3
00190	5	00770	15	01212	10	01782	4
00192	7	00790	7	01214	8	01810	3
00210	11	00792	13	01215	10	01820	3
00211	10	00794	8	01220	4	01829	3
00212	5	00796	30	01230	6	01830	3
00214	9	00797	11	01232	5	01832	6
00215	9	00800	4	01234	8	01840	6
00216	15	00802	5	01250	4	01842	6
00218	13	00811	4	01260	3	01844	6
00220	10	00812	3	01270	8	01850	3
00222	6	00813	5	01272	4	01852	4
00300	5	00820	5	01274	6	01860	3
00320	6	00830	4	01320	4	01916	5
00322	3	00832	6	01340	4	01920	7
00326	7	00834	5	01360	5	01922	7
00350	10	00836	6	01380	3	01924	5
00352	5	00840	6	01382	3	01925	7
00400	3	00842	4	01390	3	01926	8
00402	5	00844	7	01392	4	01930	5
00404	5	00846	8	01400	4	01931	7
00406	13	00848	8	01402	7	01932	6
00410	4	00851	6	01404	5	01933	7
00450	5	00860	6	01420	3	01937	4
00454	3	00862	7	01430	3	01938	4
00470	6	00864	8	01432	6	01939	4
00472	10	00865	7	01440	8	01940	4
00474	13	00866	10	01442	8	01941	5
00500	15	00868	10	01444	8	01942	5
00520	6	00870	5	01462	3	01951	3
00522	4	00872	7	01464	3	01952	5
00524	4	00873	5	01470	3	01953	1
00528	8	00880	15	01472	5	01958	5
00529	11	00882	10	01474	5	01960	5
00530	4	00902	5	01480	3	01961	7
00532	4	00904	7	01482	4	01962	8
00534	7	00906	4	01484	4	01963	8
00537	10	00908	6	01486	7	01964	4
00539	18	00910	3	01490	3	01965	4
00540	12	00912	5	01500	8	01966	4
00541	15	00914	5	01502	6	01967	5
00542	15	00916	5	01520	3	01968	2
00546	15	00918	5	01522	5	01969	5
00548	17	00920	3	01610	5	01990	7
00550	10	00921	3	01620	4	01991	3
00560	15	00922	6	01622	4	01992	5
00561	25	00924	4	01630	5	01996	3
00562	20	00926	4	01634	9	01999	IC
00563	25	00928	6	01636	15		
00566	25	00930	4	01638	10		
00567	18	00932	4	01650	6		

FIGURE 14-1 Base unit value by codes.

would be included under this charge would most likely be for drugs and anesthetic gases. Routine nonbillable supplies and anesthesia equipment charges are combined with the operating room charges. As a result, no anesthesia CPT codes are used on the facility claims. The ICD-10-CM codes that are assigned by the hospital coders for the anesthesiologist/CRNA are related to the actual surgical procedure performed.

You have already assigned surgical and diagnoses codes to cases throughout this text; therefore, no service or diagnosis codes need be assigned in this chapter. Prior to the reports are instructions that are necessary to correctly code the anesthesia services. When anesthesia is performed by an anesthesiologist, the instruction will indicate "MDA" (Medical Doctor of Anesthesiology). When anesthesia is performed by a Certified Registered Nurse Anesthetist, the instructions will indicate "CRNA." When multiple anesthesia CPT codes apply to a single case, reference the following table to determine which code has the highest base unit. The one with the highest base unit is the correct code. Assign the Qualifying Circumstances code to the directing/supervising MDA.

CASE 14-1 · *Operative Report, Flaps and Grafts*

This anesthesia service is being provided for a 76-year-old patient who has severe hypertension that the physician is having difficulty managing at the time of this procedure. Anesthesia by: MDA and CRNA. Typically one provider could manage a case such as this and it would not require the services of both the MDA and CRNA. But for practice, consider the services of both anesthesia professionals to be necessary.

LOCATION: Inpatient, Hospital

PATIENT: Josh Peterson

SURGEON: Gary Sanchez, MD

PREOPERATIVE DIAGNOSIS: Open wound, left lower extremity, with exposed tibia and exposed plate

POSTOPERATIVE DIAGNOSIS: Ulcer, left lower extremity, with exposed tibia and exposed plate

PROCEDURES PERFORMED:

1. Soleus muscle flap
2. Split-thickness skin graft 2.5 × 2.5 cm (centimeter) from the left thigh to the left lower extremity

ANESTHESIA: General endotracheal

ESTIMATED BLOOD LOSS: 130 cc (cubic centimeter)

DRAINS: One #10 Jackson-Pratt

SURGICAL FINDINGS: There was an open wound extending from the lower third of the tibia up into the middle third of the leg with an exposed plate, but tissue loss of the lower third of the leg was evident. Dr. Almaz, Orthopedics, had previously inserted antibiotic beads.

PROCEDURE: An incision was made 2.5 cm medial to the tibial border. We developed a bilobed flap and identified the separation of the soleus muscle and the gastrocnemius medial head following incision of the deep fascia. I dissected the soleus muscle free distally as far as possible and then cut it distally at the Achilles tendon insertion, transposing it through a tunnel of the bilobed flap and covering the area of soft-tissue loss by using bolsters that were tied in place with 0 Prolene. This effectively covered the open area, and then we closed the remainder of the area with 0 Prolene, closing the donor area also with 0 Prolene. We put nitro paste along the edges where there was some skin blanching and put a #10 Jackson-Pratt drain in the distal end of the wound, bringing it out through a separate stab wound incision. A split-thickness skin graft about 2.5 × 2.5 cm was taken from the left thigh, meshed with 1:1.5 mesher, and applied to the defect area measuring 2.5 × 2.5 cm with 2-0 Prolene sutures and staples. We dressed the wound with Xeroform, Kerlix fluffs, Kerlix roll, Kling, and Sof-Rol, and then a cast was applied by the orthopedic technician. The donor site was dressed with scarlet red and an ABD (Adriamycin, bleomycin, dacarbazine) pad. The patient tolerated the procedure well and left the area in good condition.

PHYSICIAN CODE: _____

CRNA CODE: _____

(Answers to every other Case are located in Appendix D . The full answer key is only available in the TEACH Instructor Resources on Evolve.)

CASE 14-2 · *Operative Report, Perirectal Fistulectomies*

Unless stated otherwise, assume "normal, healthy patient." Anesthesia by: MDA and CRNA. Anesthesiologist was medically directing 4 concurrent cases.

LOCATION: Outpatient, Hospital

PATIENT: George Papenfuss

SURGEON: Larry Friendly, MD

PREOPERATIVE DIAGNOSIS: Chronic perirectal fistulas

POSTOPERATIVE DIAGNOSIS: Perirectal fistulas

PROCEDURE PERFORMED: Perirectal fistulectomies

ANESTHESIA: General anesthetic

INDICATIONS FOR SURGERY: The patient is a 61-year-old Caucasian male who had draining perirectal fistulas, which had been incised and drained in the past. The patient is now being seen for excision of these fistulas.

DESCRIPTION OF PROCEDURE: The patient was placed in a jackknife position. He was prepped and draped in the usual manner. The patient was given a general anesthetic. The fistulous tracts were in the 2 and 11 o'clock positions. The fistulous tracts were excised; one of them had an abscessed pocket, and this was excised in its entirety. The tracts continued over the 12 o'clock midline position over into about the 2 o'clock position. All these tracts were combined into one large

Continued

CASE 14-2—cont'd

incision, and all of the inflammatory tissue was excised sharply. The rectum was also dilated up and examined. There was no evidence of any tract that could be seen directly draining into the rectum at this time and no induration. The inflammatory tissue that was present on the outer skin area was completely excised. The operative area was thoroughly irrigated. Hemostasis was obtained using Bovie cautery. The wounds were left open, a drain was placed, and dressings were applied. The patient tolerated the operation and returned to recovery in stable condition.

PHYSICIAN CODE: _____

CRNA CODE: _____

(Answers to every other Case are located in Appendix D . The full answer key is only available in the TEACH Instructor Resources on Evolve.)

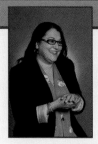

From the Trenches

"Medical coding is not for the weak! It requires tenacity, enthusiasm, attention-to-detail, and a strong work ethic."

JOHNNA FLOYD
CPMA, CPCO, CRC, CPC, CPC-P

CASE 14-3   *Operative Report, Fusion with Autograft*

The procedure is arthrodesis. Anesthesia by: CRNA. No medical direction.

LOCATION: Outpatient, Hospital

PATIENT: Rose Stich

SURGEON: Mohomad Almaz, MD

PREOPERATIVE DIAGNOSIS: Posttraumatic subtalar osteoarthritis, left hindfoot, due to old calcaneal fracture

POSTOPERATIVE DIAGNOSIS: Posttraumatic subtalar osteoarthritis, left hindfoot, due to old calcaneal fracture

PROCEDURE PERFORMED: Left subtalar fusion using moldable autograft obtained from the left iliac crest

ANESTHESIA: General

OPERATIVE PROCEDURE: The patient is a 32-year-old female. After suitable general anesthesia had been achieved, the patient's left iliac crest and left foot and ankle were prepped and draped in the usual manner. Prior to prepping, a thigh tourniquet was applied, but initially it was not inflated. Bone graft was harvested from the left iliac crest. A 10-cm (centimeter) incision was made and carried down through the subcutaneous fat. The fascia was incised in line with the crest starting about 2 cm back from the anterior-superior iliac spine. Cortical cancellous bone graft was then harvested from the inner table. Defect was packed with Gelfoam. The wound was closed in layers. The skin was closed with staples.

The leg was then elevated. The tourniquet was inflated. The incision was made from the tip of the fibula to the base of the fourth metatarsal. Distally based flap of the extensor digitorum brevis was elevated off the lateral aspect of the calcaneus. Fat pad and the sinus tarsi were split in line with the skin incision. Anterior process of the calcaneus was excised. The capsule was incised. A lot of thickened synovial tissue was removed. The joint surfaces were noted to be substantially damaged from the old calcaneal fracture. The remaining articular cartilage and scar tissue were removed with curet and rongeur. The subchondral bone was then carefully burred down to a bleeding surface. Autograft from the iliac crest was then packed in between the bone surfaces. Using image intensifier, a large fragment cannulated screw was then placed starting at the talar neck across the posterior face of the subtalar joint into the central aspect of the calcaneal body. Further gap in the fusion at the sinus tarsi area was filled with autograft and allograft. The wound was then closed. Skin was closed with 4-0 nylon. Dressing and a Robert Jones dressing with a posterior fiberglass splint were then applied. The tourniquet was released. Following tourniquet release, good circulation was noted to return to the foot. The patient tolerated the procedure well and returned to the recovery room in stable condition.

CRNA CODE: _____

(Answers to every other Case are located in Appendix D . The full answer key is only available in the TEACH Instructor Resources on Evolve.)

CASE 14-4   Operative Report, Septoplasty, Turbinate Reduction, Tonsillectomy

Anesthesia was provided for multiple procedures in this next case. Anesthesia by: MDA and CRNA. The anesthesiologist was medically directing 5 concurrent cases.

LOCATION: Inpatient, Hospital

PATIENT: Art Schear

ATTENDING PHYSICIAN: Gregory Dawson, MD

SURGEON: Loren White, MD

PREOPERATIVE DIAGNOSES:

1. Obstructive sleep apnea
2. Nasal obstruction
3. Septal deviation
4. Bilateral inferior turbinate hypertrophy
5. Hypertrophic tonsils

POSTOPERATIVE DIAGNOSES:

1. Obstructive sleep apnea
2. Nasal obstruction
3. Septal deviation
4. Bilateral inferior turbinate hypertrophy
5. Hypertrophic tonsils

PROCEDURES PERFORMED:

1. Septoplasty
2. Bilateral inferior turbinate mucosal reduction with radiofrequency
3. Tonsillectomy

ANESTHESIA: General endotracheal

INDICATION: The patient is a 16-year-old male with documented obstructive sleep apnea. He also has a prior history of severe nasal obstruction due to a traumatic injury to his nose. Examination reveals a significant septal deviation with inferior turbinate hypertrophy. He also has very hypertrophic tonsils. At this point, we will correct his nasal airway and also increase his oral airway by removing his tonsils and see if that will help his sleep apnea. If there is any residual sleep apnea, he may be treated with nasal CPAP (continuous positive airway pressure); or if he is unable to tolerate that, further airway expansion surgery will be considered.

DESCRIPTION OF PROCEDURE: After consent was obtained, the patient was taken to the operating room and placed on the operating table in the supine position. After an adequate level of general endotracheal anesthesia was obtained, the patient was turned and draped in the appropriate manner for nasal surgery. The patient's nose was packed with cotton pledgets and soaked with 4% cocaine. After several minutes, 1% Xylocaine with 1:100,000 units of epinephrine was infiltrated into the septum bilaterally. It was also infiltrated into the inferior turbinates bilaterally. The nasal hairs were trimmed. Then, utilizing a right hemitransfixion incision, the mucoperichondrium and mucoperiosteal flaps were elevated. The deviated portion of the cartilaginous bony septum was then removed. Spurs off the maxillary crest were also removed. Hemostasis was achieved with suction cautery along the maxillary crest and then with FloSeal. Attention was then focused on the inferior turbinate. The anterior mucosa was treated with a radiofrequency needle to 500 J on each side. The hemitransfixion incision was then closed with interrupted 4-0 chromic suture. A quilting suture of 4-0 plain gut was then performed. Silastic splints were then placed on both sides of the nasal septum and secured with nylon suture. The nose was then packed bilaterally with nasal packs. Packs consisted of Merocel sponge covered with a gloved finger coated with Bacitracin ointment. This was inflated with local solution. The patient was then repositioned for tonsillectomy. The McIvor mouth gag was placed allowing visualization of the tonsil. Attention was first focused on the left tonsil. The Dean retractor was placed in the superior pole, and tonsil was retracted toward the midline. Then, utilizing a harmonic scalpel at power level III, the tonsil was removed in its entirety from a superior-to-inferior direction. Hemostasis was achieved from spot suction cautery. The similar procedure was then performed on the right tonsil. The tonsillar fossa was then irrigated with saline. There was no bleeding. Tension of the mouth gag was then released. Reinspection showed no active bleeding. The anterior and posterior pillar of the superior aspect of the tonsillar fossa was then reapproximated with interrupted 3-0 chromic suture and figure-of-eight closure. Subsequent reinspection showed no active bleeding. Mouth gag was then removed. Prior to removal of mouth gag, 1% Xylocaine with 1:100,000 units of epinephrine was infiltrated into the retromolar and soft palate areas bilaterally. The patient tolerated the procedure well. There was no break in technique. The patient was extubated and taken to the post anesthesia care unit in good condition.

FLUIDS ADMINISTERED: 1800 cc (cubic centimeter) of RL

ESTIMATED BLOOD LOSS: Less than 50 cc

PREOPERATIVE MEDICATION: 1 g (gram) Ancef and 12 mg (milligram) Decadron IV (intravenous)

PHYSICIAN CODE: _____

CRNA CODE:_____

(Answers to every other Case are located in Appendix D . The full answer key is only available in the TEACH Instructor Resources on Evolve.)

CASE 14-5   Operative Report, Excision of Right Carotid Body Tumor

This patient has a mild systemic disease and is 82 years old. Anesthesia by: MDA and CRNA. Anesthesiologist was medically directing this single case.

LOCATION: Inpatient, Hospital

PATIENT: Delores Janus

SURGEON: Gary Sanchez, MD

PREOPERATIVE DIAGNOSIS: Right carotid body tumor

POSTOPERATIVE DIAGNOSIS: Frozen section confirmed a right carotid body tumor with tortuous internal and external carotids that have been displaced by tumor mass with multiple blood vessels feeding this tumor mass, rising from the external carotid, all ligated individually. The tumor was highly vascularized.

OPERATIVE PROCDURE: Excision of right carotid body tumor

ANESTHESIA: General endotracheal with EEG (electroencephalogram) monitoring

Continued

CASE 14-5—cont'd

COMPLICATIONS: Nil

NEEDLE AND SPONGE COUNTS: Needle and sponge counts appear correct. No adverse EEG changes were noted during the procedure.

ESTIMATED BLOOD LOSS: 125 cc (cubic centimeter)

No drains were placed. Incision was closed.

INDICATION FOR PROCEDURE: The patient, an 82-year-old female, upon a workup for another problem, was dubiously noted on CT (computerized tomography) scan to have what looked like a carotid body tumor; subsequently, an angiogram was done to examine this further and confirmed our suspicions and also showed that the blood supply was derived mostly from the external carotid. Consent was obtained for operative intervention. The procedure, indication, risks, benefits, and alternatives have been discussed at length with the patient. She understood and wished to proceed.

OPERATIVE TECHNIQUE: The patient was brought to the operating room and placed supine on the operating room table. General endotracheal anesthesia was administered under EEG monitoring. We then proceeded to prep the neck, lower face, and upper chest with Betadine and draped off in a sterile fashion. We proceeded with proper placement of her neck, somewhat extended to provide adequate exposure. We then proceeded with her incision anterior to the sternocleidomastoid. We extended this through skin and subcutaneous tissues and the platysma muscle down to the sternocleidomastoid and then subsequently retracted the sternocleidomastoid laterally and exposed the jugular vein, which was quite large and had many tributaries. These tributaries were doubly ligated on the large ones and also retracted laterally. The common carotid was identified, dissection carried down onto the common carotid, and a vessel loop placed around the common carotid dissection and subsequently carried distally. We identified the internal and external carotids and also placed vessel loops around this. On the external carotid, we identified the superior thyroid, placed a vessel loop around this, and followed this further. Another branch of the external carotid was noted to be feeding the tumor mass between external and internal carotid, and multiple small feeding vessels were also identified. These were individually ligated. We used bipolar cautery to dissect some of the tissues off because this was very hypervascular. The tumor was well circumscribed, although it caused a lot of hypervascularity around it. We were able to dissect this off, identify and preserve the hypoglossal nerve, and identify and preserve the vagus nerve posteriorly. Also, after taking the mass out and sending it for frozen section, this confirmed that it was a carotid body tumor. We will await permanent sections. Hemostasis was good. We then irrigated. Once satisfied with this procedure, we closed the platysma muscles with running 3-0 Vicryl sutures. We closed the skin with 4-0 Vicryl subcuticular running sutures. We applied Steri-Strips and sterile dressings. The patient tolerated the procedure well without complications. On waking up in the operating room, she was able to move all extremities. She will be transferred to the surgical critical care unit for further observation and recovery.

PHYSICIAN CODE: _____

CRNA CODE: _____

QUALIFYING CIRCUMSTANCES CODE: _____

(Answers to every other Case are located in Appendix D . The full answer key is only available in the TEACH Instructor Resources on Evolve.)

CASE 14-6   *Operative Report, Circumcision*

Sometimes one or more combinations of anesthesia types will be used during a procedure. Note that in this procedure both general anesthesia and a caudal block are used. The anesthesiologist performed the caudal block specifically for postoperative pain control as requested by the surgeon. The report does not include the procedure note for the caudal block; presume that it was performed in the holding area separate from the anesthesia for surgery and assign a code for the caudal block. This is an otherwise normal healthy 2-year-old male. Anesthesia by: MDA and CRNA. Anesthesiologist was medically directing 4 concurrent cases.

LOCATION: Outpatient, Hospital

PATIENT: Harlen Mata

SURGEON: Ira Avila, MD

PREOPERATIVE DIAGNOSIS: Recurrent balanitis and phimosis

POSTOPERATIVE DIAGNOSIS: Recurrent balanitis and phimosis

PROCEDURE PERFORMED: Circumcision

PROCEDURE: The 2-year-old male child was given general mask anesthetic as well as caudal block for postoperative pain control. He was prepped and draped in the supine position, foreskin retracted, preputial adhesions broken down. Circumcision was performed using a dorsal slit technique. Hemostasis was achieved with judicious use of electrocautery and chromic ties. Prepuce was re-anastomosed to the penile skin using 5-0 chromic catgut. Vaseline gauze dressing was applied. The patient tolerated the procedure well and transferred to the recovery room in good condition.

Pathology Report Later Indicated: Benign penile tissue

PHYSICIAN CODE: _____

CRNA CODE: _____

INJECTION CODE: _____

(Answers to every other Case are located in Appendix D . The full answer key is only available in the TEACH Instructor Resources on Evolve.)

CASE 14-7   *Operative Report, Hysteroscopy, Dilatation, and Curettage*

Unless stated otherwise, assume "normal, healthy patient." The anesthesia service was performed personally by the anesthesiologist (MDA).

LOCATION: Outpatient, Hospital

PATIENT: Mary Moore

ATTENDING PHYSICIAN: Andy Martinez, MD

SURGEON: Andy Martinez, MD

PREOPERATIVE DIAGNOSIS: Irregular uterine bleeding

POSTOPERATIVE DIAGNOSIS: Irregular uterine bleeding

OPERATIVE PROCEDURE: Hysteroscopy and dilatation and curettage of the uterus

ANESTHESIA: General

SURGICAL INDICATIONS: This patient is a 41-year-old multiparous female who had been having irregular, abnormal, and prolonged bleeding since June of this year. Ultrasound had suggested a small myoma on the right side of her uterus.

OPERATIVE FINDINGS: The uterus was 7.5 cm (centimeter) deep. The cavity was symmetrical without evidence of polyps or submucous myomas.

DESCRIPTION OF PROCEDURE: After introduction of general anesthesia, the patient was placed in the dorsolithotomy position, after which the perineum and vagina were prepped and bladder straight catheterized. The patient was then draped. The cervix was grasped with a single-tooth tenaculum, and sharp endocervical curettage was done. The endocervical canal was then dilated to 7 cm with Hegar dilators. A 5.5-mm (millimeter) Olympus hysteroscope was introduced, and the cavity was inspected. The hysteroscope was withdrawn, and then a sharp endometrial curettage was done. Blood loss was 5-10 cc (cubic centimeter). Specimen to pathology: Endocervical and endometrial curettings. The patient tolerated the procedure well and returned to the recovery room in stable condition.

Pathology Report Later Indicated: Primary endometrial carcinoma

PHYSICIAN CODE: _____

(Answers to every other Case are located in Appendix D . The full answer key is only available in the TEACH Instructor Resources on Evolve.)

CASE 14-8   *Operative Report, Osteoplastic Craniotomy*

This patient is under a constant threat of loss of life, and this procedure was performed under emergency circumstances that the operative report does not document. Anesthesia by: MDA.

LOCATION: Inpatient, Hospital

PATIENT: Arlene Samuels

ATTENDING PHYSICIAN: Timothy Pleasant, MD

SURGEON: Timothy Pleasant, MD

PREOPERATIVE DIAGNOSIS: Right temporal parietal frontal brain tumor

POSTOPERATIVE DIAGNOSIS: Glioblastoma multiforme

PROCEDURE PERFORMED: Osteoplastic craniotomy with removal of tumor in temporal lobe, frontal lobe, and middle cerebral artery complex

ANESTHESIA: General

PROCEDURE: Under general anesthesia, the patient's head was prepped and draped in the usual manner. A question mark incision was made in the front of the ear up to the frontal area. The skin flap was turned down. The temporalis muscle was incised. We then did an osteoplastic craniotomy with burr holes and craniotome. The flap was turned.

The dura was incised. We then made an incision into the superior temporal lobe. The plan was to resect the temporal lobe to get into the tumor and stay away from the middle cerebral complex and also to decompress her frontal lobe as well because the tumor was going into the frontal lobe. I got into the tumor and sent specimen for biopsy and then began the gradual dissection. I encountered some bleeding, probably from middle cerebral artery branches. I had to take a few with silver clips, perhaps two to three. Otherwise, we left the sylvian vein intact and decompressed the area. We got into the tumor cavity and took as much visual tumor as we could. The bed was then dried. I irrigated the wound well. I placed a piece of Gelfoam over the raw surface of the brain and began closure of the dura with 3-0 Vicryl. The bone flap was replaced with two straight four-holed Wurzburg plates. Hemovac was placed, and the scalp was closed in layers utilizing 3-0 Vicryl on the galea with surgical staples on the skin. Dressing was applied. The patient was discharged to PAR (postanesthesia recovery).

Pathology Report Later Indicated: Glioblastoma multiforme

PHYSICIAN CODE: _____

QUALIFYING CIRCUMSTANCES CODE: _____

(Answers to every other Case are located in Appendix D . The full answer key is only available in the TEACH Instructor Resources on Evolve.)

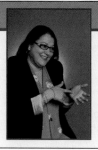

From the Trenches

"The most rewarding part of being a medical coder is when you find the information you need to translate words into codes."

JOHNNA FLOYD
CPMA, CPCO, CRC, CPC, CPC-P

CASE 14-9   *Operative Report, Nasolacrimal Duct Probing*

A certified registered nurse anesthetist provided the anesthesia service under the medical direction of an anesthesiologist who was directing three procedures at the same time. Report the CRNA and the anesthesiologist's services.

LOCATION: Outpatient, Hospital

PATIENT: Peggy Crase

ATTENDING PHYSICIAN: Rita Wimer, MD

SURGEON: Loren White, MD

PREOPERATIVE DIAGNOSIS:

1. Epiphora, both eyes
2. Nasolacrimal duct obstruction, both eyes

POSTOPERATIVE DIAGNOSIS:

1. Epiphora, both eyes
2. Nasolacrimal duct obstruction, both eyes

PROCEDURE PERFORMED: Nasolacrimal duct probing, both eyes

ANESTHESIA: General

INDICATIONS: This healthy 32-month-old white female was referred by Dr. Peterson after an allergy workup to investigate her chronic otitis media, PE (pressure equalization) tubes times two, and the chronic epiphora that she has had in both eyes. The mother was counseled as to the success of probing at this age and the possible reoperations that may be needed.

PROCEDURE: After the patient was placed under suitable anesthesia via the mask, a small punctum dilator was used to dilate the punctum inferiorly and superiorly. These were found to be very tight and occluded. A 2-0 Bowman probe could be passed only through the inferior system with difficulty on both sides. The C-loop was not irrigatable. Probing could not be attempted because there was a large bony obstruction that resisted all efforts to pass the tube. There was no fluorescein inserted in the nose. TobraDex drops were placed in the eyes. The procedure was complete, and the patient was sent to the recovery room. The patient will be referred for further ENT (ears, nose, throat) consultation and to Dr. Lorabi for the possibility of a white cell deficiency that is causing these chronic infections or other immune problems. There were no complications.

PHYSICIAN CODE: _____

CRNA CODE: _____

(Answers to every other Case are located in Appendix D . The full answer key is only available in the TEACH Instructor Resources on Evolve.)

CASE 14-10   *Operative Report, Hemithoracic Cavity Packing*

The anesthesiologist was supervising a CRNA during this procedure. The patient has well-controlled diabetes mellitus.

LOCATION: Outpatient, Hospital

PATIENT: LoriLee Putman

ATTENDING PHYSICIAN: Rita Wimer, MD

SURGEON: Loren White, MD

PREOPERATIVE DIAGNOSIS: Right empyema with bronchopleural fistula

POSTOPERATIVE DIAGNOSIS: Right empyema with bronchopleural fistula

PROCEDURE PERFORMED: Changing packing, right hemithoracic cavity

ANESTHESIA: IV (intravenous) sedation

PROCEDURE: The patient was brought to the operating room and sedated. The old packing was removed; the wound was examined and repacked with two vaginal packings soaked in 0.5% Flagyl solution. The patient tolerated the procedure well and was sent to recovery in satisfactory condition. Sponge count and needle count were correct.

PHYSICIAN CODE: _____

CRNA CODE: _____

(Answers to every other Case are located in Appendix D . The full answer key is only available in the TEACH Instructor Resources on Evolve.)

CASE 14-11 *Operative Report, Lesions*

Spinal anesthesia was used in this case. The CMA was medically directed by the anesthesiologist, who was directing four concurrent cases. The patient is a normal, healthy male.

LOCATION: Outpatient, Hospital

PATIENT: Tom Boll

SURGEON: Gary Sanchez, MD

PREOPERATIVE DIAGNOSIS: Lesions, left lower extremity

POSTOPERATIVE DIAGNOSIS: Undetermined lesion, right lower extremity, most likely benign with clear margins.

SURGICAL FINDINGS: There was a 2-cm (centimeter) diameter, raised erythematous lesion with a central pore of keratin. (This is keratosis.) Frozen section showed clear margins. Although it essentially looked benign, there is some question of well-differentiated squamous cell carcinoma, and this is reserved as a possible diagnosis.

SURGICAL PROCEDURE: Excision of lesion, left lower extremity

ANESTHESIA: Spinal

DESCRIPTION OF PROCEDURE: Under satisfactory spinal anesthesia, the patient's left leg was prepped with Betadine scrub and solution and draped in a routine sterile fashion. The lesion was excised with a 1-cm margin laterally and with a 2-cm margin proximally and distally tagging the superomedial aspect with a silk suture. Dissection was carried down to the deep layer of fascia, and bleeding was electrocoagulated. One 2-0 Monocryl suture was used subcuticularly to take tension off the wound, and then the skin was closed with interrupted vertical mattress sutures of 3-0 Prolene. We submitted the specimen for frozen section, and the frozen-section diagnosis was probably benign with the possibility of well-differentiated squamous cell carcinoma. The pathology report leaned in favor of this being a benign lesion; however, we went well around the lesion. I returned to the operating room, rescrubbed, and regloved and placed a Xeroform dressing, Kerlix fluffs over the wound, and Kerlix fluffs around the malleoli on the heels, wrapping the foot and leg from the foot to the knee with a Kerlix roll times two, Kling times two, and two Sof-Rol. The patient tolerated the procedure well and left the operating room in good condition.

Pathology Report Later Indicated: Mild hyperkeratosis with central scale crust, pseudoepitheliomatous hyperplasia, epidermal cysts, and mild chronic inflammation; margins are benign.

PHYSICIAN CODE: _____

CRNA CODE: _____

(Answers to every other Case are located in Appendix D . The full answer key is only available in the TEACH Instructor Resources on Evolve.)

CASE 14-12 *Operative Report, Breast Biopsy with Needle Localization*

This patient presents for the removal of a breast lesion that was previously marked prior to surgery with a radiological marker. The CRNA independently performed the Monitored Anesthesia Care. She is an otherwise healthy woman.

LOCATION: Outpatient, Hospital

PATIENT: Marilyn Agnes

SURGEON: Gary Sanchez, MD

PREOPERATIVE DIAGNOSIS: Right breast microcalcification by mammogram

POSTOPERATIVE DIAGNOSIS: Right breast microcalcification by mammogram

PROCEDURE PERFORMED: Right breast biopsy with needle localization

ANESTHESIA: 1% Xylocaine local; 16 cc (cubic centimeter) was used. The patient also received IV (intravenous) sedation.

INDICATIONS FOR SURGERY: The patient is a 77-year-old white female who had undergone mammography. The patient was found to have microcalcifications in her right breast. The patient was taken to the operating room for biopsy.

DESCRIPTION OF PROCEDURE: The patient had previously undergone needle localization on the right breast microcalcification. She was brought back to the operating room. The patient was then prepped and draped in the usual manner. Xylocaine was used as local anesthesia; a total of 16 cc was used. The patient also received IV sedation. An incision was made over the guidewire. The guidewire and surrounding breast tissue were incised and sent to radiology. Radiology confirmed that the microcalcifications had been removed. Hemostasis was obtained using Bovie cautery. The operative area was thoroughly irrigated. The incision was then closed with figure-of-eight 2-0 chromic sutures for the deep and superficial layers. The skin was closed with 4-0 Vicryl subcuticular stitch, and Steri-Strips were applied. The patient tolerated the operation and returned to recovery in stable condition.

Pathology Report Later Indicated: Focal fibrosis with coarse microcalcifications

CRNA CODE: _____

QUALIFYING CIRCUMSTANCES CODE: _____

(Answers to every other Case are located in Appendix D . The full answer key is only available in the TEACH Instructor Resources on Evolve.)

CASE 14-13 *Operative Report, Ulcer and Cholecystitis*

Dr. Sanchez is the general surgeon who performed the following procedures: partial gastrectomy with gastrojejunostomy, vagotomy, and cholecystectomy with cholangiogram. The anesthesiologist personally performed the anesthesia care and was not medically directing or supervising any other cases at the time. The patient has poorly controlled diabetes.

LOCATION: Inpatient, Hospital

PATIENT: Alma Kincaid

ATTENDING PHYSICIAN: Leslie Alanda, MD

SURGEON: Gary Sanchez, MD

ANESTHESIA: General endotracheal

PREOPERATIVE DIAGNOSIS: Nonhealing duodenal ulcer. Chronic cholecystitis.

POSTOPERATIVE DIAGNOSIS: Nonhealing duodenal ulcer. Chronic cholecystitis.

PROCEDURES PERFORMED:

1. Exploratory laparotomy
2. Partial gastrectomy (antrectomy)
3. Truncal vagotomy
4. Gastrojejunostomy
5. Cholecystectomy with intraoperative cholangiogram

INDICATION: The patient is a 60-year-old female who presented with a nonhealing gastric ulcer. She has had symptoms for about a year. She complains of epigastric pain. She failed medical therapy with Prilosec and therapy for *H. pylori*. Biopsy of the ulcer showed it to be benign. The patient had a negative workup for gastrinoma. Calcium level was also normal. The patient now presents for exploratory laparotomy and partial gastrectomy. The risks and benefits were discussed with the patient in detail. She understood and agreed to proceed.

PROCEDURE: The patient was brought to the operating room. Her abdomen was prepped and draped in a sterile fashion. A midline umbilical incision was made. The peritoneal cavity was entered. Initial inspection of the peritoneal cavity showed normal liver, spleen, colon, and small bowel. There was an ulcer along the first portion of the duodenum just beyond the pylorus with some scarring. There was also an ulcer in the posterior part of the duodenal bulb, which was penetrating to the pancreas. We started dissection along the greater curvature of the stomach. Vessels were ligated with 2-0 silk ties. There was an enlarged lymph node along the greater curvature of the stomach, which was sent for frozen section. It proved to be a benign lymph node. This was the only enlarged node found during dissection. We then proceeded with truncal vagotomy. The anterior vagus and posterior vagus were identified. They were clipped proximally and distally, and a segment of each nerve was excised and sent for frozen section. A segment of both vagus nerves was excised and confirmed by frozen section. An incision was made around the gastrohepatic ligament. The mesentery along the lesser curvature of the stomach was dissected. The vessels were ligated with 2-0 silk ties along the lesser curvature of the stomach. A Kocher maneuver was performed to aid mobilization. The pancreas was completely normal. No masses were seen in the pancreas. There was penetration of the ulcer in the superior part of the head of the pancreas. Dissection was continued posterior to the stomach. The adhesions posterior to the stomach were taken down. The ulcer was in the posterior segment of the duodenal bulb just beyond the pylorus, and it had penetrated the pancreas. All the posterior layer of the ulcer that was left adherent to the pancreas was shaved off. The stomach was divided with the GIA stapler so that the complete antrum would be in the specimen. The duodenum was divided between clamps. The stomach pylorus and first part of the duodenum were sent to pathology for examination. Then the duodenal stump was closed with running suture. Using 3-0 Lembert sutures, the posterior wall of the ulcer was incorporated for duodenal closure. The base of the duodenum was rolled over the ulcer, and it was all-incorporating to the duodenal closure. Our next step was to proceed with cholecystectomy. The gallbladder was separated from the liver, reflected, and taken down, and the gallbladder was divided from the liver with blunt dissection and cautery. The cystic artery was doubly ligated with silk. The cystic duct was identified. The cystic duct and gallbladder junction and gallbladder ducts were identified. Intraoperative cholangiogram was performed showing free flow of bile into the intrahepatic duct and into the duodenum. No leaks were seen. The cystic duct was doubly ligated, and the gallbladder was sent to pathology. The staple line in the proximal stomach was oversewn with 3-0 silk Lembert sutures. A retrocolic isoperistaltic Hofmeister-type gastrojejunostomy was performed on the remaining stomach and loop of jejunum. This was an isoperistaltic end-to-side two-layer anastomosis with 3-0 chromic and 3-0 silk. The stomach was secured to the transverse mesocolon with several interrupted silk sutures to prevent any herniation along the retrocolic space. The anastomosis had a good lumen and good blood supply. There was no twist along the anastomosis. Prior to finishing the anastomosis, a nasogastric tube was placed along the afferent limb of the jejunum to decompress the duodenum and prevent blowout of the duodenal stump. Extra holes were made in the NG tube to provide adequate drainage. The anastomosis was marked with two clips on each side, and a Jackson-Pratt drain was placed over the duodenal stump. The peritoneal cavity was irrigated until clear. Hemostasis was adequate. The fascia was then closed with interrupted 0 Ethibond sutures. Skin edges were approximated with staples. Subcutaneous tissues were irrigated before closure. Estimated blood loss throughout the procedure was 200 mL (milliliter), IV (intravenous) fluids: 3400 ml. Urine output: 840 ml.

FINDINGS:

1. Nonhealing benign ulcer in the posterior duodenal bulb penetrating into the head of the pancreas.
2. Partial gastrectomy (antrectomy performed) and excision of the pylorus, first portion of the duodenum along with ulcer.
3. Hofmeister-type retrocolic isoperistaltic gastrojejunostomy.
4. Posterior wall of the ulcer that was penetrating into the pancreas incorporated into closure of the duodenal stump.
5. Truncal vagotomy performed with intraoperative frozen section confirming both vagus nerves.
6. Cholecystectomy performed with normal intraoperative cholangiogram.
7. Jackson-Pratt drain placed over the duodenal stump.

Pathology Report Later Indicated: Benign antral and gastric body ulcers with acute inflammation. Multiple benign lymph nodes with mild follicular hyperplasia. Chronic cholecystitis.

PHYSICIAN CODE: _____

(Answers to every other Case are located in Appendix D . The full answer key is only available in the TEACH Instructor Resources on Evolve.)

CASE 14-14A *Operative Report, Hemicolectomy*

Anesthesia was administered by a CRNA under medical direction of an anesthesiologist directing 4 concurrent cases. The patient has well-controlled hypertension. Other than that and her cancer, she has been healthy. The surgeon ordered postoperative pain management to be provided by the anesthesiologist. See cases 14-14B and 14-14C.

LOCATION: Inpatient, Hospital

PATIENT: Sally Ortez

ATTENDING PHYSICIAN: Leslie Alanda, MD

SURGEON: Gary Sanchez, MD

PREOPERATIVE DIAGNOSIS: Adenocarcinoma of the ascending colon

POSTOPERATIVE DIAGNOSIS: Perforated adenocarcinoma of the ascending colon with attachment to the lateral abdominal wall.

PROCEDURE PERFORMED: Hemicolectomy

ANESTHESIA: General

INDICATIONS FOR SURGERY: The patient is a 56-year-old white female who is having difficulties with her bowels. The patient was found to have adenocarcinoma of the ascending colon that was proven by biopsy. The patient is taken to the operating room after a bowel prep yesterday for surgery.

PROCEDURE: The patient was prepped and draped in the usual manner. A midline abdominal incision was made. The patient has had previous surgeries, which included an appendectomy, hysterectomy, cholecystectomy, and radiation therapy to her abdomen for a lymphoma. The patient had adhesions from her multiple previous surgeries and radiation therapy. These adhesions were taken down sharply using the Bovie cautery and Metzenbaum scissors. After this was done, the right colon was elevated using the Bovie cautery to divide the peritoneum on the right lateral gutter. The colon was then brought up into the operative area. The small bowel ileum was adherent down into the pelvis from her previous surgeries. These were taken down using the Metzenbaum scissors; then the small bowel was freed up into the incision area. The dissection was carried out to the transverse colon in about the midpoint of the transverse colon. A Penrose drain was then placed around the transverse colon and also one around the ileum. During dissection of the

cancer from the lateral abdominal wall, the cancer was firmly adherent to the abdominal wall. When this was finally freed up, there was an opening in the colon that appeared to be a perforation of the area of cancer, which had been sealed by the lateral abdominal wall. There was no gross evidence of any tumor on the abdominal wall. The opening in the colon was closed with a 2-0 silk suture. Next the mesentery was scored using the Bovie cautery. The mesentery was clamped and divided using Kelly clamps and tied with interrupted 2-0 silk sutures. After this was completed, the bowel clamp was placed on the proximal ileum and also on the distal colon. Kocher clamps were placed on the specimen side of the ileum and colon. The colon and ileum were then transected and the specimen was sent to pathology. An end-to-end anastomosis was then done. A two-layer closure was done. Interrupted 3-0 silk sutures were placed on either end of the anastomosis and then the posterior layer was then placed. All sutures were placed before they were tied. After this was completed, the inner layer was then run using a running 3-0 Vicryl suture using a locking stitch for the posterior layer and a running stitch on the anterior layer. After this was completed, the bowel clamps were removed. The anterior outer layer was then placed using interrupted 3-0 silk sutures. There was an excellent anastomosis following this procedure. The opening in the mesentery was closed with a running 2-0 Vicryl suture. The operative area was thoroughly irrigated. A few small bleeders were found after the irrigation, and these were controlled by 2-0 silk ties or Bovie cautery. An additional adhesion was taken down from the omentum attached to the pelvis down into the pelvic gutter, and this was freed. After all the adhesions were taken down, the operative area was again thoroughly irrigated. The bowel was returned to the abdomen. The anastomosis was again checked and was excellent. The abdominal incision was then closed with a running no.1 looped PDS suture for the fascia and the peritoneum in a single-layer closure. The subcutaneous tissues were then thoroughly irrigated, and the skin was closed with skin clips. The patient tolerated the operation and returned to recovery in stable condition.

Pathology Report Later Indicated: Adenocarcinoma of both the colon (primary) and abdominal wall neoplasm (secondary)

PHYSICIAN CODE: _____

CRNA CODE: _____

(Answers to every other Case are located in Appendix D . The full answer key is only available in the TEACH Instructor Resources on Evolve.)

CASE 14-14B *Epidural Catheter Placement, Loss of Resistance Technique: Midline Approach*

The surgeon ordered postoperative pain management to be provided by the anesthesiologist. The anesthesiologist decided to use a continuous epidural catheter for postoperative pain. The MDA placed the catheter while the patient was in the OR (operating room) just prior to surgery.

LOCATION: Inpatient, Hospital

PATIENT: Sally Ortez

ATTENDING PHYSICIAN: Leslie Alanda, MD

ANESTHESIOLOGIST: Janice E. Larson, MD

PREOPERATIVE DIAGNOSIS: Postoperative Pain Management for Hemicolectomy due to Adenocarcinoma of the Ascending Colon

POSTOPERATIVE DIAGNOSIS: As above.

INDICATIONS FOR SURGERY: Gary Sanchez, MD, general surgeon, requested that anesthesia manage postoperative pain. This will be accomplished using continuous epidural catheter.

PROCEDURE: After checking the availability of resuscitation drugs and equipment and appropriate monitors were placed the patient was positioned. The intercristal line and midline were identified. The point of needle insertion was marked with a cruciform mark made

Continued

CASE 14-14B—cont'd

by thumbnail pressure applied in the vertical and horizontal planes. The skin was widely prepped and the field draped. A skin wheal of 1% lidocaine was made with a short 32-gauge needle. A 25-gauge 1.5-inch standard bevel needle was used to infiltrate 1% lidocaine in the supraspinous and interspinous ligaments. An 18-gauge Tuohy needle with a stylet was inserted perpendicular to the skin with the bevel facing cephalad. Depth of the needle in the supraspinous ligament was limited to 2 cm before the stylet was removed. A 5-ml saline-filled loss of resistance syringe was then attached to the needle hub. A 20-gauge epidural catheter was threaded through the needle with attention paid to the depth markings on the catheter. Moderate pressure was applied to pass the catheter tip beyond the orifice of the

needle. Light and delicate pressure was applied to advance it further to a distance in the space of 2 cm. The catheter was grasped at its entry into the skin between the thumb and index finger as the needle was removed.

The catheter was secured to the skin using benzoin and a transparent dressing. I placed a loop in the catheter where it exited the skin to prevent outward migration of the catheter. The catheter was taped lateral to the spinous processes without crossing the midline. Following a negative test dose, local anesthetic was administered in incremental doses. Morphine 50 mcg/ml and Bupivacaine 0.1% at 8 cc/hr.

INJECTION CODE: _____

(Answers to every other Case are located in Appendix D . The full answer key is only available in the TEACH Instructor Resources on Evolve.)

CASE 14-14C   *Epidural Catheter Daily Management*

The following is a note for daily management of a continuous epidural catheter.

LOCATION: Inpatient, Hospital

PATIENT: Sally Ortez

ATTENDING PHYSICIAN: Leslie Alanda, MD

ANESTHESIOLOGIST: Janice E. Larson, MD

DIAGNOSIS: Postoperative pain management for s/p hemicolectomy due to adenocarcinoma of the ascending colon

Status post hemicolectomy day 2. Epidural catheter in place. Site looks clean and intact. Receiving Morphine 50 mcg/ml and Bupivacaine 0.1% at 8 cc/hr. Denies pain at the present time. Continue with current management.

PHYSICIAN CODE: _____

(Answers to every other Case are located in Appendix D . The full answer key is only available in the TEACH Instructor Resources on Evolve.)

CASE 14-15   *Operative Report, Tendon Repair*

This patient is otherwise healthy. Anesthesia care was provided by medically directed CRNA by an MDA directing 3 concurrent cases.

LOCATION: Outpatient, Hospital

PATIENT: Melvin Brodern

ATTENDING PHYSICIAN: Mohomad Almaz, MD

SURGEON: Mohomad Almaz, MD

ANESTHESIA: Spinal

PREOPERATIVE PROCEDURE: Quadriceps tendon rupture, right knee

POSTOPERATIVE PROCEDURE: Quadriceps tendon rupture, right knee

OPERATIVE PROCEDURE: Repair of quadriceps tendon, right knee

OPERATIVE PROCEDURE: After suitable spinal anesthesia had been achieved, the patient's right knee was prepped and draped in the usual manner. Prior to prepping, a thigh tourniquet was applied. A midline skin incision was made from the inferior pole of the patella to one handbreadth above the superior pole of the patella. The patient had a thickened prepatellar bursa and chronic bursitis. This was partially

excised. The quadriceps tendon was exposed. The patient had complete rupture of the quadriceps tendon extending to the medial and lateral retinacula. The interposed clot was removed. Four blocking stitches of no. 5 Ethibond were then placed into the central aspect of the quadriceps tendon. These were passed through drill holes, going from the superior pole of the patella to the inferior pole of the patella. The sutures were then tied over a bone bridge at the inferior pole of the patella securing the main portion of the quadriceps tendon back to the patella. The medial and lateral retinacula tears were then repaired with interrupted no. 1 Panacryl. Before wound closure, a Hemovac drain was inserted into the knee joint. Subcutaneous tissue was then closed with 2-0 Vicryl, and the skin was closed with staples. A fiberglass cylinder cast was then applied. The tourniquet was released before cast application. After tourniquet release, good circulation was noted to return to the foot. The patient tolerated the procedure well and returned to the recovery room in stable condition.

PHYSICIAN CODE: _____

CRNA CODE: _____

(Answers to every other Case are located in Appendix D . The full answer key is only available in the TEACH Instructor Resources on Evolve.)

CASE 14-16   *Operative Report, Arthroplasty*

In this case the anesthesia care is provided by an anesthesiologist medically directing one CRNA. The type of anesthesia for this procedure is epidural. The surgeon has asked that anesthesia manage the painful postoperative course that is expected. Anesthesia decides to leave the epidural catheter in place for postoperative pain management. The patient is healthy.

LOCATION: Inpatient, Hospital

PATIENT: Jack Baglien

SURGEON: Mohomad Almaz, MD

PREOPERATIVE DIAGNOSIS: Osteoarthritis, right knee

POSTOPERATIVE DIAGNOSIS: Osteoarthritis, right knee

PROCEDURE PERFORMED: Right cemented posterior stabilized total knee arthroplasty

ANESTHESIA: Epidural

COMPONENTS USED: Duracon size extra-large femur, size large 2 tibia, 9-mm (millimeter) posterior stabilized tibial insert, and 33-mm symmetric patella

OPERATIVE PROCEDURE: After suitable epidural anesthesia had been achieved, the patient's right knee was prepped and draped in the usual manner. Before prepping, the thigh tourniquet was applied, but initially it was not inflated. A long anterior midline skin incision and a long anteromedial arthrotomy were performed. The patient was noted to have marked synovitis in his knee. Once the synovial bleeders, capsular bleeders, and skin bleeders were cauterized, the leg was stripped with an Esmarch, and the tourniquet inflated to 275 mmHg (millimeter of mercury).

A partial fat pad excision was performed. The patella was dislocated laterally. An entry hole was made in the distal femur for the intramedullary alignment rod. Rotation was selected off the interepicondylar axis. Anterior referencing instruments were used. Using the intramedullary alignment, the anterior shim cut and then the distal femoral cuts were performed. The tibia was then subluxed forward. The proximal tibial cut

was performed. Nine millimeters of bone was excised, referencing off the intact lateral femur. The extension gap was then measured. The flexion gap was assessed, and a mark was placed on the distal femur to reproduce the identical flexion gap. This indicated the femoral component should be extra-large sized. An extra-large 4-in-1 jig was then applied. Anterior and posterior chamfer cuts were then performed. A trial femur was then placed to fit very well. A trial tibia with a 9-mm insert was placed, and there was excellent alignment and good stability. The patella was then everted and prepared for resurfacing technique using free-hand cuts with a saw. A symmetrical 3-mm trial component was placed and fit quite well. The box was then cut for the posterior stabilized femoral component, and the slot in the tibia was cut for the keel of the tibial component. The wounds were then thoroughly irrigated and dried. Bone graft was placed into the lug holes in the distal femur and the entry hole in the distal femur. The large 2-tibial component was then cemented into place. The extra large femoral component was cemented into place. A trial tibial insert was in place, and the leg was placed into full extension. The patellar component was then cemented into place. Once the cement was hard, stability was reassessed and found to be very good. A trial component was removed. The knee was carefully examined for any cement debris, which was carefully removed. The actual 9-mm posterior stabilized insert was then placed, and a locking screw was placed. The knee was then thoroughly irrigated. Autotransfusion Hemovac drain was placed. The wound was closed in layers. The capsule was closed with no.1 Panacryl, the subcutaneous tissue with 2-0 Vicryl, and the skin with staples. A Robert Jones dressing and anterior splint were then applied. Before wound closure, an autotransfusion Hemovac drain was placed. The patient tolerated the procedure well and returned to the recovery room in stable condition.

Pathology Report Later Indicated: Benign bone.

PHYSICIAN CODE: _____

CRNA CODE: _____

(Answers to every other Case are located in Appendix D . The full answer key is only available in the TEACH Instructor Resources on Evolve.)

CASE 14-17   *Operative Report, Closed Reduction*

The sedation and regional block were provided by a medically directed CRNA. There were 4 concurrent cases. Normal, healthy patient.

LOCATION: Outpatient, Hospital

PATIENT: Scott Laranzo

SURGEON: Mohomad Almaz, MD

DIAGNOSIS: Right hand fourth metacarpal fracture, transverse and displaced. Patient was injured in a fight.

ANESTHESIA: Regional block

PROCEDURE PERFORMED: Closed reduction, percutaneous pin fixation of right fourth metacarpal fracture

PROCEDURE: Under a satisfactory level of sedation and regional block, the extremity was prepped and draped. At this time, the fracture was reducible with distraction and manipulation. This was then further augmented with intramedullary retrograde pinning.

This was demonstrated in AP (anterior posterior) lateral and oblique views to maintain virtually anatomic position. I elected, at this time, to leave the pin proud and dress the pin, and then applied an ulnar gutter spica cast, fiberglass, about the extremity, keeping free and mobile the thumb and the index finger. There were no other complicating events. Fluoroscopy photos were obtained. The patient tolerated the procedure well.

PHYSICIAN CODE: _____

CRNA CODE: _____

(Answers to every other Case are located in Appendix D . The full answer key is only available in the TEACH Instructor Resources on Evolve.)

CASE 14-18 *Operative Report, Debridement*

Anesthesia was personally performed by the MDA. Patient is noted to have severe systemic disease.

LOCATION: Outpatient, Hospital

PATIENT: Viola Reynolds

SURGEON: Mohomad Almaz, MD

ANESTHESIA: General

PREOPERATIVE DIAGNOSIS: Left frozen shoulder

POSTOPERATIVE DIAGNOSIS: Left frozen shoulder adhesive pericapsulitis

PROCEDURE PERFORMED: Arthroscopic debridement, left shoulder.

Joint manipulation, left shoulder.

CLINICAL HISTORY: This 73-year-old woman presents with a history of progressive pain and discomfort of her left shoulder. Evaluation confirmed evidence of a left frozen shoulder. After the risks and benefits of anesthesia and surgery were explained to the patient, the decision was made to undertake the procedure.

PROCEDURE: Under general anesthetic, the patient was laid in the beach-chair position on the operating room table. The left shoulder was prepped and draped in the usual fashion. A standard posterior arthroscopic portal was created, and the camera was introduced into the back of the joint. We had excellent visualization. It was immediately apparent that there was substantial inflammation and adhesions throughout the entirety of the joint. Using a switch-stick technique, an anterior portal was created and the 7-mm (millimeter) cannula was then brought in from the front. Using a 4.0 double-biter resector, the synovium was then debrided throughout the entirety of the rotator cuff over the surface of the biceps and the anterior ligamentous structures as well as inferior ligamentous structures. With this completed, the joint was then thoroughly irrigated to remove any blood. The articular surfaces were inspected and were found to be normal. The attachment of the biceps was normal, although it had been covered with synovium. Anterior ligamentum structures were free from the subscapularis. The joint was then infiltrated with 80 mg (milligram) of Depo-Medrol and 12 cc of Marcaine. The instruments were removed. The arthroscopic portal was closed with absorbable sutures and Steri-Strips. The joint was then manipulated. Before the manipulation, we had about 90 degrees of elevation passively. After manipulation, elevation was free up to 180 degrees, and external rotation in an abducted position was possible to 90 degrees, as was internal rotation. Extension was possible to 40 degrees, and adduction was possible to 50 degrees. The wounds were then dressed with Myopore dressing. The patient was then placed in a Cryo Cuff sling, awakened, placed on her hospital bed, and taken to the recovery room in good condition.

PHYSICIAN CODE: _____

QUALIFYING CIRCUMSTANCES CODE: _____

(Answers to every other Case are located in Appendix D . The full answer key is only available in the TEACH Instructor Resources on Evolve.)

CASE 14-19 *Operative Report, Entropion and Ectropion Repair*

The anesthesia care was provided by a CRNA who was medically directed by an anesthesiologist. There were 4 concurrent cases.

LOCATION: Outpatient, Hospital

PATIENT: Robert Vobr

ATTENDING PHYSICIAN: Rita Wimer, MD

PREOPERATIVE DIAGNOSIS:

1. Upper lid entropion, both eyes; lower lid ectropion, both eyes
2. Graves' disease
3. Status post chemical decompression for Graves' disease
4. Chronic exposure, keratitis secondary to diagnoses 1, 2, and 3
5. Chronic conjunctivitis secondary to diagnoses 1, 2, 3, and 4

POSTOPERATIVE DIAGNOSIS:

1. Upper lid entropion, both eyes; lower lid ectropion, both eyes
2. Graves' disease
3. Status post chemical decompression for Graves' disease
4. Chronic exposure, keratitis secondary to diagnoses 1, 2, and 3
5. Chronic conjunctivitis secondary to diagnoses 1, 2, 3, and 4

OPERATIONS PERFORMED:

1. Upper lid entropion repair, both eyes
2. Lower lid ectropion repair, both eyes

ANESTHESIA: MAC

INDICATION: The patient has had progressive increase of upper lid entropion and lower lid ectropion, ptosis, and a number of other problems secondary to eye disease related to thyroid disease. The excess tissue is now interfering with his vision.

DESCRIPTION OF PROCEDURE: After the patient was placed on the operating room table, the skin to be resected on the upper lid was marked out with a blue sterile marking pen, as was the lower lid. There was a fishtail superiorly and lateral oblique inferiorly. This was infiltrated with Xylocaine 2%, 0.75% Marcaine, and bicarbonate. It was on a 25-gauge needle, and a total of 40 cc was used throughout the procedure. The #15 Bard-Parker blade then dissected the skin to be resected superiorly on the upper lids. This was freehand dissected, and a 2-mm (millimeter) strip of orbicularis was removed. The lateral, central, and medial fat pads were isolated, clamped, cut, and cauterized on the upper lids. The wound was reapproximated without supratarsal fixation using 6-0 nylon black suture to create a 2-mm ectropion of the upper lids. The lower lids were cut out with a #15 Bard-Parker blade through the marked incision. The fat pads centrally, medially, and laterally were identified, clamped, cut, cauterized, and allowed to retract. The amount of skin to be resected inferiorly was determined by the up-eye/open-mouth position, and this was mainly a lateral resection. The wounds were then closed with 6-0 nylon sutures. Maxitrol ointment and Telfa strips were laid on all four lids and half patches so the eyes remained open. There were no complications.

PHYSICIAN CODE: _____

CRNA CODE: _____

(Answers to every other Case are located in Appendix D . The full answer key is only available in the TEACH Instructor Resources on Evolve.)

CASE 14-20   *Operative Report, Hysterectomy*

The anesthesia care was provided by a CRNA who was medically directed by an anesthesiologist. There were 4 concurrent cases. The patient is otherwise normal and healthy.

LOCATION: Inpatient, Hospital

PATIENT: Gloria Rhodes

ATTENDING PHYSICIAN: Andy Martinez, MD

SURGEON: Andy Martinez, MD

PREOPERATIVE DIAGNOSIS: Endometriosis with resultant chronic pelvic pain

POSTOPERATIVE DIAGNOSIS: Same with mild pelvic adhesions

PROCEDURES PERFORMED:

1. Total abdominal hysterectomy with bilateral salpingo-oophorectomy
2. Cystoscopy with placement of ureteral catheters (Dr. Avila)

ANESTHESIA: General endotracheal

SURGICAL INDICATIONS: This patient is a 39-year-old, gravida 2, para (to bring forth) 2, who has had multiple operations in the past for endometriosis. She had recently been tried on hormonal suppression for her symptoms of pain, and this initially worked; however, she has had breakthrough bleeding and quite bothersome discomfort. At this point in time, she had elected definitive surgery.

OPERATIVE FINDINGS: The uterus was normal size. There were a lot of anterior cul-de-sac adhesions over the bladder and anterior surface of the uterus. There were some adhesions between the left tube and ovary and the posterior aspect of the left broad ligament. The right adnexa was free of any significant adhesions. Both ovaries were small, but she had been on hormonal suppression for the past several months.

PROCEDURE: After Dr. Avila did a cystoscopy and placed ureteral catheters, the patient was placed in the supine position, and the abdominal area was prepped and draped. The abdomen was opened through a Pfannenstiel incision. A Balfour retractor was placed. The adhesions in the anterior cul-de-sac and left adnexa were separated with Metzenbaum scissors. The bowel was packed off out of the pelvis with wet lap sponges. The uterus was elevated with Pean clamps. The left round ligament was clamped, divided, and suture ligated. All sutures heretofore are 1-0 Vicryl unless otherwise indicated. The round ligament was suture ligated and tagged. The peritoneum lateral to the left infundibulopelvic ligament was opened with Metzenbaum scissors, isolating the left ovarian vasculature. This pedicle was then clamped, divided, and doubly tied, first with a free tie and then a stick tie medial to the free tie. The anterior leaf of the left broad ligament was opened with Metzenbaum scissors. These structures were treated identically on the right side. The bladder was dissected free from the lower uterine segment and cervix with blunt and sharp dissection. The uterine artery pedicles were skeletonized on both sides with Metzenbaum scissors. The uterine artery pedicles were clamped with curved Rogers clamps, cut, and suture ligated with fixation sutures of a Heaney type. The cardinal ligaments were taken with straight Heaney-Ballantine clamps, cut, and suture ligated. The vaginal angles were clamped with curved Rogers clamps and incised, and then the apex of the vagina was incised across with right-angle scissors, removing the uterus, which was then handed off. Kocher clamps were placed in the vaginal apex and mucosa for identification. Angle sutures at both right and left angles were placed and then the middle of the vagina closed with several figure-of-eight sutures of 1-0 Vicryl. There was a small bit of oozing on the underside of the bladder, and this was isolated and oversewn with 3-0 Vicryl on a GI (gastrointestinal) needle. A small piece of Hemopad was then placed over the vaginal cuff. The bladder flap was loosely approximated over the vaginal cuff with a mattress suture of 3-0 Vicryl. The pelvis was irrigated with saline. There was no bleeding noted at this time. The sponges were removed and, with sponge and needle counts correct, attention was directed toward closure. The peritoneum was closed with a running 2-0 Vicryl. A medium Hemovac drain was placed subfascially to exit below the right side of the incision. The fascia was then closed with running locked 1-0 Vicryl using two strands, one from either side to the middle. The skin was closed with staples and the drain sutured to the skin with Prolene. Blood loss estimated by Anesthesia was 175 ml (milliliter). Specimen to pathology was the uterus with attached tubes and ovaries. Final sponge and needle counts were correct.

Pathology Report Later Indicated: Mild chronic cervicitis with squamous metaplasia, adenomyosis, left and right ovaries: endometriosis

PHYSICIAN CODE: _____

CRNA CODE: _____

(Answers to every other Case are located in Appendix D . The full answer key is only available in the TEACH Instructor Resources on Evolve.)

CASE 14-21   *Operative Report, Cesarean Section*

Anesthesia care is personally performed by the anesthesiologist in this normal, healthy woman.

LOCATION: Inpatient, Hospital

PATIENT: Beth Lariat

ATTENDING PHYSICIAN: Andy Martinez, MD

SURGEON: Andy Martinez, MD

PREOPERATIVE DIAGNOSIS: Previous cesarean section

POSTOPERATIVE DIAGNOSES:

1. Previous cesarean section
2. Macrosomia
3. Breech presentation

PROCEDURE PERFORMED: Repeat low transverse cesarean section

FINDINGS: Viable infant male with Apgars of 8 and 9. The infant's weight is 4206 g (gram). Maternal anatomy normal, including uterus, ovaries, and tubes. She did have significant scarring and adhesions in the subcutaneous tissue as well as subfascially.

ESTIMATED BLOOD LOSS: Approximately 800 cc

COMPLICATIONS: None

ANESTHESIA: Spinal anesthetic with Duramorph

TECHNIQUE: The patient was prepped and draped in the usual fashion. A Pfannenstiel incision was made. I did remove a nevus that looked somewhat inflamed and was oozing. It was right on the incision. The

Continued

CASE 14-21—cont'd

nevus was removed at that time. (This nevus is also reported as a diagnosis.) This was to be sent to pathology. I sharply dissected down to the rectus fascia. The fascia was then incised in the midline. I used sharp and cautery for dissection of this subcutaneous tissue laterally and anteriorly in a U-shape. The fascia was also incised with Mayo scissors laterally and anteriorly in a U-shape. Kocher clamps were placed on the superior and inferior aspect of the fascia, removing it from the underlying rectus muscles in the midline. The fascia was removed both sharply and with cautery. I entered the peritoneum sharply by tenting the peritoneum. The peritoneal incision was extended superiorly and inferiorly by blunt lateral traction. At this point, the lower uterine segment was identified. The anterior serosa of the lower uterine segment was incised. The incision was extended laterally and anteriorly in a U-shape with Metzenbaum scissors. Bladder flap was developed at this time.

The lower uterine segment was incised. The incision was extended laterally and anteriorly in a U-shape with bandage scissors. The infant was found to be in a breech presentation with double footling presentation. (This will have an effect on the diagnosis code.) The infant was delivered through the uterine incision without problems or complications. The cord was clamped and cut. The infant was handed to the nursery team standing by. The placenta was manually removed intact with three vessels. On inspection, the placenta had appeared normal. The uterus was exteriorized and wiped clean with a moist lap. The fascial incision was then repaired in a running locking layer. There was good hemostasis. The posterior cul-de-sac was irrigated. The uterus was placed back into the abdomen. Both right and left gutters were irrigated. On inspection of the uterine incision, there was good hemostasis. The fascia was then closed in a running fashion with 0 Vicryl. The subcutaneous tissue was irrigated, and the skin was closed with staples. All needle, sponge, and instrument counts were correct. The patient was stable in the recovery room. She will be transferred to floor status when she meets criteria.

Pathology Report Later Indicated: Benign nevus

PHYSICIAN CODE: _____

(Answers to every other Case are located in Appendix D . The full answer key is only available in the TEACH Instructor Resources on Evolve.)

CASE 14-22   *Operative Report, Cesarean Section*

The anesthesia care for this delivery and sterilization was provided by a medically directed CRNA. There were 3 concurrent cases. CPT code 01961 (Anesthesia, Cesarean Delivery) has BUV of 7. CPT code 00851 (Anesthesia, Tubal ligation) has BUV of 6.

LOCATION: Inpatient, Hospital

PATIENT: Patricia Garrison

SURGEON: Andy Martinez, MD

PREOPERATIVE DIAGNOSES:

1. Intrauterine pregnancy, 33 weeks
2. Insulin-dependent diabetes with diabetic nephropathy
3. Desire for sterilization
4. Previous cesarean section

POSTOPERATIVE DIAGNOSES:

1. Intrauterine pregnancy, 33 weeks
2. Insulin-dependent diabetes with diabetic nephropathy
3. Desire for sterilization
4. Previous cesarean section

PROCEDURE PERFORMED:

1. Repeat low transverse cervical cesarean section
2. Bilateral tubal ligation

ANESTHESIA: Subarachnoid block

SURGICAL INDICATIONS: The patient is a 28-year-old gravida 2, para (to bring forth) 1 with an EDC (estimated date of conception) of 08/01 who had been hospitalized for the past several weeks with hypertension and diabetes. Her condition appeared to be worsening, her diabetes was suddenly poorly controlled, and she was having epigastric pain. Her platelet count and AST (aspartate aminotransferase [formerly SGOT]) was normal preoperatively. She had a previous C-section. She also desired permanent sterilization by tubal interruption.

OPERATIVE DESCRIPTION: After induction of subarachnoid block anesthesia, a Foley catheter was placed and the Venodynes were placed as well. The abdomen was prepped and draped. The abdomen was opened through a Pfannenstiel incision. When we separated the rectus muscles, it became apparent that there was very little room as there was so much scarring of the fascia; therefore, a Maylard incision was done by separating the bellies of the rectus muscles transversely. Retractors were placed over the bladder. There was a poor bladder flap, but we dissected some of the bladder downward. An incision was made in the low transverse part of the uterus and entering the uterus was accomplished by blunting with a Kelly clamp. A finger was introduced into the uterus to guide a bandage scissors for a low transverse incision. The infant's head was delivered through the incision, and the muscles were so tight that we were having a little difficulty extracting the head; therefore, I removed my hand and put a Murless retractor behind the head and then the baby was easily delivered. The cord was clamped and cut, and then a segment of cord was sent off for gases. The placenta was then delivered manually. The uterus was closed in two layers, first with a running locked 0 Vicryl, followed by a running horizontal Lembert 0 Vicryl. The pelvis was then irrigated with saline. A few small bleeders were bovie coagulated. The right fallopian tube was elevated and the fimbriated end identified. The mesosalpinx underneath the ampullary portion was opened with bovie, and then the lateral mesosalpinx was cross-clamped on the lateral tube. The

CASE 14-22—*cont'd*

lateral portion of the tube, including the fimbriated end, was then excised and pedicles were doubly tied with 2-0 Vicryl. An identical procedure was carried out on the left tube. With sponge and needle counts correct, attention was directed toward closure. The rectus muscles were closed with a series of mattress sutures of 0 Vicryl. A medium Hemovac drain was placed subfascially. The fascia was closed with running locked 0 Vicryl using two strands, one from either side to the middle and tied independently. The skin was then closed with staples, and the drain was sutured to the skin with silk.

BLOOD LOSS ESTIMATION: 400-500 cc (cubic centimeter)

SPECIMEN TO PATHOLOGY: Placenta

FINAL SPONGE AND NEEDLE COUNTS: Correct

The patient tolerated the procedure well and returned to the recovery room in stable condition. After the child was extracted, we did start some magnesium sulfate.

Pathology Report Later Indicated: See Case 11-9K.

PHYSICIAN CODE: _____

CRNA CODE: _____

(Answers to every other Case are located in Appendix D . The full answer key is only available in the TEACH Instructor Resources on Evolve.)

CHAPTER 14   *Auditing Review*

Audit the coding for the following reports. Provide only the anesthesia code, not the diagnosis code.

Audit Report 14.1 Operative Report, Lung Mass

One-lung ventilation was used during this procedure. This patient is critically ill and in constant threat to life.

LOCATION: Inpatient, Hospital

PATIENT: Ellen Zutz

ATTENDING PHYSICIAN: Gregory Dawson, MD

SURGEON: Gary Sanchez, MD

PREOPERATIVE DIAGNOSIS: Right lung mass

POSTOPERATIVE DIAGNOSIS: Right lung mass

PROCEDURE PERFORMED: Right upper and right middle lobectomy with biopsy of four hilar lymph nodes

INDICATIONS: This 62-year-old female with a recent cough and shortness of breath was noted on chest x-ray to have a vague right mid-lung field lesion, which was confirmed by CT scan. There was some hilar adenopathy as well.

FINDINGS AT SURGERY: Lymph nodes from the hilum were biopsied times four, all of which were negative on frozen section. The inferior pulmonary ligament area, the azygous area, and paratracheal area were all devoid of lymph nodes. The lesion was deep within the confines of the right upper lobe and appeared to cross the minor fissure into the right middle lobe.

DESCRIPTION OF PROCEDURE: The patient was brought to the operating room and placed in the supine position under general intubation anesthesia with double lumen tube. The patient was rolled in her left lateral decubitus position with the right side up. The chest was entered through the sixth intercostal space anterior axillary line with a thoracoscope. Gentle exploration of the right hemithorax showed no evidence of gross tumor implants on the parietal pleura. Retraction of the right lower lobe, however, did show evidence of what appeared to be tumor under the visceral pleura in the right upper lobe. A portion of the right middle lobe had been incorporated into this tumor mass. General exploration of all the lymph node–bearing areas really disclosed only mildly enlarged lymph nodes in the hilum. These were biopsied and sent for frozen section, and all were benign. A standard right upper and right middle lobectomy utilizing the arterial first technique was carried out. The arteries were encircled with 0 silk, ligated, and clipped. The pulmonary vein was ligated distally and stapled proximally. The fissures between the upper and lower lobe were divided by several applications of the GIA automatic stapling machine. The bronchus was then skeletonized and clamped. Forced insufflation of the endotracheal tube produced good expansion of the right lower lobe. Following this, the staples were fired and the right upper and right middle lobe removed in one piece. These were submitted for frozen-section diagnosis. Frozen section showed adenocarcinoma. The chest was then checked for hemostasis and irrigated thoroughly with antibiotic solution and closed over two, 36-French atrium chest tubes in the usual fashion. Sterile compression dressings were applied, and the patient returned to the postanesthesia care unit recovery room in satisfactory condition after application of an epidural anesthetic by Dr. Larson. Sponge count and needle count were correct times two.

One or more codes should not have been reported for this case. Indicate the code(s) incorrectly reported.

PROFESSIONAL SERVICES: Anesthesia, **00546-P4**

INCORRECTLY REPORTED CODE(S): _____

Audit Report 14.2 Operative Report, Subdural Hematoma

This anesthesia service is being provided for a 90-year-old patient. Anesthesia by: MDA and CRNA. Anesthesiologist was medically directing 3 concurrent cases. The physical status is 3.

LOCATION: Inpatient, Hospital

PATIENT: Charles Spice

SURGEON: John Hodgson, MD

PREOPERATIVE DIAGNOSIS: Chronic subdural hematoma

POSTOPERATIVE DIAGNOSIS: Subdural empyema mixed with subdural hematoma.

PROCEDURE PERFORMED: Left frontoparietal burr hole evacuation of subdural hematoma and subdural empyema.

COMPLICATIONS: None.

INDICATIONS: This is a 90-year-old female who presented with a several week history of word-finding difficulty and mild right-sided weakness. A CAT scan showed what appeared to be a subdural fluid collection consistent with blood over the left frontoparietal area. After a discussion of the options with the family, they eventually consented to surgery. The risks were discussed and they elected to proceed.

DESCRIPTION OF PROCEDURE: The patient was taken to the operating room and underwent IV sedation. The left frontoparietal area was shaved, sterilely prepped, and draped. An incision was made in the posterior left frontal area and the anterior parietal area on the left side after the skin was infiltrated with local anesthetic. The incisions were approximately 7 cm lateral to the midline and parallel to the midline. Retractors were placed. Using the craniotome, two burr holes were made. They were then curetted out of any remaining bone. The dura was first opened posteriorly with the monopolar cautery on a low setting. Chronic appearing subdural blood came forth under pressure. After approximately 10 seconds, frank pus began draining from the subdural space. I then went ahead and incised the dural also in a cruciate fashion along the anterior burr hole. The brain was definitely sunken away from the inner table of the skull by at least 2 cm over each burr hole. Again, I irrigated from the anterior bur hole to the posterior one and was able to evacuate additional amounts of pus and blood. When the irrigant returned clear, I then placed a 7 mm round Jackson-Pratt drain from the anterior hole directed posteriorly. I then brought this out through a separate stab wound in the skin. I again irrigated both burr hole sites.

Small pieces of Gelfoam were placed over each burr hole. The galea was closed with interrupted 2-0 Vicryl and the skin was closed with a running 3-0 Chromic over both holes. The drain was sutured in place. Aerobic and anaerobic cultures and a gram stain were sent when the purulent drainage was noted. The patient was taken to the recovery room in stable condition. Sponge, instrument, and needle counts were correct.

One of the following modifiers is incorrectly reported for this case. Indicate the modifier that is incorrect.

SERVICE CODE(S):   Anesthesia, **00214-QY-P3,** Extreme age of patient receiving anesthesia, **99100**

CRNA CODE: Anesthesia, **00214-QX-P3**

INCORRECT MODIFIER: _____

Audit Report 14.3 Operative Report, Laparoscopic Gastric Bypass

The physical status is 3. Anesthesia by: MDA and CRNA. Anesthesiologist was medically directing 4 concurrent cases.

LOCATION: Inpatient, Hospital

PATIENT: Krissy Morningside

SURGEON: Gary Sanchez, MD

PREOPERATIVE DIAGNOSIS: Morbid obesity.

POSTOPERATIVE DIAGNOSIS: Same.

PROCEDURE PERFORMED: 100 cm Roux-en-Y laparoscopic gastric bypass, liver biopsy.

HISTORY: The patient has morbid obesity with BMI of 40. It was elected to do a laparoscopic, possible open Roux-en-Y gastric bypass and a liver biopsy.

DESCRIPTION OF PROCEDURE: The patient was given a general anesthetic. She had been given preoperative Lovenox and antibiotics. She had SCDs (sequential compression devices) on which were functional. She was prepped and draped in the slight head up position. A curvilinear incision was made above the umbilicus, and we worked our way down to the fascia, incised the fascia, and put in retaining Vicryl stitches. We carefully worked our way in the abdomen, put in Hasson, the gas, and a 45-degree scope. We then put a 5 mm trocar in the left upper quadrant just below the rib cage and a 12 mm port below this and the Hasson. We did the same on the left side, but both of those were 12 mm trocars. We then put the Nathanson retractor through a small incision just below the xiphisternum and then we lifted up the liver. We then lifted up the stomach and went into the lesser sac. There were some adhesions posteriorly that we took down and then it completely opened up the lesser sac. We then put the taut catheter through. We then lifted up the omentum and found that there were some adhesions from her previous laparoscopic cholecystectomy. These were omentum adhesions and were stuck to the abdominal wall. I took those down with the harmonic scalpel, and this allowed us to pancake the greater omentum over the liver and stomach. We then dissected in the region of the ligament of Treitz. We went superior and to the left and worked our way into the lesser sac through the transverse mesocolon, and we found the taut catheter and brought it through. We then identified the ligament of Treitz and then went 20 cm down from it and then stapled across with the 45-2.5 stapler. We went through a little bit of mesentery with a 1.5, 45-Ethicon stapler using about ⅓ of the load.

We then marched off a 100 cm Roux limb. We then brought the two edges together and then opened up along the antimesenteric border of the biliopancreatic limb and the Roux limb and then took two fires of the 2.5, 45 stapler in and then closed what was left of the hole with the same stapler. This gave us an excellent biliopancreatic limb, common channel, and Roux limb that were of great size, under no tension with an excellent blood supply. We then closed the rent in the mesentery with a running autosuture stitch. We then sutured the proximal Roux limb to the taut catheter with the autosuture stitch. We then brought it through the lesser sac and the bowel easily came up. We then opened up the angle of His and that opened up very easily. We then put the BioEnterics tube down and put 25 cc in and then pulled it up to the esophagogastric junction. There was no hiatus hernia. We then went just below the "equator" of this and then removed the BioEnterics catheter, and then we formed our pouch using the 3.5, 45 Ethicon stapler.

We completely transected this gastric remnant from the pouch. We then put the BioEnterics tube back down. It easily went down to the bottom of the pouch and we put the snare through. We put the wire through the 14-gauge Cathelin and then we put it through the wire and brought this through the mouth. We then put the wire through the end of a 21-Stealth stapler and brought that back down through the pouch with no difficulty at all. We then removed the wire and the taut catheter. We formed our upper 12 mm port site and brought the other end of the stapler through. We then opened up the Roux limb at the staple line and then put the stapler through. We then opened it up and brought the anvil down and fired it. This gave us an excellent anastomosis under no tension. We then closed the rest of the hole with the 2.5, 45 Ethicon stapler. We then sutured at the 3 o'clock position. We then sutured at the 9 o'clock position bringing pouch down to the Roux limb to keep the tension off, and then we put this 9 o'clock stitch through a piece of fat and then put a lap tie on it. We then put the patient down flat and held the distal limb with Dorsey bowel grassers, and we put the BioEnterics tube back down, and we tested with a total of 40 cc of air after putting some fluid in. There was no leak. The stapler showed two good donuts. We then put the patient in the head-up position again and put HemaSeal in. We then went below, brought the Roux limb back down through, and then sutured the antimesenteric part of the Roux limb to the hole in the mesentery. We then straightened out the limbs and again confirmed that they were excellent quality and caliber. We then put some HemaSeal along those staple lines. We then put a flat 10 mm Jackson-Pratt drain through the right upper 12 mm port site and put it down by the jejunojejunostomy

Continued

site. We then put the colon back down, went above, and put another flat 10 mm Jackson-Pratt through the upper left 5 mm port site. We then made sure it was at the gastrojejunostomy area. We then did a liver biopsy with a Monopty biopsy device. We then confirmed we had excellent hemostasis. We removed the trocars and sutured the drains in place. We closed the umbilical fascial defect with interrupted Vicryl stitches. All skin incisions were closed with 3-0 Prolene stitches. We put in Marcaine, Steri-Strips and Op-Sites. The patient tolerated this very well and went to Recovery Room in good condition.

One or more codes should not have been reported for this case. Indicate the code(s) incorrectly reported.

SERVICE CODE(S):   Anesthesia, **00797-QK-P3**; Liver biopsy, **47001**

CRNA CODE: Anesthesia, **00797-QX-P3**

INCORRECTLY REPORTED CODE: _____

Anesthesia by: MDA and CRNA. Anesthesiologist was medically directing 4 concurrent cases.

Audit Report 14.4 Operative Report, Anesthesia

LOCATION: Inpatient, Hospital

PATIENT: Sebastian Webb

SURGEON: Larry Friendly, MD

PREOPERATIVE DIAGNOSIS: Perirectal fistula

POSTOPERATIVE DIAGNOSIS: Perirectal fistula

PROCEDURE PERFORMED: Perirectal fistulectomy

ANESTHESIA: General anesthesia

INDICATIONS FOR SURGERY: This is a normal, healthy 65-year-old male who has had a draining perirectal fistula. He is now being admitted for incision of this fistula.

DESCRIPTION OF PROCEDURE: The patient is placed in a jackknife position. He was prepped and draped in a sterile fashion. General anesthesia was given. The fistula tract was in the 3 o'clock position. This was completely excised. The tract continued over the 5 o'clock position. This tract was made into one incision, and all of the inflamed tissue was also excised. The rectum was then dilated up and examined. There was one tract that was seen directly draining into the rectum. The inflamed tissue that was on the outer skin area was also completely excised. The area was then thoroughly irrigated. Hemostasis was achieved with use of cautery. The wound was then left open and dressings were applied. The patient tolerated the procedure and was then turned over to recovery in stable condition.

One or more of the following codes are reported incorrectly for this case. Indicate the incorrect code or codes.

SERVICE CODE(S):   Anesthesia, **00902-AA**

CRNA CODE: Anesthesia, **00902-QZ**

INCORRECT/MISSING CODE(S): _____

Audit Report 14.5 Operative Report, Anesthesia

Unless stated otherwise, assume "normal, healthy patient." Anesthesia by: MDA and CRNA. Anesthesiologist was medically directing 4 concurrent cases.

INDICATIONS FOR SURGERY: This is a 28-year-old healthy male who has had some problems with sleep apnea and breathing through his nose. He is now admitted for repair of his deviated septum with bilateral inferior turbinate reduction and removal of his tonsils.

LOCATION: Inpatient, Hospital

PATIENT: Don Albet

SURGEON: Gregory Dawson, MD

PREOPERATIVE DIAGNOSIS:

1. Septal deviation
2. Bilateral inferior turbinate hypertrophy
3. Tonsillar hypertrophy

POSTOPERATIVE DIAGNOSIS:

1. Septal deviation
2. Bilateral inferior turbinate hypertrophy
3. Tonsillar hypertrophy

PROCEDURE PERFORMED:

1. Septoplasty
2. Bilateral inferior turbinate reduction
3. Tonsillectomy

ANESTHESIA: General anesthesia

SURGICAL FINDINGS: The patient had a fairly significant left septal deviation. Some of this was anterior. He also had posteriorly on the left-hand side contact between the posterior left nasal septum and the left lateral nasal wall from a bony spur. The inferior turbinates bilaterally were grossly hypertrophic. The tonsils were extremely hypertrophied. Many crypts were present.

DESCRIPTION OF PROCEDURE: After informed consent, the patient was taken to the operating room and placed in the supine position. He was draped in the usual fashion. The nose was packed bilaterally with Afrin-soaked gauze. Right and left nasal septum were each injected with 3 cc of 1% Xylocaine with Epinephrine. Some of the nose hairs were trimmed. The Afrin-soaked gauze was removed bilaterally. An incision was made at the anterior end of the right nasal septum. A mucoperichondral flap was identified. This was elevated on the right nasal septum. No perforations occurred during this. Taking care to leave a good 1 cm of anterior septal cartilage, an incision was made through the right side of the septal cartilage at its base. Through this incision, a left mucoperichondrial flap was then elevated. We also elevated a mucoperiosteal flap on the left-hand side with the freer elevator. A strip of cartilage was removed from the inferior end of the septal cartilage at its junction with the maxillary crest. A portion of the anterior inferior left-sided septal deviation was due to the deviation of the left maxillary crest. A 4-mm osteotome was used to remove this deviated portion. The bony vomer was deviated to the left-hand side with a spur in contact with the left lateral nasal wall, and I did remove this with Wilde forceps. The strip of cartilage removed was approximately 2 cm in length and 1 cm in height. At least a cm of nasal dorsal strut and anterior strut was maintained. This was to provide good tip support, which was present at the end of the case. Following removal of the cartilage and the maxillary crest, the septum was significantly straighter. There was still a small amount of anterior left septal deviation, but significantly less. The anterior inferior edges of the turbinates bilaterally were then cauterized with needlepoint cautery. Following this, a butter knife was used to out-fracture the turbinates bilaterally. This gave a significant improvement in the nasal airway. There was a small mucosal tear posteriorly on the left-hand side, which would serve as a drainage site to prevent hematoma formation beneath the mucosal flap. The anterior end of the right nasal septum was then closed using interrupted 4-0 chromic catgut. I then placed Doyle nasal splints bilaterally. The patient was then repositioned for tonsillectomy. The McIvor out gag was placed, and we were able to visualize the tonsils. They were extremely large with many crypts on them. Attention was first focused on the left tonsil. The retractor was placed in the superior pole, and the tonsil was retracted toward the midline. Then, using the harmonic scalpel at power level III, the tonsil was removed. Hemostasis was achieved from spot suction cautery. Similar procedure was then performed on the left tonsil. The tonsillar fossa was then irrigated, and hemostasis was achieved. Infiltration of 1% Xylocaine with 1:100,000 units of epinephrine was placed in the retromolar and soft palate areas bilaterally. Tension on the mouth gag was then released. Reinspection showed no active bleeding. The patient was then allowed to recover from general anesthesia. He tolerated the procedure well. He was transferred to the recovery room in good condition. He will go home on Keflex 500 mg po q.i.d. He has a prescription for Percocet for pain. He is going to be using nasal saline rinses until I see him again in 2 weeks. At that time we will be removing the stents. He will get in touch with my office if he is having any other problems.

One or more of the following codes are reported incorrectly for this case. Indicate the incorrect code or codes.

SERVICE CODE(S):   Anesthesia, **00160-QY-P2, 00170-QY-P2**

CRNA CODE: Anesthesia, **00160-QY-P2, 00170-QY-P2**

INCORRECT/MISSING CODE(S): _____

ANESTHESIA BY: CRNA.

Audit Report 14.6 Operative Report, Anesthesia

LOCATION: Outpatient, Hospital

PATIENT: Stephen Void

SURGEON: Ira Avila, MD

PREOPERATIVE DIAGNOSIS: Phimosis

POSTOPERATIVE DIAGNOSIS: Phimosis

PROCEDURE PERFORMED: Circumcision

ANESTHESIA: General mask anesthesia

PROCEDURE: This 18-month-old, normal, healthy fellow was placed on a standard circumcision board. General mask anesthesia was applied.

He was prepped in the standard procedure with Betadine. The foreskin was retracted. We then used a Gomco clamp and removed the foreskin. Vaseline gauze was applied. There were no complications. He tolerated the procedure well. The patient was transferred to the recovery room in good condition.

One or more of the following codes are reported incorrectly for this case. Indicate the incorrect code or codes.

CRNA CODE: Anesthesia, **00910-QX**

INCORRECT/MISSING CODE(S): _____

(Auditing Review answers with rationales are only available in the TEACH Instructor Resources on Evolve.)

Figure Credits

Chapter 1

Figures 2, 3, 6: Kumar: *Robbins and Cotran: Pathologic Basis of Disease*, 8th ed. 4: From Forbes CD, Jackson WF: *Color Atlas and Text of Clinical Medicine*, 3rd ed. London, Mosby, 2003, with permission. 5: From Patton KE, Thibodeau GA: *Anatomy and Physiology*, 8th ed. St. Louis, 2013, Mosby.

Chapter 2

Figures 2: Feldman: *Sleisenger & Fordtran's Gastrointestinal and Liver Disease*, 9th ed. 3: Roberts: *Clinical Procedures in Emergency Medicine*, 4th ed.

Chapter 3

Figures 9: Mettler: *Essentials of Radiology*, 2nd ed. 10: Modified from Abeloff M et al: *Clinical Oncology*, 3rd ed., Philadelphia, 2004, Churchill Livingstone. 11: Mitchell: *Grainger & Allison's Diagnostic Radiology: A Textbook of Medical Imaging*, 4th ed.

Chapter 5

Figures 1: Kumar: *Robbins and Cotran: Pathologic Basis of Disease*, 8th ed. 2: Habif: *Clinical Dermatology*, 5th ed. 5: Auerbach: *Wilderness Medicine*, 6th ed. 6: DeLee: *DeLee and Drez's Orthopaedic Sports Medicine*, 2nd ed. 8: Abeloff: *Clinical Oncology*, 4th ed. 9: From Roberts JR, Custalow CB, Thomsen TW: *Roberts and Hedges' Clinical Procedures in Emergency Medicine and Acute Care*, ed 7, Philadelphia, 2019, Elsevier. 10: Lentz: *Comprehensive Gynecology*, 6th ed.

Chapter 6

Figures 2: From Braundwald E: *Heart Disease: A Textbook of Cardiovascular Medicine*, vol 1, 6th ed., Philadelphia, 2007, WB Saunders. 6: Libby: *Braunwald's Heart Disease: A Textbook of Cardiovascular Medicine*, 8th ed. 9: Yeo: *Shackelford's Surgery of the Alimentary Tract*, 7th ed. 10: Rutherford: *Vascular Surgery*, 6th ed.

Chapter 7

Figures 3: Mettler: *Essentials of Radiology*, 2nd ed. 4: Roberts: *Clinical Procedures in Emergency Medicine*, 5th ed. 5: Marx: *Rosen's Emergency Medicine: Concepts and Clinical Practice*, 7th ed. 6: Goldman/Ausiello: *Cecil's Textbook of Medicine*, 23/e. 7: ©Elsevier Collection. 10: Feldman: *Sleisenger & Fordtran's Gastrointestinal and Liver Disease*, 9th ed. 12: Feldman: *Sleisenger & Fordtran's Gastrointestinal and Liver Disease*, 8th ed. 14: Gershenson: *Operative Gynecology*, 2nd ed.

Chapter 8

Figures 1: Elsevier: *Buck's Step-by-Step Medical Coding, 2025 Edition*, St. Louis, 2025, Elsevier. 2: Harris: *Kelley's Textbook of Rheumatology*, 7th ed. 4: Browner: *Skeletal Trauma: Basic Science, Management, and Reconstruction*, 4th ed. 5: Rakel: *Textbook of Family Medicine*, 7th ed. 6: Magee: *Orthopedic Physical Assessment*, 6th ed. 7: ©Elsevier Collection.

Chapter 9

Figures 1: Mettler: *Essentials of Radiology*, 2nd ed. 6: Spiro: *Clinical Respiratory Medicine*, 4th ed.

Chapter 10

Figures 1: Wein: *Campbell-Walsh Urology*, 10th ed. 2: Kumar: *Robbins and Cotran: Pathologic Basis of Disease*, 8th ed. 3: From Mathur, P., Porwal, K. K., Pendse, A. K., Parihar, U.S., Chittora, R. Hemangiomatous penile horn. *Journal of Urology* 155, no. 5 (1996): 1738. 4. Habif: *Clinical Dermatology*, 5th ed. 5: Townsend: *Sabiston Textbook of Surgery*, 18th ed. 9: Abeloff: *Clinical Oncology*, 4th ed. 10: Townsend: *Sabiston Textbook of Surgery*, 19th ed.

Chapter 11

Figures 2, 3: From Baggish MS: *Colposcopy of the Cervix, Vagina, and Vulva: A Comprehensive Textbook*. Philadelphia, 2003, Mosby. 4: Kumar: *Robbins and Cotran: Pathologic Basis of Disease*, 8th ed. 5: James: *High Risk Pregnancy: Management Options*, 3rd ed.

Chapter 12

Figures 2: From Patton KE, Thibodeau GA: *Anatomy and Physiology*, 8th ed., St. Louis, 2013, Mosby. 3: Cummings: *Otolaryngology: Head & Neck Surgery*, 4th ed. 4: Bradley: *Neurology in Clinical Practice*, 4th ed. 6: Modified From Applegate E: *The Anatomy and Physiology Learning System*, 4th ed., St. Louis, 2011, Saunders.

Chapter 13

Figures 3: Yanoff: *Ophthalmology*, 3rd ed. 2, 4: Yanoff: *Ophthalmology*, 2nd ed.

CMS AB-01-144

Although this memorandum specifies ICD-9-CM, it is applicable to ICD-10-CM.

Available at https://www.cms.gov/Regulations-and-Guidance/Guidance/Transmittals/Downloads/AB01144.pdf. Accessed January 26, 2024

Program Memorandum Intermediaries/Carriers
  Transmittal AB-01-144
  Department of Health
    & Human Services (DHHS)
  Centers for Medicare &
    Medicaid Services (CMS)
  Date: SEPTEMBER 26, 2001
  CHANGE REQUEST 1724
SUBJECT: ICD-9-CM Coding for Diagnostic Tests

Introduction

This Program Memorandum (PM) clarifies our current coding guidelines for reporting diagnostic tests. Specifically, this PM clarifies the reporting of the International Classification of Diseases, Ninth Revision, Clinical Modification (ICD-9-CM) codes for diagnostic tests.

As required by the Health Insurance Portability and Accountability Act (HIPAA), the Secretary published a rule designating the ICD-9-CM and its *Official ICD-9-CM Guidelines for Coding and Reporting* as one of the approved code sets for use in reporting diagnoses and inpatient procedures. This final rule requires the use of ICD-9-CM and its official coding and reporting guidelines by most health plans (including Medicare) by October 16, 2002.

The *Official ICD-9-CM Guidelines for Coding and Reporting* provides guidance on coding. The ICD-9-CM Coding Guidelines for Outpatient Services, which is part of the *Official ICD-9-CM Guidelines for Coding and Reporting*, provides guidance on diagnoses coding specifically for outpatient facilities and physician offices.

The ICD-9-CM Coding Guidelines for Outpatient Services (hospital-based and physician office) have instructed physicians to report diagnoses based on test results. The Coding Clinic for ICD-9-CM confirms this longstanding coding guideline. CMS agrees with these longstanding official coding and reporting guidelines.

Following are instructions for contractors, physicians, hospitals, and other health care providers to use in determining the use of ICD-9-CM codes for coding diagnostic test results.

The instructions below provide guidance on the appropriate assignment of ICD-9-CM diagnoses codes to simplify coding for diagnostic tests consistent with the ICD-9-CM Guidelines for Outpatient Services (hospital-based and physician office). Note that physicians are responsible for the accuracy of the information submitted on a bill.

A. Determining the Appropriate Primary ICD-9-CM Diagnosis Code for Diagnostic Tests Ordered due to Signs and/or Symptoms

1. If the physician has confirmed a diagnosis based on the results of the diagnostic test, the physician interpreting the test should code that diagnosis. The signs and/or symptoms that prompted ordering the test may be reported as additional diagnoses if they are not fully explained or related to the confirmed diagnosis.

    Example 1: A surgical specimen is sent to a pathologist with a diagnosis of "mole." The pathologist personally reviews the slides made from the specimen and makes a diagnosis of "malignant melanoma." The pathologist should report a diagnosis of "malignant melanoma" as the primary diagnosis.

    Example 2: A patient is referred to a radiologist for an abdominal CT scan with a diagnosis of abdominal pain. The CT scan reveals the presence of an abscess. The radiologist should report a diagnosis of "intra-abdominal abscess."

    Example 3: A patient is referred to a radiologist for a chest x-ray with a diagnosis of "cough." The chest x-ray reveals 3 cm peripheral pulmonary nodule. The radiologist should report a diagnosis of "pulmonary nodule" and may sequence "cough" as an additional diagnosis.

2. If the diagnostic test did not provide a diagnosis or was normal, the interpreting physician should code the sign(s) or symptom(s) that prompted the treating physician to order the study.

Example 1: A patient is referred to a radiologist for a spine x-ray due to complaints of "back pain." The radiologist performs the x-ray, and the results are normal. The radiologist should report a diagnosis of "back pain" since this was the reason for performing the spine x-ray.

Example 2: A patient is seen in the ER for chest pain. An EKG is normal, and the final diagnosis is chest pain due to suspected gastroesophageal reflux disease (GERD). The patient was told to follow-up with his primary care physician for further evaluation of the suspected GERD. The primary diagnosis code for the EKG should be chest pain. Although the EKG was normal, a definitive cause for the chest pain was not determined.

3. If the results of the diagnostic test are normal or non-diagnostic, and the referring physician records a diagnosis preceded by words that indicate uncertainty (e.g., probable, suspected, questionable, rule out, or working), then the interpreting physician should not code the referring diagnosis. Rather, the interpreting physician should report the sign(s) or symptom(s) that prompted the study. Diagnoses labeled as uncertain are considered by the ICD-9-CM Coding Guidelines as unconfirmed and should not be reported. This is consistent with the requirement to code the diagnosis to the highest degree of certainty.

Example: A patient is referred to a radiologist for a chest x-ray with a diagnosis of "rule out pneumonia." The radiologist performs a chest x-ray, and the results are normal. The radiologist should report the sign(s) or symptom(s) that prompted the test (e.g., cough).

B. Instruction to Determine the Reason for the Test

As specified in § 4317(b) of the Balanced Budget Act (BBA), referring physicians are required to provide diagnostic information to the testing entity at the time the test is ordered. As further indicated in 42 CFR 410.32, all diagnostic tests "must be ordered by the physician who is treating the beneficiary." As defined in § 15021 of the Medicare Carrier Manual (MCM), an "order" is a communication from the treating physician/practitioner requesting that a diagnostic test be performed for a beneficiary. An order may include the following forms of communication:

a. A written document signed by the treating physician/practitioner, which is hand-delivered, mailed, or faxed to the testing facility;

b. A telephone call by the treating physician/practitioner or his/her office to the testing facility; and

c. An electronic mail by the treating physician/practitioner or his/her office to the testing facility.

NOTE: If the order is communicated via telephone, both the treating physician/practitioner or his/her office and the testing facility must document the telephone call in their respective copies of the beneficiary's medical records.

On the rare occasion when the interpreting physician does not have diagnostic information as to the reason for the test and the referring physician is unavailable to provide such information, it is appropriate to obtain the information directly from the patient or the patient's medical record if it is available. However, an attempt should be made to confirm any information obtained from the patient by contacting the referring physician.

Example: A patient is referred to a radiologist for a gastrografin enema to rule out appendicitis. However, the referring physician does not provide the reason for the referral and is unavailable at the time of the study. The patient is queried and indicates that he/she saw the physician for abdominal pain, and was referred to rule out appendicitis. The radiologist performs the x-ray, and the results are normal. The radiologist should report the abdominal pain as the primary diagnosis.

C. Incidental Findings

Incidental findings should never be listed as primary diagnoses. If reported, incidental findings may be reported as secondary diagnoses by the physician interpreting the diagnostic test.

Example 1: A patient is referred to a radiologist for an abdominal ultrasound due to jaundice. After review of the ultrasound, the interpreting physician discovers that the patient has an aortic aneurysm. The interpreting physician reports jaundice as the primary diagnosis and may report the aortic aneurysm as a secondary diagnosis because it is an incidental finding.

Example 2: A patient is referred to a radiologist for a chest x-ray because of wheezing. The x-ray is normal except for scoliosis and degenerative joint disease of the thoracic spine. The interpreting physician reports wheezing as the primary diagnosis since it was the reason for the patient's visit, and may report the other findings (scoliosis and degenerative joint disease of the thoracic spine) as additional diagnoses.

Example 3: A patient is referred to a radiologist for a magnetic resonance imaging (MRI) of the lumbar spine with a diagnosis of L-4 radiculopathy. The MRI reveals degenerative joint disease at L1 and L2. The radiologist reports radiculopathy as the primary diagnosis and may report degenerative joint disease of the spine as an additional diagnosis.

D. Unrelated/Co-Existing Conditions/Diagnoses

Unrelated and co-existing conditions/diagnoses may be reported as additional diagnoses by the physician interpreting the diagnostic test.

Example: A patient is referred to a radiologist for a chest x-ray because of a cough. The result of the chest x-ray indicates the patient has pneumonia. During the performance of the diagnostic test, it was determined that the patient has hypertension and diabetes mellitus. The interpreting physician reports a primary diagnosis of pneumonia. The interpreting physician may report the hypertension and diabetes mellitus as secondary diagnoses.

E. Diagnostic Tests Ordered in the Absence of Signs and/or Symptoms (e.g., Screening Tests)

When a diagnostic test is ordered in the absence of signs/symptoms or other evidence of illness or injury, the physician interpreting the diagnostic test should report the reason for the test (e.g., screening) as the primary ICD-9-CM diagnosis code. The results of the test, if reported, may be recorded as additional diagnoses.

F. Use of ICD-9-CM to the Greatest Degree of Accuracy and Completeness

NOTE: This section explains certain coding guidelines that address diagnoses coding. These guidelines are longstanding coding guidelines that have been part of the *Official ICD-9-CM Guidelines for Coding and Reporting.*

The interpreting physician should code the ICD-9-CM code that provides the highest degree of accuracy and completeness for the diagnosis resulting from the test, or for the sign(s)/symptom(s) that prompted the ordering of the test.

In the past, there has been some confusion about the meaning of "highest degree of specificity," and in "reporting the correct number of digits." In the context of ICD-9-CM coding, the "highest degree of specificity" refers to assigning the most precise ICD-9-CM code that most fully explains the narrative description of the symptom or diagnosis.

Example 1: A chest x-ray reveals a primary lung cancer in the left lower lobe. The interpreting physician should report the ICD-9-CM code as 162.5 for malignancy of the left "lower lobe, bronchus or lung," not the code for a malignancy of "other parts of bronchus or lung" (162.8) or the code for "bronchus and lung unspecified" (162.9).

Example 2: If a sputum specimen is sent to a pathologist and the pathologist confirms growth of "streptococcus, type B," which is indicated in the patient's medical record,

the pathologist should report a primary diagnosis as 482.32 (Pneumonia due to streptococcus, Group B). However, if the pathologist is unable to specify the organism, then the pathologist should report the primary diagnosis as 486 (Pneumonia, organism unspecified).

In order to report the correct number of digits when using ICD-9-CM, refer to the following instructions:

ICD-9-CM diagnosis codes are composed of codes with 3, 4, or 5 digits. Codes with 3 digits are included in ICD-9-CM as the heading of a category of codes that may be further subdivided by the use of fourth and/or fifth digits to provide greater specificity. Assign three-digit codes only if there are no four-digit codes within that code category. Assign four-digit codes only if there is no fifth-digit subclassification for that category. Assign the fifth-digit subclassification code for those categories where it exists.

Example 3: A patient is referred to a physician with a diagnosis of diabetes mellitus. However, there is no indication that the patient has diabetic complications or that the diabetes is out of control. It would be incorrect to assign code 250 since all codes in this series have 5 digits. Reporting only three digits of a code that has 5 digits would be incorrect. One must add two more digits to make it complete. Because the type (adult onset/juvenile) of diabetes is not specified, and there is no indication that the patient has a complication or that the diabetes is out of control, the correct ICD-9-CM code would be 250.00. The fourth and fifth digits of the code would vary depending on the specific condition of the patient. One should be guided by the code book.

For the latest ICD-9-CM coding guidelines, please refer to the following website: www.cdc.gov/nchs/data/icd9/ICD9CM_guidelines_2011.pdf.

Refer to the attachment for further guidance on determining the appropriate ICD-9-CM diagnoses codes. The attachment is a listing of questions and answers that appeared in the American Hospital Association's (AHA) Coding Clinic for ICD-9-CM (1st Qtr 2000).

NOTE: Contractors are advised to make this PM available to physicians and other health care professionals. If available, immediately place this PM on your website. This PM should be distributed with your next regularly scheduled bulletin.

Online Resources

The Evolve Learning Resources offer helpful material that will extend your studies beyond the classroom.

Official Guidelines for Coding and Reporting, Content Updates, and Coding links help you stay current with this ever-changing field.

Once registered for your free Evolve resources at http://evolve.elsevier.com/Buck/next, go to the *Course Content* to reference the following:

Reference Audit Form

Coding Tips and Links
- *ICD-10-CM Official Guidelines for Coding and Reporting*
- *ICD-10-PCS Official Guidelines for Coding and Reporting*
- 1995 Guidelines for E/M Services
- 1997 Documentation Guidelines for Evaluation and Management Services
- CPT, ICD-10-CM, ICD-10-PCS, and HCPCS Update Links
- Study Tips
- WebLinks

Content Updates – Student

Abbreviations

A1 pulley	tendon on anterior surface of finger
ABD	adriamycin, bleomycin, dacarbazine
ABG	arterial blood gases
ABO	three main blood types
AC	abdominal circumference
ACL	anterior cruciate ligament
ACLS	Advanced Cardiac Life Support
ACTH	adrenocorticotropic hormone
AF	atrial fibrillation (also A Fib)
AFB	acid-fast bacillus
AFI	amniotic fluid index
A Fib	atrial fibrillation (also AF)
AFT	atrial flutter
AIC	amino-imidazole carboxamide; anti-inflammatory corticoid
AKA	above-knee amputation
Alb	albumin
Alk phos	alkaline phosphatase
ALT	alanine transaminase (formerly SGPT)
AM	acute marginal (branch of RCA)
AMA	advanced maternal age
ANA	antinuclear antibodies
ANS	autonomic nervous system
AP	anterior posterior
APTT	activated partial thromboplastin time
AR	aortic regurgitation
ARDS	acute or adult respiratory distress syndrome
AROM	artificial rupture of membranes
AS	aortic stenosis
ASCVD	arteriosclerotic cardiovascular disease
ASHD	arteriosclerotic heart disease
ASO	antistreptolysin O
AST	aspartate aminotransferase (formerly SGOT)
ASVD	arteriosclerotic vascular disease
ATN	acute tubular necrosis
AU	both ears
AV	arteriovenous
BBOW	bulging bag of water
BCP	birth control pills
b.i.d.	twice a day
Bili tot	direct bilirubin, total and direct
BiPAP	bilevel positive airway pressure
BKA	below-knee amputation
BOOP	*Bronchiolitis obliterans* organizing pneumonia
BPG	bypass graft
BSO	bilateral salpingo-oophorectomy
BTL	bilateral tubal ligation
BUN	blood urea nitrogen
BUS	Bartholin's, urethra, and Skene's glands
C	Celsius
C1-C7	cervical vertebrae
C1	first cervical vertebra
C2	second cervical vertebra
C3	third cervical vertebra
C4	fourth cervical vertebra
C5	fifth cervical vertebra
C6	sixth cervical vertebra
C7	seventh cervical vertebra
ca	cancer
Ca	calcium
CABG	coronary artery bypass graft
CAD	coronary artery disease
CAPD	continuous ambulatory peritoneal dialysis
CBC	complete blood count
Cc; cc	cubic centimeter
CCU	coronary care unit
CD	cesarean delivery
C. difficile	*Clostridium difficile*
CEA	carcinoembryonic antigen
CHD	congenital heart disease
CHF	congestive heart failure
Chol tot	total serum cholesterol
CI	chloride
CK	creatine kinase
cm	centimeter
CMP	cardiomyopathy
CMT	chiropractic manipulative treatment
CMV	cytomegalovirus
CNS	central nervous system
CO	cardiac output
CO2; CO_2	carbon dioxide
COPD	chronic obstructive pulmonary disease
COX2	cyclooxygenase-2 inhibitors
CPAP	continuous positive airway pressure
CPB	cardiopulmonary bypass

CPK	creatine phosphokinase	FEV1	forced expiratory volume in one second
CPR	cardiopulmonary resuscitation		
Creat	creatinine	FEV1:FVC	forced expiratory volume in one second to forced vital capacity ratio
CRNA	certified registered nurse anesthetist		
CSF	cerebrospinal fluid	FHR	fetal heart rate
CT	computerized tomography; CAT scan	FHT	fetal heart tones
CTS	carpal tunnel syndrome	FI	forced inspiration
CVA	stroke/cardiovascular accident	FIGO	International Federated Gynecological Oncology (staging classification for grading cancer of female genitalia)
CVD	cerebrovascular disease		
CVP	central venous pressure		
CW	clockwise	FM	fetal movements
CX	circumflex artery	FRC	functional residual capacity
Cx	cervix	FSH	follicle stimulating hormone
D&C	dilatation and curettage (also D and C)	FVC	forced vital capacity
D&E	dilatation and evacuation	g	gram (also gm)
D1	diagonal branch of the LAD artery	g/dl	gram/deciliter
D2	diagonal branch of the LAD artery	GERD	gastroesophageal reflux
D5	dextrose 5% water	GGT	gamma glutamyl transferase
D and C	dilatation and curettage (also D&C)	GI	gastrointestinal
DAT	direct antiglobulin test	Glu	glucose
DC	doctor of chiropractic	gm	gram
dl; dL	deciliter	GU	genitourinary
DLCO	diffuse capacity of lungs for carbon monoxide	GYN	gynecology
		h	hour
DM	diabetes mellitus	H/C	head circumference
DO	doctor of osteopathy	H&H	hemoglobin and hematocrit (also stated HH)
DOLV	double outlet left ventricle		
DORV	double outlet right ventricle	H_2	histamine-2
DTPA	diethylene-triamine penta-acetic acid	H and P	history and physical
DUB	dysfunctional uterine bleeding	HB3Ag	lipoprotein
DVT	deep vein thrombosis	HCG	human chorionic gonadotropin
ECA	external carotid artery	HCT; Hct	hematocrit
ECC	endocervical curettage; extracorporeal circulation (or circuit)	HDL	high-density lipoprotein
		HEENT	head, ears, eyes, nose, throat
ECG	electrocardiogram (also EKG)	HIDA	hydroxy iminodiacetic acid (imaging test)
ECHO	echocardiogram (also ECHO-C)	HGB; Hgb	hemoglobin
ECHO-C	echocardiogram (also ECHO)	HH	hematocrit and hemoglobin (also stated H&H)
ECOG	Eastern Cooperative Oncology Group		
ED	emergency department	HHN	hand-held nebulizer
EDC	estimated date of confinement; estimated date of conception	HIV	human immunodeficiency virus
		HR	heart rate
EEG	electroencephalogram	Hs	at bedtime
EF	ejection fraction; the percent of left ventricular volume ejected in a cardiac contraction	HTN	hypertension
		I&D	incision and drainage
		I&O	intake and output
EIA	enzyme immunoassay	IABP	intra-aortic balloon pump
EKG	electrocardiogram (also ECG)	IBC	iron-binding capacity
EMB	endometrial biopsy	ICA	internal carotid artery
ENA	extractable nuclear antigen	ICN	intensive care; neonatal
ENT	ear, nose, throat	ICU	intensive care unit
EOM, EOMs	extraocular movement(s)	ICS	intercostal space
EOMI	extraocular movement intact	IgM	immunoglobulin M
EP	ectopic pregnancy	IM	intramuscular
ESRD	end-stage renal disease	INR	International Normalized Ratio
ESRF	end-stage renal failure	INT	osteal ramus intermedius
FEF	forced expiratory flow	IPAP	inspiratory positive airway pressure

IUGR	intrauterine growth retardation	MMPI	Minnesota Multiphasic Personality Inventory
IUP	intrauterine pregnancy	MMRV	measles, mumps, rubella, varicella
IV	intravenous	MR	mitral regurgitation
IVC	inferior vena cava	MRI	magnetic resonance imaging
IVCD	interventricular conduction defect	ms	millisecond
IVP	intravenous pyelogram	MS	mitral stenosis
JP	jugular process, jugular pulse	MUGA	multiple gated acquisition test; a radionuclide test of myocardial performance
JVD	jugular vein distention		
K	potassium		
kg	kilogram	MV	mitral valve
KUB	kidney, ureter, bladder	MVR	mitral valve repair
L1-L5	lumbar vertebrae	MVV	maximum voluntary ventilation
L1	first lumbar vertebra	N	negative
L2	second lumbar vertebra	Na	sodium
L3	third lumbar vertebra	NC	no charge
L4	fourth lumbar vertebra	neb	nebula, a spray
L5	fifth lumbar vertebra	NG	nasogastric; nitroglycerin
LA	left atrium	NICU	neonatal intensive care unit
LAD	left anterior descending coronary artery	n.p.o.	nothing by mouth (also NPO)
LBBB	left bundle branch block	NPO	nothing by mouth (also n.p.o.)
LDH	lactate dehydrogenase	NSAID	nonsteroidal anti-inflammatory drug
LDL	low-density lipoprotein	NSVD	normal spontaneous vaginal delivery
LFT	liver function test	O_2	oxygen
LIMA	left internal mammary artery	OA	osteoarthritis
LLL	left lower lobe	OB	obstetrics
lm	lumen	OBT	occult blood test
LM	left main coronary artery	o.d.	right eye
LMCA	left main coronary artery	OM1 OM2	obtuse marginal
LMP	last menstrual period	OMT	osteopathic manipulative treatment
LP	lumbar puncture	OP	outpatient
LT C/S	low transverse C-section	OPC	outpatient clinic
LV	left ventricle	OPD	outpatient department; obstructive pulmonary disease
LVEF	left ventricle ejection fraction		
LVH	left ventricular hypertrophy	OPS	outpatient surgery
M1 tibial	tibial insert	OPV	oral poliovirus vaccine
MAA	melanoma associated antigen	OR	operating room
MAC	maximum allowable concentrate; monitored anesthesia care	os	mouth
		OTC	over-the-counter
MAP	mean aortic pressure, mean arterial pressure	OU	each eye; both eyes
		OURQ	outer upper right quadrant
MB	methylene blue, mesio-buccal; cardiac muscle	OV	office visit
		PA	pulmonary artery
mc	millicurie	PAC	premature atrial contraction
mcg	microgram	PAD	peripheral arterial disease
MCHC	mean corpuscular hemoglobin	PAR	postanesthesia recovery
MCV	mean corpuscular volume	para	to bring forth
MDI	metered dose inhaler	PAWP	pulmonary artery wedge pressure
mEq	milliequivalent	PCA	patient-controlled analgesia
mg	milligram	PCL	posterior cruciate ligament
mg/dl	milligram/deciliter	PCO	polycystic ovaries
MI	myocardial infarction; mitral insufficiency	PCO_2	partial pressure of carbon dioxide
		PCWP	pulmonary capillary wedge pressure
mL; ml	milliliter	PD	peritoneal dialysis
mm	millimeter	PDA	posterior descending artery, part of the RCA
mm/hr	millimeter/hour		
mmHg	millimeters of mercury		

PE	pressure equalization	RBC	red blood cell
PEA	pulseless electrical activity	RCA	right coronary artery
PEAP	positive end-airway pressure	RDS	respiratory distress syndrome
PEEP	positive end expiratory pressure	RDW	red cell distribution width
PERRLA	pupils equal, round, reactive to light and accommodation	RF	rheumatoid factor
		Rh	rhesus factor
PFT	pulmonary function test	Rh(D)	rhesus factor blood typing
pH; ph	potential of hydrogen	RIMA	right internal mammary artery
PID	pelvic inflammatory disease	RLQ	right lower quadrant
PIH	pregnancy induced hypertension	RPR	rapid reagin plasma
PMI	point of maximal impulse	RV	respiratory volume; right ventricle
PND	paroxysmal nocturnal dyspnea	RV:TLC	respiratory volume to total lung capacity ratio
PNS	peripheral nervous system		
p.o.	by mouth	RVH	right ventricular hypertrophy
POC	products of conception	RX	medication
PR	pulse rate	s	*sans* (without), *sigma* (sign, mark), *semis* (half)
p.r.n.	pro re nata, as needed (also prn)		
prn	pro re nata, as needed (also p.r.n.)	S1	first heart sound
PROM	premature rupture of membrane	S1 S2	sequential 1 and 2 heart sounds
Prot tot	total protein	S2	second heart sound
PSA	prostate-specific antigen	S3	third heart sound
PSVT	paroxysmal supraventricular tachycardia	S4	fourth heart sound
		Sa	saphenous
PT	prothrombin time	SAB	spontaneous abortion
PTCA	percutaneous transluminal coronary angioplasty	SBE	subacute bacterial endocarditis
		SBP	systolic blood pressure
PTH	parathyroid hormone; plasma thromboplastin antecedent; post-transfusional hepatitis	SGOT	serum glutamic oxaloacetic transaminase (AST)
		SGPT	serum glutamic pyruvic transaminase (ALT)
PTL	preterm labor		
PTT	partial thromboplastin time	SIADH	syndrome of inappropriate antidiuretic hormone
PV	pulmonary valve		
PVC	premature ventricular contraction	SIMV	synchronized intermittent mandatory ventilation
PVD	peripheral vascular disease		
q	every	SPECT	single photon emission computed tomography
q.2wk.	every 2 weeks		
q.3h.	every 3 hours	SROM	spontaneous rupture of membrane
q.4h.	every 4 hours	S tach	sinus tachycardia (also ST)
q.4wk.	every 4 weeks	ST	sinus tachycardia (also S tach)
q.a.m.	every morning	SVC	superior vena cava
q.d.	every day	SVD	spontaneous vaginal delivery
q.d.s.	four times a day	SVG	saphenous vein graft
q.h.	every hour	SV tach	supraventricular tachycardia (also SVT)
q.h.s.	each bedtime	SVT	supraventricular tachycardia (also SV tach)
q.i.d.	four times a day		
q.m.	every morning	T&A	tonsillectomy and adenoidectomy
q.o.d.	every other day	T1-T12	thoracic vertebrae
q.os.	as needed	T1	first thoracic vertebra
q.p.m.	every afternoon or every evening	T2	second thoracic vertebra
q.q.h.	every fourth hour	T3	third thoracic vertebra
q.s.	quantity sufficient	T4	fourth thoracic vertebra; tumor 4
qq.	each, every	T5	fifth thoracic vertebra
qq.h.	every hour	T6	sixth thoracic vertebra
QRS	Q-wave R-wave S-wave	T7	seventh thoracic vertebra
RA	right atrium; rheumatoid arthritis	T8	eighth thoracic vertebra
RBBB	right bundle branch block	T9	ninth thoracic vertebra

T10	tenth thoracic vertebra		TSH	thyroid stimulating hormone
T11	eleventh thoracic vertebra		TV	tricuspid valve
T12	twelfth thoracic vertebra		dl/dL	deciliter
T_4	symbol for thyroxine		UA	urine analysis
TA	therapeutic abortion		UC	uterine contraction
TAH	total abdominal hysterectomy		UPPP	uvulo-palato-pharyngoplasty
Tc-99M	technetium-99m		URI	upper respiratory infection
TCD	transcranial Doppler		UV	ultraviolet
TEE	transesophageal echocardiography		VAD	ventricular assist device
TENS	transcutaneous electrical nerve stimulator		VB	vaginal bleeding
			VBAC	vaginal birth after C-section
TH	tumor 4		VBR	ventricular branch
TIA	transient ischemic attack		VF	ventricular fibrillation (also V fib)
t.i.d.	three times a day		V fib	ventricular fibrillation (also VF)
TLC	total lung capacity		V/Q scan	ventilation/perfusion scan
TLV	total lung volume		VSD	ventricular septal defect
TMJ	temporomandibular joint		VT	ventricular tachycardia (also V tach)
TPN	total parenteral nutrition		V tach	ventricular tachycardia (also VT)
TR	tricuspid regurgitation		WBC	white blood count
Trig	triglycerides		WPW	Wolff-Parkinson-White
TS	tricuspid stenosis		ZE	Zollinger-Ellison

Answers to Every Other Case

Chapter 1

Evaluation and Management Services

Case 1-1
1-1A Initial Hospital Care
Professional Services: 99221 (Evaluation and Management, Hospital)

ICD-10-CM DX: E10.10 (Diabetes, type 1, with, ketoacidosis), **J45.909** (Asthma, asthmatic)

1-1B Discharge Summary
Professional Services: 99238 (Evaluation and Management, Hospital, Discharge)

ICD-10-CM DX: E10.10 (Diabetes, type 1, with, ketoacidosis), **E86.0** (Dehydration), **J45.909** (Asthma)

Case 1-3
1-3A Initial Hospital Service
Professional Services: 99221 (Evaluation and Management, Hospital)

ICD-10-CM DX: R10.31 (Pain[s], abdominal, lower, right quadrant), **E10.9** (Diabetes, type 1), **J01.90** (Sinusitis, acute), **J45.909** (Asthma)

1-3B Consultation
Professional Services: 99253 (Evaluation and Management, Consultation)

ICD-10-CM DX: E10.9 (Diabetes, type 1), **R10.31** (Pain[s], abdominal, lower, right quadrant)

1-3C Radiology Report
Professional Services: 76705-26 (Ultrasound, abdomen)

ICD-10-CM DX: R10.31 (Pain[s], abdominal, lower, right quadrant)

1-3D Radiology Report
Professional Services: 71046-26 (X-Ray, Chest)

ICD-10-CM DX: R05.9 (Cough), **R50.9** (Fever)

Case 1-5
1-5A Initial Hospital Care
Professional Services: 99223 (Evaluation and Management, Hospital), **99418** (Prolonged Services) or **99291** (Critical Care Services), **99292 × 3** (Critical Care Services)

ICD-10-CM DX: R00.1 (Bradycardia), **T46.0X5A** (Table of Drugs and Chemicals, Digoxin, External Cause [T-code], Adverse Effect), **T46.5X5A** (Table of Drugs and Chemicals, Antihypertensive drug NEC, Adverse Effect), **D64.9** (Anemia), **I48.91** (Fibrillation, atrial or auricular [established])

1-5B Progress Report
Professional Services: 99233 (Evaluation and Management, Hospital)

ICD-10-CM DX: R00.1 (Bradycardia), **T46.0X5A** (Table of Drugs and Chemicals, Digoxin, External Cause [T-code], Adverse Effect), **T46.5X5A** (Table of Drugs and Chemicals, Antihypertensive drug NEC, Adverse Effect), **D64.9** (Anemia), **I48.91** (Fibrillation, atrial or auricular)

Case 1-7
1-7A Progress Report
Professional Services: 99232 (Evaluation and Management, Hospital)

ICD-10-CM DX: N17.9 (Failure, failed, renal, acute), **N18.9** (Failure, failed, renal, chronic), **D63.1** (Anemia, in, chronic kidney disease), **I48.91** (Fibrillation, atrial or auricular [established])

Case 1-9
1-9A Discharge Summary
Professional Services: 99238 (Evaluation and Management, Hospital, Discharge)

ICD-10-CM DX: K26.7 (Ulcer, duodenum/duodenal, chronic)

Case 1-11
1-11A Consultation
Professional Services: 99245 (Evaluation and Management, Consultation)

ICD-10-CM DX: K27.7 (Ulcer, peptic, chronic), **F17.210** (Dependence, drug, nicotine, cigarettes)

Case 1-13
1-13A Critical Care
Professional Services: 99291 (Evaluation and Management, Critical Care), **99292** (Evaluation and Management, Critical Care)

ICD-10-CM DX: T51.0X1A (Table of Drugs and Chemicals, Alcohol, beverage, Poisoning, Accidental [Unintentional]), **R06.82** (Tachypnea), **F10.229** (Alcohol, intoxication [acute], with dependence, **I10** (Hypertension), **Z99.11** (Dependence, on, ventilator)

Case 1-15
1-15A Critical Care
Professional Services: 99291 (Evaluation and Management, Critical Care), **99292** (Evaluation and Management, Critical Care)

ICD-10-CM DX: I42.6 (Cardiomyopathy, alcoholic), **F10.188** (Abuse, alcohol, other specified disorder), **I50.9** (Failure/failed, heart, congestive), **I27.20** (Hypertension, pulmonary [artery] NEC), **N18.9** (Insufficiency, renal, chronic)

Case 1-17
1-17A Critical Care Admission
Professional Services: 99291 (Evaluation and Management, Critical Care), **99292 × 2** (Evaluation and Management, Critical Care)

ICD-10-CM DX: I95.9 (Hypotension), **J96.90** (Failure/failed, respiration/respiratory), **I50.9** (Failure/failed, heart, congestive), **N17.9** (Failure/failed, renal, acute)

Case 1-19
1-19A Office Visit
Professional Services: 99203 (Evaluation and Management, Office and Other Outpatient)

ICD-10-CM DX: J06.9 (Infection/infected/infective, respiratory, [acute] upper NOS), **R59.0** (Lymphadenopathy, localized)

1-19B Office Visit
Professional Services: 99213 (Evaluation and Management, Office and Other Outpatient)

ICD-10-CM DX: I88.9 (Lymphadenitis)

1-19C Clinic Progress Note
Professional Services: 99213 (Evaluation and Management, Office or Other Outpatient)

ICD-10-CM DX: J06.9 (Infection/infected/infective, respiratory, upper NOS), **J02.9** (Pharyngitis)

Case 1-21
1-21A Newborn Care
Professional Services: 1/1: 99460, 1/2: 99461, 1/3: 99461-25, 1/4: 99461 (Evaluation and Management, Newborn Care), **1/3: 54150** (Circumcision, Surgical Excision, Neonate), **1/5: 99238** (Evaluation and Management, Hospital, Discharge)

ICD-10-CM DX: Z38.01 (Newborn, born in hospital, by cesarean)

Case 1-23
1-23A Office Visit
Professional Services: 99395 (Evaluation and Management, Preventive Services)

ICD-10-CM DX: Z00.00 (Examination, medical, [adult]), **E03.9** (Hypothyroidism), **E66.3** (Overweight)

1-23B Office Visit
Professional Services: 99395 (Evaluation and Management, Preventive Services)

ICD-10-CM DX: Z00.00 (Examination, medical, [adult]), **E03.9** (Hypothyroidism), **E66.3** (Overweight)

1-23C Office Visit
Professional Services: 99395 (Evaluation and Management, Preventive Services)

ICD-10-CM DX: Z02.0 (Examination, medical [adult], admission to, school), **E03.9** (Hypothyroidism)

Case 1-25
1-25A Office Visit
Professional Services: 99392 (Evaluation and Management, Preventive Services)

ICD-10-CM DX: Z00.129 (Examination, child care [over 28 days old])

Chapter 2

Medicine

Case 2-1
2-1A Chart Note
Professional Services:

Substance: 90658 (Vaccines, Influenza, for Intramuscular Use)

Administration: G0008 (Vaccination, administration influenza virus)

ICD-10-CM DX: Z23 (Vaccination [prophylactic], encounter for)

Case 2-3
2-3A Chart Note
Professional Services:

Substance: 90710 (Vaccines/Measles/Mumps/Rubella/and Varicella)

Administration: 90471 (Administration, Immunization, One Vaccine/Toxoid)

ICD-10-CM DX: Z23 (Vaccination, [prophylactic], encounter for)

Case 2-5
2-5A Chart Note
Professional Services: 96372 (Injection, Intramuscular), **J0120** (Table of Drugs, Tetracycline)

ICD-10-CM DX: J06.9 (Infection, respiratory [tract], upper [acute])

Case 2-7
2-7A Hemodialysis Progress Report
Professional Services:

90960 (Dialysis, End Stage Renal Disease) (For a full month of service)

ICD-10-CM DX: Z99.2 (Status, renal dialysis [hemodialysis] [peritoneal]), **I12.0** (Hypertension, hypertensive, kidney, with, stage 5 Chronic kidney disease (CKD) or end stage renal disease) (ESRD), **N18.6** (Disease, renal, end-stage [failure], **E11.21** (Diabetes, type 2, with nephropathy), **E83.39** (Hyperphosphatemia), **E83.51** (Hypocalcemia), **E03.9** (Hypothyroidism), **Z90.5** (Absence, kidney [acquired])

Case 2-9
2-9A Duplex Carotid Artery Study
Professional Services: 93880-26 (Vascular Studies, Arterial Studies [Non-Invasive], Extracranial)

ICD-10-CM DX: I47.20 (Tachycardia, ventricular [paroxysmal])

Case 2-11
2-11A Arterial Doppler Test
Professional Services: 93922-26 (Vascular Studies, Arterial Studies [Non-Invasive], Extremities)

ICD-10-CM DX: M79.605 (Pain[s], limb, lower), **E11.9** (Diabetes, type 2)

Case 2-13
2-13A Electrical Cardioversion
Professional Services: 92960 (Cardioversion)

ICD-10-CM DX: I48.92 (Flutter, atrial or auricular)

Case 2-15
2-15A Cognitive Function Assessment
Professional Services: 96116, 96121 × 2 (Neurology, Higher Cerebral Function, Cognitive Function Tests)

ICD-10-CM DX: F03 (Dementia, senile, depressed or paranoid type)

Case 2-17
2-17A Infusion
Professional Services: 96413 (Chemotherapy, Intravenous, Infusion), **J9050** (Table of Drugs, Carmustine)

ICD-10-CM DX: Z51.11 (Encounter, chemotherapy for neoplasm), **C90.00** (Myeloma [multiple])

Case 2-19
2-19A Physical Therapy Evaluation
Professional Services: 97161 (Physical Medicine/Therapy/Occupational Therapy, Evaluation, Physical Therapy)

ICD-10-CM DX: Z51.89 (Aftercare), **M17.10** (Osteoarthritis, knee), **Z47.89** (Aftercare, following surgery, orthopedic NEC)

Case 2-21
2-21A Office Procedure
Professional Services: 11750-TA, 11750-51-T5 (Nails, Excision)

ICD-10-CM DX: L60.0 (Ingrowing, nail [finger] [toe])

2-21B Clinic Progress Note
Professional Services: 99024 (Post-Op Visit)

ICD-10-CM DX: Z48.817 (Aftercare, following surgery, skin and subcutaneous tissue)

Chapter 3

Radiology

Case 3-1
3-1A Radiology Report, Chest
Professional Services: 71045-26 (X-Ray, Chest)

ICM-10-CM DX: Z49.01 (Preparatory care for subsequent treatment NEC, for dialysis)

Case 3-3
3-3A Radiology Report, Abdomen
Professional Services: 74018-76-26 (X-Ray, Abdomen)

ICM-10-CM DX: Z46.82 (Fitting [and adjustment] [of], catheter, non-vascular), **R10.9** (Pain[s], abdominal)

Case 3-5
3-5A Radiology Report, Femur
Professional Services: 73552-26-LT (X-Ray, Femur)

ICD-10-CM DX: M79.652 (Pain[s], limb, lower, thigh)

Case 3-7
3-7A Radiology Report, Shoulder
Professional Services: 73030-26-RT (X-Ray, Shoulder), **73030-76-26-RT** (X-Ray, Shoulder)

ICD-10-CM DX: M19.011 (Osteoarthritis, shoulder)

Case 3-9
3-9A Video Swallow
Professional Services: 74230-26 (Swallowing, Imaging)
ICD-10-CM DX: R13.10 (Dysphagia)

Case 3-11
3-11A CT Scan, Sinuses
Professional Services: 70486-26 (CT Scan, without Contrast, Face), 76377-26 (CT Scan, 3D Rendering)
ICD-10-CM DX: I50.9 (Failure/failed, heart, congestive), R09.02 (Hypoxemia), Z99.11 (Dependence, on, ventilator)

Case 3-13
3-13A CT Scan, Chest
Professional Services: 71250-26 (CT Scan, without Contrast, Thorax)
ICD-10-CM DX: E85.4 and J99 (Amyloidosis, with lung involvement)

Case 3-15
3-15A CT Scan, Chest
Professional Services: 71260-26 (CT Scan, with Contrast, Thorax)
ICD-10-CM DX: J90 (Effusion, pleura/pleurisy/pleuritic/pleuropericardial), Z90.12 (Absence, breast[s] [acquired])

Case 3-17
3-17A CT Scan, Abdomen
Professional Services: 74160-26 (CT Scan, with contrast, abdomen), 76376-26 (CT Scan, 3D Rendering)
ICD-10-CM DX: R93.5 (Abnormal/abnormality/abnormalities, diagnostic imaging, abdomen/abdominal region NEC)

Case 3-19
3-19A CT-Guided Kidney Biopsy
Professional Services: 50200-50 (Biopsy, Kidney), 50200-59-RT (Biopsy, Kidney), 77012-26 (CT Scan, Guidance, Needle Placement), 76380-26 (CT Scan, Follow-Up Study)
ICD-10-CM DX: N18.9 (Insufficiency, kidney, chronic), N04.9 (Syndrome, nephrotic), D64.9 (Anemia)

Case 3-21
3-21A Ultrasound, Right Lower Quadrant
Professional Services: 76705-26 (Ultrasound, Abdomen)
ICD-10-CM DX: R10.31 (Pain[s], abdominal, lower, right quadrant), R50.9 (Fever, [with chills])

Case 3-23
3-23A Ultrasound, Renal
Professional Services: 76770-26 (Ultrasound, Kidney)
ICD-10-CM DX: N04.9 (Syndrome, nephrotic)

Case 3-25
3-25A Ultrasound, Renal
Professional Services: 76775-26 (Ultrasound, Kidney), 51798 (Urodynamic Tests, Bladder Capacity, Ultrasound)
ICD-10-CM DX: N18.9 (Failure/failed, renal, chronic), K81.1 (Cholecystitis, chronic), N28.1 (Cyst, kidney, acquired), R18.8 (Ascites [abdominal])

Case 3-27
3-27A Ultrasound, Retroperitoneal
Professional Services: 76775-26 (Ultrasound, Retroperitoneal)
ICD-10-CM DX: N10 (Pyelonephritis, acute)

Case 3-29
3-29A Radiation Oncology Consultation Note
Professional Services: 99244 (Evaluation and Management, Consultation)
ICD-10-CM DX: C79.2 (Neoplasm, skin, flank, Malignant Secondary), C61 (Neoplasm, prostate [gland], Malignant Primary), Z99.3 (Dependence, on, wheelchair)

3-29B Radiation Oncology Treatment Planning Note
Professional Services: 77263 (Radiation Therapy, Planning)
ICM-10-CM DX: C79.2 (Neoplasm, skin, flank, Malignant Secondary), C61 (Neoplasm, prostrate [gland], Malignant Primary)

3-29C Radiation Oncology Simulation Note
Professional Services: 77290-26 (Radiation Therapy, Field Setup), 77334-26 (Radiation Therapy, Treatment Device)
ICD-10-CM DX: C79.2 (Neoplasm, skin, flank, Malignant Secondary), C61 (Neoplasm, prostate [gland], Malignant Primary)

3-29D Radiation Oncology Progress Note—Week 1, 5 Days
Professional Services: 77427 (Radiation Therapy, Treatment Delivery, Weekly)
ICD-10-CM DX: C79.2 (Neoplasm, skin, flank, Malignant Secondary), C61 (Neoplasm, prostate [gland], Malignant Primary)

3-29E Radiation Oncology Progress Note—Week 2, 5 Days
Professional Services: 77427 (Radiation Therapy, Treatment Delivery, Weekly)
ICD-10-CM DX: C79.2 (Neoplasm, skin, flank, Malignant Secondary), C61 (Neoplasm, prostate [gland], Malignant Primary)

Case 3-31
3-31A Ventilation-Perfusion Lung Scan
Professional Services: 78582-26 (Lung, Nuclear Medicine, Imaging, Ventilation)

ICD-10-CM DX: R07.9 (Pain[s], chest)

Case 3-33
3-33A Gastrojejunostomy Catheter Placement
Professional Services: 49440 (Gastrostomy Tube, Obstructive Material Removal, Placement, Percutaneous), 49446-51 (Gastrostomy Tube, Conversion, to Gastro-jejunostomy Tube)

ICD-10-CM DX: E63.9 (Nutrition deficient or insufficient)

Case 3-35
3-35A Gastrojejunostomy Catheter Placement
Professional Services: 49440 (Gastrostomy Tube, Obstructive Material Removal, Placement, Percutaneous), 49446-51 (Gastrostomy Tube, Conversion, to Gastro-jejunostomy Tube)

ICD-10-CM DX: I63.9 (Stroke), J80 (Syndrome, respiratory, distress, acute, adult), Z99.11 (Dependence, on, ventilator)

Chapter 4

Pathology and Laboratory

Case 4-1
Panels

4-1A Basic Metabolic Panel (Calcium, Total)
82330

80048

Ca tot **calcium, total**

CO_2 **carbon dioxide**

Cl **chloride**

Creat **creatinine**

Glu **glucose**

K **potassium**

Na **sodium**

BUN **blood urea nitrogen**

4-1B Comprehensive Metabolic Panel
80053

Alb **albumin**

Bili tot **bilirubin, total**

Ca tot **calcium total**

CO_2 **carbon dioxide**

Cl **chloride**

Creat **creatinine**

Glu **glucose**

alk phos **alkaline phosphatase**

K **potassium**

Prot tot **protein, total**

Na **sodium**

AST **transferase, aspartate amino**

ALT **transferase, alanine amino**

BUN **blood urea nitrogen**

4-1C Hepatic Function Panel
80076

Prot tot **protein, total**

Alb **albumin**

Bili tot, dir **bilirubin, total and direct** (these are two separate tests)

alk phos **alkaline phosphatase**

AST **transferase, aspartate amino**

ALT **transferase, alanine amino**

4-1D Lipid Panel
80061

Chol tot **cholesterol, serum, total**

HDL **lipoprotein, direct measurement, high-density cholesterol**

Trig **triglycerides**

4-1E General Health Panel
80050

Comp met **comprehensive metabolic panel**

CBC **complete blood count**

TSH **thyroid stimulating hormone**

Case 4-3
4-3A Chemistry Tests
Terms in parentheses are the CPT index location of the code.

1. 82040
2. 84075
3. 84460
4. 82150
5. 82803
6. 84450
7. 82248
8. 82247
9. 84520
10. 82310
11. 82374
12. 82378
13. 82435
14. 82465

15. **82550**
16. **82565**
17. **83001**
18. **82728**
19. **82746**
20. **82977**
21. **82947**
22. **83036**
23. **84703**
24. **84702**
25. **83718**
26. **86334-90**
27. **83540**
28. **83550** NC % saturated requires iron and IBC to be ordered.
29. **83615**
30. **83002**
31. **83735**
32. **84100**
33. **84132**
34. **84146**
35. **84155**
36. **84165-90**
37. **84153**
38. **84295**
39. **84439**
40. **84443**
41. **84478**
42. **84550**
43. **82607**
44. **83525** (Insulin, Blood)
45. **83540** (Iron)
46. **83550**
47. **84590** (Vitamin A)
48. **82607** (Vitamin B$_{12}$)
49. **82570** (Creatinine, other source)
50. **82248** (Bilirubin, Blood)
51. **82247** (Bilirubin, Blood)
52. **84442** (Thyroxine Binding Globulin)
53. **84146** (Prolactin)

Case 4-5
4-5A Coagulation
1. **85730** (Thromboplastin, Partial Time)
2. **85610** (Prothrombin Time)
3. **85002** (Bleeding Time)
4. **85002** (Bleeding Time)
5. **85348** (Coagulation Time)
6. **85378** (Pathology and Laboratory, Fibrin Degradation Products, Para coagulation, D-dimer)
7. **85244** (Clotting Factor, Factor VIII, Related Antigen)
8. **85366** (Fibrin Degradation Products, Para coagulation)
9. **85384** (Fibrinogen, Activity)
10. **85730** (Thromboplastin, Partial Time)
11. **85610** (Prothrombin Time)

Case 4-7
The index locations for the codes in 406 appear in the text before the case.

4-7A Immunology
1. **86038**
2. **86225**
3. **86235 × 2**
4. **86235 × 2**
5. **86063**
6. **86430**
7. **86593**
8. **86157**
9. **87340**
10. **87340-90**
11. **86701-90**
12. **86308**
13. **86762**

Case 4-9
4-9A Office Testing
1. **81002**

Case 4-11
4-11A Evocative/Suppression Testing
1. **80434** (Evocative/Suppression Test)

   ICD-10-CM DX: R03.1 (Low, blood pressure)
2. **80418** (Evocative/Suppression Test)

   ICD-10-CM DX: H54.7 (Impaired/impairment, vision NEC), **R51.9** (Headache)

Case 4-13
4-13A Microbiology
1. **87086** (Culture, Bacteria, Urine)

   ICD-10-CM DX: R30.0 (Dysuria)
2. **87110** (Culture, Chlamydia)

   ICD-10-CM DX: A56.2 (Disease, venereal, chlamydial, genitourinary NOS)

Case 4-15
4-15A Consultations (Clinical Pathology)
1. **80500** (Consultation, Clinical Pathology)

   ICD-10-CM DX: Z51.81 (Encounter [for], therapeutic drug level monitoring)
2. **88321** (Consultation, Surgical Pathology)

   ICD-10-CM DX: C61 (Neoplasm, prostate [gland], Malignant Primary)
3. **88329** (Consultation, Surgical Pathology, Intraoperation)

   ICD-10-CM DX: C50.919 (Neoplasm, breast, female, unspecified site, Malignant Primary)

Case 4-17
4-17A Surgical Pathology Report
1. **88305 × 5** (Pathology, Surgical, Gross and Micro Exam, Level IV)

   ICD-10-CM DX: K63.5 (Polyp/polypus, colon)

Case 4-19
4-19A Pathology and Laboratory Section Review
1. **86677** (Antibody, Helicobacter Pylori)

   ICD-10-CM DX: K21.9 (Reflux, esophagus)
2. **88161** (Tzanck smear), **88312** (Pathology, Surgical, Special Stain)
3. **87252** (Culture, Tissue, Virus)
4. **86694** (Antibody, Herpes Simplex)

   ICD-10-CM DX: A60.09 (Herpes/herpes virus/ herpetic, genital/genitalis, female)
5. **86689** (Western Blot, HIV)
6. **85027** (Blood Cell Count, Hemogram, Automated)
7. **86038** (Antinuclear Antibodies)

   ICD-10-CM DX: Z11.4 (Screening [for], disease or disorder, viral, human immunodeficiency virus [HIV]), **Z72.9** (Problem, lifestyle, specified NEC)
8. **82945** (Glucose, Body Fluid)
9. **82010** (Ketone Body, Acetone)
10. **80051** (Organ or Disease-Oriented Panel, Electrolyte)
11. **82803** (Blood Gases, CO_2)

    ICD-10-CM DX: E11.9 (Diabetes/diabetic, type 2)
12. **82465** (Cholesterol, Serum)
13. **83718** (Cholesterol, Measurement, HDL)

    ICD-10-CM DX: E78.5 (Hyperlipemia/ hyperlipidemia)
14. **85027** (Complete Blood Count)
15. **84443** (Thyroid Stimulating Hormone)
16. **84146** (Prolactin)
17. **84402** (Testosterone)

    ICD-10-CM DX: N52.9 (Impotence, organic origin)
18. **85027** (Complete Blood Count)
19. **85049** (Platelet, Count), **80051** (Blood Tests, Panels, Electrolyte)
20. **82310** (Calcium, Total)
21. **83735** (Magnesium)
22. **84550** (Uric Acid, Blood)
23. **85610** (Prothrombin Time)
24. **85730** (Thromboplastin, Partial Time)

    ICD-10-CM DX: C92.10 (Leukemia/leukemic, chronic myeloid, BCR/ABL-positive)
25. **84520** (Blood Urea Nitrogen)
26. **82565** (Creatinine, Blood)
27. **85027** (Complete Blood Count)
28. **85060** (Blood Smear, Peripheral)

    ICD-10-CM DX: D75.0 (Polycythemia, benign [familial])
29. **82947** (Glucose, Blood Test)

    ICD-10-CM DX: R63.4 (Loss, weight), **R63.1** (Polydipsia), **Z83.3** (History, family [of], diabetes mellitus)
30. **82947** (Glucose, Blood Test)

    ICD-10-CM DX: R63.1 (Polydipsia), **E66.01** (Obesity, morbid)
31. **80061** (Organ or Disease-Oriented Panel, Lipid Panel)

    ICD-10-CM DX: E66.01 (Obesity, morbid)
32. **85652** (Sedimentation Rate, Blood Cell, Automated)
33. **85027** (Complete Blood Count)

    ICD-10-CM DX: I38 (Endocarditis)
34. **84520** (Blood Urea Nitrogen)
35. **81003** (Urinalysis, Automated)

    ICD-10-CM DX: N80.00 (Endometriosis, uterus)
36. **85027** (Complete Blood Count)
37. **85652** (Sedimentation Rate, Blood Cell, Automated)
38. **82947** (Glucose, Blood Test)
39. **84540** (Urea Nitrogen, Urine)
40. **84520** (Blood Urea Nitrogen)
41. **80076** (Organ or Disease-Oriented Panel, Hepatic Function Panel)
42. **82565** (Creatinine, Blood)

    ICD-10-CM DX: G51.0 (Bell's, palsy/paralysis)
43. **88305** (Pathology, Surgical, Gross and Micro Exam, Level IV), **85097** (Bone Marrow, Smear)

    ICD-10-CM DX: E85.9 (Amyloidosis)
44. **80053** (Organ or Disease-Oriented Panel, Metabolic, Comprehensive). The bilirubin total is a component of the panel test (80053) and is not reported separately.

    ICD-10-CM DX: N20.0 (Calculus/calculi/ calculous, kidney [recurrent])
45. **85049** (Platelet, Count), **85610** (Prothrombin Time), **85002** (Bleeding, Time)

    ICD-10-CM DX: D69.6 (Thrombocytopenia/ thrombocytopenic)
46. **85652** (Sedimentation Rate, Blood Cell, Automated), **84439** (Thyroxine, Free), **84443** (Thyroid Stimulating Hormone)

    ICD-10-CM DX: E05.90 (Hyperthyroidism)

47.   **84075** (Alkaline Phosphatase), **84100** (Phosphorus), **84443** (Thyroid Stimulating Hormone), **85009** (Blood Cell Count, Differential WBC Count), **85652** (Sedimentation Rate Blood cell, Automated), **81003** (Urinalysis, Automated)

   ICD-10-CM DX: M81.0 (Osteoporosis)

48.   **86593** (Syphilis Test), **80061** (Organ or Disease-Oriented Panel, Lipid Panel)

   ICD-10-CM DX: H81.09 (Ménière's disease, syndrome or vertigo)

49.   **84153** (Prostate Specific Antigen), **85008** (Blood Cell Count, Blood Smear)

   ICD-10-CM DX: N41.0 (Prostatitis, acute)

50.   **83001** (Follicle Stimulating Hormone), **83002** (Luteinizing Hormone, Gonadotropin), **84439** (Thyroxine, Free), **84443** (Thyroid Stimulating Hormone)

   ICD-10-CM DX: E22.1 (Hyperprolactinemia)

51.   **84520** (Blood Urea Nitrogen), **82565** (Creatinine, Blood)

   ICD-10-CM DX: N18.9 (Failure/failed, renal, chronic)

Chapter 5

Integumentary System

Case 5-1
5-1A Operative Report, Excision Fat Necrosis
Professional Services: 11042-78, 11045-78 × 2 (Debridement, Subcutaneous Tissue)

ICD-10-CM DX: L76.82 (Complication[s], postprocedural, specified NEC, skin and subcutaneous tissue), **L98.8** (Degeneration/degenerative, skin)

Case 5-3
5-3A Operative Report, Skin Biopsy
Professional Services: 11104 (Skin Lesion, Punch)
ICD-10-CM DX: D22.5 (Nevus, skin, chest wall)

5-3B Operative Report, Skin Tags
Professional Services: 11200 (Skin, Tags, Removal)
ICD-10-CM DX: L91.8 (Tag, skin)

Case 5-5
5-5A Operative Report, Lesions
Professional Services: 12032 (Closure), **11402-51, 11402-59** (Excision, Lesion, Skin, Benign)

ICD-10-CM DX: D23.5 (Neoplasm, skin, chest, Benign), **Z85.3** (History, personal [of], malignant neoplasm [of], breast)

Case 5-7
5-7A Operative Report, Nevus
Professional Services: 11426 (Excision, Skin, Lesion, Benign)
ICD-10-CM DX: D23.4 (Neoplasm, skin, neck, Benign)

Case 5-9
5-9A Operative Report, Keratosis Excision
Professional Services: 11443 (Excision, Skin, Lesion, Benign)
ICD-10-CM DX: L57.0 (Keratosis, actinic)

Case 5-11
5-11A Operative Report, Squamous Cell Carcinoma
Professional Services: 11644 (Excision, Skin, Lesion, Malignant)

ICD-10-CM DX: C44.329 (Neoplasm, skin, face, Squamous cell carcinoma)

Case 5-13
5-13A Clinic Progress Note
Professional Services: 11750-T5 (Excision, Nails)
ICD-10-CM DX: L60.0 (Onychocryptosis)

Case 5-15
5-15A Operative Report, Laceration
Professional Services: 13152 (Repair, Wound, Complex)

ICD-10-CM DX: S01.521A (Laceration, lip, with foreign body), **V47.6XXA** (External Cause Index, Accident, transport, car occupant, passenger, collision, [with] stationary object, [traffic])

Case 5-17
5-17A Operative Report, Umbilicoplasty
Professional Services: 13101 (Wound, Repair, Trunk, Complex), **11403-51** (Excision, Skin, Lesion, Benign), **12032-59** (Repair, Skin, Wound, Intermediate)

ICD-10-CM DX: L76.82 (Complication, postprocedural, specified NEC, skin and subcutaneous tissue), **L92.9** (Granulation Tissue [abnormal]), **M70.80** (Disorder, soft tissue, specified NEC)

Case 5-19
5-19A Operative Report, Dermabrasion
Professional Services: 13132 (Repair, Wound, Complex), **13133 × 2** (Repair, Wound, Complex)
ICD-10-CM DX: L90.5 (Scar/scarring)

Case 5-21
5-21A Operative Report, Wide Excision, Basal Cell Carcinoma
Professional Services: 11602 (Excision, Lesion, Skin, Malignant)

ICD-10-CM DX: C44.719 (Neoplasm, skin, limb, lower, basal cell carcinoma, left)

Case 5-23
5-23A Operative Report, Split-Thickness Autograft
Professional Services: 15100 (Skin, Grafts, Free)

ICD-10-CM DX: L76.82 (Complication[s], postprocedural, specified NEC, skin and subcutaneous tissue)

Case 5-25
5-25A Operative Report, Full-Thickness Skin Graft
Professional Services: 15240 (Skin, Grafts, Free)

ICD-10-CM DX: S61.002A (Wound, open, thumb, left)

Case 5-27
5-27A Operative Report, Composite Graft
Professional Services: 11643 (Excision, Lesion, Skin, Malignant), **15760-51** (Skin Graft and Flap, Composite Graft)

ICD-10-CM DX: D04.39 (Neoplasm, skin, nose [external], Ca in situ)

Case 5-29
5-29A Operative Report, Post Skin Graft
Professional Services: 15852-58 (Dressings, Change, Anesthesia)

ICD-10-CM DX: Z48.01 (Admission [for], change of, surgical dressing), **T23.321D** (Burn, finger, right, third degree)

Case 5-31
5-31A Operative Report, Breast Biopsy
Professional Services: 19101-LT (Biopsy, Breast)

ICD-10-CM DX: N63.32 (Lump, breast, axillary tail, left)

5-31B Pathology Report
Professional Services: 88305 (Pathology, Surgical, Gross and Micro Exam, Level IV), **88331** (Pathology, Surgical, Consultation, Intraoperative)

ICD-10-CM DX: N63.32 (Lump, breast, axillary tail, left)

5-31C Progress Note
Professional Services: 99024 (Post-Op Visit)

ICD-10-CM DX: Z48.02 (Suture, removal), **Z48.817** (Aftercare, following surgery, skin and subcutaneous tissue)

Case 5-33
5-33A Operative Report, Breast Biopsy with Needle Localization
Professional Services: 19125-RT (Lesion, Breast, Excision)

ICD-10-CM DX: N60.31 (Fibrosclerosis, breast)

5-33B Pathology Report
Professional Services: 88305 (Pathology, Surgical, Gross and Micro Exam, Level IV)

ICD-10-CM DX: N60.31 (Fibrosclerosis, breast)

Case 5-35
5-35A Preoperative Consultation
Professional Services: 99243 (Evaluation and Management, Consultation)

ICD-10-CM DX: N63.32 (Lump, breast, axillary tail, left), **Z85.3** (History, malignant neoplasm [of], breast)

5-35B Operative Report, Modified Radical Mastectomy
Professional Services: 19307-58-RT (Mastectomy, Modified Radical); **19101-59-RT** (Biopsy, Breast)

ICD-10-CM DX: C50.211 (Neoplasm, breast, female, upper-inner quadrant, Malignant Primary)

5-35C Pathology Report
Professional Services: 88309 (Pathology, Surgical, Gross and Micro Exam, Level VI), **88331** and **88332** (Pathology, Surgical, Consultation, Intraoperative)

ICD-10-CM DX: C50.211 (Neoplasm, breast, female, upper-inner quadrant, Malignant Primary)

5-35D Discharge Summary
Professional Services: 99238 (Evaluation and Management, Hospital, Discharge)

ICD-10-CM DX: C50.211 (Neoplasm, breast, female, upper-inner quadrant, right side, Malignant Primary)

5-35E Progress Note
Professional Services: 99024 (Post-Op Visit)

ICD-10-CM DX: Z48.3 (Aftercare, following surgery, [for], neoplasm), **C50.211** (Neoplasm, breast, female, upper-inner quadrant, right side, Malignant Primary)

Case 5-37
5-37A Operative Report, Breast Augmentation
Professional Services: 19325-50 (Breast, Augmentation)

ICD-10-CM DX: Z41.1 (Encounter, breast augmentation or reduction)

Chapter 6

Cardiovascular System

Case 6-1
6-1A Cardiothoracic Surgery Consultation
Professional Services: 99252-57 (Consultation, Inpatient)

ICD-10-CM DX: I25.10 (Arteriosclerosis/arteriosclerotic, coronary [artery]), **E11.9** (Diabetes/diabetic, type 2)

Case 6-3
6-3A Cardiology Follow-up Note
Professional Services: 99215 (Evaluation and Management, Office and Other Outpatient)

ICD-10-CM DX: I49.5 (Syndrome, sick, sinus), **I08.0** (Insufficiency, insufficient, aortic [valve], with, mitral [valve], disease), **I42.0** (Cardiomyopathy, congestive) **F03.90** (Dementia)

Case 6-5
6-5A Holter Report
Professional Services: 93224 (Electrocardiography, External Recording 48 Hours Duration)

ICD-10-CM DX: I48.91 (Fibrillation, atrial or auricular), **I42.9** (Cardiomyopathy), **I47.20** (Tachycardia, ventricular)

6-5B Radiology Report, Preimplantation
Professional Services: 71046-26 (X-Ray, Chest)

ICD-10-CM DX: I49.5 (Syndrome, sick, sinus), **I51.7** (Hypertrophy, cardiac)

6-5C Operative Report, Pacemaker Implantation
Professional Services: 33208 (Pacemaker, Heart, Insertion)

ICD-10-CM DX: I49.8 (Bradyarrhythmia, cardiac)

6-5D Radiology Report, Postimplantation
Professional Services: 71045-26 (X-Ray, Chest)

ICD-10-CM DX: Z95.0 (Status [post], pacemaker, cardiac), **R00.1** (Bradycardia)

Case 6-7
6-7A Cardiology Consultation
Professional Services: 99245 (Evaluation and Management, Consultation)

ICD-10-CM DX: R07.89 (Tightness, chest)

6-7B Hospital Service
Professional Services: No E/M code would be assigned (see rationale).

ICD-10-CM DX: I25.9 (Disease/diseased, heart, ischemic), **R01.1** (Murmur [cardiac] [heart]), **I08.0** (Insufficiency/ insufficient, aortic, with mitral [value] disease)

6-7C Radiology Report, Chest
Professional Services: 71046-26 (X-ray, chest)

ICD-10-CM DX: R07.9 (Pain[s], chest), **I25.10** (Disease/ diseased, cardiovascular [atherosclerotic])

6-7D Cardiothoracic Surgical Consultation
Professional Services: 99254 (Evaluation and Management, Consultation)

ICD-10-CM DX: I25.10 (Arteriosclerosis/arteriosclerotic, coronary [artery]), **I34.0** (Insufficiency/insufficient, mitral [valve])

6-7E Radiology Report, Chest
Professional Services: 71046-26 (X-ray, chest)

ICD-10-CM DX: R09.89 (Rales), **R05.9** (Cough)

Case 6-9
6-9A Cardiology Consultation
Professional Services: 99253 (Consultation, Inpatient)

ICD-10-CM DX: I48.91 (Fibrillation, atrial or auricular), **I97.411** (Complication, intraoperative, hemorrhage, during cardiac bypass), **D62** (Anemia, due to, blood loss, acute), **R01.1** (Murmur, [cardiac]), **L03.113** (Cellulitis, upper limb), **Z95.1** (Status, aortocoronary bypass)

Case 6-11
6-11A Hospital Admission
Professional Services: 99221 (Evaluation and Management, Hospital)

ICD-10-CM DX: R00.2 (Palpitations [heart])

6-11B General Chemistry
Professional Services: None

ICD-10-CM DX: R00.2 (Palpitations [heart])

6-11C Hematology
Professional Services: None

ICD-10-CM DX: R00.2 (Palpitations [heart])

6-11D Electrocardiography
Professional Services: 93010 (Electrocardiography, Evaluation)

ICD-10-CM DX: R00.2 (Palpitations [heart])

6-11E Radiology Report, Chest
Professional Services: 71046-26 (X-Ray, chest)

ICD-10-CM DX: R00.2 (Palpitations [heart]), **J44.9** (Disease/diseased, pulmonary, chronic obstructive)

Case 6-13
6-13A Cardioversion
Professional Services: 92960 (Cardioversion)

ICD-10-CM DX: I48.91 (Fibrillation, atrial or auricular), **I48.92** (Flutter, atrial or auricular)

Case 6-15
6-15A Operative Report, Thromboendarterectomy
Professional Services: 35301-RT (Thromboendarterectomy, Vertebral Artery)

ICD-10-CM DX: I65.21 (Occlusion, artery, carotid)

Case 6-17
6-17A Operative Report, Arteriovenous Fistula
Professional Services: **36821-RT** (Anastomosis, Arteriovenous Fistula, Direct)

ICD-10-CM DX: **N18.6** (Disease/diseased, renal, end-stage [failure])

Case 6-19
6-19A Operative Report, Femoral Artery Laceration
Professional Services: **35221-22** (Repair, Blood Vessel, Abdomen), **35221-81** (Repair, Blood Vessel, Abdomen)

ICD-10-CM DX: **I97.51** (Complication[s], puncture or laceration [accidental], circulatory system organ or structure, during circulatory system procedure), **I97.711** (Arrest, cardiac, intraoperative), **I97.418** (Complication(s), intraoperative, hemorrhage, circulatory organ or structure, during other circulatory procedure), **D65** (Coagulopathy, intravascular)

Chapter 7

Digestive System, Hemic/Lymphatic System, and Mediastinum/Diaphragm

Case 7-1
7-1A Inpatient Consultation
Professional Services: **99252** (Evaluation and Management, Consultation)

ICD-10-CM DX: **K56.609** (Obstruction/obstructed/obstructive, intestine)

Case 7-3
7-3A Operative Report, Intersphincteric Abscess
Professional Services: **46045** (Incision and Drainage, Abscess, Anal)

ICD-10-CM DX: **K61.1** (Abscess, perirectal)

Case 7-5
7-5A Operative Report, Hemorrhoidectomy
Professional Services: **46255** (Hemorrhoidectomy, Simple)

ICD-10-CM DX: **K64.1** (Hemorrhoids, 2nd degree)

Case 7-7
7-7A Operative Report, Esophagogastroduodenoscopy
Professional Services: **43239** (Endoscopy, Gastrointestinal, Upper, Biopsy)

ICD-10-CM DX: **K29.71** (Gastritis, with bleeding), **K29.81** (Duodenitis, with bleeding), **K25.4** (Ulcer/ulcerated/ulcerating/ulcerative, stomach, with hemorrhage), **K44.9** (Hernia/hernial, hiatal)

Case 7-9
7-9A Operative Report, Sigmoidoscopy
Professional Services: **45330** (Endoscopy, Colon-Sigmoid, Exploration)

ICD-10-CM DX: **R93.3** (Abnormal/abnormality/abnormalities, diagnostic imaging gastrointestinal tract)

Case 7-11
7-11A Operative Report, Colonoscopy
Professional Services: **45380** (Endoscopy, Colon, Biopsy)

ICD-10-CM DX: **C18.2** (Neoplasm, intestine/intestinal, large, colon, ascending, Malignant Primary)

7-11B Surgical Consultation
Professional Services: **99253-57** (Evaluation and Management, Consultation)

ICD-10-CM DX: **C18.2** (Neoplasm, intestine/intestinal, large, colon, ascending, Malignant Primary)

7-11C Operative Report, Hemicolectomy
Professional Services: **44160** (Colectomy, Partial, with Ileum Resection)

ICD-10-CM DX: **C18.2** (Neoplasm, intestine/intestinal, large, colon, ascending, Malignant Primary), **C78.6** (Neoplasm, mesentery/mesenteric, Malignant Secondary)

7-11D Pathology Report
Professional Services: **88309** (Pathology, Surgical, Gross and Micro Exam, Level VI)

ICD-10-CM DX: **C18.2** (Neoplasm, intestine/intestinal, large, colon, ascending, Malignant Primary), **C78.6** (Neoplasm, mesentery/mesenteric, Malignant Secondary)

Case 7-13
7-13A Operative Report, Appendectomy
Professional Services: **44950** (Appendectomy, Appendix Excision), **44602-51** (Enterorrhaphy), **49320-59** (Laparoscopy, Abdominal)

ICD-10-CM DX: **K35.80** (Appendicitis, acute), **K91.71** (Complication[s], intraoperative, puncture or laceration [accidental] [of], digestive system, during procedure on other organ), **S36.438A** (Injury, intestine, small, laceration, specified, site NEC), **Z53.31** (Laparoscopic surgical procedure converted to open procedure)

Case 7-15
7-15A Outpatient Consultation
Professional Services: **99243** (Evaluation and Management, Consultation)

ICD-10-CM DX: **K25.7** (Ulcer/ulcerated/ulcerating/ulceration/ulcerative, stomach, chronic)

7-15B Emergency and Outpatient Record

Professional Services: 99282 (Evaluation and Management, Emergency Department)

ICD-10-CM DX: R10.9 (Pain[s], abdominal), **K25.7** (Ulcer/ulcerated/ulcerating/ulceration/ulcerative, stomach, chronic)

7-15C Outpatient Consultation

Professional Services: 99245 (Evaluation and Management, Consultation), **99417** (Prolonged Services)

ICD-10-CM DX: K27.7 (Ulcer/ulcerated/ulcerating/ulceration/ulcerative, peptic, chronic)

7-15D Operative Report, Ulcer and Cholecystitis

Professional Services: 43632 (Gastrectomy, Partial, with Gastrojejunostomy), **43635** (Vagotomy, with Partial Distal Gastrectomy), **47605-51** (Cholecystectomy, with Cholangiography)

ICD-10-CM DX: K26.5 (Ulcer/ulcerated/ulcerating/ulceration/ulcerative, duodenum/duodenal, chronic, with, perforation), **K81.1** (Cholecystitis, chronic)

7-15E Intraoperative Cholangiogram

Professional Services: 74300-26 (Cholangiography, Intraoperative)

ICD-10-CM DX: K81.1 (Cholecystitis, chronic)

7-15F Pathology Report

Professional Services: 88305 × 3 (Pathology, Surgical, Gross and Micro Exam, Level IV [lymph node × 1, nerves × 2]), **88307** (Pathology, Surgical, Gross and Micro Exam, Level V [stomach, ulcer]), **88304** (Pathology, Surgical, Gross and Micro Exam, Level III [gallbladder]), **88331** (Pathology, Surgical, Consultation, Intraoperative), **88332 × 3** (Pathology, Surgical, Consultation, Intraoperative, each additional segment)

ICD-10-CM DX: K25.3 (Ulcer/ulcerated/ulcerating/ulceration/ulcerative, stomach, acute), **R59.9** (Hyperplasia/hyperplastic, lymph gland or node), **K81.1** (Cholecystitis, chronic)

7-15G Discharge Summary

Professional Services: 99238 (Evaluation and Management, Hospital, Discharge)

ICD-10-CM DX: K26.7 (Ulcer/ulcerated/ulcerating/ulceration/ulcerative, duodenum/duodenal, chronic), **K81.1** (Cholecystitis, chronic)

Case 7-17

7-17A Operative Report, Hemicolectomy

Professional Services: 44160 (Colectomy, Partial, with Ileum Removal)

ICD-10-CM DX: C18.2 (Neoplasm, intestine/intestinal, large, colon, ascending, Malignant Primary), **C79.2** (Neoplasm, abdomen/abdominal, wall, Malignant Secondary)

Case 7-19

7-19A Operative Report, Gastrojejunostomy/Tracheostomy

Professional Services: 44604 (Suture, Intestines, Large, Wound), **44015** (Catheterization, Intestine), **31600-51** (Tracheostomy, Planned)

ICD-10-CM DX: K91.71 (Complication[s], intraoperative, puncture or laceration, digestive system, during procedure on digestive system), **K50.90** (Enteritis, regional), **Z99.11** (Dependence, on, ventilator)

Case 7-21

7-21A Hospital Inpatient Service

Professional Services: 99221 (Evaluation and Management, Hospital)

ICD-10-CM DX: R19.03 (Mass, abdominal, right lower quadrant), **N39.0** (Infection/infected/infective, urinary), **I10** (Hypertension/hypertensive), **B96.20** (Infection/infected/infective, Escherichia (E.), coli in diseases classified elsewhere)

7-21B Operative Report, Cecectomy

Professional Services: 44160 (Colon, Excision, Partial), **44955** (Appendectomy, Appendix Excision)

ICD-10-CM DX: R19.03 (Mass, abdominal, right lower quadrant), **K35.201** (Appendicitis, acute, with, peritonitis, generalized [with perforation or rupture])

7-21C Discharge Summary

Professional Services: 99238 (Evaluation and Management, Hospital, Discharge)

ICD-10-CM DX: K35.201 (Appendicitis, acute, with, peritonitis, generalized [with perforation or rupture]), **I12.9** (Hypertension, kidney, with, stage I through stage IV chronic kidney disease), **N18.9** (Failure/failed, renal, chronic), **N17.9** (Failure/failed, renal, acute), **J96.90** (Failure/failed, respiration/respiratory), **K91.30** (Complication[s], gastrointestinal, postoperative, obstruction), **K46.0** (Hernia/hernial, abdominal, with, obstruction), **N39.0** (Infection/infected/infective, urinary), **B96.20** (Infection/infected/infective, Escherichia (E. coli)) **D64.9** (Anemia)

Case 7-23

7-23A Hospital Inpatient Service

Professional Services: 99221 (Evaluation and Management, Hospital)

ICD-10-CM DX: K40.90 (Hernia/hernial, inguinal)

7-23B Operative Report, Right Inguinal Hernia Repair

Professional Services: 49505-RT (Hernia Repair, Inguinal, Initial, Child 5 Years or Older)

ICD-10-CM DX: K40.90 (Hernia/hernial, inguinal)

7-23C Pathology Report

Professional Services: 88302 (Pathology, Surgical, Gross and Micro Exam, Level II)

ICD-10-CM DX: K40.90 (Hernia/hernial, inguinal)

Case 7-25

7-25A Operative Report, Axillary Node Dissection

Professional Services: 38525-LT (Lymph Nodes, Excision)

ICD-10-CM DX: C85.84 (Lymphoma, non-Hodgkin, specified, NEC axilla)

7-25B Pathology Report

Professional Services: 88305 (Pathology, Surgical, Gross and Micro Exam, Level IV), **88331** (Pathology, Surgical, Consultation, Intraoperative)

ICD-10-CM DX: C85.84 (Lymphoma, non-Hodgkin, specified, axilla)

Case 7-27

7-27A Bone Marrow Biopsy

Professional Services: 38221 (Biopsy, Bone Marrow), **38220-59-53** (Aspiration, Bone Marrow)

ICD-10-CM DX: D64.9 (Anemia), **N17.9** (Failure/failed, renal, acute), **M89.9** (Disorder, bone)

Chapter 8

Musculoskeletal System

Case 8-1

8-1A Orthopedic Consultation

Professional Services: 99241-25 (Evaluation and Management, Consultation), **20550-RT** (Injection, Tendon Sheath), **J1040** (Methylprednisolone, acetate)

ICD-10-CM DX: M77.11 (Epicondylitis [elbow], lateral)

Case 8-3

8-3A Operative Report, Hardware Removal

Professional Services: 20680 (Removal, Fixation Device)

ICD-10-CM DX: Z47.2 (Encounter, removal, internal fixation device), **S52.501D** (Fracture, radius, lower end, subsequent encounter with routine healing)

Case 8-5

8-5A Operative Report, Carbuncle Removal

Professional Services: 11400 (Excision, Lesion, Skin, Benign), **11400-59** (Excision, Lesion, Skin, Benign)

ICD-10-CM DX: L02.432 (Carbuncle, axilla), **I88.9** (Lymphadenitis)

Case 8-7

8-7A Operative Report, Nevus Removal

Professional Services: 11406 (Excision, Lesion, Skin, Benign)

ICD-10-CM DX: D23.5 (Neoplasm, skin, chest, Benign)

Case 8-9

8-9A Operative Report, Shoulder Mass Excision

Professional Services: 23075-RT (Excision, Tumor, Shoulder), **13101** (Repair, Skin, Wound, Complex), **13102x2** (Repair, Skin, Wound, Complex)

ICD-10-CM DX: D17.39 (Lipoma, subcutaneous, specified site NEC)

8-9B Pathology Report

Professional Services: 88304 (Pathology, Surgical, Gross and Micro Exam, Level III)

ICD-10-CM DX: D17.39 (Lipoma, subcutaneous, specified site NEC)

Case 8-11

8-11A Operative Report, Ganglion Cyst

Professional Services: 26160-F1 (Excision, Cyst, Finger)

ICD-10-CM DX: M67.442 (Ganglion, hand)

Case 8-13

8-13A Consultation, Tendon Rupture

Professional Services: 99221-57 (Evaluation and Management, Hospital)

ICD-10-CM DX: S46.911A (Injury, muscle, shoulder, strain), **X50.0XXA** (Overexertion), **Y93.B3** (External Cause Index, Activity [involving] [of victim at time of event], barbells), **Y99.8** (External Cause Index, Status of external cause, recreational or sport not for income or while a student)

8-13B Radiology Report, Shoulder

Professional Services: 73020-26-RT (X-Ray, Shoulder)

ICD-10-CM DX: S46.911A (Injury, muscle, shoulder, strain), **X50.0XXA** (Overexertion), **Y93.B3** (External Cause Index, Activity [involving] [of victim at time of event], barbells), **Y99.8** (External Cause Index, Status of external cause, recreational or sport not for income or while a student)

8-13C Operative Report, Open Tendon Repair

Professional Services: 24341-RT (Repair, Arm, Tendon)

ICD-10-CM DX: S46.911A (Injury, muscle, shoulder, strain), **X50.0XXA** (Overexertion), **Y93.B3** (External Cause Index, Activity [involving] [of victim at time of event], barbells), **Y99.8** (External Cause Index, Status of external cause, recreational or sport not for income or while a student)

8-13D Discharge Summary

Professional Services: 99238 (Evaluation and Management, Hospital, Discharge)

ICD-10-CM DX: S46.911A (Injury, muscle, shoulder, strain), **X50.9XXA** (Overexertion), **Y93.B3** (External Cause Index, Activity [involving] [of victim at time of event], barbells), **Y99.8** (External Cause Index, Status of external cause, recreational or sport not for income or while a student)

Case 8-15
8-15A Operative Report, Arthroplasty
Professional Services: 27447-RT (Arthroplasty, Knee)

ICD-10-CM DX: M17.11 (Osteoarthritis, Primary, Knee)

Case 8-17
8-17A Operative Report, Open Reduction
Professional Services: 25628-RT (Fracture, Scaphoid, Open Treatment), **20900-51** (Bone Graft, Harvesting)

ICD-10-CM DX: S62.001A (Fracture, traumatic, carpal bone[s], navicular), **W22.8XXA** (External Cause Index, Struck by, object)

8-17B Radiology Report, Wrist
Professional Services: 73100-26-RT (X-Ray, Wrist)

ICD-10-CM DX: S62.001A (Fracture, traumatic, carpal bone[s], navicular), **W22.8XXA** (Struck by, object)

Case 8-19
8-19A Radiology Report, Right Femur
Professional Services: 73552-26-RT (X-Ray, Femur)

ICD-10-CM DX: S72.301A (Fracture, traumatic, femur/femoral, shaft), **W18.30XA** (External Cause Index, Fall/falling [accidental], same level)

8-19B Orthopedic Consultation, Thigh Pain
Professional Services: 99253-57 (Evaluation and Management, Consultation)

ICD-10-CM DX: S72.301A (Fracture, traumatic, femur/femoral, shaft), **M81.8** (Osteoporosis, specified type NEC), **W18.30XA** (External Cause Index, Fall/falling, [accidental], same level)

8-19C Operative Report, Femur Repair, Intramedullary Nailing
Professional Services: 27506-RT (Fracture, Femur, Open Treatment [Shaft])

ICD-10-CM DX: S72.301A (Fracture, traumatic, femur/femoral, shaft), **W18.30XA** (External Cause Index, Fall/falling [accidental], same level)

8-19D Discharge Summary
Professional Services: 99238 (Evaluation and Management, Hospital, Discharge)

ICD-10-CM DX: S72.301A (Fracture, traumatic femur/femoral, shaft), **M81.8** (Osteoporosis, specified type NEC), **M83.9** (Osteomalacia), **W18.30XA** (External Cause Index, Fall/falling [accidental], same level)

Case 8-21
8-21A Operative Report, Amputation
Professional Services: 27880-LT (Amputation, Leg, Lower)

ICD-10-CM DX: E11.52 (Diabetes/diabetic, type 2, with, peripheral angiopathy, with gangrene)

Case 8-23
8-23A Operative Report, Debridement
Professional Services: 29825-LT (Arthroscopy, Surgical, Shoulder)

ICD-10-CM DX: M75.02 (Capsulitis [joint], adhesive [shoulder])

Case 8-25
8-25A Operative Report, Acromioplasty
Professional Service: 23412-RT (Repair, Shoulder, Cuff), **29826-59-RT** (Arthroscopy, Surgical, Shoulder), **29819-59-RT** (Arthroscopy, Surgical, Shoulder)

ICD-10-CM DX: M75.11 (Tear, rotator cuff, shoulder), **M19.011** (Osteoarthritis, shoulder), **M24.011** (Loose, body, joint, shoulder [region]), **Z53.33** (Conversion, closed surgical procedure to open procedure, arthroscopic)

8-25B Operative Report, Debridement and Irrigation
Professional Services: 11000-78-RT (Debridement, Skin, Infected)

ICD-10-CM DX: T81.43XA (Complication(s), surgical procedure, wound infection), **A49.01** (Infection/infected/infective, staphylococcal NEC), **T81.83XS** (Fistula, postoperative, persistent)

Case 8-27
8-27A Operative Report, Knee
Professional Services: 27331-RT (Arthrotomy, Knee), **29881-59-RT** (Arthroscopy, Surgical, Knee)

ICD-10-CM DX: S82.011A (Fracture, traumatic, patella, osteochondral [displaced]), **M23.221** (Derangement, knee, meniscus, due to old tear or injury, medial, posterior horn), **Z53.33** (Conversion, arthroscopic surgery converted to open), **X58.XXXA** (External Cause Index, Injury, injured, specified cause), **Y93.B3** (External Cause Index, Activity [involving], barbells)

Chapter 9

Respiratory System

Case 9-1
9-1A Evening Clinic, Sore Throat
Professional Services: 99213 (Evaluation and Management, Office and Other Outpatient)

ICD-10-CM DX: J00 (Nasopharyngitis [acute])

9-1B Laboratory, Respiratory Cultures
Professional Services: 87430 (Antigen Detection, Enzyme Immunoassay, Streptococcus)

ICD-10-CM DX: J00 (Nasopharyngitis [acute])

Case 9-3

9-3A Thoracic Medicine/Critical Care Consultation

Professional Services: 99221 (Evaluation and Management, Hospital)

ICD-10-CM DX: **J81.1** (Edema/edematous, lung, NOS), **J96.90** (Failure/failed, respiration/respiratory), **E11.9** (Diabetes/diabetic, type 2), **I50.9** (Failure, heart, congestive), **Z99.11** (Dependence, on, ventilator), **R78.89** (Findings, abnormal, inconclusive, without diagnosis, in blood, specified substance NEC)

9-3B Thoracic Medicine/Critical Care Progress Note

Professional Services: 99233 (Evaluation and Management, Hospital)

ICD-10-CM DX: **J81.0** (Edema, lung, acute), **J96.90** (Failure/failed, respiration/respiratory), **I42.9** (Cardiomyopathy), **E87.6** (Findings, abnormal, inconclusive, without diagnosis, potassium, deficiency), **E83.30** (Disorder, metabolism, phosphorus), **Z99.11** (Dependence, on, ventilator)

9-3C Radiology Report, Chest

Professional Services: 71045-26 (X-Ray, Chest)

ICD-10-CM DX: **I50.9** (Failure/failed, heart, congestive), **Z99.11** (Dependence, on, ventilator)

9-3D Thoracic Medicine/Critical Care Progress Note

Professional Services: 99233 (Evaluation and Management, Hospital)

ICD-10-CM DX: **J81.0** (Edema/edematous, lung, acute), **J96.90** (Failure/failed, respiration/respiratory), **I42.9** (Cardiomyopathy), **Z99.11** (Dependence, on, ventilator)

9-3E Thoracic Medicine/Critical Care Progress Note

Professional Services: 99232 (Evaluation and Management, Hospital)

ICD-10-CM DX: **I50.9** (Failure/failed, heart, congestive), **J96.90** (Failure/failed, respiration/respiratory), **J81.1** (Edema, lung), **M54.9** (Pain[s], back)

9-3F Radiology Report, Chest

Professional Services: 71045-26 (X-Ray, Chest)

ICD-10-CM DX: **I50.9** (Failure/failed, heart, congestive), **J81.1** (Edema/edematous, lung), **J96.90** (Failure/failed, respiration/respiratory)

9-3G Discharge Summary

Professional Services: 99238 (Evaluation and Management, Hospital, Discharge)

ICD-10-CM DX: **J81.0** (Edema/edematous, lung, acute), **J96.90** (Failure/failed, respiration/respiratory), **I42.9** (Cardiomyopathy), **I50.9** (Failure/failed, heart, congestive)

Case 9-5

9-5A Consultation/Transfer of Care

Professional Services: 99255 (Evaluation and Management, Consultation)

ICD-10-CM DX: **R06.2** (Wheezing), **I34.0** (Insufficiency/insufficient, mitral [valve]), **I47.20** (Tachycardia, ventricular), **R07.9** (Pain[s], chest), **R60.9** (Edema/edematous)

Case 9-7

9-7A Overnight Oxygen Desaturation Study

Professional Services: 95807-26 (Sleep Study)

ICD-10-CM DX: **R40.0** (Somnolence)

9-7B Nocturnal Polysomnogram

Professional Services: 95810-26 (Polysomnography)

ICD-10-CM DX: **R40.0** (Somnolence)

9-7C Multiple Sleep Latency Study

Professional Services: 95805-26 (Neurology, Sleep Study)

ICD-10-CM DX: **R40.0** (Somnolence), **Z72.820** (Deprivation, sleep)

Case 9-9

9-9A Pulmonary Function Study

Professional Services:

94060-26 (Pulmonology, Diagnostic, Bronchodilation)

94727-26 (Pulmonology, Diagnostic, Airway Closing Volume)

94729-26 (Pulmonology, Diagnostic, Carbon Monoxide Diffusion Capacity)

ICD-10-CM DX: **J43.9** (Disease, lung, obstructive, with, emphysema), **F17.210** (Dependence, drug, nicotine, cigarettes)

9-9B Cardiothoracic Consultation

Professional Services: 99243 (Evaluation and Management, Consultation)

ICD-10-CM DX: **R22.2** (Mass, chest)

9-9C Operative Report, Lung Mass

Professional Services: 32482-54-RT (Lobectomy, Lung)

ICD-10-CM DX: **C34.81** (Neoplasm, lung, overlapping lesion, Malignant Primary)

9-9D Pathology Report

Professional Services:

88309 (Pathology, Surgical, Gross and Micro Exam, Level VI)

88305 × 3 (Pathology, Surgical, Gross and Micro Exam, Level IV)

88331 (Pathology, Surgical, Consultation, Intraoperative)

88332 × 2 (Pathology, Surgical, Consultation, Intraoperative)

ICD-10-CM DX: C34.81 (Neoplasm, lung, overlapping lesion, Malignant Primary), **D36.0** (Neoplasm, lymph/lymphatic, gland, Benign)

9-9E Thoracic Medicine/Critical Care Note
Professional Services: 99252 (Evaluation and Management, Consultation)

ICD-10-CM DX: J43.9 (Emphysema), **Z99.11** (Dependence, on, ventilator)

9-9F Radiology Report, Chest
Professional Services: 71045-26 (X-Ray, Chest)

ICD-10-CM DX: J98.11 (Atelectasis)

9-9G Thoracic Medicine/Critical Care Progress Report
Professional Services: 32482-55-RT (Lobectomy, Lung)

ICD-10-CM DX: C34.81 (Neoplasm, lung, overlapping lesion, Malignant Primary), **J43.9** (Emphysema)

9-9H Radiology Report, Chest
Professional Services: 71045-26 (X-Ray, Chest)

ICD-10-CM DX: J96.90 (Failure/failed, respiration/respiratory)

9-9I Pulmonary Function Study
Professional Services: 94618-26 (Stress Test, Pulmonary)

ICD-10-CM DX: R06.00 (Dyspnea)

9-9J Discharge Summary
Professional Services: 99238 (Evaluation and Management, Hospital, Discharge)

ICD-10-CM DX: C34.81 (Neoplasm, lung, overlapping lesion, Malignant Primary), **I48.91** (Fibrillation, atrial or auricular), **J43.9** (Emphysema)

Case 9-11
9-11A Operative Report, Thoracentesis
Professional Services: 32555 (Thoracentesis, with Imaging Guidance)

ICD-10-CM DX: J90 (Effusion, pleura/pleurisy/pleuritic/pleuropericardial), **J13** (Pneumonia, pneumococcal)

Case 9-13
9-13A Operative Report, Septoplasty, Turbinoplasty, and Ethmoidectomy
Professional Services: 31255-LT (Ethmoidectomy, Endoscopic), **30520-51** (Septoplasty), **30130-51-50** (Turbinate, Excision)

ICD-10-CM DX: J34.2 (Deviation, septum, [nasal] [acquired]), **J34.3** (Hypertrophy/hypertrophic, mucous membrane, nose [turbinate]), **J32.2** (Sinusitis, ethmoidal)

Case 9-15
9-15A Thoracic Medicine and Critical Care Consultation
Professional Services: 99252 (Evaluation and Management, Consultation)

ICD-10-CM DX: C34.90 (Neoplasm, lung, unspecified site, Malignant Primary)

9-15B Thoracic Medicine and Critical Care Progress Report
Professional Services: 99232 (Evaluation and Management, Hospital)

ICD-10-CM DX: C80.1 (Neoplasm, unknown site or unspecified, Malignant Primary)

9-15C Thoracic Medicine and Critical Care Progress Report
Professional Services: 99232 (Evaluation and Management, Hospital)

ICD-10-CM DX: C34.90 (Neoplasm, lung, unspecified site, Malignant Primary), **C78.89** (Neoplasm, esophagus, Malignant, Secondary), **J90** (Effusion, pleura/pleurisy/pleuritic/pleuropericardial), **R07.9** (Pain[s], chest)

9-15D Radiology Report, Chest
Professional Services: 71047-26 (X-Ray, Chest)

ICD-10-CM DX: J90 (Effusion, pleura/pleurisy/pleuritic/pleuropericardial), **C34.90** (Neoplasm, lung, unspecified site, Malignant Primary)

9-15E Operative Report, Esophagogastroduodenoscopy
Professional Services: 43239 (Endoscopy, Gastrointestinal, Upper, Biopsy), **43450-59** (Dilation, Esophagus)

ICD-10-CM DX: C78.89 (Neoplasm, esophagus, upper [third], Malignant Secondary)

9-15F CT-Guided Lung Biopsy
Professional Services: 32408 (Biopsy, Lung, Needle)

ICD-10-CM DX: C34.90 (Neoplasm, lung, unspecified site, Malignant Primary)

9-15G Pathology Report
Professional Services: 88104 (Pathology and Laboratory, Cytopathology, Fluids, Washings, Brushings)

ICD-10-CM DX: C34.90 (Neoplasm, lung, unspecified site, Malignant Primary)

9-15H Ultrasound Marking for Thoracentesis
Professional Services: 76942-26 (Ultrasound, Guidance, Thoracentesis)

ICD-10-CM DX: J90 (Effusion, pleura/pleurisy/pleuritic/pleuropericardial)

9-15I Operative Report, Thoracentesis
Professional Services: **32400 × 4** (Biopsy, Pleura, Needle), **32554-59** (Thoracentesis)

ICD-10-CM DX: **C34.90** (Neoplasm, lung, unspecified site, Malignant Primary)

9-15J Pathology Report
Professional Services: **88305** (Pathology, Surgical, Gross and Micro Exam, Level IV)

ICD-10-CM DX: **C34.90** (Neoplasm, lung, unspecified site, Malignant Primary)

9-15K Oxygen Desaturation Study
Professional Services: **95807-26** (Sleep Study [oxygen, attended by technologist])

ICD-10-CM DX: **R40.0** (Somnolence)

9-15L Radiology Report, Chest
Professional Services: **71045-26** (X-Ray, Chest)

ICD-10-CM DX: **J93.9** (Pneumothorax), **J90** (Effusion, pleura/pleurisy/pleuritic/pleuropericardial)

9-15M Operative Report, Thoracostomy
Professional Services: **32551-LT** (Thoracostomy, Tube)

ICD-10-CM DX: **J90** (Effusion, pleura/pleurisy/pleuritic/pleuropericardial)

Case 9-17
9-17A Operative Report, Bronchoscopy
Professional Services: **31623** (Bronchoscopy, Brushing), **31624-51** (Bronchoscopy, Alveolar Lavage)

ICD-10-CM DX: **R91.8** (Abnormal/abnormality/abnormalities, diagnostic imaging, lung [field]), **Z99.11** (Dependence, on, ventilator)

Chapter 10

Urinary, Male Genital, and Endocrine Systems

Case 10-1
10-1A Operative Report, Kidney Biopsy
Professional Services: **50200-RT** (Biopsy, Kidney)

ICD-10-CM DX: **C64.1** (Neoplasm, kidney, unspecified site, Malignant Primary), **N18.9** (Failure/failed, renal, chronic)

Case 10-3
10-3A Operative Report, Nephrectomy
Professional Services: **50546-LT** (Nephrectomy, Laparoscopic)

ICD-10-CM DX: **N28.1** (Cyst, kidney [acquired])

Case 10-5
10-5A Urodynamic Assessment
Professional Services: **51741-26** (Urodynamic Tests, Uroflowmetry), **51726-51-26** (Cystometrogram),
51784-51-26 (Electromyography, Sphincter Muscles, Anus), **51728-51-26** (Voiding Pressure Studies, Bladder)

ICD-10-CM DX: **N18.9** (Failure/failed, renal, chronic)

Case 10-7
10-7A Operative Report, Intraperitoneal Bladder Rupture
Professional Services: **51865** (Repair, Bladder, Wound)

ICD-10-CM DX: **S37.29XA** (Injury, bladder, specified type NEC), **W11.XXXA** (External Cause Index, Fall, from/off, ladder)

Case 10-9
10-9A Operative Report, Ureteroscopic Stone Extraction
Professional Services: **52352-LT** (Cystourethroscopy, Removal, Calculus), **52332-51-LT** (Cystourethroscopy, Insertion, Indwelling Ureteral Stent), **74485-26** (X-ray, Ureter, Guide Dilation), **76000-26** (Fluoroscopy, Hourly)

ICD-10-CM DX: **N20.1** (Calculus/calculi/calculous, ureter), **N13.5** (Occlusion, ureter)

Case 10-11
10-11A Operative Report, Meatotomy
Professional Services: **52281** (Cystourethroscopy, Dilation, Urethra)

ICD-10-CM DX: **N35.919** (Stricture, urethra, male)

Case 10-13
10-13A Operative Report, Circumcision
Professional Services: **54161** (Circumcision, Surgical Excision)

ICD-10-CM DX: **N47.1** (Phimosis), **B37.42** (Balanitis, candidal)

Case 10-15
10-15A Operative Report, Vasectomy
Professional Services: **55250** (Vasectomy)

ICD-10-CM DX: **Z30.2** (Encounter [for], sterilization)

Case 10-17
10-17A Transrectal Ultrasound for Prostate Volume Determination and Biopsy
Professional Services: **55700** (Biopsy, Prostate), **76872-26** (Ultrasound, Rectal)

ICD-10-CM DX: **R97.20** (Elevated/elevation, prostate specific antigen [PSA])

Case 10-19
10-19A Operative Report, Lymphadenectomy, Prostatectomy, and Plastic Repair
Professional Services: **55845** (Prostatectomy, Retropubic, Radical)

ICD-10-CM DX: C61 (Neoplasm, prostate [gland], Malignant Primary), **C67.5** (Neoplasm, bladder, neck, Malignant Primary), **C77.5** (Neoplasm, lymph, gland, pelvic, Malignant Secondary)

Case 10-21
10-21A Operative Report, Left Thyroid Mass
Professional Services: 60240 (Thyroid Gland, Excision, Total)

ICD-10-CM DX: E04.1 (Nodule[s]/nodular, colloid [cystic], thyroid)

Chapter 11

Female Genital System and Maternity Care/Delivery

Case 11-1
11-1A Emergency Department Services
Professional Services: 99282 (Evaluation and Management, Emergency Department)

ICD-10-CM DX: R10.2 (Pain[s], adnexa [uteri])

Case 11-3
11-3A History and Physical Examination
Professional Services: 99221-57 (Evaluation and Management, Hospital)

ICD-10-CM DX: N80.9 (Endometriosis), **N94.6** (Dysmenorrhea), **R10.2** (Pain[s], pelvic [female])

11-3B Operative Report, Ureteral Stents
Professional Services: 52332-50 or **52332-RT** and **52332-LT** (Cystourethroscopy, Insertion, Indwelling Ureteral Stent)

ICD-10-CM DX: N80.00 (Endometriosis, uterus)

11-3C Operative Report, Hysterectomy
Professional Services: 58150 (Hysterectomy, Abdominal, Total)

ICD-10-CM DX: N80.03 (Adenomyosis), **N80.103** (Endometriosis, ovaries), **N72** (Cervicitis)

11-3D Pathology Report
Professional Services: 88307 (Pathology, Surgical, Gross and Micro Exam, Level V)

ICD-10-CM DX: N72 (Cervicitis), **N80.03** (Adenomyosis), **N80.103** (Endometriosis, ovaries)

11-3E Discharge Summary
Professional Services: 99238 (Evaluation and Management, Hospital, Discharge)

ICD-10-CM DX: N80.103 (Endometriosis, ovaries), **N80.03** (Adenomyosis), **N72** (Cervicitis)

Case 11-5
11-5A Operative Report, Dilatation and Curettage
Professional Services: 58558 (Hysteroscopy, Surgical with Biopsy)

ICD-10-CM DX: C54.1 (Neoplasm, uterus/uteri/uterine, endometrium, Malignant Primary)

Case 11-7
11-7A Real-Time Ultrasound
Professional Services: 76815-26 (Echography, Pregnant Uterus)

ICD-10-CM DX: O43.102 (Pregnancy, complicated by, malformation, placenta/placental)

11-7B Sonogram
Professional Services: 76816-26 (Echography, Pregnant Uterus)

ICD-10-CM DX: O43.102 (Pregnancy, complicated by, malformation, placenta/placental)

11-7C Operative Report, Cesarean Section
Professional Services: 59515 (Cesarean Delivery, Delivery with Postpartum Care)

ICD-10-CM DX: O34.219 (Delivery, cesarean [for], previous, cesarean delivery), **O64.8XX0** (Delivery, complicated by, obstruction, due to, footling presentation), **O36.60X0** (Pregnancy, complicated by, fetal, excessive growth), **D23.5** (Neoplasm, skin, abdominal, Benign), **Z37.0** (Outcome of delivery, single, liveborn)

11-7D Discharge Summary
Professional Services: 99238 (Evaluation and Management, Hospital, Discharge)

ICD-10-CM DX: O34.219 (Delivery, cesarean [for], previous, cesarean delivery), **O32.1XX0** (Delivery, cesarean [for], breech presentation), **O33.5XX0** (Delivery, complicated by, oversized fetus), **Z37.0** (Outcome of delivery, single, liveborn), **D23.5** (Neoplasm, skin, abdominal, Benign)

Case 11-9
11-9A Ob/Gyn Consultation
Professional Services: 99231 (Evaluation and Management, Hospital, [Subsequent])

ICD-10-CM DX: O21.8 (Pregnancy, complicated by, vomiting, due to diseases classified elsewhere), **O16.3** (Hypertension, complicating pregnancy), **O24.013** (Pregnancy, complicated by, diabetes [mellitus], pre-existing, type 1), **R19.7** (Diarrhea/diarrheal), **E10.21** (Diabetes/diabetic, type 1, with, nephropathy), **Z3A.30** (Gestation, 30 weeks)

11-9B Duplex Venous Examination
Professional Services: 93970-26 (Duplex Scan, Venous Studies, Extremity)

ICD-10-CM DX: O26.893 (Pregnancy, complicated by, specified condition NEC), **M79.89** (Swelling, leg)

11-9C Ultrasound
Professional Services: 76815-26 (Fetal Testing, Ultrasound, Fetal)

ICD-10-CM DX: Z36.2 (Screening [for], antenatal, of mother), **Z3A.29** (Gestation, 29 weeks)

11-9D Biophysical Profile
Professional Services: 76818-26 (Fetal Biophysical Profile)

ICD-10-CM DX: O24.013 (Pregnancy, complicated by, diabetes [mellitus], pre-existing, type 1), **E10.9** (Diabetes/diabetic, type I)

11-9E Doppler Umbilical Arterial
Professional Services: 76820-26 (Doppler Scan, Arterial Studies, Fetal, Umbilical Artery)

ICD-10-CM DX: O24.013 (Pregnancy, complicated by, diabetes [mellitus], pre-existing, type 1), **O10.213** (Hypertension, complicating pregnancy, pre-existing, with renal disease, Unspecified), **E10.21** (Diabetes/diabetic, type I, with, nephropathy)

11-9F OB Ultrasound
Professional Services: 76815-26 (Fetal Testing, Ultrasound)

ICD-10-CM DX: O47.03 (Pregnancy, complicated by, threatened, labor, before 37 completed weeks of gestation), **Z3A.32** (Gestation, 32 weeks)

11-9G OB Ultrasound
Professional Services: 76946-26 (Ultrasound, Guidance, Amniocentesis)

ICD-10-CM DX: Z36.2 (Screening [for], antenatal, of mother), **Z3A.34** (Gestation, 34 weeks)

11-9H Operative Report, Amniocentesis
Professional Services: 59000 (Amniocentesis, Diagnostic)

ICD-10-CM DX: O24.013 (Pregnancy, complicated by, diabetes [mellitus], pre-existing, type 1), **E10.21** (Diabetes/diabetic, type 1, with, nephropathy)

11-9I OB Ultrasound
Professional Services: 76816-26 (Fetal Testing, Ultrasound, Fetal)

ICD-10-CM DX: Z36.2 (Screening [for], antenatal, of mother), **Z3A.34** (Gestation, 34 weeks)

11-9J Operative Report, Cesarean Section
Professional Services: 59515 (Cesarean Delivery, Delivery with Postpartum Care), **58611** (Cesarean Delivery, with Tubal Ligation during Delivery)

ICD-10-CM DX: O24.013 (Pregnancy, complicated by, diabetes [mellitus], pre-existing, type 1), **O16.3** (Hypertension, complicating pregnancy), **E10.21** (Diabetes/diabetic, type 1, with, nephropathy), **O34.219** (Delivery, cesarean [for], previous cesarean delivery), **Z37.0** (Outcome of delivery, single, liveborn), **Z30.2** (Encounter [for], sterilization), **Z3A.33** (Pregnancy, weeks of Gestation, 33 weeks)

11-9K Pathology Report
Professional Services: 88307 (Pathology, Surgical, Gross and Micro Exam, Level V), **88302 × 2** (Surgical Pathology, Gross and Micro Exam, Level II)

ICD-10-CM DX: O24.013 (Pregnancy, complicated by, diabetes [mellitus], pre-existing, type 1), **O16.3** (Hypertension, complicating pregnancy), **E10.21** (Diabetes/diabetic, type 1, with, nephropathy)

Chapter 12

Nervous System

Case 12-1
12-1A Operative Report, Ventriculostomy
Professional Services: 61107-RT (Ventricle Puncture)

ICD-10-CM DX: I69.198 (Sequelae, hemorrhage, intracerebral, specified effect NEC), **G91.1** (Hydrocephalus, obstructive)

Case 12-3
12-3A Operative Report, Craniectomy
Professional Services: 61510 (Craniectomy, Excision, Tumor), **61781** (Stereotaxis, Computer Assisted, Brain Surgery)

ICD-10-CM DX: D33.0 (Neoplasm, brain, frontal cortex, Benign), **I66.9** (Occlusion/occluded, artery, cerebral)

12-3B Pathology Report
Professional Services: 88307 (Pathology, Surgical, Gross and Micro Exam, Level V)

ICD-10-CM DX: D33.0 (Neoplasm, brain, frontal cortex, Benign)

Case 12-5
12-5A Operative Report, Pterygocraniotomy and Cranioplasty
Professional Services: 61700-RT (Aneurysm Repair, Carotid Artery), **69990** (Operating Microscope)

ICD-10-CM DX: I67.1 (Aneurysm, brain), **I60.31** (Hemorrhage, intracranial, subarachnoid, intracranial, posterior communicating, right)

Case 12-7
12-7A Operative Report, Cranioplasty
Professional Services: 62141 (Cranioplasty, Skull Defect)

ICD-10-CM DX: M95.2 (Deformity, skull [acquired])

Case 12-9
12-9A Operative Report, Lumbar Puncture
Professional Services: 62270 (Spinal Tap, Lumbar)

ICD-10-CM DX: G44.1 (Headache, vascular NEC)

Case 12-11
12-11A Preoperative Consultation
Professional Services: 99252 (Evaluation and Management, Consultation)

ICD-10-CM DX: G80.9 (Palsy, cerebral)

12-11B Operative Report, Intrathecal Catheter Placement
Professional Services: 62361 (Insertion, Infusion Pump, Spinal Cord), **62350-51** (Catheterization, Spinal Cord)

ICD-10-CM DX: G24.2 (Dystonia, torsion, symptomatic)

12-11C Operative Report, Removal of Bard Port
Professional Services: 62362-58 (Infusion Pump, Spinal Cord)

ICD-10-CM DX: G24.2 (Dystonia, torsion, symptomatic)

12-11D Discharge Summary
Professional Services: 99238 (Evaluation and Management, Hospital, Discharge)

ICD-10-CM DX: G80.9 (Palsy, cerebral), **G24.2** (Dystonia, torsion, symptomatic), **G09** (Sequelae [of], infection, pyogenic, intracranial or intraspinal)

Case 12-13
12-13A Operative Report, Hemilaminectomy and Foraminotomy
Professional Services: 63042-LT (Hemilaminectomy), **63044-LT** (Hemilaminectomy)

ICD-10-CM DX: M54.17 (Radiculopathy, lumbosacral region)

Case 12-15
12-15A Operative Report, Cage Fusion
Professional Services: 22558 (Spine, Fusion, Anterior Approach), **22853** (Spine, Insertion, Instrumentation), **20930** (Allograft, Bone, Spine Surgery, Morselized), **95927-26** (Evoked Potential, Central Nervous System, Somatosensory Testing)

ICD-10-CM DX: M51.379 (Degeneration/degenerative, intervertebral disc, lumbosacral region)

Case 12-17
12-17A Operative Report, Discectomy
Professional Services: 63081 (Vertebral, Corpectomy), **20931** (Allograft, Bone, Structural), **22551-51** (Spine, Fusion, Anterior Approach), **22552** (Arthrodesis, Vertebral, Additional Interspace), **22845** (Spinal Instrumentation, Anterior), **95925-26** (Evoked Potentials, Central Nervous System, Somatosensory Testing [Upper Extremities])

ICD-10-CM DX: M48.02 (Stenosis/stenotic, spinal, cervical region), **M50.20** (Displacement/displaced, intervertebral disc NEC, cervical)

Case 12-19
12-19A Electroencephalogram Report
Professional Services: 95822-26 (Electroencephalography, Coma)

ICD-10-CM DX: R56.9 (Convulsions), **R40.20** (Coma), **R94.01** (Abnormal/abnormality/abnormalities, electroencephalogram [EEG])

Chapter 13

Eye and Auditory Systems

Case 13-1
13-1A Clinic Progress Note, Eye Examination
Professional Services: 92002 (Ophthalmology, Diagnostic, Eye Exam, New Patient)

ICD-10-CM DX: H26.033 (Cataract, presenile, nuclear)

Case 13-3
13-3A Clinic Progress Note, Senile Cataracts
Professional Services: 92012 (Ophthalmology, Diagnostic, Eye Exam, Established Patient)

ICD-10-CM DX: H25.9 (Cataract, senile)

Case 13-5
13-5A Clinic Progress Note, Eye Examination
Professional Services: 92002 (Ophthalmology, Eye Exam, New Patient)

ICD-10-CM DX: E10.329 (Diabetes/diabetic, type 1, with, retinopathy, nonproliferative)

13-5B Clinic Progress Note, Photocoagulation
Professional Services: 67228-LT (Destruction, Retina, Photocoagulation)

ICD-10-CM DX: E10.329 (Diabetes/diabetic, with, retinopathy, nonproliferative)

Case 13-7
13-7A Operative Report, Nasolacrimal Duct Probing
Professional Services: 68811-50 or 68811-RT and **68811-LT** (Lacrimal Duct, Exploration, with Anesthesia)

ICD-10-CM DX: Q10.5 (Obstruction/obstructed/obstructive, lacrimal [duct], congenital)

Case 13-9
13-9A Operative Report, Pressure Equalization Tube Removal
Professional Services: 69424-50 or 69424-RT and **69424-LT** (Removal, Ventilating, Tube Ear/Middle)

ICD-10-CM DX: T85.79XA (Complication[s], prosthetic device or implant, infection or inflammation)

Case 13-11
13-11A Operative Report, Tube Removal
Professional Services: 69436-LT (Tympanostomy, General Anesthesia)

ICD-10-CM DX: T85.698A (Complication[s], prosthetic device or implant, specified NEC, mechanical, obstruction)

Case 13-13
13-13A Operative Report, Tympanoplasty
Professional Services: 69633-RT (Tympanoplasty, without Mastoidectomy, with Ossicular Chain Reconstruction, and Synthetic Prosthesis)

ICD-10-CM DX: H90.11 (Deafness, conductive, unilateral), **H74.21** (Discontinuity, ossicles, ear)

Chapter 14

Anesthesia

Case 14-1
14-1A Operative Report, Flaps and Grafts
Professional Services:
PHYSICIAN CODE: 01470-AA-P3 (Anesthesia, Leg, Lower)
CRNA CODE: 01470-QZ-P3 (Anesthesia, Leg, Lower)
QUALIFYING CIRCUMSTANCES CODE: 99100 (Anesthesia, Special Circumstances, Extreme Age)

Case 14-3
14-3A Operative Report, Fusion with Autograft
Professional Services:
CRNA CODE: 01120-QZ-P1 (Anesthesia, Pelvis, Bone)

Case 14-5
14-5A Operative Report, Excision of Right Carotid Body Tumor
Professional Services:
PHYSICIAN CODE: 00320-QY-P2 (Anesthesia, Neck)
CRNA CODE: 00320-QX-P2 (Anesthesia, Neck), **36620** (Catheterization, Arterial, Percutaneous)
QUALIFYING CIRCUMSTANCES CODE: 99100 (Anesthesia, Special Circumstances, Extreme Age)

Case 14-7
14-7A Operative Report, Hysteroscopy, Dilatation, and Curettage
Professional Services:
PHYSICIAN CODE: 00952-AA-P1 (Anesthesia, Uterus)

Case 14-9
14-9A Operative Report, Nasolacrimal Duct Probing
Professional Services:
PHYSICIAN CODE: 00140-QK-P1 (Anesthesia, Eye)
CRNA CODE: 00140-QX-P1 (Anesthesia, Eye)

Case 14-11
14-11A Operative Report, Lesions
Professional Services:
PHYSICIAN CODE: 01470-QK-P1 (Anesthesia, Leg, Lower)
CRNA CODE: 01470-QX-P1 (Anesthesia, Leg, Lower)

Case 14-13
14-13A Operative Report, Ulcer and Cholecystitis
Professional Services:
PHYSICIAN CODE: 00790-AA-P3 (Anesthesia, Abdomen, Intraperitoneal)

Case 14-15
14-15A Operative Report, Tendon Repair
Professional Services:
PHYSICIAN CODE: 01320-QK-P1 (Anesthesia, Knee)
CRNA CODE: 01320-QX-P1 (Anesthesia, Knee)

Case 14-17
14-17A Operative Report, Closed Reduction
Professional Services:
PHYSICIAN CODE: 01820-QK-P1 (Anesthesia, Hand)
CRNA CODE: 01820-QX-P1 (Anesthesia, Hand)

Case 14-19
14-19A Operative Report, Entropion and Ectropion Repair
Professional Services:
PHYSICIAN CODE: 00103-QK-QS-P3 (Anesthesia, Eyelid)
CRNA CODE: 00103-QX-QS-P3 (Anesthesia, Eyelid)

Case 14-21
14-21A Operative Report, Cesarean Section
Professional Services:
PHYSICIAN CODE: 01961-AA-P1 (Anesthesia, Cesarean Delivery)

Glossary

A-mode   one-dimensional ultrasonic display reflecting the time it takes a sound wave to reach a structure and reflect back; maps the structure's outline

active immunization   injection that can either be a toxoid or a vaccine; causes an immune response to protect the patient from later infection by a specific disease

admission   attention to an acute illness or injury resulting in admission to a hospital

amputation   the removal of a limb or appendage that has been too damaged or diseased for treatment

analgesia   absence of sensibility to pain

anesthesiologist   a physician who specializes in the care of a patient before, during, and after surgery, including the evaluation and preparation of a patient for surgery

anesthetist   a registered nurse or technician trained to administer anesthetics

angioplasty   surgical or percutaneous procedure in a vessel to dilate the vessel opening; used in the treatment of atherosclerotic disease

anoscope   instrument used in an examination of the anus

antepartum   before childbirth

anteroposterior   from front to back

artery   vessel that carries oxygenated blood from the heart to body tissue

arthrocentesis   puncture and aspiration of a joint

arthroscopy   examination of the interior of a joint with an arthroscope (specialized endoscope)

atelectasis   incomplete expansion of the lung or a portion of the lung

attending physician   the physician with the primary responsibility for care of the patient

axial projection   any projection that allows an x-ray beam to pass through a body part lengthwise

B-scan   two-dimensional display of tissues and organs

balanitis   inflammation of the glans penis

benign   not progressive or recurrent

bilirubin   orange-colored pigment in bile; accumulation leads to jaundice

biopsy   removal of a small piece of living tissue for diagnostic purposes

brachytherapy   therapy using radioactive sources that are placed inside the body

bronchospasm   spasmodic contraction of the muscle of the bronchi causing constriction of the airway

cadaver   pertaining to a dead body

cardioversion   electrical shock to the heart to restore normal rhythm

cataract   opaque covering on or in the lens

catheter   tube placed into the body to put fluid in or take fluid out

cerebrovascular disease (CVD)   blockage of arteries to the brain

cholecystectomy   removal of the gallbladder

circumcision   removal of all or part of the foreskin

closed treatment   procedure in which a fracture is repaired without exposure

colposcope   scope used in colposcopy

colposcopy   examination of the cervix and vagina by means of a colposcope

comminuted fracture   one in which the bone is crushed or shattered

computed axial tomography (CAT or CT)   procedure by which selected planes of tissue are pinpointed through computer enhancement and images may be reconstructed by analysis of variance in absorption of the tissue

concurrent care   the provision of similar services (e.g., hospital visits) to the same patient by more than one physician on the same day. Each physician provides services for a separate condition not reasonably expected to be managed by the attending physician. When concurrent care is provided, the diagnoses must reflect the medical necessity of different specialties.

confirmatory consultation   type of consultation requested by patients, insurance companies, and/or third-party payers as an additional opinion and diagnosis

conscious sedation   a decreased level of consciousness in which the patient is not completely asleep

consultant   the physician providing a consultation to a requesting physician; a consultant is not an attending physician

consultation   includes those services rendered by a physician whose opinion or advice is requested by another physician or agency concerning the evaluation and/or treatment of a patient

contributory factors   counseling, coordination of care, nature of the presenting problem, and time of an E/M service

cranioplasty   surgical correction of defects in the skull

craniotomy   surgical removal of (or an incision into) the cranium

cryoablation   removal of tissue by destroying it with extreme cold

cytopathology   laboratory work done to determine whether any cellular changes are present

debridement   cleansing or removal of dead tissue from a wound

decubitus   recumbent positions where the x-ray beam is placed horizontally

dermis   second layer of skin, holding blood vessels, nerve endings, sweat glands, and hair follicles

diagnostic ultrasound   technique using high-frequency sound waves to determine the density of the outline of tissue to detect the cause of illness and disease

dialysis   mechanical cleansing of the blood; can be temporary or permanent

differential   actual count of the amount or number of blood constituents

direct face-to-face time   the time a physician spends directly with a patient during an office or outpatient visit, which can include obtaining a history, performing an examination, and/or discussing the results

discharge   release from the hospital

distal   farther from the point of attachment or origin

donor site   the site from which tissue is taken to repair another site

Doppler ultrasound   a diagnostic procedure using images that can be standard black and white or color; can be transmitted only through solid or liquids

dosimetry   scientific calculation of radiation emitted from various radioactive sources

duplex scan   one method of vascular flow analysis that uses sound waves and real-time/color-flow Doppler imaging to produce a color picture of the blood flow within the vessels

dyspnea   shortness of breath; difficult or painful breathing

echocardiography   radiographic recording of the heart or heart walls or surrounding tissues

effusion   the escape of fluid from blood vessels into a body part or tissue

ejection fraction   percentage of blood pumped with each contraction of the heart

endocrinologist   a physician who specializes in the diagnosis and treatment of conditions of the endocrine system

endometrium   inner mucous membrane of the uterus

endoscopy   inspection of body organs or cavities using a lighted scope that may be inserted through an existing opening or through a small incision

entropion   medical condition in which the lower eyelid and eyelashes roll inward toward the eye—usually the lower eyelid

epidermis   outer layer of skin

epididymitis   inflammation of the epididymis

epiphora   abnormal overflow of tears, sometimes due to a blockage of the lacrimal passages

excision   cutting or taking away (in reference to lesion removal, it is full-thickness removal of a lesion that may include simple closure)

excisional   removal of an entire lesion for biopsy

external fixation   application of a device that holds bones in place from outside the body

fistula   abnormal opening from one area to another area or to the outside of the body

foramina   a natural opening or passage

gastroenterologist   a physician who specializes in the diagnoses and treatment of the digestive system

gastrointestinal   pertaining to the stomach and intestine

global surgical procedure   a set amount of preoperative, intraoperative, and postoperative services bundled into a service code

glucose   blood sugar

graft   *autograft* is taken from the patient's own body; *allograft* is taken from another person's body, either alive or cadaver; *bilaminate graft* is made of artificial skin; *pinch graft* is a small, split-thickness repair; *split graft* is a repair that involves the epidermis and some of the dermis; *full-thickness graft* is a repair that involves the epidermis and all of the dermis; *xenograft* is one taken from another species.

gynecologist   a physician specializing in the diagnosis, treatment, and management of female genital diseases and disorders

hemangioma   benign tumor formed of blood vessels, common in infants and children

hematoma   a localized collection of blood in any body space

hemodialysis   cleansing of the blood outside of the body

hemoglobin   protein found in red blood cells that transports oxygen through the bloodstream

hemogram   graphic picture (or written record) of a detailed blood assessment

hemoptysis   expectoration of blood in sputum

hydrocele   sac or accumulation of fluid

hypertrophy   enlargement or overgrowth of an organ due to the increase in size of its cells

hypotension   abnormally low blood pressure

hypothermia   low body temperature; sometimes induced during surgical procedures

hysterectomy   surgical removal of the uterus

hysteroscope   scope used in hysteroscopy

hysteroscopy   visualization of the canal of the uterine cervix and uterine cavity using a scope placed through the vagina

implantable defibrillator   surgically placed device that directs an electric current shock to the heart to restore rhythm

incidental findings those findings that were not the reason a diagnostic test was performed; may be unrelated to the reason the test was ordered

incontinence inability to control excretory functions, such as urination

indicators written physician orders to a laboratory that set standards for any tests performed

infusion the administration of medicine over an extended period of time

inpatient one who has been formally admitted to a health care facility

internal fixation placement of hardware (rods, pins, etc.) onto or into the bone to hold it in place for repair

interstitial situated between body tissues

intracavitary within a body cavity

intralesional into a lesion

intramuscular into a muscle

intraventricular within a ventricle

ischemia deficiency of blood in a body part, usually due to constriction or obstruction of a blood vessel

ketones carbon-based compounds that are by-products of fatty acid metabolism; accumulation of ketone bodies in urine may indicate diabetes

key components the history, examination, and medical decision making complexity of an E/M service

lamina either of the pair of broad plates of bone flaring out from the pedicles of the vertebral arches

laminectomy surgical excision of the lamina

laparoscopy exploration of the abdomen and pelvic cavities using a scope placed through a small incision in the abdominal wall

lateral away from the midline of the body (to the side)

lesion abnormal or altered tissue (e.g., wound, cyst, abscess, boil)

leukocytes white blood cells

M-mode one-dimensional display of movement of structures

magnetic resonance imaging (MRI) procedure that uses nonionizing radiation to view the body in a cross-sectional view

malignant used to describe a cancerous tumor that grows worse over time

manipulation an attempt to maneuver a bone back into proper alignment

mastectomy excision (removal) of the breast

myocardial pertaining to the heart muscle

myocardial perfusion scan a radiologic procedure performed to assess the amount of blood reaching a given area of the heart

myringotomy the creation of a hole and/or incision in the tympanic membrane

nephrectomy excision of a kidney, either entirely or partially

nephrologist a physician who specializes in the diagnosis and treatment of conditions of the kidney

nephrons filtering units in the kidneys

neurologist a physician who specializes in the diagnosis and treatment of conditions of the nervous system

neurosurgeon a physician who specializes in surgical procedures of the nervous system

newborn care evaluation and determination of care management of a newborn infant

non face-to-face time time a provider spends managing the patient, without the patient present

oblique view radiographic view in which the body or part is rotated so the projection is neither frontal nor lateral

observation the classification status of a patient that requires an inpatient stay for a short period to gather further information for diagnosis and treatment; the patient does not require acute inpatient care or intensive resources

occult blood test to detect the presence of blood in stool samples

odontoid position/view with the patient's mouth open

office visit a face-to-face encounter between a physician and a patient to allow for primary management of a patient's health care status

onychectomy excision (removal) of a nail or nail bed

open treatment procedure in which a fracture site is surgically exposed and visualized

ophthalmologist a physician specializing in medical and surgical care of the eye and visual system

orthopedist a physician who specializes in the diagnosis and treatment of musculoskeletal disorders

otolaryngologist physician specializing in the management and treatment of patients with diseases and disorders of the ear, nose, and throat; often referred to as an ENT physician

outpatient a patient who receives services in an ambulatory health care facility and is currently not an inpatient

panel groups of laboratory tests that are performed together

panniculectomy removal of abdominal fat and skin

parenchyma an essential element of an organ; functional element, such as the renal parenchyma, which is the tissue that contains the nephrons

passive immunization injection of antibodies into the body to protect the patient from a specific disease; does not cause an immune response

percutaneous through the skin

peritoneal cavity the space within the abdominal lining

permanent section a specimen of tissue obtained during an operative procedure that is mounted and analyzed by a pathologist for the most definitive diagnosis

pharyngitis inflammation of the pharynx (i.e., sore throat)

phimosis constriction of the preputial orifice that does not allow the foreskin to fold back over the glans

photocoagulation procedure that uses a controlled laser to treat leaky retinal blood vessels and destroy abnormal vessels or tissues at the back of the eye

physical status modifier identifies the health status of a patient requiring anesthesia management

pleural cavity   the body cavity containing the organs and membranes of the thoracic region

position   placement of the patient during an x-ray examination

posteroanterior   from back to front

postoperative   after a surgical procedure

postpartum   after childbirth

presenting problem   a disease, condition, illness, injury, symptom, sign, finding, complaint, or any other reason for a patient encounter, with or without a diagnosis being established at the time of the patient visit

professional component   term used in describing radiology services provided by a radiologist

projection   the path of the x-ray beam

prone (ventral)   lying on the stomach

proximal   closer to the point of attachment or origin

pulmonologist   a physician specializing in treatment of diseases and disorders of the respiratory system

Qualifying Circumstances   five-digit CPT codes that describe situations or conditions that make the administration of anesthesia more difficult than is normal

qualitative   only the presence of; not an exact amount

quantitative   the exact amount present

radiologist   a physician who specializes in the use of radioactive materials in the diagnosis and treatment of disease and illnesses

radiology   branch of medicine concerned with the use of radioactive substances for diagnosis and therapy

reagent   a substance that changes color when exposed to another substance

recipient site   the site that receives tissue for repair

reconstruction   the three-dimensional image created by putting together several cross-sectional views (CT scans, MRIs, etc.)

recumbent   lying down

requesting physician   a physician asking for advice or opinion on the treatment, diagnosis, or management of a patient from another physician

ribbons   radioactive seeds embedded on a tape that is temporarily inserted into body tissues to deliver a radiation dose over time; can be cut to determine the amount of radiation the patient receives

septoplasty   surgical repair of the nasal septum

shunt   a device that diverts fluids the body cannot drain properly from one body area to another

skin graft   transplantation of tissue to repair a defect

source   a container holding a radioactive element; can be directly inserted into the body to deliver a radiation dose over time

specific gravity   weight of urine compared with an equal volume of water

sphincters   circular bands of muscles that constrict a passage or close a natural orifice

spirometry   measurement of breathing capacity

stent   mold that holds a surgically placed graft in place

stress test   a test that assesses cardiovascular health and function (by echocardiogram) after application of stress to the heart, usually exercise, but sometimes other such as atrial pacing, the cold pressor test, or specific drugs

subarachnoid   within the membranes of the brain and spinal cord

subcutaneous   tissue below the dermis, primarily fat cells that insulate the body

sulcus   a groove, trench, or valley shape

superbill (encounter form)   a form listing the most frequently used procedures and codes; the results of a patient's visit are checked off and used for billing purposes

supine (dorsal)   lying on the back

swimmers   position/view in which the arms are over the head

tangential   patient position that allows the x-ray beam to skim a body part; produces a profile of the structure of the body

thoracentesis   surgical puncture of the thoracic cavity, usually using a needle, to remove fluids

tissue expander   a sac of fluid or air or a plastic implant that is placed under the skin to stretch the skin. The stretched skin is used for grafting purposes or stretched to place an implant beneath the newly expanded skin.

tissue transfer   piece of skin for grafting that is still partially attached to the original blood supply and is used to cover an adjacent wound area

tomography   procedure that allows viewing of a single plane of the body by blurring out all but that particular level

toxoids   bacteria that cause a disease

transesophageal echocardiography (TEE)   echocardiogram performed by placing a probe down the esophagus and sending out sound waves to obtain images of the heart and its movement

tympanostomy   incision of the tympanic membrane for insertion of a pressure equalization tube for fluid drainage

ureter   tube that carries urine from the kidneys to the bladder

urinalysis   analysis of urine

urobilinogen   a colorless compound formed in the intestines by the reduction of bilirubin

urodynamics   pertaining to the flow and motion of liquids in the urinary tract

urologist   a physician who specializes in the diagnosis and treatment of conditions of the urinary system

vaccine   a small dose of a virus or bacteria that is injected into the body to produce an immune response to protect the patient from later infection by a specific disease

vasectomy   male sterilization procedure in which the vas deferens is cut, preventing the sperm from mixing with the seminal fluid

vein   vessel that carries blood to the heart from body tissues

Index

Note: Page numbers followed by *b* indicate boxes, *f* indicates figures and *t* indicate tables.

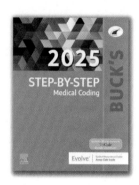

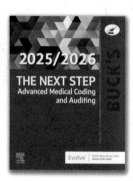
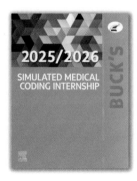
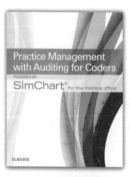
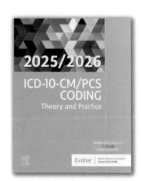